IDEAL BODY WEIGHT (IBW)

ADULTS (>18 YRS):
Male IBW (kg) = 50 + 2.3 for each inch over 60 inches
Female IBW (kg) = 45.5 + 2.3 for each inch over 60 inches

CHILDREN:
Age 1 to 18 yrs, height <60 inches: IBW (kg) = $[1.65 \times \text{height}^2 \text{ (cm)}]/1000$

CREATININE CLEARANCE CALCULATION

ADULTS (AGE >18; SERUM CREAT <5 MG/DL AND NOT CHANGING RAPIDLY):

$$\text{CrCl (ml/min)} = \frac{(140 - \text{age})\ (\text{weight in kg})}{(\text{serum creat [mg/dl]})\ (72)}$$

NOTES: 1. Multiply by 0.85 for females
2. Use the following value for weight:
   a. If actual weight <IBW, use actual weight
   b. If actual weight is 100%-130% of IBW, use IBW
   c. If actual weight >130% of IBW, easiest approximation is by using IBW + (actual weight – IBW)/3
3. Accuracy reduced in muscle wasting diseases (e.g., neuromuscular disease) and amputees

CHILDREN:
CrCl (ml/min/1.73m^2) = $[0.48 \times \text{height (cm)}]/\text{serum creat (mg/dl)}$

Mosby's

1997 Medical Drug Reference

Allan J. Ellsworth, Pharm. D.

Associate Professor of Pharmacy and Family Medicine,
University of Washington Schools of Pharmacy and Medicine,
Seattle, Washington

David C. Dugdale, M.D.

Assistant Professor of Medicine,
University of Washington School of Medicine,
Seattle, Washington

Daniel M. Witt, Pharm. D.

Clinical Pharmacy Specialist,
Kaiser Permanente,
Denver, Colorado

Lynn M. Oliver, M.D.

Assistant Professor of Family Medicine,
University of Washington School of Medicine,
Seattle, Washington

Mosby

St. Louis Baltimore Boston Carlsbad Chicago Naples New York
Philadelphia Portland London Madrid Mexico City Singapore
Sydney Tokyo Toronto Wiesbaden

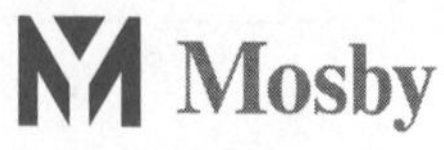

Dedicated to Publishing Excellence

A Times Mirror Company

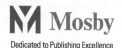

Vice President and Publisher: Anne S. Patterson
Editor: James Shanahan
Developmental Editor: Laura Berendson
Project Manager: Carol S. Weis
Senior Production Editor: Christine Carroll Schwepker
Designer: Sheilah Barrett
Cover Illustrator: Adam Cohen
Manufacturing Manager: David Graybill

A NOTE TO THE READER

The authors and publisher have made every attempt to check dosages and medical content for accuracy. Because the science of pharmacology is continually advancing, our knowledge base continues to expand. Therefore we recommend that the reader always check product information for changes in dosage or administration before administering any medication. This is particularly important with new or rarely used drugs.

Printed in the United States of America
Editing, production, and composition by Graphic World, Inc.
Printing/binding by RR Donnelley & Sons Company

Mosby–Year Book, Inc.
11830 Westline Industrial Drive
St. Louis, Missouri 63146

ISSN 1089-3202
ISBN 0-8151-3109-7

96 97 98 99 00 / 9 8 7 6 5 4 3 2 1

Instructions for Use

Mosby's 1997 Medical Drug Reference was conceived in response to the demands of physicians and other health care providers who require an authoritative, comprehensive, *portable* drug prescribing reference for use at the point of care. This compact, easily accessible manual has been created in part from the renowned and objective drug database, *Physicians GenRx,* which is updated quarterly to provide timely drug information for accurate and efficient prescribing. As a standard reference, *Physician's GenRx* is indispensible in its print and CD-ROM formats; for those situations when the demands of patient care require a portable drug prescribing guide, we proudly present *Mosby's 1997 Medical Drug Reference.*

Mosby's 1997 Medical Drug Reference is organized into several highly functional parts. The body of the book is a listing, by generic name, of more than 850 generic drugs in common clinical use, representing over 2600 trade names. The appendix of the book contains tables of comparative drug data and other information useful for choosing a drug therapy; this information will be updated and expanded in each new edition of this annual publication. The comprehensive index provides rapid reference by listing all generic and trade names; index searches are further aided by the colored index paper. The front and back covers contain formulas for calculating drug dosages and useful conversion information.

Drug monographs in *Mosby's 1997 Medical Drug Reference* are organized in a uniform fashion as follows (when there is no information in a category applicable to a given drug, the category has been deleted entirely):

Drug name (generic)
Pronunciation (phonetic)
Trade names (Canadian trade names marked with ✦, if applicable)
Chemical Class
Therapeutic Class
DEA Schedule (if applicable, see p. ix)
Clinical Pharmacology (including information about the mechanism of action and pharmacokinetics of the drug)
Indications and Uses (non–FDA-approved uses marked with *, if applicable)
Dosage
Available Forms/Cost of Therapy
Contraindications
Precautions
Pregnancy and Lactation (see p. xi)
Side Effects/Adverse Reactions (listed by organ system; *common side*

effects italicized, ***potentially life-threatening side effects bold and italicized***)

Drug Interactions (if applicable; limited to interactions that are of major clinical significance ["+" sign] and moderate clinical significance [normal type]; derived from comprehensive review of all available literature; interactions of minor clinical significance, based on poor documentation, slight potential harm, or low incidence are not included)

Lab Test Interactions (if applicable)

Special Considerations (such as patient education or monitoring parameters, if applicable)

Every possible effort has been made to ensure the accuracy and currency of the information contained within *Mosby's 1997 Medical Drug Reference.* However, drug information is constantly changing and is subject to interpretation. Neither the authors, editors, nor publishers are responsible for information that has either changed or been erroneously published, or for the consequences of such errors. Decisions regarding drug therapy for a specific patient must be based on the independent judgment of the clinician.

Allan Ellsworth
David Dugdale
Daniel Witt
Lynn Oliver

ACKNOWLEDGMENTS

We are grateful for the support, stimulus, and suggestions of our colleagues in the Departments of Family Medicine, Medicine, and Pharmacy, University of Washington, Seattle, Washington, and the Medical and Pharmacy Staff of Kaiser Permanente of Colorado, Denver, Colorado. Ann Greaney, M.D., Chief Resident, Department of Family Medicine, University of Washington, Alvin Goo, Pharm.D., Clinical Pharmacy Specialist, Kaiser Permanente of Colorado, Denver, Colorado, Tamara Marek, Pharm.D., Assistant Professor, Departments of Pharmacy and Family Medicine, University of Wyoming, Cheyenne, and Bev True, M.D., Pharm.D., Family Practice Physician, Group Health Cooperative of Puget Sound, Seattle, Washington, provided excellent editorial review. We especially appreciate the organization, coordination, computerization, and prodding of Jenny Schlieps, who contributed mightily toward the completion of the project. Finally, to our families and friends, whose support, patience, love, and understanding allowed many things to go undone during the completion of the project, we thank you all.

We wish to express our special appreciation to Linda Skidmore-Roth, R.N., M.S.N., N.P., for permission to use the database for the drug monographs from *Mosby's 1995 Nursing Drug Reference.*

Abbreviations

ABG arterial blood gas
ac before meals
ACE angiotensin–converting enzyme
AD right ear
ADH antidiuretic hormone
aer aerosol
AIDS acquired immunodeficiency syndrome
ALT alanine aminotransferase, serum
ANA antinuclear antibody
ANC absolute neutrophil count
APTT activated partial thromboplastin time
AS left ear
AST aspartate aminotransferase, serum
AU each ear
AV atrioventricular
bid twice a day
BP blood pressure
BUN blood urea nitrogen
°C degrees Celsius (centigrade)
Ca calcium
CAD coronary artery disease
cAMP cyclic adenosine monophosphate
cap capsule
cath catheterize
CBC complete blood count
cc cubic centimeter
CHF congestive heart failure
cm centimeter
C_{max} maximum concentration
CNS central nervous system
CO_2 carbon dioxide
COPD chronic obstructive pulmonary disease
CPAP continuous positive airway pressure
CPK creatine phosphokinase
CrCl creatinine clearance
cre cream
creat creatinine
CSF cerebrospinal fluid
ctb chewable tablets
CV cardiovascular
CVA cerebrovascular accident
CVP central venous pressure
CXR chest x-ray
D/C discontinue
dl deciliter
D_{LCO} diffusing capacity of carbon monoxide
DNA deoxyribonucleic acid
D_5W 5% dextrose in water
ECG electrocardiogram
ect enteric coated tablet
EDTA ethylenediamine tetraacetic acid
EEG electroencephalogram
EENT eye, ear, nose, and throat
eli elixir
EPS extra pyramidal symptoms
ESR erythrocyte sedimentation rate
EXT REL extended release
°F degrees Fahrenheit
FEV_1 forced expiratory volume in 1 second
FSH follicle-stimulating hormone
g gram
gel gelatin
GERD gastroesophageal reflux disease
GI gastrointestinal
gtt drop
GU genitourinary
H_2 histamine$_2$
HCG human chorionic gonadotropin
hct hematocrit
HEME hematologic
Hgb hemoglobin

5-HIAA 5-hydroxyindoleacetic acid
HIV human immunodeficiency virus
H_2O water
hr hour
hs at bedtime
IgG immunoglobulin G
IM intramuscular
in inch
INF infusion
INH inhalation
inj injection
IPPB intermittent positive-pressure breathing
IV intravenous
kg kilogram
L liter
L-A long acting capsule
lb pound
LDH lactate dehydrogenase
LDL low density lipoprotein
LFT liver function test
LH luteinizing hormone
liq liquid
LMP last menstrual period
loz lozenge
m meter
m^2 square meter
MAOI monoamine oxidase inhibitor
mcg microgram
mEq milliequivalent
mg milligram
Mg magnesium
MI myocardial infarction
min minute
ml milliliter
mm millimeter
mmol millimole
mo month
MS musculoskeletal
neb nebulizer
NPO nothing by mouth
NS normal saline
O_2 oxygen
OD right eye
oint ointment
ophth ophthalmic
OS left eye
OTC over-the-counter
OU each eye
oz ounce
$PaCO_2$ arterial partial pressure of carbon dioxide
PaO_2 arterial partial pressure of oxygen
pc after meals
PCWP pulmonary capillary wedge pressure
PFT pulmonary function test
P_i inorganic phosphorous
PO by mouth
PO_4 phosphate
pr per rectum
prn as needed
PT prothrombin time
PTT partial thromboplastin time
PVC premature ventricular contraction
q every
qAM every morning
qd every day
qh every hour
qid four times a day
qod every other day
qPM every night
q–h every – hour(s)
RAIU radioactive iodine uptake
RBC red blood cell or count
rect rectal
RESP respiratory
RNA ribonucleic acid
SC subcutaneous
SL sublingual
sol solution
SO_4 sulfate
ss one half
supp suppository
SUS REL sustained release
susp suspension
syr syrup
$t_{1/2}$ half life
T_3 triiodothyronine
T_4 thyroxine
tab tablet
TFT thyroid function test
tid three times a day
tinc tincture
T_{max} time to maximum concentration
top topical
trans transdermal
tro troche

TSH thyroid-stimulating hormone
TT thrombin time
U unit
UA urinalysis
UV ultraviolet
vag vaginal
V_d volume of distribution
VMA vanillylmandelic acid
vol volume
VS vital sign
WBC white blood cell or count
wk week
yr year

Federal Controlled Substances Act Schedules

SCHEDULE I: No accepted medical use in the United States and a high abuse potential. Some examples are heroin, marijuana, LSD, peyote, mescaline, psilocybin, methaqualone, and others.

SCHEDULE II: High abuse potential with severe dependence liability. Examples include opium, morphine, codeine, fentanyl, hydromorphone, methadone, meperidine, oxycodone, oxymorphone, cocaine, amphetamine, methamphetamine, phenmetrazine, methylphenidate, phencyclidine, amobarbital, pentobarbital, and secobarbital.

SCHEDULE III: Lesser abuse potential with moderate dependence liability. Examples include compounds containing limited quantities of certain narcotic drugs and nonnarcotic drugs, such as barbiturates, glutethimide, methyprylon, nalorphine, benzphetamine, chlorphentermine, clortermine, phendimetrazine, and paregoric; suppository dosage form containing amobarbital, secobarbital, or pentobarbital.

SCHEDULE IV: Low abuse potential including barbital, phenobarbital, mephobarbital, chloral hydrate, ethchlorvynol, ethinamate, meprobamate, paraldehyde, methohexital, fenfluramine, diethylpropion, phentermine, chlordiazepoxide, diazepam, oxazepam, clorazepate, flurazepam, clonazepam, prazepam, lorazepam, alprazolam, halazepam, temazepam, triazolam, mebutamate, dextropropoxyphene, and pentazocine.

SCHEDULE V: Low abuse potential, includes preparations containing limited quantities of certain narcotic drugs generally for antitussive and antidiarrheal purposes.

FDA Pregnancy Categories

A: Adequate studies in pregnant women have not demonstrated a risk to the fetus in the first trimester of pregnancy, and there is no evidence of risk in later trimesters.

B: Animal studies have not demonstrated a risk to the fetus, but there are no adequate studies in pregnant women; OR animal studies have shown an adverse effect, but adequate studies in pregnant women have not demonstrated a risk to the fetus during the first trimester of pregnancy, and there is no evidence of risk in later trimesters.

C: Animal studies have shown an adverse effect on the fetus, but there are no adequate studies in humans; OR there are no animal reproduction studies and no adequate studies in humans.

D: There is evidence of human fetal risk, but the potential benefits from the use of the drug in pregnant women may be acceptable despite its potential risks.

X: Studies in animals or humans demonstrate fetal abnormalities or adverse reaction; reports indicate evidence of fetal risk. The risk of use in a pregnant woman clearly outweighs any possible benefit.

Contents

Drugs, 1

Appendixes

A. Comparative Tables, 871
B. Bibliography, 891

Index, 893

acarbose

(a'car-bose)

Precose

Chemical Class: Complex oligosaccharide

Therapeutic Class: α-glucosidase inhibitor

CLINICAL PHARMACOLOGY

Mechanism of Action: Competitively inhibits intestinal α-glucosidase enzyme responsible for digestion of complex carbohydrates and disaccharides to absorbable monosaccharides, thus delaying postprandial absorption of glucose; results in attenuation of postprandial plasma glucose, insulin, and triglyceride peaks

Pharmacokinetics

PO: Minimally absorbed in unchanged form; 35% of dose is absorbed as metabolites; biotransformation by intestinal microorganisms; metabolites excreted by urinary and fecal routes; $t_{1/2}$ 2.7-9 hr

INDICATIONS AND USES: Diabetes mellitus, type II: first line for improving glycemic control insufficiently managed with diet alone and as adjunctive therapy in those insufficiently managed with other antidiabetic agents

DOSAGE

Adult

- *Titrated:* Initially, 25 mg tid, taken at beginning of each meal; increase after 6-8 wk to 50-100 mg tid

$ AVAILABLE FORMS/COST OF THERAPY

- Tab—Oral: 50 mg, 100's: **$45.61;** 100 mg, 100's: **$58.80**

CONTRAINDICATIONS: Inflammatory bowel disease, colonic ulceration, partial intestinal obstruction, chronic intestinal disease associated with marked disorders of absorption or digestion, conditions that might be exacerbated by increased intestinal gas or impaired hepatic function

PREGNANCY AND LACTATION: Pregnancy category B; excreted into breast milk in rats; no human data available

SIDE EFFECTS/ADVERSE REACTIONS

GI: Flatulence, abdominal distension, diarrhea, borborygmus/meteorism

METAB: Potential for hypoglycemia only with insulin or sulfonylureas

▼ DRUG INTERACTIONS

Drugs

- *Metformin:* Decreased metformin peak serum and AUC concentrations
- *Charcoal, digestive enzyme preparations:* Reduced effects of acarbose
- *Neomycin:* Enhanced reduction of postprandial blood glucose and exacerbation of adverse effects
- *Cholestyramine:* Enhanced side effects of acarbose

SPECIAL CONSIDERATIONS

PATIENT/FAMILY EDUCATION

- Because acarbose blunts the rise in blood glucose levels following ingestion of carbohydrates, take glucose rather than carbohydrate foods to abort hypoglycemic episodes
- Adverse effects tend to decrease with time and are minimized by gradual introduction of the drug and good dietary discipline (i.e., reduced sucrose)

acebutolol

(a-ce-bute'oh-lol)

Monitan, ♣ Sectral

Chemical Class: Cardioselective, hydrophilic, β-adrenoreceptor blocking agent with intrinsic sympathomimetic activity

Therapeutic Class: Antihypertensive, antianginal, antidysrhythmic

CLINICAL PHARMACOLOGY

Mechanism of Action: Competitively blocks stimulation of β_1 adrenergic receptors; produces negative chronotropic, negative inotropic activity (decreases rate of SA node discharge, increases recovery time); slows conduction of AV node; decreases heart rate, which decreases O_2 consumption in myocardium; decreases renin-aldosterone-angiotensin system at high doses; inhibits β_2 receptors in bronchial system (high doses)

Pharmacokinetics

PO: Onset 1-1½ hr; peak 2-4 hr; duration 10-12 hr; $t_{1/2}$ 6-7 hr; excreted unchanged in urine; protein binding 5%-15%

INDICATIONS AND USES: Hypertension, cardiac dysrhythmias (ventricular premature beats)

DOSAGE

Adult

• *Hypertension:* PO 400 mg qd or in 2 divided doses; increase to desired response; usual range 400-800 mg/d

• *Ventricular dysrhythmia:* PO 200 mg bid, may increase gradually; usual range 600-1200 mg daily

$ **AVAILABLE FORMS/COST OF THERAPY**

• Cap, Gel—Oral: 200 mg, 100's: **$87.96;** 400 mg, 100's: **$116.94**

CONTRAINDICATIONS: Hypersensitivity to β-blockers, cardiogenic shock, heart block (2nd, 3rd degree), sinus bradycardia, CHF, cardiac failure

PRECAUTIONS: Major surgery, diabetes mellitus, renal disease, thyroid disease, COPD, asthma, well-compensated heart failure, aortic, mitral valve disease

PREGNANCY AND LACTATION: Pregnancy category B; acebutolol and diacetolol metabolite cross placenta and appear in breast milk with a milk:plasma ratio of 7.1:12.2; use in nursing mothers not recommended

SIDE EFFECTS/ADVERSE REACTIONS

CNS: Insomnia, fatigue, dizziness, mental changes, memory loss, hallucinations, depression, lethargy, drowsiness, strange dreams, catatonia

CV: ***Profound hypotension, bradycardia, CHF,*** cold extremities, postural hypotension, ***2nd or 3rd degree heart block***

EENT: Sore throat, dry burning eyes

GI: Nausea, diarrhea, vomiting, ***mesenteric arterial thrombosis, ischemic colitis***

GU: Impotence

HEME: ***Agranulocytosis, thrombocytopenia, purpura***

METAB: Hyperglycemia; increased hypoglycemic response to insulin

RESP: ***Bronchospasm,*** dyspnea, wheezing

SKIN: Rash, fever, alopecia

▼ **DRUG INTERACTIONS**

Drugs

• *Amiodarone:* Bradycardia/ventricular dysrhythmia

• *Anesthetics, local:* Enhanced sympathomimetic effects, hypertension due to unopposed α-receptor stimulation

• *Antidiabetics:* Delayed recovery from hypoglycemia, hyperglycemia,

attenuated tachycardia during hypoglycemia, hypertension during hypoglycemia
• *Calcium channel blockers:* Bradycardia, hypotension
• *Clonidine:* Hypotension exacerbated upon withdrawal
• *Disopyramide:* Additive negative inotropic effects
• *Epinephrine:* Enhanced pressor response resulting in hypertension
• *Methyldopa:* Hypertension
• *Neuroleptics:* Increased serum levels of both resulting in accentuated pharmacologic response to both drugs
• *NSAIDs:* Reduced hypotensive effects
• *Phenylephrine:* Acute hypertensive episodes
• *Prazosin:* First-dose hypotensive response enhanced
• *Tacrine:* Additive bradycardia
• *Theophylline:* Antagonist pharmacodynamics

Labs
• *Interference:* Glucose/insulin tolerance tests
• *Increase:* Uric acid, glucose, potassium, triglyceride, lipoproteins

SPECIAL CONSIDERATIONS
• Don't discontinue abruptly, taper over 2 wk; may precipitate angina if stopped abruptly

acetaminophen

(a-seat-a-mee'noe-fen)

Acephen, Aceta, Anacin-3, Apacet, Arthritis Pain Formula, Aspirin Free Pain Relief, Atasol, ✤ Banesin, Campain, ✤ Children's Feverall, Neopap, Dapa, Datril, Dolenex, Dorcol Children's Fever and Pain Reliever, Genebs, Genapap, Halenol, Liquiprin, Meda Tab, Myapap, OraphenPD, Panadol, Panex, Phenaphen, Robigesic, ✤ Rounax, ✤ Snaplets-FR granules, St. Joseph Aspirin-Free for Children, Tempra, Tylenol, Valadol

Chemical Class: Nonsalicylate, para-aminophenol derivative
Therapeutic Class: Nonnarcotic analgesic

CLINICAL PHARMACOLOGY
Mechanism of Action: Blocks pain impulses peripherally by inhibiting cyclooxygenase and the formation of prostaglandins; no antiinflammatory properties; antipyretic action results from inhibition of prostaglandins in the CNS (hypothalamic heat-regulating center)

Pharmacokinetics
PO: Onset 10-30 min, peak ½-2 hr, duration 3-4 hr 60%-70% bioavailable
PR: Onset slow, peak 1-2 hr, duration 3-4 hr; 30%-40% bioavailable; widely distributed, $t_{1/2}$ 3-4 hr; 85%-90% metabolized by liver, excreted by kidneys

INDICATIONS AND USES: Analgesia, antipyresis; arthritic and rheumatic conditions involving musculoskeletal pain; diseases accompanied by discomfort and fever (i.e., common cold, flu, and other bacterial and viral infections)

DOSAGE

Adult and Child >14 yrs

• PO 325-650 mg q4h prn, not to exceed 4 g/day; PR 325-650 mg q4h prn, not to exceed 4 g/day

Child

• PO/PR q4-6h; 0-3 mo (2.7-5 kg) 40 mg/dose; 4-11 mo (5.1-7.7 kg) 80 mg/dose; 12-23 mo (7.8-10.5 kg) 120 mg/dose; 2-3 yr (10.6-15.9 kg) 160 mg/dose; 4-5 yr (16-21.4 kg) 240 mg/dose; 6-8 yr (21.5-26.8 kg) 320 mg/dose; 9-10 yr (26.9-32.3 kg) 400 mg/dose; 11 yr (32.4-43.2 kg) 480 mg/dose; 12-14 yr (> 43.3 kg) 650 mg/dose

$ AVAILABLE FORMS/COST OF THERAPY

• Cap—Oral: 160 mg, 30's: **$4.10;** 325 mg, 24's: **$2.62;** 500 mg, 24's: **$2.89**

• Cap, Gel—Oral: 500 mg, 100's: **$3.35**

• Drops—Oral: 80 mg/0.8 ml, 15 ml: **$1.80**

• Elixir—Oral: 160 mg/5 ml, 120 ml: **$2.08;** alcohol free, 120 ml: **$2.63**

• Geltabs—Oral: 500 mg, 24's: **$3.18**

• Suppos—Rectal: 120 mg, 12's: **$5.50;** 325 mg, 12's: **$5.75;** 650 mg, 12's: **$6.00**

• Tab—Oral: 325 mg, 100's: **$1.49;** 500 mg, 100's: **$2.49;** 650 mg, 100's: **$3.86**

• Tab, Chewable—Oral: 80 mg, 24's: **$4.10**

CONTRAINDICATIONS: Hypersensitivity

PRECAUTIONS: Anemia, hepatic disease, renal disease, chronic alcoholism, elderly

PREGNANCY AND LACTATION: Pregnancy category B; low concentrations in breast milk (1%-2% of maternal dose); compatible with breast feeding

SIDE EFFECTS/ADVERSE REACTIONS

CNS: Stimulation, drowsiness

GI: Nausea, vomiting, abdominal pain, ***hepatotoxicity***

HEME: ***Leukopenia, neutropenia, hemolytic anemia (long-term use), thrombocytopenia, pancytopenia***

SKIN: Rash, urticaria, ***angioedema***

MISC: ***Anaphylaxis;*** Toxicity: ***Cyanosis, anemia, neutropenia, jaundice, pancytopenia, CNS stimulation, delirium followed by vascular collapse, convulsions, coma, death***

▼ DRUG INTERACTIONS

Drugs

• *Barbiturates:* Enhanced hepatoxic potential of overdoses; reduced therapeutic response to acetaminophen

• *Cholestyramine:* Reduced serum acetaminophen levels with reduced therapeutic response

• *Ethanol:* Increased hepatotoxicity of acetaminophen

SPECIAL CONSIDERATIONS

PATIENT/FAMILY EDUCATION

• Do not exceed recommended dosage; acute poisoning with liver damage may result

• Acute toxicity includes symptoms of nausea, vomiting, and abdominal pain; physician should be notified immediately

• Read label on other OTC drugs; many contain acetaminophen and may cause toxicity if taken concurrently

• Urine may become dark brown as a result of phenacetin (metabolite of acetaminophen)

acetazolamide

(a-set-a-zole'-a-mide)

Acetazolam, ✦ Ak-Zol, Cetazol, Dazamide, Diamox, Diamox Sequels

Chemical Class: sulfonamide derivative; carbonic anhydrase inhibitor

Therapeutic Class: Diuretic, anticonvulsant; anti glaucomatous agent; mountain sickness

CLINICAL PHARMACOLOGY

Mechanism of Action: Inhibits carbonic anhydrase activity in proximal renal tubules to decrease reabsorption of water, sodium, potassium, bicarbonate; decreases carbonic anhydrase in CNS, increasing seizure threshold; able to decrease aqueous humor in eye, which lowers intraocular pressure; induces bicarbonate diuresis and metabolic acidosis which enhances ventilatory acclimatization and maintains oxygenation during sleep at high altitude; also counteracts fluid retention and decreases CSF pressure associated with acute mountain sickness

Pharmacokinetics

PO: Onset 1-1½ hr, peak 2-4 hr, duration 6-12 hr

PO-SUS REL: Onset 2 hr, peak 8-12 hr, duration 18-24 hr

IV: Onset 2 min, peak 15 min duration 4-5 hr

65% absorbed if fasting (oral), 75% absorbed if given with food; $t_{1/2}$ = 2½-5½ hr; excreted unchanged by kidneys (80% within 24 hr), crosses placenta

INDICATIONS AND USES: Open-angle glaucoma, narrow-angle glaucoma (preoperatively, if surgery delayed), epilepsy (petit mal, grand mal, mixed), edema in CHF, drug-induced edema, acute mountain sickness (prevention and treatment)

DOSAGE

Adult

- *Narrow-angle glaucoma:* PO/IM/IV 250 mg q4h or 250 mg bid, to be used for short-term therapy
- *Open-angle glaucoma:* PO/IM/IV 250-1000 mg/day in divided doses for amounts over 250 mg
- *Edema:* IM/IV 250-375 mg/day in AM
- *Seizures:* PO/IM/IV 8-30 mg/kg/day, usual range 375-1000 mg/day
- *Mountain sickness:* Treatment: PO 250 mg q8-12h; Prophylaxis: PO 125 mg bid; Periodic breathing at altitude: PO 62.5-125 mg with dinner or HS

Child

- *Edema:* IM/IV 5 mg/kg/day in AM
- *Seizures:* PO/IM/IV 8-30 mg/kg/day in divided doses tid or qid, or 300-900 mg/m^2/day, not to exceed 1.5 g/day

$ AVAILABLE FORMS/COST OF THERAPY

- Tab, Uncoated—Oral: 125 mg, 100's: **$6.66-$27.00;** 250 mg, 100's: **$6.38-$35.82**
- Cap, Gel, Sust Action—Oral: 500 mg, 100's: **$91.71**
- Inj, Lyphl-Sol—500 mg/5ml, 5 ml: **$16.06-$33.88**

CONTRAINDICATIONS: Hypersensitivity to sulfonamides, severe renal disease, severe hepatic disease, electrolyte imbalances (hyponatremia, hypokalemia), hyperchloremic acidosis, Addison's disease, long-term use in narrow-angle glaucoma, COPD

PRECAUTIONS: Hypercalciuria

PREGNANCY AND LACTATION: Pregnancy category D; premature delivery and congenital anomalies in humans; teratogenic (defects of the limbs) in mice, rats, hamsters, and rabbits; not recommended for nursing mothers

SIDE EFFECTS/ADVERSE REACTIONS

CNS: Drowsiness, paresthesia, anxiety, depression, headache, dizziness, confusion, stimulation, fatigue, ***seizures,*** sedation, nervousness

EENT: Myopia, tinnitus

GI: Nausea, vomiting, anorexia, constipation, diarrhea, melena, weight loss, ***hepatic insufficiency,*** taste alterations

GU: Frequency, hypokalemia, polyuria, ***uremia,*** glucosuria, hematuria, dysuria, crystalluria, renal calculi

HEME: ***Aplastic anemia, hemolytic anemia, leukopenia, agranulocytosis, thrombocytopenia, purpura, pancytopenia***

METAB: Hyperglycemia

SKIN: Rash, pruritus, urticaria, fever, ***Stevens-Johnson syndrome,*** photosensitivity

MISC: Loss of taste of carbonated beverages

▼ **DRUG INTERACTIONS**

Drugs

- *Amphetamines:* Increased amphetamine serum levels with prolonged effects
- *Ephedrine:* Increased ephedrine serum levels
- *Methenamine compounds:* Alkalinization of urine decreases antibacterial effects
- *Phenytoin:* Increased risk of osteomalacia
- *Quinidine:* Alkalinization of urine increases quinidine serum levels
- *Salicylates:* Increased serum levels of acetazolamide—CNS toxicity

Labs

- *False positive:* Urinary protein, 17 hydroxysteroid
- *Increase:* Blood glucose levels, bilirubin, blood ammonia, calcium, chloride
- *Decrease:* Urine citrate, potassium

SPECIAL CONSIDERATIONS

PATIENT/FAMILY EDUCATION

- Carbonated beverages taste flat

---

acetic acid

(a-cee'tic)

VoSol, Acetosol, Aci-Jel

Chemical Class: Organic acid

Therapeutic Class: Antibacterial, antifungal

CLINICAL PHARMACOLOGY

Mechanism of Action: Bacteriostatic, fungistatic; penetrates bacterial cells, disrupts cell membrane; restores normal vaginal acidity

INDICATIONS AND USES: Prophylactically in surgical dressings, burns, bladder/urinary catheter irrigant; therapeutically for otitis externa and vaginitis (particularly *Pseudomonas* sp., *Candida* sp., and *Aspergillus* sp.)

DOSAGE

Adult

- *Urinary bladder catheter irrigant:* 30-50 ml flush
- *Otitis externa:* Instill 4-5 drops to affected ear tid
- *Vaginitis:* Apply 1 full applicator bid

Child

- *Otitis externa:* 4-5 drops to affected ear tid

$ **AVAILABLE FORMS/COST OF THERAPY**

- Sol, bladder irrigation: 0.25%, 1000 ml: **$20.48**
- Otic drops: 2%, 15 ml: **$28**
- Gel, vag w/ applicator: 85 g: **$23.88**

SIDE EFFECTS/ADVERSE REACTIONS

EENT: Irritation, burning on instillation

GU: Irritation, local burning and stinging

SPECIAL CONSIDERATIONS

PATIENT/FAMILY EDUCATION

• Home remedy: white distilled household vinegar (5% acetic acid), diluted 50:50 with either water, propylene glycol, glycerin, or rubbing alcohol (70% isopropyl alcohol)

acetohexamide

(a-seat-oh-hex'a-mide)

Dimelor, ✤ Dymelor

Chemical Class: Sulfonylurea (1st generation)

Therapeutic Class: Antidiabetic

CLINICAL PHARMACOLOGY

Mechanism of Action: Stimulates pancreatic insulin release, leading to drop in blood glucose levels; may improve binding between insulin and insulin receptors or increase number of insulin receptors with prolonged administration; may also reduce basal hepatic glucose secretion; not effective if patient lacks functioning β-cells

Pharmacokinetics

PO: Completely absorbed, onset 1 hr, peak 2-4 hr, duration 12-24 hr, $t_{1/2}$ 6-8 hr, metabolized in liver, excreted in urine (active metabolites, unchanged drug)

INDICATIONS AND USES: Diabetes mellitus, Type II

DOSAGE

Adult

• PO 250 mg-1.5 g/day; usually given before breakfast, unless large dose is required; then dose is divided in two

$ AVAILABLE FORMS/COST OF THERAPY

• Tab, Uncoated—Oral: 250 mg, 100's: **$13.20;** 500 mg, 100's: **$25.43**

CONTRAINDICATIONS: Hypersensitivity to sulfonylureas, juvenile or brittle diabetes, renal failure

PRECAUTIONS: Elderly, cardiac disease, renal disease, hepatic disease, thyroid disease, severe hypoglycemic reactions

PREGNANCY AND LACTATION: Pregnancy category C; insulin recommended during pregnancy to maintain blood glucose levels as close to normal as possible; prolonged severe hypoglycemia in neonates; excretion into breast milk unknown, avoid during breast feeding because of potential for serious adverse effects

SIDE EFFECTS/ADVERSE REACTIONS

CNS: Headache, weakness, tinnitus, fatigue, dizziness, vertigo

GI: Nausea, vomiting, diarrhea, ***hepatotoxicity, jaundice,*** heartburn

HEME: ***Leukopenia, thrombocytopenia, agranulocytosis, aplastic anemia, hemolytic anemia***

METAB: ***Hypoglycemia,*** hyponatremia

SKIN: Rash, allergic reactions, pruritus, urticaria, eczema, photosensitivity, erythema

▼ DRUG INTERACTIONS

Drugs

• *Anabolic steroids:* Possible enhanced hypoglycemic effects

• *β-adrenergic blockers:* Altered response to hypoglycemia; may increase blood glucose

• *Clofibrate:* Enhanced hypoglycemic effects

• *Clonidine:* Diminished symptoms of hypoglycemia

• *Colestipol:* May inhibit the lipid-lowering response

• *Contraceptives, oral:* Impaired glucose tolerance

• *Corticosteroids:* Steroids increase blood glucose in diabetics

• *Dicoumarol:* Possible increased anticoagulant effect

• *Ethanol+:* Excessive alcohol increases risks of hypoglycemia; "Antabuse"-like reactions

• *Halofenate:* May increase acetohexamide serum level

• *MAO inhibitors:* Increased risk of hypoglycemia

• *Phenylbutazone+:* Increased acetohexamide serum level and hypoglycemic effects

• *Sulfonamides:* Possible enhanced hypoglycemic effects

• *Thiazide diuretics:* Thiazides increase blood glucose; may increase dosage requirements of acetohexamide

Labs

• *Increase:* AST, ALT, alk phosphatase

• *Decrease:* Uric acid

SPECIAL CONSIDERATIONS

• Additional uricosuric pharmacologic action

---

acetohydroxamic acid

(a-set′oh-hye-drox-am′ic)

Lithostat

Chemical Class: Hydroxylamine, ethyl acetate compound

Therapeutic Class: Ammonia detoxicant, reversible urease inhibitor

CLINICAL PHARMACOLOGY

Mechanism of Action: Inhibits bacterial enzyme urease, which decreases conversion of urea to ammonia; the reduced ammonia levels and decreased pH increase the effectiveness of concurrent urinary antimicrobial agents

Pharmacokinetics

PO: Peak 15-60 min; $t_{1/2}$ 3½-10 hr; hepatic metabolism; excreted in urine as unchanged drug (15%-60%)

INDICATIONS AND USES: Adjunctive treatment in chronic urea-splitting urinary tract infections

DOSAGE

Adult

• PO 250 mg q6-8h when stomach is empty, not to exceed 1.5 g/day

Child

• PO 10 mg/kg/day in 2-3 divided doses

$ AVAILABLE FORMS/COST OF THERAPY

• Tab—Oral: 250 mg, 100's: **$93.75**

CONTRAINDICATIONS: Hypersensitivity, severe renal disease, nonurease-producing organisms

PRECAUTIONS: Deep vein thrombosis, hepatic disease, renal disease, lactation

PREGNANCY AND LACTATION: Pregnancy category X: teratogenic (retarded and clubbed rear leg at 750 mg/kg and above and exencephaly and encephalocele at 1500 mg/kg) when given intraperitoneally to rats

SIDE EFFECTS/ADVERSE REACTIONS

CNS: Headache, depression, restlessness, anxiety, nervousness, malaise

CV: Phlebitis, ***deep vein thrombosis, pulmonary embolism,*** palpitations

GI: Nausea, vomiting, anorexia

HEME: ***Hemolytic anemia (Coombs negative), reticulocytosis***

SKIN: Rash on face, arms, alopecia

▼ DRUG INTERACTIONS

Drugs

• *Ethanol:* Rash

• *Heavy metals:* AHA chelates heavy metals, especially iron; reduced absorption of heavy metals

SPECIAL CONSIDERATIONS

PATIENT/FAMILY EDUCATION

• Avoid alcohol, OTC preparations that contain alcohol; skin rashes have occurred

A

• Concurrent contraception recommended during treatment

acetylcholine

(a-se-teel-koe'leen)

Miochol, Miochol-E

Chemical Class: Quaternary ammonium compound

Therapeutic Class: Miotic, cholinergic

CLINICAL PHARMACOLOGY

Mechanism of Action: Intense, immediate miosis by causing contraction of sphincter muscle of iris

Pharmacokinetics

OPHTH: Miosis occurs immediately, duration 10 min

INDICATIONS AND USES: Miosis during anterior segment surgery, cataract surgery, peripheral iridectomy, cyclodialysis

DOSAGE

Adult and Child

• INSTILL 0.5-2 ml of a 1% sol in anterior chamber of eye (instillation by physician)

$ AVAILABLE FORMS/COST OF THERAPY

• Inj, Conc—Intraocular: 20 mg/vial, 2 ml, 15 ml: **$23.52**

• Inj, Conc, w/Buff—Intraocular, Irrigation, Ophth: 1%, 2 ml: **$33.72**

• Kit—Ophth: 1%, 1's: **$23.52**

• Sol—Ophth: 1%, 2 ml: **$21.36**

CONTRAINDICATIONS: Hypersensitivity; when miosis is undesirable

PRECAUTIONS: Acute cardiac failure, bronchial asthma

SIDE EFFECTS/ADVERSE REACTIONS

CV: Hypotension, bradycardia

EENT: Blurred vision, lens opacities

acetylcysteine

(a-see-til-sis'tay-een)

Airbron, ✦ Mucomyst, Mucosil

Chemical Class: Amino acid, L-cysteine

Therapeutic Class: Mucolytic

CLINICAL PHARMACOLOGY

Mechanism of Action: Decreases viscosity of secretions by breaking disulfide links of mucoproteins; increases hepatic glutathione, which is necessary to inactivate toxic metabolites in acetaminophen overdose

Pharmacokinetics

NEB/INSTILL: Onset 1 min, duration 5-10 min

PO: peak levels within 1-2 hr (0.35-4 mg/L); 50% protein binding, terminal $t_{1/2}$ 6.25 hr, metabolized by liver, excreted in urine

INDICATIONS AND USES: Antidote for acetaminophen overdose; mucolytic: adjuvant therapy for abnormal, viscid, or inspissated mucus secretions in chronic bronchopulmonary disease (chronic bronchitis, cystic fibrosis, emphysema, tuberculosis, bronchiectasis, primary amyloidosis of lung); acute bronchopulmonary disease (pneumonia, bronchitis, tracheobronchitis); tracheostomy care, pulmonary complications associated with surgery; posttraumatic chest conditions, atelectasis due to mucus obstruction, diagnostic bronchial scans (bronchograms, bronchospirometry, bronchial wedge catheterization); keratoconjuncitivitis sicca* (as ophthalmic solution); bowel obstruction* due to meconium ileus or equivalent (PR)

DOSAGE

Adult and Child

• *Mucolytic:*INSTILL 1-2 ml (10%-

20% sol) q1-4h prn; NEB 3-5 ml (20% sol) or 6-10 ml (10% sol) tid
• *Acetaminophen toxicity*: PO 140 mg/kg, then 70 mg/kg q4h × 17 doses to total of 1330 mg/kg; (Oral administration requires dilution of the 20% solution with cola drinks, Fresca or other soft drinks, to a final concentration of 5%; 3 ml of diluent are added to each 1 ml of 20% acetylcysteine solution. Do not decrease the proportion of diluent; dilutions should be freshly prepared and utilized within one hour)

$ **AVAILABLE FORMS/COST OF THERAPY**

• Sol, Inh—Oral: 10%, 4 ml:**$2.56-$8.27;** 10 ml: **$6.52-$13.51;** 30 ml: **$16.87-$53.82**
• Sol, Inh—Oral: 20%, 1 ml:**$1.44;** 4 ml: **$5.16;** 10 ml: **$8.15-$23.77;** 30 ml: **$13.04-$67.74;** 100 ml: **$92.21**

CONTRAINDICATIONS: Hypersensitivity, increased intracranial pressure, status asthmaticus

PRECAUTIONS: Hypothyroidism, Addison's disease, CNS depression, brain tumor, asthma, hepatic disease, renal disease, COPD, psychosis, alcoholism, convulsive disorders

PREGNANCY AND LACTATION: Pregnancy category B

SIDE EFFECTS/ADVERSE REACTIONS

CNS: Dizziness, drowsiness, headache, fever, chills
CV: Hypotension
EENT: Rhinorrhea, *tooth damage*
GI: Nausea, *stomatitis, constipation, vomiting, anorexia,* ***hepatotoxicity***
RESP: ***Bronchospasm,*** *burning,* ***hemoptysis,*** *chest tightness*
SKIN: Urticaria, rash, fever, clamminess

▼ **DRUG INTERACTIONS**

• Avoid use with iron, copper, rubber

acyclovir

(ay-sye'kloe-ver)
Zovirax; Zovirax Ointment 5%; Zovirax Sterile Powder
Chemical Class: Acyclic purine nucleoside analog
Therapeutic Class: Antiviral

CLINICAL PHARMACOLOGY

Mechanism of Action: Interferes with DNA synthesis by conversion to acyclovir triphosphate, causing decreased viral replication

Pharmacokinetics

IV: Onset unknown, peak 1 hr
PO: Onset unknown, peak 1½-2 hr, absorbed minimally $t_{1/2}$ 3½ hr; distributed widely, CSF concentrations are 50% plasma, crosses placenta; metabolized by liver, excreted by kidneys as unchanged drug (95%)

INDICATIONS AND USES

• *Parenteral:* Initial and recurrent mucosal and cutaneous HSV-1, HSV-2, herpes zoster in immunocompromised patients; herpes simplex encephalitis in patients >6 months; severe initial clinical episodes of genital herpes in patients who are not immunocompromised
• *Oral:* Initial and recurrent genital herpes, acute treatment of herpes zoster and chicken pox; CMV and HSV following bone marrow or renal transplant;* disseminated primary eczema herpeticum;* herpes simplex—associated with erythremia multiforme;* herpes simplex—labialis, ocular infections, proctitis, whitlow;* herpes zoster encephalitis,* infectious mononucleosis;* varicella* pneumonia*
• *TOP:* Initial herpes genitalis and limited non-life-threatening mucocutaneous herpes simplex in immunocompromised patients

A

DOSAGE

Adult

- *Herpes simplex:* IV 5 mg/kg over 1 hr q8h × 5 days
- *Genital herpes:* PO 200 mg q4h 5 ×/day while awake for 10 days, 5 days, or 6 mo depending on whether initial, recurrent, or chronic
- *Herpes simplex encephalitis:* IV 10 mg/kg over 1 hr q8h × 10 days
- *Herpes zoster:* PO 800 mg q4h 5×/day × 7-10 days; IV 5 mg/kg over 1 hr q8h
- *Chicken pox:* PO 20 mg/kg (not to exceed 800 mg) orally, qid for 5 days; (therapy should be initiated at the earliest sign or symptom)

Child

- *Herpes simplex:* IV 250 mg/m^2 over 1 hr q8h × 5 days
- *Herpes simplex encephalitis:* Child > 6 mo: IV 500 mg/m^2 q8h × 10 days

Child > 2 yr with immunosuppression: 20 mg/kg qid × 5 days

- *Chicken Pox:* 20 mg/kg orally up to 800 mg qid for 5 days

$ **AVAILABLE FORMS/COST OF THERAPY**

- Cap, Gel—Oral: 200 mg, 100's: **$93.88**
- Inj, Lyphl-Susp—IV: 500 mg/10 ml, 10 ml: **$48.95**
- Oint—Top: 5%, 15 g: **$34.36**
- Susp—Oral: 200 mg/5 ml, 480 ml: **$80.89**
- Tab, Uncoated—Oral: 400 mg, 100's: **$182.18;** 800 mg, 100's: **$354.26**

CONTRAINDICATIONS: Hypersensitivity

PRECAUTIONS: Hepatic disease, renal disease, electrolyte imbalance, dehydration

PREGNANCY AND LACTATION: Pregnancy category C; excreted into breast milk (milk: plasma ratios 0.6-4.1); compatible with breast feeding

SIDE EFFECTS/ADVERSE REACTIONS

CNS: Tremors, confusion, lethargy, hallucinations, ***convulsions,*** *dizziness, headache,* encephalopathic changes

EENT: Gingival hyperplasia

GI: Nausea, vomiting, diarrhea, increased ALT, AST, abdominal pain, glossitis, colitis

GU: ***Oliguria, proteinuria, hematuria,*** vaginitis, moniliasis, ***glomerulonephritis, acute renal failure,*** changes in menses, polydipsia

MS: Joint pain, leg pain, muscle cramps

SKIN: Rash, urticaria, pruritus, pain or phlebitis at IV site, unusual sweating, alopecia

SPECIAL CONSIDERATIONS

- In recurrent herpes genitalis and herpes labialis in non-immunocompromised patients, no evidence of clinical benefit from topical acyclovir

---

adenosine

(ah-den'oh-seen)

Adenocard

Chemical Class: Endogenous nucleoside

Therapeutic Class: Antidysrhythmic

CLINICAL PHARMACOLOGY

Mechanism of Action: Slows conduction through AV node; can interrupt reentry pathways through AV node; restores normal sinus rhythm in patients with paroxysmal supraventricular tachycardia (PSVT)

Pharmacokinetics

IV: Cleared from plasma in <30 sec; $t_{1/2}$ 10 sec

INDICATIONS AND USES: PSVT, including PSVT associated with Wolff-Parkinson-White Syndrome. Does *not* convert atrial flutter, atrial fibrillation, or ventricular tachycardia to normal sinus rhythm; symptomatic relief of varicose vein complications with stasis dermatitis

DOSAGE AND ROUTES

Adult

- *PSVT:* IV bolus 6 mg; if conversion to normal sinus rhythm does not occur within 1-2 min, give 12 mg by rapid IV bolus; may repeat 12 mg dose again in 1-2 min
- *Varicose veins:* IM 25 mg once or twice daily until relief is obtained and then 1 ml (25 mg) 2 or 3 times weekly for maintenance

Child

- *PSVT:* IV bolus 0.05 mg/kg; if not effective within 2 min, increase dose in 0.05 mg/kg increments every 2 min to a maximum of 0.25 mg/kg or until termination of PSVT; median dose, 0.15 mg/kg; do not exceed 12 mg/dose

$ **AVAILABLE FORMS/COST OF THERAPY**

- Inj, sol—IM: 25 mg/ml, 10 ml: **$5.60-$18.50**
- Inj, sol—IV: 3 mg/ml, 2 ml: **$23.40**

CONTRAINDICATIONS: Hypersensitivity, 2nd or 3rd degree heart block, AV block, sick sinus syndrome, atrial flutter, atrial fibrillation, ventricular tachycardia

PRECAUTIONS: Asthma; may induce bronchospasm rarely

PREGNANCY AND LACTATION: Pregnancy category C

SIDE EFFECTS/ADVERSE REACTIONS

CNS: Lightheadedness, dizziness, arm tingling, numbness, apprehension, blurred vision, headache

CV: Chest pain, ***atrial tachydysrhythmia,*** sweating, palpitations, hypotension, *facial flushing*

GI: Nausea, metallic taste, throat tightness, groin pressure

RESP: Dyspnea, chest pressure, hyperventilation

▼ **DRUG INTERACTIONS**

Drug

- *Dipyridamole:* Increased serum adenosine levels, potentiates pharmacologic effects of adenosine

Labs

- *Increase:* Liver function tests

---

albuterol

(al-byoo'ter-ole)

Albuterol, Novosalmol, ✱ Proventil, Proventil Repetabs, Salbutamol, ✱ Ventolin, Ventolin Rotacaps, Volmax

Chemical Class: Adrenergic β_2 agonist

Therapeutic Class: Bronchodilator

CLINICAL PHARMACOLOGY

Mechanism of Action: Bronchodilation by action on β_2 (pulmonary) receptors by increasing levels of cAMP, which relaxes smooth muscle; produces bronchodilation, CNS, cardiac stimulation, as well as increased diuresis and gastric acid secretion; longer acting than isoproterenol

Pharmacokinetics

PO: Onset ½ hr, peak 2½ hr, duration 4-6 hr

PO EXT REL: Onset ½ hr; peak 2-3 hr; duration 12 hr

INH: Onset 5-15 min, peak 1-1½ hr, duration 4-6 hr

Metabolized in liver to inactive sulfate; 28% appears unchanged in urine; $t_{1/2}$ 2½ hr-4 hr

INDICATIONS AND USES: Prevention of exercise-induced asthma, bronchospasm

DOSAGE

Adult

- *Prevention of exercise-induced bronchospasm:* INH 2 puffs, 15 min before exercising
- *Bronchospam:* INH 1-2 puffs q4-6h; NEB 2.5 mg tid-qid; PO 2-4 mg tid-qid, not to exceed 8 mg qid

Child (6-12 years)

- *Prevention of exercise-induced bronchospasm:* INH: 2 puffs 15 min before exercising
- *Bronchospam:* PO 2 mg qid, not to exceed 24 mg per day (given in divided doses); INH 1-2 puffs q4-6h; NEB 2.5 mg tid-qid

Child (2-6 years)

- *Bronchospasm:* PO initial, 0.1 mg/kg of body weight tid, not to exceed 2 mg tid; increase to 0.2 mg/kg of body weight tid, but not to exceed a maximum of 4 mg tid

$ **AVAILABLE FORMS/COST OF THERAPY**

- Sol—Inh: 0.083%, 3 ml: **$23.00-$36.00;** 0.5%, 20 ml: **$10.25-$15.53**
- Syr—Oral: 2 mg/ml, 480 ml: **$24.75-$29.14**
- Tab, Uncoated—Oral: 2 mg, 100's: **$4.88-$34.61;** 4 mg, 100's: **$9.38-$51.62**
- Aer, Metered—Inh: 0.09 mg/inh, 17 g: **$20.33-$22.06**
- Cap, Gel—Inh: 200 μg, 100's: **$26.02**
- Tab, Coated, Sust Action—Oral: 4 mg, 100's: **$57.98**

CONTRAINDICATIONS: Hypersensitivity to sympathomimetics, tachydysrhythmias, severe cardiac disease

PRECAUTIONS: Cardiac disorders, hyperthyroidism, diabetes mellitus, hypertension, prostatic hypertrophy, narrow-angle glaucoma, seizures

PREGNANCY AND LACTATION: Pregnancy category C

SIDE EFFECTS/ADVERSE REACTIONS

CNS: *Tremors,* anxiety, insomnia, headache, dizziness, stimulation, *restlessness,* hallucinations, flushing, irritability

CV: Palpitations, tachycardia, hypertension, angina, hypotension, dysrhythmias

EENT: Dry nose, irritation of nose and throat

GI: Heartburn, nausea, vomiting

METAB: Hypokalemia

MS: Muscle cramps, inhibition of uterine contractions

SPECIAL CONSIDERATIONS

- Inhalation technique critical
- Re-educate routinely
- Consider spacer devices

alclometasone

(al-clo-met'a-sone)

Acloderm, ✤ Aclosone, ✤ Aclovate

Chemical Class: Glucocorticoid

Therapeutic Class: Low potency corticosteroid; anti-inflammatory agent

CLINICAL PHARMACOLOGY

Mechanism of Action: Anti-inflammatory, antipruritic, and vasoconstrictive actions

Pharmacokinetics

TOP: Approximately 3% absorbed during eight hours of contact with intact, normal, skin; enters pharmacokinetic pathways similarly to systemically administered corticosteroids; metabolized primarily in liver and then excreted by kidneys; also excreted into bile

INDICATIONS AND USES: Inflammatory and pruritic manifestations of corticosteroid-responsive dermatoses

DOSAGE

Adult and Child

- TOP: Apply to affected area bid

$ AVAILABLE FORMS/COST OF THERAPY

- Cre—Top: 0.05%, 15 g: **$10.31**
- Oint—Top: 0.05%, 15 g: **$10.31**

CONTRAINDICATIONS: Hypersensitivity

PRECAUTIONS: Systemic absorption has resulted in reversible HPA axis suppression, manifestations of Cushing's syndrome, hyperglycemia, and glucosuria; application of the more potent steroids, especially in children, use over large surface areas, prolonged use, and addition of occlusive dressings augments systemic absorption

PREGNANCY AND LACTATION: Pregnancy category C; systemically administered corticosteroids are secreted into breast milk in quantities not likely to have a deleterious effect on the infant

SIDE EFFECTS/ADVERSE REACTIONS

SKIN: Itching, burning, erythema, dryness, irritation, papular rashes, irritation, dryness, folliculitis, hypertrichosis, acneiform eruptions, hypopigmentation, perioral dermatitis, allergic contact dermatitis, maceration of the skin, secondary infection, skin atrophy, striae, and miliaria

▼ DRUG INTERACTIONS

Labs

- *Decreased:* Urinary free cortisol, ACTH stimulation

SPECIAL CONSIDERATIONS

PATIENT/FAMILY EDUCATION

- Caution when applied chronically to face or other thin-skinned areas

---

alfentanil

(al-fen'ta-nil)

Alfenta, Rapifen ♣

Chemical Class: Opiate, synthetic

Therapeutic Class: Narcotic analgesic

DEA Class: Controlled Substance Schedule II

CLINICAL PHARMACOLOGY

Mechanism of Action: Inhibits ascending pain pathways in limbic system, thalamus, midbrain, hypothalamus

Pharmacokinetics

IV: Duration, 30 min; $t_{1/2}$ 1-2 hr, 90% bound to plasma proteins

INDICATIONS AND USES: Adjunctive (in combination with barbiturates/nitrous oxide/oxygen) maintenance anesthesia or primary anesthetic for induction in general surgery

DOSAGE

Adult

- *Combination:* IV 8-50 μg/kg, may increase by 3-15 μg/kg
- *Anesthetic induction:* IV 130-245 μg/kg, then 0.5-1.5 μg/kg/min

$ AVAILABLE FORMS/COST OF THERAPY

- Inj, Sol—IV: 500 μg/ml, 2 ml: **$7.50**

CONTRAINDICATIONS: Children, hypersensitivity

PRECAUTIONS: Increased intracranial pressure, acute MI, severe heart disease, renal disease, hepatic disease, asthma, respiratory conditions, seizure disorders, elderly

PREGNANCY AND LACTATION: Pregnancy category C; placental transfer of the drug has been reported; significant levels detected in colostrum 4 hours after administration of 60 μg/kg, with no detectable levels present after 28 hours; no clinical significance

SIDE EFFECTS/ADVERSE REACTIONS

CNS: Drowsiness, dizziness, confusion, headache, sedation, euphoria, delirium, agitation, anxiety

CV: Palpitation, bradycardia, change in B/P, facial flushing, syncope, asystole

EENT: Tinnitus, blurred vision, miosis, diplopia

GI: Nausea, vomiting, anorexia, constipation, cramps, dry mouth

GU: Urinary retention

RESP: ***Respiratory depression, apnea***

SKIN: Rash, urticaria, bruising, flushing, diaphoresis, pruritus

▼ **DRUG INTERACTIONS**

Labs

Increase: Amylase

allopurinol

(al-oh-pure'i-nole)

Apoallopurinol, ♣ Novapurol, ♣ Lopurin, Purimol, ♣ Zyloprim

Chemical Class: Enzyme (xanthine oxidase) inhibitor

Therapeutic Class: Antigout drug

CLINICAL PHARMACOLOGY

Mechanism of Action: Inhibits the enzyme xanthine oxidase, reducing uric acid synthesis

Pharmacokinetics

PO: Peak 2-4 hr; excreted in feces and urine; $t_{1/2}$ 2-3 hr, active metabolite $t_{1/2}$ 18-30 hr

INDICATIONS AND USES: Chronic primary or secondary gout (prevention of acute attacks, tophi, joint destruction, uric acid lithiasis or nephropathy), hyperuricemia associated with malignancies, recurrent calcium oxalate calculi, prevention of fluorouracil-induced stomatitis (as mouthwash 1 mg/ml in methylcellulose*)

DOSAGE

Adult

- *Gout/hyperuricemia:* PO 200-600 mg qd depending on severity, not to exceed 800 mg/day
- *Impaired renal function:* PO 200 mg qd when CrC1 is 10-20 ml/min
- *Recurrent calculi:* PO 200-300 mg qd
- *Uric acid nephropathy prevention:* PO 600-800 mg qd × 2-3 days

Child (6-10 years)

- 300 mg qd; <6 yr: 150 mg qd

$ **AVAILABLE FORMS/COST OF THERAPY**

- Tab, Uncoated—Oral: 100 mg, 100's: **$3.38-$17.95;** 300 mg, 100's: **$10.59-$51.22**

CONTRAINDICATIONS: Hypersensitivity

PRECAUTIONS: Renal disease, hepatic disease, children; discontinue at first sign of allergy including skin rash; severe hypersensitivity reactions such as exfoliative, urticarial, and purpuric lesions as well as erythema multiforme exudativum, and generalized vasculitis, irreversible hepatotoxicity, and, on rare occasions, death may follow

PREGNANCY AND LACTATION: Pregnancy category C; allopurinol and oxypurinol have been found in the milk of a mother who was receiving allopurinol

SIDE EFFECTS/ADVERSE REACTIONS

CNS: Headache, drowsiness, neuritis, paresthesia

GI: Nausea, vomiting, anorexia, malaise, metallic taste, cramps, peptic ulcer, diarrhea, stomatitis, hepatomegaly, ***cholestatic jaundice***

EENT: Retinopathy, cataracts, epistaxis

GU: ***Renal failure***
HEME: ***Agranulocytosis, thrombocytopenia, aplastic anemia, pancytopenia, leukopenia, bone marrow depression, eosinophilia***
MS: Arthralgia, myopathy
SKIN: Dermatitis, pruritus, purpura, erythema, ecchymosis, alopecia
MISC: Fever, chills

▼ **DRUG INTERACTIONS**

Drugs

• *Angiotensin-converting enzyme inhibitors:* Predisposed to hypersensitivity reactions including Stevens-Johnson syndrome, skin eruptions, fever, and arthralgias
• *Antacids:* Aluminum hydroxide inhibits the response to allopurinol
• *Azathioprine+:* Increased toxicity of azathioprine; requires dose adjustment
• *Cyclophosphamide:* May increase cyclophosphamide toxicity—inconsistent
• *Mercaptopurine+:* Increased effect of mercaptopurine with increased risk of toxicity
• *Oral anticoagulants:* Enhanced hypothrombinemic response
• *Theophylline:* Large doses may increase serum theophylline levels

Labs

• *Increase:* AST/ALT, alk phosphatase
• *Decrease:* Hct/Hgb, leukocytes, serum glucose

SPECIAL CONSIDERATIONS

• Increased acute attacks of gout during early stages of allopurinol administration
• Maintenance doses of colchicine (0.6 mg qd-bid) should be given prophylactically along with starting with low doses of allopurinol

alprazolam

(al-pray′zoe-lam)
Apo-alpraz, ♣ Novo-alprazol, ♣ Nu-alpraz, ♣ Xanax
Chemical Class: Benzodiazepine
Therapeutic Class: Anxiolytic

CLINICAL PHARMACOLOGY

Mechanism of Action: Depresses subcortical levels of CNS, including limbic system, reticular formation

Pharmacokinetics

PO: Onset 30 min, peak 1-2 hr, duration 4-6 hr, therapeutic response 2-3 days, metabolized by liver, excreted by kidneys; crosses placenta; $t_{1/2}$ 12-15 hr

INDICATIONS AND USES: Anxiety, panic disorders, anxiety with depressive symptoms, agoraphobia with social phobia (2-8 mg/day),* depression,* premenstrual syndrome*

DOSAGE

Adult

• *Anxiety:* PO 0.25-0.5 mg tid, to 4 mg/day in divided doses
• *Panic disorder:* PO 0.5 mg tid; increase dose q3-4 days in 1 mg/d increments to 10 mg/d
• *Geriatric:* PO 0.25 mg bid-tid

$ **AVAILABLE FORMS/COST OF THERAPY**

• Tab, Plain Coated—Oral: 0.25 mg, 100's: **$33.84-$56.67;** 0.5 mg, 100's: **$38.91-$70.59;** 1 mg, 100's: **$55.38-$107.72;** 2 mg, 100's: **$88.39-$160.10**
• Sol—Oral: 0.5 mg/5ml, 500 ml: **$51.75;** 1 mg/ml w/dropper, 30 ml: **$37.50**

CONTRAINDICATIONS: Hypersensitivity to benzodiazepines, narrow-angle glaucoma

PRECAUTIONS: Elderly, debilitated, hepatic disease, renal disease

PREGNANCY AND LACTATION: Pregnancy category D; child born of a mother receiving benzodiazepines may be at some risk for withdrawal symptoms from drug during postnatal period; neonatal flaccidity and respiratory problems have been reported; since benzodiazepines are excreted in human milk, assume that alprazolam is as well; chronic administration of diazepam to nursing mothers has been reported to cause infants to become lethargic and lose weight

SIDE EFFECTS/ADVERSE REACTIONS

CNS: Dizziness, drowsiness, confusion, headache, anxiety, tremors, stimulation, fatigue, depression, insomnia, hallucinations

CV: Orthostatic hypotension, ***ECG changes, tachycardia,*** hypotension

EENT: Blurred vision, tinnitus, mydriasis

GI: Constipation, dry mouth, nausea, vomiting, anorexia, diarrhea

SKIN: Rash, dermatitis, itching

DRUG INTERACTIONS

Drugs

• *Cimetidine:* Cimetidine inhibits metabolism, increases plasma levels

• *Ethanol:* Enhanced adverse psychomotor effects; difficulty performing tasks that require alertness

• *Fluoxetine:* Increases alprazolam plasma concentrations; increases in psychomotor impairment

• *Fluvoxamine:* Increases alprazolam plasma concentration; increases in psychomotor impairment

Labs

• *Increase:* AST/ALT, serum bilirubin

• *False increase:* 17-OHCS

• *Decrease:* RAIU

SPECIAL CONSIDERATIONS

PATIENT/FAMILY EDUCATION

• Not for "everyday" stress or longer than 3 mo; avoid driving, activities that require alertness

• Caution when medication discontinued abruptly after long-term use—may precipitate withdrawal syndrome

alprostadil

(al-pros'ta-dil)

Prostin VR Pediatric,

Prostin VR ✦

Chemical Class: Prostaglandin E_1

Therapeutic Class: Hormone

CLINICAL PHARMACOLOGY

Mechanism of Action: Relaxes smooth muscle of ductus arteriosus; results in increased O_2 content throughout body

Pharmacokinetics

INTRACAVERNOSAL: Peak 5-20 min; up to 80% metabolized in lungs, excreted in urine (metabolites)

INDICATIONS AND USES: Palliative therapy to temporarily maintain patency of the ductus arteriosus until definitive surgery can be performed, erectile dysfunction

DOSAGE

Adult

• *Erectile dysfunction:* Intracavernosal 2.5-20 μg prior to intercourse, three times weekly, with at least 24 hrs between uses

Infants

• IV Inf 0.1 μg/kg/min, until desired response, then reduce to lowest effective amount, 0.4 μg/kg/min not likely to produce greater beneficial effects

AVAILABLE FORMS/COST OF THERAPY

• Inj, Sol—IV: 500 μg/ml, 1 ml: **$32.78**

• Inj, Lyoph Powder: 10 μg/ml, 6's: **$83.40;** 20 μg/ml, 6's: **$107.40**

CONTRAINDICATIONS: Hypersensitivity, respiratory distress syndrome (RDS); conditions that might predispose to priapism (eg, sickle cell anemia/trait, multiple myeloma, leukemia), patients with anatomical deformation of penis (eg, Peyronie's disease), penile implants

PRECAUTIONS: Bleeding disorders; cortical proliferation of the long bones with long-term infusions, regressed after withdrawal of the drug; men for whom sexual activity is inadvisable

SIDE EFFECTS/ADVERSE REACTIONS

CNS: Fever, ***seizures,*** cerebral bleeding, hyperextension of the neck, hyperirritability, hypothermia, jitteriness, lethargy, stiffness, ***cerebral bleeding***

CV: ***Bradycardia, tachycardia, hypotension, CHF, ventricular fibrillation, shock,*** flushing, ***cardiac arrest,*** edema

GI: Diarrhea, regurgitation, hyperbilirubinemia

GU: Oliguria, hematuria, ***anuria;*** *penile pain,* prolonged erection, penile fibrosis, injection site hematoma

HEME: ***DIC, thrombocytopenia,*** anemia, ***bleeding***

MS: Cortical proliferation of the long bones

RESP: ***Apnea, bradypnea, wheezing, respiratory depression,*** hypercapnia, tachypnea

MISC: ***Sepsis,*** hypokalemia, ***peritonitis,*** hypoglycemia, hyperkalemia

SPECIAL CONSIDERATIONS

- Instruct patient on proper storage, use, and discarding of needles and syringes

MONITORING PARAMETERS

- Infant ABG's, arterial pH, arterial pressure, continuous ECG

alteplase

(al-teep'lase)

Activase, Actilyse, ✦ TPA

Chemical Class: Tissue plasminogen activator (TPA)

Therapeutic Class: Antithrombotic

CLINICAL PHARMACOLOGY

Mechanism of Action: Promotes fibrin conversion of plasminogen to plasmin; able to bind to fibrin, convert plasminogen in thrombus to plasmin, which leads to local fibrinolysis, limited systemic proteolysis

Pharmacokinetics

IV: Cleared by liver, 80% cleared within 10 min of drug termination

INDICATIONS AND USES: Acute MI: for lysis of thrombi obstructing coronary arteries, improvement of ventricular function, and reduction in incidence of CHF; pulmonary embolism: for lysis of pulmonary embolism, defined as obstruction of flow to a lobe or multiple segments of lung or lysis accompanied by unstable hemodynamics; unstable angina pectoris*

DOSAGE

Adult

- IV a total of 100 mg (6-10 mg given IV bolus over 1-2 min, 60 mg given over first hr, 20 mg given over second hr, 20 mg given over third hr); or 1.25 mg/kg given over 3 hr for smaller patients

$ AVAILABLE FORMS/COST OF THERAPY

- Inj, Lyphl-Sol—IV: 1 mg/ml, 20 mg: **$550.00;** 1 mg/ml, 50 mg: **$1375.00;** 1 mg/ml, 100 mg: **$2750.00**

CONTRAINDICATIONS: Hypersensitivity, active bleeding, recent

CVA, severe uncontrolled hypertension, intracranial/intraspinal surgery/trauma, aneurysm, AV malformation, brain tumor, subacute bacterial endocarditis, puncture of noncompressible blood vessel within past 10 days, mitral stenosis with atrial fibrillation (left heart thrombosis concerns)

PRECAUTIONS: Recent (within 10 days) major surgery, e.g., coronary artery bypass graft, obstetrical delivery, organ biopsy; previous puncture of noncompressible vessels; cerebrovascular disease; recent gastrointestinal or genitourinary bleeding (within 10 days); recent trauma (within 10 days); hypertension (systolic BP ≥ 180 mm Hg and/or diastolic BP ≥ 110 mm Hg); high likelihood of left heart thrombus (e.g., mitral stenosis with atrial fibrillation); acute pericarditis; subacute bacterial endocarditis; hemostatic defects including those secondary to severe hepatic or renal disease; significant liver dysfunction; pregnancy; diabetic hemorrhagic retinopathy, or other hemorrhagic ophthalmic conditions; septic thrombophlebitis or occluded AV cannula at seriously infected site; advanced age (>75 yr); patients currently receiving oral anticoagulants (e.g., warfarin); any other condition in which bleeding constitutes a significant hazard or would be particularly difficult to manage because of its location; readministration

SIDE EFFECTS/ADVERSE REACTIONS

CV: ***Sinus bradycardia, ventricular tachycardia, accelerated idioventricular rhythm***

HEME: ***Intracranial, retroperitoneal bleeding, surface bleeding***

SKIN: Urticaria, rash

▼ DRUG INTERACTIONS

Drugs

- *Heparin, acetylsalicylic acid, dipyridamole:* Increased bleeding

Labs

- *Increase:* PT, APTT, TT

SPECIAL CONSIDERATIONS

- Institute therapy as soon as possible following onset of clinical symptoms

MONITORING PARAMETERS

- Prior to initiation of therapy: coagulation tests, hematocrit, platelet count
- During therapy: ECG, mental status, neurological status, vital signs; heparin (in doses sufficient to prolong the APTT to 1.5-2 times control value) is usually administered in conjunction with thrombolytic therapy; aspirin may also be administered to inhibit platelet aggregation during and/or following post-thrombolytic therapy

---

aluminum acetate

(aloo'min-um aas'a-tate)

Bluboro Powder, Boropak Powder, Burow's Solution, Domeboro, Modified Burrow's Solution, Pedi-Boro Soak Paks

Chemical Class: Aluminum salt
Therapeutic Class: Astringent

CLINICAL PHARMACOLOGY

Mechanism of Action: Maintains skin acidity, which is protective to skin surface

INDICATIONS AND USES: Skin irritation, inflammation, athlete's foot, insect bites, poison ivy, eczema, acne, rash, bruises, pruritus (anal)

DOSAGE

Adult and Child

- TOP apply for 15-30 min, q4-8h (1:10-1:40 dilution); GARGLE prn (1:10 dilution)

$ AVAILABLE FORMS/COST OF THERAPY

- Powder Packets—Top: 12's: **$7.47**
- Tab—Top: 12's: **$7.47**

CONTRAINDICATIONS: Tight, occlusive dressing

SIDE EFFECTS/ADVERSE REACTIONS

SKIN: Irritation, increasing inflammation

▼ DRUG INTERACTIONS

- *TOP collagenase oint:* Aluminum acetate inhibits action

SPECIAL CONSIDERATIONS

PATIENT/FAMILY EDUCATION

- Soap decreases the astringent actions of aluminum acetate; 1 packet or tab/1 pt water produces a modified 1:40 Burow's solution

aluminum chloride hexahydrate

Drysol, Lumicaine, Xerac Ac

Chemical Class: Aluminum salt
Therapeutic Class: Antihidrotic

CLINICAL PHARMACOLOGY

Mechanism of Action: Astrigent or increased permeability of the sweat duct causing reabsorption of sweat

INDICATIONS AND USAGE: Hyperhidrosis

DOSAGE

Adult

- TOP apply to affected area at bedtime; to help prevent irritation, area should be completely dry prior to application; wash treated area the following morning; excessive sweating may be stopped after two or more treatments; thereafter, apply once or twice weekly or as needed

$ AVAILABLE FORMS/COST OF THERAPY

- Sol—Top: 6.25%, 35 ml: **$5.78;** 20%, 35 ml: **$6.63**

PRECAUTIONS: Broken, irritated, or recently shaved skin

SIDE EFFECTS/ADVERSE REACTIONS

SKIN: Burning or prickling sensation, transient stinging or itching

SPECIAL CONSIDERATIONS

PATIENT/FAMILY EDUCATION

- Do not apply to broken or irritated skin
- Keep container tightly closed
- For maximum effect cover the treated area with saran wrap held in place by a snug fitting tee-shirt or body shirt, mitten or sock (never hold saran wrap in place with tape)
- Avoid contact with the eyes
- If irritation or sensitization occurs, discontinue use or consult physician
- May be harmful to certain metals and fabrics
- Do not use near open flame

aluminum salts

Aluminum carbonate gel
aluminum hydroxide
AlternaGEL, Alu-Cap, Alugel, ✤ Alu-Tab, Amphojel, Basalijel, ✤ Dialume

Chemical Class: Aluminum salt
Therapeutic Class: Antacid, adsorbent

CLINICAL PHARMACOLOGY

Mechanism of Action: Neutralizes gastric acidity, binds phosphates in GI tract; enhances phosphate excretion

Pharmacokinetics

PO: Onset 20-40 min; non-absorbable; excreted in feces

INDICATIONS AND USES: Antacid, (symptomatic relief of hyperacidity, GERD, peptic ulcer disease), phosphate renal stones (prevention), phosphate binder, reduction of hyperphosphatemia in chronic renal failure

DOSAGE

ALUMINUM CARBONATE

Adult

- *Urinary phosphate stones:* SUSP 5-10 ml 1 hr pc, hs; EXTRA STR SUSP 2.5-5 ml 1 hr pc, hs; PO 2-6 tabs 1 hr pc, hs
- *Antacid:* SUSP 15-45 ml 1 hr pc, hs; EXTRA STR SUSP 5-15 ml 1 hr pc, hs; PO chew 1-2 tabs or caps as needed

ALUMINUM HYDROXIDE

Adult

- *Antacid:* PO SUSP 5-15 ml 1 hr pc, hs; PO TAB 600 mg 1 hr pc, hs, chewed with milk or water
- *Hyperphosphatemia in renal failure:* PO SUSP 5-30 ml bid-qid; PO TAB 500-1800 mg bid-qid; titrate to normal serum phosphorus

Child

- *Hyperphosphatemia in renal failure:* PO SUSP 50-150 mg/kg/24 hr in divided doses q4-6 hr; titrate to normal serum phosphorus

$ AVAILABLE FORMS/COST OF THERAPY

ALUMINUM CARBONATE

- Cap—Oral: 500 mg, 100's: **$11.81**
- Susp—Oral: 400 mg/5 ml, 360 ml: **$5.34**
- Tab—Oral: 500 mg, 100's: **$10.06**

ALUMINUM HYDROXIDE

- Cap—Oral: 475 mg, 100's: **$14.70;** 500 mg, 100's: **$15.06**
- Tab—Oral: 300 mg, 100's: **$5.41;** 600 mg, 100's: **$8.56**
- Susp—Oral: 320 mg/5 ml, 360 ml: **$3.05-$5.10;** 600 mg/5 ml, 360 ml: **$5.74**
- Susp, Sugar Free—Oral: 675 mg/5 ml, 500 ml: **$6.13**

DIHYROXYALUMINUM SODIUM CARBONATE

- Tab—Chewable—Oral: 334 mg, 75's: **$4.33**

CONTRAINDICATIONS: Hypersensitivity to this drug or aluminum products, appendicitis

PRECAUTIONS: Elderly, fluid restriction, decreased GI motility, GI obstruction, dehydration, sodium-restricted diets

PREGNANCY AND LACTATION: Pregnancy category C

SIDE EFFECTS/ADVERSE REACTIONS

GI: Constipation, anorexia, ***obstruction,*** fecal impaction

METAB: Hypophosphatemia, hypercalciuria

MISC: Aluminum intoxication, osteomalacia

▼ DRUG INTERACTIONS

Drugs

- *Allopurinol:* Aluminum hydroxide inhibits the GI absorption of allopurinol and limits hyperuricemic response
- *Cefpodoxime proxetil:* Antacids reduce bioavailability and serum concentration of cefpodoxime and could reduce efficacy
- *Doxycycline:* Reduced serum doxycycline concentration and efficacy, separate doses by 1-2 hr
- *Iron:* Reduced GI absorption of iron; inhibit hematological response to iron; separate doses
- *Isoniazid:* Some antacids reduce plasma concentration of INH
- *Quinolones:* Antacids reduce the serum concentration of all the fluoroquinolones and may inhibit their efficacy
- *Salicylates:* Decreased serum salicylate concentrations, requiring salicylate dosage adjustments
- *Sodium polystyrene sulfonate resin:* Combined use may result in systemic alkalosis
- *Tacrine:* Antacids have no effect on tacrine absorption, but tacrine may increase gastric acid secretion
- *Tetracycline+:* Co-therapy with a tetracycline and an antacid containing divalent or trivalent cations can

reduce the serum concentration and efficacy of the tetracycline

SPECIAL CONSIDERATIONS

PATIENT/FAMILY EDUCATION

- Thoroughly chew chewable tablets before swallowing, follow with a glass of water
- May impair absorption of many drugs; do not take other drugs within 1-4 hr of aluminum hydroxide administration
- Stools may appear white or speckled

MONITORING PARAMETERS

- Monitor for hypophosphatemia: anorexia, weakness, fatigue, bone pain, hyporeflexia; urinary pH, Ca^{++}, electrolytes

---

amantadine

(a-man'ta-deen)

Symadine, Symmetrel

Chemical Class: Tricyclic amine

Therapeutic Class: Antiviral; antiparkinsonian agent

CLINICAL PHARMACOLOGY

Mechanism of Action: Prevents uncoating of nucleic acid in viral cell, preventing penetration of virus to host; causes release of dopamine from dopaminergic terminals in the substantia nigra

Pharmacokinetics

PO: Onset 48 hr (Parkinson's disease), $t_{1/2}$ 15-17 hr, 67% protein bound, 90% excreted unchanged in urine

INDICATIONS AND USES: Prophylaxis or treatment of influenza type A, Parkinson's disease, drug-induced extrapyramidal reactions

DOSAGE

Adult

- *Influenza type A:* PO 200 mg/day in single dose or divided bid; start treatment as soon as possible after onset of symptoms and continue for 24-48 hr after symptoms disappear; start prophylaxis in anticipation of contact or as soon as possible after exposure, continue at least 10 days following a known exposure
- *Parkinson's disease:* PO 100 mg qd for 1 wk then increase gradually to 400 mg/day in divided doses if needed
- *Drug-induced extrapyramidal reactions:* PO 100 mg bid, increase to 300 mg/day in divided doses if needed
- *Dosage with renal impairment* (based on creatinine clearance in ml/min/1.73m^2): PO (30-50) 200 mg 1st day followed by 100 mg qd thereafter; (15-29) 200 mg 1st day followed by 100 mg qod thereafter; (<15) 200 mg every 7 days

Elderly

- *Influenza type A:* 100-200 mg/day

Child

- *Influenza type A:* (1-9 yr) PO 4.4-8.8 mg/kg/day divided bid qd or bid, do not exceed 150 mg/day; (9-12 yr) PO 100 mg bid

$ AVAILABLE FORMS/COST OF THERAPY

- Cap—Oral: 100 mg, 100's: **$20.46-$84.72**
- Syr—Oral: 50 mg/5 ml, 480 ml: **$57.50-$77.52**

CONTRAINDICATIONS: Hypersensitivity, child <1 yr

PRECAUTIONS: Epilepsy, CHF, orthostatic hypotension, psychiatric disorders, hepatic disease, renal disease, peripheral edema, eczematoid rash, abrupt discontinuation

PREGNANCY AND LACTATION: Pregnancy category C; excreted in human milk, exercise caution when administering to nursing mothers because of potential for urinary retention, vomiting, and skin rash

SIDE EFFECTS/ADVERSE REACTIONS

CNS: Headache, *dizziness/light-*

A

headedness, insomnia, fatigue, anxiety, psychosis, depression, hallucinations, confusion, anorexia, ataxia, ***convulsions***

CV: Orthostatic hypotension, ***CHF,*** peripheral edema

EENT: Blurred vision

GI: Nausea, vomiting, constipation, dry mouth

GU: Urinary retention

HEME: ***Leukopenia***

SKIN: Photosensitivity, rash, eczematoid dermatitis, livedo reticularis

▼ DRUG INTERACTIONS

Drugs

• *Benztropine:* Potentiation of amantadine's CNS side effects

• *Trihexyphenidyl:* Potentiation of amantadine's CNS side effects

SPECIAL CONSIDERATIONS

PATIENT/FAMILY EDUCATION

• Administer at least 4 hr before bedtime to prevent insomnia

• Take with meals for better absorption and to decrease GI symptoms

• Divided doses may lessen CNS side effects

• Arise slowly from a reclining position; avoid hazardous activities if dizziness or blurred vision occurs

• Do not discontinue abruptly in Parkinson's disease

---

ambenonium

(am-be-noe'nee-um)

Mytelase

Chemical Class: Synthetic quaternary ammonium compound

Therapeutic Class: Cholinergics, Anticholinesterase

CLINICAL PHARMACOLOGY

Mechanism of Action: An acetylcholinesterase inhibitor, inhibits destruction of acetylcholine, which increases concentration at sites where acetylcholine is released, facilitating transmission of impulses across myoneural junction

Pharmacokinetics

PO: Onset 20-30 min, duration 3-8 hr

INDICATIONS AND USES: Myasthenia gravis (particularly useful in patients sensitive to bromides)

DOSAGE

Adult

• PO 5 mg q3-4h while awake, gradually increased q1-2 days to optimal muscle strength and no GI disturbances (range 5 mg - 75 mg per dose), doses above 200 mg/day require close supervision to avoid overdosage

$ AVAILABLE FORMS/COST OF THERAPY

• Tab, Scored—Oral: 10 mg, 100's: **$79.19**

CONTRAINDICATIONS: Obstruction of intestine, renal system; hypersensitivity

PRECAUTIONS: Seizure disorder, asthma, coronary occlusion, hyperthyroidism, dysrhythmias, peptic ulcer, bradycardia, hypotension, children, presence of other cholinergics (atropine sulfate should be available for cholinergic crisis)

PREGNANCY AND LACTATION: Pregnancy category C; would not be expected to cross placenta or be excreted into breast milk because it is ionized at physiologic pH; although apparently safe for the fetus, may cause transient muscle weakness in the newborn

SIDE EFFECTS/ADVERSE REACTIONS

CNS: Dizziness, headache, ***convulsions,*** incoordination, ***paralysis, loss of consciousness,*** drowsiness

CV: Tachycardia, dysrhythmias, bradycardia, hypotension, AV block, nodal rhythm, nonspecific ECG changes, ***cardiac arrest,*** syncope

EENT: Miosis, blurred vision, lacrimation, visual changes, spasm of accommodation, diplopia, conjunctival hyperemia

GI: Nausea, diarrhea, vomiting, cramps, increased salivation, increased gastric secretions, dysphagia, increased peristalsis, flatulence

GU: Frequency, incontinence, urgency

MS: Weakness, fasciculation, muscle cramps and spasms, arthralgia

RESP: ***Respiratory depression, bronchospasm, constriction, laryngospasm, respiratory arrest,*** increased secretions, dyspnea

SKIN: Rash, urticaria, sweating

SPECIAL CONSIDERATIONS

PATIENT/FAMILY EDUCATION

- Notify physician of nausea, vomiting, diarrhea, sweating, increased salivation, irregular heartbeat, muscle weakness, severe abdominal pain or difficulty in breathing occurs
- Administer on an empty stomach

MONITORING PARAMETERS

- Therapeutic response: Increased muscle strength, improved gait, absence of labored breathing (if severe)
- Appearance of side effects: Narrow margin between first appearance of side effects and serious toxicity

amcinonide

(am-sin'oh-nide)

Cyclocort

Chemical Class: Synthetic fluorinated agent, high potency

Therapeutic Class: Topical corticosteroid

CLINICAL PHARMACOLOGY

Mechanism of Action: Depresses formation, release and activity of the endogenous mediators of inflammation such as prostaglandins, kinins, histamine, liposomal enzymes, and the complement system resulting in decreased edema, erythema, and pruritus

Pharmacokinetics

Absorbed through the skin (increased by inflammation and occlusive dressings), metabolized primarily in the liver

INDICATIONS AND USES: Psoriasis, eczema, contact dermatitis, pruritus

DOSAGE

Adult and Child

- Apply to affected area bid; rub completely into skin

$ AVAILABLE FORMS/COST OF THERAPY

- Cre—Top: 0.1%, 15, 30 and 60 g: **$15.34-$38.38**
- Lotion—Top: 0.1%, 20 and 60 ml: **18.48-$36.54**
- Oint—Top: 0.1%, 15, 30 and 60 g: **$15.34-$38.38**

CONTRAINDICATIONS: Hypersensitivity to corticosteroids, fungal infections, use on face, groin or axilla

PRECAUTIONS: Viral infections, bacterial infections, children

PREGNANCY AND LACTATION: Pregnancy category C; unknown whether topical application could result in sufficient systemic absorption to produce detectable amounts in breast milk (systemic corticosteroids are secreted into breast milk in quantities not likely to have detrimental effects on infant)

SIDE EFFECTS/ADVERSE REACTIONS

SKIN: Burning, dryness, itching, irritation, acne, folliculitis, hypertrichosis, perioral dermatitis, hypopigmentation, atrophy, striae, miliaria, allergic contact dermatitis, secondary infection

MISC: Systemic absorption of topical corticosteroids has produced reversible HPA axis suppression (more likely with occlusive dressings, prolonged administration, application to large surface areas, liver failure, and in children)

SPECIAL CONSIDERATIONS

PATIENT/FAMILY EDUCATION

- Apply sparingly only to affected area
- Avoid contact with the eyes
- Do not put bandages or dressings over the treated area unless directed by physician
- Do not use on weeping, denuded, or infected areas
- Discontinue drug, notify physician if local irritation or fever develops

---

amikacin

(am-i-kay'sin)
Amikin
Chemical Class: Aminoglycoside
Therapeutic Class: Antibiotic

CLINICAL PHARMACOLOGY

Mechanism of Action: Interferes with protein synthesis in bacterial cell by binding to ribosomal subunit, which causes misreading of genetic code, inaccurate peptide sequence forms in protein chain, causing bacterial death

Pharmacokinetics

IM: Onset rapid, peak 1-2 hr
IV: Onset immediate
Plasma $t_{1/2}$ 2-3 hr, not metabolized, excreted unchanged in urine

INDICATIONS AND USES: Severe systemic infections of CNS, respiratory, GI, urinary tract, bone, skin, soft tissues caused by susceptible organisms

Antibacterial spectrum usually includes:

- Gram-positive organisms: *Staphylococcus* sp. including methicillin-resistant strains (in general has a low order of activity against other Gram-positive organisms)
- Gram-negative organisms: *Pseudomonas* sp., *E. coli, Proteus* sp. (indole-positive and indole-negative), *Providencia* sp., *Klebsiella, Enterobacter,* and *Serratia* sp., *Acinetobacter* sp., *Citrobacter freundii*

DOSAGE

Adult

- *Severe systemic infections:* IV INF 15 mg/kg/day (use ideal body weight) in 2-3 divided doses q8-12h in 100-200 ml diluent over 30-60 min, not to exceed 1.5 g/day; decreased doses are needed in poor renal function as determined by blood levels and renal function studies; IM 15 mg/kg/day in divided doses q8-12h
- *Uncomplicated urinary tract infections:* IM 250 mg bid
- *In patient with poor renal function:* 7.5 mg/kg initially, then adjusted as determined by blood levels and renal function studies

Child

- *Severe systemic infections:* IV INF 15 mg/kg/day (use ideal body weight) in 2-3 divided doses q8-12h in 100-200 ml diluent over 30-60 min, not to exceed 1.5 g/day; decreased doses are needed in poor renal function as determined by blood levels and renal function studies; IM 15 mg/kg/day in divided doses q8-12h

Neonate

- IV INF 10 mg/kg initially, then 7.5 mg/kg q12h in diluent over 1-2 hr

$ AVAILABLE FORMS/COST OF THERAPY

- Inj, Sol—IM, IV: 50 mg/ml, 2 ml: **$35.25-$36.99;** 250 mg/ml, 2 ml:

\$58.75-\$68.56; 250 mg/ml, 4 ml: **\$116.10-\$126.92**

CONTRAINDICATIONS: Hypersensitivity to aminoglycosides

PRECAUTIONS: Neonates, renal disease, myasthenia gravis, hearing deficits, Parkinson's disease, elderly, sulfite sensitivity (contains sodium bisulfite), dehydration

PREGNANCY AND LACTATION: Pregnancy category C; ototoxicity has not been reported as an effect of *in utero* exposure; 8th cranial nerve toxicity in the fetus is well known following exposure to other aminoglycosides and could potentially occur with amikacin; excreted into breast milk in low concentrations, poor oral bioavailability reduces potential for ototoxicity for the infant, may modify bowel flora or interfere with interpretation of culture results if fever workup is required

SIDE EFFECTS/ADVERSE REACTIONS

CNS: Confusion, depression, numbness, tremors, ***convulsions,*** muscle twitching, ***neurotoxicity,*** dizziness, vertigo

CV: Hypotension or hypertension, palpitations

EENT: Ototoxicity: hearing loss, deafness; visual disturbances, tinnitus

GI: Nausea, vomiting

GU: ***Oliguria,*** hematuria, ***renal damage,*** azotemia, ***renal failure,*** nephrotoxicity

HEME: ***Agranulocytosis, thrombocytopenia, leukopenia,*** eosinophilia, anemia

SKIN: *Rash,* urticaria, dermatitis, alopecia

▼ **DRUG INTERACTIONS**

Drugs

- *Amphotericin B:* Synergistic nephrotoxicity
- *Cephalosporins:* Increased potential for nephrotoxicity in patients with pre-existing renal disease
- *Cyclosporine:* Additive renal damage
- *Ethacrynic acid+:* Increased risk of ototoxicity
- *Extended spectrum penicillins:* Potential for inactivation of amikacin in patients with renal failure
- *Methoxyflurane:* Enhanced renal toxicity
- *Neuromuscular blocking agents+:* Potentiation of respiratory suppression produced by neuromuscular blocking agents
- *NSAIDs:* Reduced renal clearance of aminoglycosides in premature infants

SPECIAL CONSIDERATIONS

PATIENT/FAMILY EDUCATION

- Report headache, dizziness, loss of hearing, ringing, roaring in ears or feeling of fullness in head

MONITORING PARAMETERS

- Urinalysis for proteinuria, cells, casts; urine output
- Serum peak, drawn at 30-60 min after IV inf or 60 min after IM inj, trough level drawn just before next dose, adjust dosage per levels (usual therapeutic plasma levels; peak 20-35 mg/L, trough ≤10 mg/L)
- Serum creatinine for CrCl calculation

amiloride

(a-mill'oh-ride)

Midamor

Chemical Class: Pyrazine

Therapeutic Class: Potassium-sparing diuretic

CLINICAL PHARMACOLOGY

Mechanism of Action: Inhibits sodium reabsorption at the distal convoluted tubule, cortical collecting tubule, and collecting duct which decreases the net negative potential of the tubular lumen and reduces both potassium and hydrogen secretion and their subsequent excretion

Pharmacokinetics

PO: Onset 2 hr, peak 6-10 hr, duration 24 hr, excreted unchanged in urine (60%), feces (40%), $t_{1/2}$ 6-9 hr

INDICATIONS AND USES: Adjunctive treatment with thiazide or loop diuretics in congestive heart failure or hypertension to help restore potassium balance; lithium-induced polyuria;* aerosolized administration (drug dissolved in 0.3% saline delivered by nebulizer) in cystic fibrosis*

DOSAGE

Adult

- PO 5 mg qd, may be increased to 10-20 mg qd if needed

$ AVAILABLE FORMS/COST OF THERAPY

- Tab, Uncoated—Oral: 5 mg, 100's: **$17.03-$44.65**

CONTRAINDICATIONS: Hypersensitivity, hyperkalemia (serum potassium >5.5 mEq/L), impaired renal function

PRECAUTIONS: Dehydration, diabetes, acidosis, hepatic function impairment, children

PREGNANCY AND LACTATION: Pregnancy category B; excretion into breast milk unknown, use caution in nursing mothers

SIDE EFFECTS/ADVERSE REACTIONS

CNS: Headache, dizziness, fatigue, weakness, paresthesias, tremor, depression, anxiety, encephalopathy, vertigo, nervousness, mental confusion, insomnia, decreased libido

CV: Orthostatic hypotension, dysrhythmias, angina

EENT: Loss of hearing, tinnitus, blurred vision, nasal congestion, increased intraocular pressure

GI: Nausea, diarrhea, dry mouth, *vomiting, anorexia,* cramps, constipation, abdominal pain, jaundice, GI bleeding, dyspepsia, flatulence

GU: Polyuria, dysuria, frequency, impotence

HEME: ***Agranulocytopenia, leukopenia, thrombocytopenia*** (rare)

METAB: Acidosis, hyponatremia, ***hyperkalemia,*** hypochloremia

MS: Cramps, joint pain

SKIN: Rash, pruritus, alopecia, urticaria

▼ DRUG INTERACTIONS

Drugs

- *ACE inhibitors:* Hyperkalemia in predisposed patients
- *Potassium+:* Hyperkalemia in predisposed patients

Labs

- *Interfere:* GTT

SPECIAL CONSIDERATIONS

PATIENT/FAMILY EDUCATION

- Notify physician of muscle cramps, weakness, nausea, dizziness, blurred vision
- Take with food or milk for GI symptoms
- Take early in day to prevent nocturia
- Avoid large quantities of potassium-rich foods: oranges, bananas, salt substitutes

MONITORING PARAMETERS

- BP: postural hypotension may occur
- Electrolytes: potassium, sodium, chloride
- Glucose (serum), BUN, serum creatinine

aminocaproic acid

(a-mee-noe-ka-proe′ik)

Amicar

Chemical Class: Synthetic monoaminocarboxylic acid

Therapeutic Class: Hemostatic

CLINICAL PHARMACOLOGY

Mechanism of Action: Inhibits fibrinolysis by inhibiting plasminogen activator substances and, to a lesser degree, by antiplasmin activity

Pharmacokinetics

PO: Rapidly absorbed, peak 2 hr; excreted by kidneys as unmetabolized drug, $t_{1/2}$ 2 hr

INDICATIONS AND USES: Hemorrhage from systemic hyperfibrinolysis and urinary fibrinolysis; adjunctive therapy in hemophilia;* recurrent subarachnoid hemorrhage;* amegakaryocytic thrombocytopenia*

DOSAGE

Adult

• IV 4-5 g in 250 ml NS, D_5W or LR, infused over 1 hr, followed by continuous infusion at the rate of 1 g/hr diluted in 50-100 ml of compatible solution, not to exceed 30 g/day; use infusion pump; do not give by direct IV; PO 5 g loading dose during first hour, then 1-1.25 g qh if needed, not to exceed 30 g/day

Child

• IV 100 mg/kg or 3 g/m^2 loading dose followed by continuous infusion at the rate of 33.3 mg/kg/hr or 1 g/m^2/hr, do not exceed 18 g/m^2/day; PO 100-200 mg/kg loading dose followed by 100 mg/kg/dose q6h, not to exceed 30 g/day

$ AVAILABLE FORMS/COST OF THERAPY

• Inj, Sol—IV: 250 mg/ml, 96 ml: **$26.34-$74.04**

• Syr—Oral: 1.25 g/5 ml, 480 ml: **$391.27**

• Tab, Uncoated—Oral: 500 mg, 100's: **$156.75**

CONTRAINDICATIONS: Hypersensitivity, DIC, upper urinary tract bleeding, neonates (injectable contains benzyl alcohol)

PRECAUTIONS: Renal disease, hepatic disease, thrombosis, cardiac disease

PREGNANCY AND LACTATION: Pregnancy category C; excretion in milk unknown, use caution in nursing mothers

SIDE EFFECTS/ADVERSE REACTIONS

CNS: Headache, dizziness, hallucinations, delirium, psychosis, ***convulsions***

CV: ***Dysrhythmias,*** hypotension, bradycardia

EENT: Tinnitus, nasal congestion, conjunctival suffusion

GI: Nausea, vomiting, abdominal cramps, diarrhea

GU: Dysuria, frequency, oliguria, ***renal failure,*** ejaculatory failure, menstrual irregularities

HEME: ***Thrombosis***

MS: Myopathy, fatigue, malaise, weakness, ***rhabdomyolysis***

SKIN: Rash

▼ DRUG INTERACTIONS

Labs

• *Increased:* K^+, CPK

SPECIAL CONSIDERATIONS

PATIENT/FAMILY EDUCATION

• Report any signs of bleeding (gums, under skin, urine, stools, emesis) or myopathy

• Change position slowly to decrease orthostatic hypotension

MONITORING PARAMETERS

• Do **not** administer without a definite diagnosis and laboratory findings indicative of hyperfibrinolysis

• Blood studies including coagulation factors, platelets, protamine coagulation test for extravascular clotting, thrombophlebitis; CPK, urinalysis

aminoglutethimide

(a-meen-noe-gloo-teth'i-mide)

Cytadren

Chemical Class: Hormone

Therapeutic Class: Adrenal steroid inhibitor; antineoplastic, adjuvant

CLINICAL PHARMACOLOGY

Mechanism of Action: Inhibits the enzymatic conversion of cholesterol to Δ^5-pregnenolone, resulting in a decrease in the production of adrenal glucocorticoids, mineralocorticoids, androgens, and estrogens

Pharmacokinetics

PO: Peak 1.5 hr, $t_{1/2}$ 13 hr, metabolized in liver, excreted in urine

INDICATIONS AND USES: Suppression of adrenal function in Cushing's syndrome (usually as an interim measure until surgery or in cases where more definitive therapy is not appropriate); postmenopausal patients with advanced breast cancer; metastatic prostate cancer

DOSAGE

Adult

- PO 250 mg qid at 6 hr intervals, may increase by 250 mg/day q1-2 wk, not to exceed 2 g/day

$ AVAILABLE FORMS/COST OF THERAPY

- Tab, Uncoated—Oral: 250 mg, 100's: **$100.34**

CONTRAINDICATIONS: Hypersensitivity to glutethamide or aminoglutethamide

PRECAUTIONS: Condition of stress (e.g., surgery, trauma, acute illness), hypothyroidism, hypotension

SIDE EFFECTS/ADVERSE REACTIONS

CNS: Drowsiness, dizziness, headache, lethargy

CV: ***Hypotension, tachycardia***

GI: Nausea, vomiting, anorexia, ***hepatotoxicity***

HEME: (Rare) ***neutropenia, leukopenia, pancytopenia, thrombocytopenia, agranulocytosis***

METAB: Adrenal insufficiency, hypothyroidism

SKIN: Rash, pruritus, hirsutism

▼ DRUG INTERACTIONS

Drugs

- *Corticosteroids:* Enhanced elimination leading to reduction in corticosteroid response
- *Digitoxin:* Reduced serum digitoxin concentration
- *Medroxyprogesterone:* Reduced plasma medroxyprogesterone concentrations
- *Oral anticoagulants:* Reduced hypoprothrombinemic response
- *Tamoxifen:* Reduced serum tamoxifen concentration

SPECIAL CONSIDERATIONS

PATIENT/FAMILY EDUCATION

- May cause drowsiness or dizziness, rash, fainting, weakness, headache, nausea and loss of appetite

MONITORING PARAMETERS

- BUN, serum uric acid, urine CrCl, electrolytes before, during therapy
- Temperature may indicate infection
- Liver function tests before, during therapy (bilirubin, AST, ALT, LDH)
- CBC

aminophylline (theophylline ethylenediamine)

(am-in-off'i-lin)

Corophyllin, ✤ Palaron, ✤ Phyllocontin, Truphylline

Chemical Class: Xanthine, ethylenediamine

Therapeutic Class: Bronchodilator

CLINICAL PHARMACOLOGY

Mechanism of Action: Activity due to theophylline; directly relaxes the smooth muscle of bronchi and pulmonary blood vessels, stimulates respiration and increases diaphragmatic contractility, probably via inhibition of extracellular adenosine (which causes bronchoconstriction); stimulation of endogenous catecholamines, antagonism of prostaglandins, direct effect on mobilization of intracellular calcium, and inhibition of cGMP metabolism (inhibition of phosphodiesterase with resultant increases in cAMP does not occur to an appreciable extent at therapeutic concentrations)

Pharmacokinetics

PO: Well absorbed, onset ¼ hr, peak 1-2 hr, duration 6-8 hr

PO-ER: Onset unknown, peak 4-7 hr, duration 8-12 hr

IV: Onset rapid, duration 6-8 hr

PR: Absorption slow and erratic, onset erratic, peak 3-5 hr, duration 6-8 hr

Metabolized by liver; excreted in urine; $t_{1/2}$ 3-12 hr, $t_{1/2}$ increased in geriatric patients, hepatic disease, cor pulmonale and CHF, decreased in children and smoking

INDICATIONS AND USES: Asthma, reversible bronchospasm associated with COPD; apnea and bradycardia of prematurity,* essential tremor,* pulmonary edema

DOSAGE

Adult and Child

• *PO acute therapy (patients not currently receiving theophylline products):* Following a 6.3 mg/kg loading dose, maintenance dose follows: children age 1-9 yr, 5.1 mg/kg q6h; children age 9-16 yr and smokers, 3.8 mg/kg q6h; otherwise healthy non-smoking adults, 3.8 mg/kg q8h; older patients/patients with CHF, cor pulmonale, 2.5 mg/kg q8h

• *PO acute therapy (patients currently receiving theophylline products):* Defer loading dose if serum theophylline concentration can be rapidly obtained; base loading dose on the principle that each 0.63 mg/kg of aminophylline will increase serum theophylline concentration by 1 µ/ml; if this is not possible and sufficient respiratory distress is present use 3.1 mg/kg of aminophylline administered in a rapidly available form; will likely increase serum theophylline concentration 5 µg/ml (administer only if theophylline toxicity is not present); maintenance dosage as described above

• *PO chronic therapy:* Initial dose 20.3 mg/kg/24 hr or 500 mg/24 hr (whichever is less) divided q6-8h; increase q 3 days by 25% as tolerated until clinical response or maximum dose is reached (below); monitor serum theophylline concentrations. Do not exceed the following (or 1140 mg, whichever is less without serum level monitoring): Age 1-9 yr, 30.4 mg/kg/day; age 9-12 yr, 25.3 mg/kg/day; age 12-16 yr, 22.8 mg/kg/day; age 16 yr and older, 16.5 mg/kg/day

• *IV (patients not currently receiving theophylline products):* Following a 6.3 mg/kg IV loading dose, maintenance dose follows: Children age 1-9 yr, 1 mg/kg/hr; children age 9-16 yr and smokers, 0.8 mg/kg/hr; otherwise healthy nonsmoking adults, 0.5 mg/kg/hr; older patients/patients with cor pulmonale, 0.3 mg/kg/hr; patients with CHF, 0.1-0.2 mg/kg/hr

• *IV (patients currently receiving theophylline products):* Defer loading dose if serum theophylline concentration can be rapidly obtained. Base loading dose on the principle that each 0.63 mg/kg of aminophylline will increase serum theophylline concentration by 1 μg/ml. If this is not possible and sufficient respiratory distress is present use 3.1 mg/kg of aminophylline; will likely increase serum theophylline concentration 5 μg/ml (administer only if theophylline toxicity is not present); maintenance dosage as described above

$ AVAILABLE FORMS/COST OF THERAPY

- Inj, Sol—IV: 25 mg/ml, 10 ml: **$2.05-$18.44**
- Sol—Oral: 105 mg/5 ml, 240 ml: **$5.69-$12.13**
- Tab, Uncoated—Oral: 100 mg, 100's: **$1.50-$8.26;** 200 mg, 100's: **$3.02-$8.96**
- Tab, Uncoated, Sust Action—Oral: 225 mg, 100's: **$33.22**
- Supp—Rect: 250 mg, 10's: **$7.50-$13.12;** 500 mg, 10's: **$8.50-$14.48**

CONTRAINDICATIONS: Hypersensitivity to xanthines or ethylenediamine, underlying seizure disorder (not on anticonvulsant therapy); suppositories are contraindicated in the presence of irritation or infection of the rectum or lower colon

PRECAUTIONS: Elderly, CHF, cor pulmonale, hepatic disease, preexisting arrhythmias, hypertension, infants <1 yr, hypoxemia, sustained high fever, history of peptic ulcer, alcoholism

PREGNANCY AND LACTATION: Pregnancy category C; pharmacokinetics of theophylline may be altered during pregnancy, monitor serum concentrations carefully; excreted into breast milk, may cause irritability in the nursing infant, otherwise compatible with breast feeding

SIDE EFFECTS/ADVERSE REACTIONS

CNS: Anxiety, restlessness, insomnia, *dizziness,* ***convulsions,*** headache, lightheadedness, muscle twitching, reflex hyperexcitability

CV: Palpitations, sinus tachycardia, hypotension, flushing, ventricular arrhythmias, circulatory failure, extrasystoles

GI: Nausea, vomiting, anorexia, diarrhea, bitter taste, dyspepsia, anal irritation (suppositories), epigastric pain, hematemesis, esophageal reflux

GU: Urinary frequency, proteinuria

METAB: Hyperglycemia, SIADH (consider ethylenediamine)

RESP: Tachypnea

SKIN: Urticaria, alopecia

▼ DRUG INTERACTIONS

Drugs

- *Allopurinol, Cimetidine+, Ciprofloxacin, Disulfiram, Fluvaxamine, Mexiletine, Pefloxacin, Pentoxifylline, Propafenone, Radioactive iodine, Thiabendazole, Ticlopidine, Troleandomycin:* Increased serum theophylline concentrations
- *Barbiturates, Carbamazepine, Rifampin:* Reduced serum theophylline concentrations
- *β-adrenergic blockers:* Antagonistic pharmacologic effects, propranolol increases serum theophylline concentrations in a dose-dependent manner
- *Calcium channel blockers:* Increased serum theophylline concentrations with verapamil and possibly diltiazem
- *Enoxacin:* Markedly increased serum theophylline concentrations
- *Erythromycin:* Increased serum theophylline concentrations; reduced erythromycin concentrations
- *Interferon:* Increased serum theophylline concentrations, especially in smokers and other patients with high pre-existing theophylline clearance
- *Lithium:* Reduced lithium concentrations

• *Phenytoin:* Reduced serum theophylline concentrations; decreased serum phenytoin concentrations
• *Smoking:* Increased theophylline dosing requirements

SPECIAL CONSIDERATIONS

PATIENT/FAMILY EDUCATION

• Take doses as prescribed; do not change doses without consulting physician
• Avoid large amounts of caffeine-containing products (tea, coffee, chocolate, colas)
• If GI upset occurs, take with 8 oz water
• Notify physician if nausea, vomiting, insomnia, jitteriness, headache, rash, palpitations occur

MONITORING PARAMETERS

• Serum theophylline concentrations (therapeutic level is 10-20 μg/ml); toxicity may occur with small increase above 20 μg/ml, especially in the elderly

---

aminosalicylate

(a-mee-noe-sal-i'si-late)
Sodium P.A.S.
Chemical Class: Salicylate
Therapeutic Class: Antituberculosis agent

CLINICAL PHARMACOLOGY

Mechanism of Action: Prevents synthesis of folic acid by competitively blocking the conversion of aminobenzoic acid to dihydrofolic acid; bacteriostatic against *Mycobacterium tuberculosis;* inhibits onset of bacterial resistance to isoniazid and streptomycin

Pharmacokinetics

PO: Peak 0.5-1 hr; concentrates in pleural and caseous tissue; metabolized by liver, excreted in urine; $t_{1/2}$ 1 hr

INDICATIONS AND USES: Alternative treatment of tuberculosis (always in combination with streptomycin, isoniazid, or both)

DOSAGE

Adult

PO 14-16 g/day in 2-3 divided doses

Child

PO 275-420 mg/kg/day in 3-4 divided doses

$ AVAILABLE FORMS/COST OF THERAPY

• Tab, Coated—Oral: 0.5 g, 100's: **$9.60**

CONTRAINDICATIONS: Severe hypersensitivity to aminosalicylate sodium and its congeners; G-6-PD deficiency

PRECAUTIONS: Impaired renal or hepatic function, acidic urine, gastric ulcer, CHF and other situations in which excess sodium is potentially harmful

PREGNANCY AND LACTATION: Pregnancy category C; excreted into breast milk, use caution in nursing mothers

SIDE EFFECTS/ADVERSE REACTIONS

GI: Nausea, vomiting, diarrhea, abdominal pain, hepatitis, jaundice
HEME: ***Leukopenia, agranulocytosis, thrombocytopenia, hemolytic anemia***
METAB: Goiter with or without myxedema
SKIN: Skin eruptions
MISC: Fever, infectious mononucleosis-like syndrome, encephalopathy, Loffler's syndrome, vasculitis

▼ DRUG INTERACTIONS

Drugs

• *Digitalis glycosides:* Small reduction in serum digoxin concentrations
• *Probenecid:* Increased serum aminosalicylic acid concentrations
• *Rifampin:* Reduced serum rifampin concentrations

SPECIAL CONSIDERATIONS

PATIENT/FAMILY EDUCATION

- Administer with food to decrease stomach upset
- Protect from moisture and extremes of temperature
- Notify physician if fever, sore throat, unusual bleeding or bruising, or skin rashes occur

---

amiodarone

(a-mee′oh-da-rone)

Cordarone

Chemical Class: Iodinated benzofuran derivative

Therapeutic Class: Antidysrhythmic (Class III)

CLINICAL PHARMACOLOGY

Mechanism of Action: Prolongs action potential duration, and effective refractory period, noncompetitive α- and β-adrenergic inhibition

Pharmacokinetics

PO: Slowly and variably absorbed; onset 1-3 wk; extensive distribution; $t_{1/2}$ 26-107 days; eliminated via hepatic excretion into bile

INDICATIONS AND USES: Life-threatening recurrent ventricular fibrillation and hemodynamically unstable ventricular tachycardia unresponsive to adequate doses of other antiarrhythmics; refractory sustained or paroxysmal atrial fibrillation and paroxysmal supraventricular tachycardia,* symptomatic atrial flutter,* CHF (low dose)*

DOSAGE

Adult

- PO loading dose 800-1600 mg/day for 1-3 wk; then 600-800 mg/day for1 mo; maintenance 200-600 mg/day

Child

- PO loading dose 10-15 mg/kg/day or 600-800 mg/1.73 m^2/day for 4-14 days or until adequate control of dysrhythmia or prominent adverse effects occur; maintenance 5 mg/kg/day or 200-400 mg/1.73 m^2/day qd for several weeks, reduce to lowest effective dosage possible

$ AVAILABLE FORMS/COST OF THERAPY

- Tab, Uncoated—Oral: 200 mg, 60's: **$163.71**

CONTRAINDICATIONS: Severe sinus-node dysfunction, with resultant marked sinus bradycardia; 2nd and 3rd degree AV block; syncope caused by episodes of bradycardia (except when used in conjunction with a pacemaker); hypersensitivity

PRECAUTIONS: Thyroid disease, 2nd or 3rd degree AV block, electrolyte imbalances, bradycardia, pulmonary disease (poorer prognosis should pulmonary toxicity develop)

PREGNANCY AND LACTATION: Pregnancy category C; due to a very long $t_{1/2}$, amiodarone should be discontinued several months prior to conception to avoid early gestational exposure, reserve for refractory dysrhythmias; newborns exposed to amiodarone should have TFTs; excreted into breast milk, contains high proportions of iodine, breastfeeding not recommended

SIDE EFFECTS/ADVERSE REACTIONS

Adverse reactions occur in about 75% of patients receiving doses ≥400 mg/day and cause discontinuation in 7%-18%

CNS: Headache, dizziness, involuntary movements, tremors, peripheral neuropathy, malaise, fatigue, ataxia, paresthesias, insomnia, lack of coordination

CV: Hypotension, bradycardia, ***sinus arrest,*** CHF, ***dysrhythmias, SA node dysfunction, cardiac conduction abnormalities***

EENT: Blurred vision, halos, photophobia, corneal microdeposits, dry eyes

GI: Nausea, vomiting, diarrhea, abdominal pain, anorexia, constipation, ***hepatotoxicity***

METAB: Hyperthyroidism or hypothyroidism

MS: Weakness, pain in extremities

RESP: ***Pulmonary fibrosis,*** pulmonary inflammation

SKIN: Rash, photosensitivity, blue-gray skin discoloration, alopecia, spontaneous ecchymosis

MISC: Flushing, abnormal taste or smell, edema, abnormal salivation, coagulation abnormalities

▼ **DRUG INTERACTIONS**

Drugs

• *β-adrenergic blockers:* Bradycardia, cardiac arrest, or ventricular arrhythmia shortly after initiation of β-adrenergic blockers that undergo extensive hepatic metabolism

• *Calcium channel blockers:* Cardiotoxicity with bradycardia and decreased cardiac output with diltiazem and potentially verapamil

• *Cyclosporine:* Increased cyclosporine concentrations

• *Digitalis glycosides:* Accumulation of digoxin

• *Flecainide:* Increased flecainide serum concentrations

• *Oral anticoagulants+:* Enhanced hypoprothrombinemic response to warfarin

• *Phenytoin:* Increased serum phenytoin concentrations, decreased amiodarone concentrations

• *Procainamide:* Increased procainamide concentrations

• *Quinidine:* Increased quinidine plasma concentrations

Labs

• *Increase:* Serum T4 and serum reverse T3

• *Decrease:* Serum T3

SPECIAL CONSIDERATIONS

Should be administered only by physicians experienced in treatment of life-threatening dysrhythmias who are thoroughly familiar with the risks and benefits of amiodarone therapy

PATIENT/FAMILY EDUCATION

• Take with food and/or divide doses if GI intolerance occurs

• Use sunscreen or stay out of sun to prevent burns

• Report side effects immediately

• Skin discoloration is usually reversible

MONITORING PARAMETERS

• Chest x-ray and PFTs (baseline and q3mo)

• Electrolytes

• LFTs

• ECG (measure PR, QRS, QT intervals, check for PVCs, other dysrhythmias)

• TFTs

• CNS symptoms

amitriptyline

(a-mee-trip′ti-leen)

Elavil, Endep, Enovil, Levate, ♣ Meravil, ♣ Novo-triptyn, ♣ Rolavil ♣

Chemical Class: Tertiary amine

Therapeutic Class: Antidepressant–tricyclic

CLINICAL PHARMACOLOGY

Mechanism of Action: Inhibits the reuptake of norepinephrine and serotonin at the presynaptic neuron, prolonging neuronal activity; inhibits histamine and acetylcholine activity; mild peripheral vasodilator effects and possible "quinidine-like" actions

Pharmacokinetics

PO/IM: Onset 45 min, peak 2-4 hr, therapeutic response 2-4 wk once adequate dosage achieved; metabolized by liver (active metabolite, nortriptyline), excreted in urine/feces, crosses placenta, $t_{1/2}$ 10-50 hr

INDICATIONS AND USES: Depression, chronic pain (chronic tension headache, migraine, diabetic neuropathy, cancer pain, postherpetic neuralgia),* panic disorder,* eating disorders,* myofacial pain syndromes*

DOSAGE

Adult

• PO 50-100 mg hs, may increase to 200 mg/day, not to exceed 300 mg/day (chronic pain doses usually at lower end of range); IM (do not administer IV) 20-30 mg qid, or 80-120 mg hs

Adolescent/Geriatric

• PO 30 mg/day in divided doses, may be increased to 150 mg/day

Child

• *Chronic pain management:* PO 0.1 mg/kg/day in 3 divided doses initially, advance as tolerated over 2-3 weeks to 0.5-2 mg/kg qhs

• *Depression:* PO 1 mg/kg/day in 3 divided doses initially with increases to 1.5 mg/kg/day

$ **AVAILABLE FORMS/COST OF THERAPY**

• Inj, Sol—10 mg/ml, 10 ml: **$4.00-$8.54**

• Tab, Coated—Oral: 10 mg, 100's: **$1.43-$17.87;** 25 mg, 100's: **$1.65-$39.31;** 50 mg, 100's: **$2.40-$66.34;** 75 mg, 100's: **$2.93-$87.26;** 100 mg, 100's: **$3.38-$110.34;** 150 mg, 100's: **$7.05-$157.01**

CONTRAINDICATIONS: Hypersensitivity to tricyclic antidepressants, acute recovery phase of MI, concurrent use of MAO inhibitors

PRECAUTIONS: Suicidal patients, convulsive disorders, prostatic hypertrophy, psychiatric disease, severe depression, increased intraocular pressure, narrow-angle glaucoma, urinary retention, cardiac disease (2° or 3° heart block or sick sinus syndrome), hepatic disease/renal disease, hyperthyroidism, electroshock therapy, elective surgery, elderly, abrupt discontinuation

PREGNANCY AND LACTATION: Pregnancy category D; excreted into breast milk, effect on nursing infant unknown but may be of concern

SIDE EFFECTS/ADVERSE REACTIONS

CNS: Dizziness, drowsiness, confusion (especially in elderly), headache, anxiety, nervousness, panic, tremors, stimulation, weakness, fatigue, insomnia, nightmares, extra pyramidal symptoms (elderly), increased psychiatric symptoms, memory impairment

CV: Orthostatic hypotension, ***ECG changes, tachycardia, dysrhythmias,*** hypertension, palpitations, syncope

EENT: Blurred vision, tinnitus, mydriasis, ophthalmoplegia, nasal congestion

GI: Constipation, dry mouth, nausea, vomiting, ***paralytic ileus,*** increased appetite, weight gain, cramps, epigastric distress, jaundice, ***hepatitis,*** stomatitis, diarrhea

GU: Urinary retention

HEME: ***Agranulocytosis, thrombocytopenia, eosinophilia, leukopenia***

SKIN: Rash, urticaria, sweating, pruritus, photosensitivity

▼ **DRUG INTERACTIONS**

Drugs

• *Amphetamines:* Theoretical increase in effect of amphetamines, clinical evidence lacking

• *Anticholinergics:* Excessive anticholinergic effects

• *Barbiturates:* Reduced serum concentrations of cyclic antidepressants

• *Bethanidine:* Reduced antihypertensive effect of bethanidine

• *Carbamazepine:* Reduced antidepressant serum concentrations
• *Clonidine:* Reduced antihypertensive response to clonidine; enhanced hypertensive response with abrupt clonidine withdrawal
• *Debrisoquin:* Inhibited antihypertensive response of debrisoquin
• *Epinephrine+:* Markedly enhanced pressor response to IV epinephrine
• *Ethanol:* Additive impairment of motor skills; abstinent alcoholics may eliminate cyclic antidepressants more rapidly than non-alcoholics
• *Fluoxetine:* Marked increases in cyclic antidepressant plasma concentrations
• *Guanethidine:* Inhibited antihypertensive response to guanethidine
• *MAO inhibitors:* Excessive sympathetic response, mania, or hyperpyrexia possible
• *Moclobemide+:* Potential association with fatal or non-fatal serotonin syndrome
• *Neuroleptics:* Increased therapeutic and toxic effects of both drugs
• *Norepinephrine+:* Markedly enhanced pressor response to norepinephrine
• *Phenylephrine:* Enhanced pressor response to IV phenylephrine
• *Phenytoin:* Altered seizure control; decreased cyclic antidepressant serum concentrations
• *Propoxyphene:* Enhanced effect of cyclic antidepressants
• *Quinidine:* Increased cyclic antidepressant serum concentrations

Labs

• *Increase:* Serum bilirubin, blood glucose, alk phosphatase
• *Decrease:* VMA, 5-HIAA
• *False increase:* Urinary catecholamines

SPECIAL CONSIDERATIONS

PATIENT/FAMILY EDUCATION

• Therapeutic effects may take 2-3 wk
• Use caution in driving or other activities requiring alertness
• Avoid rising quickly from sitting to standing, especially elderly
• Avoid alcohol ingestion, other CNS depressants
• Do not discontinue abruptly after long-term use
• Wear sunscreen or large hat to prevent photosensitivity
• Increase fluids, bulk in diet if constipation occurs
• Gum, hard sugarless candy, or frequent sips of water for dry mouth

MONITORING PARAMETERS

• CBC
• Weight
• ECG
• Mental status: mood, sensorium, affect, suicidal tendencies
• Determination of amitriptyline plasma concentrations is not routinely recommended but may be useful in identifying toxicity, drug interactions, or noncompliance (adjustments in dosage should be made according to clinical response not plasma concentrations)
• Therapeutic plasma levels 125-250 μg/L (including active metabolites)

amlodipine

(am-loh-dih'peen)

Norvasc

Chemical Class: Dihydropyridine

Therapeutic Class: Calcium channel blocker

CLINICAL PHARMACOLOGY

Mechanism of Action: Inhibits calcium ion influx across cell membrane in vascular smooth muscle and cardiac muscle; produces relaxation of coronary vascular smooth muscle, peripheral vascular smooth muscle; reduces total peripheral resistance (afterload); increases myocardial oxygen delivery

Pharmacokinetics

PO: Onset not determined (ionized at physiologic pH resulting in gradual association and disassociation with receptor binding site and gradual onset of action), peak 6-12 hr, $t_{1/2}$ 30-50 hr, metabolized by liver, excreted in urine (90% as metabolites)

INDICATIONS AND USES: Chronic stable angina pectoris, hypertension, vasospastic (Prinzmetal's or variant) angina

DOSAGE

Adult

- *Angina:* PO 5-10 mg qd
- *Hypertension:* PO 5 mg qd initially, may increase up to 10 mg/day (small, fragile or elderly patients or patients with hepatic insufficiency may be started on 2.5 mg qd)

$ AVAILABLE FORMS/COST OF THERAPY

- Tab, Uncoated—Oral: 2.5 mg, 100's: **$113.35;** 5 mg, 100's: **$113.35;** 10 mg, 100's: **$196.13**

CONTRAINDICATIONS: Hypersensitivity

PRECAUTIONS: CHF, hypotension, hepatic insufficiency, aortic stenosis, elderly

PREGNANCY AND LACTATION: Pregnancy category C; unknown if excreted into milk, use caution in nursing mothers

SIDE EFFECTS/ADVERSE REACTIONS

CNS: Headache, fatigue, dizziness, anxiety, depression, insomnia, paresthesia, somnolence, asthenia, nervousness, malaise, tremor

CV: Dysrhythmia, *peripheral edema,* bradycardia, hypotension, palpitations, syncope, tachycardia

GI: Nausea, vomiting, diarrhea, gastric upset, constipation, abdominal cramps, flatulence, dry mouth

GU: Nocturia, polyuria

SKIN: Rash, pruritus, urticaria, hair loss

MISC: Flushing, nasal congestion, sweating, shortness of breath, sexual dysfunction, muscle cramps, cough, weight gain, tinnitus, epistaxis

▼ DRUG INTERACTIONS

Drugs

- *Barbiturates:* Reduced plasma concentrations of amlodipine
- *β-adrenergic blockers:* Enhanced effects of β-adrenergic blockers, hypotension
- *Cimetidine:* Increased amlodipine concentrations possible
- *Neuromuscular blocking agents:* Prolongation of neuromuscular blockade

SPECIAL CONSIDERATIONS

PATIENT/FAMILY EDUCATION

- Notify physician of irregular heart beat, shortness of breath, swelling of feet and hands, pronounced dizziness, hypotension

ammonium chloride

Chemical Class: Ammonium ion
Therapeutic Class: Acidifier

CLINICAL PHARMACOLOGY

Mechanism of Action: Lowers urinary pH, conversion to urea by the liver liberates hydrogen and chloride ions in blood and extracellular fluid with decreased pH and correction of alkalosis

Pharmacokinetics

PO: Absorption occurs in 3-6 hr, metabolized in liver to urea and HCl, excreted in urine and feces

INDICATIONS AND USES: Hypochloremic states and metabolic alkalosis, systemic and urinary acidifier, expectorant (usually in combination with other expectorants and cough mixtures), diuretic (particularly in edematous conditions associated with hypochloremia)

DOSAGE

Adult

- *Alkalosis:* IV Add contents of 1-2 vials (100-200 mEq) to 500 or 1000 ml of 0.9% sodium chloride inj, do not exceed concentration of 1%-2% ammonium chloride or an infusion rate of 5 ml/min; monitor dosage by repeated serum bicarbonate determinations
- *Acidifier:* PO 4-12 g/day in divided doses
- *Expectorant:* PO 250-500 mg q2-4h as needed

Child

- *Acidifier:* PO 75 mg/kg/day in 4 divided doses

$ **AVAILABLE FORMS/COST OF THERAPY**

- Tab, Delayed Release, Enteric Coated—Oral: 500 mg, 100's: **$3.04**
- Inj, Conc-Sol—IV: 5.35 g/20 ml (100 mEq), 20 ml: **$4.68**

CONTRAINDICATIONS: Hypersensitivity, severe hepatic disease, severe renal disease, metabolic alkalosis due to vomiting of hydrochloric acid when accompanied by loss of sodium (excretion of sodium bicarbonate in the urine)

PRECAUTIONS: Severe respiratory disease, cardiac edema, respiratory acidosis, infants, children, elderly

PREGNANCY AND LACTATION: Pregnancy category B; when consumed in large quantities near term may cause acidosis in mother and fetus; no data available regarding use in nursing mothers

SIDE EFFECTS/ADVERSE REACTIONS

CNS: Drowsiness, headache, confusion, stimulation, tremors, *twitching, hyperreflexia,* ***tetany, tonic convulsions, coma, EEG changes***

CV: Bradycardia, dysrhythmias, bounding pulse

GI: Gastric irritation, nausea, vomiting, anorexia, diarrhea, thirst

GU: Glycosuria

METAB: Metabolic acidosis, hypokalemia, hyperchloremia, hyperglycemia

RESP: ***Apnea,*** irregular respirations, hyperventilation

SKIN: Rash, pain and irritation at infusion site (minimized by slow infusion), pallor, sweating

▼ **DRUG INTERACTIONS**

Labs

- *Increase:* Blood ammonia, LFTs
- *Decrease:* Serum magnesium, urine urobilinogen

SPECIAL CONSIDERATIONS

PATIENT/FAMILY EDUCATION

- Administer with meals if GI symptoms occur

MONITORING PARAMETERS:

- Electrolytes and CO_2
- Chloride before and during treatment
- Urine pH, urinary output, urine glucose, specific gravity during beginning treatment
- ABGs

amobarbital

(am-oh-bar'bi-tal)

Amytal Sodium

Chemical Class: Amylobarbitone

Therapeutic Class: Sedative/hypnotic-barbiturate (intermediate acting)

DEA Class: Schedule II

CLINICAL PHARMACOLOGY

Mechanism of Action: Depresses activity in brain cells primarily in reticular activating system in brain stem; also selectively depresses neurons in posterior hypothalamus, limbic structures; able to decrease seizure activity in hypnotic doses by inhibition of impulses in CNS; depresses REM sleep

Pharmacokinetics

PO: Onset 45-60 min, duration 6-8 hr

IV: Onset 5 min, duration 3-6 hr

Metabolized by liver, excreted by kidneys (inactive metabolites), highly protein bound, $t_{1/2}$ 16-40 hr

INDICATIONS AND USES: Sedation, preanesthetic sedation, short-term (up to 2 weeks) treatment of insomnia, anticonvulsant (status epilepticus),* adjunct in psychiatry*

DOSAGE

Adult

- *Preanesthetic sedation:* PO/IM 200 mg 1-2 hr preoperatively
- *Anticonvulsant/psychiatry:* IV 65-500 mg given over several min, not to exceed 100 mg/min; not to exceed 1 g
- *Insomnia:* PO/IM 65-200 mg hs

Child >6 yr

- *Sedation:* PO 2 mg/kg/day in 4 divided doses
- *Anticonvulsant/psychiatry:* IV 65-500 mg given over several min, not to exceed 100 mg/min; not to exceed 1 g
- *Insomnia:* IM 2-3 mg/kg hs

$ AVAILABLE FORMS/COST OF THERAPY

- Cap, Gel—Oral: 200 mg, 100's: **$22.53**
- Inj, Lyphl-Sol—IM; IV: 0.5 g/vial, 10's: **$82.49**
- Inj, Sol—IV: 250 mg, 10's: **$47.01**

CONTRAINDICATIONS: Hypersensitivity to barbiturates, respiratory depression, severe liver impairment, porphyria

PRECAUTIONS: Anemia, addiction to barbiturates, hepatic disease, COPD/emphysema, renal disease, hypertension, elderly, acute/chronic pain, mental depression, history of drug abuse, abrupt discontinuation

PREGNANCY AND LACTATION: Pregnancy category D; small amount excreted in breast milk, use caution in nursing mothers

SIDE EFFECTS/ADVERSE REACTIONS

CNS: Lethargy, drowsiness, hangover, dizziness, stimulation in the elderly and children, lightheadedness, physical dependence, CNS depression, mental depression, slurred speech, vertigo, headache

CV: Hypotension, bradycardia

GI: Nausea, vomiting, diarrhea, constipation

HEME: ***Agranulocytosis, thrombocytopenia, megaloblastic anemia*** (long-term treatment)

RESP: ***Depression, apnea, laryngospasm, bronchospasm***

SKIN: Rash, urticaria, erythema multiforme, pain, abscesses at injection site, ***angioedema,*** thrombophlebitis, ***Stevens-Johnson syndrome***

MISC: Rickets, osteomalacia (prolonged use)

▼ DRUG INTERACTIONS

Drugs

- *Acetaminophen:* Enhanced hepatotoxic potential of acetaminophen overdoses
- *Antidepressants:* Reduced serum concentration of cyclic antidepressants
- *β-adrenergic blockers:* Reduced serum concentrations of β-blockers which are extensively metabolized
- *Calcium channel blockers:* Reduced concentrations of verapamil and nifedipine

• *Central nervous system depressants:* Excessive CNS depression
• *Chloramphenicol:* Increased barbiturate concentrations; reduced serum chloramphenicol concentrations
• *Corticosteroids:* Reduced serum concentrations of corticosteroids, may impair therapeutic effect
• *Disopyramide:* Reduced serum concentrations of disopyramide
• *Doxycycline:* Reduced serum doxycycline concentrations
• *Ethanol:* Excessive CNS depression
• *Methoxyflurane:* Enhanced nephrotoxic effect
• *MAO inhibitors:* Prolonged effect of some barbiturates
• *Narcotic analgesics:* Increased toxicity of meperidine; reduced effect of methadone; additive CNS depression
• *Neuroleptics:* Reduced effect of either drug
• *Oral anticoagulants+:* Decreased hypoprothrombinemic response to oral anticoagulants
• *Oral contraceptives:* Reduced efficacy of oral contraceptives
• *Quinidine:* Reduced quinidine plasma concentrations
• *Theophylline:* Reduced serum theophylline concentrations

SPECIAL CONSIDERATIONS

PATIENT/FAMILY EDUCATION

• Indicated only for short-term treatment of insomnia and is probably ineffective after 2 wk; physical dependency may result when used for extended time (45-90 days depending on dose)
• Avoid driving or other activities requiring alertness
• Avoid alcohol ingestion or CNS depressants
• Do not discontinue medication abruptly after long-term use

MONITORING PARAMETERS

• CBC
• Serum folate, vitamin D (if on long-term therapy)
• PT in patients receiving anticoagulants
• LFTs
• Mental status, vital signs

amoxapine

(a-mox'a-peen)
Asendin
Chemical Class: Dibenzoxazepine derivative, secondary amine
Therapeutic Class: Antidepressant, tricyclic

CLINICAL PHARMACOLOGY

Mechanism of Action: Inhibits reuptake of norepinephrine and serotonin at the presynaptic neuron prolonging neuronal activity; blocks postsynaptic dopamine receptors; inhibits activity of histamine and acetylcholine; mild peripheral vasodilator effects and possible "quinidine-like" actions

Pharmacokinetics

PO: Steady state 7 days, metabolized by liver, excreted by kidneys, $t_{1/2}$ 8 hr

INDICATIONS AND USES: Depression in patients with neurotic or reactive depressive disorders; endogenous and psychotic depressions; depression accompanied by anxiety or agitation

DOSAGE

Adult

• PO 50 mg bid-tid, may increase to 100 mg bid-tid by the end of the first week, not to exceed 300 mg/day unless lower doses have been given for at least 2 wk, may be given daily dose hs, not to exceed 600 mg/day in hospitalized patients

Adolescents

• PO 25-50 mg/day, increase gradually to 100 mg/day (divided or as single hs dose)

Child

- Not recommended for patients <16 yr

$ AVAILABLE FORMS/COST OF THERAPY

- Tab, Uncoated—Oral: 25 mg, 100's: **$41.33-$72.33;** 50 mg, 100's: **$64.43-$121.29;** 100 mg, 100's: **$112.43-$196.27;** 150 mg, 30's: **$53.25-$92.82**

CONTRAINDICATIONS: Hypersensitivity, acute recovery phase of MI, concurrent use of MAO inhibitors

PRECAUTIONS: Suicidal patients, severe depression, increased intraocular pressure, narrow-angle glaucoma, urinary retention, cardiac disease, hepatic disease, hyperthyroidism, electroshock therapy, elective surgery, elderly, convulsive disorders, prostatic hypertrophy

PREGNANCY AND LACTATION: Pregnancy category C; excreted into breast milk, effect on nursing infant unknown but may be of concern

SIDE EFFECTS/ADVERSE REACTIONS

CNS: Dizziness, drowsiness, confusion, headache, anxiety, tremor, stimulation, weakness, insomnia, nightmares, EPS, increased psychiatric symptoms, paresthesia, impairment of sexual functioning, ***neuroleptic malignant syndrome, tardive dyskinesia, seizures,*** ataxia

CV: Orthostatic hypotension, ***ECG changes,*** *tachycardia,* ***hypertension,*** palpitations, syncope

EENT: Blurred vision, tinnitus, mydriasis, ophthalmoplegia

GI: Dry mouth, constipation, nausea, vomiting, ***paralytic ileus,*** increased appetite, cramps, epigastric distress, jaundice, ***hepatitis,*** stomatitis, diarrhea, peculiar taste

GU: Urinary retention

HEME: ***Agranulocytosis, thrombocytopenia, eosinophilia, leukopenia***

METAB: Menstrual irregularity, breast enlargement, galactorrhea, SIADH

SKIN: Rash, urticaria, sweating, pruritus, photosensitivity

▼ DRUG INTERACTIONS

Drugs

- *Amphetamines:* Theoretical increase in effect of amphetamines, clinical evidence lacking
- *Anticholinergics:* Excessive anticholinergic effects
- *Barbiturates:* Reduced serum concentrations of cyclic antidepressants
- *Bethanidine:* Reduced antihypertensive effect of bethanidine
- *Carbamazepine:* Reduced cyclic antidepressant serum concentrations
- *Clonidine:* Reduced antihypertensive response to clonidine; enhanced hypertensive response with abrupt clonidine withdrawal
- *Debrisoquin:* Inhibited antihypertensive response of debrisoquin
- *Epinephrine+:* Markedly enhanced pressor response to IV epinephrine
- *Ethanol:* Additive impairment of motor skills; abstinent alcoholics may eliminate cyclic antidepressants more rapidly than nonalcoholics
- *Fluoxetine:* Marked increases in cyclic antidepressant plasma concentrations
- *Guanethidine:* Inhibited antihypertensive response to guanethidine
- *Moclobemide+:* Potential association with fatal or non-fatal serotonin syndrome) MAO inhibitors (excessive sympathetic response, mania or hyperpyrexia possible
- *Neuroleptics:* Increased therapeutic and toxic effects of both drugs
- *Norepinephrine+:* Markedly enhanced pressor response to norepinephrine

• *Phenylephrine:* Enhanced pressor response to IV phenylephrine
• *Phenytoin:* Altered seizure control; decreased cyclic antidepressant serum concentrations
• *Propoxyphene:* Enhanced effect of cyclic antidepressants
• *Quinidine:* Increased cyclic antidepressant serum concentrations

Labs

• *False increase:* Urinary catecholamines
• *Decrease:* VMA, 5-HIAA

SPECIAL CONSIDERATIONS

PATIENT/FAMILY EDUCATION

• Therapeutic effects may take 2-3 wk
• Use caution in driving or other activities requiring alertness
• Avoid rising quickly from sitting to standing, especially elderly
• Avoid alcohol ingestion, other CNS depressants
• Do not discontinue abruptly after long-term use
• Wear sunscreen or large hat to prevent photosensitivity
• Increase fluids, bulk in diet if constipation occurs
• Use gum, hard sugarless candy, or frequent sips of water for dry mouth
• Potential for tardive dyskinesia

MONITORING PARAMETERS

• CBC
• Weight
• ECG
• Mental status: mood, sensorium, affect, suicidal tendencies

amoxicillin

(a-mox-i-sill'in)

Amoxil, Biomox, Polymox, Trimox, Wymox

Chemical Class: Aminopenicillin

Therapeutic Class: Antibiotic

CLINICAL PHARMACOLOGY

Mechanism of Action: Inhibits the biosynthesis of cell wall mucopeptide in susceptible organisms; bacteriocidal

Pharmacokinetics

PO: Peak 1 hr, duration 6-8 hr, $t_{1/2}$ 1-1.3 hr, excreted largely unchanged in urine by glomerular filtration and active tubular secretion (can be delayed by concomitant administration of probenecid)

INDICATIONS AND USES: Infections of the ear, nose, throat, GU tract, skin and soft tissues, lower respiratory tract caused by susceptible organisms; gonococcal infections; prevention of bacterial endocarditis; *Chlamydia trachomatis* in pregnancy*

Antibacterial spectrum usually includes:

• Gram negative organisms - *Haemophilus influenzae, E. coli, Proteus mirabilis* and *Neisseria gonorrhoeae*
• Gram positive organisms - Streptococci (including *S. faecalis, S. pyogenes, S. pneumoniae)* and non-penicilinase-producing staphylococc

DOSAGE

Adult

• *Systemic infections:* PO 250-500 mg q8h
• *Gonorrhea:* PO 3 g given with 1 g probenecid as a single dose (not first line), follow with doxycycline
• *Bacterial endocarditis prophylaxis:* PO 3 g 1 hr before procedure, then 1.5 g 6 hr after initial dose

Child

• *Systemic infections:* PO 20-40 mg/kg/day in divided doses q8h

$ AVAILABLE FORMS/COST OF THERAPY

• Cap, Gel—Oral: 250 mg, 100's: **$8.03-$24.95;** 500 mg, 100's: **$15.75-$40.40**
• Powder, Reconst—Oral: 125 mg/5

ml, 150 ml: **$2.22-$4.11;** 250 mg/5 ml, 150 ml: **$2.94-$7.06**

- Tab, Chewable—Oral: 125 mg, 60's: **$8.85;** 250 mg, 100's: **$22.82-$25.35**

CONTRAINDICATIONS: Hypersensitivity to penicillins

PRECAUTIONS: Hypersensitivity to cephalosporins, renal insufficiency, prolonged or repeated therapy, mononucleosis

PREGNANCY AND LACTATION: Pregnancy category B; excreted into breast milk in low concentrations, no adverse effects have been observed but potential exists for modification of bowel flora in nursing infant, allergy/sensitization and interference with interpretation of culture results if fever workup required

SIDE EFFECTS/ADVERSE REACTIONS

CNS: Headache, fever

GI: Nausea, vomiting, diarrhea, increased AST, ALT, abdominal pain, glossitis, colitis, ***pseudomembranous colitis***

HEME: Anemia, increased bleeding time, ***bone marrow depression, granulocytopenia, leukopenia, eosinophilia***

RESP: ***Anaphylaxis, respiratory distress***

SKIN: Urticaria, rash, erythema multiforme

▼ **DRUG INTERACTIONS**

Drugs

- *Chloramphenicol:* Inhibited antibacterial activity of amoxicillin, ensure adequate amounts of both agents are given and administer amoxicillin a few hours before chloramphenicol
- *Methotrexate:* Increased serum methotrexate concentrations
- *Oral contraceptives:* Occasional impairment of oral contraceptive efficacy, consider use of supplementary contraception during cycles in which amoxicillin is used
- *Tetracyclines:* Inhibited antibacterial activity of amoxicillin, ensure adequate amounts of both agents are given and administer amoxicillin a few hours before tetracycline

Labs

False positive: Urine glucose, urine protein

SPECIAL CONSIDERATIONS

PATIENT/FAMILY EDUCATION

- Complete entire course of medication
- May administer on a full or empty stomach
- Administer at even intervals
- Report sore throat, fever, fatigue, excessive diarrhea, skin rash, itching, hives, shortness of breath, wheezing
- Shake oral suspensions well before administering, discard after 14 days

---

amoxicillin/clavulanate

(a-mox-i-sill'in clav-u-lan'ate)

Augmentin, Clavulin ♣

Chemical Class: Aminopenicillin/β-lactamase inhibitor

Therapeutic Class: Antibiotic

CLINICAL PHARMACOLOGY

Mechanism of Action: Inhibits biosynthesis of cell wall mucopeptide in susceptible organisms; bacteriocidal; clavulanate protects amoxicillin from degredation by β-lactamase enzymes effectively extending the spectrum of activity

Pharmacokinetics

PO: Peak 2 hr, duration 6-8 hr, $t_{1/2}$ 1-1.3 hr, excreted largely unchanged in urine

INDICATIONS AND USES: Infections of the lower respiratory tract, ear, sinuses, skin and soft tissues, urinary tract caused by susceptible organisms

Antibacterial spectrum usually includes:

• Gram-positive organisms: *Staphylococcus aureus, S. epidermidis, S. saprophyticus, Streptococcus faecalis (Enterococcus), Str. pneumoniae, Str. pyogenes, Str. viridans*

• Gram-negative organisms: *Hemophilus influenzae, Moraxella catarrhalis, Escherichia coli, Klebsiella* sp., *Enterobacter* sp., *Proteus mirabilis, P. vulgaris, Neisseria gonorrhoeae, Legionella* sp

• Anaerobes: *Clostridium* sp., *Peptococcus* sp., *Peptostreptococcus* sp., *Bacteroides* sp., including *B. fragilis*

DOSAGE

Adult

• PO 250-500 mg (amoxicillin) q8h depending on severity of infection

Child

• PO 20-40 mg/kg/day (amoxicillin) in divided doses q8h

$ **AVAILABLE FORMS/COST OF THERAPY**

• Powder, Reconst—Oral: 125 mg/31.25 mg/5 ml, 150 ml: **$26.25;** 250 mg/62.5 mg/5 ml, 150 ml: **$50.00**

• Tab, Chewable—Oral: 125 mg/31.25 mg, 30's: **$26.25;** 250 mg/62.5 mg, 30's: **$50.00**

• Tab, Uncoated—Oral: 250 mg/125 mg, 30's: **$55.95;** 500 mg/125 mg, 30's: **$78.00**

• Note: due to clavulanate strength, 2 × 250 mg tablets do not equal a 500 mg tablet

CONTRAINDICATIONS: Hypersensitivity to penicillins

PRECAUTIONS: Hypersensitivity to cephalosporins, renal insufficiency, prolonged or repeated therapy, mononucleosis

PREGNANCY AND LACTATION: Pregnancy category B; excreted into breast milk in low concentrations, no adverse effects have been observed but potential exists for modification of bowel flora in nursing infant, allergy/sensitization and interference with interpretation of culture results if fever workup required

SIDE EFFECTS/ADVERSE REACTIONS

CNS: Headache, fever

GI: Nausea, diarrhea, vomiting, increased AST, ALT, abdominal pain, glossitis, colitis, black tongue, ***pseudomembranous colitis***

GU: Vaginitis, moniliasis

HEME: Anemia, increased bleeding time, ***bone marrow depression, granulocytopenia, leukopenia, eosinophilia***

METAB: Hyperkalemia, hypokalemia, alkalosis, hypernatremia

RESP: ***Anaphylaxis, respiratory distress***

SKIN: Urticaria, rash, erythema multiforme

▼ **DRUG INTERACTIONS**

Drugs

• *Chloramphenicol:* Inhibited antibacterial activity of amoxicillin, ensure adequate amounts of both agents are given and administer amoxicillin a few hours before chloramphenicol

• *Methotrexate:* Increased serum methotrexate concentrations

• *Oral contraceptives:* Occasional impairment of oral contraceptive efficacy, consider use of supplementary contraception during cycles in which amoxicillin is used

• *Tetracyclines:* Inhibited antibacterial activity of amoxicillin, ensure adequate amounts of both agents are given and administer amoxicillin a few hours before tetracycline

Labs

• *False positive:* Urine glucose, urine protein

SPECIAL CONSIDERATIONS
PATIENT/FAMILY EDUCATION
• Complete entire course of medication
• Administer with food
• Administer at even intervals
• Report sore throat, fever, fatigue, excessive diarrhea, skin rash, itching, hives, shortness of breath, wheezing
• Shake oral suspensions well before administering, discard after 14 days

amphetamine

(am-fet'a-meen)
Chemical Class: Amphetamine
Therapeutic Class: Cerebral stimulant
DEA Class: Schedule II

CLINICAL PHARMACOLOGY
Mechanism of Action: Increases release of norepinephrine from central noradrenergic neurons, at higher doses dopamine may be released in the mesolimbic system
Pharmacokinetics
PO: Onset 30 min, peak 1-3 hr, duration 4-20 hr, metabolized by liver, excreted by kidneys, crosses placenta, $t_{1/2}$ dependent on urinary pH, at urinary pH <5.6 $t_{1/2}$ is 7-8 hr (increases with alkinization of urine)
INDICATIONS AND USES: Narcolepsy, short-term adjunct to caloric restriction in exogenous obesity **(high potential for abuse, use only when alternative therapies have failed),** attention deficit disorder
DOSAGE
Adult
• *Narcolepsy:* PO 5-60 mg qd in divided doses
• *Obesity:* PO 5-30 mg in divided doses 30-60 min before meals
Child
• *Narcolepsy:* >12 yr: PO 10 mg qd increasing by 10 mg/day at weekly intervals; 6-12 yr: PO 5 mg qd increasing by 5 mg/wk (max 60 mg/day)
• *Attention deficit disorder:* ≥6 yr: PO 5 mg qd-bid increasing by 5 mg/day at weekly intervals (will rarely exceed 40 mg/day); 3-5 yr: PO 2.5 mg qd increasing by 2.5 mg/day at weekly intervals (usual range 0.1-0.5 mg/kg/dose)

$ **AVAILABLE FORMS/COST OF THERAPY**
• Tab, Plain Coated—Oral: 5 mg, 1000's: **$40.27;** 10 mg, 1000's: **$55.16**

CONTRAINDICATIONS: Hypersensitivity to sympathomimetic amines, hyperthyroidism, moderate to severe hypertension, glaucoma, severe arteriosclerosis, history of drug abuse, cardiovascular disease, agitated states, within 14 days of MAO inhibitor administration
PRECAUTIONS: Mild hypertension, child <3 yr, Tourette's syndrome, motor and phonic tics
PREGNANCY AND LACTATION: Pregnancy category C; use of amphetamine for medical indications not a significant risk to the fetus for congenital anomalies, mild withdrawal symptoms may be observed in the newborn; illicit maternal use presents significant risks to the fetus and newborn, including intrauterine growth retardation, premature delivery and the potential for increased maternal, fetal, and neonatal morbidity; concentrated in breast milk, contraindicated during breast feeding
SIDE EFFECTS/ADVERSE REACTIONS
CNS: Hyperactivity, insomnia, restlessness, talkativeness, dizziness, headache, chills, overstimulation, dysphoria, euphoria, irritability, aggressiveness, tremor, dependence,

addiction, dyskinesia, changes in libido, psychotic episodes
CV: Palpitations, tachycardia, hypertension, dysrhythmias, reflex decrease in heart rate, dysryhthmias (at larger doses)
GI: Nausea, vomiting, anorexia, dry mouth, diarrhea, constipation, weight loss, metallic taste, cramps
GU: Impotence
METAB: Reversible elevations in serum thyroxine (T_4) with heavy use
SKIN: Urticaria

▼ **DRUG INTERACTIONS**

Drugs

- *Acetazolamide:* Increased serum amphetamine concentrations and prolonged amphetamine effects
- *Antidepressants:* Increased effect of amphetamines, clinical evidence lacking
- *Furazolidone:* Hypertensive reactions
- *Guanadrel:* Inhibition of the antihypertensive response to guanadrel
- *Guanethidine:* Inhibition of the antihypertensive response to guanethidine
- *MAO inhibitors+:* Severe hypertensive reactions possible
- *Sodium bicarbonate:* Large doses of sodium bicarbonate inhibit the elimination and increase the effect of amphetamines

Labs

- *Increase:* Plasma corticosteroid
- *Altered:* Urinary steroid

SPECIAL CONSIDERATIONS

PATIENT/FAMILY EDUCATION

- Take early in the day
- Do not discontinue abruptly
- Avoid hazardous activities until stabilized on medication
- Avoid OTC preparations unless approved by physician
- Notify physician if pronounced nervousness, restlessness, insomnia, dizziness, anorexia, dry mouth, or GI disturbances occur

amphotericin B

(am-foe-ter'i-sin)
Fungizone IV
Fungizone (topical)
Chemical Class: Amphoteric polyene
Therapeutic Class: Antifungal

CLINICAL PHARMACOLOGY

Mechanism of Action: Binds to sterols in the cell membrane of susceptible fungi with a resultant change in cell permeability allowing leakage of intracellular components; fungistatic or fungicidal depending on the concentration obtained in body fluids and on the susceptibility of the fungus

Pharmacokinetics

IV: Peak 1-2 hr, initial $t_{1/2}$ 24 hr, elimination $t_{1/2}$ of approximately 15 days, metabolic pathways are not known, very slowly excreted by the kidneys (metabolites), highly bound to plasma proteins; poorly penetrates CSF, bronchial secretions, aqueous humor, muscle, bone, brain, pancreas

INDICATIONS AND USES: TOP: Cutaneous and mucocutaneous mycotic infections caused by *Candida* sp. IV: Potentially life-threatening fungal infections: aspergillosis *(A. fumigatus),* cryptococcosis (torulosis), North American blastomycosis, systemic moniliasis, coccidiomycosis and histoplasmosis, mucormycosis due to susceptible species of the genera *Absidia* sp., *Mucor* sp., *Rhizopus* sp., *Entomophthora* sp., and *Basidiobolus* sp., sporthrichosis *(S. schenckii);* American mucocutaneous leishmaniasis (not drug of choice as primary therapy)

Do not use IV form to treat noninvasive fungal infections, such as

oral thrush, vaginal candidiasis and esophageal candidiasis in patients with normal neutrophil counts

DOSAGE

Adult and child

• TOP: bid-qid for 7-21 days or longer if needed

• IV INF (minimum dilution 0.1 mg/ml) infuse 1 mg test dose slowly over 20-30 min to determine patient tolerance; initial therapeutic dose (if test dose tolerated) 0.25 mg/kg/day over 4-6 hr; individualize subsequent doses by increasing in 0.25 mg/kg/day increments (usual range 0.25-1 mg/kg/day); do not exceed 1.5 mg/kg/day; INTRATHECAL 25-100 μg q48-72 hr; increase to 500 μg as tolerated; BLADDER IRRIGATION 5-15 mg/100 ml of sterile water irrigation solution at 100-300 ml/day; instill into bladder, clamp catheter for 60-120 minutes then drain; repeat 3-4 times/day for 2-5 days

$ **AVAILABLE FORMS/COST OF THERAPY**

• Cre—Top: 3%, 20 g: **$30.43**
• Lotion—Top: 3%, 30 ml: **$41.74**
• Oint—Top: 3%, 20 g: **$29.25**
• Inj, Lyphl, Sol—IV: 50 mg/15 ml vial, 1's: **$30.88-$38.60**

CONTRAINDICATIONS: Hypersensitivity

PRECAUTIONS: Renal disease, rapid IV infusion, prior total body irradiation, leukocyte infusions, avoid eye contact

PREGNANCY AND LACTATION: Pregnancy category B; excretion in human milk unknown, due to the potential toxicity consider discontinuing nursing

SIDE EFFECTS/ADVERSE REACTIONS

Severe reactions may be lessened by giving acetaminophen, antihistamines, and antiemetics before infusion and by maintaining sodium balance

CNS: Headache, fever, chills, peripheral nerve pain, paresthesias, peripheral neuropathy, ***convulsions,*** dizziness

CV: Dysrhythmias, ventricular fibrillation, cardiac arrest, hypertension, hypotension

EENT: Tinnitus, deafness, diplopia, blurred vision

GI: Nausea, vomiting, anorexia, diarrhea, cramps, epigastric pain, ***hemorrhagic gastroenteritis, acute liver failure***

GU: Hypokalemia, azotemia, hyposthenuria, ***renal tubular acidosis,*** nephrocalcinosis, ***permanent renal impairment, anuria, oliguria***

HEME: Normochromic, normocytic anemia, ***thrombocytopenia, agranulocytosis, leukopenia, eosinophilia,*** hyponatremia, hypomagnesemia

MS: ***Arthralgia, myalgia,*** generalized pain, weakness, weight loss

SKIN: Burning, irritation, pain, necrosis at injection site with extravasation, flushing, urticaria, stinging, dry skin, pruritus, contact dermatitis, erythema, staining of nail lesions

▼ **DRUG INTERACTIONS**

Drugs

• *Aminoglycosides:* Synergistic nephrotoxicity
• *Cyclosporine:* Increased nephrotoxicity of both drugs
• *Neuromuscular blocking agents:* Prolonged muscle relaxation due to hypokalemia

SPECIAL CONSIDERATIONS

PATIENT/FAMILY EDUCATION

• Long-term therapy may be needed to clear infection (2 wk-3 mo depending on type of infection)

MONITORING PARAMETERS

• BUN, serum creatinine weekly; if BUN exceeds 40 mg/dl or serum creatinine exceeds 3 mg/dl discon-

tinue the drug or reduce dosage until renal function improves
- Weekly CBC, K, Na, Mg
- Total dosage
- Periodic LFTs

ampicillin

(am-pi-sill'in)

Amicill, D-Amp, ♣ Nu-Amp, ♣ Omnipen, Omnipen–N, Polycillin, Polycillin-N, Totacillin, Totacillin-N

Chemical Class: Aminopenicillin

Therapeutic Class: Antibiotic

CLINICAL PHARMACOLOGY

Mechanism of Action: Inhibits the biosynthesis of cell wall mucopeptide in susceptible organisms; bacteriocidal

Pharmacokinetics

PO: Peak 2 hr

IV: Peak 5 min

IM: Peak 1 hr

$t_{1/2}$ 50-110 min, excreted largely unchanged in urine by glomerular filtration and active tubular secretion (can be delayed by concomitant administration of probenecid)

INDICATIONS AND USES: Infections of the respiratory tract and soft tissues caused by susceptible organisms; bacterial meningitis caused by susceptible organisms; septicemia; gonococcal infections; prevention of bacterial endocarditis; prophylaxis in cesarean section*

Antibacterial spectrum usually includes:
- Gram-positive organisms: α- and β-hemolytic streptococci, *Streptococcus pneumoniae,* nonpenicillinase-producing staphylococci, *Bacillus anthracis,* and most strains of enterococci and clostridia
- Gram-negative organisms: *Haemophilus influenzae, Neisseria gonorrhoeae, N. meningitidis, N. catarrhalis, Escherichia coli, Proteus mirabilis, Bacteroides funduliformis, Salmonellae* sp. and *Shigellae* sp.

DOSAGE

Adult
- *Systemic infections:* PO 250-500 mg q6h; IV/IM 500 mg-3 g q4-6h
- *Meningitis:* IV 8-14 g/day in divided doses q3-4h
- *Gonorrhea:* PO 3.5 g given with 1 g probenecid as a single dose
- *Renal impairment:* CrCl 10-30 ml/min: administer q6-12h; CrCl <10 ml/min: administer q12h

Child
- *Systemic infections:* PO 50-100 mg/kg/day in divided doses q6h; IV/IM 100-200 mg/kg/day in divided doses q4-6h; max 2-3 g/day
- *Meningitis:* IV 200-400 mg/kg/day in divided doses q4-6h; max 12 g/day

$ AVAILABLE FORMS/COST OF THERAPY
- Inj, Dry-Sol—IM; IV: 125 mg/vial, 10's: **$12.13-$19.68;** 250 mg/vial, 10's: **$14.20-$22.74;** 500 mg/vial, 10's: **$18.61-$43.10;** 1 g/vial, 10's: **$23.82-$48.60;** 2 g/vial, 10's: **$46.80-$69.00**
- Cap, Gel—Oral: 250 mg, 100's: **$7.37-$14.86;** 500 mg, 100's: **$13.43-$26.51**
- Powder, Reconst—Oral: 125 mg/5ml, 200 ml: **$2.95-$4.64;** 250 mg/5ml, 200 ml: **$2.70-$6.69**

CONTRAINDICATIONS: Hypersensitivity to penicillins

PRECAUTIONS: Hypersensitivity to cephalosporins, renal insufficiency, prolonged or repeated therapy, mononucleosis, neonates

PREGNANCY AND LACTATION: Pregnancy category B; excreted into breast milk in low concentrations, no adverse effects have been observed but potential exists for modification of bowel flora in nursing infant, allergy/sensitization and interference with interpretation of culture results if fever workup required

SIDE EFFECTS/ADVERSE REACTIONS

CNS: Lethargy, hallucinations, anxiety, depression, twitching, ***coma, convulsions***

GI: Nausea, vomiting, diarrhea, glossitis, stomatitis, black "hairy" tongue, ***pseudomembranous colitis***

GU: Oliguria, proteinuria, hematuria, *vaginitis, moniliasis,* ***glomerulonephritis***

HEME: Anemia, increased bleeding time, ***bone marrow depression, granulocytopenia***

RESP: ***Anaphylaxis, respiratory distress***

SKIN: Rash, urticaria, erythema multiforme

▼ **DRUG INTERACTIONS**

Drugs

• *Chloramphenicol:* Inhibited antibacterial activity of amoxicillin, ensure adequate amounts of both agents are given and administer amoxicillin a few hours before chloramphenicol

• *Methotrexate:* Increased serum methotrexate concentrations

• *Oral contraceptives:* Occasional impairment of oral contraceptive efficacy, consider use of supplementary contraception during cycles in which amoxicillin is used

• *Tetracyclines:* Inhibited antibacterial activity of amoxicillin, ensure adequate amounts of both agents are given and administer amoxicillin a few hours before tetracycline

Labs

• *False positive:* Urine glucose, urine protein

SPECIAL CONSIDERATIONS

PATIENT/FAMILY EDUCATION

• Complete entire course of medication

• Administer on an empty stomach

• Administer at even intervals

• Report sore throat, fever, fatigue, excessive diarrhea, skin rash, itching, hives, shortness of breath, wheezing

• Shake oral suspensions well before administering, discard after 14 days

amrinone

(am′ri-none)

Inocor

Chemical Class: Bipyrimidine derivative

Therapeutic Class: Cardiac inotropic agent

CLINICAL PHARMACOLOGY

Mechanism of Action: Cardiac inotrope distinct from digitalis glycosides or catecholamines; direct vasodilator which reduces preload and afterload; not a beta-adrenergic agonist; inhibits myocardial c-AMP phosphodiesterase activity and increases cellular levels of c-AMP. Following single IV bolus in patients with congestive heart failure, dose-related increases in cardiac output occur (28% at 0.75 mg/kg to about 61% at 3 mg/kg); pulmonary capillary wedge pressure, total peripheral resistance, and diastolic and mean arterial pressures show dose-related decreases; heart rate generally unchanged. Changes in hemodynamic parameters are maintained during continuous IV inf and for several hours thereafter. Improved left ventricular function and relief of congestive heart failure in patients with ischemic heart disease occur without symptoms or ECG signs of myocardial ischemia

Pharmacokinetics

Onset of action 2-5 min, peak 10

min, duration variable; $t_{1/2}$ 4-6 hr, metabolized in liver, 60%-90% excreted in urine as drug and metabolites. In patients with compromised renal and hepatic perfusion, plasma levels of amrinone may rise during the infusion period

INDICATIONS AND USES: Short-term management of congestive heart failure unresponsive to other medication

DOSAGE

Adult

- IV bolus 0.75 mg/kg over 2-3 min; start infusion of 5-10 μg/kg/min; may give another 0.75 mg/kg bolus 30 min after start of therapy; daily dose should not exceed 10 mg/kg. The above dosing regimen will yield a plasma concentration of amrinone of 3 μg/ml. Increases in cardiac index show a linear relationship to plasma concentration in a range of 0.5 μg/ml to 7 μg/ml

$ AVAILABLE FORMS/COST OF THERAPY

- Inj: 20 ml (5 mg/ml), 25: **$1448.66**

CONTRAINDICATIONS: Hypersensitivity to this drug or bisulfites, severe aortic or pulmonic obstructive valvular disease, acute MI

PRECAUTIONS: Patients who have received vigorous diuretic therapy may have insufficient cardiac filling pressure to respond adequately to amrinone lactate injection. While amrinone has not been shown to be dysrhythmogenic, supraventricular and ventricular dysrhythmias have been observed

PREGNANCY AND LACTATION: Pregnancy category C

SIDE EFFECTS/ADVERSE REACTIONS

CV: ***Dysrhythmias (3%), hypotension (1.3%),*** headache, chest pain

GI: Nausea, vomiting, anorexia, abdominal pain, ***hepatotoxicity,*** hiccups

HEME: ***Thrombocytopenia (2.4%); dose dependent***

RESP: Pleuritis

SKIN: Allergic reactions, burning at injection site

MISC: Fever, hypersensitivity reaction manifested by pleuritis, pericarditis, myositis, or interstitial pulmonary infiltrates

▼ DRUG INTERACTIONS

Drugs

- *Furosemide:* Precipitates when furosemide is injected into an IV line infusing amrinone

SPECIAL CONSIDERATIONS

MONITORING PARAMETERS

- BP and pulse q5min during infusion; if BP drops 30 mm Hg, stop infusion
- Cardiac output and pulmonary capillary wedge pressure
- Monitor platelet count and serum K, Na, Cl, Ca, BUN, creatinine, ALT, AST, and bilirubin daily

amyl nitrite

(am′il)

Amyl nitrite

Chemical Class: Nitrite

Therapeutic Class: Coronary vasodilator

CLINICAL PHARMACOLOGY

Mechanism of Action: Relaxes vascular smooth muscle; may dilate coronary blood vessels; reduces preload and afterload, which decreases left ventricular end diastolic pressure and cardiac output; converts hemoglobin to methemoglobin, which is able to bind cyanide

Pharmacokinetics

INH: Onset 30 sec, duration 3-5 min; metabolized by liver, ⅓ excreted in urine

INDICATIONS AND USES: Acute angina pectoris, cyanide poisoning, diagnostic aid in cardiac auscultation*

DOSAGE: With the patient seated or recumbent, a capsule of amyl nitrite is crushed with the fingers and held to the nostrils for inhalation of the vapors

Adult

- *Angina pectoris, cardiac diagnostic aid:* Inhalation 0.18-0.3 ml cap as needed, 1-6 inhalations from 1 cap, may repeat in 3-5 min
- *Cyanide poisoning:* Inhalation 0.3 ml cap inhaled for 15 sec until sodium nitrite infusion is ready

$ AVAILABLE FORMS/COST OF THERAPY

- Caps—Inh: 0.18 ml, 12's: **$21.40;** 0.3 ml, 12's: **$3.85-$6.00**

CONTRAINDICATIONS: Hypersensitivity to nitrites, severe anemia, increased intracranial pressure, hypertension, cerebral hemorrhage

PRECAUTIONS: Volatile nitrites abused for sexual stimulation; tolerance to nitrites may develop with repeated use; transient dizziness, weakness, or other signs of cerebral hypoperfusion may develop following inhalation

PREGNANCY AND LACTATION: Pregnancy category C

SIDE EFFECTS/ADVERSE REACTIONS

CNS: Headache, dizziness, weakness, syncope

CV: Postural hypotension, ***tachycardia, cardiovascular collapse,*** palpitations

GI: Nausea, vomiting, abdominal pain

GU: Urinary incontinence

HEME: ***Hemolytic anemia, methemoglobinemia***

MS: Muscle twitching

SKIN: Flushing, pallor, sweating

SPECIAL CONSIDERATIONS

PATIENT/FAMILY EDUCATION

- This drug should be inhaled while the patient is seated or lying down
- Taking it after drinking alcohol may worsen its side effects
- Amyl nitrite is very flammable

---

anisindione

(ay-nis-in'die-own)

Miradon

Chemical Class: Inandione

Therapeutic Class: Anticoagulant

CLINICAL PHARMACOLOGY

Mechanism of Action: Interferes with the hepatic synthesis of vitamin K-dependent clotting factors which results in a depletion of factors II, VII, IX and X; has no effect on an established thrombus, but may prevent further extension of the formed clot and prevent secondary thromboembolic complications

Pharmacokinetics

PO: Peak activity 2-3 days, 97%-99% protein bound, $t_{1/2}$ 3-5 days, metabolized by liver and excreted in the urine and feces as inactive metabolites; anticoagulant effects are dependent on the half-lives of the vitamin K-dependent clotting factors, although factor VII is quickly depleted and an initial prolongation of the prothrombin time (PT) is seen in 8-12 hr, maximum anticoagulation is not approached for 3-5 days as the other factors are depleted and the drug achieves steady state

INDICATIONS AND USES: Venous thrombosis and its extension, atrial fibrillation, pulmonary embolism, adjunctive treatment of coronary occlusion, prevention of recurrent transient ischemic attacks and recurrent MI* (warfarin is generally the oral anticoagulant of choice due to higher incidence of serious adverse reactions including cutaneous, hepatic and hematologic effects with anisindione)

DOSAGE

Adult

• PO 300 mg the first day, 200 mg the second day, 100 mg the third day and 25-250 mg qd for maintenance based on the results of PT monitoring

$ AVAILABLE FORMS/COST OF THERAPY

• Tab, Uncoated—Oral: 50 mg, 100's: **$35.82**

CONTRAINDICATIONS: Active bleeding; hemorrhagic blood dyscrasias; hemorrhagic tendencies (e.g., hemophilia, polycythemia vera, purpura, leukemia); history of bleeding diathesis; recent cerebral hemorrhage; active ulceration of the GI tract; ulcerative colitis; open traumatic or surgical wounds; recent or contemplated brain, eye, spinal cord surgery or prostatectomy; regional or lumbar block anesthesia; continuous tube drainage of the small intestine; severe renal or hepatic disease; subacute bacterial endocarditis; pericarditis; polyarthritis; diverticulitis; visceral carcinoma; severe or malignant hypertension; eclampsia or preeclampsia; threatened abortion; emaciation; malnutrition; vitamin C or K deficiencies; pregnancy; breastfeeding

PRECAUTIONS: Trauma, infection, renal insufficiency, hypertension, vasculitis, indwelling catheters, severe diabetes, active tuberculosis, postpartum, protein C deficiency, hepatic insufficiency, elderly, children, hyperthyroidism, hypothyroidism, CHF

PREGNANCY AND LACTATION: Pregnancy category X; may be excreted in breast milk in amounts sufficient to cause prothrombopenic state and bleeding in the nursing infant, contraindicated in breastfeeding

SIDE EFFECTS/ADVERSE REACTIONS

CNS: Headache

EENT: Sore throat, blurred vision, paralysis of accommodation

GI: Steatorrhea, ***hepatitis, liver damage,*** nausea, diarrhea, sore mouth, mouth ulcers

GU: ***Renal tubular necrosis,*** albuminuria, anuria

HEME: ***Hemorrhage,*** myeloid immaturity, leukocyte agglutinins, red cell aplasia, atypical mononuclear cells, ***leukopenia,*** leukocytosis, anemia, ***thrombocytopenia,*** eosinophilia, ***agranulocytosis***

SKIN: Dermatitis, urticaria, alopecia

▼ DRUG INTERACTIONS

Drugs

• Little is known about interactions with other drugs

SPECIAL CONSIDERATIONS

PATIENT/FAMILY EDUCATION

• Dosing is highly individual and may have to be adjusted several times based on lab test results

• Strict adherence to prescribed dosage schedule is necessary

• Do not take or discontinue any other medication, except on advice of physician or pharmacist

• Avoid alcohol, salicylates, and drastic changes in dietary habits

• Notify physician if unusual bleeding or bruising, red or dark brown urine, red or tarry black stools or diarrhea occurs

• Consult physician before undergoing dental work or elective surgery

MONITORING PARAMETERS

• International normalized ratio (INR), CBC, stool guaiac, urinalysis

anistreplase (anisoylated plasminogen streptokinase activator complex, APSAC)

(an-ih-strep'layz)

Eminase

Chemical Class: Anisoylated plasminogen streptokinase activator complex

Therapeutic Class: Thrombolytic enzyme

CLINICAL PHARMACOLOGY

Mechanism of Action: Inactive derivative of a fibrinolytic enzyme with the catalytic center of the activator complex temporarily blocked by an anisoyl group; when activated, it promotes thrombolysis by promoting conversion of plasminogen to plasmin; made *in vitro* from lys-plasminogen and streptokinase; activation of anistreplase occurs with release of the anisoyl group by deacylation which starts immediately; the enzymatically active lys-plasminogen-streptokinase activator complex is then progressively formed; the production of plasmin from plasminogen by deacylated anistreplase can take place in the bloodstream or within the thrombus; reperfusion rates are 50%-68% for patients receiving anistreplase within 6 hours of symptom onset

Pharmacokinetics

IV: Onset immediate; $t_{1/2}$ of fibrinolytic activity of circulating anistreplase 70-120 min

INDICATIONS AND USES: Acute MI (lysis of obstructing coronary artery thrombi)

DOSAGE

Adult

• *IV:* 30 U over 4-5 min as soon as possible after onset of symptoms

$ AVAILABLE FORMS/COST OF THERAPY

• Powder for inj: 30 U/vial, 1 vial: **$2,233.70**

CONTRAINDICATIONS: History of severe allergic reactions to anistreplase or streptokinase, active internal bleeding, intraspinal or intracranial surgery within 2 months, neoplasms of CNS, severe hypertension, cerebral embolism/thrombosis/hemorrhage, known bleeding diathesis

PRECAUTIONS: ***Bleeding:*** Anistreplase has 2 types of bleeding complications: 1. Internal bleeding involving the GI or GU tract, or retroperitoneal, ocular, or intracranial sites 2. Superficial or surface bleeding, mainly at invaded or disturbed sites (e.g., venous cutdowns, arterial punctures, sites of recent surgical intervention). As fibrin is lysed during anistreplase therapy, bleeding from recent puncture sites may occur. Avoid IM injections during treatment with anistreplase. Perform venipunctures carefully. For arterial punctures following administration of anistreplase, use an upper-extremity vessel that is accessible to manual compression; use a pressure dressing.

In the following conditions, the risks of anistreplase therapy may be increased:

• Recent (within 10 days) major surgery (e.g., coronary artery bypass graft, obstetrical delivery, organ biopsy, puncture of noncompressible vessels)
• Cerebrovascular disease
• Recent GI or GU bleeding (within 10 days)
• Recent trauma (within 10 days) including cardiopulmonary resuscitation

• Hypertension: systolic BP ≥180 mm Hg and/or diastolic BP ≥110 mm Hg
• High likelihood of left heart thrombus (e.g., mitral stenosis with atrial fibrillation)
• Bacterial endocarditis
• Acute pericarditis
• Hemostatic defects including those secondary to hepatic or renal disease
• Pregnancy
• Age > 75 years (use of anistreplase in patients over 75 years old has not been adequately studied)
• Hemorrhagic diabetic retinopathy or other hemorrhagic ophthalmic conditions
• Septic thrombophlebitis or occluded arteriovenous cannula at seriously infected site
• Patients currently receiving oral anticoagulants (e.g., warfarin sodium)
• Any other condition in which bleeding constitutes a significant hazard or would be particularly difficult to manage because of its location

Arrhythmias
Coronary thrombolysis may result in sinus bradycardia, accelerated idioventricular rhythm, ventricular premature depolarizations, and ventricular tachycardia associated with reperfusion; these arrhythmias may be managed with standard antiarrhythmic measures

Readministration
Because of the increased likelihood of resistance due to antistreptokinase antibody, anistreplase may not be effective if administered more than 5 days after prior anistreplase or streptokinase therapy, particularly between 5 days and 12 months after prior therapy; risk of allergic reactions also increased following readministration

PREGNANCY AND LACTATION: Pregnancy category C

SIDE EFFECTS/ADVERSE REACTIONS

CNS: Headache, fever, sweating, agitation, dizziness, paresthesia, tremor, vertigo

CV: ***Hypotension (10%), dysrhythmias and conduction disorders (38%)***

EENT: Epistaxis

GI: Nausea, vomiting, elevated transaminase levels

GU: Hematuria

HEME: GI (2%), GU (2%), ***intracranial (1%), retroperitoneal,*** *or surface bleeding (total incidence 15%),* thrombocytopenia

MS: Low back pain, arthralgia

RESP: Hemoptysis, dyspnea, ***bronchospasm, lung edema***

SKIN: Rash, urticaria, phlebitis at infusion site, itching, flushing

MISC: ***Anaphylaxis (0.2%)***

▼ **DRUG INTERACTIONS**

Labs
• *Increase:* PT, APTT, TT
• *Decrease:* Fibrinogen, plasminogen

anthralin

(anth-rah'lin)

Anthra-Derm, Dritho-Scalp, Drithocreme, Lasan

Chemical Class: 1,8,9-anthratriol

Therapeutic Class: Anti-psoriatic agent

CLINICAL PHARMACOLOGY

Mechanism of Action: Reduces the mitotic rate and proliferation of epidermal cells in psoriasis by inhibiting the synthesis of nucleic protein

Pharmacokinetics
Absorption in man has not been determined

INDICATIONS AND USES: Psoriasis

DOSAGE

Adult

Begin with the lowest concentration (0.1%) and gradually increase until desired effect is obtained

• *Skin:* TOP apply at bedtime to plaque sites, wash off remaining drug in the morning

• *Scalp:* TOP massage into affected areas, shampoo in the morning

$ **AVAILABLE FORMS/COST OF THERAPY**

• Cre—Top: 0.1%, 50 g: **$19.80;** 0.25%, 50 g: **$21.33-$22.09;** 0.5%, 50 g: **$23.83-$24.48;** 1%, 50 g: **$27.96**

• Oint—Top: 0.1%, 45 g: **$23.12;** 0.25%, 45g: **$23.12;** 0.4%, 60 g: **$12.94;** 0.5%, 45 g: **$24.52;** 1%, 45 g: **$24.95**

• Powder—Top: 25 g: **$45.50-$85.95**

CONTRAINDICATIONS: Acute psoriasis, hypersensitivity

PRECAUTIONS: Excessive irritation, renal and hepatic impairment, inflammation, application to face, genitalia or intertriginous skin

PREGNANCY AND LACTATION: Pregnancy category C; excretion into human milk unknown, because of the potential for tumorigenicity shown in animal studies, use with caution in nursing mothers

SIDE EFFECTS/ADVERSE REACTIONS

SKIN: Irritation of normal skin, sensitivity reaction, discoloration of fingernails, staining of hair

SPECIAL CONSIDERATIONS

PATIENT/FAMILY EDUCATION

• Use plastic gloves for application and wear a plastic cap over treated scalp at bedtime to avoid staining

• Apply a protective film of petrolatum to areas surrounding plaque

• May stain fabrics

MONITORING PARAMETERS

• Perform periodic urine tests for albuminuria in patients with renal impairment

---

antipyrine and benzocaine

(an-tee-pye'reen)

A/B Otic, Allergen, Auralgan, Aurodex, Auroto, Benzotic, Decon Otic Ear Drops, Rx Otic Drops

Chemical Class: Pyrazolon derivative (antipyrine); aminobenzoate derivative (benzocaine)

Therapeutic Class: Otic agent; analgesic; cerumenolytic

CLINICAL PHARMACOLOGY

Mechanism of Action: Relieves pressure, reduces inflammation and congestion, and alleviates pain and discomfort in acute otitis media

INDICATIONS AND USES: Temporary relief of pain and reduction of inflammation associated with acute congestive and serous otitis media; facilitates ear wax removal; swimmer's ear;* otitis externa*

DOSAGE

Adult and Child

• *Acute otitis media:* OTIC Instill permitting the solution to run along the wall of the canal until it is filled, moisten a cotton pledget and insert into external ear; repeat every 1-2 hr until pain and congestion are relieved

• *Removal of cerumen:* OTIC Instill tid for 2-3 days to help detach cerumen from wall of canal and facilitate removal

$ **AVAILABLE FORMS/COST OF THERAPY**

• Sol—Otic: 54 mg/14 mg, 10-15 ml: **$1.47-$12.73**

CONTRAINDICATIONS: Hypersensitivity to any components, perforated tympanic membrane
PRECAUTIONS: May mask symptoms of fulminating middle ear infection, not intended for prolonged use
PREGNANCY AND LACTATION: Pregnancy category C
SIDE EFFECTS/ADVERSE REACTIONS
EENT: Burning, stinging, tenderness, edema
MISC: Hypersensitivity

SPECIAL CONSIDERATIONS

PATIENT/FAMILY EDUCATION

- Do not rinse dropper after use
- Protect the solution from light and heat, store at room temperature; do not use if it is brown or contains a precipitate
- Discard this product six months after dropper is first placed in the drug solution

---

apraclonidine

(ap-raa-kloe'ni-deen)
Iopidine
Chemical Class: Selective α-adrenergic agonist
Therapeutic Class: Topical ophthalmic agent

CLINICAL PHARMACOLOGY
Mechanism of Action: Reduces intraocular pressure by reducing aqueous formation; exact mechanism of action unknown
Pharmacokinetics
Onset 1 hr, peak 3-5 hr
INDICATIONS AND USES: Controls or prevents elevations of intraocular pressure after laser iridotomy or trabeculoplasty; short-term adjunctive therapy in patients requiring additional reduction of intraocular pressure

DOSAGE
Adult
- Instill 1 gtt 1 hr before laser surgery, second gtt at completion of surgery (1%); for short-term adjunctive therapy instill 1-2 gtt 0.5% sol tid

Child
- Safety and efficacy not established

$ AVAILABLE FORMS/COST OF THERAPY
- Sol—Ophth: 0.5%, 5 ml: **$33.75;** 1%, 0.2 ml × 12: **$142.50**

CONTRAINDICATIONS: Hypersensitivity to this drug or clonidine
PRECAUTIONS: Severe cardiovascular disease, history of vasovagal attack
PREGNANCY AND LACTATION: Pregnancy category C; excretion into breast milk unknown, consider discontinuing nursing on day apraclonidine is used
SIDE EFFECTS/ADVERSE REACTIONS
CNS: Insomnia, irritability, restlessness, headache, dream disturbances
CV: Bradycardia, palpitations, vasovagal attack, orthostatic episode
EENT: Upper lid elevation, conjunctival blanching, mydriasis, burning, dryness, itching, blurred vision, conjunctival microhemorrhage, foreign body sensation, taste abnormalities, nasal dryness/burning
GI: Abdominal pain, diarrhea, cramps, emesis, dry mouth
MISC: Shortness of breath, head cold sensation, sweaty palms, fatigue, paresthesia, pruritus

SPECIAL CONSIDERATIONS

PATIENT/FAMILY EDUCATION

- May cause burning, itching, blurring, dryness of eye area
- Store at room temperature, away from light

A

aprobarbital

(ape-roh-bar'bi-tal)

Alurate

Chemical Class: Barbituric acid derivative

Therapeutic Class: Sedative/hypnotic-barbiturate (intermediate acting)

DEA Class: Schedule III

CLINICAL PHARMACOLOGY

Mechanism of Action: Depresses activity in brain cells primarily in reticular activating system in brain stem; also selectively depresses neurons in posterior hypothalamus, limbic structures; able to decrease seizure activity in hypnotic doses by inhibition of impulses in CNS; depresses REM sleep

Pharmacokinetics

PO: Peak 3 hr, 35% bound to plasma proteins, $t_{1/2}$ 14-40 hr, partially metabolized by liver, excreted in urine as unchanged drug and inactive metabolites

INDICATIONS AND USES: Routine sedation; hypnotic in the short-term treatment of insomnia for periods up to 2 weeks (may lose efficacy for sleep induction and maintenance after this period of time)

DOSAGE

Adult

- *Sedative:* PO 40 mg tid
- *Mild insomnia:* PO 40-80 mg before retiring
- *Pronounced insomnia:* PO 80-160 mg before retiring

$ AVAILABLE FORMS/COST OF THERAPY

- Elixir—Oral: 40 mg/5 ml, 480 ml: **$28.11**

CONTRAINDICATIONS: Hypersensitivity to barbiturates, respiratory depression, addiction to barbiturates, severe liver impairment, porphyria

PRECAUTIONS: Anemia, hepatic disease, renal disease, hypertension, elderly, acute/chronic pain, mental depression, history of drug abuse, abrupt discontinuation

PREGNANCY AND LACTATION: Pregnancy category D; small amount excreted in breast milk, use caution in nursing mothers

SIDE EFFECTS/ADVERSE REACTIONS

CNS: Lethargy, drowsiness, hangover, dizziness, stimulation in the elderly and children, light-headedness, physical dependence, CNS depression, mental depression, slurred speech, vertigo, headache

CV: Hypotension, bradycardia

GI: Nausea, vomiting, diarrhea, constipation

HEME: ***Agranulocytosis, thrombocytopenia, megaloblastic anemia*** (long-term treatment)

RESP: ***Depression, apnea, laryngospasm, bronchospasm***

SKIN: Rash, urticaria, erythema multiforme, pain, ***angioedema,*** thrombophlebitis, ***Stevens-Johnson syndrome***

MISC: Rickets, osteomalacia (prolonged use)

▼ DRUG INTERACTIONS

Drugs

- *Acetaminophen:* Enhanced hepatotoxic potential of acetaminophen overdoses
- *Antidepressants:* Reduced serum concentration of cyclic antidepressants
- *β-adrenergic blockers:* Reduced serum concentrations of β-blockers which are extensively metabolized
- *Calcium channel blockers:* Reduced concentrations of verapamil and nifedipine
- *Central nervous system depressants:* Excessive CNS depression

• *Chloramphenicol:* Increased barbiturate concentrations; reduced serum chloramphenicol concentrations
• *Corticosteroids:* Reduced serum concentrations of corticosteroids may impair therapeutic effect
• *Disopyramide:* Reduced serum concentrations of disopyramide
• *Doxycycline:* Reduced serum doxycycline concentrations
• *Ethanol:* Excessive CNS depression
• *MAO inhibitors:* Prolonged effect of some barbiturates
• *Methoxyflurane:* Enhanced nephrotoxic effect
• *Narcotic analgesics:* Increased toxicity of meperidine; reduced effect of methadone; additive CNS depression
• *Neuroleptics:* Reduced effect of either drug
• *Oral anticoagulants+:* Inhibited hypoprothrombinemic response to oral anticoagulants
• *Oral contraceptives:* Reduced efficacy of oral contraceptives
• *Quinidine:* Reduced quinidine plasma concentrations
• *Theophylline:* Reduced serum theophylline concentrations

SPECIAL CONSIDERATIONS

• Indicated only for short-term treatment of insomnia and is probably ineffective after 2 wk; physical dependency may result when used for extended time (45-90 days depending on dose)

PATIENT/FAMILY EDUCATION

• Avoid driving or other activities requiring alertness
• Avoid alcohol ingestion or CNS depressants
• Do not discontinue medication abruptly after long-term use

MONITORING PARAMETERS

• CBC
• Serum folate, vitamin D (if on long-term therapy)
• PT in patients receiving anticoagulants
• LFTs
• Mental status, vital signs

ascorbic acid (vitamin C)

(a-skor′bic)

Apo-C, ✦Ascorbicap, Cecon, Cenolate, Cetane, Cevalin, Cevi-Bid, Ce-Vi-Sol, C-Crystals, Cebid Timecelles, Dull-C, Flavorcee, N'ice Vitamin C Drops, Redoxon, ✦Vita-C

Chemical Class: Water soluble vitamin

Therapeutic Class: Urinary acidifying agent; vitamin

CLINICAL PHARMACOLOGY

Mechanism of Action: Needed for wound healing, collagen synthesis, carbohydrate metabolism; antioxidant, involved in some oxidation-reduction reactions as well as many other metabolic reactions

Pharmacokinetics

PO: Readily absorbed, metabolized in liver by oxidation and sulfation, unused amounts excreted in urine (unchanged) and as metabolites

INDICATIONS AND USES: Prevention and treatment of scurvy, urinary acidifying agent, dietary supplementation

DOSAGE

Adult

• *Scurvy:* PO/SC/IM/IV 100 mg-500 mg qd for at least 2 wk, then 50 mg or more qd
• *Urinary acidification:* PO/SC/IM/IV 4-12 g qd in divided doses
• *Dietary supplementation:* PO/SC/IM/IV 50-200 mg qd

Child

• *Scurvy:* PO/SC/IM/IV 100-300 mg qd for at least 2 wk, then 35 mg or more qd

• *Urinary acidification:* PO/SC/IM/IV 500 mg q6-8h
• *Dietary supplementation:* PO/SC/IM/IV 35-100 mg qd

$ AVAILABLE FORMS/COST OF THERAPY

• Inj, Sol—IM, IV, SC: 250 mg/ml, 30 ml: **$4.20-$6.80;** 500 mg/ml, 50 ml: **$3.80-$12.75**
• Syr—Oral: 500 mg/5 ml, 480 ml: **$12.00**
• Sol—Oral: 100 mg/ml, 50 ml: **$11.84**
• Tab—Oral: 100 mg, 100's: **$1.30-$1.75;** 250 mg, 100's: **$1.50-$2.95;** 500 mg, 100's: **$1.80-$4.88;** 1000 mg, 100's: **$3.50-$6.27**
• Tab, Chewable—Oral: 250 mg, 100's: **$1.90;** 500 mg, 100's: **$2.70**

CONTRAINDICATIONS: None significant

PRECAUTIONS: Gout, excessive doses for prolonged periods of time (diabetics, patients with recurrent renal calculi, patients undergoing anticoagulant therapy), tatrazine sensitivity, sulfite sensitivity

PREGNANCY AND LACTATION: Pregnancy category A if doses do not exceed the RDA, otherwise pregnancy category C; excreted into breast milk via a saturable process, the RDA during lactation is 90-100 mg, maternal supplementation up to the RDA is needed only in those women with poor nutritional status

SIDE EFFECTS/ADVERSE REACTIONS

CNS: Headache, insomnia, dizziness, fatigue, flushing
GI: Nausea, vomiting, diarrhea, anorexia, heartburn, cramps
GU: Polyuria, urine acidification, oxalate or urate renal stones
HEME: ***Hemolysis*** (after large doses in patients with G-6-PD deficiency), sickle-cell crisis

▼ DRUG INTERACTIONS

Labs

• *False negative:* amine-dependent stool occult blood, urine glucose determinations

SPECIAL CONSIDERATIONS

PATIENT/FAMILY EDUCATION

• Do not exceed recommended doses

aspirin

(as'pir-in)

A.S.A., Ancasal, ♣ Aspergum, Bayer, Bayer Children's Aspirin, Easprin, Ecotrin, Ecotrin Maximum Strength, 8-Hour Bayer Timed Release, Empirin, Genprin, Maximum Bayer, Norwich Extra-Strength, St. Joseph Children's, Supasa, ♣ Therapy Bayer, ZORprin

Chemical Class: Salicylate
Therapeutic Class: Nonnarcotic analgesic; antiinflammatory; antiplatelet; antipyretic

CLINICAL PHARMACOLOGY

Mechanism of Action: Inhibits prostaglandin synthesis and release; acts on the hypothalamus heat-regulating center to reduce fever; blocks prostaglandin synthetase action which prevents formation of the platelet-aggregating substance thromboxane A_2

Pharmacokinetics

PO: Well absorbed, enteric coated product may exhibit erratic absorption, onset 15-30 min (delayed with enteric coated), peak 1-2 hr, duration 4-6 hr
PR: Absorption erratic, onset slow, duration 4-6 hr
Metabolized by liver, metabolites excreted by kidneys, $t_{1/2}$ 3 hr at lower doses (300-600 mg), 5-6 hr (1000 mg) up to 30 hrs in larger doses (due to saturable metabolic pathways)

INDICATIONS AND USES: Mild to moderate pain and fever; various inflammatory conditions such as rheumatic fever, rheumatoid arthritis and osteoarthritis; thromboembolic disorders; reducing risk of recurrent transient ischemic attacks; reducing the risk of death or nonfatal MI in patients with previous MI or unstable angina; low doses may be useful in preventing toxemia of pregnancy*

DOSAGE

Adult

- *Arthritis:* PO 2.6-5.2 g/day in divided doses q4-6h
- *Pain/fever:* PO/PR 325-650 mg q4h prn, not to exceed 4 g/day
- *Transient ischemic attacks:* PO 325-650 mg qd or bid (325 mg/day may be as effective as larger doses and associated with fewer side effects)
- *MI prophylaxis:* PO 165-325 mg/day

Child

- *Arthritis:* PO 60-90 mg/kg/day in divided doses; usual maintenance dose 80-100 mg/kg/day divided q6-8h; maintain serum salicylate level of 150-300 µg/ml
- *Pain/fever:* PO/PR 10-15 mg/kg/dose q4-6h prn

$ AVAILABLE FORMS/COST OF THERAPY

- Tab, Chewable—Oral: 81 mg, 36's: **$0.69-$2.18**
- Tab, Enteric Coated—Oral: 165 mg, 60's: **$3.20;** 325 mg, 100's: **$1.55-$6.25;** 500 mg, 60's: **$1.55-$6.26;** 650 mg, 100's: **$3.70-$4.51**
- Gum Tab, Chewable—Oral: 227.5 mg, 16's: **$2.26**
- Tab, Film Coated—Oral: 325 mg, 100's: **$0.75-$2.10;** 500 mg, 100's: **$1.29**
- Tab, Enteric Coated, Sust Action—Oral: 800 mg, 100's: **$9.00-$31.56;** 975 mg, 100's: **$11.48-$34.88**
- Supp—Rect: 120 mg, 12's: **$1.80-$2.10;** 200 mg, 12's: **$1.85;** 300 mg, 12's: **$1.90-$2.25;** 600 mg, 12's: **$2.00-$2.70**

CONTRAINDICATIONS: Hypersensitivity to salicylates, NSAIDs, or tartrazine (FDC yellow dye #5); GI bleeding; hemophilia; hemorrhagic states

PRECAUTIONS: Anemia, hepatic disease, renal disease, Hodgkin's disease, pre/postoperatively, children or teenagers with flulike symptoms (may be associated with the development of Reye's syndrome), gout, history of coagulation defects, bleeding disorders

PREGNANCY AND LACTATION: Pregnancy category C (category D if full-doses used in 3rd trimester); use in pregnancy should generally be avoided; in pregnancies at risk for the development of pregnancy-induced hypertension and preeclampsia, and in fetuses with intrauterine growth retardation, low-dose aspirin (40-150 mg/day) may be beneficial, but more studies are required; excreted into breast milk in low concentrations, use with caution in nursing mothers due to potential adverse effects in the nursing infant

SIDE EFFECTS/ADVERSE REACTIONS

CNS: Drowsiness, dizziness, confusion, headache

EENT: Tinnitus, reversible hearing loss, dimness of vision

GI: Nausea, dyspepsia, ***GI bleeding,*** diarrhea, heartburn, epigastric discomfort, anorexia, ***acute reversible hepatotoxicity***

HEME: ***Thrombocytopenia, leukopenia,*** prolonged bleeding time, decreased plasma iron concentration, shortened erythrocyte survival time

METAB: Hypoglycemia, hyponatremia, hypokalemia

A

RESP: Wheezing, hyperpnea
SKIN: Rash, hives, angioedema, urticaria, bruising
MISC: Fever, thirst

▼ DRUG INTERACTIONS

Drugs

- *Acetazolamide:* Increased concentrations of acetazolamide, possibly leading to CNS toxicity
- *Antacids:* Decreased serum salicylate concentrations
- *Antidiabetics:* Enhanced hypoglycemic response to sulfonylureas, particularly chlorpropamide
- *Corticosteroids:* Increased incidence and/or severity of GI ulceration
- *Ethanol:* Enhanced aspirin-induced GI mucosal damage and aspirin-induced prolongation of bleeding time
- *Heparin:* Increased risk of bleeding
- *Methotrexate+:* Increased serum methotrexate concentrations and enhanced methotrexate toxicity
- *Oral anticoagulants+:* Increased risk of bleeding by inhibiting platelet function and possibly by producing gastric erosions
- *Phenytoin:* Large doses of salicylates may reduce total serum phenytoin concentrations, but free serum concentrations do not appear to be affected
- *Probenecid:* Salicylates inhibit the uricosuric activity of probenecid
- *Sulfinpyrazone:* Salicylates inhibit the uricosuric activity of sulfinpyrazone
- *Valproic acid:* Salicylates may increase unbound serum valproic acid concentrations sufficiently to result in toxicity

Labs

- *Increase:* Serum uric acid (small doses), protein bound iodine
- *Decrease:* Serum uric acid (large doses)
- *Interfere:* Urine catecholamines, urine glucose tests (Clinistix, Tes-Tape), urine ketone tests

SPECIAL CONSIDERATIONS

PATIENT/FAMILY EDUCATION

- Report any symptoms of hepatotoxicity (dark urine, clay-colored stools, yellowing of skin, sclera, itching, abdominal pain, fever, diarrhea), renal toxicity (decreased urine output), visual changes, ototoxicity (tinnitus, ringing, roaring in ears), allergic reactions, bleeding (long-term therapy)
- Administer with food
- Do not exceed recommended doses
- Read label on other OTC drugs, many contain aspirin
- Therapeutic response may take 2 wk (arthritis)
- Avoid alcohol ingestion, GI bleeding may occur
- **Not to be given to children with flu-like symptoms, Reye's syndrome may develop**

MONITORING PARAMETERS

- AST, ALT, bilirubin, creatinine, CBC, hematocrit if patient is on long-term therapy

---

astemizole

(a-stem'mi-zole)
Hismanal
Chemical Class: Benzimidazole
Therapeutic Class: Antihistamine

CLINICAL PHARMACOLOGY

Mechanism of Action: Competitively antagonizes most of the pharmacologic effects of histamine by preferentially binding to peripheral rather than central H_1-receptors; has little sedative or anticholinergic effects

Pharmacokinetics

PO: Absorption reduced by 60%

when taken with food, peak 1-2 hr (does not correlate with onset of effect), 97% bound to plasma proteins, metabolized in the liver, terminal $t_{1/2}$ 7-11 days

INDICATIONS AND USES: Seasonal allergic rhinitis; chronic idiopathic urticaria (should not be used as a prn product for immediate relief of symptoms)

DOSAGE

Adult and Child >12 yr

- PO 10 mg qd on an empty stomach

Child 6-12 yr

- PO 5 mg qd on an empty stomach

Child <6 yr

- PO 0.2 mg/kg qd on an empty stomach

$ AVAILABLE FORMS/COST OF THERAPY

- Tab, Uncoated—Oral: 10 mg, 100's: **$177.02**

CONTRAINDICATIONS: Hypersensitivity; severe hepatic disease; concomitant erythromycin, ketoconazole, or itraconazole therapy

PRECAUTIONS: Conditions leading to QT prolongation, hepatic dysfunction

PREGNANCY AND LACTATION: Pregnancy category C; to avoid early exposure during pregnancy remember that metabolites may remain in the body for as long as 4 months after end of dosing; excretion into breast milk unknown, use caution in nursing mothers

SIDE EFFECTS/ADVERSE REACTIONS

CNS: Headache, drowsiness, fatigue, increased appetite, nervousness

CV: ***Dysrrhythmias*** (rare)

EENT: Dry mouth, pharyngitis, conjunctivitis

GI: Nausea, diarrhea, abdominal pain

MISC: Increased weight

▼ DRUG INTERACTIONS

Drugs

- *Erythromycin+:* QT interval prolongation and arrhythmia
- *Fluvoxamine:* Increased astemizole concentrations, potential for QT interval prolongation and arrhythmia
- *Ketoconazole+:* QT interval prolongation and arrhythmia

Labs

- *False negative:* skin allergy tests (may persist for prolonged periods due to long $t_{1/2}$)

SPECIAL CONSIDERATIONS

PATIENT/FAMILY EDUCATION

- Administer on empty stomach, 1 hr before or 2 hr after meals
- Do not increase the dose in an attempt to accelerate the onset of action
- Do not exceed recommended dose, dysrrhythmias may occur
- Do not use as needed for immediate relief of symptoms

atenolol

(a-ten'oh-lol)

Apo-Atenol, ♣ Tenormin

Chemical Class: β_1-selective (cardioselective) adrenoreceptor blocking agent

Therapeutic Class: Antihypertensive, antianginal

CLINICAL PHARMACOLOGY

Mechanism of Action: Preferentially competes with β-adrenergic agonists for available β_1-receptor sites inhibiting the chronotropic and inotropic responses to β_1-adrenergic stimulation (cardioselective); slows conduction of AV node, decreases heart rate, decreases O_2 consumption in myocardium, also decreases renin-aldosterone-angiotensin system at higher doses; blocks β_2-receptors in bronchial system at higher doses; lacks membrane stabilizing or intrinsic sympathomimetic (partial agonist) activities

Pharmacokinetics

PO: Peak 2-4 hr, $t_{1/2}$ 6-7 hr, excreted unchanged in urine, protein binding 6%-16%

INDICATIONS AND USES: Angina pectoris due to coronary atherosclerosis; hypertension; acute MI; migraine headache prophylaxis;* alcohol withdrawal syndrome;* esophageal varices in cirrhotic patients;* situational anxiety;* ventricular dysrhythmias;* rate control in atrial fibrillation*

DOSAGE

Adult

- IV 5 mg over 5 min, repeat in 10 min if initial dose is well tolerated, then start PO dose 10 min after last IV dose; PO 50 mg qd, increasing q1-2 wk to 100 mg qd; may increase to 200 mg qd for angina

Child

- PO Initial 1-1.2 mg/kg/dose given daily, maximum 2 mg/kg/day

Dose in renal impairment:

CREATININE CLEARANCE	MAXIMUM DOSE	DOSING INTERVAL
15-35 ml/min	50 mg or 1 mg/kg/dose	Daily
<15 ml/min	50 mg or 1 mg/kg/dose	Every other day

$ AVAILABLE FORMS/COST OF THERAPY

- Tab, Uncoated—Oral: 25 mg, 100's: **$11.39-$85.01;** 50 mg, 100's: **$8.48-$86.74;** 100 mg, 100's: **$12.90-$130.10**
- Inj, Sol—IV, Buffered: 5 mg/10 ml, 10 ml × 6: **$17.70**

CONTRAINDICATIONS: Hypersensitivity to β-blockers, cardiogenic shock, 2nd or 3rd degree heart block, sinus bradycardia, CHF unless secondary to a tachyarrhythmia treatable with β-blockers, overt cardiac failure

PRECAUTIONS: Major surgery, diabetes mellitus, renal disease, thyroid disease, COPD, asthma, well-compensated heart failure, abrupt withdrawal, peripheral vascular disease

PREGNANCY AND LACTATION: Pregnancy category C; safe use for the treatment of hypertension in pregnant women has been demonstrated, no fetal malformations have been reported, but experience during the first trimester is lacking; excreted into breast milk, monitor nursing infants closely for bradycardia and other signs and symptoms of β-blockade

SIDE EFFECTS/ADVERSE REACTIONS

CNS: Insomnia, *fatigue, dizziness,* mental changes, memory loss, hallucinations, depression, *lethargy,* drowsiness, strange dreams

CV: Profound hypotension, ***bradycardia,*** CHF, cold extremities, postural hypotension, ***2nd or 3rd degree heart block***

EENT: Sore throat, dry burning eyes, visual disturbances

GI: Nausea, diarrhea, vomiting, dry mouth, ***mesenteric arterial thrombosis, ischemic colitis***

GU: Impotence, sexual dysfunction

HEME: ***Agranulocytosis, thrombocytopenia***

METAB: Masked hypoglycemic response to insulin (sweating excepted), hyperlipidemia (increase TG, total cholesterol, LDL; decrease HDL)

RESP: ***Bronchospasm,*** dyspnea, wheezing

SKIN: Rash, pruritis, alopecia

▼ DRUG INTERACTIONS

Drugs

- *Antidiabetics:* Altered response to hypoglycemia, prolonged recovery of normoglycemia, hypertension, blockade of tachycardia; may increase blood glucose and impair peripheral circulation

• *Clonidine:* Exacerbation of rebound hypertension upon discontinuation of clonidine

• *Dihydropyridines:* Additive hemodynamic effects

• *Diltiazem:* Enhanced effects of both drugs, particularly atrioventricular conduction slowing

• *Dipyridamole:* Bradycardia

• *Disopyramide:* Additive negative inotropic effects

• *Epinephrine+:* Enhanced pressor response to epinephrine; less likely with cardioselective agents like atenolol

• *Isoproterenol:* Potential reduction in effectiveness of isoproterenol in the treatment of asthma; less likely with cardioselective agents like atenolol

• *Lidocaine:* Increased lidocaine concentrations possible

• *Local anesthetics:* Use of local anesthetics containing epinephrine may result in hypertensive reactions in patients taking β-blockers

• *Methyldopa:* Development of hypertension during situations resulting in release of catecholamines

• *NSAIDs:* Reduced hypotensive effects of β-blockers

• *Phenylephrine:* Enhanced pressor response to phenylephrine, particularly when it is administered IV

• *Prazosin:* First-dose response to prazosin may be enhanced by β-blockade

• *Tacrine:* Additive bradycardia

• *Theophylline:* Antagonistic pharmacodynamic effects

• *Verapamil:* Enhanced effects of both drugs, particularly antrioventricular conduction slowing

Labs

• *Interference:* Glucose/insulin tolerance tests

SPECIAL CONSIDERATIONS

PATIENT/FAMILY EDUCATION

• Do not discontinue drug abruptly, may precipitate angina

• Report bradycardia, dizziness, confusion, depression, fever, shortness of breath, swelling of the extremities

• Take pulse at home, notify physician if <50 beats/min

• Avoid hazardous activities if dizziness, drowsiness, lightheadedness are present

• May mask the symptoms of hypoglycemia, except for sweating, in diabetic patients

MONITORING PARAMETERS

• Blood pressure, pulse

---

atovaquone

(a-toe'va-kwone)

Mepron

Chemical Class: Hydroxy-napthoquinone

Therapeutic Class: Antiprotozoal

CLINICAL PHARMACOLOGY

Mechanism of Action: Inhibits synthesis of nucleic acid and ATP; possibly cidal against susceptible organisms

Pharmacokinetics

PO: Double peak, 1-8 hr and 24-96 hr (13.9 μg/ml) (Note correlation between plasma levels and the likelihood of successful treatment and survival: <5 μg/mL more likely to die than those with concentrations ≥5 μg/mL); low/variable bioavailability (increases 3-fold when administered with meals), highly lipophilic, with low aqueous solubility (CSF:plasma ratio <1%); 99.9%

protein bound; $t_{1/2}$, 2.2-2.9 days, fecal elimination

INDICATIONS AND USES: Acute oral treatment of mild to moderate *Pneumocystis carinii* pneumonia (PCP) in patients who are intolerant to co-trimoxazole

DOSAGE

Adult

• PO 750 mg tid with food for 21 days

$ AVAILABLE FORMS/COST OF THERAPY

• Susp—Oral: 750 mg/5 ml, 210 ml: **$523.51**

• Tab, Coated—Oral: 250 mg, 200's: **$553.98**

CONTRAINDICATIONS: Hypersensitivity, GI disorders that may inhibit absorption

PREGNANCY AND LACTATION: Pregnancy category C; human breast milk studies not available; in rats, concentrations in milk was 30% of maternal serum

SIDE EFFECTS/ADVERSE REACTIONS

CNS: Headache, insomnia

GI: Diarrhea, nausea, vomiting

METAB: Fever

RESP: Cough

SKIN: Skin rash

SPECIAL CONSIDERATIONS

PATIENT/FAMILY EDUCATION

• Should be taken with a high-fat meal to enhance absorption

atropine

(a'troe-peen)

Atropair, Atropen, Atropisol, I-Tropine, Isopto Atropine, Minims-Atropine, ♣ Ocu-Tropine, Sal-Tropine, Spectro-Atropine

Chemical Class: Belladonna alkaloid

Therapeutic Class: Anticholinergic, parasympatholytic, mydriatic

CLINICAL PHARMACOLOGY

Mechanism of Action: Blocks acetylcholine at parasympathetic neuroeffector sites; increases cardiac output and heart rate by blocking vagal stimulation in heart; dries secretions by blocking vagus; blocks response of iris sphincter muscle, muscle of accommodation of ciliary body to cholinergic stimulation, resulting in dilation, paralysis of accommodation

Pharmacokinetics

PO/IM/SC: Well absorbed

PO: Onset ½ hr; peak ½-1 hr; duration 4-6 hr

IM/SC: Onset 15-50 min; peak 30 min, duration 4-6 hr

IV: Peak 2-4 min, duration 4-6 hr

OPHTH: Peak 30-40 min (mydriasis), 60-180 min (cycloplegia), duration 6-12 days $t_{1/2}$ 13-40 hr, excreted by kidneys unchanged (70%-90% in 24 hr); metabolized in liver, 40%-50% crosses placenta, excreted in breast milk

INDICATIONS AND USES: Bradycardia, bradydysrhythmia; anticholinesterase insecticide poisoning; blockade of cardiac vagal reflexes; antisialagogue (preanesthetic to prevent or reduce secretions of the respiratory tract and end of life comfort measure); rigidity and tremor of parkinsonism; antispasmodic with GU, biliary surgery; bronchodilator, mydriasis/cycloplegia, for iritis, cycloplegic refraction, INH via nebulizer for bronchospasm with COPD* (replaced with ipratropium bromide)

DOSAGE

Adult

- *Bradycardia/bradydysrhythmias:* IV BOL 0.5-1 mg given q3-5 min, not to exceed 2 mg
- *Insecticide poisoning:* IM/IV 2 mg qh until muscarinic symptoms disappear, may need 6 mg qh
- *Pre-surgery:* SC/IM/IV 0.4-0.6 mg before anesthesia
- *Iritis/cycloplegic refraction:* INSTILL SOL 1-2 gtt of a 1% sol qd-tid for iritis or 1 hr before refracting

Child

- *Bradycardia/bradydysrhythmias:* IV BOL 0.01-0.03 mg/kg up to 0.4 mg or 0.3 mg/m^2; may repeat q4-6h
- *Insecticide poisoning:* IM/IV 2 mg qh until muscarinic symptoms disappear, may need 6 mg qh
- *Pre-surgery:* SC 0.1-0.4 mg 30 min before surgery
- *Iritis/cycloplegic refraction:* INSTILL SOL 1-2 gtt of a 0.5% sol qd-tid for iritis or bid × 1-3 days before exam (cycloplegic refraction); INSTILL OINT qd-bid 2-3 days before exam

$ AVAILABLE FORMS/COST OF THERAPY

- Inj, Sol—IM, IV, SC: 0.1 mg/ml, 5 ml: **$11.74;** 10 ml: **$12.12;** 0.4 mg/ml, 2 ml × 25: **$12.60;** 20 ml: **$4.78;** 0.5 mg/ml, 5 ml: **$9.29;** 1 mg/ml, 2 ml × 25: **$12.30**
- Oint—Ophth: 1%, 3.5 g: **$2.30-$4.79**
- Sol—Ophth: 0.5%, 5 ml **$9.38;** 1%, 1 ml × 12: **$25.80;** 2 ml: **$2.20-$3.31;** 5 ml: **$2.52-$10.13;** 15 ml: **$2.31-$13.75;** 3%, 5 ml: **$10.00**

CONTRAINDICATIONS: Hypersensitivity to belladonna alkaloids, angle-closure glaucoma, GI obstructions, myasthenia gravis, thyrotoxicosis, ulcerative colitis, prostatic hypertrophy, tachycardia/tachydysrhythmias, asthma, acute hemorrhage, hepatic disease, myocardial ischemia

PRECAUTIONS: Renal disease, lactation, CHF, hyperthyroidism, COPD, hepatic disease, child <6 yr, hypertension, elderly, intraabdominal infections, Down syndrome, spastic paralysis, gastric ulcer

PREGNANCY AND LACTATION: Pregnancy category C; passage into breast milk still controversial; neonates particularly sensitive to anticholinergic agents; compatible with breast feeding

SIDE EFFECTS/ADVERSE REACTIONS

CNS: Headache, dizziness, involuntary movement, confusion, psychosis, anxiety, coma, flushing, drowsiness, insomnia, weakness

CV: Hypotension, paradoxical bradycardia, angina, PVCs, hypertension, tachycardia, ectopic ventricular beats

EENT: Blurred vision, photophobia, glaucoma, eye pain, pupil dilation, nasal congestion

GI: Dry mouth, nausea, vomiting, abdominal pain, anorexia, constipation, paralytic ileus, abdominal distension, altered taste

GU: Retention, hesitancy, impotence, dysuria

SKIN: Rash, urticaria, contact dermatitis, dry skin, flushing

MISC: Suppression of lactation, decreased sweating

▼ DRUG INTERACTIONS

Drugs

- β-*blockers:* Anticholinergic drugs can block β-blocker-induced brady-

* = non-FDA-approved use

+ = major clinical significance

cardia and may increase atenolol concentration

auranofin

(aur-an'oh-fin)

Ridaura

Chemical Class: Heavy metal; active gold compound (29%)
Therapeutic Class: Gold salt, slowly-acting antiarthritic drug; disease-modifying arthritis drug (DMARD)

CLINICAL PHARMACOLOGY

Mechanism of Action: Antiinflammatory action unknown; may decrease phagocytosis, lysosomal activity or decrease prostaglandin synthesis; decreases concentration of rheumatoid factor, immunoglobulins

Pharmacokinetics

PO: 25% of the gold absorbed by GI tract, peak 2 hr, steady state 8-16 wk; excreted in urine (60% of the absorbed gold) and feces; terminal plasma $t_{1/2}$ (steady state), 26 days; terminal body $t_{1/2}$, 80 days

INDICATIONS AND USES: Rheumatoid arthritis, alternative or adjuvant to corticosteroids in treatment of pemphigus,* psoriatic arthritis*

DOSAGE

Adult

• PO 6 mg qd or 3 mg bid, may increase to 9 mg/day after 3 mo

Child

• PO (initial) 0.1 mg/kg/day; (maintenance) 0.15 mg/kg/day; (max) 0.2 mg/kg/day

$ AVAILABLE FORMS/COST OF THERAPY

• Cap, Gel—Oral: 3 mg, 60's: **$69.00**

CONTRAINDICATIONS: Hypersensitivity to gold, necrotizing enterocolitis, bone marrow aplasia, child <6 yr, lactation, pulmonary fibrosis, exfoliative dermatitis, blood dyscrasias, recent radiation therapy, renal/hepatic disease, marked hypertension, uncontrolled CHF

PRECAUTIONS: Elderly, CHF, diabetes mellitus, allergic conditions, ulcerative colitis, renal disease, liver disease

PREGNANCY AND LACTATION: Pregnancy category C; nursing not recommended, gold appears in breast milk

SIDE EFFECTS/ADVERSE REACTIONS

CNS: Dizziness, confusion, hallucinations, ***seizures,*** EEG abnormalities

EENT: Iritis, corneal ulcers, gold deposits in ocular tissues

GI: Diarrhea, abdominal cramping, stomatitis, nausea, vomiting, enterocolitis, anorexia, flatulence, metallic taste, dyspepsia, jaundice, increased AST/ALT, glossitis, gingivitis, melena, constipation

GU: ***Proteinuria, hematuria,*** increased BUN/creatinine, vaginitis

HEME: ***Thrombocytopenia, agranulocytosis, aplastic anemia, leukopenia, eosinophilia, neutropenia***

RESP: ***Interstitial pneumonitis, fibrosis,*** cough, dyspnea

SKIN: Rash, pruritus, dermatitis, ***exfoliative dermatitis,*** urticaria, alopecia, photosensitivity

MISC: Gold toxicity: decreased Hgb, WBC <4000/mm^3, granulocytes <1500/mm^3, platelets <150,000/mm^3, severe diarrhea, stomatitis, hematuria, rash, itching, proteinuria

▼ DRUG INTERACTIONS

Labs

• *False positive:* TB test

SPECIAL CONSIDERATIONS

MONITORING PARAMETERS

• Urinalysis (hematuria, proteinuria)
• CBC with platelets
• Skin for rash, qmo

aurothioglucose/gold sodium thiomalate

(aur-oh-thye-oh-gloo'kose/gold sodium thye-oh'maa-late)

Solganal/Myochrysine, Aurolate

Chemical Class: Heavy metal, active gold compound (50%)
Therapeutic Class: Gold salt, slowly-acting antiarthritic drug, disease-modifying arthritis drug (DMARD)

CLINICAL PHARMACOLOGY

Mechanism of Action: Antiinflammatory action unknown; may decrease phagocytosis, lysosomal activity, prostaglandin synthesis

Pharmacokinetics

IM: Peak 4-6 hr; excreted in urine, feces; $t_{1/2}$ 3-27 days; increases up to 168 days with 11th dose

INDICATIONS AND USES: Rheumatoid arthritis, psoriatic arthritis,* pemphigus*

DOSAGE

Adult

- *Aurothioglucose:* IM administer weekly; 1st dose 10 mg; 2nd, 3rd doses 25 mg; then 50 mg qwk up to 0.8-1.0 g; continue 25-50 mg q3-4wk if improvement without toxicity
- *Gold sodium thiomalate:* IM 10 mg, then 25 mg after 1 wk, then 50 mg qwk for total of 14-20 doses, then 50 mg q2wk × 4, then 50 mg q3wk × 4, then 50 mg qmo for maintenance

Child 6-12 yr

- *Aurothioglucose:* IM 1 mg/kg/wk × 20 wk, or ¼ of adult dose
- *Gold sodium thiomalate:* IM 1 mg/kg/wk × 20 wk, then q3-4wk if improvement without toxicity; not to exceed 50 mg/dose

$ AVAILABLE FORMS/COST OF THERAPY

Aurothioglucose

- Inj, susp in oil—IM: 50 mg/ml, 10 ml: **$107.30**

Gold Sodium Thiomalate

- Inj, Sol—IM: 25 mg/ml, 1 ml × 6: **$43.41;** 50 mg/ml, 1 ml × 6: **$55.04-$62.80;** 50 mg/ml, 10 ml: **$85.75-$98.04**

CONTRAINDICATIONS: Hypersensitivity to gold, systemic lupus erythematosus, uncontrolled diabetes mellitus, marked hypertension, recent radiation therapy, CHF, lactation, renal disease, liver disease

PRECAUTIONS: Decreased tolerance in elderly, children, blood dyscrasias

PREGNANCY AND LACTATION: Pregnancy category C; gold has been demonstrated in breast milk and in the serum and red blood cells of a nursing infant; the slow excretion and persistence of gold in the mother, even after discontinuing therapy must also be considered

SIDE EFFECTS/ADVERSE REACTIONS

CNS: Dizziness, EEG abnormalities, ***encephalitis,*** confusion, hallucinations

CV: Bradycardia, rapid pulse

EENT: Iritis, corneal ulcers

GI: Stomatitis, nausea, vomiting, metallic taste, jaundice, ***hepatitis,*** diarrhea, cramping, flatulence

GU: Proteinuria, hematuria, ***nephrosis, tubular necrosis***

HEME: Thrombocytopenia, ***agranulocytosis, aplastic anemia, leukopenia, eosinophilia, neutropenia***

RESP: Interstitial pneumonitis, pharyngitis, ***pulmonary fibrosis***

SKIN: Rash, pruritus, dermatitis, urticaria, alopecia, photosensitivity, ***exfoliative dermatitis, angioedema***

MISC: ***Anaphylaxis;*** *"nitritoid" reaction* (vasomotor reaction manifests as nausea, weakness, flushing, tachycardia, and/or syncope in 5% of patients receiving gold sodium thiomalate; not reported with aurothioglucose, hence probably related to vehicle or preservative in alternative product); gold toxicity (decreased Hgb, WBC <4000/mm^3, granulocytes <1500/mm^3, platelets <150,000/mm^3, severe diarrhea, stomatitis, hematuria, rash, itching, proteinuria)

▼ DRUG INTERACTIONS

Labs

- *False positive:* TB test

SPECIAL CONSIDERATIONS

MONITORING PARAMETERS

- *Urinalysis:* Hematuria, proteinuria
- CBC with platelets
- Skin for rash qmo

---

azatadine

(a-za'ta-deen)

Optimine

Chemical Class: Piperidine H_1-receptor antagonist

Therapeutic Class: Antihistamine

CLINICAL PHARMACOLOGY

Mechanism of Action: Competitive with histamine for H_1-receptor sites in blood vessels, GI tract, and respiratory system; decreases allergic response as histamine blocker

Pharmacokinetics

PO: Peak 4 hr; metabolized in liver, excreted by kidneys, crosses placenta, crosses blood-brain barrier, minimally bound to plasma proteins, $t_{1/2}$ 9-12 hr

INDICATIONS AND USES: Allergy symptoms, rhinitis, chronic urticaria

DOSAGE

Adult

- PO 1-2 mg bid, not to exceed 4 mg/day

Child >12 years

- PO 1-2 mg bid

$ AVAILABLE FORMS/COST OF THERAPY

- Tab, uncoated—Oral: 1 mg, 100's: **$81.94**

CONTRAINDICATIONS: Hypersensitivity to H_1-receptor antagonists, concurrent acute asthma attack, lower respiratory tract disease, child <12 yr

PRECAUTIONS: Increased intraocular pressure, renal disease, cardiac disease, bronchial asthma, seizure disorder, stenosed peptic ulcers, hyperthyroidism, prostatic hypertrophy, bladder neck obstruction, elderly

PREGNANCY AND LACTATION: Pregnancy category B

SIDE EFFECTS/ADVERSE REACTIONS

CNS: Dizziness, drowsiness, poor coordination, fatigue, anxiety, euphoria, confusion, paresthesia, neuritis, sweating, chills

CV: Hypotension, palpitations, tachycardia

EENT: Blurred vision, dilated pupils, tinnitus, dry nose, throat, mouth

GI: Constipation, dry mouth, nausea, vomiting, anorexia

GU: Retention, dysuria, frequency, impotence

HEME: ***Thrombocytopenia, agranulocytosis, hemolytic anemia***

RESP: Increased thick secretions, wheezing, chest tightness

SKIN: Rash, urticaria, photosensitivity

▼ DRUG INTERACTIONS

Labs

- *False negative:* Skin allergy tests

SPECIAL CONSIDERATIONS

PATIENT/FAMILY EDUCATION

- Avoid driving or other hazardous activities if drowsiness occurs
- Avoid concurrent use of alcohol or other CNS depressants

---

azathioprine

(ay-za-thye'oh-preen)

Imuran

Chemical Class: Purine analog; derivative of 6-mercaptopurine

Therapeutic Class: Immunosuppressive antimetabolite

CLINICAL PHARMACOLOGY

Mechanism of Action: Immunosuppressive by inhibiting purine synthesis in cells

Pharmacokinetics

PO: peaks 1-2 hr; metabolized in liver (cleaved to mercaptopurine then inactivated by xanthine oxidase); 30% bound to serum proteins; excreted in urine (both parent and metabolite) rapidly, crosses placenta

INDICATIONS AND USES: Renal homotransplantation to prevent graft rejection, refractory rheumatoid arthritis, refractory ITP,* glomerulonephritis,* nephrotic syndrome,* bone marrow transplant,* ulcerative colitis,* myasthenia gravis* (2-3 mg/kg/day), Behçet's syndrome,* Crohn's disease*

DOSAGE

Adult

- *Prevention of rejection:* PO/IV 3-5 mg/kg/day, then maintenance (PO) of at least 1-2 mg/kg/day
- *Refractory rheumatoid arthritis:* PO 1 mg/kg/day, may increase dose after 2 mo by 0.5 mg/kg/day, not to exceed 2.5 mg/kg/day

Child

- *Prevention of rejection:* PO/IV 3-5 mg/kg/day, then maintenance (PO) of at least 1-2 mg/kg/day

$ AVAILABLE FORMS/COST OF THERAPY

- Inj, Lyphl-Soln—IV: 10 mg/ml, 20 ml: **$62.21;** 100 mg/ml, 20 ml: **$88.42**
- Tab, Uncoated—Oral: 50 mg, 100's: **$113.35**

CONTRAINDICATIONS: Hypersensitivity

PRECAUTIONS: Severe leukopenia and/or thrombocytopenia may occur as well as macrocytic anemia and bone marrow depression; fungal, viral, bacterial and protozoal infections may be fatal; may increase the patient's risk of neoplasia via mutagenic and carcinogenic properties (skin cancer and reticulum cell or lymphomatous tumors); temporary depression in spermatogenesis

PREGNANCY AND LACTATION: Pregnancy category D

SIDE EFFECTS/ADVERSE REACTIONS

GI: Nausea, vomiting, stomatitis, esophagitis, ***pancreatitis, hepatotoxicity, jaundice***

HEME: ***Leukopenia, thrombocytopenia, anemia (macrocytic), pancytopenia***

MS: Arthralgia, muscle wasting

SKIN: Rash

MISC: Fungal, viral, bacterial, and protozoal infections

▼ DRUG INTERACTIONS

Drugs

- *Allopurinol+:* Allopurinol may increase toxicity of azathioprine; dosage adjustment is necessary

SPECIAL CONSIDERATIONS

MONITORING PARAMETERS

- Hgb, WBC, platelets monthly
- DC if leukocytes are <3000/mm^3
- Therapeutic response may take 3-4 mo in rheumatoid arthritis

---

azithromycin

(ay-zi-thro-mye'sin)

Zithromax

Chemical Class: Macrolide (azalide) antibiotic

Therapeutic Class: Antibacterial

CLINICAL PHARMACOLOGY

Mechanism of Action: Binds to 50S ribosomal subunits of susceptible bacteria and suppresses protein synthesis

Pharmacokinetics

PO: Peak 12 hr, duration 24 hr; Rapidly absorbed and widely distributed into tissues (higher concentrations in tissues than in plasma); $t_{1/2}$ 11-57 hr, excreted in bile, feces, urine primarily as unchanged drug

INDICATIONS AND USES: Mild to moderate infections of the upper and lower respiratory tract, uncomplicated skin and skin structure infections, and nongonococcal urethritis or cervicitis caused by susceptible organisms

Antibacterial spectrum usually includes:

- Gram-positive organisms: *Staphylococcus aureus, Streptococcus pneumoniae, S. pyogenes, S. agalactiae,* streptococci (Groups C,F, G), *S. viridans* group streptococci
- Gram-negative organisms: *Moraxella catarrhalis, Haemophilus influenzae, Bordetella pertussi, Campylobacter jejuni, H. ducreyi, Legionella pneumophilia*
- Anaerobes: *Bacteroides bivivu, Clostridium perfringens,* other *Clostridium* sp., *Peptostreptococcus* sp.

Misc: *Chlamydia trachomatis, Borrelia burgdorferi, Mycoplasma pneumoniae, Treponema pallidum, Ureaplasma urealyticum*

DOSAGE

Adult

PO 500 mg on day 1, then 250 mg qd on days 2-5 for a total dose of 1.5 g

- *Nongonococcal urethritis or cervicitis:* 1 g single PO dose for chlamydial infections
- *Chancroid:* 1 g as a single dose

Child

- Acute otitis media: PO 10 mg/kg × 1, then 5 mg/kg qd for next 4 days

$ AVAILABLE FORMS/COST OF THERAPY

- Cap—Oral: 250 mg, 6's: **$48.75**
- Sachet—Oral: 1 g: **$18.75**
- Susp—Oral: 100 mg/5 ml, 15 ml: **$25.55;** 200 mg/5 ml, 15 mg: **$25.55**

CONTRAINDICATIONS: Hypersensitivity to azithromycin or erythromycin

PRECAUTIONS: Hepatic, renal, cardiac disease

PREGNANCY AND LACTATION: Pregnancy category B; excretion into breast milk unknown

SIDE EFFECTS/ADVERSE REACTIONS

CV: Palpitations, chest pain

CNS: Dizziness, headache, vertigo, somnolence

GI: Nausea, vomiting, diarrhea, ***hepatotoxicity,*** abdominal pain, stomatitis, heartburn, dyspepsia, flatulence, melena, ***cholestatic jaundice***

GU: Vaginitis, moniliasis, nephritis

SKIN: Rash, urticaria, pruritus, photosensitivity

▼ DRUG INTERACTIONS

Labs

- *False increase:* 17-OHCS/17-KS, AST, ALT
- *Decrease:* Folate assay

SPECIAL CONSIDERATIONS

PATIENT/FAMILY EDUCATION

- Take on empty stomach (1 hr before or 2 hr after meals; do not take with fruit juices)

azlocillin

(az-loe-sill'in)

Azlin

Chemical Class: Semi-synthetic, β-lactam antibiotic

Therapeutic Class: Broad-spectrum, extended spectrum, penicillin

CLINICAL PHARMACOLOGY

Mechanism of Action: Interferes with synthesis of cell wall components of susceptible organisms; bactericidal

Pharmacokinetics

IV: Peak, 239 μg/ml 5 min after completing 2 g infusion; $t_{1/2}$ 55-70 min; metabolized in liver; excreted in urine, bile, breast milk (small amount), crosses placenta

INDICATIONS AND USES: Lower respiratory and urinary tract infections, infections of the skin and bone, bacterial septicemia, and yaws caused by susceptible organisms Antibacterial spectrum usually includes:

- Gram-positive organisms: *Staphylococcus aureus, Streptococcus pyogenes, S. faecalis,* β-hemolytic streptococci (Groups A and B), *S. pneumoniae, Listeria monocytogenes*
- Gram-negative organisms: *Pseudomonas aeruginosa, E. coli, Haemophilus influenzae, Proteus vulgaris, P. mirabilis, Enterobacter* sp., *Shigella* sp., *Morganella morganii, H. parainfluenzae, Providencia rettgeri, Neisseria* sp., *Providencia stuartii, Citrobacter* sp., *Klebsiella* sp., *Serratia* sp., *Salmonella* sp., and *Acinetobacter* sp.
- Anaerobes: *Peptococcus* sp., *Fusobacterium* sp., *Peptostreptococcus* sp., *Veillonella* sp., *Clostridium* sp., *Eubacterium* sp., *Bacteroides* sp. (including *B. fragilis* group).

DOSAGE

Adult

- IV 100-350 mg/kg/day in 4-6 divided doses, max 24 g/day

Child

- IV 75 mg/kg q4h, up to a max of 24 g/day
- *Cystic fibrosis:* IV 75 mg/kg q4h max 24 g/day

$ **AVAILABLE FORMS/COST OF THERAPY**

- Inj, Dry-Soln—IV: 2 g/vial, 30 ml: **$95.98;** 3 g/vial, 50 ml: **$141.90,** 100 ml: **$149.10;** 4 g/vial, 50 ml: **$180.07**

CONTRAINDICATIONS: Hypersensitivity to penicillins

PRECAUTIONS: Hypersensitivity to cephalosporins; neonates

PREGNANCY AND LACTATION: Pregnancy category B; crosses the placenta, found in cord blood and amniotic fluid; low concentrations in milk of nursing mothers

SIDE EFFECTS/ADVERSE REACTIONS

CNS: Lethargy, hallucinations, anxiety, depression, twitching, ***coma, convulsions***

GI: Nausea, vomiting, diarrhea, increased AST, ALT, abdominal pain, glossitis, colitis

GU: Oliguria, proteinuria, hematuria, *vaginitis, moniliasis,* ***glomerulonephritis***

HEME: Anemia, increased bleeding time, ***bone marrow depression, granulocytopenia***

METAB: Hypokalemia, alkalosis, hypernatremia

MISC: Hypersensitivity (anaphylactic) reactions

▼ **DRUG INTERACTIONS**

Drugs

- *Aminoglycosides:* Some penicillins inactivate certain aminoglycosides *in vitro* and, in certain situations, *in vivo,* thus reducing the effect of the aminoglycoside

Labs

- *False positive:* Urine glucose, urine protein
- *Decrease:* Uric acid

aztreonam

(az-tree'oo-nam)

Azactam

Chemical Class: Monobactam

Therapeutic Class: Expanded spectrum penicillin antibiotic

CLINICAL PHARMACOLOGY

Mechanism of Action: Inhibits bacterial cell wall synthesis, bactericidal

Pharmacokinetics

IV: Peak, following single 1 g dose 204 μg/ml; trough, at 8 hr 3 μg/ml; $t_{1/2}$ 1.7 hr; $t_{1/2}$ prolonged in renal disease; protein binding 56%; metabolized by liver; excreted in urine; small amounts appear in breast milk, placenta

INDICATIONS AND USES: Infections of the respiratory, urinary, and gynecologic tracts, skin, muscle, and bone; intra-abdominal septicemia caused by susceptible organisms Antibacterial spectrum usually includes:

Gram-negative organisms: *E. coli, Klebsiella pneumoniae, Proteus mirabilis, P. aeruginosa, Enterobacter* sp., *K. oxytoca, Citrobacter* and *S. marcescens; Haemophilus influenzae*

DOSAGE

Adult

- *Urinary tract infections:* IV/IM 500 mg-1 g q8-12h
- *Systemic infections:* IV/IM 1-2 g q8-12h
- *Severe systemic infections:* IV/IM 2 g q6-8h; do not exceed 8 g/day; continue treatment for 48 hr after negative culture or until patient is asymptomatic

Child

- Postnatal age <7 days, <2000 g: IM/IV 30 mg/kg q12h; >2000 g 30 mg/kg q8h
- Postnatal age >7 days, <2000 g: 30 mg/kg q8h; >2000 g: 30 mg/kg q6h
- Children >1 mo: 90-120 mg/kg/day divided q6-8h
- *Cystic Fibrosis:* 50 mg/kg/dose q6-8h (max 6-8 g/day)

$ **AVAILABLE FORMS/COST OF THERAPY**

- Inj, Lyphl-Soln—IM, IV: 1 g/vial, 10's: **$143.50;** 2 g/vial, 10's: **$286.63;** 500 mg/vial, 10's: **$75.13**

CONTRAINDICATIONS: Hypersensitivity

PRECAUTIONS: Children; impaired renal, hepatic function; elderly; hypersensitivity to penicillins, cephalosporins

PREGNANCY AND LACTATION: Pregnancy category B; excreted in breast milk in concentrations <1% of maternal serum concentrations

SIDE EFFECTS/ADVERSE REACTIONS

CNS: Lethargy, hallucinations, anxiety, depression, twitching, ***coma, convulsions,*** malaise

EENT: Tinnitus, diplopia, nasal congestion

GI: Nausea, vomiting, diarrhea, increased AST/ALT, abdominal pain, glossitis, colitis

GU: Vaginal candidiasis, vaginitis, breast tenderness

HEME: Anemia, increased bleeding time, ***bone marrow depression, granulocytopenia***

SPECIAL CONSIDERATIONS

- Minimal cross reactivity between aztreonam and penicillins and cephalosporins; aztreonam and aminoglycosides have been shown to be synergistic in vitro against most strains of *P. aeruginosa,* many strains of *Enterobacteriaceae,* and other gram-negative aerobic bacilli

bacampicillin

(ba-kam′pi-sill′in)

Penglobe, ✤ Spectrobid

Chemical Class: Aminopenicillin

Therapeutic Class: Ampicillin class of semi-synthetic penicillins, expanded spectrum antibiotic

CLINICAL PHARMACOLOGY

Mechanism of Action: Inhibits bacterial cell wall synthesis, bactericidal

Pharmacokinetics

PO: Peak 30-60 min (400 mg provides peak serum concentrations ampicillin, 7.9 μg/ml), duration 5-6 hr; hydrolyzed to ampicillin during absorption; $t_{1/2}$ ½-1 hr, metabolized in liver, excreted in urine

INDICATIONS AND USES: Infections of the upper and lower respiratory tract, including acute exacerbations of chronic bronchitis, skin and skin structure, urinary tract infections, and gonorrhea (acute uncomplicated urogenital infections) due to susceptible organisms

Antibacterial spectrum usually includes:

- Gram-positive organisms: *Streptococcus faecalis, S. pneumoniae,* β-hemolytic streptococci, *S. pyogenes,* non-penicillinase-producing staphylococci
- Gram-negative organisms: *Neisseria gonorrhoeae, E. coli, Haemophilus influenzae, Proteus mirabilis*

DOSAGE

Adult

- Usual dosage PO 400-800 mg q12h
- *Gonorrhea:* (acute uncomplicated urogenital infections due to *N. gonorrhoeae,* males and females) 1.6 grams (4 × 400 mg tablet plus 1 g probenecid) as a single oral dose

Child

- Usual dosage PO 25-50 mg/kg/day in divided doses q12h

$ AVAILABLE FORMS/COST OF THERAPY

- Tab, Uncoated—Oral: 400 mg, 100's: **$209.75**
- Susp—Oral: 125 mg/5 ml, 100 ml: **$15.99**

CONTRAINDICATIONS: Hypersensitivity to penicillins

PRECAUTIONS: Superinfections with mycotic or bacterial pathogens; concomitant mononucleosis (high percentage develop a skin rash)

PREGNANCY AND LACTATION: Pregnancy category B; excreted in milk; milk:plasma ratios up to 0.2

SIDE EFFECTS/ADVERSE REACTIONS

CNS: Lethargy, hallucinations, anxiety, depression, twitching, ***coma, convulsions***

GI: Nausea, vomiting, diarrhea, increased AST/ALT, gastritis, stomatitis, glossitis, black "hairy" tongue, enterocolitis, and ***pseudomembranous colitis***

GU: Oliguria, proteinuria, hematuria, *vaginitis, moniliasis,* ***glomerulonephritis***

HEME: Anemia, increased bleeding time, ***bone marrow depression, granulocytopenia, thrombocytopenia, thrombocytopenic purpura, eosinophilia, leukopenia, and agranulocytosis*** (hypersensitivity phenomena)

MISC: Hypersensitivity reactions (skin rashes, urticaria, erythema multiforme, and an occasional case of exfoliative dermatitis; skin rash when given with allopurinol); serious and occasional fatal hypersensitivity (anaphylactic)

▼ **DRUG INTERACTIONS**

Drugs

- *Chloramphenicol:* Chloramphenicol may inhibit the antibacterial activity of penicillins
- *Methotrexate:* Amoxicillin administration to a patient on methotrexate will increase plasma concentration of methotrexate and may lead to the development of toxicity
- *Oral anticoagulants:* Altered hypoprothrombinemic response when penicillins administered with oral anticoagulants
- *Oral contraceptives:* Oral Ampicillin occasionally impairs oral contraceptive efficacy
- *Tetracyclines:* Tetracycline administration may impair the efficacy of penicillin therapy

Labs

- *False positive:* Urine glucose, urine protein
- *Decrease:* Uric acid

SPECIAL CONSIDERATIONS

- A 400 mg tablet of bacampicillin and 125 mg/5 ml of the oral suspension is chemically equivalent to 280 mg and 87.5 mg of ampicillin, respectively

PATIENT/FAMILY EDUCATION

- Administer 1 hr before or 2 hr after meals

bacitracin

(bass-i-tray′sin)

Ak-Tracin, Baci-Rx, Bacticin, Ocu-Tracin, Spectro-Bacitracin

Chemical Class: Bacillus subtilis derivative

Therapeutic Class: Antibacterial

CLINICAL PHARMACOLOGY

Mechanism of Action: Inhibits bacterial cell wall synthesis (bactericidal)

Pharmacokinetics

IM: Peak 1-2 hr duration >12 hr; widely distributed (demonstrable in ascitic and pleural fluids after IM injection); metabolized in liver, excreted in urine

INDICATIONS AND USES: OPHTH superficial ocular infections involving the conjunctiva and/or cornea caused by susceptible organisms; IM infants with pneumonia and empyema caused by susceptible staphylococci; PO antiobiotic-associated colitis (Orphan Drug status); TOP treatment of impetigo due to *Staphylococcus aureus*

DOSAGE

Adult

- OPHTH: Apply to conjunctival sac bid-qid; IM: 20,000-25,000 U q6h × 7-10 days; PO: 25,000 U qid × 10 days

Child

- OPHTH: Apply to conjunctival sac bid-qid; IM: Infants <2.5 kg 900 U/kg/day in divided doses q8-12h; Infants >2.5 kg 1000 U/kg/day in divided doses q8-12h

$ **AVAILABLE FORMS/COST OF THERAPY**

- Inj, Lyphl-Soln—IM: 50,000 U/vial: **$6.25-$9.26**
- Oint—Ophth: 500 unit/g, 3.5 g: **$1.40-$4.95**
- Powder: 5,000,000 U: **$120.04**

CONTRAINDICATIONS: Hypersensitivity, severe renal disease

PRECAUTIONS: Overgrowth of non-susceptible organisms

PREGNANCY AND LACTATION: Pregnancy category C

SIDE EFFECTS/ADVERSE REACTIONS

EENT: Poor corneal wound healing, visual haze (temporary)

GI: Nausea, vomiting, diarrhea

GU: Albuminuria, cylindruria, ***pro-***

teinuria, casts, renal failure due to tubular and glomerular necrosis
SKIN: Rash
MISC: Pain at injection site

SPECIAL CONSIDERATIONS

• Administer IM in deep muscle mass; rotate injection site; do *not* give IV/SC

baclofen

(bak'loe-fen)
Lioresal, Lioresal DS, Lioresal Intrathecal
Chemical Class: GABA chlorophenyl derivative
Therapeutic Class: Skeletal muscle relaxant, central acting

CLINICAL PHARMACOLOGY

Mechanism of Action: Inhibits synaptic responses at the spinal level by decreasing excitatory neurotransmitter release, which decreases neurotransmitter function; decreases frequency, severity of muscle spasms; structural analog of the inhibitory neurotransmitter gamma-aminobutyric acid (GABA) and may exert its effects by stimulation of the $GABA_{\beta}$ receptor subtype; general CNS depressant properties as indicated by the production of sedation with tolerance, somnolence, ataxia, and respiratory and cardiovascular depression

Pharmacokinetics

PO: Peak 2-3 hr, duration >8 hr
INTRATHECAL: (CSF levels with plasma levels 100 times oral route); Bolus: onset ½-1 hr; peak 4 hr; duration 4-8 hr; Continuous infusion: peak, 24-48 hr; $t_{1/2}$ 2½-4 hr, partially metabolized in liver, excreted in urine (unchanged)

INDICATIONS AND USES: Spasticity with spinal cord injury, spasticity in multiple sclerosis, intractable spasticity in children with cerebral palsy,* trigeminal neuralgia,* tardive dyskinesia in combination with neuroleptics*

DOSAGE

Adult

• PO 5 mg tid × 3 days, then 10 mg tid × 3 days, then 15 mg tid × 3 days, then 20 mg tid × 3 days, then titrated to response, not to exceed 80 mg/day;
• INTRATHECAL use implantable intrathecal INF pump; use screening trial of 3 separate bolus doses if needed (50 μg/ml, 75 μg/1.5 ml, 100 μg/2 ml); Initial: double screening dose that produced result and give over 24 hr, increase by 10%-30% q24h only; Maintenance: 12-1500 μg/day

Child

• 2-7 years initial: PO 10-15 mg/24 hr divided q8h; titrate dose every 3 days in increments of 5-15 mg/day to a max of 40 mg/day;
• ≥8 years: PO max 60 mg/day in 3 divided doses

$ AVAILABLE FORMS/COST OF THERAPY

• Tab, Uncoated—Oral: 10 mg, 100's: **$22.43-$47.08;** 20 mg, 100's: **$41.93-$86.23**
• Kit—IT: 500 μg/ml: **$187.20;** 2000 μg/ml: **$393.60-$732.00**

CONTRAINDICATIONS: Hypersensitivity

PRECAUTIONS: Peptic ulcer disease, renal disease, hepatic disease, stroke, seizure disorder, diabetes mellitus, elderly

PREGNANCY AND LACTATION: Pregnancy category C; present in breast milk, 0.1% of mother's dose; compatible with breast feeding

SIDE EFFECTS/ADVERSE REACTIONS

CNS: Dizziness, weakness, fatigue, drowsiness, headache, disorientation, insomnia, paresthesias, tremors; ***seizures*** (decreased seizure threshold)

CV: Hypotension, chest pain, palpitations, edema

EENT: Nasal congestion, blurred vision, mydriasis, tinnitus

GI: Nausea, constipation, vomiting, increased AST, alk phosphatase, abdominal pain, dry mouth, anorexia

GU: Urinary frequency

SKIN: Rash, pruritus

▼ DRUG INTERACTIONS

Labs

Increase: AST, alk phosphatase, blood glucose

SPECIAL CONSIDERATIONS

• Abrupt discontinuation may lead to hallucinations, spasticity, tachycardia; drug should be tapered off over 1-2 wk

---

beclomethasone

(be-kloe-meth'a-sone)

INH: Beclovent, Vanceril;
NASAL: Beconase AQ, Beconase, Vancenase AQ, Vancenase

Chemical Class: Halogenated synthetic glucocorticoid

Therapeutic Class: Antiinflammatory corticosteroid, synthetic

CLINICAL PHARMACOLOGY

Mechanism of Action: Antiinflammatory via inhibition of migration of polymorphonuclear leukocytes, fibroblasts, reversal of increased capillary permeability and lysosomal stabilization

Pharmacokinetics

INH: Despite inhaled routes, systemic absorption occurs; absorption occurs rapidly from all respiratory and gastrointestinal tissues; metabolized in lungs, liver, GI system; excreted in feces (with metabolites), less than 10% excreted in urine; $t_{1/2}$ 3-15 hr, crosses placenta

INDICATIONS AND USES: INH Chronic asthma; NASAL seasonal or perennial rhinitis; prevention of recurrence of nasal polyps; nonallergic (vasomotor) rhinitis

DOSAGE

Adult

• INH 2-4 puffs tid-qid, not to exceed 20 inh/day; NASAL 1-2 sprays in each nostril bid-qid

Child (6-12 yr)

• INH 1-2 puffs tid-qid, not to exceed 10 inh/day

Child (>12 yr)

• NASAL 1-2 sprays in each nostril bid-qid

$ AVAILABLE FORMS/COST OF THERAPY

• MDI Aer—Inh: 42 μg/inh, 6.7-7 g: **$17.23-$28.72;** 16.8 g: **$28.72**

• MDI Aer—Nasal Inh: 16.8 g: **$26.51-$28.72**

• Spray—Nasal: 42 μg/spray: 25 g: **$31.01**

CONTRAINDICATIONS: Hypersensitivity; primary treatment for status asthmaticus; nonasthmatic bronchial disease; bacterial, fungal, or viral infections of mouth, throat, or lungs; children <3 yr

PRECAUTIONS: Nasal disease/surgery, children <12 (potential reduction in bone growth velocity), nasal ulcers, recurrent epistaxis; suppression of HPA-axis observed when administered at doses of 2000 μg/day by oral aerosol; not a bronchodilator; not indicated for rapid relief of bronchospasm; systemic effects such as mental disturbances, increased bruising, weight gain, cushingoid features, and cataracts

PREGNANCY AND LACTATION: Pregnancy category C; breast milk excretion unknown; other corticosteroids excreted in low concentrations with systemic administration; compatible with breast feeding

SIDE EFFECTS/ADVERSE REACTIONS

CNS: Headache, paresthesia
EENT: *Dryness, nasal irritation, burning, sneezing,* secretions with blood, nasal ulcerations, ***perforation of nasal septum, Candidal infection,*** sore throat, earache
GI: Dry mouth, dysphonia
METAB: Adrenal suppression
RESP: ***Bronchospasm***
SKIN: Urticaria, pruritus

SPECIAL CONSIDERATIONS

PATIENT/FAMILY EDUCATION

- Rinse mouth with water following INH to decrease possibility of fungal infections, dysphonia
- Review proper MDI administration technique regularly
- Systemic corticosteroid effects from inhaled and nasal steroids inadequate to prevent adrenal insufficiency in patients withdrawn from corticosteroids abruptly

belladonna alkaloids

(bell-a-don'a)
Bellafoline

Chemical Class: Belladonna alkaloid
Therapeutic Class: Gastrointestinal anticholinergic/antispasmodic

CLINICAL PHARMACOLOGY

Mechanism of Action: Inhibits muscarinic actions of acetylcholine at postganglionic parasympathetic neuroeffector sites including smooth muscle, secretory glands and CNS sites

Pharmacokinetics

PO: Duration 4-6 hr, metabolized by liver, excreted in urine

INDICATIONS AND USES: Gastrointestinal spasm, peptic ulcer, pylorospasm, spastic colitis, intestinal and biliary colic, dysmenorrhea, renal colic, nocturnal enuresis, postencephalitic parkinsonism, motion sickness

DOSAGE

Adult

- PO 0.25-0.5 mg tid

Child >6 yr

- PO 0.125-0.25 mg tid

$ AVAILABLE FORMS/COST OF THERAPY

- Tab, Uncoated—Oral: 0.25 mg: Available only in combination or as tincture

CONTRAINDICATIONS: Hypersensitivity to anticholinergics, narrow angle glaucoma, GI obstruction, myasthenia gravis, paralytic ileus, GI atony, toxic megacolon, obstructive uropathy

PRECAUTIONS: Hyperthyroidism, coronary artery disease, dysrhythmias, CHF, ulcerative colitis, hypertension, hiatal hernia, hepatic disease, renal disease, elderly, children, prostatic hypertrophy, chronic lung disease, high environmental temperatures

PREGNANCY AND LACTATION: Pregnancy category C; excretion into breast milk is controversial, neonates may be particularly sensitive to anticholinergic agents; use caution in nursing mothers

SIDE EFFECTS/ADVERSE REACTIONS

CNS: Confusion, stimulation in elderly, headache, insomnia, dizziness, drowsiness, anxiety, nervousness, weakness, hallucination
CV: Palpitations, tachycardia
EENT: *Blurred vision,* photophobia, mydriasis, cycloplegia, increased ocular pressure
GI: *Dry mouth, constipation,* ***paralytic ileus,*** heartburn, nausea, vomiting, dysphagia, altered taste
GU: *Hesitancy, retention,* impotence
SKIN: Urticaria, rash, pruritus, anhidrosis, allergic reactions, flushing

▼ DRUG INTERACTIONS

Drugs

- *Amantadine:* Anticholinergic drugs may potentiate the side effects of amantadine
- *Cyclic antidepressants:* Excessive anticholinergic effects
- *Neuroleptics:* Inhibition of therapeutic response to neuroleptics; excessive anticholinergic effects

SPECIAL CONSIDERATIONS

PATIENT/FAMILY EDUCATION

- Avoid driving or other hazardous activities until stabilized on medication
- Alcohol or other CNS depressants will enhance sedating properties of this drug
- Avoid hot environments, heat stroke may occur
- Use sunglasses when outside to prevent photophobia

belladonna and opium

(bell-a-don'a)

B & O Suppositories

Chemical Class: Belladonna alkaloid/opiate

Therapeutic Class: Antispasmodic; narcotic analgesic

DEA Class: Schedule II

CLINICAL PHARMACOLOGY

Mechanism of Action: Belladonna inhibits muscarinic actions of acetylcholine at postganglionic parasympathetic neuroeffector sites including smooth muscle, secretory glands and CNS sites; opium contains many narcotic alkaloids including morphine which inhibit gastric motility and provide sedation and analgesic properties

Pharmacokinetics

PR: Onset 30 min (opium), 1-2 hr (belladonna), opium metabolized in the liver

INDICATIONS AND USES: Ureteral spasm not responsive to non-narcotic analgesics; rectal or bladder tenesmus occurring in postoperative states and neoplastic situations

DOSAGE

Adult

- PR 1 suppository 1-2 times daily, up to 4 doses/day

Child

- Not recommended for children <12

$ AVAILABLE FORMS/COST OF THERAPY

- Supp—Rect: 16.2 mg/30 mg, 12's: **$29.87;** 16.2 mg/60 mg, 12's: **$16.50-$34.00**

CONTRAINDICATIONS: Hypersensitivity to anticholinergics or opium, narrow angle glaucoma, severe hepatic or renal disease, bronchial asthma, respiratory depression, seizure disorders, acute alcoholism, delirium tremens, premature labor

PRECAUTIONS: Elderly, debilitated patients, increased intracranial pressure, toxic psychosis, myxedema

PREGNANCY AND LACTATION: Pregnancy category C; excretion of belladonna into breast milk is controversial, neonates may be particularly sensitive to anticholinergic agents, therefore use caution in nursing mothers

SIDE EFFECTS/ADVERSE REACTIONS

CNS: CNS depression, *drowsiness,* sedation, memory loss, weakness, tiredness, headache, confusion

CV: Hypotension, bradycardia, peripheral vasodilation, increased intracranial pressure, flushing, tachycardia, palpitations, arrhythmia, orthostatic hypotension

EENT: Dry mouth, blurred vision,

intraocular pain, mydriasis, photophobia
GI: Nausea, vomiting, *constipation,* bloated feeling
GU: Retention, *hesitancy*
RESP: ***Respiratory depression***
SKIN: Decreased sweating, rash
MISC: Physical and psychological dependence

▼ **DRUG INTERACTIONS**

Labs

- *Increase:* Aminotransferase (ALT, AST)

SPECIAL CONSIDERATIONS

PATIENT/FAMILY EDUCATION

- Moisten finger and suppository with water before inserting
- May cause drowsiness, dry mouth and blurred vision
- Store at room temperature, DO NOT refrigerate

---

benazepril

(ben-a-ze′pril)
Lotensin
Chemical Class: Angiotensin-converting enzyme (ACE) inhibitor
Therapeutic Class: Antihypertensive

CLINICAL PHARMACOLOGY

Mechanism of Action: Selectively suppresses renin-angiotensin-aldosterone system; inhibits ACE preventing the conversion of angiotensin I to angiotensin II; results in dilation of arterial, venous vessels

Pharmacokinetics

PO: Peak ½-1 hr, serum protein binding 97%, $t_{1/2}$ 10-11 hr, metabolized by liver to active metabolite (benazeprilat) which is excreted by the kidneys

INDICATIONS AND USES: Hypertension, CHF,* diabetic nephropathy*

DOSAGE

Adult

- PO 10 mg qd initially, increase as needed to 20-40 mg/day divided bid or qd
- *Renal impairment:* PO 5 mg qd with Cl_{cr} <30 ml/min/1.73 m^2, increase as needed to maximum of 40 mg/day

$ **AVAILABLE FORMS/COST OF THERAPY**

- Tab, Uncoated—Oral: 5 mg, 100's: **$63.63;** 10 mg, 100's: **$63.63;** 20 mg, 100's: **$63.63;** 40 mg, 100's: **$63.63**

CONTRAINDICATIONS: Hypersensitivity to ACE inhibitors

PRECAUTIONS: Impaired renal and liver function, dialysis patients, hypovolemia, diuretic therapy, collagen-vascular diseases, CHF, elderly, bilateral renal artery stenosis

PREGNANCY AND LACTATION: Pregnancy category C (first trimester), category D (second and third trimesters); ACE inhibitors can cause fetal and neonatal morbidity and death when administered to pregnant women, when pregnancy is detected, discontinue ACE inhibitors as soon as possible; detectable in breast milk in trace amounts, a newborn would receive <0.1% of the mg/kg maternal dose; effect on nursing infant has not been determined, use with caution in nursing mothers

SIDE EFFECTS/ADVERSE REACTIONS

CNS: Anxiety, insomnia, paresthesia, *headache, dizziness, fatigue*
CV: Hypotension, postural hypotension, syncope (especially with first dose), palpitations, angina
GI: Nausea, constipation, vomiting, melena, abdominal pain
GU: Increased BUN/creatinine, decreased libido, impotence, urinary tract infection

HEME: ***Neutropenia, agranulocytosis***
METAB: Hyperkalemia, hyponatremia
MS: Arthralgia, arthritis, myalgia
RESP: *Cough,* asthma, bronchitis, dyspnea, sinusitis
SKIN: ***Angioedema,*** rash, flushing, sweating

DRUG INTERACTIONS

Drugs

- *Lithium:* Increased risk of serious lithium toxicity
- *Loop diuretics:* Initiation of ACE inhibitor therapy in the presence of intensive diruetic therapy results in a precipitous fall in blood pressure in some patients; ACE inhibitors may induce renal insufficiency in the presence of diuretic-induced sodium depletion
- *NSAIDs:* Inhibition of the antihypertensive response to ACE inhibitors
- *Potassium sparing diuretics:* Increased risk for hyperkalemia

SPECIAL CONSIDERATIONS

PATIENT/FAMILY EDUCATION

- Do not use salt substitutes containing potassium without consulting physician
- Rise slowly to sitting or standing position to minimize orthostatic hypotension
- Notify physician of mouth sores, sore throat, fever, swelling of hands or feet, irregular heartbeat, chest pain
- Dizziness, fainting, light-headedness may occur during 1st few days of therapy

MONITORING PARAMETERS

- BUN, creatinine (watch for increased levels that may indicate acute renal failure)
- Potassium levels, although hyperkalemia rarely occurs

benzalkonium chloride

(benz-al-koe'nee-um)
Benasept, Benza, Germicin, Zephiran
Chemical Class: Quaternary ammonium cationic surfactant
Therapeutic Class: Disinfectant

CLINICAL PHARMACOLOGY

Mechanism of Action: Inhibits and destroys bacteria and some viruses by enzyme inactivation (bactericidal/bacteriostatic depending on solution concentration)

INDICATIONS AND USES: Irrigation of eye, vagina, bladder, urethra, body cavities; disinfection of skin before surgery; treatment of minor skin wounds and abrasions

DOSAGE

Adult and child

- TOP 1:750 for minor wounds, disinfection before surgery; 1:3,000-20,000 deep infected wounds; 1:2,000-5,000 vaginal douche/irrigation; 1:5,000-10,000 denuded skin, eye, mucous membrane irrigation; 1:5,000-20,000 bladder, urethral irrigation; 1:20,000-40,000 bladder retention lavage

$ **AVAILABLE FORMS/COST OF THERAPY**

- Conc—Top: 17%, 120 ml: **$21.45**
- Sol—Top: 1:750, 240 ml: **$11.79**
- Tincture—Top: 1:750, 240 ml: **$11.79;** gallon: **$125.26**
- Tissue—Top: single use packets, 100's: **$49.41**

CONTRAINDICATIONS: Hypersensitivity, occlusive dressing, casts, anal or vaginal packs

PRECAUTIONS: Prolonged contact, inflammed/irritated tissues, eyes (solutions stronger than 1:3,000), mucous membranes (solutions stronger than 1:5,000, except the vaginal mucosa)

SIDE EFFECTS/ADVERSE REACTIONS

CNS: Confusion, restlessness

GI: Nausea, vomiting (if ingested)

RESP: Dyspnea, ***respiratory paralysis, coma*** (if ingested)

SKIN: Irritation, contact dermatitis, hypersensitivity, rash, burning

SPECIAL CONSIDERATIONS

PATIENT/FAMILY EDUCATION

- Store at room temperature no longer than 1 wk
- Use applicator, insert high into vagina
- Notify physician of itching, discharge, burning

benzocaine

(ben-zoe'kane)

Americaine, Anacaine, Otocain

Chemical Class: Ethyl aminobenzoate

Therapeutic Class: Topical local anesthetic

CLINICAL PHARMACOLOGY

Mechanism of Action: Reversibly stabilizes the neuronal membranae which decreases its permeability to sodium ions; depolarization of the neuronal membrane is inhibited thereby blocking the initiation and conduction of nerve impulses

Pharmacokinetics

TOP: Peak 1 min, duration 0.5-1 hr

INDICATIONS AND USES: Lubricant and topical anesthetic on intratracheal catheters, nasogastric and endoscopic tubes, urinary catheters, laryngoscopes, proctoscopes, sigmoidoscopes, vaginal specula; topical anesthetic for pharyngeal and nasal airways to obtund the pharyngeal and tracheal reflexes; relief of pain and pruritis in acute congestive and serous otitis media, acute swimmer's ear, and other forms of otitis externa

DOSAGE

Adult and Child >1 yr

- *Anesthetic Lubricant:* TOP apply evenly to exterior of tube or instrument prior to use
- *Otic Drops:* Instill 4-5 gtts in the external auditory canal, then insert a cotton pledget into the external ear, repeat every 1-2 hr if necessary

$ AVAILABLE FORMS/COST OF THERAPY

- Sol—Otic: 20%, 15 ml: **$10.04-$12.76**
- Lubricant—Top: 20%, 30 g: **$13.09**

CONTRAINDICATIONS: Hypersensitivity, perforated tympanic membrane or ear discharge (otic drops)

PREGNANCY AND LACTATION: Pregnancy category C; excretion in breast milk unknown, use caution in nursing mothers

SIDE EFFECTS/ADVERSE REACTIONS

EENT: Itching, irritation in ear

HEME: Methemoglobinemia in infants

SKIN: Burning, stinging, pruritis, tenderness, erythema, rash, urticaria, edema

SPECIAL CONSIDERATIONS

PATIENT/FAMILY EDUCATION

- (Otic Solution) not to rinse dropper after use
- Protect the solution from light and heat, do not use if it is brown or contains a precipitate
- Discard this product six months after dropper is first placed in the drug solution
- Store at room temperature

benzonatate

(ben-zoe′na-tate)
Tessalon Perles
Chemical Class: Tetracaine derivative
Therapeutic Class: Antitussive, nonnarcotic

CLINICAL PHARMACOLOGY
Mechanism of Action: Acts peripherally by anesthetizing the stretch receptors located in the respiratory passages, lungs, and pleura; reduces cough reflex at its source; has no inhibitory effect on the respiratory center in recommended dosage
Pharmacokinetics
PO: Onset 15-20 min, duration 3-8 hr
INDICATIONS AND USES: Symptomatic relief of cough
DOSAGE
Adult and Child (>10 yr)
• PO 100 mg tid, not to exceed 600 mg/day
$ AVAILABLE FORMS/COST OF THERAPY
• Cap, Elastic—Oral: 100 mg, 100's: **$45.16-$75.91**
CONTRAINDICATIONS: Hypersensitivity to benzonatate or related compounds (e.g. tetracaine)
PREGNANCY AND LACTATION: Pregnancy category C; excretion into breast milk unknown, use with caution in nursing mothers
SIDE EFFECTS/ADVERSE REACTIONS
CNS: Dizziness, drowsiness, headache
CV: Chest numbness
EENT: Nasal congestion, burning eyes
GI: Nausea, constipation, upset stomach
SKIN: Urticaria, rash, pruritus

SPECIAL CONSIDERATIONS
PATIENT/FAMILY EDUCATION
• Avoid driving, other hazardous activities until stabilized on this medication
• Do not chew or break capsules, will anesthetize mouth

benzoyl peroxide

(ben′zoe-ill per-ox′ide)
Acne-10, Acnigel, Ben-Aqua, Benzac, Benzagel, Benzashave, Brevoxyl, Clearplex, Desquam-E, Desquam-X, PanOxyl, Peroxin, Persa-Gel, Syoxin, Theroxide, Zeroxin
Chemical Class: Benzoic acid derivative
Therapeutic Class: Antiacne medication

CLINICAL PHARMACOLOGY
Mechanism of Action: Antibacterial activity against *Propionibacterium acnes,* the predominant organism in sebaceous follicles and comedones; aided by mild drying action, removal of excess sebum, mild desquamation and sebostatic effects
Pharmacokinetics
TOP: 50% absorbed through skin, metabolized to benzoic acid, excreted in urine as benzoate
INDICATIONS AND USES: Mild-moderate acne
DOSAGE
Adult and Child
• TOP apply to affected area qd or bid
$ AVAILABLE FORMS/COST OF THERAPY
• Bar—Top: 10%, 4 oz: **$7.34**
• Cre—Top: 5%, 120 g: **$9.50-$14.24;** 10%, 120 g: **$11.50-$15.54**
• Gel—Top: 2.5%, 45, 60, 90 g: **$7.60-$14.25;** 4%, 42.5, 90 g: **$11.24-$15.75;** 5%, 45, 60, 90

g: **$1.73-$16.12;** 10%, 45, 60, 90 g: **$2.40-$16.88**
• Liq—Top: 2.5%, 240 ml: **$16.75;** 5%, 120, 150, 240 ml: **$9.19-$18.87;** 10%, 150, 240 ml: **$8.50-$20.94**
• Lotion—Top: 4%, 297 ml: **$16.57;** 5%, 30, 120, 240 ml: **$2.77-$10.00;** 10%, 30 ml: **$1.69-$3.15**
• Soap/Det—Top: 5%, 5 oz: **$12.03;** 10%, 5 oz: **$12.87**

CONTRAINDICATIONS: Hypersensitivity to benzoic acid derivatives

PREGNANCY AND LACTATION: Pregnancy category C; excretion into milk unknown

SIDE EFFECTS/ADVERSE REACTIONS

SKIN: Local skin irritation, stinging, dryness, scaling, erythema, edema, allergic and contact dermatitis

▼ DRUG INTERACTIONS

Drugs

• *Tretinoin:* Increased skin irritation

SPECIAL CONSIDERATIONS

PATIENT/FAMILY EDUCATION

• Keep away from eyes, mouth, inside of nose and other mucous membranes
• May cause transitory feeling of warmth or slight stinging
• Expect dryness and peeling, discontinue use if rash or irritation develops
• Avoid contact with hair or clothing, may bleach
• Water-based cosmetics may be used over drug
• Avoid other sources of skin irritation (e.g. sunlamps, sunlight, other topical acne medications) unless directed by physician

benzquinamide

(benz-kwin'a-mide)
Emete-Con
Chemical Class: Benzoquinolize amide
Therapeutic Class: Antiemetic

CLINICAL PHARMACOLOGY

Mechanism of Action: Has antiemetic, antihistaminic, mild anticholinergic and sedative actions in animals, the mechanism of action in humans is unknown

Pharmacokinetics

IM/IV: Onset 15 min, duration 3-4 hr, metabolized by liver, excreted in urine and bile, $t_{1/2}$ 40 min

INDICATIONS AND USES: Prevention and treatment of nausea and vomiting associated with anesthetic, surgery

DOSAGE

Adult

• IM 50 mg or 0.5-1 mg/kg, may be repeated in 1 hr, then q3-4 hr prn; IV 25 mg or 0.2-0.4 mg/kg as a one-time dose at a rate not to exceed 1 ml/0.5 to 1 min, give subsequent doses IM

Child

• Not recommended for children <12

$ AVAILABLE FORMS/COST OF THERAPY

• Inj, Sol—IV; IM: 50 mg/vial: **$5.76**

CONTRAINDICATIONS: Hypersensitivity

PRECAUTIONS: IV administration (associated with hypertension and transient arrhythmias)

PREGNANCY AND LACTATION: Safety for use during pregnancy has not been established, not recommended

SIDE EFFECTS/ADVERSE REACTIONS

CNS: Drowsiness, fatigue, restlessness, tremor, headache, stimulation,

dizziness, insomnia, excitement, nervousness, extrapyramidal symptoms
CV: ***Premature atrial or ventricular contractions,*** atrial fibrillation, hypertension, hypotension
EENT: Dry mouth, blurred vision, hiccups, salivation
GI: Nausea, anorexia
MS: Shivering, chills, twitching
SKIN: Rash, urticaria, flushing, hives, sweating

▼ **DRUG INTERACTIONS**

Drugs

• Pressor agents: Increased risk for hypertension

---

benztropine

(benz'troe-peen)
Bensylate, ✤ Cogentin
Chemical Class: Tertiary amine
Therapeutic Class: Anticholinergic, antiparkinson agent

CLINICAL PHARMACOLOGY

Mechanism of Action: Blockade of striatal cholinergic receptors which helps balance cholinergic and dopaminergic activity

Pharmacokinetics

IM/IV: Onset 15 min, duration 6-10 hr
PO: Onset 1 hr, duration 6-10 hr

INDICATIONS AND USES: Adjunctive treatment of all forms of Parkinson's disease; treatment of drug-induced extrapyramidal effects and acute dystonic reactions

DOSAGE

Adult

• *Parkinsonism:* PO 0.5-6 mg/day in 1-2 divided doses, begin with 0.5 mg/day and increase in 0.5 mg increments at 5-6 day intervals to achieve desired effect

• *Drug-induced extrapyramidal reaction:* PO/IM/IV 1-4 mg/dose 1-2 times/day, switch to PO as soon as possible

Child (>3 yr)

• *Drug-induced extrapyramidal reaction:* PO/IM/IV 0.02-0.05 mg/kg/dose 1-2 times/day

$ **AVAILABLE FORMS/COST OF THERAPY**

• Tab, Uncoated—Oral: 0.5 mg, 100's: **$2.40-$17.66;** 1 mg, 100's: **$2.63-$20.19;** 2 mg, 100's: **$3.30-$25.45**

• Inj, Sol—IM; IV: 1 mg/ml, 2 ml, 6's: **$40.46**

CONTRAINDICATIONS: Hypersensitivity, narrow-angle glaucoma, myasthenia gravis, GI/GU obstruction, child <3 yr, peptic ulcer, megacolon, prostatic hypertrophy

PRECAUTIONS: Elderly, tachycardia, liver/kidney disease, drug abuse history, dysrhythmias, hypotension, hypertension, psychiatric patients, children, tardive dyskinesia

PREGNANCY AND LACTATION: Pregnancy category C; an inhibitory effect on lactation may occur, infants may be particularly sensitive to anticholinergic effects

SIDE EFFECTS/ADVERSE REACTIONS

CNS: Confusion, anxiety, restlessness, irritability, delusions, hallucinations, headache, sedation, depression, incoherence, dizziness, memory loss
CV: Palpitations, tachycardia, hypotension, mild bradycardia, postural hypotension
EENT: Blurred vision, photophobia, dilated pupils, difficulty swallowing, dry eyes, mydriasis, increased intraocular tension, angle-closure glaucoma
GI: *Dry mouth, constipation,* nausea, vomiting, abdominal distress, ***paralytic ileus,*** epigastric distress
GU: Hesitancy, retention, dysuria
MS: Muscular weakness, cramping

SKIN: Rash, urticaria, other dermatoses

MISC: Increased temperature, flushing, decreased sweating, hyperthermia, heat stroke, numbness of fingers, erectile dysfunction

▼ **DRUG INTERACTIONS**

Drugs

- *Antihistamines, phenothiazines, amantadine:* Increased anticholinergic effect
- *Haloperidol:* Increased schizophrenic symptoms
- *Levodopa, phenothiazines:* Decreased effect of levodopa, phenothiazines

SPECIAL CONSIDERATIONS

PATIENT/FAMILY EDUCATION

- Do not discontinue this drug abruptly
- Avoid driving or other hazardous activities, drowsiness may occur
- Use hard candy, frequent drinks, sugarless gum to relieve dry mouth
- Administer with or after meals to prevent GI upset
- Use caution in hot weather drug may increase susceptibility to heat stroke
- May cause constipation; increase fluids, bulk, exercise if this occurs

---

benzylpenicilloyl-polylysine

(ben′-zill-pen-i-cill′-oyl-poly-ly′-seen)

Pre-Pen

Chemical Class: Penicillin

Therapeutic Class: Penicillin allergy skin test

CLINICAL PHARMACOLOGY

Mechanism of Action: Elicits IgE antibodies which produce type I accelerated urticarial reactions to penicillins

INDICATIONS AND USES: Adjunct in assessing the risk of administering penicillin (benzylpenicillin or penicillin G) when it is the preferred drug of choice in patients who have a history of clinical penicillin hypersensitivity

DOSAGE

Adult and Child

- *Scratch Test* (always perform first): A sterile 20 gauge needle should be used to make a 3-5 mm scratch of the epidermis; apply a small drop of Pre-Pen solution to the scratch and rub gently with an applicator, toothpick, or the side of the needle; a positive reaction consists of the development within 10 minutes of a pale wheal, usually with pseudopods, surrounding the scratch site and varying in diameter from 5 to 15 mm (or more)
- *Intradermal Test* (use only if scratch test completely negative): Use a tuberculin syringe with a 26 to 30 gauge, short bevel needle to inject a volume of 0.01-0.02 ml; use a separate syringe and needle to inject a like amount of saline as a control at least 1.5 inches removed from the test site; most skin reactions will develop within 5-15 minutes; a positive reaction consists of itching and marked increase in size of original bleb, wheal may exceed 20 mm in diameter and exhibit pseudopods; the control site should be completely reactionless

$ **AVAILABLE FORMS/COST OF THERAPY**

- Inj, Sol—Intradermal: 0.25 ml, 5's: **$67.33**

CONTRAINDICATIONS: Extreme hypersensitivity

PRECAUTIONS: Repeated skin testing; does not identify those patients who react to a minor antigenic determinant; does not reliably predict the ocurrence of late reactions;

patients with a negative skin test may still have allergic reactions to therapeutic penicillin

PREGNANCY AND LACTATION: Pregnancy category C

SIDE EFFECTS/ADVERSE REACTIONS

SKIN: Pruritus, erythema, wheal, urticaria, edema

MISC: Systemic allergic reactions occur rarely

---

bepridil

(beh'prih-dill)

Vascor

Chemical Class: Calcium channel blocker

Therapeutic Class: Antianginal

CLINICAL PHARMACOLOGY

Mechanism of Action: Inhibits both slow calcium and fast sodium inward currents across the cell membrane during cardiac depolarization; produces relaxation of coronary vascular smooth muscle, dilates coronary arteries, decreases SA/AV node conduction, dilates peripheral arteries

Pharmacokinetics

PO: Peak 2-3 hr, 99% bound to plasma proteins, $t_{1/2}$ 24 hr, completely metabolized in the liver, excreted in urine and feces

INDICATIONS AND USES: Chronic stable angina; has caused serious ventricular arrhythmias, including torsades de pointes type ventricular tachycardia, and has also been associated with agranulocytosis, should therefore be reserved for patients who have failed to respond optimally to, or are intolerant of, other anti-anginal medication; may be used alone or in combination with beta blockers and/or nitrates

DOSAGE

Adult

- PO 200 mg qd initially, increase after 10 days depending on response, max 400 mg/day

$ AVAILABLE FORMS/COST OF THERAPY

- Tab, Plain Coated—Oral: 200 mg, 100's: **$257.08;** 300 mg, 100's: **$313.56;** 400 mg, 100's: **$353.63**

CONTRAINDICATIONS: Sick sinus syndrome, 2nd or 3rd degree heart block, Wolff-Parkinson-White syndrome, hypotension <90 mm Hg systolic, uncompensated cardiac insufficiency, history of serious ventricular dysrhythmias, congenital QT interval prolongation or taking other drugs that prolong QT interval

PRECAUTIONS: CHF, renal disease, hepatic disease, children, hypokalemia, left bundle branch block, sinus bradycardia, recent MI

PREGNANCY AND LACTATION: Pregnancy category C; excreted in breast milk, use caution in nursing mothers

SIDE EFFECTS/ADVERSE REACTIONS

CNS: Headache, asthenia, fatigue, drowsiness, *dizziness,* anxiety, depression, weakness, insomnia, confusion, light-headedness, nervousness, tremor

CV: ***Dysrhythmia,*** edema, CHF, bradycardia, hypotension, palpitations, AV block

EENT: Blurred vision, tinnitus

GI: Nausea, gastric upset, vomiting, *diarrhea,* constipation, dry mouth, increased liver function studies

GU: Nocturia, polyuria

HEME: ***Agranulocytosis*** (rare)

RESP: Shortness of breath

SKIN: Rash

▼ **DRUG INTERACTIONS**

Drugs

• *Digoxin:* Increased serum digoxin concentrations

Labs

• *Increase:* Liver function tests, aminotransferase

SPECIAL CONSIDERATIONS

PATIENT/FAMILY EDUCATION

• ECGs will be necessary during initiation of therapy and after dosage changes

• Notify physician immediately for irregular heartbeat, shortness of breath, pronounced dizziness, constipation or hypotension

• May be taken with food or meals

MONITORING PARAMETERS

• Blood pressure, pulse, respiration, ECG intervals (PR, QRS, QT)

• Serum potassium

---

beractant

(ber-akt′ant)

Survanta

Chemical Class: A mixture containing phospholipids, neutral lipids, fatty acids, and surfactant-associated proteins to which colfosceril palmitate (dipalmitoylphosphatidylcholine), palmitic acid, and tripalmitin are added to standardize the composition and to mimic surface-tension lowering properties of natural lung surfactant

Therapeutic Class: Lung surfactant

CLINICAL PHARMACOLOGY

Mechanism of Action: Prevents the alveoli from collapsing during expiration by lowering surface tension between air and alveolar surfaces in neonates with deficient or ineffective endogenous lung surfactant

Pharmacokinetics

Most of the dose probably becomes lung-associated within hours of administration, the lipids enter endogenous surfactant pathways of reutilization and recycling

INDICATIONS AND USES: Prevention and treatment (rescue) of respiratory distress syndrome (RDS) in premature infants

DOSAGE

Infant

• Administer through a number 5 French end-hole catheter inserted into the endotracheal tube with the tip protruding just beyond the end of the endotracheal tube, divide each dose into quarters and administer with infant in different positions

• *Prophylactic treatment:* INTRATRACHEAL 4 ml/kg as soon as possible (preferably within 15 min of birth), as many as 4 doses may be administered during the first 48 hr of life no more frequently than q6h

• *Rescue treatment:* INTRATRACHEAL 4 ml/kg as soon as diagnosis of RDS is made (preferably by 8 hr of age)

$ AVAILABLE FORMS/COST OF THERAPY

• Susp—Intratracheal: 25 mg phospholipids/ml, 8 ml: **$688.82**

PRECAUTIONS: Use in infants <600 g birth weight or >1750 g birth weight has not been evaluated in controlled trials; use only in highly supervised clinical settings with immediate availability of clinicians experienced with intubation, ventilator management, and general care of premature infants

SIDE EFFECTS/ADVERSE REACTIONS

CV: Transient bradycardia, vasoconstriction, hypotension, hypertension

RESP: Oxygen desaturation, endotracheal tube reflux and blockage, hypopcarbia, hypercarbia, apnea

SKIN: Pallor

SPECIAL CONSIDERATIONS
MONITORING PARAMETERS
- Continuous ECG and transcutaneous oxygen saturation during instillation
- Frequent ABG sampling is necessary to prevent postdosing hyperoxia and hypocarbia

Storage
- Refrigerate unopened vials (2-8°C), protect from light

betamethasone

(bay-ta-meth'a-sone)
Systemic: Celestone, Cel-U-Jec, Selestoject, Celstone Soluspan
Topical: Uticort, Alphatrex, Diprosone, Maxivate, Psorion, Teladar, Betatrex, Beta-Val, Valison

Chemical Class: Corticosteroid, synthetic; medium potency: benzoate (cream, gel, lotion), dipropionate (lotion), valerate (cream); high potency: dipropionate (cream, ointment), valerate (ointment)
Therapeutic Class: Antiinflammatory, glucocorticoid, topical corticosteroid

CLINICAL PHARMACOLOGY
Mechanism of Action: Controls the rate of protein synthesis, depresses the migrations of polymorphonuclear leukocytes and fibroblasts, reverses capillary permeability, and causes lysosomal stabilization at the cellular level to prevent or control inflammation
Pharmacokinetics
Extensive metabolism in liver, $t_{1/2}$ 300+ minutes, duration 36-54 hr
INDICATIONS AND USES:
Systemic: Antiinflammatory or immunosuppressant agent in the treatment of a variety of diseases including those of hematologic, allergic, inflammatory, neoplastic, and autoimmune origin; prevention of neonatal respiratory distress syndrome (by administration to mother)*
Topical: Psoriasis, eczema, contact dermatitis, pruritus, corticosteroid responsive dermotoses
DOSAGE
Adult
- PO 0.6-7.2 mg/day; IM 0.5-9 mg/day divided q12h (usually ⅓-½ the oral dose); IV (sodium phosphate salt only) up to 9 mg; intra-articular and soft tissue (sodium phosphate/acetate salt): large joints 6-12 mg (1-2 ml), smaller joints 1.5-3 mg (0.25-1 ml), bursitis 6 mg, ganglia 3 mg, tendonitis 1.5-3 mg; TOP Apply to affected area bid-tid

Child
- PO 0.0175-0.25 mg/kg/day divided q6-8h or 0.5-7.5 mg/m^2/day divided q6-8h; IM 0.0175-0.125 mg base/kg/day divided q6-12h or 0.5-7.5 mg/m^2/day divided q6-12h; TOP Apply to affected area bid-tid

$ AVAILABLE FORMS/COST OF THERAPY
- Syr—Oral: 0.6 mg/5 ml, 120 ml: **$31.02**
- Tab, Uncoated—Oral: 0.6 mg, 100's: **$124.18**
- Inj, Susp (sodium phosphate/acetate)—Intra-Articular; Intradermal; IM: 3 mg/ml, 5 ml: **$18.47**
- Inj, Sol (sodium phosphate)—IM; IV: 3 mg/ml, 5 ml: **$4.25-$20.50**
- Cre (benzoate)—Top: 0.025%, 60 g: **$36.72**
- Gel (benzoate)—Top: 0.025%, 15, 60 g: **$13.81-$36.72**
- Lotion (benzoate)—Top: 0.025%, 60 g: **$28.10**
- Cre (dipropionate)—Top: 0.05%, 15, 45 g: **3.38-$34.61**
- Lotion (dipropionate)—Top: 0.05%, 20, 60 ml: **$4.30-$43.32**

• Oint (dipropionate)—Top: 0.05%, 15, 45 g: **$4.69-$32.81**
• Aer, Spray (dipropionate)—Top: 0.1%, 85 g: **$18.86**
• Cre, Augmented (dipropionate)—Top: 0.05%, 15, 45 g: **$21.92-$44.11**
• Gel (dipropionate)—Top: 0.05%, 15, 45 g: **$21.92-$44.11**
• Lotion, Augmented (dipropionate)—Top: 0.05%, 30, 60 ml: **$25.14-$49.55**
• Oint, Augmented (dipropionate)—Top: 0.05%, 15, 45 g: **$21.92-$44.11**
• Cre (valerate)—Top: 0.01%, 15, 60 g: **$9.11-$21.00;** 0.1%, 15, 45, 110, 430 g: **$1.95-$160.92**
• Lotion (valerate)—Top: 0.1%, 20, 60 ml: **$2.20-$37.27**
• Oint (valerate)—Top: 0.1%, 15, 45, 454 g: **$2.16-$98.06**
• Powder (valerate): 5 g: **$106.88**

CONTRAINDICATIONS: Systemic fungal infection, hypersensitivity, idiopathic thrombocytopenic purpura (IM); use on face, groin, or axilla (topical)

PRECAUTIONS: Psychosis, acute glomerulonephritis, amebiasis, cerebral malaria, child <2 yr, elderly, AIDS, tuberculosis, diabetes mellitus, glaucoma, osteoporosis, ulcerative colitis, CHF, myasthenia gravis, renal disease, esophagitis, peptic ulcer, ocular herpes simplex, live virus vaccines, hypertension; viral infections, bacterial infections, children (topical)

PREGNANCY AND LACTATION: Pregnancy category C; used in patients with premature labor at about 24-36 weeks gestation to stimulate fetal lung maturation; may appear in breast milk and could suppress growth, interfere with endogenous corticosteroid production or cause unwanted effects in the nursing infant

SIDE EFFECTS/ADVERSE REACTIONS

CNS: Depression, vertigo, ***convulsions,*** headache, *mood changes*
CV: Hypertension, thrombophlebitis, ***thromboembolism,*** tachycardia, CHF
EENT: Increased intraocular pressure, blurred vision, cataract
GI: Diarrhea, nausea, abdominal distention, ***GI hemorrhage,*** increased appetite, ***pancreatitis***
METAB: Cushingoid state, growth suppression in children, HPA suppression, decreased glucose tolerance
MS: Fractures, osteoporosis, aseptic necrosis of femoral and humeral heads, weakness, muscle mass loss
SKIN: Acne, poor wound healing, ecchymosis, bruising, petechiae, striae, thin fragile skin, suppression of skin test reactions; burning, dryness, itching, irritation, acne, folliculitis, hypertridosis, perioral dermatitis, hypopigmentation, atrophy, striae, miliaria, allergic contact dermatitis, secondary infection (topical)

▼ DRUG INTERACTIONS

Drugs

• *Aminoglutethamide:* Enhanced elimination of corticosteroids, diminished corticosteroid response
• *Antidiabetics:* Increased blood glucose
• *Barbiturates:* Reduced serum concentrations and therapeutic response of corticosteroids
• *Carbamazepine:* Reduced serum concentrations and therapeutic response of corticosteroids
• *Cholestyramine:* May lower plasma concentrations of orally administered corticosteroids
• *Estrogens:* Enhanced effects of corticosteroids
• *Isoniazid:* Reduced plasma concentrations of isoniazid

• *Phenytoin:* Reduced serum concentrations and therapeutic response of corticosteroids
• *Rifampin:* Reduced serum concentrations and therapeutic response of corticosteroids
• *Salicylates:* Enhanced elimination of salicylates

Labs

• *Increase:* Cholesterol, blood glucose, urine glucose
• *Decrease:* Calcium, potassium, T_4, T_3, thyroid ^{131}I uptake test
• *False negative:* Skin allergy tests

SPECIAL CONSIDERATIONS

PATIENT/FAMILY EDUCATION

• May cause GI upset, take with meals or snacks
• Take single daily doses in AM
• Notify physician if unusual weight gain, swelling of lower extremities, muscle weakness, black tarry stools, vomiting of blood, puffing of the face, menstural irregularities, prolonged sore throat, fever, cold or infection occurs
• Signs of adrenal insufficiency include fatigue, anorexia, nausea, vomiting, diarrhea, weight loss, weakness, dizziness and low blood sugar, notify physician if these signs and symptoms appear following dose reduction or withdrawal of therapy
• Avoid abrupt withdrawal of therapy following high dose or long-term therapy
• Do not use top products on weeping, denuded, or infected areas

MONITORING PARAMETERS

• Potassium and blood sugar during long-term therapy
• Edema, blood pressure, cardiac symptoms, mental status, weight
• Observe growth and development of infants and children on prolonged therapy

betaxolol

(bay-tax'oh-lol)
Kerlone, Betoptic, Betoptic S
Chemical Class: β_1-selective (cardioselective) adrenoreceptor blocking agent
Therapeutic Class: Antihypertensive; antiglaucoma agent

CLINICAL PHARMACOLOGY

Mechanism of Action: Preferentially competes with β-adrenergic agonists for available β_1-receptor sites inhibiting the chronotropic and inotropic responses to β_1-adrenergic stimulation (cardioselective); blocks β_2-receptors in bronchial system at higher doses; weak membrane stabilizing activity; lacks intrinsic sympathomimetic (partial agonist) activity; the exact mechanism of ocular antihypertensive action is not established, but appears to be a reduction of aqueous production, does not produce miosis or accommodative spasm which are frequently seen with miotic agents

Pharmacokinetics

PO: Peak 1.5-6 hr
OPHTH: Onset 30 min, duration 12 hr
50% protein bound, metabolized by liver, excreted in urine as metabolites and unchanged drug, $t_{1/2}$ 14-22 hr

INDICATIONS AND USES: Hypertension; chronic open-angle glaucoma

DOSAGE

Adult

• PO 10 mg qd, increased to 20 mg qd after 7-14 days if desired response is not achieved; doses >20 mg/day have not produced additional antihypertensive effect
• OPHTH 1 gtt bid

Elderly

• PO reduce initial dose to 5 mg qd

$ **AVAILABLE FORMS/COST OF THERAPY**

- Susp—Ophth: 0.25%, 2.5, 5, 10, 15 ml: **$9.63-$51.62**
- Sol—Ophth: 0.5%, 2.5, 5, 10, 15 ml: **$9.63-$51.62**
- Tab, Plain Coated—Oral: 10 mg, 100's: **$69.37;** 20 mg, 100's: **$104.04**

CONTRAINDICATIONS: Hypersensitivity to β-blockers, cardiogenic shock, 2nd or 3rd degree heart block, sinus bradycardia, CHF unless secondary to a tachydysrhythmia treatable with β-blockers, overt cardiac failure

PRECAUTIONS: Major surgery, diabetes mellitus, renal disease, thyroid disease, COPD, asthma, well-compensated heart failure, abrupt withdrawal, peripheral vascular disease; ophthalmic preparations can be absorbed systemically

PREGNANCY AND LACTATION: Pregnancy category C; excretion into breast milk unknown, use caution in nursing mothers

SIDE EFFECTS/ADVERSE REACTIONS

CNS: Insomnia, *fatigue, dizziness,* mental changes, memory loss, hallucinations, depression, *lethargy,* drowsiness, strange dreams

CV: Profound hypotension, ***bradycardia,*** CHF, cold extremities, postural hypotension, ***2nd or 3rd degree heart block***

EENT: Sore throat, dry burning eyes, visual disturbances, keratitis, blepharoptosis, diplopia, ptosis

GI: Nausea, diarrhea, vomiting, dry mouth, ***mesenteric arterial thrombosis, ischemic colitis***

GU: Impotence, sexual dysfunction

HEME: ***Agranulocytosis, thrombocytopenia***

METAB: Masked hypoglycemic response to insulin (sweating excepted), hyperlipidemia (increase TG, total cholesterol, LDL; decrease HDL)

RESP: ***Bronchospasm,*** dyspnea, wheezing

SKIN: Rash, pruritis, alopecia

▼ **DRUG INTERACTIONS**

Drugs

- *Antidiabetics:* Altered response to hypoglycemia, prolonged recovery of normoglycemia, hypertension, blockade of tachycardia; may increase blood glucose and impair peripheral circulation
- *Clonidine:* Exacerbation of rebound hypertension upon discontinuation of clonidine
- *Dihydropyridines:* Additive hemodynamic effects
- *Diltiazem:* Enhanced effects of both drugs, particularly antrioventricular conduction slowing
- *Dipyridamole:* Bradycardia
- *Disopyramide:* Additive negative inotropic effects
- *Epinephrine+:* Enhanced pressor response to epinephrine; less likely with cardioselective agents like betaxolol
- *Isoproterenol:* Potential reduction in effectiveness of isoproterenol in the treatment of asthma; less likely with cardioselective agents like betaxolol
- *Lidocaine:* Increased lidocaine concentrations possible
- *Local anesthetics:* Use of local anesthetics containing epinephrine may result in hypertensive reactions in patients taking β-blockers
- *Methyldopa:* Development of hypertension during situations resulting in release of catecholamines
- *NSAIDs:* Reduced hypotensive effects of β-blockers
- *Phenylephrine:* Enhanced pressor response to phenylephrine, particularly when it is administered IV
- *Prazosin:* First-dose response to

prazosin may be enhanced by β-blockade
- *Tacrine:* Additive bradycardia
- *Theophylline:* Antagonistic pharmacodynamic effects
- *Verapamil:* Enhanced effects of both drugs, particularly antrioventricular conduction slowing

Labs
- *Interference:* Glucose/insulin tolerance tests

SPECIAL CONSIDERATIONS

PATIENT/FAMILY EDUCATION
- Do not discontinue drug abruptly, may precipitate angina
- Report bradycardia, dizziness, confusion, depression, fever, shortness of breath, swelling of the extremities
- Take pulse at home, notify physician if <50 beats/min
- Avoid hazardous activities if dizziness, drowsiness, lightheadedness are present
- May mask the symptoms of hypoglycemia, except for sweating, in diabetic patients
- Transient stinging/discomfort is relatively common with ophthalmic preparations, notify physician if severe

MONITORING PARAMETERS
- Blood pressure, pulse, intraocular pressure

bethanechol

(be-than'e-kole)
Duvoid, Myotonachol, Urecholine
Chemical Class: Synthetic choline ester
Therapeutic Class: Cholinergic stimulant

CLINICAL PHARMACOLOGY
Mechanism of Action: Stimulates muscarinic acetylcholine receptors directly mimicking the effects of parasympathetic nervous system stimulation; stimulates gastric motility, and micturition

Pharmacokinetics
PO: Onset 30-90 min, duration 1-6 hr
SC: Onset 5-15 min, duration 1 hr

INDICATIONS AND USES: Acute postoperative and postpartum nonobstructive (functional) urinary retention; neurogenic atony of the urinary bladder with retention; gastric atony or stasis;* congenital megacolon;* gastroesophageal reflux*

DOSAGE
Adult
- PO 10-50 mg bid-qid; SC 2.5-5 mg tid-qid, up to 7.5-10 mg q4h for neurogenic bladder

Child
- *Abdominal distention or urinary retention:* PO 0.6 mg/kg/day divided tid-qid
- *Gastroesophageal reflux:* PO 0.1-0.2 mg/kg/dose given 30 min to 1 hr before each meal, max qid; SC 0.12-0.2 mg/kg/day divided tid-qid

$ **AVAILABLE FORMS/COST OF THERAPY**
- Tab, Uncoated—Oral: 5 mg, 100's: **$2.10-$34.43;** 10 mg, 100's: **$2.25-$68.24;** 25 mg, 100's: **$3.15-$109.26;** 50 mg, 100's: **$6.75-$169.00**
- Inj, Sol—SC: 5 mg/ml, 1 ml, 6's: **$29.89**

CONTRAINDICATIONS: Hypersensitivity, severe bradycardia, asthma, severe hypotension, hypertension, hyperthyroidism, peptic ulcer, parkinsonism, seizure disorders, coronary artery disease, coronary occlusion, mechanical bladder neck obstruction, possible GI obstruction, peritonitis, recent urinary or GI surgery, atrio-ventricular conduction defects, vasomotor instability, IM/IV inj

PRECAUTIONS: Child <8 yr, urinary retention

PREGNANCY AND LACTATION: Pregnancy category C; abdominal pain and diarrhea have been reported in a nursing infant exposed to bethanechol in milk, use caution in nursing mothers

SIDE EFFECTS/ADVERSE REACTIONS

More common after SC injection

CNS: Headache, dizziness

CV: Fall in blood pressure with reflex tachycardia, vasomotor response

EENT: Lacrimation, miosis

GI: Abdominal cramps, colicky pain, *nausea, belching, diarrhea,* borborygmi, salivation

GU: Urinary urgency

RESP: ***Bronchial constriction, asthmatic attacks***

SKIN: Flushing producing a feeling of warmth, sensation of heat about the face, sweating

MISC: Malaise

SPECIAL CONSIDERATIONS

PATIENT/FAMILY EDUCATION

- To avoid nausea and vomiting, take on an empty stomach
- May cause abdominal discomfort, salivation, sweating or flushing; notify physician if these effects are pronounced
- Dizziness, lightheadedness or fainting may occur, especially when getting up from a lying or sitting position

biperiden

(bye-per′-i-den)

Akineton

Chemical Class: Tertiary amine

Therapeutic Class: Anticholinergic

CLINICAL PHARMACOLOGY

Mechanism of Action: Centrally acting competitive anticholinergic

Pharmacokinetics

IM/IV: Onset 15 min, duration 6-10 hr

PO: Onset 1 hr, duration 6-10 hr

INDICATIONS AND USES: Parkinsonian symptoms, extrapyramidal symptoms secondary to neuroleptic drug therapy

DOSAGE

Adult

- *Parkinson symptoms:* PO 2 mg tid-qid; max 16 mg/24 hr
- *Extrapyramidal symptoms:* PO 2 mg qd-tid; IM/IV 2 mg q30min, if needed; max 8 mg/24 hr

$ AVAILABLE FORMS/COST OF THERAPY

- Inj—IM; IV: 5 mg/ml, 1 ml, 10's: **$33.30**
- Tab, Uncoated—Oral: 2 mg, 100's: **$23.99**

CONTRAINDICATIONS: Hypersensitivity, narrow-angle glaucoma, myasthenia gravis, GI/GU obstruction, megacolon, stenosing peptic ulcers, prostatic hypertrophy

PRECAUTIONS: Elderly, tachycardia, dysrhythmias, liver or kidney disease, drug abuse, hypotension, hypertension, psychiatric patients, give parenteral dose with patient recumbent to prevent postural hypotension; isolated instances of mental confusion, euphoria, agitation and disturbed behavior have been reported in susceptible patients

PREGNANCY AND LACTATION: Pregnancy category C

SIDE EFFECTS/ADVERSE REACTIONS

CNS: Confusion, anxiety, restlessness, irritability, delusions, hallucinations, headache, sedation, depression, incoherence, dizziness, euphoria, tremors, memory loss

CV: Palpitations, tachycardia, postural hypotension, bradycardia

EENT: Blurred vision, photophobia, dilated pupils, difficulty swallowing, mydriasis, increased intraocular tension, angle-closure glaucoma

GI: Dryness of mouth, constipation, nausea, vomiting, abdominal distress, ***paralytic ileus***

GU: Hesitancy, retention, dysuria

MS: Weakness, cramping

SKIN: Rash, urticaria, dermatoses

MISC: Increased temperature, flushing, decreased sweating, hyperthermia, heat stroke, numbness of fingers

▼ **DRUG INTERACTIONS**

Drugs

- *Amantadine:* Increased anticholinergic effect
- *Antihistamines:* Increased anticholinergic effect
- *Haloperidol:* Increased psychotic symptoms
- *Opiates, phenothiazines, and tricyclic antidepressants:* Increased anticholinergic effect

SPECIAL CONSIDERATIONS

PATIENT/FAMILY EDUCATION

- May increase susceptibility to heatstroke
- Do not discontinue drug abruptly; taper off over 1 wk
- Avoid driving or other hazardous activities
- Avoid nonprescription medications with alcohol or antihistamines unless directed by physician

---

bisacodyl

(bis-a-koe′-dill)

Apo-Bisacodyl, ✦ Bisac-Evac, Bisacodyl Uniserts, Bisco-Lax, Carter's Little Pills, Dulcolax, Fleet Bisacodyl Laxit ✦

Chemical Class: Diphenylmethane derivative

Therapeutic Class: Stimulant laxative

CLINICAL PHARMACOLOGY

Mechanism of Action: Acts directly on intestine by increasing motor activity; irritates colonic intramural plexus

Pharmacokinetics

PO: Onset 6-8 hr

PR: Onset 15-60 min

Absorption is minimal; absorbed drug metabolized by liver; excreted in urine, bile, feces, breast milk

INDICATIONS AND USES: Short-term treatment of constipation; bowel or rectal preparation for surgery, examination

DOSAGE

Adult

- PO 5-15 mg; up to 30 mg for bowel or rect preparation; PR 10 mg, 30 mL enema

Child

- PO 5-10 mg (or 0.3 mg/kg) for age >3 yr; PR 5-10 mg for age 2-11 yr; 5 mg for age <2 yr

$ **AVAILABLE FORMS/COST OF THERAPY**

- Enteric Coated Tabs—Oral: 5 mg, 25's: **$1.55-$3.27**
- Supp—Rect: 5 mg, 12's: **$2.00;** 10 mg, 12's: **$1.90-$8.37**
- Susp—Rect (enema): 10 mg/1.25 oz: **$11.38**

CONTRAINDICATIONS: Hypersensitivity, rectal fissures, abdominal pain, nausea, vomiting, appendicitis, acute surgical abdomen, ulcerated hemorrhoids, acute hepatitis, fecal impaction, intestinal/biliary tract obstruction.

PREGNANCY AND LACTATION: Pregnancy category B; excreted in breast milk

SIDE EFFECTS/ADVERSE REACTIONS

GI: Nausea, vomiting, anorexia, cramps, diarrhea, rectal burning (suppositories)

METAB: Protein-losing enteropathy, alkalosis, hypokalemia, ***tetany***

MS: Muscle weakness

SPECIAL CONSIDERATIONS
PATIENT/FAMILY EDUCATION
- Do not take within 1 hr of antacids or milk
- Swallow tabs whole

bismuth subsalicylate

(bis'-meth)
Pepto-Bismol, Pink Bismuth
Chemical Class: Salicylate
Therapeutic Class: Antidiarrheal

CLINICAL PHARMACOLOGY
Mechanism of Action: Inhibits prostaglandin synthesis responsible for GI hypersecretion and hypermotility (salicylate moiety); bismuth moiety may have direct antimicrobial effect
Pharmacokinetics
PO: Onset 1 hr, peak 2 hr, duration 4 hr; salicylate moiety absorbed (262 mg bismuth subsalicylate yields 102 mg salicylate)
INDICATIONS AND USES: Diarrhea (cause undetermined); prevention of travelers' diarrhea, as part of combination therapy for *Helicobacter pylori**
DOSAGE
Adult
- *Diarrhea:* PO 30 ml or 2 tabs q30-60 min, not to exceed 8 doses for >2 days
- *Prevention of travelers' diarrhea:* PO 30 ml or 2 tabs qid

Child
- *Diarrhea:* Age 9-12 yr PO 15 ml or 1 tab q30-60 min, not to exceed 8 doses for >2 days; Age 6-9 yr PO 10 ml or ⅔ tab q30-60 min, not to exceed 8 doses for >2 days; Age 3-6 yr PO 5 ml or ⅓ tab q30-60 min, not to exceed 8 doses for >2 days

$ AVAILABLE FORMS/COST OF THERAPY
- Tab, Chewable—Oral: 262 mg, 30's: **$2.00-$3.75**
- Susp—Oral: 262 mg/15 ml, 240 ml: **$2.90-$34.99;** 524 mg/15 ml, 240 ml: **$3.15-$49.10**
- Powder—Oral: 125 g: **$28.15**

CONTRAINDICATIONS: Child <3 yr, hypersensitivity to salicylates or bismuth
PRECAUTIONS: Anticoagulant therapy; stop use if symptoms do not improve within 2 days or become worse, or if diarrhea is accompanied by high fever or severe abdominal pain
PREGNANCY AND LACTATION: Pregnancy category C; salicylate excreted in breast milk
SIDE EFFECTS/ADVERSE REACTIONS
CNS: Confusion, twitching
EENT: Hearing loss, tinnitus, metallic taste, blue gums
GI: Fecal impaction (high doses), *dark stools*
HEME: Increased bleeding time
▼ DRUG INTERACTIONS
Drugs
- *Acetazolamide:* Increased serum level of acetazolamide; increased serum level of salicylate
- *Antacids:* Decreased salicylate level
- *Chlorpropamide:* Increased chlorpropamide effect
- *Corticosteroids:* Decreased salicylate concentration
- *Ethanol:* Increased GI toxicity of salicylate
- *Heparin +:* Increased bleeding risk
- *Methotrexate +:* Increased serum level of methotrexate
- *Phenytoin:* Increased serum level of phenytoin
- *Probenecid:* Decreased uricosuric effect of probenecid
- *Sulfinpyrazone:* Decreased uricosuric effect of sulfinpyrazone
- *Tetracyclines:* Decreased absorption of tetracyclines

* = non-FDA-approved use
+ = major clinical significance

• *Tolbutamide:* Increased tolbutamide effect
• *Valproic acid:* Increased serum level of valproic acid
• *Warfarin +:* Increased anticoagulant effect

Labs

• *Interfere:* Radiographic studies of GI tract

SPECIAL CONSIDERATIONS

PATIENT/FAMILY EDUCATION

• Chew or dissolve in mouth; do not swallow whole
• Shake suspension before using
• Stools may turn gray or black
• Tongue may darken

---

bisoprolol

(bis-o-prole′-lole)
Zebeta
Chemical Class: β_1 adrenergic blocker
Therapeutic Class: Antihypertensive

CLINICAL PHARMACOLOGY

Mechanism of Action: Selective β_1 adrenergic blocker; blocks β_2 receptors at doses above 20 mg per day

Pharmacokinetics

PO: Peak plasma level 2-4 hr; plasma $t_{1/2}$ 9-12 hr, 50% excreted unchanged in urine, protein binding 30%; metabolized in liver to inactive metabolites; full antihypertensive effect after 1 week of therapy; if creatinine clearance <40 ml/min, plasma $t_{1/2}$ tripled; in cirrhotics, plasma $t_{1/2}$ is 8.3 to 21.7 hours

INDICATIONS AND USES: Mild to moderate hypertension

DOSAGE

Adult

• PO 2.5-5.0 mg qd; max dose 20 mg qd; reduce dose in renal or hepatic impairment

$ AVAILABLE FORMS/COST OF THERAPY

• Tab, Plain Coated—Oral: 5 mg, 30's: **$25.32;** 10 mg, 30's: **$25.32**

CONTRAINDICATIONS: Hypersensitivity to beta blockers, cardiogenic shock, heart block (2nd, 3rd degree), sinus bradycardia, overt cardiac failure

PRECAUTIONS: Major surgery, diabetes mellitus, renal or hepatic disease, thyroid disease, COPD, asthma, well-compensated heart failure, aortic or mitral valve disease, peripheral vascular disease, myasthenia gravis; do not stop therapy abruptly, taper over 2 weeks

PREGNANCY AND LACTATION: Pregnancy category C; excreted in breast milk

SIDE EFFECTS/ADVERSE REACTIONS

CNS: Vertigo, *headache,* insomnia, *fatigue, dizziness,* mental changes, memory loss, hallucinations, depression, lethargy, drowsiness, strange dreams, catatonia, peripheral neuropathy

CV: ***Ventricular dysrhythmias, profound hypotension, bradycardia, CHF,*** cold extremities, postural hypotension, ***2nd or 3rd degree heart block***

EENT: Sore throat, dry burning eyes, *rhinitis,* sinusitis

GI: Nausea, *diarrhea,* vomiting, mesenteric arterial thrombosis, ischemic colitis, flatulence, gastritis, gastric pain, increased AST/ALT (1-2 times normal in 4%)

GU: Impotence, decreased libido

HEME: ***Agranulocytosis, thrombocytopenia,*** purpura, ***eosinophilia***

METAB: Increased hypoglycemic response to insulin, hypertriglyceridemia; hyperuricemia, hyperkalemia, hyperglycemia, azotemia

MS: Joint pain, arthralgia

RESP: Bronchospasm, dyspnea, wheezing, cough,
SKIN: Rash, fever, alopecia, pruritus, sweating
MISC: Facial swelling, weight gain, decreased exercise tolerance, *edema*

▼ **DRUG INTERACTIONS**

Drugs

- *Amiodarone:* Increased bradycardic effect of bisoprolol
- *Antidiabetics:* Bisoprolol reduces response to hypoglycemia
- *Barbiturates:* Enhanced bisoprolol metabolism
- *Calcium channel blockers:* Decreased bisoprolol metabolism
- *Cimetidine:* Decreased bisoprolol metabolism
- *Disopyramide:* Increased negative inotropic effect
- *Methyldopa:* May promote hypertension if used together
- *Neuroleptics:* Decreased bisoprolol metabolism; decreased neuroleptic metabolism
- *NSAIDs:* Reduced antihypertensive effect
- *Prazosin:* Enhanced 1st dose response to prazosin
- *Propafenone:* Decreased bisoprolol metabolism
- *Propoxyphene:* Decreased bisoprolol metabolism
- *Quinidine:* Decreased bisoprolol metabolism
- *Rifampin:* Enhanced bisoprolol metabolism
- *Theophylline:* Decreased metabolism of theophylline

Labs

- Positive anti-nuclear antibody (ANA) in 15% receiving long-term; one-third of these become ANA negative while continuing therapy

SPECIAL CONSIDERATIONS

PATIENT/FAMILY EDUCATION

- Do not stop drug abruptly (may cause/precipitate angina); taper over 2 weeks
- Do not use products containing alpha adrenergic stimulants (such as nasal decongestants, OTC cold preparations) unless directed by physician

---

bitolterol

(bye-tole′-ter-ol)
Tornalate

Chemical Class: Acid ester of colterol
Therapeutic Class: β_2 adrenergic agonist

CLINICAL PHARMACOLOGY

Mechanism of Action: Stimulates β_2 receptors causing increased synthesis of cAMP and bronchial smooth muscle relaxation; inhibits mast cell degranulation; stimulates cilia to remove secretions. Mean maximum increase in FEV_1 is 40%; bitolterol is a pro-drug which is hydrolyzed by esterases in tissue and blood to the active moiety colterol

Pharmacokinetics

INH: Onset 3 min, peak 30-60 min, duration 5-8 hr

INDICATIONS AND USES: Asthma, bronchospasm (prophylaxis and treatment)

DOSAGE

Adult and Child >12 yr

- *Bronchospasm:* INH 1-3 puffs at intervals of 1-3 min, not to exceed 3 INH q6h or 2 INH q4h
- *Prophylaxis of bronchospasm:* INH 2 puffs at intervals of 1-3 min q8h

$ **AVAILABLE FORMS/COST OF THERAPY**

- Aer—Inh: 0.37 mg/0.05 ml, 15 ml in metered dose inhaler: **$34.01**
- Sol—Inh: 0.37 mg/0.05 ml, 30 ml: **$12.09;** 0.37 mg/0.05 ml, 60 ml: **$22.89**

CONTRAINDICATIONS: Hypersensitivity to sympathomimetics
PRECAUTIONS: Ischemic heart disease, cardiac dysrhythmias, hyperthyroidism, diabetes mellitus, hypertension
PREGNANCY AND LACTATION: Pregnancy category C
SIDE EFFECTS/ADVERSE REACTIONS
CNS: *Tremors,* nervousness, headache, dizziness, lightheadedness, insomnia, hyperkinesia, hallucinations
CV: Palpitations, chest discomfort, tachycardia
EENT: Throat irritation
GI: Nausea, heartburn
MS: Muscle cramps
RESP: Coughing, bronchospasm, dyspnea

SPECIAL CONSIDERATIONS

PATIENT/FAMILY EDUCATION

- After shaking, exhale, place mouthpiece 1-2 cm from open mouth, inhale slowly while activating inhaler, hold breath then exhale slowly
- Wash inhaler in warm water and dry qd

---

bretylium

(bre-til′-ee-um)
Bretylate, ✤ Bretylol
Chemical Class: Quaternary ammonium compound
Therapeutic Class: Antidysrhythmic (Class III)

CLINICAL PHARMACOLOGY
Mechanism of Action: Causes an early release of norepinephrine from postganglionic nerve terminals then selectively accumulates in sympathetic ganglia and their postganglionic adrenergic neurons where it inhibits norepinephrine release; suppresses ventricular fibrillation and ventricular arrhythmias; increases action potential duration and effective refractory period without changes in heart rate
Pharmacokinetics
IV: Onset 5 min for suppression of ventricular fibrillation, onset 20-120 min for suppression of ventricular tachycardia
IM: Onset 20-120 min for suppression of ventricular tachycardia; duration 6-24 hr; 80% excreted unchanged by kidneys in 24 hr
INDICATIONS AND USES: Ventricular tachycardia, cardioversion, ventricular fibrillation
DOSAGES
Adult

- *Ventricular fibrillation:* IV bolus 5 mg/kg, then 10 mg/kg repeated q15 min, up to total 30-35 mg/kg; maintenance therapy is IV inf 1-2 mg/min or 5-10 mg/kg over 10 min q6h
- *Ventricular dysrhythmias:* IV inf 500 mg diluted in 50 ml D_5W or NS, infuse over 10-30 min, may repeat in 1 hr, maintain with 1-2 mg/min or 5-10 mg/kg over 10-30 min q6h; IM 5-10 mg/kg undiluted; repeat in 1-2 hr if needed; maintain with same dose q6-8h

Child

- *Ventricular fibrillation:* IV bolus 5 mg/kg; then 10 mg/kg if ventricular fibrillation persists

$ AVAILABLE FORMS/COST OF THERAPY

- Inj, Sol—IM; IV: 50 mg/ml, 10 ml: **$6.00-$34.12**
- Premixed for IV inf: 250 ml, 2 mg/ml, 4 mg/ml: **$28.01-$75.66**

CONTRAINDICATIONS: Hypersensitivity, digitalis toxicity (initial release of norepinephrine caused by bretylium may aggravate digitalis toxicity), aortic stenosis, pulmonary hypertension
PRECAUTIONS: Renal disease, postural hypotension, hypertension

or increased frequency of PVCs and other dysrhythmias may occur transiently in some patients

PREGNANCY AND LACTATION: Pregnancy category C

SIDE EFFECTS/ADVERSE REACTIONS

CNS: ***Syncope,*** dizziness, confusion, psychosis, anxiety

CV: ***Hypotension, postural hypotension (50%),*** bradycardia, angina, PVCs, transient hypertension

GI: Nausea, vomiting

RESP: ***Respiratory depression***

---

bromocriptine

(broe-moe-krip′-teen)

Parlodel

Chemical Class: Ergot alkaloid derivative

Therapeutic Class: Dopamine receptor agonist; ovulation stimulant

CLINICAL PHARMACOLOGY

Mechanism of Action: Inhibits prolactin release by activating postsynaptic dopamine receptors; activation of striatal dopamine receptors may be reason for improvement in Parkinson's disease

Pharmacokinetics

PO: Peak 1-3 hr, duration 4-8 hr; 90%-96% protein bound, $t_{1/2}$ 3 hr, metabolized by liver (inactive metabolites), 85%-98% of dose excreted in feces

INDICATIONS AND USES: Hyperprolactinemia-associated dysfunctions (including amenorrhea with or without galactorrhea, infertility, or hypogonadism); prolactin-secreting adenomas (may be used to reduce the tumor mass prior to surgery); female infertility associated with hyperprolactinemia; acromegaly; Parkinson's disease; prevention of physiological lactation* (after parturition when the mother elects not to breastfeed the infant, when breastfeeding is contraindicated, after stillbirth or abortion), neuroleptic malignant syndrome,* cocaine addiction*

DOSAGE

Adult

- *Hyperprolactinemic indications:* PO 1.25-2.5 mg with meals; may increase by 2.5 mg q3-7 days, usual 5-7.5 mg/day with range from 2.5-15 mg/day
- *Acromegaly:* PO 1.25-2.5 mg with food × 3 days; may increase by 1.25-2.5 mg q3-7 days until optimal therapeutic benefit; usual range 20-30 mg/day, max 100 mg/day (monitor growth hormone levels)
- *Parkinson's disease:* PO 1.25 mg bid with meals, may increase q2-4 wk by 2.5 mg/day, not to exceed 100 mg qd
- *Postpartum lactation:* (after vital signs have stabilized and no sooner than 4 hours after delivery) PO 2.5 mg bid with meals × 14 days; an additional 7 days may be necessary

$ **AVAILABLE FORMS/COST OF THERAPY**

- Cap, Gel—Oral: 5 mg, 100's: **$166.55-$219.24**
- Tab, Uncoated—Oral: 2.5 mg, 100's: **$108.47-$143.58**

CONTRAINDICATIONS: Hypersensitivity to ergot, severe ischemic disease, uncontrolled hypertension, toxemia of pregnancy, sensitivity to any ergot alkaloids, severe peripheral vascular disease

PRECAUTIONS: Hepatic disease, renal disease, children, pituitary tumors, hypotension, concurrent blood pressure lowering medications

PREGNANCY AND LACTATION: Pregnancy category D; since it prevents lactation, should not be administered to mothers who elect to breastfeed infants

SIDE EFFECTS/ADVERSE REACTIONS

CNS: Headache, depression, restlessness, anxiety, nervousness, confusion, ***convulsions,*** hallucinations, dizziness, fatigue, drowsiness, abnormal involuntary movements, "on-off" phenomenon, visual disturbance, ataxia, insomnia, psychosis, cerebrospinal fluid rhinorrhea (treatment of prolactinomas)

CV: Orthostatic hypotension, decreased B/P, palpitation, extra systole, ***stroke, shock,*** dysrhythmias, bradycardia

EENT: Blurred vision, diplopia, burning eyes, nasal congestion

GI: Nausea, vomiting, anorexia, cramps, constipation, diarrhea, dry mouth, GI hemorrhage

GU: Frequency, retention, incontinence, diuresis

SKIN: Rash on face, arms, alopecia

▼ **DRUG INTERACTIONS**

Drugs

- *Isometheptene+:* Case report of hypertension and ventricular tachycardia with combination
- *Neuroleptics:* Neuroleptic drugs probably inhibit the ability of bromocriptine to lower serum prolactin concentrations in patients with pituitary adenomas; theoretically, bromocriptine should inhibit the antipsychotic effects of neuroleptic agents, but clinical evidence suggests that this may be uncommon
- *Phenylpropanolamine+:* Increased risk of hypertension and seizures

Labs

- *Increase:* Growth hormone, AST/ALT, CPK, BUN, uric acid, alk phosphatase, GGTP

SPECIAL CONSIDERATIONS

PATIENT/FAMILY EDUCATION

- Use measures to prevent orthostatic hypotension

brompheniramine

(brome-fen-ir'a-meen)

Bromphen, Codimal-A, Cophene-B, Dehist, Diamine T.D., Dimetane, Dimetane Extentabs, Histaject, ND Stat, Nasahist-B, Oraminic II, Veltane

Chemical Class: Alkylamine derivative

Therapeutic Class: Antihistamine

CLINICAL PHARMACOLOGY

Mechanism of Action: Competes with histamine for H_1-receptor sites on effector cells in the GI tract, blood vessels, and respiratory tract

Pharmacokinetics

PO: Peak 2-5 hr, metabolized in liver, excreted in urine as inactive metabolites, $t_{1/2}$ 12-34 hr

INDICATIONS AND USES: Perennial and seasonal allergic rhinitis and other allergic symptoms including urticaria; combination therapy with H_2-receptor antagonist in chronic idiopathic urticaria*

DOSAGE

Adult

- PO 4-8 mg tid-qid, not to exceed 24 mg/day; PO TIME REL 8-12 mg bid-tid or 12 mg q12h, not to exceed 24 mg/day; IM/IV/SC 5-20 mg q6-12h, not to exceed 40 mg/day

Child (6-12 yr)

- PO 2-4 mg q4-6h, not to exceed 16 mg/day; IM/IV/SC 0.5 mg/kg/day divided q6-8h

Child (<6 yr)

- PO 0.125 mg/kg/dose q6h, not to exceed 8 mg/day

$ **AVAILABLE FORMS/COST OF THERAPY**

- Tab, Uncoated—Oral: 4 mg, 100's: **$2.95-$4.05**
- Tab, Ext Rel—Oral: 8 mg, 100's: **$17.66**

• Elixir—Oral: 2 mg/5 ml, 120, 480 ml: **$3.12-$10.28**
• Inj, Sol—IM; IV; SC: 10 mg/ml, 10 ml: **$6.00-$19.90**

CONTRAINDICATIONS: Hypersensitivity, narrow-angle glaucoma, bladder neck obstruction

PRECAUTIONS: Liver disease, elderly, increased intraocular pressure, hyperthyroidism, cardiovascular disease, hypertension, urinary retention, newborn or premature infants, renal disease, stenosed peptic ulcers

PREGNANCY AND LACTATION: Pregnancy category C; an association between first trimester exposure and congenital defects has been found in humans; excreted into breast milk, compatible with breastfeeding

SIDE EFFECTS/ADVERSE REACTIONS

CNS: Dizziness, drowsiness, poor coordination, fatigue, anxiety, euphoria, confusion, paresthesia, neuritis

CV: Hypotension, palpitations, tachycardia

EENT: Blurred vision, dilated pupils, tinnitus, nasal stuffiness, dry nose, throat

GI: Dry mouth, nausea, vomiting, anorexia, *constipation,* diarrhea

GU: Retention, dysuria, frequency, impotence

HEME: ***Thrombocytopenia, agranulocytosis, hemolytic anemia***

RESP: Increased thick secretions, wheezing, chest tightness

SKIN: Photosensitivity

▼ **DRUG INTERACTIONS**

Drugs

• *Barbiturates:* Excessive CNS depression

Labs

• *False negative:* Skin allergy tests

SPECIAL CONSIDERATIONS

PATIENT/FAMILY EDUCATION

• Do not crush or chew sustained release forms
• Notify physician if confusion/sedation/hypotension occurs
• Avoid driving or other hazardous activities if drowsiness occurs
• Avoid use of alcohol or other CNS depressants while taking drug
• Use hard candy, gum, frequent rinsing of mouth for dryness

buclizine

(byoo'kli-zeen)

Bucladin-S Softabs

Chemical Class: Piperazine, H_1-receptor antagonist

Therapeutic Class: Antiemetic; antihistamine; anticholinergic

CLINICAL PHARMACOLOGY

Mechanism of Action: Acts centrally by blocking chemoreceptor trigger zone, which in turn acts on vomiting center

Pharmacokinetics

PO: Duration 4-6 hr, other pharmacokinetics not known

INDICATIONS AND USES: Motion sickness, dizziness, nausea, vomiting

DOSAGE

Adult

• *Nausea:* PO 50 mg bid, not to exceed 150 mg/day
• *Motion sickness:* PO 50 mg 0.5 hr before beginning travel, a 2nd 50 mg dose may be taken after 4-6h for extended travel

$ **AVAILABLE FORMS/COST OF THERAPY**

• Tab, Soft/Chewable—Oral: 50 mg, 100's: **$47.20**

CONTRAINDICATIONS: Hypersensitivity

PRECAUTIONS: Children, narrow-angle glaucoma, prostatic hypertro-

phy, elderly, tartrazine sensitivity
PREGNANCY AND LACTATION: Pregnancy category C; the manufacturer considers the drug to be contraindicated in early pregnancy; excretion into breast milk unknown
SIDE EFFECTS/ADVERSE REACTIONS
CNS: Drowsiness, dizziness, fatigue, restlessness, headache, insomnia
GI: Nausea, anorexia
EENT: Dry mouth, blurred vision

SPECIAL CONSIDERATIONS

PATIENT/FAMILY EDUCATION

- Can be taken without water, place the Softab tablet in the mouth and allow it to dissolve, or the tablet may be chewed
- Avoid hazardous activities or activities requiring alertness; dizziness may occur
- Avoid alcohol and other CNS depressants

---

bumetanide

(byoo-met′a-nide)
Bumex
Chemical Class: Sulfonamide derivative
Therapeutic Class: Loop diuretic

CLINICAL PHARMACOLOGY
Mechanism of Action: Inhibits sodium and chloride reabsorption in the ascending limb of the loop of Henle; potassium excretion is increased in a dose-related fashion; may have an additional action in the proximal tubule
Pharmacokinetics
PO: Onset 0.5-1 hr, duration 4 hr
IM: Onset 40 min, duration 4 hr
IV: Onset 5 min, duration 2-3 hr
94-96% bound to plasma proteins, excreted by kidneys, $t_{1/2}$ 1-1.5 hr
INDICATIONS AND USES: Edema associated with congestive heart failure, hepatic and renal disease, including the nephrotic syndrome; hypertension; adult nocturia*
DOSAGE
Adult

- PO 0.5-2.0 mg qd, may give 2nd or 3rd dose at 4-5 hr intervals up to max of 20 mg/day; may be given on alternate days or intermittently; IV/IM 0.5-1.0 mg/day; may give 2nd or 3rd dose at 2-3 hr intervals up to max of 10 mg/day

Child (>6 months)

- PO/IM/IV 0.015 mg/kg/dose qd or qod, maximum 0.1 mg/kg/day or 10 mg

$ **AVAILABLE FORMS/COST OF THERAPY**

- Inj, Sol—IM; IV: 0.25 mg/ml, 2 ml, 10's: **$17.22**
- Tab, Uncoated—Oral: 0.5 mg, 100's: **$29.33;** 1 mg, 100's: **$41.19;** 2 mg, 100's: **$69.64**

CONTRAINDICATIONS: Hypersensitivity, anuria, hepatic coma, severe electrolyte depletion
PRECAUTIONS: Dehydration, ascites, severe renal disease, hepatic cirrhosis, volume depletion, allergy to sulfonamides, thrombocytopenia, diabetes
PREGNANCY AND LACTATION: Pregnancy category C; excretion into milk unknown
SIDE EFFECTS/ADVERSE REACTIONS
CNS: Headache, *dizziness,* fatigue, weakness, vertigo
CV: Hypotension, ECG changes
EENT: Ototoxicity, ear pain, tinnitus, blurred vision
GI: Nausea, diarrhea, dry mouth, vomiting, anorexia, cramps, upset stomach, abdominal pain
GU: Polyuria, ***renal failure,*** glycosuria, sexual dysfunction
HEME: ***Thrombocytopenia***
METAB: Hypokalemia, hypochloremic alkalosis, hypomagnesemia,

hyperuricemia, hypocalcemia, hyponatremia, hyperglycemia
MS: Muscular cramps, arthritis, stiffness, tenderness
SKIN: Rash, pruritus, purpura, ***Stevens-Johnson syndrome,*** sweating, photosensitivity

▼ **DRUG INTERACTIONS**

Drugs

- *ACE inhibitors:* hypotension, renal insufficiency
- *Digitalis glycosides:* Diuretic-induced hypokalemia may increase the risk of digitalis toxicity
- *Indomethacin:* Reduced diuretic and antihypertensive efficacy of bumetanide

Labs

- *Increase:* BUN, creatinine, ammonia, amylase, glucose, uric acid
- *Decrease:* Sodium, calcium, chloride, potassium

SPECIAL CONSIDERATIONS

Cross-sensitivity with furosemide rare. May substitute bumetanide at a 1:40 ratio with furosemide in patients allergic to furosemide

PATIENT/FAMILY EDUCATION

- May cause GI upset, take with food
- Take early in the day
- Arise slowly from a reclining position
- Photosensitivity may occur

MONITORING PARAMETERS

- Electrolytes: potassium, sodium, chloride
- BUN, glucose, CBC, serum creatinine
- Uric acid, calcium, magnesium
- Weight, I&O

bupivacaine

(byoo-piv′a-caine)
Marcaine, Sensorcaine
Chemical Class: Amide, aminoacyl derivative
Therapeutic Class: Local anesthetic

CLINICAL PHARMACOLOGY

Mechanism of Action: Blocks the generation and conduction of nerve impulses, presumably by increasing the threshold for electrical excitation in the nerve, slowing the propagation of the nerve impulse, and reducing the rate rise of the action potential; the progression of anesthesia is related to the diameter, myelination, and conduction velocity of affected nerve fibers; the order of loss of nerve function is as follows: (1) pain, (2) temperature, (3) touch, (4) proprioception, and (5) skeletal muscle tone

Pharmacokinetics

INJ: Peak 30-45 min, duration 3-6 hr, 96% bound to plasma proteins, metabolized in liver, excreted in urine, $t_{1/2}$ 3.5 hr

INDICATIONS AND USES: Local or regional anesthesia; analgesia for surgery, oral surgical procedures, diagnostic and therapeutic procedures, obstetrical procedures

DOSAGE

Dose varies with procedure, depth of anesthesia, vascularity of tissues, duration of anesthesia, and condition of patient

Adult

- *Caudal block:* INJ 15-30 ml of 0.25% or 0.5%
- *Epidural block:* INJ 10-20 ml of 0.25% or 0.5%
- *Peripheral nerve block:* INJ 5 ml of 0.25% or 0.5% (12.5-25 mg), max 2.5 mg/kg or 400 mg/day

• *Sympathetic nerve block:* INJ 20-50 ml of 0.25%

Child

• *Caudal block:* INJ 1-3.7 mg/kg
• *Epidural block:* INJ 1.25 mg/kg/dose

$ AVAILABLE FORMS/COST OF THERAPY

• Inj, Sol—Caudal Block, Epidural: 0.25%, 30 ml: **$4.43-$6.34;** 0.5%, 30 ml: **$4.79-$12.67;** 0.75%, 30 ml: **$5.00-$7.17**

CONTRAINDICATIONS: Obstetrical paracervical block anesthesia, hypersensitivity to amide local anesthetics

PRECAUTIONS: Obstetrical anesthesia (0.75% concentration), intravenous regional anesthesia, hypotension, heart block, hepatic disease, impaired cardiovascular function, use in head and neck area, retrobulbar blocks, elderly

PREGNANCY AND LACTATION: Pregnancy category C; excretion into breast milk unknown, regional use may prolong labor and delivery

SIDE EFFECTS/ADVERSE REACTIONS

CNS: Anxiety, restlessness, ***convulsions, loss of consciousness,*** drowsiness, disorientation, tremors, shivering

CV: ***Myocardial depression, cardiac arrest, dysrhythmias,*** bradycardia, hypotension, hypertension, fetal bradycardia

EENT: Blurred vision, tinnitus, pupil constriction

GI: Nausea, vomiting

RESP: ***Respiratory arrest, anaphylaxis***

SKIN: Rash, urticaria, allergic reactions, edema, burning, skin discoloration at injection site, tissue necrosis

▼ DRUG INTERACTIONS

Drugs

• *β-adrenergic blockers:* Hypertensive reactions possible; acute discontinuation of β-blockers before local anesthesia may increase the risk of side effects due to anesthetic

SPECIAL CONSIDERATIONS

MONITORING PARAMETERS

• Blood pressure, pulse, respiration during treatment, ECG
• Fetal heart tones if drug is used during labor

---

buprenorphine

(byoo-pre-nor′feen)
Buprenex

Chemical Class: Opiate, thebaine derivative
Therapeutic Class: Narcotic agonist-antagonist analgesic
DEA Class: Schedule V

CLINICAL PHARMACOLOGY

Mechanism of Action: Produces analgesia via high affinity binding to μ subclass opiate receptors in the CNS; narcotic antagonist activity is approximately equipotent to naloxone

Pharmacokinetics

IM: Onset 15 min, peak 1 hr, duration 6 hr

IV: Onset 1 min, peak 5 min, duration 2-5 hr

Metabolized by liver, excreted predominantly in feces, 96% bound to plasma proteins, $t_{1/2}$ 2-3 hr

INDICATIONS AND USES: Moderate to severe pain

DOSAGE

Adult

• IM/IV 0.3 mg q6h prn (reduce dosage by half in the elderly, debilitated patients, or in the presence of respiratory disease); repeat once (up to 0.3 mg) prn, 30-60 min after initial dose

Child >2 yr

• IM/IV 2 μg/kg/dose q6-8h prn

$ AVAILABLE FORMS/COST OF THERAPY

• Inj, Sol—IM; IV: 0.3 mg/ml, 10's: **$23.10**

CONTRAINDICATIONS: Hypersensitivity

PRECAUTIONS: Addictive personality, narcotic dependent patients (may cause withdrawal), increased intracranial pressure, respiratory depression, hepatic disease, renal disease, hypothyroidism, biliary tract dysfunction, prostatic hyertrophy

PREGNANCY AND LACTATION: Pregnancy category C; safe use in labor and delivery has not been established; excretion into breast milk unknown

SIDE EFFECTS/ADVERSE REACTIONS

CNS: Sedation, dizziness, headache, confusion, psychosis, euphoria, weakness, nervousness, slurred speech, paresthesia, depression, hallucinations, tremor, ***coma***

CV: Hypotension, hypertension, tachycardia, bradycardia

EENT: Miosis, blurred vision, diplopia, conjunctivitis, visual abnormalities, tinnitus

GI: Nausea, constipation, dry mouth, dyspepsia, flatulence, loss of appetite

GU: Urinary retention

RESP: Hypoventilation, dyspnea, cyanosis, apnea

SKIN: Sweating, pruritus, injection site reaction, rash, pallor, urticaria

▼ DRUG INTERACTIONS

Drugs

• *Barbiturates:* Additive CNS depression

• *Cimetidine:* Enhanced CNS and respiratory depression

• *Neuroleptics:* Hypotension; excessive CNS depression

SPECIAL CONSIDERATIONS

PATIENT/FAMILY EDUCATION

• May cause dizziness or drowsiness; avoid other CNS depressant (e.g. alcohol, benzodiazepines)

---

bupropion

(byoo-proe′pee-on)
Wellbutrin

Chemical Class: Aminoketone
Therapeutic Class: Antidepressant

CLINICAL PHARMACOLOGY

Mechanism of Action: Inhibits neuronal reuptake of dopamine, serotonin, norepinephrine

Pharmacokinetics

PO: Peak 2 hr, onset 2-4 wk, $t_{1/2}$ 12-14 hr, metabolized by liver

INDICATIONS AND USES: Depression

DOSAGE

Adult

• PO 100 mg bid initially, increase based on clinical response to 100 mg tid no sooner than 3 days after initiating therapy, may increase after 1 month to 150 mg tid; **no single dose should exceed 150 mg, at least 6 hr should elapse between doses**

$ AVAILABLE FORMS/COST OF THERAPY

• Tab, Coated—Oral: 75 mg, 100's: **$54.13;** 100 mg, 100's: **$72.22**

CONTRAINDICATIONS: Hypersensitivity, seizure disorder, prior or current diagnosis of bulemia or anorexia nervosa (increased risk of seizure), concurrent use of MAO inhibitor

PRECAUTIONS: Renal and hepatic disease, recent MI, unstable heart disease, history of drug abuse or dependence, bipolar affective disorder

PREGNANCY AND LACTATION: Pregnancy category B; excretion into breast milk unknown

SIDE EFFECTS/ADVERSE REACTIONS

CNS: Dry mouth, sweating, *headache/migraine, insomnia,* tremor, *agitation, anxiety, confusion,* decreased libido, ***seizures***

CV: Cardiac arrhythmias, dizziness, hypertension, hypotension, palpitations, syncope, tachycardia, edema

EENT: Auditory disturbance, blurred vision

GI: Appetite increase, constipation, dyspepsia, *nausea/vomiting*

GU: Impotence, menstrual complaints, urinary frequency

METAB: Gynecomastia, glycosuria

MS: Arthritis

SKIN: Pruritus, rash

SPECIAL CONSIDERATIONS

PATIENT/FAMILY EDUCATION

- Take in equally divided doses 3 or 4 times daily to minimize risk of seizures
- May impair ability to perform tasks requiring judgment or motor and cognitive skills
- Avoid alcohol
- Therapeutic effects may take 2-4 wk
- Do not discontinue medication quickly after long-term use

---

buspirone

(byoo-spir'own)

BuSpar

Chemical Class: Azaspirodecanedione

Therapeutic Class: Antianxiety agent

CLINICAL PHARMACOLOGY

Mechanism of Action: The mechanism of action of buspirone is unknown; does not exert anticonvulsant or muscle relaxant effects; in vitro, has a high affinity for serotonin (5-HT_{1A}) receptors; has no significant affinity for benzodiazepine receptors and does not affect GABA binding in vitro or in vivo; has moderate affinity for brain D_2-dopamine receptors; some studies suggest indirect effects on other neurotransmitter systems

Pharmacokinetics

PO: Peak 40-90 min, 95% bound to plasma proteins, metabolized by liver, excreted in urine and feces, $t_{1/2}$ 2-3 hr

INDICATIONS AND USES: Anxiety disorders, premenstrual syndrome*

DOSAGE

Adult

- PO 5 mg tid, may increase by 5 mg/day q2-3d, not to exceed 60 mg/day

$ AVAILABLE FORMS/COST OF THERAPY

- Tab, Uncoated—Oral: 5 mg, 100's: **$57.23;** 10 mg, 100's: **$99.84**

CONTRAINDICATIONS: Hypersensitivity

PRECAUTIONS: Liver disease, renal disease, elderly, children <18 yr

PREGNANCY AND LACTATION: Pregnancy category B; excretion into breast milk unknown, use caution in nursing mothers

SIDE EFFECTS/ADVERSE REACTIONS

CNS: Dizziness, drowsiness, headache, depression, stimulation, insomnia, nervousness, light-headedness, numbness, paresthesia, incoordination, tremors, excitement, involuntary movements, confusion, akathisia

CV: Bradycardia, palpitations, ***hypotension,*** hypertension, nonspecific chest pain

EENT: Sore throat, tinnitus, blurred vision, nasal congestion, red, itching eyes, altered taste, altered smell

GI: Nausea, dry mouth, diarrhea, constipation, flatulence, increased appetite, rectal bleeding, dyspepsia

GU: Frequency, hesitancy, menstrual irregularity, change in libido
MS: Pain, weakness, muscle cramps, spasms
RESP: Hyperventilation, chest congestion, shortness of breath
SKIN: Rash, edema, pruritus, alopecia, dry skin
MISC: Sweating, fatigue, weight gain, fever

SPECIAL CONSIDERATIONS

PATIENT/FAMILY EDUCATION

- May cause drowsiness and dizziness, use caution while driving or performing other tasks requiring alertness
- Avoid alcohol and other CNS depressants
- Optimal results may take 3-4 weeks of treatment, some improvement may be seen after 7-10 days

---

butabarbital

(byoo-tah-bar'bi-tal)

Barbased, Butisol Sodium, Buticaps, Butatran, Sarisol, Butalan

Chemical Class: Barbituric acid derivative
Therapeutic Class: Sedative/hypnotic-barbiturate (intermediate acting)
DEA Class: Schedule III

CLINICAL PHARMACOLOGY

Mechanism of Action: Depresses activity in brain cells primarily in reticular activating system in brain stem; also selectively depresses neurons in posterior hypothalamus, limbic structures; able to decrease seizure activity in anesthetic doses by inhibition of impulses in CNS; depresses REM sleep

Pharmacokinetics

PO: Onset 0.5-1 hr, $t_{1/2}$ 66-140 hr, metabolized by liver, excreted in urine as metabolites

INDICATIONS AND USES: Routine sedation; hypnotic in the short-term treatment of insomnia for periods up to 2 weeks in duration (may lose efficacy for sleep induction and maintenance after this period of time)

DOSAGE

Adult

- *Daytime sedation:* PO 15-30 mg, tid-qid
- *Bedtime hypnotic:* PO 50-100 mg
- *Preoperative sedation:* PO 50-100 mg, 60-90 min before surgery

Child

- *Preoperative sedation:* PO 2-6 mg/kg, max 100 mg
- *Daytime sedation:* PO 7.5-30 mg, depending on age, weight and sedation desired

$ **AVAILABLE FORMS/COST OF THERAPY**

- Elixir—Oral: 30 mg/5 ml, 480 ml: **$5.93-$76.37**
- Tab, Uncoated—Oral: 15 mg, 100's: **$40.78;** 30 mg, 100's: **$54.17;** 50 mg, 100's: **$70.44;** 100 mg, 100's: **$83.62**

CONTRAINDICATIONS: Hypersensitivity to barbiturates, respiratory depression, addiction to barbiturates, severe liver impairment, porphyria

PRECAUTIONS: Anemia, hepatic disease, renal disease, hypertension, elderly, acute/chronic pain, mental depression, history of drug abuse, abrupt discontinuation

PREGNANCY AND LACTATION: Pregnancy category D; small amounts excreted in breast milk, use caution in nursing mothers

SIDE EFFECTS/ADVERSE REACTIONS

CNS: Lethargy, drowsiness, hangover, dizziness, stimulation in the elderly and children, lightheadedness, physical dependence, CNS depression, mental depression,

slurred speech, vertigo, headache
CV: ***Hypotension,*** bradycardia
GI: Nausea, vomiting, diarrhea, constipation
HEME: ***Agranulocytosis, thrombocytopenia, megaloblastic anemia*** (long-term treatment)
MS: Rickets, osteomalacia (prolonged use)
RESP: ***Depression, apnea, laryngospasm, bronchospasm***
SKIN: *Rash,* urticaria, erythema multiforme, pain, abscesses at injection site, ***angioedema,*** thrombophlebitis, ***Stevens-Johnson syndrome***

▼ **DRUG INTERACTIONS**

Drugs

- *Acetaminophen:* Enhanced hepatotoxic potential of overdoses, and potentially large therapeutic doses of acetaminophen; possible reduced therapeutic response to acetaminophen
- *Antidepressants:* Reduced serum concentrations and therapeutic response of cyclic antidepressants
- *Antihistamines:* Excessive CNS depression
- *β-adrenergic blockers:* Reduced serum concentrations of β-blockers that are extensively metabolized
- *Calcium channel blockers:* Reduced plasma concentrations of verapamil and nifedipine
- *CNS depressants:* Excessive CNS depression
- *Chloramphenicol:* Increased serum barbiturate concentrations; reduced serum chloramphenicol concentrations
- *Corticosteroids:* Reduced serum concentrations and therapeutic response of corticosteroids
- *Disopyramide:* Reduced serum concentrations of disopyramide
- *Doxycycline:* Reduced serum doxycycline concentrations
- *Ethanol:* Excessive CNS depression
- *Methoxyflurane:* Enhanced nephrotoxicity of methoxyflurane
- *MAO inhibitors:* Prolonged effect of barbiturates
- *Narcotic analgesics:* Increased toxicity of meperidine; reduced effect of methadone; excessive CNS depression
- *Neuroleptics:* Possible reduction in neuroleptic effect
- *Oral contraceptives:* Reduced efficacy of oral contraceptives, menstrual irregularities and unintended pregnancies may occur
- *Oral anticoagulants+:* Inhibited hypoprothrombinemic response to oral anticoagulants; fatal bleeding episodes have occurred when barbiturates were discontinued in patients stabilized on an anticoagulant
- *Quinidine:* Reduced serum quinidine plasma concentrations
- *Theophylline:* Reduced serum theophylline concentrations; potential reduced therapeutic response to theophylline

SPECIAL CONSIDERATIONS

PATIENT/FAMILY EDUCATION

- Indicated only for short-term treatment of insomnia and is probably ineffective after 2 wk
- Physical dependency may result when used for extended time (45-90 days depending on dose)
- Avoid driving or other activities requiring alertness
- Avoid alcohol ingestion or CNS depressants
- Do not discontinue medication abruptly after long-term use

MONITORING PARAMETERS

- CBC, serum folate, vitamin D (if on long-term therapy)
- PT in patients receiving anticoagulants LFTs
- Mental status, vital signs

butalbital compound

(byoo-tal'bih-tall)

Butalbital/acetaminophen/caffeine: Algesic, Amaphen, Americet, Anolor 300, Anoquan, Butace, Dolmar, Endolor, Equi-Cet, Esgic, Esgic-Plus, Ezol, Fembutal, Femcet, Fioricet, G-1, Geone, Ide-Cet, Isocet, Isopap, Margesic, Medigesic, Minotal, Mygracet, Pacaps, Pharmagesic, Repan, Rogesic, Tacet, Tencet, Triad, Two-Dyne

Butalbital/aspirin/caffeine: B-A-C, Butal Compound, Butalbital Compound, Butalgen, Farbital, Fembutal, Fiorex, Fiorgen, Fiorinal, Fiormor, Fortabs, Idenal, Isobutal, Isolin, Isollyl, Laniroif, Lanorinal, Marnal, Vibutal

Chemical Class: Barbituric acid derivative (butalbital)

Therapeutic Class: Nonnarcotic analgesic; barbiturate combination

DEA Class: Schedule III (aspirin-containing products)

CLINICAL PHARMACOLOGY

Mechanism of Action: Combines the analgesic properties of acetaminophen, aspirin, and caffeine with the anxiolytic and muscle relaxant properties of butalbital

INDICATIONS AND USES: Tension (muscle contraction) headache

DOSAGE

Adult

- PO 1-2 tabs q4h as needed, max 6 tabs/day

$ AVAILABLE FORMS/COST OF THERAPY

Butalbital/Acetaminophen/Caffeine

- Cap, Gel—Oral: 50 mg/325 mg/40 mg, 100's: **$11.93-$72.73**
- Tab, Uncoated—Oral: 50 mg/325 mg/40 mg, 100's: **$5.93-$77.14;** 50 mg/500 mg/40 mg, 100's: **$62.59**

Butalbital/Aspirin/Caffeine

- Cap, Gel—Oral: 50 mg/325 mg/40 mg, 100's: **$33.75-$45.06**
- Tab, Uncoated—Oral: 325 mg/50 mg/40 mg, 100's: **$3.00-$43.32**

CONTRAINDICATIONS: Hypersensitivity to acetaminophen, aspirin, caffeine, or barbiturates; porphyria

PRECAUTIONS: History of drug abuse, elderly, children

PREGNANCY AND LACTATION: Pregnancy category C (category D if used for prolonged periods or in high doses at term); excretion into breast milk unknown (see also aspirin, acetaminophen, and caffeine)

SIDE EFFECTS/ADVERSE REACTIONS (see also aspirin, acetaminophen and caffeine)

CNS: Drowsiness, dizziness, lightheadedness, mental confusion, depression, chronic daily headache

GI: Nausea, vomiting, flatulence

▼ DRUG INTERACTIONS

Drugs

- *Oral anticoagulants+:* Barbiturates inhibit the hypoprothrombinemic response to oral anticoagulants; fatal bleeding episodes have occurred when barbiturates were discontinued in patients stabilized on an anticoagulant (see also aspirin, acetaminophen and caffeine)

SPECIAL CONSIDERATIONS

PATIENT/FAMILY EDUCATION

- May cause psychological and/or physical dependence
- May cause drowsiness, use caution driving or operating machinery
- Avoid alcohol and other CNS depressants

B

butoconazole

(byoo-toe-ko'na-zole)

Femstat

Chemical Class: Imidazole derivative of azole antimycotic agents

Therapeutic Class: Local antifungal

CLINICAL PHARMACOLOGY

Mechanism of Action: Binds sterols in fungal cell membrane, resulting in a reduced osmotic resistance and viability of the fungus

Pharmacokinetics

PV: 5.5% of dose absorbed; peak plasma levels at 24 hr; $t_{1/2}$ 21-24 hr

INDICATIONS AND USES: Vulvovaginal infections caused by susceptible organisms; antifungal spectrum usually includes: *Candida* sp., *Trichophyton, Microsporum,* and *Epidermophyton*

DOSAGE

Adult

- VAG 1 applicator hs × 3 days (nonpregnant), 6 days (2nd/3rd trimester pregnancy)

$ AVAILABLE FORMS/COST OF THERAPY

- Cre—Vag: 2%, 3 applicators: **$19.40**; 28 g: **$18.35**

CONTRAINDICATIONS: Hypersensitivity

PREGNANCY AND LACTATION: Pregnancy category C

SIDE EFFECTS/ADVERSE REACTIONS

GU: Rash, stinging, burning, vulvovaginal itching, soreness, swelling, discharge, finger itching

butorphanol

(byoo-tor'fa-nole)

Stadol

Chemical Class: Synthetically derived opioid agonist-antagonist analgesic of the phenanthrene series

Therapeutic Class: Narcotic analgesic

CLINICAL PHARMACOLOGY

Mechanism of Action: Mixed agonist-antagonist action at opioid receptors; acts centrally to depress respirations and cough, stimulate emetic center and cause sedation

Pharmacokinetics

IM: Onset 10-30 min, peak ½ hr, duration 3-4 hr

IV: Onset 1 min, peak 5 min, duration 2-4 hr

PR: Onset slow, duration 4-6 hr

NASAL: 15 min; peak 30-60 min

80% protein bound; extensively metabolized by liver; excreted by kidneys (reduce dose to 75% for Cl_{cr} 10-50 ml/min, to 50% for $Cl_{cr} < 10$ ml/min); $t_{1/2}$ 2½-3½ hr

INDICATIONS AND USES: Moderate to severe pain, including postoperative analgesia, preoperative or preanesthetic medication, as a supplement to balanced anesthesia, and for the relief of pain during labor

DOSAGE

Adult

- IM 1-4 mg q3-4h prn (2 mg IM is approximately equivalent to 10 mg morphine or 80 mg meperidine); IV 0.5-2 mg q3-4h prn; NASAL 1 mg (1 spray in one nostril); may repeat in 60-90 minutes if adequate pain relief is not achieved; initial two dose sequence may be repeated in 3-4 hours as needed; depending on the severity of the pain, an initial dose of 2 mg (1 spray in each nostril) may be given

- *Geriatric:* Half the usual dose at twice the usual interval

$ AVAILABLE FORMS/COST OF THERAPY

- Aer, Spray—Nasal: 10 mg/ml, 2.5 ml: **$55.75**
- Inj, Sol—IM; IV: 1 mg/ml, 1 ml: **$6.93;** 2 mg/ml, 1 ml: **$7.23**

CONTRAINDICATIONS: Hypersensitivity, narcotic addiction (may precipitate withdrawal), CHF, MI

PRECAUTIONS: Hypotension, addictive personality, head injuries, increased intracranial pressure, respiratory depression, hepatic disease, renal disease; child <18 yr

PREGNANCY AND LACTATION: Pregnancy category B; crosses placenta; excreted in breast milk, though probably clinically insignificant

SIDE EFFECTS/ADVERSE REACTIONS

CNS: Drowsiness, dizziness, confusion, headache, sedation, euphoria, asthenia/lethargy, hallucinations, drug abuse and dependence

CV: Palpitations, bradycardia, hypotension, hypertension

EENT: Tinnitus, blurred vision, miosis, diplopia, *nasal congestion, epistaxis, nasal irritation, sinus congestion*

GI: Nausea, vomiting, anorexia, constipation, dry mouth, cramps

GU: Increased urinary output, dysuria, urinary retention

RESP: ***Respiratory depression,*** pulmonary hypertension

SKIN: Rash, urticaria, bruising, flushing, diaphoresis, pruritus

▼ DRUG INTERACTIONS

Drugs

- *Nasal vasoconstrictors:* slower onset of action of butorphanol

Labs

- *Increase:* Amylase

SPECIAL CONSIDERATIONS

Chronic use can precipitate withdrawal symptoms of anxiety, agitation, mood changes, hallucinations, dysphoria, weakness, and diarrhea

caffeine

(kaf'-een)

Caffedrine, Caffeine, Citrated Caffeine, Dexitac, No-Doz, Quick Pep, Tirend, Vivarin; also available in a number of OTC analgesic combinations

Chemical Class: Xanthine
Therapeutic Class: Analeptic

CLINICAL PHARMACOLOGY

Mechanism of Action: Increases calcium permeability in sarcoplasmic reticulum; promotes accumulation of cAMP; competitively blocks adenosine receptors; stimulates the CNS, produces diuresis, relaxes smooth bronchial muscle

Pharmacokinetics

PO: Onset 15 min, peak ½-1 hr; metabolized by liver, less than 5% excreted unchanged by kidneys, crosses placenta, $t_{1/2}$ 3-4 hr

INDICATIONS AND USES: Respiratory depression associated with overdose; CNS stimulation; aid in staying awake and restoring mental alertness, adjuvant with analgesics, diuretic for fluid retention associated with menstruation, neonatal apnea;* headaches associated with spinal puncture,* orthostatic hypotension*

DOSAGE

Adult

- PO 100-200 mg q4h prn; timed rel 200-250 mg q4-6h; IM 500 mg

Child

- Neonatal apnea: PO 10-20 mg/kg as caffeine citrate (5-10 mg/kg as caffeine base). Maintenance 5-10 mg/kg as caffeine citrate based on response and serum levels

$ AVAILABLE FORMS/COST OF THERAPY

• Tab—Oral: 100 mg, 12's: **$1.58;** 150 mg, 12's: **$1.07;** 200 mg, 12's: **$1.69**
• Caplets/Caps—Oral: 200 mg, 12's: **$1.67**
• Inj, Sol—IM; IV: 250 mg/ml, 2 ml: **$6.81**

CONTRAINDICATIONS: Hypersensitivity

PRECAUTIONS: Dysrhythmias, Gilles de la Tourette's disorder, renal, psychologic disorders, depression, ulcers, diabetes mellitus

PREGNANCY AND LACTATION: Pregnancy category B; amounts in breast milk after maternal ingestion of caffeinated beverages not clinically significant; accumulation can occur in heavy using mothers

SIDE EFFECTS/ADVERSE REACTIONS

CNS: Hyperactivity, insomnia, restlessness, talkativeness, dizziness, headache, *stimulation,* irritability, aggressiveness, tremors, twitching, mild delirium, tinnitus, scintillating scotoma

CV: Tachycardia, extrasystole, dysrhythmias, palpitations

GI: Nausea, vomiting, anorexia, gastric irritation, diarrhea

GU: Diuresis

HEME: Hypoglycemia

SKIN: Hyperesthesia

▼ DRUG INTERACTIONS

Drugs

• *Ciprofloxacin:* Increases caffeine concentrations and may enhance its side effects
• *Pipemidic acid:* Produces a large increase in caffeine concentrations and may increase side effects

Labs

• *Increase:* Urinary catecholamines
• *False positive:* Serum urate

SPECIAL CONSIDERATIONS

PATIENT/FAMILY EDUCATION

• Gradual taper if used long-term to prevent withdrawal syndrome, especially headache

calcifediol

(kal-si-fe-dye'ole)

Calderol

Chemical Class: Sterol

Therapeutic Class: Vit D analog

CLINICAL PHARMACOLOGY

Mechanism of Action: Increases intestinal absorption of calcium; increases renal tubular absorption of phosphate; increases mobilization of calcium from bones, bone resorption

Pharmacokinetics

PO: Peak 4 hr, duration 15-20 days; rapid absorption from small intestine, activated in kidneys, stored in liver and fat, $t_{1/2}$ 12-22 days, excreted via bile in feces

INDICATIONS AND USES: Management of metabolic bone disease or hypocalcemia in patients with chronic renal failure

DOSAGE

Adult

• PO: 300-350 μg qwk divided into qd or qod doses; may increase q4wk

$ AVAILABLE FORMS/COST OF THERAPY

• Cap, Elastic, Sust Action—Oral: 20 μg, 60's: **$48.37;** 50 μg, 60's: **$110.32**

CONTRAINDICATIONS: Hypersensitivity, hyperphosphatemia, hypercalcemia, Vit D toxicity

PRECAUTIONS: Renal calculi, CV disease

PREGNANCY AND LACTATION: Pregnancy category C; excreted in breast milk and may cause infant hypercalcemia

SIDE EFFECTS/ADVERSE REACTIONS

CNS: Drowsiness, headache, vertigo, fever, lethargy

CV: ***Dysrhythmias***

EENT: Tinnitus, conjunctivitis, photophobia, rhinorrhea

GI: Nausea, diarrhea, vomiting, jaundice, anorexia, dry mouth, constipation, cramps, metallic taste

GU: Polyuria, hypercalciuria, hyperphosphatemia, hematuria

MS: Myalgia, arthralgia, decreased bone development

▼ DRUG INTERACTIONS

Drugs

- *Cholestyramine:* Decreased absorption of calcifediol
- *Colestipol:* Decreased absorption of calcifediol
- *Corticosteroids:* Decreased vitamin D effects
- *Mineral oil:* Decreased absorption of calcifediol
- *Thiazide diuretics:* Hypercalcemia

Labs

- *Increase:* Serum calcium, alkaline phosphatase, parathyroid hormone levels
- *False increase:* Cholesterol

SPECIAL CONSIDERATIONS

MONITORING PARAMETERS

- Blood Ca, P determinations must be made every 2 weeks, or more frequently if necessary
- Vit D levels also helpful, although less frequently
- Height and weight in children

calcitonin (human; salmon)

(kal-si-toe′ nin)

Human: Cibacalcin

Salmon: Calcimar, Miacalcin

Chemical Class: Polypeptide hormone

Therapeutic Class: Parathyroid agents (calcium regulator)

CLINICAL PHARMACOLOGY

Mechanism of Action: Decreases bone resorption and blood calcium levels; increases deposits of calcium in bones; analgesic effect thought to be related to prostaglandin inhibition

Pharmacokinetics

IM/SC: Onset 15 min, peak 4 hr, duration 8-24 hr; metabolized by kidneys, excreted as inactive metabolites

INDICATIONS AND USES: Hypercalcemia, postmenopausal osteoporosis, Paget's disease, analgesia secondary to vertebral fracture

DOSAGE

- *Skin test* (salmon calcitonin): 1 unit/0.1 mg (0.1 ml of 10 IU dilution) intradermally; observe for 15 min for significant erythema

Adult

- *Osteoporosis:* Salmon SC/IM 100 IU qd; NASAL 200 IU QD alternating nostrils
- *Hypercalcemia:* Salmon IM 4-8 IU/kg q6-12h
- *Paget's disease:* Human SC 0.5 mg/day initially maintenance range 0.5 mg bid to 0.25-0.5 mg 2-3 ×/week; Salmon SC/IM 100 IU qd initially; usual maintenance 50 IU qd or qod
- *Analgesic doses:* Same as above, salmon 100 IU SC/IM qd × 2-4 wk, then 50 IU qod-tiw as maintenance

(effect should be noticeable within 2 wk)

$ AVAILABLE FORMS/COST OF THERAPY

• Inj, Sol—IM; SC: 200 U/ml, 2 ml: **$26.40-$42.45** (salmon)
• Spray, Sol—Nasal: 200 IU/metered dose, 14 doses/2 ml: **$28.50** (salmon)
• Inj, Sol—SC: 0.5 mg/syringe, 1 ml: **$8.78** (human)

CONTRAINDICATIONS: Hypersensitivity (skin test recommended for salmon calcitonin), children

PRECAUTIONS: Hypocalcemia

PREGNANCY AND LACTATION: Pregnancy category C; inhibits lactation in animals

SIDE EFFECTS/ADVERSE REACTIONS

CNS: Headache, flushing, ***tetany,*** chills, weakness, dizziness
CV: Chest pressure
ENT: Nasal irritation, dryness, redness, itching, bleeding
GI: Nausea, diarrhea, vomiting, anorexia, abdominal pain, salty taste, epigastric pain
GU: Diuresis
MS: Swelling, tingling of hands
RESP: Dyspnea
SKIN: Rash, flushing, pruritus of ear lobes, edema of feet

SPECIAL CONSIDERATIONS

MONITORING PARAMETERS

• Monitor serum Ca

calcitriol (1,25-dihydroxycholecalciferol)

(kal-si-trye'ole)

Rocaltrol, Calcijex

Chemical Class: Vitamin D hormone

Therapeutic Class: Parathyroid agents (calcium regulator)

CLINICAL PHARMACOLOGY

Mechanism of Action: 1,25-(OH) 2D3 (calcitriol), the active form of vitamin D3; active in regulation of the absorption of calcium from the gastrointestinal tract and its utilization in the body; increases renal tubular resorption of phosphate

Pharmacokinetics

PO: Peak 3-6 hr, duration 3-5 days, $t_{1/2}$ 3-6 hr; rapid oral absorption, metabolized and excreted via bile in feces, 4-6% excreted in urine

INDICATIONS AND USES: Hypocalcemia in chronic renal disease, hypoparathyroidism, osteoporosis; pseudohypoparathyroidism

DOSAGE

Adult

• *Hypocalcemia:* PO 0.25 µg qd, may increase by 0.25 µg/day q4-8wk, maintenance 0.25-3 µg qd
• *Hypoparathyroidism/pseudohypoparathyroidism:* PO 0.25 µg qd, may be increased by 0.25 µg/day q2-4wk maintenance 0.25-2 µg qd
• *Osteoporosis:* 0.25 µg qd

Child (>1 yr)

• *Hypoparathyroidism/pseudohypoparathyroidism:* PO 0.25 µg qd, may be increased q2-4 wk; maintenance 0.25-2 µg qd

$ AVAILABLE FORMS/COST OF THERAPY

• Cap, Elastic—Oral: 0.25 µg, 30's: **$30.21;** 0.5 µg, 100's: **$158.72**

• Inj, Sol—IV: 1 μg/ml, 1 ml: **$588.75;** 2 μg/ml, 1 ml: **$1010.00**

CONTRAINDICATIONS: Hypersensitivity, hyperphosphatemia, hypercalcemia, Vit D toxicity

PRECAUTIONS: Renal calculi, CV disease

PREGNANCY AND LACTATION: Pregnancy category C; may be excreted in breast milk

SIDE EFFECTS/ADVERSE REACTIONS

CNS: Drowsiness, headache, vertigo, fever, lethargy

GI: Nausea, diarrhea, vomiting, jaundice, anorexia, dry mouth, constipation, cramps, metallic taste

GU: Polyuria, hypercalciuria, hyperphosphatemia, hematuria

MS: Myalgia, arthralgia, decreased bone development

▼ DRUG INTERACTIONS

Drugs

• *Barbiturates, phenytoin, corticosteroids:* Anti-vitamin D effects

• *Cholestyramine, colestipol, mineral oil:* Decreased absorption

• *Digoxin:* Cardiac arrhythmias with hypercalcemia

• *Thiazide diuretics*: Hypercalcemia

• *Verapamil:* Cardiac arrhythmias with hypercalcemia

Labs

• *False increase:* Cholesterol

SPECIAL CONSIDERATIONS

MONITORING PARAMETERS

• Blood Ca and P determinations must be made every week until stable, or more frequently if necessary

• Vit D levels also helpful, although less frequently

• Height and weight in children

• Avoid magnesium-containing antacids

calcium salts

Calcium acetate: PhosLo, Phos-Ex

Calcium carbonate: Alka-Mints, Amitone, Biocal, Cal Carb-HD, Calci-Chew, Calci-Mix, Cal Carb-HD, Calciday, Cal-Guard, Cal-Plus, Caltrate, Caltrate Jr., Chooz, Dicarbosil, Equilet, Florical, Gelcalc, Mallamint, Nephro-Calci, Os-Cal, Oyster-cal, Oysco, Oyst-Cal, Oyster Shell Calcium, Rolaids, Titralac, Tums

Calcium chloride: Cal Plus

Calcium citrate: Citracal

Calcium glubionate: Neo-Calglucon

Calcium gluconate: Kalcinate

Tricalcium phosphate: Posture

Therapeutic Class: Cation electrolyte, calcium supplement, antacid

CLINICAL PHARMACOLOGY

Mechanism of Action: Neutralizes gastric acidity; cation needed for maintenance of nervous, muscular, skeletal, enzyme reactions, normal cardiac contractility, coagulation of blood; effects secretory activity of endocrine, exocrine glands: Percentage elemental calcium content of various calcium salts: calcium acetate (25), calcium carbonate (40), calcium chloride (27.2), calcium citrate (21), calcium glubionate (6.5), calcium gluceptate (8.2), calcium gluconate (9.3), calcium lactate (13), tricalcium phosphate, (39)

Pharmacokinetics

PO: 30% absorbed (variably) depending on needs, demands, etc.; Vitamin D dependent; bioavailability not significantly different between different salts

IV: Rapid increase in serum levels, with return to pre-drug level within

30 min-2 hr; 80% excreted in the feces as insoluble salts; urinary excretion accounts for the remaining 20%

INDICATIONS AND USES: Prevention and treatment of hypocalcemia, hypermagnesemia, hypoparathyroidism, osteoporosis, neonatal tetany, cardiac toxicity caused by hyperkalemia, cardiac arrest (adjunct), lead colic, hyperphosphatemia, Vit D deficiency; hyperacidity (antacid)

DOSAGE

Adult

• Calcium acetate

Hyperphosphatemia: PO initial, 1334 mg/2 tabs with meals; increase gradually to bring phosphate below 6 mg/dl (usually 3-4 tabs per meal)

• Calcium carbonate

Hypocalcemia (replenish electrolytes): PO 1.25 g (500 mg Ca^{++}) 4-6 per day, chewed with water

Antacid: PO tabs 500 mg-1 g (250-500 mg Ca^{++}) 1 hr pc, hs; SUSP 1.25 g (500 mg Cat^{++}), 1 hr pc, hs

• Calcium chloride

Hypocalcemia (replenish electrolytes): IV 500 mg-1 g (6.8-13.6 mEq Ca^{++}) q1-3 days as indicated by serum calcium levels; give at <1 ml/min

Cardiotonic: IV 500 mg-1 g (6.8-13.6 mEq Ca^{++}); give at <1 ml/min; Intraventricular 200-800 mg (2.72-9.6 mEq Ca^{++}) inj as single dose

• Calcium citrate

Hypocalcemia (replenish electrolytes): PO: 950 mg-1.9 g (200-400 mg Ca^{++}) tid-qid, pc

• Calcium glubionate

Hypocalcemia (replenish electrolytes): 5.4 g (345 mg Ca^{++}) tid-qid

• Calcium gluceptate

Hypocalcemia (replenish electrolytes): IM 440 mg-1.1 g (1.8-4.5 mEq Ca^{++}); IV 1.1-4.4 g (1.8-4.5 mEq Ca^{++}), slowly (rate not to exceed 2 mL/min)

• Calcium gluconate

Hypocalcemia, hyperkalemia, hypermagnesemia (replenish electrolytes): PO 11 g (1 g Ca^{++})/day in divided doses; IV 1 g (4.72 mEq Ca^{++}) at 0.5 ml/min (10% sol)

• Calcium lactate

Hypocalcemia: PO 325 mg-1.3 g (1 g Ca^{++}/day) tid with meals

• Tribasic calcium phosphate:

Hypocalcemia: PO 1.6 mg (600 mg Ca^{++}) bid after meals

Child

• Calcium chloride: IV 25 mg/kg over several min

• Calcium glubionate

Infants up to 1 yr PO 1.8 g (115 mg Ca^{++}) 5 times daily before meals

Children 1-4 yr PO 3.6 g (230 mg Ca^{++}) tid, ac

Children > 4 yr PO see adult dose

• Calcium gluceptate

Newborn

Hypocalcemia: IM 440 mg-1.1 g (1.8-4.5 mEq Ca^{++}); IV 440 mg-1.1 g (1.8-4.5 mEq Ca^{++}) as single dose, rate not to exceed 2 mL/min

Exchange transfusions in newborns: IV 110 mg (approx. 0.45 mEq Ca^{++}) after every 100 ml of blood transfused

• Calcium gluconate: PO 500 mg/kg/day in divided doses, pc

• Calcium lactate: PO 500 mg/kg/day in divided doses

$ **AVAILABLE FORMS/COST OF THERAPY**

Calcium acetate

• Inj, Sol—IV: 0.5 mEq/ml, 10 ml: **$0.99-$3.34**

• Tab, Uncoated—Oral: 667 mg, 200's: **$17.94**

Calcium carbonate

• Tab, Uncoated—Oral/Chewable: 500 mg, 60's: **$2.00;** 650 mg, 60's: **$2.95**

Calcium chloride

• Inj, Sol—IV: 10%, 10 ml: **$4.53-$12.80**

Calcium citrate
• Tab: 950 mg, 100's: **$2.98-$6.87**
Calcium glubionate
• Syr—Oral: 1.8 g/5 ml, 480 ml: **$16.00-$21.48**
Calcium gluceptate
• Inj, Sol—IM; IV: 90 mg/5 ml, 50 ml: **$11.90**
Calcium gluconate
• Inj, Sol—IV: 10%, 10 ml: **$1.75**
• Tab: 500 mg, 100's: **$5.00-$6.91;** 650 mg, 100's: **$2.16-$3.49;** 975 mg, 100's: **$7.95**
Calcium lactate
• Tab: 325 mg, 100's: **$1.50;** 650 mg, 100's: **$1.55-$5.25**
Tribasic calcium phosphate
• Tab: 600 mg, 60's: **$7.81**

CONTRAINDICATIONS: Hypersensitivity, hypercalcemia, hypercalciuria, hyperparathyroidism, bone tumors, digitalis toxicity, ventricular fibrillation, renal calculi, sarcoidosis, renal insufficiency (tribasic calcium phosphate)

PRECAUTIONS: Elderly, fluid restriction, decreased GI motility, GI obstruction, dehydration

PREGNANCY AND LACTATION: Pregnancy category C; some oral supplemental calcium may be excreted in breast milk (chloride, gluconate, unknown); concentrations not sufficient to produce an adverse effect in neonates

SIDE EFFECTS/ADVERSE REACTIONS

CV: Hemorrhage, ***rebound hypertension,*** shortened Q-T, heart block, hypotension, bradycardia, dysrhythymias, ***cardiac arrest***

GI: Constipation, anorexia, ***obstruction,*** nausea, vomiting, flatulence, diarrhea, rebound hyperacidity, eructation

GU: Renal dysfunction, renal stones, ***renal failure***

METAB: Hypercalcemia (drowsiness, lethargy, muscle weakness, headache, constipation, ***coma,*** anorexia, nausea, vomiting, polyuria, thirst), metabolic alkalosis; milk-alkali syndrome (nausea, vomiting, disorientation, headache)

MISC: Pain, burning at IV site, severe venous thrombosis, necrosis, extravasation

▼ **DRUG INTERACTIONS**

Drugs

• *Amphetamines:* Alkalinization of urine inhibits the elimination and increases the effects of amphetamines
• *Cefpodoxime proxetil:* Antacids reduce the bioavailability and serum concentrations of cefpodoxime
• *Ciprofloxacin, enoxacin, lomefloxacin, norfloxacin, ofloxacin:* Antacids reduce the serum concentrations of quinolones and may inhibit efficacy
• *Doxycycline+:* Co-therapy with a tetracycline and a divalent or trivalent cation can reduce the serum concentration and efficacy of the tetracycline
• *Iron:* Some calcium antacids reduce the GI absorption of iron; inhibition of the hematological response to iron has been reported
• *Quinidine:* Calcium antacids capable of increasing urine pH may increase serum quinidine concentrations
• *Salicylates:* Antacids (large doses) can decrease serum salicylate concentrations in patients receiving large doses of salicylates, requiring salicylate dosage adjustment
• *Sodium polystyrene sulfonate resin:* Combined use with calcium-containing antacid may result in systemic alkalosis
• *Tetracycline+:* Co-therapy with a tetracycline and a divalent or triva-

lent cation can reduce the serum concentration and efficacy of the tetracycline

Labs

- *Increase:* 11-OHCS
- *False decrease:* Magnesium
- *Decrease:* 17-OHCS

SPECIAL CONSIDERATIONS

MONITORING PARAMETERS

- Serum calcium or serum ionized calcium concentrations (ionized calcium concentrations are preferable to determine free and bound calcium, especially with concurrent low serum albumin)
- Alternatively, ionized calcium can be estimated using the following rule: total serum calcium will fall by 0.8 mg/dL for each 1.0 g/dL decrease in serum albumin concentration

---

capreomycin

(kap-ree-oh-mye′sin)

Capastat

Chemical Class: S. capreolus polypeptide antibiotic

Therapeutic Class: Antibacterial (antimycobacterial)

CLINICAL PHARMACOLOGY

Mechanism of Action: Inhibits RNA synthesis, decreases mycobacterial bacilli replication

Pharmacokinetics

IM: Peak 1-2 hr, mean 28-32 μg/mL (range 20-47 μg/mL after 1 g dose) mean urine concentrations after 1 g dose, 1680 μg/mL; $t_{1/2}$ 4-6 hr (prolonged with decreased renal function); excreted in urine unchanged (small amount in bile)

INDICATIONS AND USES: Pulmonary tuberculosis caused by *Mycobacterium tuberculosis* after failure or intolerability with primary medications; concurrently with other antituberculars

DOSAGE

Adult

- IM 1 g or 13.9 mg/kg (not to exceed 20 mg/kg/day) qd × 2-4 mo, then 1 g 2-3 ×/wk × 18-24 mo, not to exceed 20 mg/kg/day; *must* be given with another antitubercular medication; dosage reduction necessary with declining renal function, as follows (dose in mg/kg/day designed to achieve steady state levels of 10 mg/L: if CrCl = 50 ml/min, give 7 mg/kg q24h; if CrCl = 20 ml/min, give 3.6 mg/kg q24h; if CrCl = 10 ml/min, give 2.4 mg/kg q24h; if CrCl = 0 ml/min, give 1.3 mg/kg q24h

$ AVAILABLE FORMS/COST OF THERAPY

- Inj, Sol—IM: 1 g/5 ml, 10 ml: **$20.86**

CONTRAINDICATIONS: Hypersensitivity

PRECAUTIONS: Renal disease, hearing impairment, allergy history, hepatic disease, myasthenia gravis, parkinsonism

PREGNANCY AND LACTATION: Pregnancy category C; breast milk excretion is unknown, however, problems in humans have not been documented (poorly absorbed from GI tract)

SIDE EFFECTS/ADVERSE REACTIONS

CNS: Vertigo, fever, headache

EENT: Tinnitus, deafness, ototoxicity

GU: ***Proteinuria,*** decreased CrCl, increased BUN, serum Cr, ***tubular necrosis,*** hypokalemia, alkalosis, hematuria, ***albuminuria, nephrotoxicity***

HEME: ***Eosinophilia, leukocytosis, leukopenia***

SKIN: Pain, irritation, sterile abscess at injection site, rash, urticaria

▼ **DRUG INTERACTIONS**

Drugs

- *Amphotericin B:* Additive nephrotoxicity risk
- *Cephalosporins:* Additive nephrotoxicity
- *Cyclosporine:* Additive nephrotoxicity
- *Ethacrynic acid+:* Additive ototoxicity
- *Methoxyflurane:* Enhanced nephrotoxicity
- *Neuromuscular blocking agents+:* Potentiate the respiratory suppression produced by neuromuscular blocking agents
- *Oral anticoagulants:* Enhanced hypothrombinemic response

SPECIAL CONSIDERATIONS

MONITORING PARAMETERS

- Liver and renal function studies
- Blood levels of drug
- Audiometric testing before, during, after treatment
- Serum K (hypokalemia may occur)
- When used in renal insufficiency or preexisting auditory impairment, risks of additional eighth-nerve impairment or renal injury should be weighed against the benefits of therapy

---

captopril

(kap'toe-pril)

Capoten

Chemical Class: Angiotensin-converting enzyme inhibitor

Therapeutic Class: Antihypertensive, afterload reducer

CLINICAL PHARMACOLOGY

Mechanism of Action: Selectively suppresses renin-angiotensin-aldosterone system; inhibits angiotensin-converting enzyme (ACE); prevents conversion of angiotensin I to angiotensin II; results in dilation of arterial and venous vessels

Pharmacokinetics

PO: Peak 1 hr (presence of food reduces absorption by 3-40%); duration 2-6 hr; $t_{1/2}$ <2-3 hr; metabolized by liver (metabolites), excreted in urine (40-50% unchanged); crosses placenta; excreted in breast milk

INDICATIONS AND USES: Hypertension, heart failure, left ventricular dysfunction after MI, diabetic nephropathy (proteinuria >500 mg/day) in type I patients; hypertensive crises,* neonatal and childhood hypertension,* rheumatoid arthritis,* diagnosis of anatomic renal artery stenosis,* diagnosis of primary aldosteronism, idiopathic edema, Barter's syndrome (improves K metabolism and corrects hypokalemia)*

DOSAGE

Adult

- *Malignant hypertension:* PO 25 mg increasing q2h until desired response, not to exceed 450 mg/day
- *Hypertension:* Initial dose 12.5 mg bid-tid (consider discontinuing previous antihypertensive therapy, especially diuretics prior to starting); may increase to 50 mg bid-tid at 1-2 wk intervals; usual range 25-150 mg bid-tid; max 450 mg/day
- *Diabetic nephropathy:* Initial dose 12.5 mg bid-tid; may increase to 50 mg bid-tid at 1-2 wk intervals; usual range: 25-150 mg bid-tid
- *Congestive heart failure:* 12.5 mg bid-tid (consider smaller doses in patients vigorously pretreated with diuretics and who may be hyponatremic and/or hypovolemic, i.e., a starting dose of 6.25); may increase to 50 mg bid-tid; after 14 days, may increase to 150 mg tid if needed

Child

- *Hypertension:* Initiate 0.15 mg/

kg/dose; double at intervals of approx. 2 hr until BP controlled (max 6 mg/kg/24 hr)

$ AVAILABLE FORMS/COST OF THERAPY

- Tab, Uncoated—Oral: 12.5 mg, 100's: **$63.63;** 25 mg, 100's: **$68.78;** 50 mg, 100's: **$117.94;** 100 mg, 100's: **$160.86**

CONTRAINDICATIONS: Hypersensitivity, heart block, K-sparing diuretics, bilateral renal artery stenosis

PRECAUTIONS: Dialysis patients, hypovolemia, leukemia, scleroderma, lupus erythematosus, blood dyscrasias, thyroid disease, COPD, asthma, impaired renal function, severe renal artery stenosis, CHF, hyperkalemia, cough, aortic stenosis, pediatric use (limited experience; infants, especially newborns, may be more susceptible to the adverse hemodynamic effects)

PREGNANCY AND LACTATION: Pregnancy category C (first trimester) and D (second and third trimesters—fetal and neonatal hypotension, neonatal skull hypoplasia, anuria, reversible or irreversible renal failure, death, oligohydramnios); excreted into breast milk in small amounts (average milk:plasma ratio = 0.012); compatible with breast feeding

SIDE EFFECTS/ADVERSE REACTIONS

CNS: Fever, chills

CV: Hypotension, postural hypotension, tachycardia, chest pain, palpitations

GI: Loss of taste

GU: Impotence, dysuria, nocturia, proteinuria, ***nephrotic syndrome, acute reversible renal failure,*** polyuria, oliguria, frequency

HEME: ***Neutropenia,*** agranulocytosis

METAB: Hyperkalemia, hyponatremia

RESP: Bronchospasm, dyspnea, cough, ***angioedema***

SKIN: Rash

▼ DRUG INTERACTIONS

Drugs

- *Allopurinol:* Increased risk of hypersensitivity reactions including Stevens-Johnson syndrome, skin eruptions, fever, and arthralgias
- *Loop diuretics:* Initiation of ACE inhibition therapy with concurrent intensive diuretic therapy may cause significant hypotension, renal insufficiency
- *Indomethacin:* Inhibits the antihypertensive response to ACE inhibition; other NSAIDs probably have similar effect
- *Lithium:* Increased risk of lithium toxicity
- *Potassium:* ACE inhibition tends to increase potassium; increased risk of hyperkalemia in predisposed patients
- *Potassium sparing diuretics:* ACE inhibition tends to increase potassium; increased risk of hyperkalemia in predisposed patients

Labs

- *Increase:* Potassium, BUN/creatinine (transient, especially in renovascular hypertension, volume depleted patients and those with rapid BP reduction)
- *Decrease:* Sodium (especially in patients on diuretics or low sodium diet)
- *False positive:* Urine acetone, ANA (0.5 mEq/dl)

SPECIAL CONSIDERATIONS

ACE inhibition can account for approximately 0.5 mEq/L rise in serum potassium

carbachol

(kar'ba-kole)

Miostat; Isopto Carbachol

Chemical Class: Parasympathomimetic agent

Therapeutic Class: Antiglaucoma agent

CLINICAL PHARMACOLOGY

Mechanism of Action: Cholinergic (parasympathomimetic) agent, stimulates the motor endplate of the muscle cell, and also partially inhibits cholinesterase; contracts sphincter muscle of iris; causes spasms of ciliary muscle, deepening of anterior chamber

Pharmacokinetics

OPHTH: Onset of miosis, 10-20 min; peak reduction in intraocular pressure 4 hr; duration of miosis 4-8 hr; decreased intraocular pressure 8 hr

INTRAOCULAR: peak miosis within 2-5 min; duration miosis 24 hr

INDICATIONS AND USES: Miosis induction, ocular surgery, glaucoma (open-angle, narrow-angle)

DOSAGE

• *Ocular surgery:* INTRAOCULAR 0.5 ml 0.01% sol in anterior chamber of eye (done by physician) for miosis during surgery

• *Glaucoma:* INSTILL 1-2 gtt (topical) of 0.75%-3% sol into eye bid-tid

$ **AVAILABLE FORMS/COST OF THERAPY**

• Sol—Ophth: 0.75%, 15 ml: **$16.25;** 1.5%, 15 ml: **$17.06;** 2.25%, 15 ml: **$17.87;** 3%, 15 ml: **$18.62**

CONTRAINDICATIONS: Hypersensitivity; when miosis is undesirable; corneal abrasions

PRECAUTIONS: Bradycardia, CAD, hyperthyroidism, asthma, pregnancy, obstruction of GI or urinary tract, peptic ulcer, parkinsonism, epilepsy, peritonitis; retinal detachment reported in susceptible individuals

PREGNANCY AND LACTATION: Pregnancy category C

SIDE EFFECTS/ADVERSE REACTIONS

CV: ***Marked hypotension,*** bradycardia, headache

EENT: Blurred vision, myopia, decreased visual acuity in dim light, conjunctival hyperemia, eye ache

GI: Nausea, vomiting, abdominal discomfort, diarrhea, salivation

RESP: ***Bronchospasm***

SPECIAL CONSIDERATIONS

PATIENT/FAMILY EDUCATION

• Blurred vision will decrease with repeated use of drug

• Caution if driving during first few days of treatment

carbamazepine

(kar-ba-maz'e-peen)

Apo-Carbamazepine, ✤ Epitol, Mazepine, ✤ Novocarbamaz, ✤ PMS Carbamazepine, ✤ Tegretol

Chemical Class: Imino stilbene derivative

Therapeutic Class: Anticonvulsant, antineuralgic, antimanic, antidiuretic, antipsychotic

CLINICAL PHARMACOLOGY

Mechanism of Action: Anticonvulsant action by inhibition of influx of sodium ions across nerve cell membrane in motor cortex, reducing polysynaptic response and blocking the posttetanic potentiation; antineuralgic may involve $GABA_B$ receptors, which may be linked to calcium channels; antimanic/antipsychotic effects on neurotransmitter modulator systems

Pharmacokinetics

PO: Anticonvulsant onset varies hrs

to days; anineuralgic onset 8-72 hr; antimanic onset 7-10 days; peak concentrations: susp 1.5 hr; tabs 4-5 hr; therapeutic serum concentrations 4-12 μg/mL; absorption slow (suspension faster than tablets), metabolized by liver (autoinduction); excreted in urine and feces; crosses placenta; excreted in breast milk; $t_{1/2}$ variable, 14-16 hr after repeated dosing

INDICATIONS AND USES: Tonic-clonic, complex-partial, mixed seizures; trigeminal neuralgia, glossopharyngeal neuralgia; manic depressive disorder, chronic neurogenic pain syndromes,* diabetes insipidus (central),* alcohol withdrawal,* psychotic disorders,* restless legs syndrome*

DOSAGE

Adult

- *Seizures:* PO 200 mg bid, may be increased by 200 mg/day in divided doses q6-8h; maintenance 800-1200 mg/day; max 1200 mg/day
- *Trigeminal neuralgia:* PO 100 mg bid, may increase 100 mg q12h until pain subsides, not to exceed 1.2 g/day; maintenance is 200-400 mg bid
- *Antidiuretic:* 300-600 mg/day, as sole therapy; 200-400 mg/day if concurrent with other antidiuretic agents
- *Antipsychotic:* PO 200-400 mg/day divided tid-qid; max 1600 mg/day

Child

- *Seizures:* >12 years PO 200 mg bid, may be increased by 200 mg/day in divided doses q6-8h, maintenance 800-1200 mg/day; max 1200 mg/day; <12 yr PO 10-20 mg/kg/day in 2-3 divided doses

$ AVAILABLE FORMS/COST OF THERAPY

- Tab, Chewable—Oral: 100 mg, 100's: **$14.50-$18.00**
- Tab, Uncoated—Oral: 200 mg, 100's: **$17.27-$34.66**
- Susp—Oral: 100 mg/5 ml, 450 ml: **$22.32**

CONTRAINDICATIONS: Hypersensitivity to carbamazepine or tricyclic antidepressants, bone marrow depression, concomitant use of MAOIs

PRECAUTIONS: Glaucoma, hepatic disease, renal disease, cardiac disease, psychosis, child <6 yr

PREGNANCY AND LACTATION: Pregnancy category C; concentration in milk approximately 60% of maternal plasma concentration, compatible with breast feeding

SIDE EFFECTS/ADVERSE REACTIONS

CNS: Ataxia, drowsiness, dizziness, confusion, fatigue, ***paralysis,*** headache, hallucinations

CV: Hypertension, ***CHF,*** hypotension, aggravation of coronary artery disease

EENT: Tinnitus, dry mouth, blurred vision, diplopia, nystagmus, conjunctivitis

GI: Nausea, *constipation, diarrhea,* anorexia, vomiting, abdominal pain, stomatitis, glossitis, increased liver enzymes, ***hepatitis***

GU: Frequency, urinary retention, albuminuria, glycosuria, impotence

HEME: ***Thrombocytopenia, agranulocytosis, leukocytosis, neutropenia, aplastic anemia, eosinophilia***

RESP: Pulmonary hypersensitivity (fever, dyspnea, pneumonitis)

SKIN: Rash, ***Stevens-Johnson syndrome,*** urticaria

▼ DRUG INTERACTIONS

Drugs

- *Antidepressants, tricyclic:* Carbamazepine reduces serum concentrations of imipramine and probably other cyclic antidepressants
- *Calcium channel blockers:* Verapamil and diltiazem reduce the me-

tabolism, of carbamazepine leading to increased carbamazepine toxicity when these CCBs are added to chronic carbamazepine therapy; enzyme induction by carbamazepine can reduce the bioavailability of CCBs that undergo extensive first-pass hepatic clearance, like felodipine (94% reduction)

• *Cimetidine, danazol, erythromycin, fluoxetine, isoniazid+, propoxyphene+, quinine, troleandomycin:* These drugs cause increased carbamazepine levels, with increased risk of toxicity (with cimetidine, dissipates after one wk; with erythromycin, marked increase via inhibition of hepatic oxidative metabolism)

• *Clozapine, corticosteroids, cyclosporine, doxycycline, haloperidol, methadone, theophylline, thyroid hormone:* Reduced concentrations of and therapeutic response to these drugs

• *Lithium:* Increased potential for neurotoxicity with normal lithium concentrations; reverses carbamazepine-induced leukopenia; additive antithyroidal effects

• *Mebendazole:* Carbamazepine decreases mebendazole levels, significant only when large doses given

• *Oral anticoagulants:* Increased prothrombin time

• *Oral contraceptives:* Carbamazepine induced metabolic induction may lead to menstrual irregularities and unplanned pregnancies

• *Valproic acid:* Valproic acid can increase, decrease, or have no effect on carbamazepine, monitor serum levels; carbamazepine decreases levels of valproic acid

SPECIAL CONSIDERATIONS

PATIENT/FAMILY EDUCATION

• Caution about driving and other activities that require alertness, at least initially

• Seizures may result from alcohol ingestion

• Drug may turn urine pink to brown

MONITORING PARAMETERS

• CBC—aplastic anemia and agranulocytosis have been reported 5-8 times greater than in the general public

• Liver function tests, serum drug levels (therapeutic 3-9 μg/ml) during initial treatment

---

carbamide peroxide

(kar′ba-mide per-ox′ide)

Auro Ear Drops, Debrox, Murine Ear Drops

Chemical Class: Urea compound and hydrogen peroxide

Therapeutic Class: Otic wax remover

CLINICAL PHARMACOLOGY

Mechanism of Action: Foaming action facilitates removal of impacted cerumen

INDICATIONS AND USES: Impacted cerumen, prevention of ceruminosis

DOSAGE

Adult and Child

• INSTILL 5-10 gtt affected ear bid × 3-4 days

$ AVAILABLE FORMS/COST OF THERAPY

• Sol—Drops: 6.5%, 30 ml: **$3.51**

CONTRAINDICATIONS: Hypersensitivity, otic surgery, perforated eardrum

PREGNANCY AND LACTATION: Pregnancy category C

SIDE EFFECTS/ADVERSE REACTIONS

EENT: Itching, irritation in ear, redness

carbenicillin

(car-ben'a-sillin)

Geopen, Geocillin, Geopen Oral, ✦ Pyopen ✦

Chemical Class: Expanded spectrum, semisynthetic penicillin

Therapeutic Class: Antibiotic

CLINICAL PHARMACOLOGY

Mechanism of Action: Interferes with final cell wall synthesis of susceptible bacteria

Pharmacokinetics

PO: Peak serum concentration, 9.6 µg/ml, 1 hr after 764 mg dose; peak urine concentration within 3 hr, 1428 µg/ml (therapeutic concentrations *only* in urine)

IM: Peak serum concentration, 15-20 µg/ml after 1 g; urine peak, >2000 µg/ml

IV: Peak serum concentration, 124 µg/ml, after 1 g in 30 min inf

Rapidly absorbed PO from the small intestine (40% bioavailable), distributed to bile, 50% protein bound; $t_{1/2}$ 1-1.5 hr; excreted in the urine (85-90% unchanged), crosses placenta

INDICATIONS AND USES: PO acute and chronic infections of the upper and lower urinary tract and in asymptomatic bacteriuria due to susceptible strains of the following organisms: *Escherichia coli, Proteus mirabilis, Morganella morganii, Providencia rettgeri, Proteus vulgaris, Pseudomonas, Enterobacter* and enterococci; prostatitis due to susceptible strains of the following organisms: *E. coli, S. faecalis, P. mirabilis, Enterobacter* sp; IV infections of the genitourinary tract, lower respiratory tract, urinary tract, skin and soft tissue and septicemia caused by susceptible organisms

Aerobic antibacterial spectrum usually includes:

- Gram-negative organisms: *Neisseria gonorrhoeae, Enterobacter* sp, *Enterococcus faecalis, E. coli, Haemophilus influenzae, Klebsiella* sp, *Pseudomonas aeruginosa, Serratia* sp
- Anaerobes: *Bacteroides* sp

DOSAGE

Adult

- *UTI:* PO 382-764 mg q6h; IM/IV 1-2 g q6h up to 50 mg/kg/day
- *Prostatitis:* 764 mg q6h
- *Other indications:* IM/IV 50-83.3 mg/kg q4h

Child

- *UTI:* IM/IV 1-2 g q6h up to 50 mg/kg/day
- *Other indications:* IM/IV 50-83.3 mg/kg q4h
- *Neonates:* 100 mg stat, then 75-100 mg/kg q8h

$ AVAILABLE FORMS/COST OF THERAPY

- Tab, Uncoated—Oral: 382 mg, 100's: **$173.21**
- Powder for inj—IM; IV: 1 g: **$1.85;** 2 g: **$4.43;** 5 g: **$8.11**

CONTRAINDICATIONS: Penicillin allergy

PRECAUTIONS: Allergic responses, including anaphylaxis possible; superinfections with nonsusceptible organisms

PREGNANCY AND LACTATION: Pregnancy category B

SIDE EFFECTS/ADVERSE REACTIONS

GI: Nausea, bad taste, diarrhea, vomiting, flatulence, glossitis, mild SGOT elevations

HEME: Anemia, thrombocytopenia, leukopenia, neutropenia, eosinophilia

SKIN: Hypersensitivity reactions (skin rash, urticaria, pruritus)

MISC: Hyperthermia, headache, itchy eyes, vaginitis, and loose stools

▼ **DRUG INTERACTIONS**

Drug

- *Aminoglycosides:* Chemically inactivated by carbenicillin
- *Methotrexate:* Increased methotrexate serum concentration

SPECIAL CONSIDERATIONS

- **NOTE:** When high and rapid blood and urine levels of antibiotic are indicated, alternative parenteral therapy should be used. Sodium content: 4.7-5.3 mEq per gram of carbenicillin.

---

carbidopa-levodopa

(kar-bee-doe'pa- lee-voe-doe'pa)

Sinemet, Sinemet CR

Chemical Class: Catecholamine precursor

Therapeutic Class: Anti Parkinson's agent, antidyskinetic

CLINICAL PHARMACOLOGY

Mechanism of Action: Carbidopa inhibits peripheral decarboxylation of levodopa; thus more levodopa is made available for transport to brain and conversion to dopamine; carbidopa reduces the amount of levodopa required by about 75%, increases both plasma levels and the plasma $t_{1/2}$ of levodopa, and decreases plasma and urinary dopamine. Pyridoxine hydrochloride (vitamin B6), in oral doses of 10 mg to 25 mg may reverse the effects of levodopa by increasing the rate of aromatic amino acid decarboxylation. Carbidopa inhibits the action of pyridoxine.

Pharmacokinetics

PO: peak concentration tabs, 0.7 hr; time-release, 2.4 hr; tabs rapid and complete within 2-3 hr; time-release: gradual and continuous over 4-6 hr, widely distributed, 36% protein bound, $t_{1/2}$ 1-2 hr; excreted in urine (metabolites)

INDICATIONS AND USES: Parkinson's disease, restless legs syndrome*

DOSAGE

Adult

- PO 3-6 tabs of 25 mg carbidopa/250 mg levodopa daily, in divided doses, not to exceed 8 tabs/day; time-release 1 tab bid at intervals of not less than 6 hr; usual: 2-8 tabs/day at intervals of 4-8 hr; conversion from levodopa therapy: discontinue levodopa for at least 8 hr; patients requiring <1.5 g of levodopa/day: Sinemet 10/100 or 25/100 tid-qid; for patients requiring ≥1.5 g of levodopa/day; Sinemet 25/250 mg tid.

$ **AVAILABLE FORMS/COST OF THERAPY**

- Tab, Uncoated—Oral: 10 mg/100 mg, 100's: **$51.40-$59.88;** 25 mg/100 mg, 100's: **$51.95-$66.63;** 25 mg/250 mg, 100's: **$62.50-$85.63**
- Tab, Time-Rel—Oral: 50 mg/100 mg, 100's: **$68.06;** 50 mg/200 mg, 100's: **$136.13**

CONTRAINDICATIONS: Hypersensitivity, narrow-angle glaucoma, undiagnosed skin lesions

PRECAUTIONS: Renal disease, cardiac disease, hepatic disease, respiratory disease, MI with dysrhythmias, convulsions, peptic ulcer

PREGNANCY AND LACTATION: Pregnancy category C; should not be given to nursing mothers

SIDE EFFECTS/ADVERSE REACTIONS

CV: Orthostatic hypotension, tachycardia, hypertension, palpitation

CNS: Involuntary choreiform movements, hand tremors, fatigue, headache, anxiety, twitching, numbness, weakness, confusion, agitation, insomnia, nightmares, psychosis, hallucination, hypomania, severe depression, dizziness

EENT: Blurred vision, diplopia, dilated pupils
GI: Nausea, vomiting, anorexia, abdominal distress, dry mouth, flatulence, dysphagia, bitter taste, diarrhea, constipation
GU: Urinary retention, incontinence, dark urine
HEME: ***Hemolytic anemia, leukopenia, agranulocytosis***
METAB: Weight change
SKIN: Rash, sweating, alopecia

▼ DRUG INTERACTIONS

Drugs

- *Food:* High protein diets inhibit the efficacy of levodopa
- *MAO inhibitors:* May result in hypertensive response
- *Methionine:* Inhibits the clinical response to levodopa
- *Neuroleptics:* Phenothiazines block dopamine receptors, can produce extrapyramidal symptoms, and inhibit the antiparkinsonian effect of levodopa
- *Papaverine:* Inhibits the therapeutic response to levodopa in parkinsonian patients
- *Phenytoin:* May inhibit the antiparkinsonian effect of levodopa
- *Pyridoxine:* Inhibits the antiparkinsonian effect of levodopa; concurrent carbidopa negates the interaction
- *Spiramycin:* Reduces the plasma concentration of levodopa, with reduction of antiparkinson efficacy

Labs

- *False positive:* Urine ketones
- *False negative:* Urine glucose
- *False increase:* Uric acid, urine protein
- *Decrease:* VMA, BUN, creatinine

SPECIAL CONSIDERATIONS

- Caution with use until after MAOIs have been discontinued for 2 wk
- If previously on levodopa, discontinue for at least 8 hr before change to levodopa-carbidopa

PATIENT/FAMILY EDUCATION

- Limit protein taken with drug
- Measures to prevent orthostasis

carbinoxamine/ pseudoephedrine

(kar-bi-nox'-a-meen)
Formerly Clistin, now available only in combination
Chemical Class: Ethanolamine
Therapeutic Class: Antihistamine

CLINICAL PHARMACOLOGY

Mechanism of Action: Carbinoxamine is a competitive antagonist of histamine at the H_1 receptor site; anticholinergic (drying), antipruritic, and sedative effects

Pharmacokinetics (carbinoxamine)

PO: onset of action, 15-30 min; duration 6 hr; $t_{1/2}$ 10-20 hr; metabolized in liver; excreted in urine as inactive metabolites

INDICATIONS AND USES: Symptomatic relief of perennial and seasonal allergic rhinitis, vasomotor rhinitis, allergic conjunctivitis, common cold, allergic and non-allergic pruritic symptoms, urticaria and angioedema

DOSAGE

Adult

- 4-8 mg tid-qid

Child

- 0.2 to 0.4 mg/kg/day

$ AVAILABLE FORMS/COST OF THERAPY

Available in combination with pseudoephedrine with or without dextromethorphan:

- Syr—Oral: 4 mg/25 mg, 480 ml: **$10.12-$19.49**
- Tab, Coated, Sust Action— Oral: 8 mg/120 mg, 100's: **$24.29- $87.44**

• Tab, Uncoated—Oral: 4 mg/60 mg, 100's: **$16.23-$37.64**

CONTRAINDICATIONS: Hypersensitivity or idiosyncrasy to any ingredients, patients taking MAO inhibitors, patients with narrow-angle glaucoma, urinary retention, severe hypertension or CAD, or patients undergoing an asthmatic attack

PRECAUTIONS: Patients sensitive to antihistamines may experience moderate to severe drowsiness; patients sensitive to sympathomimetic amines may note mild CNS stimulation

PREGNANCY AND LACTATION: Pregnancy category C

SIDE EFFECTS/ADVERSE REACTIONS (CARBINOXAMINE)

CNS: Sedation, dizziness, diplopia, headache, nervousness, weakness, excitability in children

GI: Vomiting, diarrhea, dry mouth, nausea, anorexia, heartburn

GU: Polyuria, dysuria

SPECIAL CONSIDERATIONS

PATIENT/FAMILY EDUCATION

• Avoid concurrent alcohol and other CNS depressants

carboprost

(kar'boe-prost)

Prostin/15 M

Chemical Class: Prostaglandin F2(α)

Therapeutic Class: Abortifacient; uterine stimulant; antihemorrhagic (post partum and postabortal uterine bleeding)

CLINICAL PHARMACOLOGY

Mechanism of Action: Stimulates uterine contractions, usually sufficient to cause abortion

Pharmacokinetics

IM: Peak concentration 2060 pg/ml after 250 μg at 30 min; mean abortion time, 16 hr; metabolized in lungs, liver; excreted in urine (metabolites)

INDICATIONS AND USES: Abortion between 13-20 wk gestation as calculated from the first day of the last normal menstrual period and in the following conditions related to second trimester abortion:

• Failure of expulsion of the fetus during the course of treatment by another method

• Premature rupture of membranes using intrauterine methods with loss of drug and insufficient or absent uterine activity

• Requirement of a repeat intrauterine instillation of drug for expulsion of the fetus

• Inadvertent or spontaneous rupture of membranes in the presence of a previable fetus and absence of adequate activity for expulsion

Postpartum hemorrhage due to uterine atony which has not responded to conventional methods of management

DOSAGE

Adult

• *Abortion:* IM 250 μg, then 250 μg q1 ½-3 ½ hr, may increase to 500 μg if no response, not to exceed 12 mg total dose

• *Refractory postpartum uterine bleeding:* IM 250 μg single inj (75% response); selected cases multiple dosing at intervals of 15 to 90 min; max dose, 2 mg (total)

$ AVAILABLE FORMS/COST OF THERAPY

• Inj, Sol—IM: 250 μg/ml, 1 ml: **$27.38**

CONTRAINDICATIONS: Hypersensitivity, severe hepatic disease, severe renal disease, PID, respiratory disease, cardiac disease

PRECAUTIONS: Asthma, anemia, jaundice, diabetes mellitus, convulsive disorders, past uterine surgery

PREGNANCY AND LACTATION: Pregnancy category C; any dose which produces increased uterine tone could put the embryo or fetus at risk.

SIDE EFFECTS/ADVERSE REACTIONS

CNS: Fever, chills, headache

GI: Nausea, vomiting, diarrhea

SPECIAL CONSIDERATIONS

- Antiemetic, analgesic, and antidiarrheal medications should be considered concurrently to counter adverse GI effects

---

carisoprodol

(kar'i-so-pro'dol)

Rela, Soma, Soprodol ✤

Chemical Class: Meprobamate congener

Therapeutic Class: Skeletal muscle relaxant, central acting

CLINICAL PHARMACOLOGY

Mechanism of Action: Muscle relaxation by blocking interneuronal activity in the descending reticular formation and spinal cord; produces sedation

Pharmacokinetics

PO: Onset 1/2 hr, duration 4-6 hr; metabolized by liver; excreted in urine; $t_{1/2}$ 8 hr

INDICATIONS AND USES: Adjunct to rest, physical therapy, and other measures for the relief of discomfort associated with acute, painful, musculoskeletal conditions; does not directly relax tense skeletal muscles

DOSAGE

Adult and child >12 yr

- PO 350 mg tid and hs

$ **AVAILABLE FORMS/COST OF THERAPY**

- Tab, Uncoated—Oral: 350 mg, 100's: **$6.75-$149.22**

CONTRAINDICATIONS: Hypersensitivity (including related compounds, such as meprobamate, mebutamate, or tybamate), child <12 yr, intermittent porphyria

PRECAUTIONS: Renal disease, hepatic disease, addictive personality, elderly

PREGNANCY AND LACTATION: Pregnancy category C; crosses placenta; excreted in breast milk (2-4 × maternal plasma)

SIDE EFFECTS/ADVERSE REACTIONS

CNS: Dizziness, weakness, drowsiness, headache, tremor, depression, insomnia, ataxia, irritability, vertigo, agitation, syncope, insomnia

CV: Postural hypotension, tachycardia, facial flushing

EENT: Diplopia, temporary loss of vision

GI: Nausea, vomiting, hiccups, epigastric discomfort

SKIN: Rash, pruritus, fever, facial flushing, erythema multiforme, eosinophilia, and fixed drug eruptions

SPECIAL CONSIDERATIONS

- May impair mental and/or physical abilities required for the performance of *potentially* hazardous tasks such as driving a motor vehicle or operating machinery
- Additive with alcohol and other CNS depressants
- Caution when used in addiction-prone individuals
- Abrupt cessation may precipitate mild withdrawal symptoms such as abdominal cramps, insomnia, chills, headache, and nausea
- Psychological dependence and abuse also reported
- Abused on the street in conjunction with narcotics

carteolol

(kar-tee'-oe-lole)

Cartrol, Ocupress

Chemical Class: Nonselective β blocker

Therapeutic Class: Antihypertensive, antiglaucoma agent

CLINICAL PHARMACOLOGY

Mechanism of Action: Nonselective β-adrenergic blocker with intrinsic sympathomimetic activity

Pharmacokinetics

PO: Onset 1-2 hr, peak 2-4 hr, duration 8-12 hr, $t_{1/2}$ 6-8 hr; food slows absorption but does not lower total absorption; metabolized by liver (metabolites inactive); excreted in urine, bile; crosses placenta

INDICATIONS AND USES: Chronic open-angle glaucoma, hypertension (does not alter serum cholesterol or triglycerides)

DOSAGE

Adult

- *Hypertension:* PO 2.5-10 mg qd (if CrCl>60 ml/min); in renal impairment, CrCl 20-60 ml/min, dosage interval is 48 hrs; CrCl <20 ml/min, dosage interval is 72 hrs
- *Chronic open angle glaucoma:* Ophth sol, 1%, 1 gtt in affected eye bid

$ **AVAILABLE FORMS/COST OF THERAPY**

- Sol—Ophth: 1%, 5 ml: **$15.26;** 1%, 10 ml: **$28.78**
- Tab, Plain Coated—Oral: 2.5 mg, 100's: **$95.02;** 5 mg, 100's: **$95.02**

CONTRAINDICATIONS: Hypersensitivity to β-blockers, heart block (2nd or 3rd degree), sinus bradycardia, overt CHF, bronchial asthma

PRECAUTIONS: Major surgery, diabetes mellitus, renal disease, thyroid disease, COPD, well-compensated heart failure, nonallergic bronchospasm; exacerbation of angina or MI may occur following abrupt discontinuation of β-blockers; ophth carteolol may be absorbed systemically; adverse reactions found with systemic administration may occur with ophth administration

PREGNANCY AND LACTATION: Pregnancy category C; excreted in breast milk

SIDE EFFECTS/ADVERSE REACTIONS

CNS: Dizziness, mental changes, drowsiness, *Fatigue (7%),* headache, catatonia, depression, anxiety, nightmares, paresthesia, lethargy, insomnia, decreased concentration

CV: Orthostatic hypotension, ***bradycardia, CHF, chest pain, ventricular dysrhythmias, AV block, peripheral vascular insufficiency,*** palpitations

EENT: Tinnitus, visual changes, sore throat, double vision, dry burning eyes

GI: Nausea, vomiting, diarrhea, dry mouth, flatulence, constipation, anorexia

GU: Impotence, dysuria, ejaculatory failure, urinary retention

HEME: ***Agranulocytosis, thrombocytopenic purpura (rare)***

MS: Joint pain, arthralgia, muscle cramps (3%)

RESP: ***Bronchospasm,*** dyspnea, wheezing, nasal stuffiness, pharyngitis

SKIN: Rash, alopecia, urticaria, pruritus, fever

MISC: Facial swelling, decreased exercise tolerance, weight change, Raynaud's disease

▼ **DRUG INTERACTIONS**

Drugs

- *Amiodarone:* Increased bradycardic effect of carteolol
- *Antidiabetics:* Carteolol reduces response to hypoglycemia

• *Barbiturates:* Enhanced carteolol metabolism
• *Calcium channel blockers:* Decreased carteolol metabolism
• *Cimetidine:* Decreased carteolol metabolism
• *Disopyramide:* Increased negative inotropic effect
• *Epinepherine+:* Enhanced pressor response; resulting in hypertension and bradycardia
• *Methyldopa:* May promote hypertension if used together
• *Neuroleptics:* Decreased carteolol metabolism; decreased neuroleptic metabolism
• *Nonsteroidal anti-inflammatory drugs:* Reduced antihypertensive effect
• *Prazosin:* Enhanced 1st dose response to prazosin
• *Propafenone:* Decreased carteolol metabolism
• *Propoxyphene:* Decreased carteolol metabolism
• *Quinidine:* Decreased carteolol metabolism
• *Rifampin:* Enhanced carteolol metabolism
• *Theophylline:* Decreased metabolism of theophylline

Labs

• *False positive:* Urinary catecholamines
• *Interference:* Glucose tolerance test

SPECIAL CONSIDERATIONS

PATIENT/FAMILY EDUCATION

• Do not stop drug abruptly; taper over 2 wk
• Do not use OTC products containing alpha-adrenergic stimulants (nasal decongestants, cold remedies) unless directed by physician

cascara sagrada

(kas-kar′-a)
Cascara
Chemical Class: Anthraquinone
Therapeutic Class: Stimulant laxative

CLINICAL PHARMACOLOGY

Mechanism of Action: Direct chemical irritation in colon; increases propulsion of stool

Pharmacokinetics

PO: Peak 6-12 hr; only slightly absorbed; metabolized by liver; excreted by kidneys and in feces

INDICATIONS AND USES: Constipation; bowel or rectal preparation for surgery or examination

DOSAGE

Adult

• PO (powder, tab) 325-1000 mg hs; FLUID 0.5-1.5 ml qd; AROMATIC FLUID 2-6 ml qd

Child

• Age >12 yr: PO (powder, tab) 325-1000 mg hs; FLUID 0.5-1.5 ml qd; AROMATIC FLUID 2-6 ml qd; Age 2-12 yr: PO/FLUID/AROMATIC FLUID ½ adult dose; Age <2 yr: PO/FLUID/AROMATIC FLUID ¼ adult dose

$ AVAILABLE FORMS/COST OF THERAPY

• Powder—Oral: 125 g: **$8.40**
• Tab—Oral: 325 mg, 100's: **$3.75-$4.72**
• Sol (fluid extract): 1 g cascara/1 ml fluid extract, 120 ml: **$2.20-$3.60**
• Sol (aromatic fluid): 1 g cascara/1 ml aromatic fluid, 120 ml: **$2.10-$3.00**

CONTRAINDICATIONS: Hypersensitivity, GI bleeding, obstruction, appendicitis, acute surgical abdomen

PRECAUTIONS: CHF, abdominal pain, nausea/vomiting, alcoholism (aromatic form)

PREGNANCY AND LACTATION: Pregnancy category C; excreted in breast milk

SIDE EFFECTS/ADVERSE REACTIONS

GI: *Nausea, vomiting, anorexia, cramps,* diarrhea, melanosis coli

GU: Discoloration of urine (pink, red, brown)

METAB: Hypocalcemia, ***tetany,*** alkalosis, hypokalemia

SPECIAL CONSIDERATIONS

- Stimulant laxatives are habit forming
- Long term use may lead to colonic atony

---

castor oil

Alphamul, Emulsoil, Fleet Castor Oil, Neoloid

Chemical Class: Fatty acid ester
Therapeutic Class: Stimulant laxative

CLINICAL PHARMACOLOGY

Mechanism of Action: Increases motor activity of small intestine and colon; causes fluid secretion in colon

Pharmacokinetics

PO: Peak effect 2-3 hr; ester hydrolyzed in small intestine and partially absorbed

INDICATIONS AND USES: Constipation; bowel preparation for surgery or examination

DOSAGE

Adult

- PO LIQ 15-60 ml

Child

- Age >2 yr: PO LIQ 5-15 ml; Age <2 yr: PO LIQ 1.25-7.5 ml

$ **AVAILABLE FORMS/COST OF THERAPY**

- Oil—Oral: 60 ml: **$0.95-$2.00**
- Liq—Oral: 36.4% oil, 120 ml: **$3.60;** 67% oil, 45 ml: **$9.89;** 95% oil, 60 ml: **$2.10**

CONTRAINDICATIONS: Hypersensitivity, fecal impaction, GI bleeding, appendicitis, intestinal obstruction

PRECAUTIONS: Abdominal pain, nausea/vomiting, laxative dependence; colonic atony from prolonged use

PREGNANCY AND LACTATION: Pregnancy category X; excreted in breast milk

SIDE EFFECTS/ADVERSE REACTIONS

GI: *Nausea, vomiting, anorexia, cramps,* diarrhea, rebound constipation, colon irritation, flatus

METAB: Alkalosis, hypokalemia, fluid or electrolyte imbalance

---

cefaclor

(sef'-a-klor)

Ceclor

Chemical Class: Cephalosporin (2nd generation)
Therapeutic Class: Antibiotic

CLINICAL PHARMACOLOGY

Mechanism of Action: Inhibits bacterial cell wall synthesis, bactericidal

Pharmacokinetics

PO: Peak ½-1 hr (15 μg/ml after 500 mg), $t_{1/2}$ 36-54 min; 25% bound by plasma proteins; 60%-85% eliminated unchanged in urine in 8 hr; crosses placenta; total absorption unaffected by food but when taken with food peak concentration is 50%-75% of that when taken fasting; serum $t_{1/2}$ slightly prolonged in renal insufficiency; $t_{1/2}$ 2.3-2.8 hr if anephric; hemodialysis shortens $t_{1/2}$ by 25%-30%

INDICATIONS AND USES: Pharyngitis, tonsillitis, otitis media, bronchitis, pneumonia, skin and urinary tract infections caused by susceptible organisms.

Antibacterial spectrum usually includes:

• Gram-negative organisms: *H. influenzae, Moraxella catarrhalis, E. coli, P. mirabilis, Klebsiella* sp

• Gram-positive organisms: *S. pneumoniae, S. pyogenes, S. aureus*

• Anaerobes: *Peptococci, Peptostreptococci*

• β-lactamase-producing strains of the above pathogens are usually susceptible.

DOSAGE

Adult

• PO 250-500 mg q8h, double dose in serious infections and pneumonia

Child >1 mo

• PO 20-40 mg/kg qd in divided doses q8h, not to exceed 1 g/day (use higher dose in serious infections and otitis media)

$ AVAILABLE FORMS/COST OF THERAPY

• Cap, Gel—Oral: 250 mg, 15's: **$32.68;** 500 mg, 15's: **$62.02**

• Powder, Reconst—Oral: 125 mg/5 ml, 75 ml: **$14.97;** 187 mg/5 ml, 50 ml: **$14.97;** 250 mg/5 ml, 75 ml: **$27.78;** 375 mg/5 ml, 50 ml: **$27.78**

CONTRAINDICATIONS: Hypersensitivity to cephalosporins, infants <1 mo

PRECAUTIONS: Hypersensitivity to penicillins, renal disease

PREGNANCY AND LACTATION: Pregnancy category B; excreted in breast milk

SIDE EFFECTS/ADVERSE REACTIONS

CNS: Headache, dizziness, weakness, paresthesia, fever, chills

GI: Nausea, vomiting, diarrhea, anorexia, pain, glossitis, bleeding, increased AST, increased ALT, increased bilirubin, increased LDH, increased alkaline phosphatase, abdominal pain, ***pseudomembranous colitis***

GU: Proteinuria, vaginitis, pruritus, candidiasis, ***nephrotoxicity***

HEME: ***Leukopenia, neutropenia, agranulocytosis, thrombocytopenia,*** anemia, ***hemolytic anemia, pancytopenia,*** lymphocytosis, eosinophilia, thrombocytosis.

RESP: Dyspnea

SKIN: Rash, urticaria, dermatitis

MISC: Serum sickness-like syndrome, ***anaphylaxis***

▼ DRUG INTERACTIONS

Drugs

• *Aminoglycosides:* Increased risk of nephrotoxicity due to aminoglycoside

• *Warfarin:* Hypoprothrombinemic response enhanced

Labs

• *False positive:* Urine 17-ketosteroids, urine protein, urine glucose, direct Coombs' test

• *Increase:* Urine/serum creatinine (not by alkaline picrate method)

• *Interference:* Cross-matching

SPECIAL CONSIDERATIONS

• Last choice 2nd generation cephalosporin given decreased activity against *S. pneumonia*

cefadroxil

(sef-a-drox'ill)

Cefadroxil, Duricef, Ultracef

Chemical Class: Cephalosporin (1st generation)

Therapeutic Class: Antibiotic

CLINICAL PHARMACOLOGY

Mechanism of Action: Inhibition

of bacterial cell wall synthesis; bacteriocidal

Pharmacokinetics

PO: Peak serum levels, 1-1 ½ hr following single doses of 500 and 1000 mg: 16 and 28 μg/ml, respectively; measurable levels persist for 12 hr; 90% excreted unchanged in urine within 24 hr; peak urine concentration, 1800 μg/ml following a single 500 mg oral dose; $t_{1/2}$, 1-2 hr; 20% bound by plasma proteins

INDICATIONS AND USES: Infections of the upper and lower respiratory tract, tonsils, otitis media, urinary tract, and skin caused by susceptible organisms

Antibacterial spectrum usually includes:

- Gram-negative bacilli: *E. coli, P. mirabilis, Klebsiella*
- Gram-positive organisms: *S. pneumoniae, S. pyogenes, S. aureus*

DOSAGE

Adult

- PO 1-2 g qd or q12h, give a loading dose of 1 g initially; dosage reduction appropriate in renal impairment (CrCl <50 ml/min)

Child

- PO 30 mg/kg/day

$ AVAILABLE FORMS/COST OF THERAPY

- Cap, Gel—Oral: 500 mg, 100's: **$306.02**
- Powder, Reconst—Oral: 125 mg/5 ml: **$12.24-$24.88;** 250 mg/5 ml: **$23.00-$43.40;** 500 mg/5 ml, 100 ml: **$31.85**
- Tab, Uncoated—Oral:1 g, 100's: **$591.53**

CONTRAINDICATIONS: Hypersensitivity to cephalosporins, infants <1 mo

PRECAUTIONS: Hypersensitivity to penicillins

PREGNANCY AND LACTATION: Pregnancy category B; low concentrations in milk; M:P ratio at 1 hr = 0.011

SIDE EFFECTS/ADVERSE REACTIONS

CNS: Headache, dizziness, weakness, paresthesia, fever, chills

GI: Nausea, vomiting, *diarrhea, anorexia,* pain, glossitis, bleeding, increased AST, ALT, bilirubin, LDH, alk phosphatase, abdominal pain, ***pseudomembranous colitis***

GU: Proteinuria, vaginitis, pruritus, candidiasis, increased BUN, ***nephrotoxicity, renal failure***

HEME: ***Leukopenia, thrombocytopenia, agranulocytosis,*** anemia, ***neutropenia, lymphocytosis, eosinophilia, pancytopenia, hemolytic anemia***

RESP: Dyspnea

SKIN: Rash, urticaria, dermatitis, ***anaphylaxis***

▼ DRUG INTERACTIONS

Drugs

- *Oral anticoagulants:* Enhanced hypoprothrombinemia

Labs

- *Increase (false):* Creatinine (serum, urine), urinary 17-KS
- *False positive:* Urinary protein, direct Coombs' test, urine glucose
- *Interference:* Cross-matching

---

cefamandole

(sef-a-man'dole)

Mandol

Chemical Class: Cephalosporin (2nd generation)

Therapeutic Class: Antibiotic

CLINICAL PHARMACOLOGY

Mechanism of Action: Inhibition of cell wall synthesis; bacteriocidal

Pharmacokinetics

IM/IV: Peak serum levels 1-1 ½ hr (IM: 25 μg/ml; IV: 139 μg/ml, after 1 gm); $t_{1/2}$, ½-1 hr; 60%-75% bound by plasma proteins; distributed to pleura, joint fluids, bile, and bone; 85% excreted by kidneys over 8 hr

INDICATIONS AND USES: Infections of the lower respiratory tract, urinary tract, skin and skin-structure, and bone and joints; peritonitis, septicemia, and presurgical prophylactic therapy caused by susceptible organisms. Antibacterial spectrum usually includes:

- Gram-positive organisms: *S. pneumoniae, S. aureus* (penicillinase and non-penicillinase-producing), β-hemolytic streptococci, *S. epidermidis, S. pyogenes*
- Gram-negative organisms: *H. influenzae, Klebsiella* sp, *P. mirabilis E. coli, Proteus* sp, *Enterobacter* sp.
- Anaerobes: *Peptostreptococcus, Peptococcus* sp., *Clostridium* sp

DOSAGE

Adult

- IM/IV 500 mg-1g q4-8h; may give up to 2 g q4h for severe infections; 1 or 2 g IM/IV ½-1 hr prior to surgery, followed by 1 or 2 g q6h after surgery for 24-48 hr for prophylaxis

Child >1 mo

- IM/IV 50-150 mg/kg/day in divided doses q4-8h, not to exceed adult dose; 50 to 100 mg/kg/day in equally divided doses ½-1 hr before surgery and q6h for 24-48 hr after surgery for prophylaxis

Dosage reduction indicated in severe renal impairment (CrCl <5 ml/min): 1 g q12h

$ AVAILABLE FORMS/COST OF THERAPY

- Inj, Dry-Sol—IM; IV: 500 mg/vial: **$4.53;** 1 g/vial: **$2.06;** 2 g/vial: **$18.65**

CONTRAINDICATIONS: Hypersensitivity to cephalosporins, infants <1 mo

PRECAUTIONS: Hypersensitivity to penicillins, renal disease (nephrotoxicity, especially with co-administration of aminoglycoside antibiotics), superinfection; hypoprothrombinemia, with or without bleeding, especially in elderly, debilitated, depleted vitamin K stores

PREGNANCY AND LACTATION: Pregnancy category B; low milk concentrations; M:P ratio at 1 hr = 0.02

SIDE EFFECTS/ADVERSE REACTIONS

CNS: Headache, dizziness, weakness, paresthesia, fever, chills

GI: Nausea, vomiting, diarrhea, anorexia, pain, glossitis, bleeding, increased AST, ALT, bilirubin, LDH, alk phosphatase, abdominal pain, (pseudomembranous colitis, transient hepatitis and cholestatic jaundice)

GU: Proteinuria, vaginitis, pruritus, candidiasis, increased BUN, ***nephrotoxicity, renal failure***

HEME: ***Leukopenia, thrombocytopenia, agranulocytosis,*** anemia, ***neutropenia, lymphocytosis, eosinophilia, pancytopenia, hemolytic anemia (Coombs positive),*** bleeding, ***hypoprothrombinemia***

RESP: Dyspnea

SKIN: Maculopapular rash, urticaria, dermatitis, ***anaphylaxis***

MISC: Pain on IM inj (infrequent), thrombophlebitis (rare), anaphylaxis, drug fever

▼ DRUG INTERACTIONS

Drugs

- *Aminoglycosides:* Potential additive nephrotoxicity
- *Ethanol:* Disulfiram-like reactions secondary to acetaldehyde accumulation
- *Oral anticoagulants:* Additive hypoprothrombinemia

Labs

- *Increase (false):* Urinary 17-KS
- *False positive:* Urinary protein, direct Coombs', urine glucose

- *Interference:* Cross-matching blood products

SPECIAL CONSIDERATIONS

- Caution with alcohol, disulfiram reaction possible

MONITORING PARAMETERS

- If severe diarrhea occurs, pseudomembranous colitis should be considered
- Bleeding: ecchymosis, bleeding gums, hematuria, stool guaiac daily

---

cefazolin sodium

(sef-a'zoe-lin)

Ancef, Kefzol, Zolicef ✦

Chemical Class: Cephalosporin (1st generation)

Therapeutic Class: Antibiotic

CLINICAL PHARMACOLOGY

Mechanism of Action: Inhibition of bacterial cell wall synthesis; bacteriocidal

Pharmacokinetics

IM: Peak ½-2 hr (37 μg/ml and 3 μg/ml after 500 mg doses, 64 μg/ml and 7 μg/ml after 1 g doses at 1 and 8 hr, respectively)

IV: Peak 10 min (188 μg/ml after 1 g) $t_{1/2}$, 1½-2¼ hr; distribution (70% to 86% protein bound) to bile, without obstructive biliary disease levels can reach or exceed serum levels by up to five times; with obstructive biliary disease, bile levels considerably lower than serum levels (<1.0 μg/ml); to synovial fluid, comparable to levels reached in serum at about 4 hr after administration; eliminated unchanged in urine

INDICATIONS AND USES: Infections of the lower respiratory tract, urinary tract, biliary tract, and genitourinary tract; infections of the skin and skin structure, bones and joints; endocarditis, surgical prophylaxis, septicemia. Antibacterial spectrum usually includes:

- Gram-negative bacilli: *E. coli, P. mirabilis, Klebsiella*
- Gram-positive organisms: *S. pneumoniae, S. pyogenes, S. aureus*
- Anaerobes: *Peptostreptococcus, Peptococcus* sp

DOSAGE

Adult

- *Life-threatening infections:* IM/IV 1-2 g q6h
- *Mild/moderate infections:* IM/IV 250-500 mg q8h

Child >1 mo

- *Life-threatening infections:* IM/IV 100 mg/kg in 3-4 equal doses
- *Mild/moderate infections:* IM/IV 25-50 mg/kg in 3-4 equal doses

Dosage reduction appropriate in renal impairment (CrCl <50 ml/min)

$ AVAILABLE FORMS/COST OF THERAPY

- Inj, Dry-Sol—IM; IV: 1 g/vial: **$2.48-$6.00**

CONTRAINDICATIONS: Hypersensitivity to cephalosporins, infants <1 mo

PRECAUTIONS: Hypersensitivity to penicillins, renal disease

PREGNANCY AND LACTATION: Pregnancy category B; low milk concentrations; M:P ratio average over 4 hr = 0.02

SIDE EFFECTS/ADVERSE REACTIONS

CNS: Headache, dizziness, weakness, paresthesia, fever, chills

GI: Nausea, vomiting, *diarrhea, anorexia,* pain, glossitis, bleeding, increased AST, ALT, bilirubin, LDH, alk phosphatase, abdominal pain, oral candidiasis

GU: Proteinuria, vaginitis, pruritus, candidiasis, increased BUN, ***nephrotoxicity, renal failure***

HEME: ***Leukopenia, thrombocytopenia, agranulocytosis,*** anemia, ***neutropenia, lymphocytosis, eosinophilia, pancytopenia, hemolytic anemia***

SKIN: Rash, urticaria, dermatitis, ***anaphylaxis***

▼ **DRUG INTERACTIONS**

Drugs

• *Aminoglycosides:* Additive nephrotoxicity

• *Colistin:* Additive nephrotoxicity

Labs

• *Increase (false):* Urinary 17-KS

• *False positive:* urinary protein, direct Coombs' test, urine glucose

• *Interference:* Cross-matching blood

cefixime

(sef-ix'ime)

Suprax

Chemical Class: Oral cephalosporin (3rd generation)

Therapeutic Class: Antibiotic

CLINICAL PHARMACOLOGY

Mechanism of Action: Inhibition of bacterial cell wall synthesis; bacteriocidal

Pharmacokinetics

PO: Peak 1 hr; $t_{1/2}$ 3-4 hr, 65% bound by plasma proteins, 50% eliminated unchanged in urine; crosses placenta

INDICATIONS AND USES: Infections of the upper and lower respiratory tract (including pharyngitis, tonsillitis), genitourinary tract (including uncomplicated UTI and gonorrhea, cervical and urethral due to *N. gonorrhoeae*)

Antibacterial spectrum usually includes:

• Gram-negative bacilli: *E. coli, P. mirabilis, Klebsiella; H. influenzae, M. catarrhalis*

• Gram-positive organisms: *S. pneumoniae, S. pyogenes*

• Anaerobes: *Peptostreptococcus, Peptococcus* sp

Note: No *S. aureus* coverage

DOSAGE

Adult

• PO 400 mg qd as a single dose or 200 mg q12h; for uncomplicated cervical/urethral GC infections, single 400 mg oral dose

Child >50 kg or >12 yrs

• PO use adult dosage

Child <50 kg or <12 years

• PO 8 mg/kg/day as a single dose or 4 mg/kg q12h

$ **AVAILABLE FORMS/COST OF THERAPY**

• Susp—Oral: 100 mg/5 ml, 100 ml: **$59.35**

• Tab, Plain Coated—Oral: 200 mg, 100's: **$309.81;** 400 mg, 100's: **$607.16**

CONTRAINDICATIONS: Hypersensitivity to cephalosporins, infants <6 mo

PRECAUTIONS: Hypersensitivity to penicillins

PREGNANCY AND LACTATION: Pregnancy category B; excreted in breast milk

SIDE EFFECTS/ADVERSE REACTIONS

CNS: Headache, dizziness, paresthesia, fever, chills, lethargy, fatigue, confusion

GI: Nausea, vomiting, diarrhea, pseudomembranous colitis, anorexia, pain, glossitis, bleeding, increased AST, ALT, bilirubin, LDH, alk phosphatase, heartburn, dysgeusia, flatulence

GU: ***Proteinuria,*** vaginitis, pruritus, increased BUN, ***nephrotoxicity, renal failure,*** pyuria, dysuria, candidiasis

HEME: ***Leukopenia, thrombocytopenia, agranulocytosis,*** anemia, ***neutropenia, lymphocytosis, eosinophilia, pancytopenia, hemolytic anemia***

RESP: ***Bronchospasm,*** dyspnea, tight chest

SKIN: Rash, urticaria, ***exfoliative dermatitis, anaphylaxis***

▼ **DRUG INTERACTIONS**

Labs

• *Increase (false):* Urinary 17-KS
• *False positive:* Urinary protein, direct Coombs', urine glucose
• *Interference:* Cross-matching blood for transfusion

SPECIAL CONSIDERATIONS

• No *S. aureus* coverage

---

cefmetazole

(sef-met'a-zole)
Zefazone
Chemical Class: Cephalosporin (2nd generation)
Therapeutic Class: Antibiotic

CLINICAL PHARMACOLOGY

Mechanism of Action: Inhibition of bacterial cell wall synthesis; bacteriocidal

Pharmacokinetics

IV: Peak, 86 μg/ml after 1 g inf; 68% bound by plasma proteins; excreted by kidneys; $t_{1/2}$ 1-3 hr

INDICATIONS AND USES: Infections of the lower respiratory tract, urinary tract, skin and skin structure, bones and joints; septicemia, and intra-abdominal infections.

Antibacterial spectrum usually includes:

• Gram-negative organisms: *H. influenzae, E. coli, Proteus, Klebsiella*
• Gram-positive organisms: *S. pneumoniae, S. pyogenes, S. aureus*
• Anaerobes: *B. fragilis, Clostridium* sp

DOSAGE

Adult

• *Uncomplicated gonorrhea:* Single dose IM 1 g (with 1 g of probenecid given by mouth at the same time or up to ½ hour before)
• *UTI:* IV 2 g q12h
• *Mild to moderate infections:* IV 2 g q8h
• *Severe to life-threatening infections:* IV 2 g q6h
• *Postoperative prophylaxis:* Following vaginal hysterectomy, abdominal hysterectomy, cesarean section, colorectal surgery, or cholecystectomy (high risk) in adults, 2 g given as a single dose 30-90 min before surgery or 1 g doses given 30-90 min before surgery and repeated 8 and 16 hr later (if surgery lasts more than 4 hours, the preoperative dose should be repeated) Dosage reduction appropriate with impaired renal function.

$ **AVAILABLE FORMS/COST OF THERAPY**

• Inj, Lyphl-Sol—IV: 1 g/vial: **$7.19;** 2 g/vial: **$14.34**

CONTRAINDICATIONS: Hypersensitivity to cephalosporins, infants <1 mo

PRECAUTIONS: Hypersensitivity to penicillins

PREGNANCY AND LACTATION: Pregnancy category B; trace milk concentrations

SIDE EFFECTS/ADVERSE REACTIONS

CNS: Headache, dizziness, paresthesia, fever, chills, lethargy, fatigue, confusion
CV: Shock, hypotension
EENT: Periorbital edema
GI: Nausea, vomiting, diarrhea (4%), anorexia, pain, glossitis, bleeding, increased AST, ALT, bilirubin, LDH, alk phosphatase, heartburn, flatulence, pseudomembranous colitis
GU: ***Proteinuria,*** vaginitis, pruritus, candidiasis, increased BUN, ***nephrotoxicity, renal failure***
HEME: ***Leukopenia, thrombocytopenia, agranulocytosis,*** anemia, ***neutropenia, lymphocytosis, eosinophilia, pancytopenia, hemolytic anemia***

SKIN: Rash, urticaria, ***exfoliative dermatitis,*** thrombophlebitis ***angioedema,*** erythema, pruritus
MISC: ***Anaphylaxis,*** pain and/or swelling at inj site, phlebitis, thrombophlebitis, superinfection

▼ DRUG INTERACTIONS

Drugs

- *Aminoglycosides:* Additive nephrotoxicity
- *Colistin:* Additive nephrotoxicity
- *Oral anticoagulants:* Additive hypoprothrombinemia, enhanced anticoagulation effect

Labs

- *Increase (false):* Creatinine (serum urine), urinary 17-KS
- *False positive:* Urinary protein, direct Coombs' test, urine glucose
- *Interference:* Cross-matching for blood transfusions

cefonicid

(se-fon'i-sid)
Monocid
Chemical Class: Cephalosporin (2nd generation)
Therapeutic Class: Antibiotic

CLINICAL PHARMACOLOGY

Mechanism of Action: Inhibition of bacterial cell wall synthesis; bacteriocidal

Pharmacokinetics

IV: Peak, 5 min, 221.3 μg/ml
IM: Peak, 1 hr, 98.6 μg/ml; $t_{1/2}$, 4½ hr; 98% protein bound; although reaches therapeutic levels in bile, levels lower than those seen with other cephalosporins, and amounts released into the GI tract are minute; *not* metabolized; 99% is excreted unchanged in the urine in 24 hr; excreted in breast milk

INDICATIONS AND USES: Infections of the lower respiratory and urinary tracts; skin and skin structure infections, septicemia, bone and joint infections, and preoperative prophylaxis, due to susceptible organisms.
Antibacterial spectrum usually includes:

- Gram-positive organisms: *S. aureus, S. epidermidis* (Note: Methicillin-resistant staphylococci are resistant to cephalosporins, including cefonicid.); *S. pneumoniae, S. pyogenes* (Group A beta-hemolytic Streptococcus), and *S. agalactiae* (Group B Streptococcus)
- Gram-negative organisms: *E. coli; K. pneumoniae; Providencia rettgeri; Proteus vulgaris; Morganella morganii; Proteus mirabilis; H. influenzae; Moraxella catarrhalis; K. oxytoca; Enterobacter aerogenes; N. gonorrhoeae*
- Anaerobes: *C. perfringens; Peptostreptococcus anaerobius; Peptococcus magnus; P. prevotii; Propionibacterium acnes; C. freundii; C. diversus, Fusobacterium nucleatum*

DOSAGE

Adult

- IM/IV BOL or INF 1-2 g/24 hr; (divide in two doses if giving 2 g) Dosage reduction appropriate in renal impairment (CrCl <50 ml/min)

$ AVAILABLE FORMS/COST OF THERAPY

- Inj, Lyphl-Sol—IM; IV: 0.5 g: **$13.10;** 1 g: **$27.11**

CONTRAINDICATIONS: Hypersensitivity to cephalosporins, infants <1 mo

PRECAUTIONS: Hypersensitivity to penicillins, renal disease

PREGNANCY AND LACTATION: Pregnancy category B; excreted in breast milk in low concentrations (milk levels 1 hr after 1 g IM dose averaged 0.16 μg/ml)

SIDE EFFECTS/ADVERSE REACTIONS

CNS: Headache, dizziness, weakness, paresthesia, fever, chills

GI: Nausea, vomiting, diarrhea, anorexia, pain, glossitis, bleeding, increased AST, ALT, bilirubin, LDH, alk phosphatase, abdominal pain
GU: Proteinuria, vaginitis, pruritus, candidiasis, increased BUN, ***nephrotoxicity***
HEME: ***Leukopenia, thrombocytopenia, agranulocytosis,*** anemia, ***neutropenia, lymphocytosis, eosinophilia, pancytopenia, hemolytic anemia***
SKIN: Rash, urticaria, dermatitis
MISC: Anaphylaxis

▼ **DRUG INTERACTIONS**

Drugs

• *Aminoglycosides:* Increased risk of nephrotoxicity

Labs

• *Increase (false):* Urinary 17-KS
• *False positive:* Urinary protein, direct Coombs' test, urine glucose
• *Interference:* Cross-matching blood

cefoperazone

(sef-oh-per'a-zone)
Cefobid
Chemical Class: Cephalosporin (3rd generation)
Therapeutic Class: Antibiotic broad-spectrum

CLINICAL PHARMACOLOGY

Mechanism of Action: Inhibition of bacterial cell wall synthesis; bacteriocidal

Pharmacokinetics

IV: peak 5 min, 153 μg/ml after 1 g, duration 6-8 hr
IM: Peak 1-2 hr, 57 μg/ml after 1 g, duration 6-8 hr
$t_{1/2}$, 2 hr; 70%-75% is eliminated unchanged in bile; 20%-30% unchanged in urine

INDICATIONS AND USES: Infections of the lower respiratory tract, urinary tract, skin, bone infections, bacterial septicemia, peritonitis, PID caused by susceptible organisms. Antibacterial spectrum usually includes:

• Gram-negative organisms: *H. influenzae, E. coli, Proteus mirabilis, P. vulgaris, Klebsiella, Enterobacter, Serratia, Citrobacter, Morganella morganii, N. gonorrhoeae, Providencia, Pseudomonas aeruginosa*
• Gram-positive organisms: *S. aureus,* (penicillinase and non-penicillinase-producing strains), *S. epidermidis, Streptococcus pneumoniae, S. pyogenes,* Group A beta-hemolytic streptococci, *S. agalactiae,* Group B beta-hemolytic streptococci, *Enterococcus, Streptococcus faecalis, S. faecium* and *S. durans;* anaerobic organisms
• Gram-positive cocci (including *Peptococcus* and *Peptostreptococcus*), *Clostridium* sp, *Bacteroides fragilis,* and other *Bacteroides* species

DOSAGE

Adult

• *Mild/moderate infections:* IM/IV 1-2 g q12h
• *Severe infections:* IM/IV 6-12 g/day divided in 2-4 equal doses

Child

• Neonates 50 mg/kg/dose q12h; children 100-150 mg/kg/day divided q8-12h; up to 12 g/day

$ **AVAILABLE FORMS/COST OF THERAPY**

• Inj, Sol—IM; IV: 1 g: **$15.79-$31.57**

CONTRAINDICATIONS: Hypersensitivity to cephalosporins, infants <1 mo

PRECAUTIONS: Hypersensitivity to penicillins

PREGNANCY AND LACTATION: Pregnancy category B; low concentrations excreted in human milk (IV, 1 g dose produced levels ranging from 0.4-0.9 μg/ml)

SIDE EFFECTS/ADVERSE REACTIONS

CNS: Headache, dizziness, weakness, paresthesia, fever, chills
GI: Nausea, vomiting, diarrhea, anorexia, pain, glossitis, bleeding, increased AST, ALT, bilirubin, LDH, alk phosphatase, abdominal pain, pseudomembranous colitis
GU: Proteinuria, vaginitis, pruritus, candidiasis, increased BUN, ***nephrotoxicity, renal failure***
HEME: Leukopenia, ***thrombocytopenia, agranulocytosis,*** *anemia,* ***neutropenia, lymphocytosis, eosinophilia, pancytopenia, hemolytic anemia, bleeding, hypoprothrombinemia***
RESP: Dyspnea
SKIN: Rash, urticaria, dermatitis, ***anaphylaxis***

▼ **DRUG INTERACTIONS**

Drugs

- *Aminoglycosides:* Increased risk of nephrotoxicity
- *Ethanol:* Disulfiram-like reactions as a result of acetaldehyde accumulation
- *Oral anticoagulants:* Via hypoprothrombinemia, may enhance anticoagulant effects

Labs

- *Increase (false):* Urinary 17-KS
- *False positive:* Urinary protein, direct Coombs' test, urine glucose
- *Interference:* Cross-matching blood

SPECIAL CONSIDERATIONS

PATIENT/FAMILY EDUCATION

- Avoid alcohol during or for 3 days after use

ceforanide

(sef-or'aa-nide)
Precef
Chemical Class: Cephalosporin (2nd generation)
Therapeutic Class: Antibiotic

CLINICAL PHARMACOLOGY

Mechanism of Action: Inhibition of bacterial cell wall synthesis; bacteriocidal

Pharmacokinetics

IV: Peak concentration with 1.0 g, 125 μg/ml, declining to 5.9 μg/ml in 12 hr
IM: Peak concentration with 0.5 g, 40 μg/ml at 1 hr, declining to 3.9 μg/ml at 12 hr; $t_{1/2}$, 2½-3 hr; 80% bound to plasma proteins; reaches therapeutic levels in the gall bladder, myocardium, bone, skeletal muscle, and vaginal tissue, pericardial fluid, and synovial fluid; 90% eliminated unchanged in urine; 1 g IV doses produced mean urinary conc of 2550 and 190 μg/ml, within 2 and 12 hr after administration

INDICATIONS AND USES: Infections of the lower respiratory tract, urinary tract, skin, bone infections, bacterial septicemia, endocarditis, and perioperative prophylaxis, caused by susceptible organisms. Antibacterial spectrum usually includes:

- Gram-negative organisms: *H. influenzae, E. coli, P. mirabilis, Klebsiella*
- Gram-positive organisms: *S. pneumoniae, S. aureus*

DOSAGE

Adult

- IM/IV 0.5-1 g q12h

Child

- IM/IV 20-40 mg/kg/day in 2 equal doses q12h

Dosage reduction appropriate in renal impairment (CrCl <50 ml/min)

$ AVAILABLE FORMS/COST OF THERAPY

- Inj, Dry-Sol—IM; IV: 500 mg/vial: **$7.20;** 1 g/vial: **$11.94**

CONTRAINDICATIONS: Hypersensitivity to cephalosporins, infants <1 mo

PRECAUTIONS: Hypersensitivity

to penicillins, renal disease

PREGNANCY AND LACTATION: Pregnancy category B

SIDE EFFECTS/ADVERSE REACTIONS

CNS: Headache, dizziness, weakness, paresthesia, fever, chills

GI: Nausea, vomiting, diarrhea, anorexia, pain, glossitis, bleeding, increased AST, ALT, bilirubin, LDH, alk phosphatase, abdominal pain

GU: Proteinuria, vaginitis, pruritus, increased BUN, ***nephrotoxicity, renal failure***

HEME: ***Leukopenia, thrombocytopenia, agranulocytosis,*** anemia, ***neutropenia, lymphocytosis, eosinophilia, pancytopenia, hemolytic anemia***

RESP: Dyspnea

SKIN: Rash, urticaria, dermatitis, ***anaphylaxis***

▼ **DRUG INTERACTIONS**

Drugs

• *Aminoglycosides:* Additive nephrotoxicity
• *Colistin:* Additive nephrotoxicity

Labs

• *Increase (false):* Urinary 17-KS
• *False positive:* Urinary protein, direct Coombs' test, urine glucose
• *Interference:* Cross-matching for blood transfusion

---

cefotaxime

(sef-oh-taks'eem)

Claforan

Chemical Class: Cephalosporin (3rd generation)

Therapeutic Class: Antibiotic, broad-spectrum

CLINICAL PHARMACOLOGY

Mechanism of Action: Inhibition of bacterial cell wall synthesis; bacteriocidal.

Pharmacokinetics

IV: Onset 5 min; 500 mg, 1 g, and 2 g doses produced peak levels of 38.9, 101.7, and 214.4 μg/ml, respectively

IM: Onset 30 min; peak levels of 11.7 and 20.5 μg/ml respectively, following 500 mg or 1 g doses $t_{1/2}$, 1 hr; 35%-65% protein bound; 40%-65% is eliminated unchanged in urine in 24 hr; 25% metabolized to active and inactive metabolites

INDICATIONS AND USES: Infections of the lower respiratory tract, genitourinary tract (including UTI, uncomplicated gonorrhea, PID, endometritis, pelvic cellulitis), skin and skin structure, bone and joints, CNS, e.g., meningitis and ventriculitis; bacteremia/septicemia, intra-abdominal infections including peritonitis, and perioperative prophylaxis around certain surgical procedures (e.g., abdominal or vaginal hysterectomy, gastrointestinal and genitourinary tract surgery).

Antibacterial spectrum usually includes:

• Gram-positive organisms: Group A streptococci *(S. pneumoniae, S. pyogenes)* and other streptococci (excluding enterococci, e.g. *S. faecalis*), *Staphylococcus aureus* (penicillinase and non-penicillinase producing), *Enterococcus* sp, *S. epidermidis*

• Gram-negative organisms: *E. coli, Klebsiella* sp, *H. influenzae* (including ampicillin resistant strains), *H. parainfluenzae, P. mirabilis, S. marcescens, Enterobacter* sp, indole positive *Proteus* and *Pseudomonas* sp (including *P. aeruginosa, Citrobacter* sp, *Morganella morganii, Providencia rettgeri, N. gonorrhoeae,* including penicillinase producing strains

• Anaerobes: *Bacteroides* sp (including *Bacteroides fragilis*) *Clostridium* sp, and anaerobic cocci including *Peptostreptococcus* sp, *Peptococcus* sp, and *Fusobacterium* sp including *F. nucleatum*

DOSAGE

Adult

- IM/IV 1 g q8-12h
- *Severe infections:* IM/IV 2 g q4h, not to exceed 12 g/day
- *Uncomplicated gonorrhea:* 1 g IM
- *Perioperative prophylaxis:* 1 g IM or IV administered 30 to 90 min prior to start of surgery, followed by doses at 6 and 12 hr post surgery
- Dosage reduction appropriate for severe renal impairment (CrCl <10 ml/min)

Child

- Neonates: 0-1 week of age 50 mg/kg IV q12h; 1-4 weeks of age 50 mg/kg IV q8h (it is not necessary to differentiate between premature and normal-gestational age infants); infants and children (1 month to 12 years): For body weights <50 kg 50 to 180 mg/kg IM or IV of body weight divided into four to six equal doses; for body weights >50 kg the usual adult dosage should be used; max daily dosage should not exceed 12 g

$ AVAILABLE FORMS/COST OF THERAPY

- Inj, Dry-Sol—IM; IV: 1 g/vial: **$11.18;** 2 g/vial: **$20.95**

CONTRAINDICATIONS: Hypersensitivity to cephalosporins

PRECAUTIONS: Hypersensitivity to penicillins; colitis

PREGNANCY AND LACTATION: Pregnancy category B; low milk concentrations; M:P ratio, 0.09 at 1 hr

SIDE EFFECTS/ADVERSE REACTIONS

CNS: Headache, dizziness, weakness, paresthesia, fever, chills

GI: Nausea, vomiting, diarrhea, anorexia, pain, glossitis, bleeding, increased AST, ALT, bilirubin, LDH, alk phosphatase, abdominal pain, pseudomembranous colitis

GU: Proteinuria, vaginitis, pruritus, candidiasis, increased BUN, ***renal failure***

HEME: ***Leukopenia, thrombocytopenia, agranulocytosis,*** anemia, ***neutropenia, lymphocytosis, eosinophilia, pancytopenia, hemolytic anemia***

SKIN: Rash, urticaria, dermatitis, ***anaphylaxis,*** pain, induration (IM), inflammation (IV)

▼ DRUG INTERACTIONS

Drugs

- *Aminoglycosides:* Additive nephrotoxicity
- *Colistin:* Additive nephrotoxicity

Labs

- *Increase (false): Urinary 17-KS*
- *False positive:* Urinary protein, direct Coombs' test, urine glucose
- *Interference:* Cross-matching for blood transfusions

---

cefotetan

(sef'oh-tee-tan)

Cefotan

Chemical Class: Cephalosporin (2nd generation)

Therapeutic Class: Antibiotic

CLINICAL PHARMACOLOGY

Mechanism of Action: Inhibition of bacterial cell wall synthesis; bacteriocidal

Pharmacokinetics

IV: Peak, 158 µg/ml at end of inf

IM: Peak, 71 µg/ml at 1 hr

$t_{1/2}$, 3-5 hr, 88% bound by plasma proteins; wide distribution; no active metabolites; 50%-80% eliminated unchanged in urine over 24 hr (peak urinary concentration 1 hr after 1 g IV dose, 1700 µg/ml)

INDICATIONS AND USES: Lower respiratory tract, urinary tract, skin and skin structure, gynecologic, intra-abdominal, bone and joint infections as well as perioperative prophylaxis of susceptible organisms.

Antibacterial spectrum usually includes:

• Gram-positive organisms: *Streptococcus pneumoniae, S. pyogenes, S. agalactiae, Staphylococcus aureus* (penicillinase- and non-penicillinase-producing strains), *S. epidermidis*

• Gram-negative organisms: *E. coli, Klebsiella* sp, *Proteus* sp, *H. influenzae* (including ampicillin-resistant strains), *Serratia marcescens, N. gonorrhoeae;* anaerobes: *Peptococcus niger, Peptostreptococcus* sp, *Bacteroides* sp (excluding *B. distasonis, B. ovatus, B. thetaiotaomicron*), *Fusobacterium* sp

DOSAGE

Adult

• IV/IM 1-2g q12h

• *Perioperative prophylaxis:* IV 1-2 g ½-1 hr before surgery

Child

• IV/IM 20-40 mg/kg q12h

$ AVAILABLE FORMS/COST OF THERAPY

• Inj, Lyphl-Sol—IM; IV: 1 g/vial: **$11.58;** 2 g/vial: **$22.32**

CONTRAINDICATIONS: Hypersensitivity to cephalosporins; children

PRECAUTIONS: Hypersensitivity to penicillins

PREGNANCY AND LACTATION: Pregnancy category B; small amounts excreted into breast milk; M:P ratio average over 10 hr = 0.05

SIDE EFFECTS/ADVERSE REACTIONS

CNS: Headache, dizziness, weakness, paresthesia, fever, chills

CV: Hypotension

GI: Nausea, vomiting, diarrhea, anorexia, pain, glossitis, bleeding, increased AST, ALT, bilirubin, LDH, alk phosphatase, abdominal pain, ***pseudomembranous colitis***

GU: Proteinuria, vaginitis, pruritus, candidiasis, increased BUN

HEME: ***Leukopenia, thrombocytopenia, agranulocytosis,*** anemia, ***neutropenia, lymphocytosis, eosinophilia, pancytopenia, hemolytic anemia***

SKIN: Rash, ***exfoliative dermatitis,*** urticaria, dermatitis, pruritus, thrombophlebitis

MISC: ***Anaphylaxis***

▼ DRUG INTERACTIONS

Drugs

• *Aminoglycosides:* Additive nephrotoxicity

• *Colistin:* Additive nephrotoxicity

• *Ethanol:* disulfiram-like reaction

• *Oral anticoagulants:* Additive hypoprothrombinemia, enhanced anticoagulant effects

Labs

• *Increase (false): Urinary 17-KS*

• *False positive:* Urinary protein, direct Coombs' test, urine glucose

• *Interference:* Cross-matching for blood transfusion

cefoxitin sodium

(se-fox'i-tin)

Mefoxin

Chemical Class: Cephamycin (2nd generation)

Therapeutic Class: Antibiotic

CLINICAL PHARMACOLOGY

Mechanism of Action: Inhibition of bacterial cell wall synthesis; bacteriocidal

Pharmacokinetics

IV: Peak 5 min after 1 g infusion 110 µg/ml, declining to less than 1 µg/ml at 4 hr

IM: Peak 20-30 min after 1 g dose 24 µg/ml

$t_{1/2}$ 1 hr; 55%-75% bound by plasma proteins; passes into pleural and joint fluids and is detectable in antibacterial concentrations in bile; 85% eliminated unchanged in urine, 3000 µg/ml observed following an IM 1 g dose; not metabolized; crosses blood-brain barrier

INDICATIONS AND USES: Lower respiratory tract, urinary tract, skin and skin structure, gynecologic, intra-abdominal, bone and joint infections as well as perioperative prophylaxis of susceptible organisms. Antibacterial spectrum usually includes:

- Gram-positive organisms: *Streptococcus pneumoniae, S. pyogenes, S. agalactiae, Staphylococcus aureus* (penicillinase- and nonpenicillinase-producing strains), *S. epidermidis*
- Gram-negative organisms: *E. coli, Klebsiella* sp, *Proteus* sp, *H. influenzae* (including ampicillin-resistant strains), *Serratia marcescens, N. gonorrhoeae, Morganella morganii, Providencia* sp
- Anaerobes: *Peptococcus niger, Peptostreptococcus* sp, *Bacteroides* sp (excluding *B. distasonis, B. ovatus, B. thetaiotaomicron*), *Fusobacterium* sp

DOSAGE

Adult

- IM/IV 1-2 g q6-8h
- *Uncomplicated gonorrhea:* 2 g IM as single dose with 1 g PO probenecid
- *Severe infections:* IM/IV 2 g q4h
- Dose reduction appropriate in renal impairment (CrCl <50 ml/min)

Child (3 months and older)

- IM/IV 80 to 160 mg/kg of body weight per day divided into four to six equal doses, not to exceed 12 g/day.

$ AVAILABLE FORMS/COST OF THERAPY

- Inj, Dry-Sol—IM; IV: 1 g: **$8.52;** 2 g: **$16.99**

CONTRAINDICATIONS: Hypersensitivity to cephalosporins

PRECAUTIONS: Hypersensitivity to penicillins

PREGNANCY AND LACTATION: Pregnancy category B; low milk concentrations

SIDE EFFECTS/ADVERSE REACTIONS

CNS: Headache, dizziness, weakness, paresthesia, fever, chills

CV: Hypotension

GI: Nausea, vomiting, diarrhea, anorexia, pain, glossitis, bleeding, increased AST, ALT, bilirubin, LDH, alk phosphatase, abdominal pain, pseudomembranous colitis

GU: Proteinuria, vaginitis, pruritus, candidiasis, increased BUN

HEME: ***Leukopenia, thrombocytopenia, agranulocytosis,*** anemia, ***neutropenia, lymphocytosis, eosinophilia, pancytopenia, hemolytic anemia***

SKIN: Rash, ***exfoliative dermatitis;*** urticaria, dermatitis, pruritus, thrombophlebitis

MISC: ***Anaphylaxis***

▼ DRUG INTERACTIONS

Drugs

- *Aminoglycosides:* Additive nephrotoxicity
- *Colistin:* Additive nephrotoxicity
- *Oral anticoagulants:* Additive hypoprothrombinemia, enhanced anticoagulant effects

Labs

- *Increase (false):* Creatinine (serum urine), urinary 17-KS
- *False positive:* Urinary protein, direct Coombs' test, urine glucose
- *Interference:* Cross-matching blood transfusions

cefpodoxime

(sef-pod'-ox-ime)

Vantin

Chemical Class: Cephalosporin (2nd generation)

Therapeutic Class: Antibiotic

CLINICAL PHARMACOLOGY
Mechanism of Action: Inhibition of bacterial cell wall synthesis; bacteriocidal
Pharmacokinetics
PO: Peak levels 2.3 μg/ml after 200 mg at 2-3 hr; absorbed as prodrug, de-esterified to its active metabolite, cefpodoxime (approximately 50% of the administered dose is systemically absorbed); minimal metabolism; $t_{1/2}$ 2-3 hr; 25% bound by plasma proteins; 30% eliminated unchanged in urine in 12 hr
INDICATIONS AND USES: Upper and lower respiratory tract, skin and skin structure, urinary tract infections and sexually transmitted diseases (acute, uncomplicated urethral and cervical gonorrhea) caused by susceptible organisms.
Antibacterial spectrum usually includes:
- Gram-positive organisms: *Streptococcus pneumoniae, S. pyogenes, Staphylococcus aureus* (including penicillinase-producing strains)
- Gram-negative organisms: *H. influenzae* (non-β-lactamase-producing strains only), *N. gonorrhoeae* (including penicillinase-producing strains), *Moraxella catarrhalis, E. coli, Klebsiella pneumoniae, Proteus mirabilis, S. saprophyticus*

DOSAGE
Adult
- *Pneumonia:* 200 mg q12h for 14 days
- *Uncomplicated gonorrhea:* 200 mg single dose
- *Skin and skin structure:* 400 mg q12h for 7-14 days
- *Pharyngitis and tonsillitis:* 100 mg q12h for 10 days
- *Uncomplicated UTI:* 100 mg q12h for 7 days

Child
- *Acute otitis media:* 5 mg/kg q12h for 14 days
- *Uncomplicated gonorrhea:* 200 mg single dose
- *Skin and skin structure:* 400 mg q12h for 7-14 days
- *Pharyngitis and tonsillitis:* 100 mg q12h (max 200 mg/dose or 400 mg/day) for 10 days
- *Pharyngitis/tonsillitis:* 5 mg/kg q12h (max 100 mg/dose or 200 mg/day) for 10 days

$ **AVAILABLE FORMS/COST OF THERAPY**
- Susp—Oral: 50 mg/5 ml, 100 ml: **$29.59;** 100 mg/5 ml, 100 ml: **$56.30**
- Tab, Uncoated—Oral: 100 mg, 100's: **$172.13;** 200 mg, 100's: **$327.86**

CONTRAINDICATIONS: Hypersensitivity to cephalosporins; infants
PRECAUTIONS: Hypersensitivity to penicillins, renal disease
PREGNANCY AND LACTATION: Pregnancy category B; excreted into breast milk; average 2% of serum levels at 4 hr following 200 mg dose
SIDE EFFECTS/ADVERSE REACTIONS
CNS: Headache, dizziness, lethargy, fatigue, paresthesia, fever, chills
GI: Nausea, vomiting, diarrhea, anorexia, pain, glossitis, bleeding, increased AST, ALT, bilirubin, LDH, alk phosphatase, ***pseudomembranous colitis***
GU: Proteinuria, vaginitis, pruritus, candidiasis, increased BUN
HEME: ***Leukopenia, thrombocytopenia, agranulocytosis,*** anemia, ***neutropenia, lymphocytosis, eosinophilia, pancytopenia, hemolytic anemia***
RESP: ***Dyspnea***
SKIN: Rash, urticaria, dermatitis, ***anaphylaxis***
▼ **DRUG INTERACTIONS**
Drugs
- *Antacids*: Reduced bioavailabil-

ity and serum cefpodoxime levels
Labs
• *Increased (false)*: Creatinine (serum urine), urinary 17-KS
• *False positive:* Urinary protein, direct Coombs' test, urine glucose
• *Interference:* Cross-matching for blood transfusions

cefprozil

(sef-pro'zil)
Cefzil
Chemical Class: Cephalosporin, second generation
Therapeutic Class: Antibiotic

CLINICAL PHARMACOLOGY
Mechanism of Action: Inhibition of bacterial cell wall synthesis; bacteriocidal
Pharmacokinetics
PO: Peak serum and urine concentration, 1.5 and 4 hr after 500 mg dose, 10.5 μg/ml and 1000 μg/ml, respectively; 95% absorbed (no food effect observed); plasma protein binding, 36%; $t_{1/2}$, 1.3 hr
INDICATIONS AND USES: Infections of the upper and lower respiratory tract, skin and skin structure due to susceptible organisms.
Antibacterial spectrum usually includes:
• Gram-positive organisms: *Staphylococcus aureus* including penicillinase-producing strains
NOTE: Cefprozil is inactive against methicillin-resistant staphylococci, *Streptococcus pneumoniae*, *S. pyogenes*
• Gram-negative organisms: *Moraxella catarrhalis*, *H. influenzae* (including penicillinase-producing strains)
DOSAGE
Adult
• *Upper respiratory infections:* PO 500 mg qd × 10 days
• *Lower respiratory infections:* PO 500 mg bid × 10 days
• *Skin/skin structure infections:* PO 250-500 mg q12h × 10 days
Child (6 mo-12 yr)
• *Otitis media:* PO 15mg/kg q12h × 10 days
$ AVAILABLE FORMS/COST OF THERAPY
• Susp—Oral: 125 mg/5 ml, 100 ml: **$26.15;** 250 mg/5 ml, 100 ml: **$47.40**
• Tab, Uncoated—Oral: 250 mg, 100's: **$273.73;** 500 mg, 100's: **$537.89**
CONTRAINDICATIONS: Hypersensitivity to cephalosporins
PRECAUTIONS: Elderly, hypersensitivity to penicillins
PREGNANCY AND LACTATION: Pregnancy category B
SIDE EFFECTS/ADVERSE REACTIONS
CNS: Dizziness, headache, weakness, paresthesia, fever, chills
GI: Diarrhea, nausea, vomiting, pain, glossitis, anorexia, bleeding, increased AST, ALT, bilirubin, LDH, alk phosphatase, abdominal pain, ***pseudomembranous colitis,*** flatulence
GU: ***Nephrotoxicity, proteinuria, increased BUN, renal failure, hematuria,*** vaginitis, genitoanal pruritus, candidiasis
HEME: ***Leukopenia, thrombocytopenia, agranulocytosis,*** anemia, ***neutropenia, lymphocytosis, eosinophilia, pancytopenia, hemolytic anemia***
SKIN: Rash, urticaria, dermatitis
RESP: ***Anaphylaxis,*** dyspnea
▼ DRUG INTERACTIONS
Labs
• *Increase (false):* Urinary 17-KS
• *False positive:* Urinary protein, direct Coombs' test, urine glucose
• *Interference:* Cross-matching

blood for transfusion

ceftazidime

(sef-taz'i-deem)
Ceptaz, Fortaz, Pentacef, Tazicef, Tazidime
Chemical Class: Cephalosporin (3rd generation)
Therapeutic Class: Antibiotic, broad-spectrum

CLINICAL PHARMACOLOGY
Mechanism of Action: Inhibition of bacterial cell wall synthesis; bacteriocidal
Pharmacokinetics
IV: Peak, 60 µg/ml, 1 gm over 20 min
IM: 1 g peak, 39 µg/ml at 1 hr
$t_{1/2}$ 1.9 hr; <10% bound to plasma proteins; 80% eliminated unchanged in urine
INDICATIONS AND USES: Upper and lower respiratory tract, urinary tract, skin and skin structure, gonococcal, and intraabdominal infections; septicemia, meningitis caused by susceptible organisms.
Antibacterial spectrum usually includes:
• Gram-positive organisms: *Streptococcus pneumoniae, S. pyogenes, S. agalactiae* (group B streptococci), *Staphylococcus aureus*
• Gram-negative organisms: *H. influenzae, E. coli, E. aerogenes, P. aeruginosa, P. mirabilis, P. vulgaris, Klebsiella, Citrobacter, Enterobacter, Salmonella, Shigella, Acinetobacter, B. fragilis, Neisseria, Serratia*
DOSAGE
Adult
• IV/IM 1 g q8-12h
Child
• IV 30-50 mg/kg/day q8h, not to exceed 6 g/day
Neonates
• IV 30 mg/kg q8-12h
$ **AVAILABLE FORMS/COST OF THERAPY**
• Inj, Dry-Sol—IV; IM: 500 mg/vial: **$7.11;** 1 g/vial: **$14.59-$15.66;** 2 g/vial: **$28.93**
CONTRAINDICATIONS: Hypersensitivity to cephalosporins, children
PRECAUTIONS: Hypersensitivity to penicillins, renal disease
PREGNANCY AND LACTATION: Pregnancy category B; excreted in human milk in low concentrations (mean milk concentrations 1 hr post-2 gm dose, 5.2 µg/ml, with no accumulation)
SIDE EFFECTS/ADVERSE REACTIONS
CNS: Headache, dizziness, weakness, paresthesia, fever, chills
GI: Nausea, vomiting, diarrhea, anorexia, pain, glossitis, bleeding, increased AST, ALT, bilirubin, LDH, alk phosphatase
GU: Proteinuria, vaginitis, pruritus, candidiasis, increased BUN, ***nephrotoxicity, renal failure***
HEME: ***Leukopenia, thrombocytopenia, agranulocytosis***, *anemia,* ***neutropenia, lymphocytosis, eosinophilia, pancytopenia, hemolytic anemia***
RESP: Dyspnea
SKIN: Rash, urticaria, dermatitis, ***anaphylaxis***
▼ **DRUG INTERACTIONS**
Drugs
• *Aminoglycosides:* Increased risk of nephrotoxicity
• *Colistin:* Additive nephrotoxicity
Labs
• *Increase (false)*: Urinary 17-KS
• *False positive*: Urinary protein, direct Coombs' test, urine glucose
• *Interference*: Cross-matching blood

ceftizoxime

(sef-ti-zox'eem)
Cefizox
Chemical Class: Cephalosporin (3rd generation)
Therapeutic Class: Antibiotic, broad-spectrum

CLINICAL PHARMACOLOGY
Mechanism of Action: Inhibition of bacterial cell wall synthesis; bacteriocidal
Pharmacokinetics
IV: Peak, 60.5 µg/ml, following 1 g inf
IM: Peak, 1 hr 39 µg/ml
$t_{1/2}$, 1.7 hr; 30% bound by plasma proteins; not metabolized; eliminated unchanged in urine in 24 hr; crosses placenta
INDICATIONS AND USES: Infections of the lower respiratory tract, urinary tract, gonorrhea, pelvic inflammatory disease, septicemia, skin and skin structure, bone and joint infections, meningitis caused by susceptible organisms.
Antibacterial spectrum usually includes:
• Gram-positive organisms: *Streptococcus pneumoniae, S. pyogenes, S. agalactiae, Staphylococcus aureus; S. epidermis*
• Gram-negative organisms: *Acinetobacter, H. influenzae, E. coli, E. aerogenes, P. mirabilis, P. vulgaris, Providencia rettgeri, P. aeruginosa, Serratia, Klebsiella, Enterobacter, Morganella morganii, N. gonorrhoeae*
• Anaerobes: *Bacteroides, Peptococcus, Peptostreptococcus*
DOSAGE
Adult
• IM/IV 1-2 g q8-12h, may give up to 2g q4h in life-threatening infections
• *PID:* IV 2 g q8h
• *Uncomplicated gonorrhea:* single, 1 g IM dose, may increase to 2 g q4h in severe infections
Child (≥6 mo)
• 150-200 mg/kg/day divided q6-8h
• Dosage reduction appropriate in renal impairment (CrCl < 50 ml/min)

$ AVAILABLE FORMS/COST OF THERAPY
• Inj, Sol—IV: 1 g: **$11.86;** 2 g: **$22.03;** 500 mg: **$6.75**
CONTRAINDICATIONS: Hypersensitivity to cephalosporins, infants <1 mo
PRECAUTIONS: Hypersensitivity to penicillins, renal disease
PREGNANCY AND LACTATION: Pregnancy category B; excreted in human milk in low concentrations (mean levels following single 2 g dose <0.5 µg/ml)
SIDE EFFECTS/ADVERSE REACTIONS
CNS: Headache, dizziness, paresthesia, fever
GI: Nausea, vomiting, diarrhea, anorexia, pain, glossitis, bleeding, increased AST, ALT, bilirubin, LDH, alk phosphatase, abdominal pain, ***pseudomembranous colitis***
GU: Proteinuria, vaginitis, pruritus, candidiasis
HEME: ***Leukopenia, thrombocytopenia, agranulocytosis,*** *anemia,* ***neutropenia, eosinophilia, hemolytic anemia***
RESP: Dyspnea
SKIN: Rash, urticaria, dermatitis
MISC: ***Anaphylaxis***

▼ DRUG INTERACTIONS
Drugs
• *Aminoglycosides:* Increased risk of nephrotoxicity
• *Oral anticoagulants:* Via hypoprothrombinemia, may enhance anticoagulant effects
Labs
• *Increase (false):* Urinary 17-KS

• *False positive:* Urinary protein, direct Coombs' test, urine glucose
• *Interference:* Cross-matching blood

ceftriaxone

(sef-try-ax'-one)
Rocephin
Chemical Class: Cephalosporin (3rd generation)
Therapeutic Class: Antibiotic

CLINICAL PHARMACOLOGY
Mechanism of Action: Inhibits bacterial cell wall synthesis; bacteriocidal
Pharmacokinetics
IV: Peak 30 min (123 μg/ml for 1 g)
IM: Peak 1.5-4 hr (83 μg/ml for 1 g)
$t_{1/2}$ 5-8 hr; 90% bound by plasma proteins; 35%-60% eliminated unchanged in urine, remainder secreted in bile; crosses placenta; elimination $t_{1/2}$ in elderly and in renal or hepatic disease, healthy subjects, 7.2 hr; elderly subjects 8.9 hr; patients with liver disease 8.8 hr; hemodialysis patients 14.7 hr; CrCl 5-15 ml/min 15.7 hr; CrCl 16-30 ml/min 11.4 hr; CrCl 31-60 ml/min 12.4 hr
INDICATIONS AND USES: Infections of the lower respiratory tract, urinary tract, skin, bone, joint; intra-abdominal infections; septicemia, or meningitis caused by susceptible organisms; localized and disseminated gonococcal infections.
Antibacterial spectrum usually includes:
• Gram-negative organisms: *H. influenzae, E. coli, E. aerogenes, E. cloacae, P. mirabilis, P. vulgaris, Serratia marcescens, Providencia rettgeri, Klebsiella* sp, *Citrobacter* sp, *Salmonella* sp (including *S. typhi*), *Shigella* sp, *Acinetobacter* sp, *Neisseria* sp; some strains of *Pseudomonas aeruginosa*
• Gram-positive organisms: *Streptococcus pneumoniae, S. pyogenes, Staphylococcus aureus*
• Anaerobes: *B. fragilis, B. bivivus, B. melaninogenicus, Peptostreptococcus* sp
DOSAGE
Adult
• *Infections of the lower respiratory tract, urinary tract, skin, bone, joint; intra-abdominal infections; septicemia:* IM/IV 1-2 g qd or in two equal doses not to exceed 4 g qd
• *Uncomplicated gonorrhea:* IM 125-250 mg as single dose (reduce dose if CrCl < 10 ml/min)
• *Meningitis:* IM/IV 100 mg/kg/day in equal doses q12h not to exceed 4 g qd
• *Surgical prophylaxis:* IV 1 g ½-2 hr preop
Child
• *Infections of the lower respiratory tract, urinary tract, skin, bone, joint; intra-abdominal infections; septicemia:* IM/IV 50-75 mg/kg/day in equal doses q12h; not to exceed 2 g qd
• *Meningitis:* IM/IV 100 mg/kg/day in equal doses q12h not to exceed 4 g qd

$ AVAILABLE FORMS/COST OF THERAPY
• Inj, Dry-Sol—IM; IV: 250 mg/vial, 10's: **$102.96;** 500 mg/vial, 10's: **$177.15;** 1 g/vial, 10's: **$323.53;** 2 g/vial, 10's: **$641.67**
CONTRAINDICATIONS: Hypersensitivity to the cephalosporin class of antibiotics
PRECAUTIONS: Hypersensitivity to penicillins, renal disease
PREGNANCY AND LACTATION: Pregnancy category B; excreted in breast milk
SIDE EFFECTS/ADVERSE REACTIONS
CNS: Headache, dizziness, weakness, paresthesia, fever, chills

GI: Nausea, vomiting, diarrhea, anorexia, pain, glossitis, bleeding, increased AST, ALT, bilirubin, LDH, alkaline phosphatase, abdominal pain, ***pseudomembranous colitis***
GU: Proteinuria, vaginitis, pruritus, candidiasis, ***nephrotoxicity***
HEME: ***Leukopenia (2%), neutropenia, agranulocytosis, thrombocytopenia, agranulocytosis,*** anemia, ***hemolytic anemia, pancytopenia,*** lymphocytosis, eosinophilia, thrombocytosis, ***increased prothrombin time***
RESP: Dyspnea
SKIN: Rash, urticaria, dermatitis, pain, induration or tenderness at injection site
MISC: ***Anaphylaxis***

▼ **DRUG INTERACTIONS**

Drugs

• *Aminoglycosides:* Increased risk of nephrotoxicity due to aminoglycoside
• *Warfarin:* Hypoprothrombinemic response enhanced

Labs

• *False positive:* Urine 17-KS, urine protein, urine glucose, direct Coombs' test
• *Interference:* Cross-matching

---

cefuroxime

(sef-yoor-ox'-eem)
Zinacef, Kefurox (as sodium); Ceftin (as axetil)
Chemical Class: Cephalosporin (2nd generation)
Therapeutic Class: Antibiotic

CLINICAL PHARMACOLOGY

Mechanism of Action: Inhibits bacterial cell wall synthesis; bacteriocidal

Pharmacokinetics

PO: Hydrolyzed to cefuroxime, peak level 2 hr (7 µg/ml after 500 mg); *IV:* Peak 30 min (100 µg/ml after 1g) *IM:* Peak 15-60 min (36 µg/ml after 1 g)
Absorption greater after food (absolute bioavailability increases from 37% to 52%); bioavailability of suspension 91% of tab; peak plasma concentration for suspension 71% of peak plasma concentration for tablets; $t_{1/2}$ 1-2 hr; 33%-50% bound by plasma proteins; 70%-100% eliminated unchanged in urine; crosses placenta, blood-brain barrier; not metabolized

INDICATIONS AND USES: Pharyngitis, tonsillitis, otitis media, bronchitis, pneumonia, infections of the skin and urinary tract, localized and disseminated gonococcal infections, bone or joint infections, septicemia, or meningitis caused by susceptible organisms.
Antibacterial spectrum usually includes:
• Gram-negative organisms: *H. influenzae, H. parainfluenzae, Moraxella catarrhalis* (including ampicillin- and cephalothin-resistant strains), *E. coli, P. mirabilis, Neisseria* sp, *Klebsiella* sp
• Gram-positive organisms: *Streptococcus pneumoniae, S. pyogenes, Staphylococcus aureus*
• Anaerobes: *Peptococcus* and *Peptostreptococcus* sp; β-lactamase-producing strains of these pathogens are usually susceptible

DOSAGE

Adult

• *Pharyngitis, tonsillitis, bronchitis, skin infections:* PO (tab) 250-500 mg q12h
• *UTI:* PO (tab) 125-250 mg q12h
• *Urethral/cervical gonorrhea:* PO 1,000 mg single dose
• *Uncomplicated urinary tract infections, skin infections, disseminated gonococcal infections, and uncomplicated pneumonia:* IM/IV 750

mg-1.5 g q8h

• *Bone and joint infections:* IM/IV 1.5 g q8h

• *Surgical prophylaxis:* IV 1.5 g ½-1 hr preop

• *Severe infections including meningitis:* IM/IV 1.5 g q6h; may give up to 3 g q8h for bacterial meningitis

• *Uncomplicated gonorrhea:* 1.5 g IM as single dose, 2 sites, with 1 g oral probenecid

• *Dosage in renal impairment:* CrCl >20 ml/min, use 750 mg-1.5 g q8h; CrCl 10-20 ml/min, use 750 mg q12h; CrCl <10 ml/min, use 750 mg q24h; since cefuroxime sodium is dialyzable, patients on hemodialysis should be given a further dose at the end of the dialysis

Child

• *Pharyngitis, tonsillitis, bronchitis:* Age >12 yr PO (tab) 250-500 mg q12h; age 3 mo-12 yr PO (susp) 20 mg/kg/day, divided bid, max dose 500 qd

• *Skin infections:* Age >12 yr PO (tab) 250-500 mg q12h; age 3 mo-12 yr PO (susp) 30 mg/kg/day, divided bid, 1,000 mg qd

• *Otitis media:* Age 2 yr-12 yr PO (tab) 250 mg bid, PO (susp) 30 mg/kg/day, divided bid, max dose 1,000 mg qd; age 3 mo-12 yr PO (tab) 125 mg bid, PO (susp) 30 mg/kg/day, divided bid, max dose 1,000 mg qd

• *Uncomplicated urinary tract infections, skin infections, disseminated gonococcal infections, and uncomplicated pneumonia:* Age > 3 mo IM/IV 50-100 mg/kg qd (not to exceed the max adult dosage) in equally divided doses q8h

• *Bone and joint infections:* Age >3 mo IM/IV 150 mg/kg qd (not to exceed the max adult dosage) in equally divided doses q8h

• *Severe infections including meningitis:* Age >3 mo IM/IV 50-100 mg/kg qd in equally divided doses q6-8h; may give up to 200-240 mg/kg/day IV in divided doses for bacterial meningitis

$ AVAILABLE FORMS/COST OF THERAPY

• Powder, Reconst—Oral: 125 mg/5 ml, 100 ml: **$28.58**

• Tab, Coated—Oral: 125 mg, 20's: **$34.86;** 250 mg, 20's: **$65.35;** 500 mg, 20's: **$123.98**

• Inj, Dry-Sol—IM; IV: 750 mg/vial, 10's: **$60.88-$73.80;** 1.5 g/vial, 10's: **121.12-$139.39;** 7.5 g/vial, 10's: **$593.52**

CONTRAINDICATIONS: Hypersensitivity to cephalosporins, infants <1 mo

PRECAUTIONS: Hypersensitivity to penicillins, renal disease

PREGNANCY AND LACTATION: Pregnancy category B; excreted in breast milk

SIDE EFFECTS/ADVERSE REACTIONS

CNS: Headache, dizziness, weakness, paresthesia, fever, chills

GI: Nausea, vomiting, diarrhea, anorexia, pain, glossitis, bleeding, increased AST, ALT, bilirubin, LDH; abdominal pain, ***pseudomembranous colitis***

GU: Proteinuria, vaginitis, pruritus, candidiasis, ***nephrotoxicity***

HEME: ***Leukopenia, neutropenia, agranulocytosis, thrombocytopenia,*** anemia, ***hemolytic anemia, pancytopenia,*** lymphocytosis, eosinophilia, thrombocytosis

RESP: Dyspnea

SKIN: Rash, urticaria, dermatitis

MISC: ***Anaphylaxis***

▼ DRUG INTERACTIONS

Drugs

• *Aminoglycosides:* Increased risk of nephrotoxicity due to aminoglycoside

• *Antacids:* Decreased absorption of cefuroxime axetil

• *H_2 blockers:* Decreased absorption of cefuroxime axetil
• *Omeprazole:* Decreased absorption of cefuroxime axetil
• *Warfarin:* Hypoprothrombinemic response enhanced

Labs

• *False positive:* Urine 17-KS, urine protein, urine glucose, direct Coombs' test; increase urine/serum creatinine (not by alkaline picrate method)
• *Interference:* Cross-matching

SPECIAL CONSIDERATIONS

• Oral tabs and oral susp not bioequivalent
• Take with food

---

cellulose sodium phosphate (CSP)

Calcibind

Chemical Class: Phosphorylated cellulose

Therapeutic Class: Antihypercalcemic

CLINICAL PHARMACOLOGY

Mechanism of Action: Decreases hypercalciuria by binding with calcium in bowel; reduces urinary calcium by approximately 50 mg/5 g qd of CSP

Pharmacokinetics

Not absorbed

INDICATIONS AND USES: Absorptive hypercalciuria type I with recurrent calcium oxalate or calcium phosphate renal stones

DOSAGE

Adult

• PO 15 g qd divided between each meal, then 10 g qd (5 g with supper, 2.5 g with each remaining meal) when 24 hr urine Ca excretion <150 mg. For each 15 g qd of CSP, give 1.5 g Mg gluconate bid (at least 1 hr before or after a dose of CSP)

$ **AVAILABLE FORMS/COST OF THERAPY**

• Powder, Reconst—Oral: 2.5 g/scoop, 300 g: **$75.00**

CONTRAINDICATIONS: Hypersensitivity, hyperparathyroidism, hypomagnesemia, enteric hyperoxaluria, metabolic bone disease, hypocalcemia

PRECAUTIONS: CHF, ascites, liver disease, children, elderly

PREGNANCY AND LACTATION: Pregnancy category C

SIDE EFFECTS/ADVERSE REACTIONS

GI: Nausea, anorexia, diarrhea, dyspepsia

GU: Hypomagnesuria, hyperoxaluria, hyperphosphaturia

METAB: Hypomagnesemia, depletion of trace metals (copper, zinc, iron)

▼ **DRUG INTERACTIONS**

• *Ascorbic acid:* Increased hyperoxaluria due to CSP
• M*agnesium-containing preparations:* Decreased action of CSP

SPECIAL CONSIDERATIONS

MONITORING PARAMETERS: Serum Ca, Mg, copper, zinc, iron, parathyroid hormone, and CBC every 3 to 6 mo

• Serum parathyroid hormone should be obtained at least once between the first 2 wk to 3 mo of treatment

---

cephalexin

(sef-a-lex′-in)

Keftab, Biocef, Cefanex, Cephalexin, Ceporex, ♣ Keflex, Novolexin, ♣ Nu-Cephalex ♣

Chemical Class: Cephalosporin (1st generation)

Therapeutic Class: Antibiotic

CLINICAL PHARMACOLOGY

Mechanism of Action: Inhibits bacterial cell wall synthesis; bacteriocidal

Pharmacokinetics

PO: Peak 1 hr (15 µg/ml after 500 mg), duration 6-8 hr, t½ 30-72 min; 5%-15% bound by plasma proteins; 90%-100% eliminated unchanged in urine within 8 hr; crosses placenta; may be given without regard to meals

INDICATIONS AND USES: Pharyngitis, tonsillitis, otitis media, bronchitis, pneumonia, skin and urinary tract infections caused by susceptible organisms.

Antibacterial spectrum usually includes:

- Gram-negative organisms: *H. influenzae, E. coli, P. mirabilis, Moraxella catarrhalis, Klebsiella* sp
- Gram-positive organisms: *Streptococcus pneumoniae, S. pyogenes, Staphylococcus aureus*

DOSAGE

Adult

- *Bronchitis, pneumonia, urinary tract infections:* PO 250-500 mg q6h
- *Pharyngitis, tonsillitis, cystitis, mild to moderate skin infections:* PO 500 mg q12h
- *Severe infections:* PO 500 mg-1 g q6h
- Dosage in renal impairment: CrCl 11-40 ml/min, max adult dose 500 mg q8-12h; CrCl 5-10 ml/min, max adult dose 250 mg q12h; CrCl <5 ml/min, max adult dose 250 mg q12-24h

Child

- *Bronchitis, pneumonia, urinary tract infections:* PO 25-50 mg/kg/day in 4 equal doses
- *Pharyngitis, tonsillitis, cystitis, mild to moderate skin infections:* Age >15 yr PO 500 mg q12h; age >1 yr PO 25-50 mg/kg qd in 2 equal doses
- *Severe infections:* PO 50-100 mg/kg/day in 4 equal doses
- *Otitis media:* PO 75-100 mg/kg/day in 4 equal doses

$ **AVAILABLE FORMS/COST OF THERAPY**

- Cap, Gel—Oral: 250 mg, 100's: **$19.43-$133.16;** 500 mg, 100's: **$38.18-$257.49**
- Powder, Reconst—Oral: 125 mg/5 ml, 200 ml: **$9.62-$25.25;** 250 mg/5 ml, 200 ml: **$18.15-$47.53**
- Tab, Plain Coated—Oral: 250 mg, 100's: **$32.33-$95.41;** 500 mg, 100's: **$44.49-$87.52**

CONTRAINDICATIONS: Hypersensitivity to cephalosporins, infants <1 mo

PRECAUTIONS: Hypersensitivity to penicillins, renal disease

PREGNANCY AND LACTATION: Pregnancy category B, excreted in breast milk

SIDE EFFECTS/ADVERSE REACTIONS

CNS: Headache, dizziness, weakness, paresthesia, fever, chills

GI: Nausea, vomiting, *diarrhea,* anorexia, pain, glossitis, bleeding, increased AST, ALT, bilirubin, LDH, alkaline phosphatase; abdominal pain, ***pseudomembranous colitis***

GU: Proteinuria, vaginitis, pruritus, candidiasis, ***nephrotoxicity***

HEME: ***Leukopenia, neutropenia, agranulocytosis, thrombocytopenia,*** anemia, ***hemolytic anemia, pancytopenia,*** lymphocytosis, eosinophilia, thrombocytosis

RESP: Dyspnea

SKIN: Rash, urticaria, dermatitis

MISC: Serum sickness-like syndrome, ***anaphylaxis***

▼ **DRUG INTERACTIONS**

Drugs

- *Aminoglycosides:* Increased risk of nephrotoxicity due to aminoglycoside
- *Colistin:* Increased risk of nephrotoxicity due to colistin
- *Warfarin:* Hypoprothrombinemic response enhanced

Labs

- *False positive:* Urine 17-KS, urine protein, urine glucose, direct Coombs' test; increase urine/serum creatinine (not by alkaline picrate method)
- *Interference:* Cross-matching

cephalothin

(sef-a-loe'thin)

Keflin, Seffin ♣

Chemical Class: Cephalosporin (1st generation)

Therapeutic Class: Antibiotic

CLINICAL PHARMACOLOGY

Mechanism of Action: Inhibits the biosynthesis of cell wall mucopeptide in susceptible organisms; bacteriocidal when adequate concentrations are reached

Pharmacokinetics

IM: Peak 0.5 hr, excreted by the kidneys (inhibited by probenecid), $t_{1/2}$ ½-1hr, 65%-80% bound by plasma proteins

INDICATIONS AND USES: Infections of the respiratory tract, skin and skin structures, genitourinary tract, gastrointestinal tract, bones and joints; endocarditis, septicemia; meningitis (NOTE: Inasmuch as only low levels are found in the cerebrospinal fluid, cannot be recommended for treatment of meningitis; has, however, proved to be effective in a number of cases of meningitis and may be considered for unusual circumstances in which other, more reliably effective antibiotics cannot be used); perioperative prophylaxis for contaminated or potentially contaminated procedures; all approved indications caused by susceptible organisms. Antibacterial spectrum usually includes:

- Gram-positive organisms: group A β-hemolytic streptococci, Staphylococci (including coagulase-positive, coagulase-negative, and penicillinase-producing strains [not MRSA]), *Streptococcus pneumoniae*
- Gram-negative organisms: *Haemophilus influenzae, Escherichia coli* and other coliform bacteria, *Klebsiella* sp, *Proteus mirabilis, Salmonella* sp, *Shigella* sp

DOSAGE

Adult

- IM/IV 500 mg-1 g q4-6h
- *Uncomplicated gonorrhea:* IM 2 g as single dose
- *Severe infections:* IM/IV 1-2 g q4h
- Dosage reduction indicated in renal impairment (CrCl <50 ml/min)

Child

- IM/IV 14-27 mg/kg q4h or 20-40 mg/kg q6h

$ **AVAILABLE FORMS/COST OF THERAPY**

- Inj, Dry-Sol—IV: 1 g/vial, 25's: **$85.53,** 2 g/vial, 10's: **$61.20**

CONTRAINDICATIONS: Hypersensitivity to cephalosporins

PRECAUTIONS: Hypersensitivity to penicillins, renal disease, prolonged use, colitis

PREGNANCY AND LACTATION: Pregnancy category B; excreted into breast milk in low concentrations, no adverse effects have been observed but potential exists for modification of bowel flora in nursing infant, allergy/sensitization and interference with interpretation of culture results if fever workup required

SIDE EFFECTS/ADVERSE REACTIONS

CNS: Headache, dizziness, weakness, paresthesia, fever, chills

GI: Nausea, vomiting, *diarrhea,* anorexia, pain, glossitis, bleeding, increased AST, ALT, bilirubin, LDH, alk phosphatase, abdominal pain, ***pseudomembranous colitis***

GU: ***Proteinuria,*** vaginitis, pruritus, candidiasis, increased BUN, ***nephrotoxicity, renal failure***

HEME: ***Leukopenia, thrombocytopenia, agranulocytosis,*** anemia, ***neutropenia, lymphocytosis, eosinophilia, pancytopenia, hemolytic anemia***

RESP: Dyspnea, ***anaphylaxis***

SKIN: Rash, urticaria, dermatitis

▼ DRUG INTERACTIONS

Drugs

- *Aminoglycosides:* Possible development of renal failure in patients with pre-existing renal disease
- *Colistin:* Increased renal toxicity of colistin
- *Oral anticoagulants:* Potential increase in hypoprothrombinemic response to oral anticoagulants

Labs

- *False positive:* Urinary protein; urinary glucose by Benedict's or Fehling's solution, Clinitest tabs
- *Increase (False):* Creatinine (serum, urine), urinary 17-KS

cephapirin

(sef-a-peer'in)

Cefadyl

Chemical Class: Cephalosporin (1st generation)

Therapeutic Class: Antibiotic

CLINICAL PHARMACOLOGY

Mechanism of Action: Inhibits the biosynthesis of cell wall mucopeptide in susceptible organisms; bacteriocidal when adequate concentrations are reached

Pharmacokinetics

IM: Peak 30 min, $t_{1/2}$ 21-47 min, 44-50% bound by plasma proteins, metabolized in liver, 40%-70% eliminated unchanged in urine

INDICATIONS AND USES: Infections of the respiratory tract, skin and skin structures, urinary tract; septicemia; endocarditis; osteomyelitis; perioperative prophylaxis for contaminated or potentially contaminated procedures; all approved indications caused by susceptible organisms.

Antibacterial spectrum usually includes:

- Gram-positive organisms: Group A, β-hemolytic streptococci, staphylococci (including coagulase-positive, coagulase-negative, and penicillinase-producing strains [not MRSA]), *Streptococcus pneumoniae*
- Gram-negative organisms: *Haemophilus influenzae, Escherichia coli, Klebsiella* sp, *Proteus mirabilis*

DOSAGE

Adult

- IM/IV 500 mg-1 g q4-6h, maximum 12 g/day
- Renal function impairment (serum creatinine > 5 mg/dl): IM/IV 7.5-15 mg/kg q12h

Child

- IM/IV 40-80 mg/kg q6h

$ AVAILABLE FORMS/COST OF THERAPY

- Inj, Dry-Sol—IM; IV: 1 g/vial, 10's: **$35.70;** 2 g/vial, 10's: **$68.78;** 4 g/vial, 10's: **$133.88;** 500 mg/vial, 25's: **$51.17**

CONTRAINDICATIONS: Hypersensitivity to cephalosporins

PRECAUTIONS: Hypersensitivity to penicillins, renal disease, prolonged use, colitis

PREGNANCY AND LACTATION: Pregnancy category B; excreted into breast milk in low concentrations, no adverse effects have been observed but potential exists for modification of bowel flora in nursing infant, allergy/sensitization and interference with interpretation of culture results if fever workup required

SIDE EFFECTS/ADVERSE REACTIONS

CNS: Headache, dizziness, weakness, paresthesia, fever, chills

GI: Nausea, vomiting, *diarrhea,* anorexia, pain, glossitis, bleeding, increased AST, ALT, bilirubin, LDH, alk phosphatase, abdominal pain, ***pseudomembranous colitis***

GU: ***Proteinuria,*** vaginitis, pruritus, candidiasis, increased BUN, ***nephrotoxicity, renal failure***

HEME: ***Leukopenia, thrombocytopenia, agranulocytosis,*** anemia, ***neutropenia, lymphocytosis, eosinophilia, pancytopenia, hemolytic anemia***

RESP: Dyspnea, ***anaphylaxis***

SKIN: Rash, urticaria, dermatitis

▼ DRUG INTERACTIONS

Drugs

- *Aminoglycosides:* Possible development of renal failure in patients with pre-existing renal disease
- *Oral anticoagulants:* Potential increase in hypoprothrombinemic response to oral anticoagulants

Labs

- *False positive:* Urinary protein; urinary glucose by Benedict's or Fehling's solution, Clinitest tabs; Coombs' test
- Increase (False): Urinary 17-KS

cephradine

(sef′ra-deen)

Velosef

Chemical Class: Cephalosporin (1st generation)

Therapeutic Class: Antibiotic

CLINICAL PHARMACOLOGY

Mechanism of Action: Inhibits the biosynthesis of cell wall mucopeptide in susceptible organisms; bacteriocidal when adequate concentrations are reached

Pharmacokinetics

PO: Peak 1 hr

IM: Peak 1 hr

$t_{1/2}$ 0.75-1.5 h, 8%-17% bound to plasma proteins, 80%-90% eliminated unchanged in urine

INDICATIONS AND USES: Infections of the respiratory tract, skin and skin structure, urinary tract; otitis media; osteomyelitis; septicemia (parenteral only); perioperative prophylaxis for contaminated or potentially contaminated procedures (parenteral only); all approved indications caused by susceptible organisms.

Antibacterial spectrum usually includes:

- Gram-positive organisms: Group A β-hemolytic streptococci, Staphylococci (including coagulase-positive, coagulase-negative, and penicillinase-producing strains [not MRSA]), *Streptococcus pneumoniae*
- Gram-negative organisms: *Escherichia coli, Proteus mirabilis, Klebsiella* sp, *Hemophilus influenzae*

DOSAGE

Adult

- IM/IV 500 mg-1 g q4-6h not to exceed 8 g/day; PO 250 mg-1 g q6-12h

Child >1 yr

- IM/IV 12-25 mg/kg q6h; PO 6-12 mg/kg q6h

▼ AVAILABLE FORMS/COST OF THERAPY

- Cap, Gel—Oral: 250 mg, 100's: **$33.38-$85.99;** 500 mg, 100's: **$65.93-$168.89**
- Powder, Reconst—Oral:125 mg/5 ml, 100 ml: **$7.49-$9.43;** 250 mg/5 ml, 100 ml: **$12.74-$17.69;** 500 mg/5 ml, 100 ml: **$14.25**
- Inj, Dry-Sol—IM; IV: 250 mg/vial, 10's: **$23.36**
- Inj, Dry-Sol—IV: 2 g/bottle, 100

ml: **$15.45**

• Inj, Lyphl-Sol—IM; IV: 1 g/vial, 10's: **$77.76**

• Inj, Lyphl-Susp—IM; IV: 500 mg/vial, 10's: **$41.34**

CONTRAINDICATIONS: Hypersensitivity to cephalosporins

PRECAUTIONS: Hypersensitivity to penicillins, renal disease, prolonged use, colitis

PREGNANCY AND LACTATION: Pregnancy category B; excreted into breast milk in low concentrations, no adverse effects have been observed but potential exists for modification of bowel flora in nursing infant, allergy/sensitization and interference with interpretation of culture results if fever workup required

SIDE EFFECTS/ADVERSE REACTIONS

CNS: Headache, dizziness, weakness, paresthesia, fever, chills

GI: Nausea, vomiting, *diarrhea,* anorexia, pain, glossitis, bleeding, increased AST, ALT, bilirubin, LDH, alk phosphatase, abdominal pain, ***pseudomembranous colitis***

GU: ***Proteinuria,*** vaginitis, pruritus, candidiasis, increased BUN, ***nephrotoxicity, renal failure***

HEME: ***Leukopenia, thrombocytopenia, agranulocytosis,*** anemia, ***neutropenia, lymphocytosis, eosinophilia, pancytopenia, hemolytic anemia***

RESP: Dyspnea, ***anaphylaxis***

SKIN: Rash, urticaria, dermatitis

▼ **DRUG INTERACTIONS**

Drugs

• *Aminoglycosides:* Possible development of renal failure in patients with pre-existing renal disease

• *Oral anticoagulants:* Potential increase in hypoprothrombinemic response to oral anticoagulants

Labs

• *False positive:* Urinary protein; urinary glucose by Benedict's or Fehling's solution, Clinitest tabs; Coombs' test

• *Increase (False):* Urinary 17-KS

SPECIAL CONSIDERATIONS

PATIENT/FAMILY EDUCATION

• Complete full course of therapy

• May cause GI upset; take with food or milk

• Notify physician of nausea, vomiting or diarrhea (especially if the diarrhea is severe or contains blood, mucus or pus)

---

charcoal/activated charcoal

(char'coal)

Oral tablets: CharcoCaps

Oral suspensions (activated): Arm-a-char, Actidose-Aqua, Liqu-Char, Charcoaide, Charcodote

Oral powders (activated): Superchar

Therapeutic Class: Antiflatulent; antidote (activated)

CLINICAL PHARMACOLOGY

Mechanism of Action: Adsorbent, detoxicant, soothing; reduces volume of intestinal gas; binds poisons, toxins, irritants in GI tract; bound toxins inactive until excreted

Pharmacokinetics

PO: Insoluble in water; excreted in feces

INDICATIONS AND USES: Flatulence, emergency treatment in most poisonings, dyspepsia, abdominal distention, deodorant in wounds, diarrhea

DOSAGE

Adult

• *Flatulence/dyspepsia:* PO 520-975 mg p.c. up to 4.16 g/day

• *Poisoning:* PO 5-10 × weight of substance ingested, minimum dose 50 g/250 ml of water (range 25-100 g as single dose), may give 20-40 g q6h for 1-2 days in severe poisoning; co-administration of cathartic or in combination with sorbitol (1.5g/kg)

Child (< 1 yr)

• *Poisoning:* 1 g/kg as single dose

Child (1-12 yrs)

• *Poisoning:* 25-50 g as single dose

▼ **AVAILABLE FORMS/COST OF THERAPY**

• Powder (activated)—Oral: 125 g: **$7.00**

• Susp (activated)—Oral: 25 g/120 ml: **$3.40-$5.92**

• Caps—Oral: 260 mg, 12's: **$.75-$1.50**

• Tab—Oral: 325 mg, 100's: **$1.05**

CONTRAINDICATIONS: Hypersensitivity to drug, unconsciousness, semiconsciousness, poisoning of cyanide, mineral acids, alkalies

PRECAUTIONS: Absence of bowel sounds

SIDE EFFECTS/ADVERSE REACTIONS

GI: Nausea, black stools, vomiting, constipation, diarrhea

▼ **DRUG INTERACTIONS**

• *Acetaminophen+:* Reduced acetaminophen levels

• *Digitalis glycosides+:* Reduced digoxin levels; less effect on digitoxin

• *Acetylcysteine:* Reduced effect

• *Ipecac:* Reduced effect

SPECIAL CONSIDERATIONS:

• Administer activated charcoal for adsorption in emergency management of poisonings as a slurry with water, a saline cathartic, or sorbitol

chenodiol

(kee-noe-dye'ole)

Chenix

Chemical Class: Chenodeoxycholic acid

Therapeutic Class: Cholelitholytic

CLINICAL PHARMACOLOGY

Mechanism of Action: Suppresses hepatic synthesis of cholesterol and cholic acid, replacing cholic acid with drug metabolite; contributes to biliary cholesterol desaturation and gradual dissolution of radiolucent cholesterol gallstones; has no effects on radiopaque (calcified) gallstones or on radiolucent bile pigment stones

Pharmacokinetics

PO: Extensive enterohepatic recirculation, 80% excreted in feces as metabolite

INDICATIONS AND USES: Dissolution of gallstones in patients with radiolucent stones in well-opacifying gallbladders, in whom effective surgery would be undertaken except for the presence of increased surgical risk due to systemic disease or age (the likelihood of successful dissolution is far greater if the stones are floatable or small)

DOSAGE

Adult

• PO 250 mg bid for 2 wk, then increased by 250 mg/day, not to exceed 16 mg/kg/day

▼ **AVAILABLE FORMS/COST OF THERAPY**

• Tab, Plain Coated—Oral: 250 mg, 100's: **$107.98**

CONTRAINDICATIONS: Hypersensitivity, hepatic disease, bile duct abnormalities, biliary GI fistula

PRECAUTIONS: Children, atherosclerosis, elderly, colon cancer

PREGNANCY AND LACTATION: Pregnancy category X; excretion into breast milk unknown, use extreme caution in nursing mothers

SIDE EFFECTS/ADVERSE REACTIONS

GI: Diarrhea, fecal urgency, heartburn, *nausea,* cramps, increased ALT, AST, LDH, vomiting, dysphagia, absence of taste, ***hepatotox-***

icity, flatulence, dyspepsia, *biliary pain*

HEME: ***Leukopenia***

METAB: Increased total cholesterol and LDL

SPECIAL CONSIDERATIONS

PATIENT/FAMILY EDUCATION

• Periodic blood tests for liver function tests will be required during therapy

• Report nonspecific abdominal pain, severe right upper quadrant pain, nausea, vomiting to physician immediately

MONITORING PARAMETERS

• Monthly aminotransferase levels for 3 mo then q3mo

• Serum cholesterol, cholecystogram or ultrasonogram, CBC

---

chloral hydrate

(klor-al hye'drate)

Aquachloral Supprettes, Noctec, Novochlorhydrate ♣

Chemical Class: Chloral derivative

Therapeutic Class: Sedative-hypnotic

DEA Class: Schedule IV

CLINICAL PHARMACOLOGY

Mechanism of Action: CNS depressant effects are due to active metabolite trichloroethanol, mechanism unknown

Pharmacokinetics

PO: Onset 30 min-1 hr, duration 4-8 hr

PR: Onset slow, duration 4-6 hr

Metabolized by liver to trichloroethanol, excreted by kidneys and feces, $t_{1/2}$ (trichloroethanol) 8-11 hr

INDICATIONS AND USES: Nocturnal sedation, preoperative sedation, sedation prior to EEG evaluations; adjunct to opiates and analgesics in postoperative care and pain control; alcohol withdrawal

DOSAGE

Adult

• *Sedation:* PO/PR 250 mg tid pc

• *Hypnotic:* PO/PR 500 mg-1g 0.5 hr before bedtime or 0.5 hr before surgery

Child

• *Sedative:* PO 8 mg/kg tid, not to exceed 500 mg tid

• *Hypnotic:* PO/PR 50 mg/kg in one dose, not to exceed 1 g

▼ **AVAILABLE FORMS/COST OF THERAPY**

• Cap, Gel—Oral: 250 mg, 100's: **$7.61;** 500 mg, 100's: **$7.31-$12.25**

• Supp—Rect: 500 mg, 12's: **$26.25**

• Syr—Oral: 250 mg/5ml, 10 ml × 40: **$23.81;** 500 mg/5 ml, 480 ml: **$6.40-$11.55**

CONTRAINDICATIONS: Hypersensitivity to chloral derivatives, severe renal disease, severe hepatic disease, severe cardiac disease, gastritis

PRECAUTIONS: Cardiac disease, GI conditions, acute intermittant porphyria, history of drug abuse, tartrazine sensitivity, elderly

PREGNANCY AND LACTATION: Pregnancy category C; excreted into breast milk, may cause mild drowsiness in infant, otherwise compatible with breast feeding

SIDE EFFECTS/ADVERSE REACTIONS

CNS: Drowsiness, dizziness, stimulation, nightmares, ataxia, hangover (rare), light-headedness, headache, paranoia, mental confusion, hallucinations (rare), disorientation, somnambulism

GI: Nausea, vomiting, flatulence, diarrhea, unpleasant taste, gastric irritation

HEME: ***Eosinophilia, leukopenia***

SKIN: Rash, urticaria, hives, erythema, eczematoid dermatitis, scarlatiniform exanthems

▼ DRUG INTERACTIONS

Drugs

- *Ethanol:* Additive CNS-depressant effects
- *Warfarin:* Transient increase in the hypoprothrombinemic response to warfarin

Labs

- *Interference:* Urine catecholamines, urinary 17-OHCS
- *False Positive:* Urine glucose (copper sulfate test)

SPECIAL CONSIDERATIONS

PATIENT/FAMILY EDUCATION

- May cause GI upset, take capsules with full glass of water or fruit juice, dilute syrup in a half glass of water or fruit juice
- Swallow capsules whole, do not chew
- May cause drowsiness, use caution when performing tasks requiring alertness
- Avoid alcohol and other CNS depressants
- May be habit forming, do not discontinue abruptly

chloramphenicol

(klor-am-fen′i-kole)

Systemic: Chloromycetin Kapseals, Chloromycetin Sodium Succinate, Chloromycetin Palmitate; Topical: Chloromycetin; Ophthalmic: AK-Chlor, Chloromycetin Ophthalmic, Chloroptic, Chloroptic S.O.P.; Otic: Chloromycetin Otic

Chemical Class: Dichloroacetic acid derivative

Therapeutic Class: Antibacterial; antirickettsial

CLINICAL PHARMACOLOGY

Mechanism of Action: Reversibly binds to 50S ribosomal subunits of susceptible organisms, preventing amino acids from being transferred to growing peptide chains thus inhibiting protein synthesis

Pharmacokinetics

PO/IV: Peak 1-2 hr, duration 8 hr, 60% bound to plasma proteins, $t_{1/2}$ 1.5-4 hr, conjugated in liver, excreted in urine (up to 15% as free drug) and feces (in neonates, 6%-80% of drug excreted unchanged in the urine, $t_{1/2}$ 10-24 hr)

INDICATIONS AND USES Meningitis, paratyphoid fever, Q fever, rickettsial pox, Rocky Mountain spotted fever, septicemia, typhoid fever, typhus infections; serious infections due to organisms resistant to other less toxic antibiotics or when its penetration into the site of infection is clinically superior to other antibiotics to which the organisms are sensitive.

Antibacterial spectrum usually includes:

- Gram-positive organisms: *Streptococcus pneumoniae* and other streptococci
- Gram-negative organisms: *Haemophilus influenzae, Neisseria meningitidis, Salmonella, Proteus mirabilis, Pseudomonas mallei, P. cepacia, Vibrio cholerae, Francisella tularensis, Yersinia pestis, Brucella,* and *Shigella*
- Anaerobes: *Prevotella melaninogenica, B. fragilis, Clostridium, Fusobacterium,* and *Veillonella;* other: *Rickettsia, Chlamydia,* and *Mycoplasma*

DOSAGE

Adult

- PO/IV 50-100 mg/kg/day divided q6h, max 4 g/day; OPHTHAL apply 1 gtt or small amount of ointment q3-6h, increase interval between applications after 48 hr; TOP gently rub into affected area tid-qid; OTIC instill 2-3 gtt into the ear tid

Child

- *Meningitis:* IV 75-100 mg/kg/

day divided q6h, max dose 4 g/day
- *Other infections:* PO/IV 50-75 mg/kg/day divided q6h, max 4 g/day

Neonates
- IV 20 mg/kg loading dose, maintenance dose based on postnatal age (given 12 hr after loading dose); ≤7 days or ≤2,000 g 25 mg/kg/day q24h; >7 days and >2,000 g 50 mg/kg/day q12h

$ AVAILABLE FORMS/COST OF THERAPY
- Cap, Gel—Oral: 250 mg, 100's: **$38.70-$125.42**
- Oint—Ophth: 1%, 3.5 g: **$2.44-$12.69**
- Sol—Ophth: 0.5%, 15 ml: **$4.13-$9.96**
- Sol—Otic: 5 mg/ml, 15 ml: **$21.04**
- Inj, Lyphl-Sol—IV: 10%, 1 g: **$41.48**

CONTRAINDICATIONS: Hypersensitivity, trivial infections, prophylaxis

PRECAUTIONS: Neonates (use in reduced dosages to avoid "gray baby syndrome" toxicity), repeated courses, prolonged therapy, impaired hepatic or renal function, acute intermittent porphyria, G-6-PD deficiency, bone marrow depression (drug-induced)

PREGNANCY AND LACTATION: Pregnancy category C; use caution at term due to potential for "gray baby syndrome" toxicity; excreted into breast milk, milk levels are too low to precipitate the "gray baby syndrome", but a theoretical risk does exist for bone marrow depression

SIDE EFFECTS/ADVERSE REACTIONS

CNS: Headache, mild depression, confusion, delirium, peripheral neuropathy

CV: ***Gray baby syndrome in newborns (failure to feed, pallor, cyanosis, abdominal distention, irregular respiration, vasomotor collapse)***

EENT: Optic neuritis (prolonged therapy); poor corneal wound healing, temporary visual haze, overgrowth of nonsusceptible organisms (ophthalmic preparations); itching, irritation in ear (otic preparations)

GI: Nausea, vomiting, diarrhea, glossitis, enterocolitis

HEME: ***Serious and fatal blood dyscrasias (aplastic anemia, hypoplastic anemia, thrombocytopenia and granulocytopenia)***

SKIN: Itching, urticaria, contact dermatitis, rash, stinging, burning, ***angioedema***

▼ DRUG INTERACTIONS

Drugs
- *Antidiabetics:* Increased hypoglycemic effects of tolbutamide and chlorpropamide
- *Barbiturates:* Increased serum barbiturate concentrations; reduced serum chloramphenicol concentrations
- *Dicumarol:* Enhanced hypoprothrombinemic response to dicumarol and possibly other oral anticoagulants
- *Penicillins:* Inhibited antibacterial activity of penicillins
- *Phenytoin+:* Predictable increases in serum phenytoin concentrations, toxicity has occurred
- *Rifampin:* Reduced chloramphenicol concentrations

SPECIAL CONSIDERATIONS

PATIENT/FAMILY EDUCATION
- Preferably take on an empty stomach, can take with food if GI upset occurs
- Notify physician if fever, sore throat, tiredness or unusual bruising/bleeding occurs

MONITORING PARAMETERS
- AST, ALT, urinalysis, protein, blood, BUN, creatinine before and occasionally during therapy

• CBC with platelets and reticulocytes before and frequently during therapy (discontinue drug if bone marrow depression occurs), serum iron and iron-binding globulin saturation may also be useful
• Serum drug level (peak 10-20 μg/ml, trough 5-10 μg/ml) weekly (more often in impaired hepatic, renal systems)
• Early signs of "gray baby syndrome" (cyanosis, abdominal distension, irregular respiration, failure to feed), ***drug should be discontinued immediately***

chlordiazepoxide

(klor-dye-az-e-pox′ide)
Libritabs, Librium, Medilium, ✤ Mitran, ✤ Resposans-10, ✤ Solium ✤
Chemical Class: Benzodiazepine
Therapeutic Class: Antianxiety agent
DEA Class: Schedule IV

CLINICAL PHARMACOLOGY
Mechanism of Action: Potentiates the effects of γ-aminobutyric acid (GABA) and other inhibitory transmitters by binding to specific benzodiazepine receptor sites
Pharmacokinetics
PO: Onset 30 min, peak ½-4 hr
IM: Slow erratic absorption and lower peak plasma levels than oral or IV administration
Metabolized by liver to active metabolites, excreted by kidneys, $t_{1/2}$ 5-30 hr
INDICATIONS AND USES: Anxiety disorders, acute alcohol withdrawal, preoperative apprehension and anxiety; familial, senile or essential action tremors;* tension headache,* panic disorders*

DOSAGE
Adult
• *Mild anxiety:* PO 5-10 mg tid-qid
• *Severe anxiety:* PO 20-25 mg tid-qid; IM/IV 50-100 mg initially, then 25-50 mg tid-qid prn
• *Preoperative apprehension and anxiety:* PO 5-10 mg tid-qid on days before surgery; IM 50-100 mg 1 hr before surgery
• *Acute alcohol withdrawal:* PO/IM/IV 50-100 mg initially, repeat in 2-4 hr prn, not to exceed 300 mg/day
Geriatric or debilitated patients
• PO 5 mg bid-qid
Child >6 yr
• PO 5 mg bid-qid, not to exceed 10 mg bid-tid

$ **AVAILABLE FORMS/COST OF THERAPY**
• Inj, Conc, w/buf—IM; IV: 100 mg/ampul, 5 ml: **$7.61**
• Cap, Gel—Oral: 5 mg, 100's: **$5.03-$34.73;** 10 mg, 100's: **$3.83-$50.56;** 25 mg, 100's: **$5.40-$88.78**
• Tab, Plain Coated—Oral: 5 mg, 100's: **$33.38;** 10 mg, 100's: **$48.11;** 25 mg, 100's: **$83.32**
CONTRAINDICATIONS: Hypersensitivity to benzodiazepines, narrow-angle glaucoma, psychosis
PRECAUTIONS: Elderly, debilitated, hepatic disease, renal disease, long-term use, history of drug abuse
PREGNANCY AND LACTATION: Pregnancy category D; excreted into breast milk, drug and metabolites may accumulate to toxic levels in nursing infant
SIDE EFFECTS/ADVERSE REACTIONS
CNS: Dizziness, *drowsiness, confusion,* headache, anxiety, tremors, stimulation, fatigue, depression, insomnia, hallucinations, anterograde amnesia, slurred speech, ataxia, hysteria, psychosis
CV: Orthostatic hypotension, tachy-

cardia, bradycardia, hypertension, hypotension, ***cardiovascular collapse***

EENT: Blurred vision, mydriasis, nystagmus, auditory disturbances

GI: Constipation, dry mouth, nausea, vomiting, anorexia, diarrhea

GU: Incontinence, changes in libido, urinary retention, menstrual irregularities

SKIN Rash, dermatitis, itching, urticaria, hair loss, hirsutism

▼ **DRUG INTERACTIONS**

Drugs

- *Cimetidine:* Increased plasma levels of chlordiazepoxide and/or active metabolites
- *Clozapine:* Isolated cases of cardiorespiratory collapse have been reported; causal relationship to benzodiazepines has not been established
- *Disulfiram:* Increased serum chlordiazepoxide concentrations
- *Ethanol:* Enhanced adverse psychomotor side effects of benzodiazepines
- *Rifampin:* Reduced serum chlordiazepoxide concentrations

SPECIAL CONSIDERATIONS

PATIENT/FAMILY EDUCATION

- Do not use for everyday stress or use longer than 4 mo, unless directed by physician
- Do not take more than prescribed amount, may be habit-forming
- Avoid OTC preparations unless approved by physician
- Avoid driving, activities that require alertness; drowsiness may occur
- Avoid alcohol ingestion or other CNS depressants
- Do not discontinue medication abruptly after long-term use

chlorhexidine

(klor-hex'ih-deen)

Peridex, Periogard

Chemical Class: Bis-biguanide

Therapeutic Class: Antimicrobial mouth rinse

CLINICAL PHARMACOLOGY

Mechanism of Action: Adsorbed during oral rinsing on the surfaces of teeth, plaque, and oral mucosa; gradually released from these sites by diffusion for up to 24 hr; adsorbed onto the cell walls of microorganisms, which causes leakage of intracellular components

Pharmacokinetics

PO: Poorly absorbed, 30% retained in oral cavity following rinsing and is slowly released into the oral fluids; excreted primarily through the feces

INDICATIONS AND USES: Gingivitis, prophylaxis of mouth infections,* stomatitis,* reduction of dental plaque*

DOSAGE

Adult

- Use 15 ml as oral rinse for 30 sec bid after toothbrushing (not intended for ingestion, expectorate after rinsing)

$ **AVAILABLE FORMS/COST OF THERAPY**

- Mouthwash—Oral: 0.12%, 480 ml: **$11.82**

CONTRAINDICATIONS: Hypersensitivity

PREGNANCY AND LACTATION: Pregnancy category B; excretion into breast milk unknown, use caution in nursing mothers

SIDE EFFECTS/ADVERSE REACTIONS

GI: Staining of teeth and other oral surfaces, increase in calculus formation, altered taste perception, irritation of oral mucosa, transient parotitis

SPECIAL CONSIDERATIONS
PATIENT/FAMILY EDUCATION
• Do not swallow
• Do not rinse after use
• May cause reduced taste sensation, which is generally reversible
• May cause discoloration of teeth

chlormezanone
(klor-mehz'ah-non)
Trancopal
Chemical Class: Substituted metathiazonone
Therapeutic Class: Antianxiety agent

CLINICAL PHARMACOLOGY
Mechanism of Action: Unknown, but animal studies have shown activity on subcortical levels of the CNS similar to those of meprobamate
Pharmacokinetics
PO: Peak 1-2 hr, onset 15-30 min, duration 6 hr, metabolized in the liver, excreted in the urine and feces, $t_{1/2}$ 24 hr
INDICATIONS AND USES: Anxiety and tension states
DOSAGE
Adult
• PO 100-200 mg tid-qid
Child (5-12 yr)
• PO 50-100 mg tid-qid
$ AVAILABLE FORMS/COST OF THERAPY
• Tab, Uncoated—Oral: 100 mg, 100's: **$93.67;** 200 mg, 100's: **$107.35**
CONTRAINDICATIONS: Hypersensitivity
PRECAUTIONS: Potentially hazardous tasks
PREGNANCY AND LACTATION: Safety during pregnancy and lactation has not been established
SIDE EFFECTS/ADVERSE REACTIONS
CNS: Dizziness, drowsiness, depression, weakness, excitement, tremor, confusion, headache
GI: Dry mouth, cholestatic jaundice
GU: Inability to void
SKIN: Rash, erythema multiforme, ***Stevens-Johnson syndrome (rare)***

SPECIAL CONSIDERATIONS
PATIENT/FAMILY EDUCATION
• May cause drowsiness, use caution when performing tasks requiring alertness
• Avoid alcohol
• Notify physician if skin rash, sore throat or fever occurs

chloroprocaine
(klor-oh-pro'kane)
Nesacaine, Nesacaine-MPF
Chemical Class: Ester
Therapeutic Class: Local anesthetic

CLINICAL PHARMACOLOGY
Mechanism of Action: Blocks the generation and the conduction of nerve impulses, presumably by increasing the threshold for electrical excitation in the nerve, by slowing the propagation of the nerve impulse and by reducing the rate of rise of the action potential
Pharmacokinetics
INJ: Rapid onset, 6-12 min, duration of anesthesia, up to 60 min
Widely distributed; $t_{1/2}$ 21-25 sec (adults); metabolized by pseudocholinesterase to metabolites which inhibit sulfonamides; excreted renally (NOTE: Altered by the presence of hepatic or renal disease, addition of epinephrine, factors affecting urinary pH, renal blood flow, the route of administration, and age)
INDICATIONS AND USES: Infiltration and peripheral nerve block,

central nerve block, including caudal and epidural blocks (without preservatives)

DOSAGE

Adult

- Max single recommended doses without epinephrine, 11 mg/kg, not to exceed a max total dose of 800 mg; with epinephrine (1:200,000) 14 mg/kg, not to exceed a max total dose of 1000 mg
- *Caudal and lumbar epidural block:* 15 to 25 ml of a 2% or 3% solution; repeated doses may be given at 40 to 60 min intervals
- *Infiltration and peripheral nerve block (1-2%):* Mandibular 2-3 ml; infraorbital 0.5-1 ml; brachial plexus 30-40 ml; digital (without epinephrine) 3-4 ml; pudendal 10 ml each side; paracervical 3 per each of up to 4 sites
- *Lumbar epidural anesthesia:* 15 to 25 ml, repeated doses 10-20 ml at 40 to 50 min intervals

Child

- Max single recommended dose 11 mg/kg

$ AVAILABLE FORMS/COST OF THERAPY

- Inj, Sol-Caudal Block, Epidural—Inf: 2%, 30 ml: **$7.88-$16.95;** 3%, 30 ml: **$9.61-$17.80**

CONTRAINDICATIONS: Hypersensitivity to drugs of the PABA ester group

PRECAUTIONS: Lumber and caudal epidural anesthesia should be used with extreme caution in persons with the following conditions: existing neurological disease, spinal deformities, septicemia, and severe hypertension

PREGNANCY AND LACTATION: Pregnancy category C

SIDE EFFECTS/ADVERSE REACTIONS

CNS: Anxiety, restlessness, ***convulsions, loss of consciousness,*** drowsiness, disorientation, tremors, shivering

CV: ***Myocardial depression, cardiac arrest, dysrhythmias,*** bradycardia, hypotension, hypertension, fetal bradycardia

EENT: Blurred vision, tinnitus, pupil constriction

GI: Nausea, vomiting

RESP: ***Status asthmaticus, respiratory arrest, anaphylaxis***

SKIN: Rash, urticaria, allergic reactions, edema, burning, skin discoloration at inj site, tissue necrosis

▼ DRUG INTERACTIONS

Drugs

- *β-adrenergic blockers:* Enhanced sympathomimetic effects, hypertension (acute discontinuation of β-blocker before local anesthetic side effects)

---

chloroquine

(klor′oh-kwin)

Aralen, Novochloroquine ♣

Chemical Class: Synthetic 4-aminoquinoline derivative

Therapeutic Class: Antimalarial

CLINICAL PHARMACOLOGY

Mechanism of Action: Inhibits parasite replication, via an interaction with DNA transcription

Pharmacokinetics

PO: Peak 1-6 hr, $t_{1/2}$ 3-5 days

Rapidly and completely absorbed; 55% protein bound; deposited in brain, spinal cord, liver, spleen, kidney, lungs, and leukocytes (from 30 to 700 times the plasma concentration); metabolized in the liver; excretion slow (enhanced via acidification of urine) in urine, feces; crosses placenta

INDICATIONS AND USES: Malaria caused by susceptible strains, including *P. vivax, P. malariae, P.*

ovale, P. falciparum (some strains); and extraintestinal amebiasis

DOSAGE

NOTE: The dosage of chloroquine is often expressed or calculated as the base: 500 mg tab of chloroquine phosphate is equivalent to 300 mg base; 50 mg of chloroquine hydrochloride is equivalent to 40 mg base.

Adult

- *Malaria suppression:* PO 5 mg/kg/wk on same day of wk, not to exceed 300 mg (base); treatment should begin 1-2 wk before exposure and for 8 wk after; if treatment begins after exposure, 600 mg (base) in 2 divided doses 6 hr apart
- *Extraintestinal amebiasis:* IM 200-250 mg qd (HCl) up to 12 days, then 1 g (phosphate) qd × 2 days, then 500 mg qd × 2-3 wk

Child

- *Malaria suppression:* PO 5 mg/kg/wk on same day of wk, not to exceed 300 mg (base); treatment should begin 1-2 wk before exposure and for 8 wk after; if treatment begins after exposure, 10 mg/kg (base) in 2 divided doses 6 hr apart
- *Extraintestinal amebiasis:* IM/PO 10 mg/kg qd (HCl) × 2-3 wk, not to exceed 300 mg/day

$ AVAILABLE FORMS/COST OF THERAPY

- Tab, Uncoated—Oral: 250 mg, 100's: **$7.80;** 500 mg, 100's: **$171.00**
- Inj, Sol—IV; IM: 50 mg/ml, 5 ml: **$14.43**

CONTRAINDICATIONS: Hypersensitivity, retinal field changes, porphyria

PRECAUTIONS: Children, blood dyscrasias, severe GI disease, neurologic disease, alcoholism, hepatic disease, G-6-PD deficiency, psoriasis, eczema, lactation, porphyria

PREGNANCY AND LACTATION: Pregnancy category C; excreted into breast milk; following 5 mg/kg IM, mean milk conc, 0.227 µg/ml (range 0.163-0.319 µg/ml); mean ratio was 0.358; based on 500 ml of milk/day average infant consumption, considered safe; NOTE: doesn't protect infant against malaria

SIDE EFFECTS/ADVERSE REACTIONS

CNS: Headache, stimulation, fatigue, ***convulsion,*** psychosis

CV: Hypotension, heart block, asystole with syncope, ECG changes

EENT: Blurred vision, corneal changes, retinal changes, difficulty focusing, tinnitus, vertigo, deafness, photophobia, corneal edema

GI: Nausea, vomiting, anorexia, diarrhea, cramps

HEME: ***Thrombocytopenia, agranulocytosis, hemolytic anemia, leukopenia***

SKIN: Pruritus, pigmentary changes, skin eruptions, lichen planus like eruptions, eczema, ***exfoliative dermatitis***

▼ DRUG INTERACTIONS

Drugs

- *Cyclosporine:* Elevates cyclosporine levels, toxicity possible

SPECIAL CONSIDERATIONS

MONITORING PARAMETERS

- Ophthalmic test if long-term treatment or drug dosage >150 mg/day

chlorothiazide

(klor-oh-thye'a-zide)

Diachlor, Diuril

Chemical Class: Thiazide; sulfonamide derivative

Therapeutic Class: Diuretic

CLINICAL PHARMACOLOGY

Mechanism of Action: Acts on distal tubule by increasing excretion of water, sodium, chloride, potassium, magnesium

Pharmacokinetics

PO: Onset 2 hr, peak 4 hr, duration 6-12 hr

IV: onset 15 min, maximal action 30 min

Not well absorbed PO; eliminated unchanged by the kidneys, crosses placenta, but not blood-brain barrier, excreted in breast milk; $t_{1/2}$ 45-120 min

INDICATIONS AND USES: Edema, hypertension, diuresis

DOSAGE

Adult

• *Edema, hypertension:* PO/IV 500 mg-2 g qd in 2 divided doses

Child

• *Diuresis, hypertension:* PO/IV 10-20 mg/kg/day in 2 divided doses not to exceed 375 mg per day in infants up to 2 yr of age or 1 g per day in children 2 to 12 yr of age; infants less than 6 mo of age, up to 30 mg/kg/day in 2 divided doses

$ **AVAILABLE FORMS/COST OF THERAPY**

• Tab, Uncoated—Oral: 250 mg, 100's: **$3.35;** 500 mg, 100's: **$5.76**

• Susp—Oral: 250 mg/5 ml, 237 ml: **$9.31**

• Inj—IV: 500 mg: **$8.39**

CONTRAINDICATIONS: Hypersensitivity to thiazides or sulfonamides, anuria, renal decompensation, lactation

PRECAUTIONS: Fluid or electrolyte imbalance (including sodium, potassium, magnesium, calcium), hyperuricemia, renal disease, hepatic disease, gout, COPD, lupus erythematosus, diabetes mellitus, elderly, post sympathectomy, hyperparathyroidism, elevated cholesterol/triglycerides

PREGNANCY AND LACTATION: Pregnancy category D; excreted in low concentrations (<1 μg/ml after 500 mg dose) in breast milk; pharmacologic effects remote

SIDE EFFECTS/ADVERSE REACTIONS

CNS: Drowsiness, paresthesia, anxiety, depression, headache, *dizziness, fatigue, weakness*

CV: Irregular pulse, orthostatic hypotension, palpitations, volume depletion

EENT: Blurred vision

ELECTROLYTES: Hypokalemia, hypercalcemia, hyponatremia, hypochloremia, hypophosphatemia, hypomagnesemia

GI: Nausea, vomiting, anorexia, constipation, diarrhea, cramps, pancreatitis, GI irritation, ***hepatitis***

GU: Frequency, polyuria, ***uremia,*** glucosuria

HEME: ***Aplastic anemia, hemolytic anemia, leukopenia, agranulocytosis, thrombocytopenia, neutropenia***

METAB: Hyperglycemia, *hyperuricemia,* hypomagnesemia, increased creatinine, BUN

SKIN: Rash, urticaria, purpura, photosensitivity, fever

▼ **DRUG INTERACTIONS**

Drugs

• *Antidiabetics:* Thiazides increase blood sugar, thus dose requirements

• *Cholestyramine:* Reduced thiazide concentration and effect

• *Colestipol:* Reduced thiazide concentration and effect

• *Diazoxide:* Hyperglycemia

• *Digitalis glycosides:* Diuretic-induced hypokalemia may increase the risk of digitalis toxicity

• *Lithium:* Increased lithium levels, potential toxicity

Labs

• *False negative:* Phentolamine and tyramine tests

• *Interference:* Urine steroid tests

• *Increase:* BSP retention, Ca, amylase, parathyroid test

• *Decrease:* PBI, PSP

SPECIAL CONSIDERATIONS
MONITORING PARAMETERS
- Electrolytes, i.e., sodium, chloride, potassium, BUN, creatinine, glucose, magnesium
- Minimal doses (125-250 mg qd) may provide optimal blood pressure control without added metabolic and electrolyte disturbance

chlorotrianisene

(klor-oh-trye-an'i-seen)
TACE
Chemical Class: Nonsteroidal synthetic estrogen
Therapeutic Class: Estrogen

CLINICAL PHARMACOLOGY
Mechanism of Action: Development and maintenance of female reproductive hormone and secondary sex characteristics; through feedback loops, affect release of pituitary gonadotropins; inhibits ovulation; conserves calcium and phosphorus, stimulates bone formation, capillary dilation, fluid retention, protein anabolism
Pharmacokinetics
PO: Some effect after the 14th day after administration; stored in fat tissues, with delayed and prolonged duration of action; effect persists after discontinuance; metabolized to more active metabolite in liver; excreted in urine; crosses placenta
INDICATIONS AND USES: Postpartum breast engorgement, moderate to severe vasomotor symptoms associated with menopause, atrophic vaginitis and kraurosis vulvae, female hypogonadism, prostatic carcinoma
DOSAGE
Adult
- *Prostatic cancer:* PO 12-25 mg qd
- *Menopause:* PO 12-25 mg qd × 30 days or 3 wk on 1 wk off
- *Female hypogonadism:* PO cycle 12-25 mg × 21 days, then progesterone 100 mg IM or coadminister 5 days of progesterone PO during last 5 days of cycle
- *Vaginitis:* PO 12-25 mg qd × 30-60 days

$ AVAILABLE FORMS/COST OF THERAPY
- Cap, Gel—Oral: 12 mg, 100's: **$98.46**

CONTRAINDICATIONS: Breast cancer, thromboembolic disorders, reproductive cancer, genital bleeding (abnormal, undiagnosed)
PRECAUTIONS: Hypertension, blood dyscrasias, gallbladder disease, CHF, diabetes mellitus, bone disease, depression, migraine headache, convulsive disorders, hepatic disease, renal disease, family history of cancer of the breast or reproductive tract
PREGNANCY AND LACTATION: Pregnancy category X; excreted into milk; associated with shortened duration of lactation, decreased infant weight gain, decreased milk production, decreased nitrogen and protein content of milk
SIDE EFFECTS/ADVERSE REACTIONS
CNS: Dizziness, headache, migraines, depression
CV: Hypotension, ***thrombophlebitis***, edema, ***thromboembolism***, stroke, pulmonary embolism, MI
EENT: Contact lens intolerance, increased myopia, astigmatism
GI: Nausea, vomiting, diarrhea, anorexia, pancreatitis, cramps, constipation, increased appetite, increased weight, ***cholestatic jaundice***
GU: Amenorrhea, cervical erosion, breakthrough bleeding, dysmenorrhea, vaginal candidiasis, breast

changes, *gynecomastia, testicular atrophy, impotence*
METAB: Folic acid deficiency, hypercalcemia, hyperglycemia
SKIN: Rash, urticaria, acne, hirsutism, alopecia, oily skin, seborrhea, purpura, melasma

▼ **DRUG INTERACTIONS**

Drugs

• *Corticosteroids:* Increased action of corticosteroids

Labs

• *Increase:* BSP retention test, PBI, T_4, serum sodium, platelet aggregation, thyroxine-binding globulin (TBG), prothrombin, factors VII, VIII, IX, X, triglycerides
• *Decrease:* Serum folate, serum triglyceride, T_3 resin uptake test, glucose tolerance test, antithrombin III, pregnanediol, metyrapone test
• *False positive:* LE prep, antinuclear antibodies

SPECIAL CONSIDERATIONS

PATIENT/FAMILY EDUCATION

• Encourage SBE
• Report unusual vaginal bleeding, edema, headache, blurred vision, abdominal pain, numbness, stiffness, or pain in legs, chest pain

chloroxine

(klor-ox′ine)
Capitrol
Chemical Class: 5,7-dichloro-8-hydroxyquinoline
Therapeutic Class: Synthetic antibacterial

CLINICAL PHARMACOLOGY

Mechanism of Action: Presumed reduction in scaling via effects on mitotic activity; antibacterial and antifungal role in seborrheic dermatitis speculated as *S. aureus* and *Pityrosporon* sp are often present in increased numbers

INDICATIONS AND USES: Dandruff and mild-to-moderately severe seborrheic dermatitis

DOSAGE

Adult

• TOP rub into wet scalp, allow to remain × 3 min before rinse, repeat; two treatments/wk

$ **AVAILABLE FORMS/COST OF THERAPY**

• Shampoo—Top: 120 ml: **$16.60**

CONTRAINDICATIONS: Hypersensitivity to ingredients, acute inflammation

PRECAUTIONS: External use only; avoid contact with eyes

PREGNANCY AND LACTATION: Pregnancy category C

SIDE EFFECTS/ADVERSE REACTIONS

SKIN: Irritation and burning, discoloration of light colored (blond, gray, bleached) hair

chlorphenesin

(klor-fen′e-sin)
Maolate, Rinlaxer ♣
Chemical Class: Carbamate
Therapeutic Class: Skeletal muscle relaxant, central acting

CLINICAL PHARMACOLOGY

Mechanism of Action: Unknown; related to central sedative properties; does not directly relax muscle or depress nerve conduction

Pharmacokinetics

PO: Onset ½ hr, peak 1-2 hr, duration 4-6 hr; metabolized by liver; excreted in urine; crosses placenta; $t_{1/2}$ 4 hr

INDICATIONS AND USES: Adjunct for relieving pain in acute, painful musculoskeletal conditions

DOSAGE

Adult

• PO 800 mg tid, maintenance 400 mg qid, not to exceed 8 wk

$ **AVAILABLE FORMS/COST OF THERAPY**

- Tab, Uncoated—Oral: 400 mg, 50's: **$36.40**

CONTRAINDICATIONS: Hypersensitivity, child <12 yr, intermittent porphyria

PRECAUTIONS: Renal disease, hepatic disease, addictive personality, elderly, hypersensitivity to FD&C Yellow No. 5 (tartrazine), or aspirin hypersensitivity

PREGNANCY AND LACTATION: Pregnancy category C; excreted in breast milk (large amounts), safety not established

SIDE EFFECTS/ADVERSE REACTIONS

CV: Postural hypotension, tachycardia

CNS: Dizziness, weakness, drowsiness, headache, tremor, depression, insomnia, confusion

EENT: Diplopia, temporary loss of vision

GI: Nausea, vomiting, hiccups

HEME: ***Blood dyscrasias***

MISC: ***Anaphylaxis***

SKIN: Rash, pruritus, fever, facial flushing

SPECIAL CONSIDERATIONS

PATIENT/FAMILY EDUCATION

- Possible lowered seizure threshold, poor seizure control has occurred with concurrent use
- Avoid concurrent alcohol, other CNS depressants, hazardous activities if drowsiness/dizziness occurs
- Abrupt withdrawal can precipitate symptoms (insomnia, nausea, headache, spasticity, tachycardia); taper over 1-2 wk

chlorpheniramine

(klor-fen-eer'a-meen)

Aller-Chlor, Chlo-Amine, Chlor-100, Chlor-Pro, Chlorate, Chlor-Pro 10, Chlorspan-12, Chlortab-B, Chlortab-4, Chlor-Trimeton, Chlor-Trimeton Repetabs, Pedia Care Allergy Formula, Pfeiffer's Allergy, Phenetron, Telachlor, Teldrin

Chemical Class: Alkylamine, H_1-receptor antagonist

Therapeutic Class: Antihistamine

CLINICAL PHARMACOLOGY

Mechanism of Action: Acts on blood vessels, GI system, respiratory system, by competing with histamine for H_1-receptor site; decreases allergic response by blocking actions of histamine

Pharmacokinetics

PO: Onset 20-60 min, duration 8-12 hr; detoxified in liver; excreted by kidneys (metabolites/free drug); $t_{1/2}$ 20-24 hr

INDICATIONS AND USES: Symptomatic relief of allergy symptoms, rhinitis, URI symptoms, pruritis symptoms

DOSAGE

Adult

- PO 2-4 mg tid-qid, not to exceed 36 mg/day; TIME-REL 8-12 mg bid-tid, not to exceed 36 mg/day; IM/IV/SC 5-40 mg/day

Child

- 2-5 yr: PO 1 mg q6h, not to exceed 6 mg/day
- 6-12 yr: PO 2 mg q4-6h, not to exceed 12 mg/day; SUS REL 8 mg hs or qd, (not recommended for child <6 yr)

$ **AVAILABLE FORMS/COST OF THERAPY**

- Tab, Uncoated—Oral: 4 mg, 100's: **$0.85**

• Cap, Gel, Sust Action—Oral: 4 mg, 100's: **$4.49;** 8 mg, 100's: **$6.25;** 12 mg, 100's: **$7.15**
• Inj, Sol—IV: 100 mg/ml, 10 ml: **$4.00;** 10 mg/ml, 1 ml: **$0.60-$2.34**
• Syr—Oral: 2 mg/5 ml, 480 ml: **$4.60**

CONTRAINDICATIONS: Hypersensitivity to H_1-receptor antagonists, acute asthma attack, lower respiratory tract disease

PRECAUTIONS: Increased intraocular pressure (angle closure glaucoma), renal disease, cardiac disease, hypertension, bronchial asthma, seizure disorder, stenosed peptic ulcers, hyperthyroidism, prostatic hypertrophy, bladder neck obstruction, elderly

PREGNANCY AND LACTATION: Pregnancy category B

SIDE EFFECTS/ADVERSE REACTIONS

CNS: Dizziness, drowsiness, poor coordination, fatigue, anxiety, euphoria, confusion, paresthesia, neuritis
EENT: Blurred vision, dilated pupils, tinnitus, dry nose, throat
GI: Dry mouth, nausea, anorexia, diarrhea
GU: Retention, dysuria, frequency
HEME: ***Thrombocytopenia, agranulocytosis, hemolytic anemia***
RESP: Increased thick secretions, wheezing, chest tightness
SKIN: Photosensitivity

▼ **DRUG INTERACTIONS**

Labs

• *False negative:* Skin allergy tests

SPECIAL CONSIDERATIONS

PATIENT/FAMILY EDUCATION

• Avoid driving or other hazardous activity if drowsiness occurs
• Avoid concurrent use of alcohol or other CNS depressants
• Diazepam and/or physostigmine for seizures associated with overdosage

---

chlorpromazine

(klor-proe'ma-zeen)
Chlorpromanyl, ♣ Ormazine, Thorazine
Chemical Class: Aliphatic phenothiazine
Therapeutic Class: Antipsychotic/neuroleptic

CLINICAL PHARMACOLOGY

Mechanism of Action: Depresses cerebral cortex, hypothalamus, limbic system, which control activity, aggression; blocks neurotransmission produced by dopamine at synapse; exhibits a strong α-adrenergic, anticholinergic blocking action; mechanism for antipsychotic effects is unclear

Pharmacokinetics

PO: Absorption variable, onset erratic 30-60 min, duration 4-6 hr
IM: Well absorbed; peak 15-20 min, duration 4 to 8 hr
IV: Onset 5 min, peak 10 min, duration unknown
PO-ER: Onset 30-60 min, peak unknown, duration 10-12 hr
REC: Onset erratic, duration 3 hr
Widely distributed; metabolized by liver, excreted in urine (metabolites), crosses placenta, 95% bound to plasma proteins; elimination $t_{1/2}$ 10-30 hr

INDICATIONS AND USES: Psychotic disorders, mania, schizophrenia, anxiety, intractable hiccups, nausea, vomiting; preoperatively for relaxation; acute intermittent porphyria, behavioral problems in children, adjunct in treatment of tetanus, treatment of PCP psychosis,* migraine headaches*

DOSAGE

Adult

• *Psychosis:* PO/IM 10-50 mg q1-4h

initially, then increase up to 2 g/day PRN

• *Nausea and vomiting:* PO 10-25 mg q4-6h prn; IM 25-50 mg q3h prn; REC 50-100 mg q6-8h prn, not to exceed 400 mg/day; IV 25-50 mg qd-qid

• *Intractable hiccups:* PO 25-50 mg tid-qid; IM 25-50 mg (used only if PO dose does not work); IV 25-50 mg in 500-1000 ml saline (only for severe hiccups)

Child

• Not to exceed 40 mg/day (<5 yr) or 75 mg/day (5-12 yr)

• *Psychosis:* PO 0.25 mg/kg q4-6h prn; IM 0.25 mg/kg q6-8h; REC 1 mg/kg q6-8h

• *Nausea and vomiting:* PO 0.55 mg/kg q4-6h prn, IM 0.55 mg/kg q6-8h prn; REC 1.1 mg/kg: q6-8h prn; IV 0.55 mg/kg q6-8h

$ **AVAILABLE FORMS/COST OF THERAPY**

• Conc—Oral: 30 mg/ml, 120 ml: **$5.33-$29.25;** 100 mg/ml, 240 ml: **$22.75-$158.10**

• Inj, Sol—IM; IV: 25 mg/ml, 1 ml: **$6.91-$9.76**

• Syr—Oral: 10 mg/5 ml, 120 ml: **$15.95-$20.85**

• Cap, Gel, Sust Action—Oral: 30 mg, 50's: **$47.10;** 75 mg, 50's: **$63.30;** 150 mg, 50's: **$85.30;** 200 mg, 50's: **$90.50**

• Supp—Rect: 25 mg, 12's: **$33.80;** 100 mg, 12's: **$42.85**

• Tab, Plain Coated—Oral: 10 mg, 100's, **$3.40-$31.70;** 25 mg, 100's: **$5.65-$47.75;** 50 mg, 100's: **$6.50-$59.60;** 100 mg, 100's: **$8.92-$76.90;** 200 mg, 100's: **$9.30-$97.70**

CONTRAINDICATIONS: Hypersensitivity, circulatory collapse, liver damage, cerebral arteriosclerosis, coronary disease, severe hypertension/hypotension, blood dyscrasias, coma, child <2 years, brain damage, bone marrow depression, alcohol and barbiturate withdrawal

PRECAUTIONS: Seizure disorders, hypertension, hepatic disease, cardiac disease, elderly (orthostasis upon arising)

PREGNANCY AND LACTATION: Pregnancy category C; enters breast milk in small concentrations (following 1200 mg dose [20 mg/kg], 0.29 μg/ml measured at 2 hr); M:P ratio <0.5; report of drowsy and lethargic infant who consumed milk with 92 ng/ml concentration

SIDE EFFECTS/ADVERSE REACTIONS

CNS: Extrapyramidal symptoms: pseudoparkinsonism, akathisia, dystonia, tardive dyskinesia, seizures, *headache*

CV: Orthostatic hypotension, hypertension, ***cardiac arrest,*** ECG changes, ***tachycardia***

EENT: Blurred vision, glaucoma, dry eyes

GI: Dry mouth, nausea, vomiting, anorexia, constipation, diarrhea, jaundice, weight gain

GU: Urinary retention, urinary frequency, enuresis, impotence, amenorrhea, gynecomastia, breast engorgement

HEME: Anemia, ***leukopenia, leukocytosis, agranulocytosis***

MISC: ***Neuroleptic malignant syndrome (NMS)***

RESP: ***Laryngospasm,*** dyspnea, ***respiratory depression***

SKIN: Rash, photosensitivity, dermatitis

▼ **DRUG INTERACTIONS**

Drugs

• *Anticholinergics:* May inhibit neuroleptic response, excess anticholinergic effects

• *Antidepressants:* Potential for increased therapeutic and toxic effects from increased levels of both drugs

• *Barbiturates:* Decreased neuroleptic levels
• *Epinephrine:* Blunted pressor response to epinephrine
• *Lithium:* Lowered levels of both drugs, rarely neurotoxicity in acute mania
• *Narcotic analgesics:* Hypotension and increased CNS depression
• *Orphenadrine:* Lower neuroleptic concentrations, excessive anticholinergic effects, hypoglycemia(?)
• *Propranolol:* Increased plasma levels of both drugs with accentuated responses

Labs

• *Increase:* Liver function tests, cardiac enzymes, cholesterol, blood glucose, prolactin, bilirubin, PBI, cholinesterase, alk phosphatase, leukocytes, granulocytes, platelets
• *False positive:* Pregnancy tests, PKU
• *False negative:* Urinary steroids, 17-OHCS

SPECIAL CONSIDERATIONS

PATIENT/FAMILY EDUCATION

• Orthostasis on rising, especially in elderly
• Avoid hot tubs, hot showers, tub baths
• Extrapyramidal symptoms including akathisia (inability to sit still, no pattern to movements), tardive dyskinesia (bizarre movements of the jaw, mouth, tongue, extremities), pseudoparkinsonism (rigidity, tremors, pill rolling, shuffling gait); responds to antiparkinsonian agent
• Meticulous oral hygiene; frequent rinsing of mouth, sugarless gum for dry mouth
• Avoid hazardous activities until drug response is determined
• Use a sunscreen and sunglasses
• Urine may turn pink or red

chlorpropamide

(klor-proe'pa-mide)

Chloronase, ♣ Chlorpropamide, Diabinese, Novopropamide ♣

Chemical Class: Sulfonylurea (1st generation)

Therapeutic Class: Antidiabetic

CLINICAL PHARMACOLOGY

Mechanism of Action: Stimulates functioning pancreatic β-cells to release insulin; improves/increases insulin binding to receptors/number of insulin receptors; reduces basal hepatic glucose secretion; ineffective without functioning β-cells

Pharmacokinetics

PO: Onset 1 hr, peak 3-6 hr, duration 60 hr; completely absorbed by GI route, $t_{1/2}$ 36 hr; 90%-95% plasma protein bound; metabolized in liver; excreted in urine (metabolites and unchanged drug)

INDICATIONS AND USES: Diabetes mellitus (type II), neurogenic diabetes insipidus,* adjuncts to insulin to improve control in selected patients*

DOSAGE

Adult

• PO 100-250 mg qd, initially, then 100-500 mg maintenance according to response; max 750 mg/day

$ **AVAILABLE FORMS/COST OF THERAPY**

• Tab, Uncoated—Oral: 100 mg, 100's: **$1.79-$34.11;** 250 mg, 100's: **$2.93-$69.62**

CONTRAINDICATIONS: Hypersensitivity to sulfonylureas, juvenile or brittle diabetes, renal failure

PRECAUTIONS: Elderly, cardiac disease, thyroid disease, renal disease, hepatic disease, severe hypoglycemic reactions

PREGNANCY AND LACTATION: Pregnancy category D; excreted

into breast milk, following 500 mg oral dose, milk concentration at 5 hrs was 5 µg/ml; significance unestablished

SIDE EFFECTS/ADVERSE REACTIONS

CNS: Headache, weakness, dizziness, drowsiness, tinnitus, fatigue, vertigo

GI: ***Hepatotoxicity, cholestatic jaundice,*** nausea, vomiting, diarrhea, anorexia, hunger

HEME: ***Leukopenia, thrombocytopenia, agranulocytosis, aplastic anemia, pancytopenia, hemolytic anemia***

METAB: ***Hypoglycemia,*** hyponatremia, disulfiram-like reactions, hepatic porphyria, SIADH

SKIN: Rash, allergic reactions, pruritus, urticaria, eczema, photosensitivity, erythema multiforme, ***exfoliative dermatitis***

▼ **DRUG INTERACTIONS**

Drugs

- *Anabolic steroids:* Enhanced hypoglycemic effect
- *β-adrenergic blockers:* Altered response to hypoglycemia, β-blockers also increase blood glucose levels and impair peripheral circulation
- *Chloramphenicol:* Increased hypoglycemic effects
- *Clonidine:* Diminished symptoms of hypoglycemia
- *Colestipol:* Sulfonylureas inhibit lipid lowering response
- *Corticosteroids:* Increased blood glucose concentrations
- *Dicoumarol (but not warfarin):* Enhanced hypoglycemic response; no effect on hypoprothrombinemic response to anticoagulants
- *Ethanol+:* Altered glycemic control, most commonly hypoglycemia; disulfiram-like reaction may occur
- *Fibric acid derivatives:* Enhanced hypoglycemic effects
- *Halofenate:* Increased sulfonylurea concentrations
- *MAOI inhibitors:* Excessive hypoglycemia
- *NSAIDs+:* Excessive hypoglycemic action, especially phenylbutazone and salicylates
- *Oral contraceptives:* OC's impair glucose tolerance
- *Phenformin+:* Additive hypoglycemia
- *Salicylates:* Enhanced hypoglycemic response
- *Smoking:* Increased glucose concentrations
- *Sulfonamides:* Potential for enhanced hypoglycemic actions
- *Thiazide diuretics:* Increased glucose concentrations, may increase dose requirements

SPECIAL CONSIDERATIONS

PATIENT/FAMILY EDUCATION

- Teach symptoms and management of hypo/hyperglycemia
- Consider glucagon kit, Medic-Alert ID for emergency purposes
- Avoid alcohol

---

chlorprothixene

(klor-pro-thix'een)

Taractan

Chemical Class: Thioxanthene derivative of phenothiazines

Therapeutic Class: Neuroleptic antipsychotic/antimanic

CLINICAL PHARMACOLOGY

Mechanism of Action: Blocks postsynaptic dopamine receptors (both D_1 and D_2) in basal ganglia, hypothalamus, limbic system, brain stem and medulla; depresses reticular activating system involving control of basal metabolism, body temperature, wakefulness, vasomotor tone, emesis and hormonal balance; exerts anticholinergic and α-adrenergic blocking effects; like other neuroleptics, diminishes conditional behavioral responses, selectively dampens neurophysiologic effects of peripheral stimuli on the forebrain, and has limited ability to induce generalized sedation; causes lack of initiative and interest in the environment, minimizes display of emotion and affect

Pharmacokinetics

PO: Onset 2-4 hr

IM: Onset 1 hr

Oral absorption erratic and variable (liquid > tab); wide distribution (CNS > plasma); 91-99% protein bound; lipophilic, thus persists; extensive hepatic metabolism with active metabolites; $t_{1/2}$ 10-20 hr

INDICATIONS AND USES: Psychotic disorders

DOSAGE

Adult

• PO 25-50 mg tid-qid, initially, increase PRN (max 600 mg/day); IM 25-50 mg up to tid-qid, then individualize

Child (>6 years)

• PO 10-25 mg tid-qid

$ AVAILABLE FORMS/COST OF THERAPY

• Inj, Sol—IM: 25 mg/2 ml, 2 ml: **$5.13**

• Susp, Conc—Oral: 100 mg/5 ml, 480 ml: **$74.30**

• Tab, Sugar Coated—Oral: 10 mg, 100's: **$42.60;** 25 mg, 100's: **$58.63;** 50 mg, 100's: **$69.70;** 100 mg, 100's: **$87.80**

CONTRAINDICATIONS: Comatose or severely depressed states, hypersensitivity, large amounts of concurrent CNS depressants, bone marrow depression, blood dyscrasias, circulatory collapse, subcortical brain damage, liver damage, cerebral arteriosclerosis, severe hypotension or hypertension

PRECAUTIONS: Epilepsy, coronary artery disease, respiratory impairment, FD&C Yellow No. 5 (tartrazine) or aspirin hypersensitivity

PREGNANCY AND LACTATION: Pregnancy category C; excreted into breast milk, M:P ratios vary between 1.2-2.6, metabolite, 0.5-0.8, effects unknown, but may be of concern

SIDE EFFECTS/ADVERSE REACTIONS

CNS: Pseudoparkinsonism, akathisia, dystonias, tardive dyskinesia (persistent), dizziness, ***neuroleptic malignant syndrome,*** lowering of seizure threshold

CV: Orthostatic hypotension

EENT: Nasal congestion, cornea and lens changes, pigmentary retinopathy

GI: Constipation, nausea and vomiting, stomach pain, cholestatic jaundice, hepatotoxicity

GU: Difficulty in urination, ejaculatory disturbances, changes in libido, priapism

HEME: ***Agranulocytosis,*** leukopenia

METAB: Menstrual cycle changes, weight gain, temperature control impairment, galactorrhea, breast pain

MS: Finger tremor

SKIN: Decreased sweating, photosensitivity, discoloration (blue-gray)

▼ DRUG INTERACTIONS

Drugs

• *Anticholinergics:* Anticholinergics inhibit therapeutic response to neuroleptics, excess anticholinergic effects

• *Antidepressants:* Increased levels of both classes of drugs, with increased therapeutic and toxic effects of both drugs possible

• *β-adrenergic blockers:* Increased levels of both classes of drugs, with increased therapeutic and toxic effects of both drugs possible

• *Bromocriptine:* Bromocriptine ability to lower serum prolactin lev-

els blunted; theoretically bromocriptine should inhibit the antipsychotic effects, but clinical evidence doesn't confirm
- *Epinephrine:* Blunted pressor response to epinephrine
- *Levodopa:* Neuroleptics inhibit antiparkinsonian effects of levodopa
- *Orphenadrine:* Lower neuroleptic levels and excessive anticholinergic effects

SPECIAL CONSIDERATIONS

PATIENT/FAMILY EDUCATION
- Prominent uricosuric effect when used at usual therapeutic doses
- Discuss the development of tardive dyskinesia with patient and/or guardian prior to therapy

chlortetracycline

(klor-te-tra-sye'kleen)

Aureomycin

Chemical Class: Tetracycline; prepared from *Streptomyces* sp

Therapeutic Class: Broad-spectrum antibacterial

CLINICAL PHARMACOLOGY

Mechanism of Action: Bacteriostatic via interference with bacterial protein cell synthesis

INDICATIONS AND USES: Minor pyogenic skin infections caused by susceptible organisms; antibacterial spectrum usually includes a wide variety of both Gram-positive and Gram-negative organisms

DOSAGE

Adult and child
- TOP rub into affected area bid-qid

$ **AVAILABLE FORMS/COST OF THERAPY**
- Oint—Ophth: 1%, 3.5 g: **$14.35**

CONTRAINDICATIONS: Hypersensitivity

PRECAUTIONS: Lactation

PREGNANCY AND LACTATION: Pregnancy category D; theoretical only risk of dental staining and inhibition of bone growth

SIDE EFFECTS/ADVERSE REACTIONS

SKIN: Rash, urticaria, stinging, burning, dry skin, photosensitivity, yellow-brown staining

SPECIAL CONSIDERATIONS

Fluoresces under ultraviolet light

chlorthalidone

(klor-thal'i-done)

Hygroton, Hylidone, Novothalidone, ♣ Thalitone

Chemical Class: Thiazide-like; phthalimidine derivative

Therapeutic Class: Diuretic

CLINICAL PHARMACOLOGY

Mechanism of Action: Blocks sodium/water reabsorption in distal tubule, increases excretion of water, sodium, chloride, potassium, magnesium, bicarbonate

Pharmacokinetics

PO: Onset 2 hr, peak 6 hr, duration 48-72 hr; $t_{1/2}$ 40 hr; excreted unchanged by kidneys; crosses placenta; enters breast milk

INDICATIONS AND USES: Edema associated with CHF, hepatic cirrhosis, renal dysfunction (i.e., nephrotic syndrome, acute glomerulonephritis) and corticosteroid and estrogen therapy; hypertension; calcium nephrolithiasis;* osteoporosis;* diabetes insipidus*

DOSAGE

Adult
- PO 25-100 mg/day or 100 mg every other day

Child
- PO 2 mg/kg 3 ×/wk

$ **AVAILABLE FORMS/COST OF THERAPY**
- Tab, Uncoated—Oral: 25 mg, 100's: **$3.11;** 50 mg, 100's: **$3.48**

CONTRAINDICATIONS: Hypersensitivity to thiazides or sulfonamides, anuria, renal decompensation, lactation

PRECAUTIONS: Hypokalemia, renal disease (CrCl <35 ml/min), hepatic disease, gout, diabetes mellitus, elderly

PREGNANCY AND LACTATION: Pregnancy category D; low M:P ratio, 0.05; compatible with breast feeding

SIDE EFFECTS/ADVERSE REACTIONS

CNS: Drowsiness, paresthesia, anxiety, depression, headache, *dizziness, fatigue, weakness*

CV: Irregular pulse, orthostatic hypotension, palpitations, volume depletion

EENT: Blurred vision

GI: Nausea, vomiting, anorexia, constipation, diarrhea, cramps, pancreatitis, GI irritation, ***hepatitis***

GU: Frequency, polyuria, ***uremia,*** glucosuria, impotence

HEME: ***Aplastic anemia, hemolytic anemia, leukopenia, agranulocytosis, thrombocytopenia, neutropenia***

METAB: Hyperglycemia, hyperuremia, increased creatinine, BUN, gout, *hypokalemia,* hypomagnesemia, hypercalcemia, hyponatremia, hypochloremia

SKIN: Rash, urticaria, purpura, photosensitivity, fever

▼ **DRUG INTERACTIONS**

Drugs

- *Antidiabetics:* Increased dosage requirements due to increased glucose levels
- *Carbenoxolone:* Additive potassium wasting, severe hypokalemia
- *Cholestyramine/colestipol:* Reduced absorption
- *Diazoxide:* Hyperglycemia
- *Digitalis glycosides:* Diuretic-induced hypokalemia increases risk of digitalis toxicity
- *Lithium+:* Increased lithium levels, potential toxicity

Labs

- *Increase:* Ca, cholesterol, triglycerides, amylase
- *Decrease:* Parathyroid test

---

chlorzoxazone

(klor-zox'a-zone)

Chlorzoxazone, Paraflex, Parafon Forte DSC, Remular-S

Chemical Class: Benzoxazole derivative

Therapeutic Class: Skeletal muscle relaxant

CLINICAL PHARMACOLOGY

Mechanism of Action: Inhibition of multisynaptic reflex arcs involved in producing and maintaining skeletal muscle spasm of varied etiology at the level of the spinal cord and subcortical areas of the brain; mode of action may be related to its sedative properties

Pharmacokinetics

PO: Onset 30 min, peak 1-2 hr, duration 6 hr; metabolized in liver; excreted in urine (glucuronide metabolites), $t_{1/2}$ 1 hr

INDICATIONS AND USES: Adjunct for the relief of discomfort associated with acute, painful musculoskeletal conditions; does not directly relax tense skeletal muscles

DOSAGE

Adult

- PO 250-750 mg tid-qid

Child

- PO 20 mg/kg/day in divided doses bid-tid

$ **AVAILABLE FORMS/COST OF THERAPY**

- Tab, Uncoated—Oral: 250 mg, 100's: **$5.99;** 500 mg, 100's: **$10.73-$90.66**

CONTRAINDICATIONS: Hypersensitivity, impaired hepatic function

PRECAUTIONS: Lactation, hepatic disease, elderly

PREGNANCY AND LACTATION: Pregnancy category C

SIDE EFFECTS/ADVERSE REACTIONS

CNS: Dizziness, drowsiness, headache, insomnia, stimulation, malaise

GI: Nausea, vomiting, anorexia, diarrhea, constipation, ***hepatotoxicity, jaundice,*** gastrointestinal bleeding

GU: Urine discoloration

HEME: ***Granulocytopenia, anemia***

SKIN: Rash, pruritus, petechiae, ecchymoses, ***angioedema***

MISC: ***Anaphylaxis***

SPECIAL CONSIDERATIONS

PATIENT/FAMILY EDUCATION

- May lower seizure threshold, use caution in epileptic patients
- Potential for psychologic dependency
- Avoid hazardous activities if drowsiness, dizziness occurs
- Avoid concurrent alcohol, other CNS depressants

cholestyramine

(koe-less-tir′a-meen)

Cholybar, Questran, Questran Light

Chemical Class: Basic anion exchange resin

Therapeutic Class: Bile acid sequestrant; antilipemic

CLINICAL PHARMACOLOGY

Mechanism of Action: Absorbs, combines with bile acids to form insoluble complex that is excreted via feces; loss of bile acids lowers cholesterol levels

Pharmacokinetics

PO: Excreted in feces, max effect in 2 wk

INDICATIONS AND USES: Primary hypercholesterolemia, pruritus associated with biliary obstruction, diarrhea caused by excess bile acid, digitalis toxicity, xanthomas

DOSAGE

Adult

- PO 4 g ac, and hs, not to exceed 32 g/day

Child

- PO 240 mg/kg/day in 3 divided doses

$ AVAILABLE FORMS/COST OF THERAPY

- Powder—Oral: 4 g/9 g, 60 pkts: **$79.40;** 378 g: **$34.78** (Questran)
- Powder, Reconst—Oral: 4 g/5 g, 60 pkts: **$79.40;** 210 g: **$34.78** (Questran Light)

CONTRAINDICATIONS: Hypersensitivity, biliary obstruction

PRECAUTIONS: Lactation, children

PREGNANCY AND LACTATION: Pregnancy category C

SIDE EFFECTS/ADVERSE REACTIONS

CNS: Headache, dizziness, drowsiness, vertigo, tinnitus

MS: Muscle, joint pain

GI: Constipation, abdominal pain, nausea, fecal impaction, hemorrhoids, flatulence, vomiting, steatorrhea, peptic ulcer

SKIN: Rash, irritation of perianal area, tongue, skin

HEME: Decreased Vit A, D, K, red cell folate content, ***hyperchloremic acidosis, bleeding,*** decreased pro-time

▼ DRUG INTERACTIONS

Drugs

- *Acetaminophen, corticosteroids, diclofenac, digitalis glycosides, furosemide, methotrexate, thiazide diuretics, thyroid hormones:* Cholestyramine reduces interacting drug concentrations and probably subsequent therapeutic response

• *Oral anticoagulants:* Inhibition of hypoprothrombinemic response; colestipol might be less likely to interact

Labs

• *Increase:* Liver function studies, Cl, PO_4

SPECIAL CONSIDERATIONS

PATIENT/FAMILY EDUCATION

• Give all other medications 1 hr before, or 4 hr after cholestyramine to avoid poor absorption

• Drug mixed with applesauce or stirred into beverage (2-6 oz), do not take dry, let stand for 2 min

---

choline magnesium trisalicylate

(koe'leen/mag-nees'ee-um/tri-sal'eh-cye'late)

Trilisate

Chemical Class: Salicylate

Therapeutic Class: Nonnarcotic analgesic, nonsteroidal antiinflammatory agent

CLINICAL PHARMACOLOGY

Mechanism of Action: Inhibits prostaglandin synthesis; analgesic, antiinflammatory, antipyretic actions

Pharmacokinetics

PO: Onset 15-30 min, peak 1.5-2 hrs (33 μg/ml following 500 mg dose); rapid absorption, metabolized by liver; excreted by kidneys

INDICATIONS AND USES: Mild to moderate pain, inflammation or fever including osteoarthritis, rheumatoid arthritis, juvenile rheumatoid arthritis; consider for patients with GI intolerance to aspirin or in patients in whom interference with normal platelet function by aspirin or other NSAIDs is undesirable

DOSAGE

(NOTE: Each 500 mg of choline magnesium trisalicylate contains 500 mg of salicylate [equivalent to 650 mg aspirin]; dosage based on total salicylate content)

Adult

• PO 1.5-4.0 g of salicylate daily in single dose or in 2-3 divided doses (based on response, tolerance, and serum salicylate concentration)

Child

• PO 50 mg/kg/day divided into two doses

$ **AVAILABLE FORMS/COST OF THERAPY**

• Liq—Oral: 500 mg/5 ml, 240 ml: **$28.67**

• Tab, Uncoated—Oral: 500 mg, 100's: **$27.70-$62.92;** 750 mg, 100's: **$34.40-$74.87;** 1000 mg, 100's: **$44.80-$96.54**

CONTRAINDICATIONS: Hypersensitivity to salicylates, GI bleeding, bleeding disorders, children <3 yr, Vit K deficiency, children with flu-like symptoms

PRECAUTIONS: Anemia, hepatic disease, renal disease, Hodgkin's disease, lactation

PREGNANCY AND LACTATION: Pregnancy category C; excreted into breast milk (peak 1.1-10 μg/ml)

SIDE EFFECTS/ADVERSE REACTIONS

CNS: Stimulation, drowsiness, dizziness, confusion, ***convulsion,*** headache, flushing, hallucinations, ***coma***

CV: Rapid pulse, pulmonary edema

EENT: Tinnitus, hearing loss

GI: Nausea, vomiting, GI bleeding, diarrhea, heartburn, anorexia, ***hepatitis***

HEME: ***Thrombocytopenia, agranulocytosis, leukopenia, neutropenia, hemolytic anemia,*** increased pro-time

METAB: Hypoglycemia, hyponatremia, hypokalemia
SKIN: *Rash,* urticaria, bruising
RESP: Wheezing, hyperpnea

▼ **DRUG INTERACTIONS**

Drugs

• *Acetazolamide:* Increased acetazolamide plasma concentrations with CNS toxicity
• *Antacids:* Decreased salicylate concentrations
• *Antidiabetics:* Enhanced hypoglycemic response, especially chlorpropamide
• *Corticosteroids:* Steroids markedly enhance the elimination of salicylates; discontinuing steroids during high-dose salicylate therapy may result in salicylate toxicity
• *Ethanol:* Enhanced salicylate-induced gastric mucosal damage
• *Methotrexate+:* Increased methotrexate serum concentrations and enhanced toxicity
• *Phenytoin:* Large doses of salicylates may reduce total serum phenytoin concentrations; free serum phenytoin concentrations do not appear to be affected
• *Probenecid:* Salicylates inhibit the uricosuric activities of probenecid, but not the ability to inhibit the renal elimination of penicillins
• *Sulfinpyrazone:* Salicylates inhibit uricosuric effects
• *Valproic acid:* Combination increases unbound serum valproic acid concentrations sufficiently to produce toxicity

Labs

• *Increase:* Coagulation studies, liver function studies, serum uric acid, amylase, CO_2, urinary protein
• *Decrease:* Serum potassium, PBI, cholesterol
• *Interference:* Urine catecholamines, pregnancy test

SPECIAL CONSIDERATIONS

MONITORING PARAMETERS

• Liver and renal function studies, stool for occult blood and Hct if long-term therapy

C

---

choline salicylate

(koe'leen sa-lis'i-late)
Arthropan, Teejel ✤
Chemical Class: Salicylate
Therapeutic Class: Nonnarcotic analgesic, nonsteroidal antiinflammatory agent

CLINICAL PHARMACOLOGY

Mechanism of Action: Inhibits prostaglandin synthesis; analgesic, antiinflammatory, antipyretic actions

Pharmacokinetics

PO: Onset 15-30 min; rapid absorption, metabolized by liver; excreted by kidneys

INDICATIONS AND USES: Mild to moderate pain, inflammation or fever including osteoarthritis, rheumatoid arthritis, juvenile rheumatoid arthritis; consider for patients with GI intolerance to aspirin or in patients in whom interference with normal platelet function by aspirin or other NSAIDs is undesirable

DOSAGE

(NOTE: dosage based on total salicylate content)

Adult

• Arthritis: PO 987-1740 mg qid; max 6 g/day
• Pain/fever: PO 870 mg q3-4h prn

Child

• PO 50 mg/kg/day in 2 divided doses for children weighing up to 37 kg and 2250 mg/day for larger children

$ **AVAILABLE FORMS/COST OF THERAPY**

• Liq—Oral: 870 mg/5 ml, 480 ml: **$35.73**

CONTRAINDICATIONS: Hypersensitivity to salicylates, GI bleeding, bleeding disorders, children <3 yr, Vit K deficiency, children with flu-like symptoms

PRECAUTIONS: Anemia, hepatic disease, renal disease, Hodgkin's disease, lactation

PREGNANCY AND LACTATION: Pregnancy category C; excreted into breast milk (peak 1.1-10 μg/ml)

SIDE EFFECTS/ADVERSE REACTIONS

CNS: Stimulation, drowsiness, dizziness, confusion, ***convulsion,*** headache, flushing, hallucinations, ***coma***

CV: Rapid pulse, pulmonary edema

EENT: Tinnitus, hearing loss

GI: Nausea, vomiting, GI bleeding, diarrhea, heartburn, anorexia, ***hepatitis***

HEME: ***Thrombocytopenia, agranulocytosis, leukopenia, neutropenia, hemolytic anemia,*** increased pro-time

METAB: Hypoglycemia, hyponatremia, hypokalemia

SKIN Rash, urticaria, bruising

RESP: Wheezing, hyperpnea

▼ **DRUG INTERACTIONS**

Drugs

• *Acetazolamide:* Increased acetazolamide plasma concentrations with CNS toxicity

• *Antacids:* Decreased salicylate concentrations

• *Antidiabetics:* Enhanced hypoglycemic response, especially chlorpropamide

• *Corticosteroids:* Steroids markedly enhance the elimination of salicylates; discontinuing steroids during high-dose salicylate therapy may result in salicylate toxicity

• *Ethanol:* Enhanced salicylate-induced gastric mucosal damage

• *Methotrexate+:* Increased methotrexate serum concentrations and enhanced toxicity

• *Phenytoin:* Large doses of salicylates may reduce total serum phenytoin concentrations; free serum phenytoin concentrations do not appear to be affected

• *Probenecid:* Salicylates inhibit the uricosuric activities of probenecid, but not the ability to inhibit the renal elimination of penicillins

• *Sulfinpyrazone:* Salicylates inhibit uricosuric effects

• *Valproic acid:* Combination increases unbound serum valproic acid concentrations sufficiently to produce toxicity

Labs

• *Increase:* Coagulation studies, liver function studies, serum uric acid, amylase, CO_2, urinary protein

• *Decrease:* Serum potassium, PBI, cholesterol

• *Interference:* Urine catecholamines, pregnancy test

SPECIAL CONSIDERATIONS

MONITORING PARAMETERS

• Liver and renal function studies, stool for occult blood and Hct if long-term therapy

ciclopirox

(sye-kloe-peer'ox)

Loprox

Therapeutic Class: Synthetic, broad-spectrum, antifungal agent

CLINICAL PHARMACOLOGY

Mechanism of Action: Interferes with fungal cell membrane, which increases permeability, leaking of cell nutrients

INDICATIONS AND USES: Topical dermal infections (Tinea cruris, Tinea corporis, Tinea pedis, Tinea versicolor, cutaneous candidiasis) caused by susceptible organisms. Antifungal spectrum usually includes *Trichophyton mentagrophytes, Epidermophyton floccosum, Trichophyton rubrum,* and *Microsporum canis; Candida albicans;* and *Malassezia furfur*

DOSAGE

Adult and Child >(10 yr)

- TOP apply bid

$ AVAILABLE FORMS/COST OF THERAPY

- Cre—Top: 1%, 15 g: **$10.18**
- Lotion—Top: 1%, 30 ml: **$20.00**

CONTRAINDICATIONS: Hypersensitivity

PREGNANCY AND LACTATION: Pregnancy category B

SIDE EFFECTS/ADVERSE REACTIONS

SKIN: Rash, urticaria, stinging, burning, pruritus, pain

SPECIAL CONSIDERATIONS

PATIENT/FAMILY EDUCATION

- Continue medication for several days after condition clears

---

cimetidine

(sye-met'i-deen)

Tagamet, Tagamet HB, Peptol, ✤ Novocimetine ✤

Chemical Class: Imidazole derivative

Therapeutic Class: H_2 Histamine receptor antagonist

CLINICAL PHARMACOLOGY

Mechanism of Action: Competitively inhibits the action of histamine at the histamine H_2 receptors of the parietal cells (H_2-receptor antagonist); inhibits gastric acid secretion

Pharmacokinetics

IM/IV: Onset 10 min, peak ½ hr, duration 4-5 hr

PO: Peak 1-1½ hr, $t_{1/2}$ 1½-2 hr

Well absorbed (PO, IM); 30%-40% metabolized by liver (sulfoxide, major metabolite), excreted in urine (75% unchanged after 24 hr), crosses placenta

INDICATIONS AND USES: Short-term treatment of duodenal and benign gastric ulcers; maintenance therapy for duodenal ulcer (reduced dosage); erosive gastroesophageal reflux disease (GERD); prevention of upper gastrointestinal bleeding in critically ill patients; treatment of pathological hypersecretory conditions (i.e., Zollinger-Ellison Syndrome, systemic mastocytosis, multiple endocrine adenomas); heartburn, acid indigestion, and sour stomach (OTC only)

DOSAGE

Adult and Child (>16 yrs)

- *Treatment:* PO 300 mg qid with meals, hs × 8 wk or 400 mg bid or 800 mg hs; after 8 wk give 300-400 mg hs dose only; IV BOL 300 mg/20 ml 0.9% NaC1 over 1-2 min q6h; IV INF 300 mg/50 ml D_5W over 15-20 min; IM 300 mg q6h, not to exceed 2400 mg
- *Prophylaxis of duodenal ulcer:* 400 mg hs

$ AVAILABLE FORMS/COST OF THERAPY

- Inj, Sol—IM; IV: 300 mg/2 ml, 8 ml: **$12.86**
- Inj, Sol—IV: 300 mg/2 ml: **$1.81-$3.96;** 300 mg/50 ml: **$5.58**
- Liq—Oral: 300 mg/5 ml, 240 ml: **$86.25-$99.75**
- Tab, Coated—Oral: 200 mg, 100's: **$54.45-$84.70;** 300 mg, 30's: **$17.10-$44.90;** 400 mg, 30's: **$28.37-$88.25;** 800 mg, 30's: **$55.33-$78.20**

CONTRAINDICATIONS: Hypersensitivity

PRECAUTIONS: Organic brain syndrome, hepatic disease, renal disease, elderly

PREGNANCY AND LACTATION: Pregnancy category B; excreted into breast milk and may accumulate (single dose M:P ratio 1:6; multiple oral doses of 200 and 400 mg result in M:P ratio 4.6-7.44), theoretically, adversely affects the nursing infant's gastric acidity, inhibits drug metabolism, and produces CNS stimulation—all not reported; compatible with breast feeding

SIDE EFFECTS/ADVERSE REACTIONS

CNS: Confusion, headache, depression, dizziness, anxiety, weakness, psychosis, tremors, ***convulsions***

CV: Bradycardia, tachycardia

GI: Diarrhea, abdominal cramps, paralytic ileus, jaundice

GU: Gynecomastia, galactorrhea, impotence, increase in BUN, creatinine

HEME: ***Agranulocytosis, thrombocytopenia, neutropenia, aplastic anemia, increase in pro-time***

SKIN: Urticaria, rash, alopecia, sweating, flushing, ***exfoliative dermatitis***

▼ DRUG INTERACTIONS

Drugs

- *Benzodiazepines:* Cimetidine increases plasma levels of several benzodiazepines and/or metabolites; potential for increased CNS adverse effects
- *β-adrenergic blockers:* Plasma concentrations of β-blockers that undergo significant hepatic metabolism, e.g., propranolol, may be increased
- *Calcium channel blockers:* Increased serum concentration of calcium channel blockers, variably
- *Carmustine:* Increased myelotoxicity of carmustine
- *Clozapine:* Increased clozapine concentrations and evidence of clozapine toxicity
- *Desipramine:* Increased serum desipramine concentrations
- *Doxepin:* Substantially increased serum concentrations of doxepin
- *Ketoconazole:* Reduced ketoconazole concentrations
- *Lidocaine:* Modestly increases lidocaine serum concentrations
- *Narcotic analgesics:* Increased effects of narcotic analgesics; morphine may be less likely to interact than other narcotics
- *Nortriptyline:* Increased serum nortriptyline concentrations
- *Oral anticoagulants:* Increased hypoprothrombinemic response to oral anticoagulants
- *Phenytoin:* Increased phenytoin concentrations; phenytoin intoxication occurs in some patients
- *Procainamide:* Significantly increased procainamide serum concentrations, with toxicity
- *Propranolol:* Plasma concentrations of β-blockers that undergo significant hepatic metabolism, e.g., propranolol, may be increased
- *Quinidine:* Elevated quinidine concentrations
- *Tacrine:* Increased tacrine plasma concentrations
- *Theophylline:* Increased theophylline concentrations; potential toxicity
- *Warfarin:* Increased hypoprothrombinemic response to oral anticoagulants

Labs

- *Increase:* Alk phosphatase, AST, creatinine
- *False positive:* Gastric bleeding test

SPECIAL CONSIDERATIONS

PATIENT/FAMILY EDUCATION

- Smoking decreases the effectiveness of cimetidine

cinoxacin

(sin-ox'a-sin)

Cinobac, Cinoxacin

Chemical Class: Synthetic organic acid, quinolone (related to nalidixic acid)

Therapeutic Class: Urinary tract antibacterial

CLINICAL PHARMACOLOGY

Mechanism of Action: Inhibits DNA replication; DNA gyrase inhibitor

Pharmacokinetics

PO: Peak 2 hr (15 μg/ml after 500 mg dose), duration 6-8 hr; $t_{1/2}$ 1½ hr; excreted in urine (unchanged/inactive metabolites)

INDICATIONS AND USES: Infections of the urinary tract caused by susceptible organisms. Antibacterial spectrum usually includes: *E. coli, Klebsiella, Enterobacter, P. mirabilis, P. vulgaris, M. morganii, Serratia, Citrobacter*

DOSAGE

Adult and Child >12 yr

• PO 1 g/day in 2-4 divided doses × 1-2 wk

$ AVAILABLE FORMS/COST OF THERAPY

• Cap, Gel—Oral: 250 mg, 40's: **$35.70;** 500 mg, 50's: **$77.60-$95.30**

CONTRAINDICATIONS: Hypersensitivity to this drug, anuria, CNS damage

PRECAUTIONS: Renal disease, hepatic disease

PREGNANCY AND LACTATION: Pregnancy category B

SIDE EFFECTS/ADVERSE REACTIONS

CNS: Dizziness, headache, agitation, insomnia, confusion

EENT: Sensitivity to light, visual disturbances, blurred vision, tinnitus

GI: Nausea, vomiting, anorexia, abdominal cramps, diarrhea

SKIN: Pruritus, rash, urticaria, photosensitivity, edema

▼ **DRUG INTERACTIONS**

Labs

• *Increase:* AST/ALT, BUN, creatinine, alk phosphatase

ciprofloxacin

(sip-ro-floks'a-sin)

Cipro, Cipro IV

Chemical Class: Fluoroquinolone antibacterial

Therapeutic Class: Urinary anti-infective

CLINICAL PHARMACOLOGY

Mechanism of Action: Interferes with the enzyme DNA gyrase which is needed for the synthesis of bacterial DNA; with 60-minute IV inf of 200 mg and 400 mg ciprofloxacin to normal volunteers, the mean max serum concentrations achieved were 2.1 and 4.6

Pharmacokinetics

PO: Peak 1-2 hr (2.4 μg/ml following 500 mg dose)

IV: Peak 4.6 μg/ml (following 400 mg 60 min inf)

60%-85% bioavailable PO with minimal 1st pass; widely distributed; 30-50% excreted in urine as active drug (2 hr following 250 mg oral dose, 200 μg/ml), 20-40% of dose excreted in feces (biliary excretion); $t_{1/2}$ 4 hr; metabolites less active

INDICATIONS AND USES: Infections of the lower respiratory tract, skin and skin structure, bone and joints, urinary tract, external auditory canal, infectious diarrhea, and superficial ocular infections caused by susceptible organisms.

Antibacterial spectrum usually includes:

• Gram-positive organisms: *Enterococcus faecalis,* (many strains are only moderately susceptible), *Staphylococcus aureus, S. epidermidis, Streptococcus pneumoniae* (minimally), *S. pyogenes*
• Gram-negative organisms: *Campylobacter jejuni, Citrobacter diversus, C. freundii, Enterobacter cloacae, Escherichia coli, H. influenzae, H. parainfluenzae, Klebsiella pneumoniae, Morganella morganii, Proteus mirabilis, P. vulgaris, Providencia rettgeri, P. stuartii, Pseudomonas aeruginosa, Serratia marcescens, Shigella flexneri, S. sonnei*
• Most strains of *Pseudomonas cepacia* and some strains of *Pseudomonas maltophilia* are *resistant* to ciprofloxacin as are most anaerobic bacteria, including *Bacteroides fragilis* and *Clostridium difficile*

DOSAGE

Adult

• *Uncomplicated UTI:* PO 250 mg q12h; IV 200 mg q12h × 7 days
• *Complicated/severe urinary tract infections:* PO 500 mg q12h × 14 days; IV 400 mg q12h
• *Respiratory, skin, bone, and joint infections:* (Bone and joint infections may require treatment for 4 to 6 wk or longer) PO 500-750 mg q12h × 7-14 days
• *Infectious diarrhea:* 500 mg q12h × 5-7 days
• *Ocular:* 1 gtt 5-6 times/day
• *Renal impairment:* CrCl 10-50 ml/min 50% of dose; CrCl <10 ml/min 30% of dose

$ AVAILABLE FORMS/COST OF THERAPY

• Inj, Sol—IV: 200 mg/100 ml: **$15.60;** 400 mg/200 ml × 24s: **$30.01**
• Sol, Ophth—Top: 0.3%, 2.5 ml: **$10.31**
• Tab, Uncoated—Oral: 250 mg, 100's: **$270.53;** 500 mg, 100's: **$313.07;** 750 mg, 50's: **$271.50**

CONTRAINDICATIONS: Hypersensitivity to quinolones

PRECAUTIONS: Children (arthropathy in juvenile animals), renal disease, excessive sunlight, caution with known or suspected CNS disorders

PREGNANCY AND LACTATION: Pregnancy category C; appears in breast milk at levels similar to serum; allow 48 hr to elapse after last dose, before resuming breast feeding

SIDE EFFECTS/ADVERSE REACTIONS

CNS: Headache, dizziness, fatigue, insomnia, depression, restlessness, nightmares, hallucinations
EENT: Blurred vision, tinnitus
GI: Abdominal pain/discomfort, nausea, constipation, increased ALT, AST, flatulence, insomnia, heartburn, vomiting, diarrhea, oral candidiasis, dysphagia
SKIN: Rash, pruritus, urticaria, photosensitivity, flushing, fever, chills

▼ DRUG INTERACTIONS

Drugs

• *Antacids:* Reduced absorption, serum levels and efficacy; bismuth subsalicylate does not alter plasma concentrations
• *Caffeine:* Increases caffeine levels, may enhance side effects
• *Didanosine:* Buffers in didanosine markedly reduce ciprofloxacin serum levels; separate by 2 hrs
• *H_2-receptor antagonists:* Cimetidine increases levels minimally
• *Iron:* Lowers antibiotic levels, may reduce efficacy
• *Oral anticoagulants:* Enhanced hypoprothrombinemic response
• *Sucralfate:* Markedly reduces ciprofloxacin levels
• *Tacrine:* Ciprofloxacin moderate inhibitor of CYP1A2, potential for increased cholinergic side effects
• *Theophylline:* Increased theophyl-

line levels and toxicity
• *Zinc:* Multivits with zinc will reduce ciprofloxacin levels
Labs
• *Increase:* AST, ALT, BUN, creatinine, alk phosphatase

SPECIAL CONSIDERATIONS

PATIENT/FAMILY EDUCATION
• Do not take antacids containing magnesium or aluminum with this drug or within 2 hr of drug
• Crystalluria related to ciprofloxacin avoidable by patient being well hydrated and minimizing alkaline urine

---

cisapride

(sis'-eh-pride)
Propulsid
Chemical Class: Substituted methoxybenzamide
Therapeutic Class: GI prokinetic agent

CLINICAL PHARMACOLOGY
Mechanism of Action: Enhances acetylcholine release at the myenteric plexus
Pharmacokinetics
• Onset 30-60 min, peak 1-1.5 hr, duration 6 hr; bioavailability less when gastric acidity reduced; 98% protein bound, mainly to albumin; 90% metabolized by N-dealkylation; terminal $t_{1/2}$ 6-12 hr, longer in elderly and renal or hepatic impairment
INDICATIONS AND USES: Gastroesophageal reflux disease, dyspepsia;* irritable bowel syndrome,* gastroparesis*
DOSAGE
Adult
• PO 10-20 mg qid, 15-60 min ac and hs; no dose adjustment in elderly, renal, hepatic impairment
Child
• PO 0.15-0.3 mg/kg ac and hs

$ AVAILABLE FORMS/COST OF THERAPY
• Tab, Uncoated—Oral: 10 mg, 100's: **$60.00;** 20 mg, 100's: **$116.40**
CONTRAINDICATIONS: GI hemorrhage, obstruction, or perforation; known intolerance of the drug.
PRECAUTIONS: Sedative effects of benzodiazepines or alcohol may be accelerated by cisapride; accelerated gastric emptying may change the rate of absorption of other drugs; anticholinergic drugs may reduce benefit of cisapride
PREGNANCY AND LACTATION: Pregnancy category C; excreted in breast milk
SIDE EFFECTS/ADVERSE REACTIONS
CNS: Headache (19%), seizures, extrapyramidal syndromes, insomnia (2%), anxiety (1%)
CV: Palpitation, sinus tachycardia
EENT: Rhinitis (7%), sinusitis (4%), abnormal vision (1%)
GI: Diarrhea (14%), abdominal pain (10%), nausea (8%), constipation (7%), flatulence (3%), dyspepsia (3%)

---

clarithromycin

(clare-i-thro-mye'sin)
Biaxin
Chemical Class: Macrolide antibiotic
Therapeutic Class: Antibacterial

CLINICAL PHARMACOLOGY
Mechanism of Action: Binds to 50S ribosomal subunits of susceptible bacteria and suppresses protein synthesis
Pharmacokinetics
PO: Peak 2-4 hr, 65% bound to plasma proteins, extensively metabolized in liver (14-OH metabo-

lite twice as active as parent compound vs *Haemophilus influenzae*), $t_{1/2}$ 3-7 hr (metabolite 5-7 hr)

INDICATIONS AND USES: Infections of upper and lower respiratory tract, skin and skin structures; disseminated mycobacterial infections due to *Mycoplasma avium* and *M. intracellulare*

Antibacterial spectrum usually includes: gram-positive organisms: *Staphylococcus aureus, Streptococcus pneumoniae, S. pyogenes, S. agalactiae,* streptococci (Groups C, F, G), Viridans group streptococci, *Listeria monocytogenes*

• Gram-negative organisms: *Haemophilus influenzae, Moraxella catarrhalis, Bordetella pertussis, Campylobacter jejuni, Legionella pneumophila, Neisseria gonorrhoeae, Pasteurella multocida*

• Anaerobes: *Clostridium perfringens, Peptococcus niger, Propionibacterium acnes, Bacteriodes melaninogenicus*

• Other organisms: *Mycoplasma pneumoniae, M. avium* complex (MAC) consisting of *M. avium* and *M. intracellulare; Chlamydia trachomatis*

DOSAGE

Adult

• *Acute maxillary sinusitis:* PO 500 mg bid for 14 days

• *Acute exacerbation of chronic bronchitis:* (due to *Haemophilus influenzae*) PO 500 mg bid for 7-14 days

• *Mycobacterial infections:* PO 500 mg bid

• *Other infections:* PO 250 mg bid for 7-14 days

• Dosing adjustment in renal impairment (CrCl <30 ml/min) decrease dose by 50%

Child

• *Mycobacterial infections:* PO 7.5 mg/kg bid, do not exceed 500 mg bid

$ AVAILABLE FORMS/COST OF THERAPY

• Powder, Reconst—Oral: 125 mg/5 ml, 100 ml: **$24.93;** 250 mg/5 ml, 100 ml: **$47.48**

• Tab, Coated—Oral: 250, 500 mg, 60's: **$178.30**

CONTRAINDICATIONS Hypersensitivity to any macrolide antibiotic

PRECAUTIONS: Renal impairment, children

PREGNANCY AND LACTATION: Pregnancy category C; excretion into breast milk unknown, use caution in nursing mothers; potential exists for modification of bowel flora in nursing infant, allergy/sensitization and interference with interpretation of culture results if fever workup required

SIDE EFFECTS/ADVERSE REACTIONS

CNS: Headache

GI: Nausea, vomiting, diarrhea, ***hepatotoxicity,*** abdominal pain, stomatitis, heartburn, anorexia, abnormal taste

GU: Vaginitis, moniliasis

SKIN: Rash, urticaria, pruritus

▼ DRUG INTERACTIONS

Drugs

• *Cyclosporine:* Increased cyclosporine concentrations; renal toxicity may result

• *Tacrolimus:* Increased tacrolimus concentrations; nephrotoxicity could result

• *Terfenadine:* Elevated terfenadine and terfenadine carboxylate plasma concentrations; cardiac arrhythmias could result

SPECIAL CONSIDERATION

PATIENT/FAMILY EDUCATION

• May be given without regard to meals

• Complete full course of prescribed medication

clemastine

(klem′as-teen)

Tavist

Chemical Class: Ethanolamine derivative

Therapeutic Class: Antihistamine

CLINICAL PHARMACOLOGY

Mechanism of Action: Competes with histamine for H_1-receptor sites on effector cells in GI tract, blood vessels, and respiratory tract

Pharmacokinetics

PO: Peak 5-7 hr, duration 10-12 hr, metabolized by liver, excreted by kidneys

INDICATIONS AND USES: Perennial and seasonal allergic rhinitis and other allergic symptoms including urticaria

DOSAGE

Adult and Child >12 yr

• PO 1.34-2.68 mg bid-tid, not to exceed 8.04 mg/d

$ **AVAILABLE FORMS/COST OF THERAPY**

• Syr—Oral: 0.67 mg/5 ml, 120 ml: **$16.50-$22.68**

• Tab, Uncoated—Oral: 1.34 mg, 100's: **$31.17-$63.84;** 2.68 mg, 100's: **$72.50-$95.22**

CONTRAINDICATIONS: Hypersensitivity, narrow-angle glaucoma, bladder neck obstruction

PRECAUTIONS: Liver disease, elderly, increased intraocular pressure, hyperthyroidism, cardiovascular disease, hypertension, urinary retention, renal disease, stenosed peptic ulcers

PREGNANCY AND LACTATION: Pregnancy category C; excreted into breast milk, may cause drowsiness and irritability in nursing infant, use with caution during breast feeding

SIDE EFFECTS/ADVERSE REACTIONS

CNS: Dizziness, drowsiness, poor coordination, fatigue, anxiety, euphoria, confusion, paresthesia, neuritis

CV: Hypotension, palpitations, tachycardia

EENT: Blurred vision, dilated pupils, tinnitus, nasal stuffiness, dry nose, throat

GI: Dry mouth, nausea, vomiting, anorexia, *constipation,* diarrhea

GU: Retention, dysuria, frequency, impotence

HEME: ***Thrombocytopenia, agranulocytosis, hemolytic anemia***

RESP: Increased thick secretions, wheezing, chest tightness

SKIN: Photosensitivity, rash, urticaria

▼ **DRUG INTERACTIONS**

Drugs

• *Barbiturates:* Excessive CNS depression

Labs

• *False negative:* Skin allergy tests

SPECIAL CONSIDERATIONS

PATIENT/FAMILY EDUCATION

• Notify physician if confusion/sedation/hypotension occurs

• Avoid driving or other hazardous activities if drowsiness occurs

• Avoid use of alcohol or other CNS depressants while taking drug

• Use hard candy, gum, frequent rinsing of mouth for dryness

clidinium

(kli-din′ee-um)

Quarzan

Chemical Class: Synthetic quaternary ammonium antimuscarinic

Therapeutic Class: GI anticholinergic; antispasmodic

CLINICAL PHARMACOLOGY

Mechanism of Action: Inhibits gastrointestinal motility and diminishes gastric acid secretion

Pharmacokinetics

PO: Onset 1 hr, duration 3 hr, ionized, excreted in urine

INDICATIONS AND USES: Peptic ulcer disease (in combination with other drugs); functional GI disorders (diarrhea, pylorospasm, hypermotility, neurogenic colon);* irritable bowel syndrome (spastic colon, mucous colitis);* acute enterocolitis,* ulcerative colitis,* diverticulitis,* mild dysenteries,* pancreatitis,* splenic flexure syndrome*

DOSAGE

Adult

• PO 2.5-5 mg tid-qid ac, hs (use lower dose for elderly or debilitated patients)

$ AVAILABLE FORMS/COST OF THERAPY

• Cap, Gel—Oral: 2.5 mg, 100's: **$19.42;** 5 mg, 100's: **$26.46**

CONTRAINDICATIONS: Hypersensitivity to anticholinergic drugs, narrow-angle glaucoma, obstructive uropathy (e.g. bladder neck obstruction due to prostatic hypertrophy), obstructive disease of the GI tract (e.g. pyloroduodenal stenosis), paralytic ileus, intestinal atony, unstable cardiovascular status in acute hemorrhage, severe ulcerative colitis, toxic megacolon complicating ulcerative colitis, myasthenia gravis

PRECAUTIONS: Hyperthyroidism, coronary artery disease, dysrhythmias, CHF, ulcerative colitis, hypertension, hiatal hernia, hepatic disease, renal disease, urinary retention, prostatic hypertrophy, elderly

PREGNANCY AND LACTATION: Pregnancy category C; excretion into breast milk unknown, although would be expected to be minimal due to quaternary structure (see also atropine)

SIDE EFFECTS/ADVERSE REACTIONS

CNS: Confusion, stimulation (especially in elderly), headache, insomnia, dizziness, drowsiness, anxiety, weakness, hallucination

CV: Palpitations, tachycardia

EENT: Blurred vision, photophobia, mydriasis, cycloplegia, increased ocular tension

GI: Dry mouth, constipation, ***paralytic ileus,*** heartburn, nausea, vomiting, dysphagia, absence of taste

GU: Hesitancy, retention, impotence

SKIN: Urticaria, rash, pruritus, anhidrosis, fever, allergic reactions

SPECIAL CONSIDERATIONS

PATIENT/FAMILY EDUCATION

• Avoid driving or other hazardous activities until stabilized on medication

• Avoid alcohol or other CNS depressants, will enhance sedating properties of this drug

• Avoid hot environments, drug suppresses perspiration, heat stroke may occur

• Use sunglasses when outside to prevent photophobia, may cause blurred vision

• Drink plenty of fluids, increase bulk, exercise to decrease constipation

• Use gum, hard candy, frequent rinsing of mouth for dry mouth

clindamycin

(klin-da-mye'sin)

Cleocin, Cleocin-T, Clinda-Derm

Chemical Class: Lincomycin derivative

Therapeutic Class: Antibiotic

CLINICAL PHARMACOLOGY

Mechanism of Action: Inhibits bacterial protein synthesis by preferentially binding to the 50S ribosomal subunit and affecting the process of peptide chain initiation

Pharmacokinetics

PO: Peak 45 min, duration 6 hr
IM: Peak 3 hr, duration 8-12 hr
VAG: Peak 16 hr
$t_{1/2}$ 2.5 hr, 90% bound to plasma proteins; metabolized in liver; excreted in urine, bile, feces as active/inactive metabolites

INDICATIONS AND USES: Infections of the respiratory tract (e.g. empyema, anaerobic pneumonitis, lung abscess), skin and soft tissues, female pelvis and genital tract; septicemia; intra-abdominal infections (e.g. peritonitis, abscess); bone and joint infections; CNS toxoplasmosis in AIDS patients (in combination with pyrimethamine);* *Pneumocystis carinii** pneumonia *(in combination with primaquine);** *Chlamydia trachomatis* infections in women;* acne vulgaris (TOP formulations); rosacea (TOP formulations);* bacterial vaginosis (VAG formulation)

Antibacterial spectrum usually includes:

- Gram-positive organisms: *Staphylococcus aureus, S. epidermidis* (penicillinase and nonpenicillinase-producing strains), streptococci (except *Str. faecalis*), pneumococci
- Anaerobes: *Bacteroides* sp. (including *B. fragilis* and *B. melaninogenicus*), *Fusobacterium, Propionibacterium, Eubacterium, Actinomyces* sp, *Peptococcus, Peptostreptococcus, Clostridium perfringens, C. tetani, Veillonella*

DOSAGE

Adult

- PO 150-450 mg q6-8h, not to exceed 1.8 g/d; IM/IV 1.2-1.8 g/d in 2-4 divided doses, not to exceed 4.8 g/d; VAG insert 1 applicatorful qhs for 7 days; TOP apply bid

Child

- PO 10-30 mg/kg/d divided q6h; IM/IV 25-40 mg/kg/d divided q6-8h; TOP apply bid

$ AVAILABLE FORMS/COST OF THERAPY

- Inj, Sol—IM; IV: 150 mg/ml, 4 ml: **$14.71-$260.94**
- Sol—Top: 1%, 60 ml: **$13.44-$23.12**
- Gel—Top: 1%, 30 g: **$19.16**
- Lotion—Top: 1%, 60 ml: **$26.63**
- Swab, Medicated—Top: 1%, 60's: **$27.50**
- Cre—Vag: 2%, 40 g: **$29.22**
- Cap, Gel—Oral: 75, 150, 300 mg, 100's: **$44.50-$221.44**
- Granule, Reconst—Oral: 75 mg/5 ml, 100 ml: **$12.35**

CONTRAINDICATIONS: Hypersensitivity to this drug or lincomycin, regional enteritis, ulcerative colitis, antibiotic-associated colitis

PRECAUTIONS: History of GI disease, liver disease, renal disease, atopic individuals, tartrazine sensitivity (75 and 150 mg caps), elderly, prolonged therapy

PREGNANCY AND LACTATION: Pregnancy category B; excreted into breast milk, compatible with breast feeding, however may cause modification of bowel flora in nursing infant, allergy/sensitization and interference with interpretation of culture results if fever workup required

SIDE EFFECTS/ADVERSE REACTIONS

*GI: Nausea, vomiting, abdominal pain, diarrhea, **pseudomembranous colitis,*** anorexia, weight loss, increased AST/ALT, bilirubin, alk phosphatase, jaundice

GU: Vaginitis, urinary frequency, vulvar irritation

HEME: ***Leukopenia, eosinophilia,***

agranulocytosis, thrombocytopenia

SKIN: Rash, urticaria, pruritus, erythema, pain, abscess at inj site

SPECIAL CONSIDERATIONS

PATIENT/FAMILY EDUCATION

- Notify physician if diarrhea occurs, do not treat without notifying physician
- Take each dose with a full glass of water
- Report sore throat, fever, fatigue; may indicate superimposed infection

MONITORING PARAMETERS

- AST, ALT, CBC, urinalysis, BUN, creatinine

---

clioquinol (iodochlorhydroxyquin)

(klee-oh-kwee′nole)

Vioform

Chemical Class: Halogenated hydroxyquinoline

Therapeutic Class: Local anti-infective

CLINICAL PHARMACOLOGY

Mechanism of Action: Increases cell membrane permeability in susceptible organisms by binding sterols; decreases potassium, sodium, and nutrients in cell; inhibits the growth of various mycotic organisms such as Microsporons, Trichophytons, and *Candida albicans* and gram positive cocci such as staphylococci and enterococci

Pharmacokinetics

Some absorbed through the skin, excreted in urine (conjugated form), the rest excreted slowly

INDICATIONS AND USES: Inflamed conditions of the skin such as eczema, athlete's foot, and other fungal infections

DOSAGE

Adult

- Top apply to affected area bid-tid, not for use >1 wk

$ AVAILABLE FORMS/COST OF THERAPY

- Cre—Top: 3%, 30 g: **$2.05-$3.00**

CONTRAINDICATIONS: Hypersensitivity, lesions of the eye, tuberculosis of the skin, most viral skin lesions (including herpes simplex, vaccinia, and varicella), children <2 years of age, diaper rash

PRECAUTIONS: Sensitized skin, deep or puncture wounds, serious burns

PREGNANCY AND LACTATION: Pregnancy category C

SIDE EFFECTS/ADVERSE REACTIONS

SKIN: Rash, urticaria, stinging, burning, dry skin, pruritus, contact dermatitis, erythema, redness, staining of hair and skin

SPECIAL CONSIDERATIONS

PATIENT/FAMILY EDUCATION

- For external use only
- Avoid contact with eyes
- If itching, redness, irritation, stinging, or swelling persists or increases, discontinue use
- May stain fabric, skin, or hair

---

clobetasol

(klo-bet′a-sol)

Temovate

Chemical Class: Synthetic fluorinated agent, very high potency

Therapeutic Class: Topical corticosteroid

CLINICAL PHARMACOLOGY

Mechanism of Action: Depresses formation, release, and activity of endogenous mediators of inflammation such as prostaglandins, kinins, histamine, liposomal enzymes, and the complement system resulting in decreased edema, erythema, and pruritus

Pharmacokinetics

Absorbed through the skin (increased by inflammation and occlusive dressings), metabolized primarily in the liver

INDICATIONS AND USES: Psoriasis, eczema, contact dermatitis, pruritus (usually reserved for severe dermatoses that have not responded to less potent formulation)

DOSAGE

Adult and Child >12 yr

- TOP apply to affected area bid, do not use for >2 wk or exceed total dosage of 50 g

$ AVAILABLE FORMS/COST OF THERAPY

- Cre—Top: 0.05%, 15, 30, 60 g: **$20.45-$51.36**
- Gel—Top: 0.05%, 15, 30, 60 g: **$20.45-$51.36**
- Liq—Top: 0.05%, 25, 50 ml: **$23.40-$45.02**

CONTRAINDICATIONS: Hypersensitivity to corticosteroids, fungal infections, use on face, groin or axilla

PRECAUTIONS: Viral infections, bacterial infections, children, use >2 weeks

PREGNANCY AND LACTATION: Pregnancy category C; unknown whether top application could result in sufficient systemic absorption to produce detectable amounts in breast milk (systemic corticosteroids are secreted into breast milk in quantities not likely to have detrimental effects on infant)

SIDE EFFECTS/ADVERSE REACTIONS

SKIN: Burning, dryness, itching, irritation, acne, folliculitis, hypertrichosis, perioral dermatitis, hypopigmentation, atrophy, striae, miliaria, allergic contact dermatitis, secondary infection

MISC: Systemic absorption of topical corticosteroids has produced reversible HPA axis suppression (more likely with occlusive dressings, prolonged administration, application to large surface areas, liver failure, and in children)

SPECIAL CONSIDERATIONS

PATIENT/FAMILY EDUCATION

- Apply sparingly only to affected area
- Avoid contact with eyes
- Do not put bandages or dressings over treated area unless directed by physician
- Do not use on weeping, denuded, or infected areas
- Discontinue drug, notify physician if local irritation or fever develops

clocortolone

(klo-kort'o-lone)

Cloderm

Chemical Class: Synthetic fluorinated agent, medium potency

Therapeutic Class: Topical corticosteroid

CLINICAL PHARMACOLOGY

Mechanism of Action: Depresses formation, release, and activity of endogenous mediators of inflammation such as prostaglandins, kinins, histamine, liposomal enzymes, and the complement system resulting in decreased edema, erythema, and pruritus

Pharmacokinetics

Absorbed through the skin (increased by inflammation and occlusive dressings), metabolized primarily in the liver

INDICATIONS AND USES: Psoriasis, eczema, contact dermatitis, pruritus

DOSAGE

Adult and Child

- TOP apply to affected area tid or qid

$ **AVAILABLE FORMS/COST OF THERAPY**

- Cre—Top: 0.1%, 15, 45 g: **$12.25-$24.50**

CONTRAINDICATIONS: Hypersensitivity to corticosteroids, fungal infections, use on face, groin, or axilla

PRECAUTIONS: Viral infections, bacterial infections, children

PREGNANCY AND LACTATION: Pregnancy category C; unknown whether topical application could result in sufficient systemic absorption to produce detectable amounts in breast milk (systemic corticosteroids are secreted into breast milk in quantities not likely to have detrimental effects on infant)

SIDE EFFECTS/ADVERSE REACTIONS

SKIN: Burning, dryness, itching, irritation, acne, folliculitis, hypertrichosis, perioral dermatitis, hypopigmentation, atrophy, striae, miliaria, allergic contact dermatitis, secondary infection

MISC: Systemic absorption of topical corticosteroids has produced reversible HPA axis suppression (more likely with occlusive dressings, prolonged administration, application to large surface areas, liver failure, and in children)

SPECIAL CONSIDERATIONS

PATIENT/FAMILY EDUCATION

- Apply sparingly only to affected area
- Avoid contact with eyes
- Do not put bandages or dressings over treated area unless directed by physician
- Do not use on weeping, denuded, or infected areas
- Discontinue drug, notify physician if local irritation or fever develops

---

clofazimine

(kloe-faz'i-meen)

Lamprene

Chemical Class: Iminophenazine dye

Therapeutic Class: Leprostatic

CLINICAL PHARMACOLOGY

Mechanism of Action: Exerts a slow bactericidal effect on *Mycobacterium leprae* (Hansen's bacillus); inhibits mycobacterial growth and binds preferentially to mycobacterial DNA, also exerts antiinflammatory properties in controlling erythema nodosum leprosum reactions; precise mechanisms of action are unknown

Pharmacokinetics

PO: Deposited in fatty tissue and reticuloendothelial system, $t_{1/2}$ 70 days, small amount excreted in feces, sputum, sweat

INDICATIONS AND USES: Lepromatous leprosy (including dapsone-resistant lepromatous leprosy and lepromatous leprosy complicated by erythema nodosum leprosum); combination therapy with other antiinfectives in *Mycobacterium avium-intracellulare* (MAI) infections*

DOSAGE

Adult

- *Dapsone-resistant leprosy:* PO 100 mg qd in combination with 1 or more other antileprosy drugs for 3 yr, followed by monotherapy with 100 mg clofazamine qd
- *Dapsone-sensitive multibacillary leprosy:* PO 50-100 mg qd in combination with 2 or more other antileprosy drugs for 2 yr, followed by single drug therapy with an appropriate agent

• *Erythema nodosum leprosum:* PO 100-200 mg qd for up to 3 mo or longer, then taper dose to 100 mg qd when possible
• *MAI infections:* PO 100 mg qd-tid in combination with other mycobacterial agents

Child

• *Leprosy:* PO 1 mg/kg q24h in combination with dapsone and rifampin

$ AVAILABLE FORMS/COST OF THERAPY

• Cap, Elastic—Oral: 50 mg, 100's: **$13.02;** 100 mg, 100's: **$23.19**

CONTRAINDICATIONS: None known

PRECAUTIONS: Children, abdominal pain, diarrhea, depression

PREGNANCY AND LACTATION: Pregnancy category C; excreted into breast milk, do not administer to nursing mother unless clearly indicated

SIDE EFFECTS/ADVERSE REACTIONS

CNS: Dizziness, drowsiness, fatigue, headache, giddiness, neuralgia, taste disorder, depression (secondary to skin discoloration)

EENT: Conjunctival and corneal pigmentation, dry, burning, itching, irritated eyes

GI: Abdominal/epigastric pain, diarrhea, nausea, vomiting, *GI intolerance,* anorexia, constipation, weight loss, hepatitis, jaundice, eosinophilic enteritis, enlarged liver

HEME: Eosinophilia

METAB: Hypokalemia

SKIN: Pigmentation (pink to brownish black), ichthyosis, dryness, rash, pruritus, phototoxicity, erythroderma, acneiform eruptions, monilial cheilosis

▼ DRUG INTERACTIONS

Labs

• *Increase:* Albuminm, bilirubin, AST

SPECIAL CONSIDERATIONS

PATIENT/FAMILY EDUCATION

• Take with meals
• Compliance with dosage schedule and length of treatment is necessary
• May discolor skin from pink to brownish black, as well as discoloring the conjunctivae, lacrimal fluid, sweat, sputum, urine, and feces; skin discoloration may take several months or years to disappear after discontinuation of therapy

MONITORING PARAMETERS

• Periodic LFTs, potassium

---

clofibrate

(kloe-fye'brate)

Atromid-S, Claripen, ♣ Claripex ♣

Chemical Class: Aryloxisobutyric acid derivative

Therapeutic Class: Antilipemic

CLINICAL PHARMACOLOGY

Mechanism of Action: Acts to lower elevated serum lipids by reducing the very low-density lipoprotein fraction rich in triglycerides; serum cholesterol may be decreased, particularly in those patients whose cholesterol elevation is due to the presence of IDL as a result of Type III hyperlipoproteinemia; the exact mechanism of action has not been established

Pharmacokinetics

PO: Peak 2-6 hr, >90% bound to plasma proteins, $t_{1/2}$ 18-22 hr, metabolized in liver, excreted in urine

INDICATIONS AND USES: Primary dysbetalipoproteinemia (Type III hyperlipidemia); Type IV and V hyperlipidemia (in patients at risk of abdominal pain and pancreatitis)

DOSAGE

Adult

• PO 2 g/d in 4 divided doses

$ AVAILABLE FORMS/COST OF THERAPY

• Cap, Elastic—Oral: 500 mg, 100's: **$13.13-$84.60**

CONTRAINDICATIONS: Severe hepatic disease, severe renal disease, primary biliary cirrhosis

PRECAUTIONS: Peptic ulcer

PREGNANCY AND LACTATION: Pregnancy category C; animal data suggest that the drug is excreted into breast milk, use caution in nursing mothers

SIDE EFFECTS/ADVERSE REACTIONS

CNS: Fatigue, weakness, drowsiness, dizziness, headache

CV: Angina, dysrhythmias, thrombophlebitis

GI: Nausea, vomiting, diarrhea, loose stools, dyspepsia, increased liver enzymes, stomatitis, flatulence, bloating, abdominal distress, hepatomegaly, gastritis, increased cholelithiasis, weight gain

GU: Decreased libido, impotence, dysuria, proteinuria, oliguria, hematuria

HEME: ***Leukopenia,*** anemia, ***eosinophilia,*** bleeding

MS: Myalgias, arthralgias

SKIN: Rash, urticaria, pruritus, dry hair and skin, alopecia

MISC: Polyphagia

▼ DRUG INTERACTIONS

Drugs

• *Antidiabetics:* Enhanced effect of oral hypoglycemic drugs in some patients

• *Furosemide:* Enhanced effects of both drugs in patients with hypoalbuminemia

• *Oral anticoagulants+:* Increased hypoprothrombinemic response to warfarin and possibly other oral anticoagulants; serious bleeding episodes have occurred

Labs

• *Increase:* Liver function studies, CPK, BSP, thymol turbidity

SPECIAL CONSIDERATIONS

No evidence substantiates a beneficial effect from clofibrate on cardiovascular mortality (a 36% increase in incidence of noncardiovascular deaths was reported in one study)

PATIENT/FAMILY EDUCATION

• May be taken with food if GI upset occurs

• Notify physician of chest pain, shortness of breath, irregular heartbeat, severe stomach pain with nausea and vomiting, fever and chills, sore throat, blood in urine, decrease in urination, swelling of lower extremities, weight gain

MONITORING PARAMETERS

• Fasting lipid profile, LFTs, CBC

clomiphene

(kloe'mi-feen)

Clomid, Milophene, Serophene

Chemical Class: Nonsteroidal antiestrogenic

Therapeutic Class: Ovulation stimulant

CLINICAL PHARMACOLOGY

Mechanism of Action: Decreases the number of estrogenic receptors in the cytoplasm, stimulating the secretion of luteinizing hormone (LH), follicle stimulating hormone (FSH), and gonadotropins, which in turn stimulate the maturation and endocrine activity of the ovarian follicle and the subsequent development and function of the corpus luteum

Pharmacokinetics

PO: Metabolized in liver, excreted in feces

INDICATIONS AND USES: Ovulatory failure in patients desiring pregnancy who meet the following conditions: normal liver function, good levels of endogenous estrogen (reduced levels are less favorable but do not preclude successful therapy), and whose partners have adequate sperm; male infertility*

DOSAGE

Adult

- *Ovulatory failure:* PO 50-100 mg qd for 5 days beginning on day 5 of cycle, may be repeated until conception occurs or 3 cycles of therapy have been completed
- *Male infertility:* PO 25 mg qd for 25 days with 5 days rest, or 100 mg every Monday, Wednesday, and Friday

$ AVAILABLE FORMS/COST OF THERAPY

- Tab, Uncoated—Oral: 50 mg, 30's: **$163.29-$217.92**

CONTRAINDICATIONS: Hypersensitivity, hepatic disease, undiagnosed vaginal bleeding

PRECAUTIONS: Hypertension, depression, convulsions, diabetes mellitus, ovarian cyst, polycystic ovary syndrome

PREGNANCY AND LACTATION: Pregnancy category X; each new course of drug should be started only after pregnancy has been excluded

SIDE EFFECTS/ADVERSE REACTIONS

CNS: Nervousness, insomnia, dizziness, lightheadedness

CV: Vasomotor flushing

EENT: Blurred vision, diplopia, photophobia

GI: Nausea, vomiting, constipation, abdominal pain, bloating

GU: Polyuria, frequency, birth defects, spontaneous abortions, multiple ovulation, breast pain, oliguria, abnormal uterine bleeding, abnormal ovarian enlargement

SKIN: Rash, dermatitis, urticaria, alopecia

▼ DRUG INTERACTIONS

Labs

- *Increase:* FSH/LH, BSP, thyroxine, TBG

SPECIAL CONSIDERATIONS

PATIENT/FAMILY EDUCATION

- Multiple births are common after drug is taken
- Notify physician if low abdominal pain occurs (may indicate ovarian cyst, cyst rupture)
- If dose is missed, double at next time, if more than one dose is missed, call physician
- Response usually occurs 4-10 days after last day of treatment
- Record basal body temperature to determine whether ovulation has occurred; if ovulation can be determined (there is a slight decrease in temperature, then a sharp increase for ovulation), attempt coitus 3 days before and qod until after ovulation
- If pregnancy is suspected, notify physician immediately

MONITORING PARAMETERS

- Ovarian size in patients who complain of pelvic pain after receiving clomiphine

clomipramine

(klom-ip'ra-meen)

Anafranil

Chemical Class: Dibenzazepine tricyclic antidepressant

Therapeutic Class: Antiobsessional agent

CLINICAL PHARMACOLOGY

Mechanism of Action: The actual neurochemical mechanism is unknown, but the capacity to inhibit the reuptake of serotonin (5-HT) is thought to be important

Pharmacokinetics

PO: Peak 4.7 hr, extensively bound to tissue and plasma proteins, demethylated in liver, active metabolites excreted in urine; $t_{1/2}$ 32 hr (parent compound), 69 hr (metabolite)

INDICATIONS AND USES: Obsessive-compulsive disorder (OCD), depression,* anxiety disorders*

DOSAGE

Adult

- *OCD:* PO 25 mg hs, increase gradually over 4 wk to a dose of 75-250 mg/d in divided doses, after titration, the entire dose may be given hs
- *Depression:* PO 50-150 mg/d in a single or divided dose
- *Anxiety/Agoraphobia:* PO 25-75 mg/d

Child

- PO 25 mg hs, increase gradually over several wk to 3 mg/kg/d or 100 mg whichever is smaller

$ **AVAILABLE FORMS/COST OF THERAPY**

- Cap, Gel—Oral: 25, 50, 75 mg, 100's: **$78.29-$138.97**

CONTRAINDICATIONS: Hypersensitivity, administration within 14 days of MAOI therapy, acute recovery period following MI

PRECAUTIONS: Seizures, suicidal patients, elderly, cardiac disease

PREGNANCY AND LACTATION: Pregnancy category C; withdrawal symptoms, including jitteriness, tremor, and seizures have been reported in neonates whose mothers had taken clomipramine until delivery; has been found in human milk, use caution in nursing mothers

SIDE EFFECTS/ADVERSE REACTIONS

CNS: Somnolence, tremor, dizziness, headache, insomnia, libido change, nervousness, myoclonus, increased appetite, paresthesia, memory impairment, anxiety, twitching, impaired concentration, depression, hypertonia, sleep disorder, psychosomatic disorder, yawning, confusion, speech disorder, abnormal dreaming, agitation, migraine, depersonalization, irritability, emotional lability, panic reaction

CV: Postural hypotension, palpitations, ***tachycardia,*** syncope, abnormal ECG, ***dysrhythmia, bradycardia, cardiac arrest,*** extrasystoles, pallor

EENT: Abnormal vision, tinnitus

GI: Dry mouth, constipation, nausea, dyspepsia, diarrhea, anorexia, abdominal pain, vomiting, flatulence, tooth disorder, gastrointestinal disorder, dysphagia, esophagitis, ulcerative stomatitis

GU: Ejaculation disorder, impotence, micturition disorder

MS: Myalgia, arthralgia, back pain

RESP: Pharyngitis, rhinitis, sinusitis, coughing, ***bronchospasm***

SKIN: Increased sweating, rash, pruritus, dermatitis, acne, dry skin, urticaria, abnormal skin odor

▼ **DRUG INTERACTIONS**

Drugs

- *Amphetamines:* Theoretical increase in effect of amphetamines, clinical evidence lacking
- *Anticholinergics:* Excessive anticholinergic effects
- *Barbiturates:* Reduced serum concentrations of cyclic antidepressants
- *Bethanidine:* Reduced antihypertensive effect of bethanidine
- *Carbamazepine:* Reduced cyclic antidepressant serum concentrations
- *Clonidine:* Reduced antihypertensive response to clonidine; enhanced hypertensive response with abrupt clonidine withdrawal
- *Debrisoquin:* Inhibited antihypertensive response of debrisoquin
- *Epinephrine+:* Markedly enhanced pressor response to IV epinephrine
- *Ethanol:* Additive impairment of motor skills; abstinent alcoholics may eliminate cyclic antidepres-

sants more rapidly than nonalcoholics

- *Fluoxetine:* Marked increases in cyclic antidepressant plasma concentrations
- *Guanethidine:* Inhibited antihypertensive response to guanethidine
- *MAOIs:* Excessive sympathetic response, mania, or hyperpyrexia possible
- *Moclobemide+:* Potential association with fatal or non-fatal serotonin syndrome
- *Neuroleptics:* Increased therapeutic and toxic effects of both drugs
- *Norepinephrine+:* Markedly enhanced pressor response to norepinephrine
- *Phenylephrine:* Enhanced pressor response to IV phenylephrine
- *Phenytoin:* Altered seizure control; decreased cyclic antidepressant serum concentrations
- *Propoxyphene:* Enhanced effect of cyclic antidepressants
- *Quinidine:* Increased cyclic antidepressant serum concentrations

Labs

- *Increase:* Serum bilirubin, blood glucose, alk phosphatase
- *Decrease:* VMA, 5-HIAA
- *False increase:* Urinary catecholamines

SPECIAL CONSIDERATIONS

PATIENT/FAMILY EDUCATION

- Beneficial effects may take 2-3 wk
- May cause drowsiness, use caution driving or other activities requiring alertness
- Avoid alcohol and other CNS depressants
- Do not discontinue abruptly

clonazepam

(kloe-na'zi-pam)

Klonopin

Chemical Class: Benzodiazepine
Therapeutic Class: Anticonvulsant
DEA Class: Schedule IV

CLINICAL PHARMACOLOGY

Mechanism of Action: Limits the spread of seizure activity, possibly due to benzodiazepine enhancement of the inhibitory neurotransmitter, γ-aminobutyric acid (GABA)

Pharmacokinetics

PO: Peak 1-3 hr, 88% bound to plasma proteins, metabolized by liver (principal metabolite is inactive), excreted in urine, $t_{1/2}$ 18-50 hr

INDICATIONS AND USES: Lennox-Gastaut syndrome (petit mal variant), akinetic and myoclonic seizures, absence seizures (petit mal) in patients who have failed to respond to succinimides, restless legs,* Parkinsonian dysarthria,* multifocal tic disorders,* acute manic episodes of bipolar affective disorder,* deafferentation pain syndromes,* schizophrenia (adjunctive therapy)*

DOSAGE

Adult

- PO 1.5 mg/d in 3 divided doses initially, may be increased 0.5-1 mg q3d until desired response or side effects, max 20 mg/d

Child (<10 yr or <30 kg)

- PO 0.01-0.03 mg/kg/d in 2-3 divided doses, not to exceed 0.05 mg/kg/d, may be increased 0.25-0.5 mg q3d until desired response, not to exceed 0.1-0.2 mg/kg/d

$ AVAILABLE FORMS/COST OF THERAPY

- Tab, Uncoated—Oral: 0.5, 1, 2 mg, 100's: **$69.84-$110.40**

CONTRAINDICATIONS: Hypersensitivity to benzodiazepines, severe liver disease, acute narrow-angle glaucoma

PRECAUTIONS: COPD, impaired renal function, abrupt discontinuation (may precipitate withdrawal), status epilepticus, elderly

PREGNANCY AND LACTATION: Pregnancy category C; episodes of prolonged apnea in the newborn, apparently related to clonazepam, have been reported; excreted into breast milk, monitor closely for CNS depression or apnea in nursing infant

SIDE EFFECTS/ADVERSE REACTIONS

CNS: ***Drowsiness,*** dizziness, confusion, behavioral changes, tremors, insomnia, headache, suicidal tendencies, slurred speech, ataxia

CV: Palpitations, bradycardia, hypotension

EENT: Nystagmus, diplopia, abnormal eye movements, blurred vision

GI: Nausea, constipation, polyphagia, anorexia, xerostomia, diarrhea, gastritis, sore gums

GU: Dysuria, enuresis, nocturia, retention

HEME: ***Thrombocytopenia, leukocytosis, eosinophilia,*** anemia

RESP: ***Respiratory depression,*** dyspnea, congestion

SKIN: Rash

▼ **DRUG INTERACTIONS**

Drugs

- *Cimetidine:* Increased plasma levels of clonazepam
- *Clozapine:* Isolated cases of cardiorespiratory collapse have been reported; causal relationship to benzodiazepines has not been established
- *Disulfiram:* Increased serum clonazepam concentrations
- *Ethanol:* Enhanced adverse psychomotor side effects of benzodiazepines
- *Rifampin:* Reduced serum clonazepam concentrations

Labs

- *Increase:* AST, alk phosphatase

SPECIAL CONSIDERATIONS

Up to 30% of patients have shown a loss of anticonvulsant activity, often within three mo of administration, dosage adjustment may reestablish efficacy

PATIENT/FAMILY EDUCATION

- Do not take more than prescribed amount, may be habit-forming
- Avoid OTC preparations unless approved by physician
- Avoid driving, activities that require alertness, drowsiness may occur
- Avoid alcohol ingestion or other CNS depressants unless prescribed by physician
- Do not discontinue medication abruptly after long-term use

MONITORING PARAMETERS

- Although relationship between serum concentrations and seizure control is not well established, proposed therapeutic concentrations are 20-80 ng/ml, potentially toxic concentrations >80 ng/ml
- Close attention to seizure frequency is important in order to detect the emergence of tolerance

clonidine

(klon′i-deen)

Catapres, Catapres-TTS, Dixarit 🍁

Chemical Class: Imidazoline derivative

Therapeutic Class: Antihypertensive

CLINICAL PHARMACOLOGY

Mechanism of Action: Stimulates α_2-adrenergic receptors in the brain stem, resulting in reduced sympathetic outflow from the CNS and a decrease in peripheral resistance

Pharmacokinetics

PO: Peak 3-5 hr

TOP: Therapeutic plasma levels 2-3 days after initial application, drug released at constant rate for approximately 7 days, following removal plasma levels persist for 8 hr then decline slowly over several days Metabolized in liver, excreted in urine (50% unchanged), $t_{1/2}$ 12-16 hr

INDICATIONS AND USES: Hypertension, alcohol withdrawal,* diabetic diarrhea,* Gilles de la Tourette syndrome,* hypertensive urgencies,* menopausal flushing,* opiate detoxification,* postherpetic neuralgia,* smoking cessation,* ulcerative colitis*

DOSAGE

Adult

• PO 0.1 mg bid initially, increase 0.1-0.2 mg/d if needed, max 2.4 mg/d (minimize sedation by giving majority of daily dose hs); TOP apply patch to hairless area of intact skin on upper arm or torso once q7d, rotate sites, start with TTS-1 (0.1 mg/24 hr) and increase after 1-2 wk if needed (using >2 TTS-3 systems usually does not improve efficacy)

Child

• PO 5-25 µg/kg/d in divided doses q6h, increase at 5-7 day intervals

$ AVAILABLE FORMS/COST OF THERAPY

• Tab, Uncoated—Oral: 0.1, 0.2, 0.3 mg, 100's: **$2.03-$107.76**

• Film, Cont Rel—Percutaneous: 2.5 mg/unit (TTS-1), 3 × 4: **$90.11;** 5 mg/unit (TTS-2), 3 × 4: **$152.15;** 7.5 mg/unit (TTS-3), 4's: **$70.14**

CONTRAINDICATIONS: Hypersensitivity to clonidine or any component of adhesive layer of transdermal system

PRECAUTIONS: Severe coronary insufficiency, recent MI, cerebrovascular disease, chronic renal failure, abrupt discontinuation (PO)

PREGNANCY AND LACTATION: Pregnancy category C; secreted into breast milk, hypotension has not been observed in nursing infants, although clonidine was found in the serum of the infants

SIDE EFFECTS/ADVERSE REACTIONS

Less severe with transdermal systems

CNS: Constipation, drowsiness, dizziness, sedation, dreams or nightmares, insomnia, hallucinations, delirium, nervousness, agitation, restlessness, anxiety, depression, headache

CV: CHF, orthostatic hypotension, palpitations, tachycardia and bradycardia, Raynaud's phenomenon, ECG abnormalities, conduction disturbances, dysrhythmias

GI: Dry mouth, constipation, anorexia, nausea, vomiting, parotid pain, mild transient abnormalities in LFTs

GU: Impotence, loss of libido, nocturia, difficulty urinating, urinary retention

METAB: Weight gain, transient elevation of blood glucose, gynecomastia

MS: Weakness, fatigue, muscle or joint pain, cramps of the lower limbs

SKIN: Rash, angioneurotic edema, hives, urticaria, hair thinning and alopecia, pruritus, transient localized skin reactions (TOP)

▼ DRUG INTERACTIONS

Drugs

• *Antidepressants:* Cyclic antidepressants may inhibit the antihypertensive response to clonidine

• *Beta blockers:* Rebound hypertension from clonidine withdrawal exacerbated by noncardioselective beta blockers

• *Piribedil:* Inhibited antiparkinsonian effect of piribedil

Labs

• *Increase:* Blood glucose

• *Decrease:* VMA, catecholamines, aldosterone

SPECIAL CONSIDERATIONS

PATIENT/FAMILY EDUCATION

• Avoid hazardous activities, since drug may cause drowsiness

• Do not discontinue oral drug abruptly, or withdrawal symptoms may occur (anxiety, increased B/P, headache, insomnia, increased pulse, tremors, nausea, sweating)

• Do not use OTC (cough, cold, or allergy) products unless directed by physician

• Rise slowly to sitting or standing position to minimize orthostatic hypotension, especially elderly

• May cause dizziness, fainting, light-headedness may occur during 1st few days of therapy

• May cause dry mouth: use hard candy, saliva product, or frequent rinsing of mouth

• Response may take 2-3 days if drug is given transdermally

• Apply patch to hairless area of intact skin on upper arm or torso, rotate sites

clorazepate

(klor-az'e-pate)

Gen-Xene, Novoclopate, ♣ Tranxene, Tranxene-SD, Tranxene-SD Half Strength

Chemical Class: Benzodiazepine

Therapeutic Class: Antianxiety agent, anticonvulsant

DEA Class: Schedule IV

CLINICAL PHARMACOLOGY

Mechanism of Action: Potentiates the effects of γ-aminobutyric acid (GABA) and other inhibitory transmitters by binding to specific benzodiazepine receptor sites

Pharmacokinetics

PO: Onset 15 min, peak 1-2 hr, duration 4-6 hr, metabolized by liver to active metabolites, excreted by kidneys, $t_{1/2}$ 30-100 hr

INDICATIONS AND USES: Anxiety disorders, acute alcohol withdrawal, partial seizures (adjunctive therapy)

DOSAGE

Adult

• *Anxiety:* PO 7.5-15 mg bid-qid, or as single qhs dose of 15-22.5 mg, lower doses may be indicated for elderly or debilitated patients

• *Alcohol withdrawal:* PO 30 mg initially, then 15 mg bid-qid on first day, gradually decrease dose over subsequent days

• *Seizure disorders:* PO 7.5 mg tid; may increase by 7.5 mg/wk or less, not to exceed 90 mg/d

Child 9-12 yr

• *Seizure disorders:* PO 3.75-7.5 mg bid, increase by 3.75 mg at weekly intervals, max 60 mg/d in 2-3 divided doses

$ **AVAILABLE FORMS/COST OF THERAPY**

• Tab, Uncoated—Oral: 3.75, 7.5, 15 mg, 100's: **$3.57-$188.63**

• Tab, Uncoated, Sus Action—Oral: 11.25 mg, 100's: **$295.74;** 22.5 mg, 100's: **$378.74**

CONTRAINDICATIONS: Hypersensitivity to benzodiazepines, narrow-angle glaucoma, psychosis

PRECAUTIONS: Elderly, debilitated, hepatic disease, renal disease, long-term use, history of drug abuse

PREGNANCY AND LACTATION: Pregnancy category D; excreted into breast milk, drug and metabolites may accumulate to toxic levels in nursing infant

SIDE EFFECTS/ADVERSE REACTIONS

CNS: Dizziness, *drowsiness, confusion,* headache, anxiety, tremors, stimulation, fatigue, depression, insomnia, hallucinations, anterograde amnesia, slurred speech, ataxia, hysteria, psychosis

CV: Orthostatic hypotension, tachycardia, bradycardia, hypertension, hypotension, ***cardiovascular collapse***

EENT: Blurred vision, mydriasis, nystagmus, auditory disturbances

GI: Constipation, dry mouth, nausea, vomiting, anorexia, diarrhea

GU: Incontinence, changes in libido, urinary retention, menstrual irregularities

SKIN: Rash, dermatitis, itching, urticaria, hair loss, hirsutism

▼ DRUG INTERACTIONS

Drugs

- *Cimetidine:* Increased plasma levels of clorazepate and/or active metabolites
- *Clozapine:* Isolated cases of cardiorespiratory collapse have been reported; causal relationship to benzodiazepines has not been established
- *Disulfiram:* Increased serum clorazepate concentrations
- *Ethanol:* Enhanced adverse psychomotor side effects of benzodiazepines
- *Rifampin:* Reduced serum clorazepate concentrations

SPECIAL CONSIDERATIONS

PATIENT/FAMILY EDUCATION

- Do not use for everyday stress or for longer than 4 mo, unless directed by physician
- Do not take more than prescribed amount, may be habit-forming
- Avoid OTC preparations unless approved by physician
- Avoid driving, activities that require alertness, drowsiness may occur
- Avoid alcohol ingestion or other CNS depressants unless prescribed by physician
- Do not discontinue medication abruptly after long-term use

---

clotrimazole

(kloe-trim′a-zole)

Mycelex Troches, Lotrimin, Lotrimin AF, Mycelex, Mycelex OTC, Canesten, ✦ FemCare, Gyne-Lotrimin, Mycelex-G, Mycelex-7, Mycelex Twin Pack

Chemical Class: Imidazole derivative

Therapeutic Class: Local antifungal

CLINICAL PHARMACOLOGY

Mechanism of Action: Broad-spectrum antifungal agent that inhibits growth of pathogenic dermatophytes, yeasts, and *Malassezia furfur;* exhibits fungistatic and fungicidal activity against isolates of *Trichophyton rubrum, T. mentagrophytes, Epidermophyton floccosum, Microsporum canis,* and *Candida* sp., including *C. albicans;* interferes with fungal DNA replication by binding sterols in fungal cell membrane, which increases permeability and causes leaking of cell nutrients

Pharmacokinetics Well absorbed following oral administration, eliminated mainly as inactive metabolites, minimally absorbed following topical and vaginal administration

INDICATIONS AND USES: Tinea pedis, tinea cruris, tinea corporis, tinea versicolor; *C. albicans* infection of the vagina, vulva, throat, mouth

DOSAGE

Adult and Child >3 yr

• PO 10 mg troche dissolved slowly 5 times/d; TOP apply bid

Adult and Child >12 yr

• VAG 100 mg qhs for 7 days or 200 mg qhs for 3 days or 500 mg × 1 or 5 g (1 applicatorful) of 1% VAG cream qhs for 7-14 days

$ AVAILABLE FORMS/COST OF THERAPY

• Cre—Top: 1%, 15, 30, 45 g: **$7.85-$22.80**

• Cre—Vag: 1%, 45, 90 g: **$14.00-$24.44**

• Sol—Top: 1%, 10, 30 ml: **$7.82-$20.28**

• Lotion—Top: 1%, 30 ml: **$21.23**

• Tab, Uncoated, Sust Action—Vag: 100 mg, 7's: **$14.71;** 500 mg, 1's: **$12.71**

• Troche—Buccal: 10 mg, 70's: **$52.59**

CONTRAINDICATIONS: Hypersensitivity

PREGNANCY AND LACTATION: Pregnancy category B; excretion in breast milk unknown

SIDE EFFECTS/ADVERSE REACTIONS

GI: Abdominal cramps, bloating

GU: Urinary frequency, dyspareunia

SKIN: Rash, urticaria, stinging, burning, peeling, blistering, skin fissures

SPECIAL CONSIDERATIONS

PATIENT/FAMILY EDUCATION

• Use medication for the full treatment time even though symptoms may have improved

• Notify physician if there is no improvement after 4 wk of treatment

• Inform physician if the area of application shows signs of increased irritation (redness, itching, burning, blistering, oozing) indicative of possible sensitization

• Avoid sources of infection or reinfection

• Abstain from sexual intercourse during vaginal/vulvular treatment

• Use vaginal preparations continuously even during menstrual period

cloxacillin

(klox-a-sill'in)

Cloxapen, Novocloxin, ♣ Nuclox, ♣ Tegopen

Chemical Class: Isoxazolyl penicillin

Therapeutic Class: Penicillinase-resistant antibiotic

CLINICAL PHARMACOLOGY

Mechanism of Action: Inhibits the biosynthesis of cell wall mucopeptide in susceptible organisms; the cell wall, rendered osmotically unstable, swells and bursts from osmotic pressure; highly resistant to inactivation by staphylococcal penicillinase and active against penicillinase producing and non-penicillinase producing strains of *Staphylococcus aureus* (except methicillin resistant strains)

Pharmacokinetics

PO: Peak 1 hr, duration 6 hr, $t_{1/2}$ 30-60 min, metabolized in liver, excreted in urine and bile

INDICATIONS AND USES: Infections of the respiratory tract, skin and skin structure, bones and joints. Antibacterial spectrum usually includes:

• Gram-positive organisms: most gram-positive aerobic cocci, *Staphylococcus aureus, S. epidermidis* (except methicillin resistant strains)

• Gram-negative organisms: Most gram-negative aerobic cocci

DOSAGE

Adult

• PO 250-500 mg q6h

Child

• PO 50-100 mg/kg/d in divided doses q6h, max 4 g/d

AVAILABLE FORMS/COST OF THERAPY

• Cap, Gel—Oral: 250, 500 mg, 100's: **$20.95-$150.69**

• Powder, Reconst—Oral: 125 mg/5 ml, 100, 200 ml: **$3.25-$11.04**

CONTRAINDICATIONS: Hypersensitivity to penicillins

PRECAUTIONS: Hypersensitivity to cephalosporins, prolonged or repeated therapy

PREGNANCY AND LACTATION: Pregnancy category B; potential exists for modification of bowel flora in nursing infant, allergy/sensitization and interference with interpretation of culture results if fever workup required

SIDE EFFECTS/ADVERSE REACTIONS

CNS: Headache, fever, hallucinations, anxiety, depression, twitching

GI: Nausea, vomiting, diarrhea, increased AST/ALT, abdominal pain, glossitis, colitis

GU: Hematuria, vaginitis

HEME: Anemia, increased bleeding time, ***bone marrow depression, granulocytopenia, leukopenia, eosinophilia***

RESP: ***Anaphylaxis, respiratory distress***

SKIN: Urticaria, rash

▼ DRUG INTERACTIONS

Drugs

• *Chloramphenicol:* Potential inhibition of the antibacterial activity of penicillins

• *Methotrexate:* Increased methotrexate concentrations, toxicity

• *Oral anticoagulants:* Decreased hypoprothrombinemic response to warfarin or other anticoagulants

• *Tetracyclines:* Impaired efficacy of penicillin therapy

Labs

• *False positive:* Urine glucose, urine protein

• *Decreased:* Uric acid

SPECIAL CONSIDERATIONS

PATIENT/FAMILY EDUCATION

• Complete entire course of medication

• Administer on an empty stomach (1 hr before or 2 hr after meals)

• Administer at even intervals

• Report sore throat, fever, fatigue, excessive diarrhea, skin rash, itching, hives, shortness of breath, wheezing

• Shake oral suspensions well before administering, discard after 14 days

MONITORING PARAMETERS

• BUN, serum creatinine, urinalysis, LFTs

• Additional information: sodium content of 250 mg cap = 0.6 mEq; sodium content of 125 mg susp = 0.24 mEq

clozapine

(klo'za-peen)

Clozaril

Chemical Class: Tricyclic dibenzodiazepine derivative

Therapeutic Class: Antipsychotic

CLINICAL PHARMACOLOGY

Mechanism of Action: Interferes with the binding of dopamine at both D_{-1} and D_{-2} receptors, but is preferentially more active at limbic than at striatal dopamine receptors, which may explain the relative freedom from extrapyramidal side effects; also acts as an antagonist at adrenergic, cholinergic, histaminergic, and serotonergic receptors

Pharmacokinetics

PO: Peak 2.5 hr, 95% protein bound, completely metabolized by the liver, excreted in urine and feces (metabolites), $t_{1/2}$ 8-12 hr

INDICATIONS AND USES: Severely ill schizophrenic patients who fail to respond adequately to standard antipsychotic drug treatment

DOSAGE

Adult

• PO 12.5 mg qd-bid initially, increase by 25-50 mg/d to achieve a target range of 300-450 mg/d after 2 wk; increase prn by no more than 100 mg in 2 wk intervals, do not exceed 900 mg/d; use lowest dose to control symptoms

$ AVAILABLE FORMS/COST OF THERAPY

• Tab, Uncoated—Oral: 25 mg, 100's: **$132.00;** 100 mg, 100's: **$342.00**

CONTRAINDICATIONS: Myeloproliferative disorders, uncontrolled epilepsy, history of clozapine-induced agranulocytosis or severe granulocytopenia, severe CNS depression, comatose states, hypersensitivity, narrow-angle glaucoma

PRECAUTIONS: Cardiovascular disease, pulmonary disease, elderly, prostatic enlargement, hepatic disease, renal disease, general anesthesia, seizures

PREGNANCY AND LACTATION: Pregnancy category B; may be excreted in breast milk, avoid breastfeeding during clozapine therapy

SIDE EFFECTS/ADVERSE REACTIONS

CNS: Drowsiness/sedation, dizziness/vertigo, headache, tremor, syncope, disturbed sleep/nightmares, restlessness, hypokinesia/akinesia, agitation, seizures, rigidity, akathisia, confusion, fatigue, insomnia, hyperkinesia, weakness, lethargy, ataxia, slurred speech, depression, epileptiform movements/myoclonic jerks, anxiety

CV: Tachycardia, hypotension, hypertension, chest pain/angina, ECG change/cardiac abnormality

EENT: Blurred vision

GI: Constipation, nausea, abdominal discomfort/heartburn, nausea, vomiting, diarrhea, liver test abnormality, anorexia, dry mouth, *salivation*

GU: Urinary abnormalities, incontinence, abnormal ejaculation, urinary urgency/frequency, urinary retention

HEME: ***Neutropenia, leukopenia, agranulocytosis, eosinophilia***

SKIN: Rash

MISC: Fever, weight gain

▼ DRUG INTERACTIONS

Drugs

• *Benzodiazepines:* Isolated cases of cardiorespiratory collapse have been reported

• *Carbamazepine:* Considerable reduction in plasma clozapine concentrations

• *Cimetidine:* Increased serum clozapine concentrations

• *Erythromycin:* Increased serum clozapine concentrations

• *Fluvoxamine:* Marked increase in plasma clozapine concentrations

Labs

• *Increase:* Liver function tests, cardiac enzymes, cholesterol, blood glucose, bilirubin, PBI, cholinesterase, ^{131}I

• *False positive:* Pregnancy tests, PKU

• *False negative:* Urinary steroids, 17-OHCS

SPECIAL CONSIDERATIONS

The risk of agranulocytosis and seizures limits use to patients who have failed to respond or were unable to tolerate treatment with appropriate courses of standard antipsychotics

PATIENT/FAMILY EDUCATION

• Rise from sitting or lying position gradually

• Avoid hot tubs, hot showers, or tub baths, hypotension may occur
• Avoid abrupt withdrawal of this drug
• Avoid OTC preparations (cough, hay fever, cold) unless approved by physician
• Avoid use with alcohol or CNS depressants
• Compliance with drug regimen and blood monitoring are essential
• Report sore throat, malaise, fever, bleeding, mouth sores
• Take extra precautions to stay cool in hot weather
• Avoid driving or other hazardous activities

MONITORING PARAMETERS

• WBC at baseline and then qwk for the duration of treatment and for 4 wk after discontinuation
• Blood pressure, LFTs

co-trimoxazole (sulfamethoxazole and trimethoprim)

(koe-trye-mox′a-zole)

Apo-sulfatrim, ♣ Bactrim, Bactrim DS, Cotrim, Cotrim DS, Comoxol, Septra, Septra DS, Sulfatrim, Sulfatrim DS, Bethaprim, Uroplus SS, Uroplus DS, Sulfamethoprim

Chemical Class: Sulfonamide derivative; dihydrofolate reductase inhibitor
Therapeutic Class: Antibiotic

CLINICAL PHARMACOLOGY

Mechanism of Action: Sulfamethoxazole (SMX) inhibits bacterial synthesis of dihydrofolic acid by competing with paraaminobenzoic acid; trimethoprim (TMP) blocks the production of tetrahydrofolic acid by inhibiting the enzyme dihydrofolate reductase; the combination blocks two consecutive steps in the bacterial biosynthesis of essential nucleic acids and proteins

Pharmacokinetics

PO: Rapidly absorbed, peak 1-4 hr, $t_{1/2}$ (SMX) 10-12 hr (TMP) 8-11 hr, excreted in urine (metabolites and unchanged), 70% (SMX) 44% (TMP) bound to plasma proteins

INDICATIONS AND USES: Infections of the urinary tract; otitis media; acute exacerbation of chronic bronchitis; enteritis; *Pneumocystis carinii* pneumonia (treatment and prophylaxis); traveler's diarrhea; cholera,* salmonella-type infections,* nocardiosis,* prostatitis.* Antibacterial spectrum usually includes:

• Gram-positive organisms: *Streptococcus pneumoniae, Staphylococcus aureus,* group A β-hemolytic streptococci (some strains may not respond to co-trimoxazole in tonsillopharyngeal infections), *Nocardia*
• Gram-negative organisms: *Acinetobacter, Enterobacter, Escherichia coli, Klebsiella pneumoniae, Proteus mirabilis, Salmonella, Shigella, Haemophilus influenzae, H. ducreyi, Neisseria gonorrhoeae,* indole-positive *Proteus* (70% of isolates), *Providencia* and *Serratia* (50% of isolates)
• Protozoa: *Pneumocystis carinii*

DOSAGE

Adult

• *UTIs, shigellosis, acute exacerbations of chronic bronchitis, acute otitis media:* PO 160 mg TMP/800 mg SMX q12h for 10-14 days (3 days for uncomplicated cystitis in otherwise healthy females, 5 days for shigellosis); IV 8-10 mg TMP/kg/d in 2-4 divided doses q6,8, or 12h for up to 14 days (5 days for shigellosis)

• *Traveler's diarrhea:* PO 160 mg TMP/800 mg SMX q12h for 5 days
• *Pneumocystis carinii* pneumonitis: PO 20 mg TMP/kg/d divided q6h for 14 days; IV 15-20 mg TMP/kg/d divided q6-8h for 14 days
• *Pneumocystic carinii* pneumonia prophylaxis: PO 160 mg TMP/800 mg SMX qd or 3× week
• Dosage adjustment for impaired renal function: CrCl >30 ml/min, usual regimen; CrCl 15-30 ml/min, ½ usual regimen; CrCl <15 ml/min, not recommended

Child >2 months

• *UTIs, shigellosis, and acute otitis media:* PO 8 mg TMP/kg/d divided q12h (1 ml/kg susp divided q12h)
• *Pneumocystis carinii* pneumonitis: PO/IV 15-20 mg TMP/kg/d divided q6h for 14 days

$ AVAILABLE FORMS/COST OF THERAPY

• Inj, Conc-Sol—IV: 80 mg TMP/400 mg SMX/5 ml, 5 ml × 10: **$26.76-$74.05**
• Susp—Oral: 200 mg SMX/40 mg TMP/5 ml, 100, 480 ml: **$3.76-$42.33**
• Tab, Uncoated—Oral: 400 mg SMX/80 mg TMP, 100's: **$7.43-$72.59;** 800 mg SMX/160 mg TMP, 100's: **$8.93-$114.89**

CONTRAINDICATIONS: Hypersensitivity to TMP or SMX, megaloblastic anemia due to folate deficiency, infants <2 mo

PRECAUTIONS: Streptococcal pharyngitis, elderly patients receiving diuretics, renal and hepatic function impairment, possible folate deficiency (elderly, chronic alcoholics, anticonvulsant therapy, malabsorption syndrome, malnutrition), G-6-PD deficiency

PREGNANCY AND LACTATION: Pregnancy category C; **Do not use at term,** may cause kernicterus in the neonate; not recommended in the nursing period because sulfonamides excreted in breast milk may cause kernicterus

SIDE EFFECTS/ADVERSE REACTIONS

CNS: Headache, insomnia, hallucinations, depression, vertigo, fatigue, anxiety, ***convulsions,*** drug fever, chills, aseptic meningitis, ataxia

GI: Nausea, vomiting, abdominal pain, stomatitis, ***hepatitis,*** glossitis, pancreatitis, diarrhea, ***pseudomembranous enterocolitis,*** anorexia

GU: ***Renal failure, toxic nephrosis,*** increased BUN and creatinine, crystalluria

HEME: ***Leukopenia, neutropenia, thrombocytopenia, agranulocytosis, hemolytic anemia, hypoprothrombinemia, methemoglobinemia, eosinophilia***

SKIN: Rash, dermatitis, urticaria, ***Stevens-Johnson syndrome,*** erythema, *photosensitivity,* pain and inflammation at inj site

RESP: Cough, shortness of breath

▼ DRUG INTERACTIONS

Drugs

• *Cyclosporine:* Sulfonamides may produce additive nephrotoxicity with cyclosporine; reduced plasma concentrations of cyclosporine
• *Methotrexate:* Elevated methotrexate concentrations and toxicity
• *Oral anticoagulants+:* Enhanced hypoprothrombinemic response to warfarin and possibly other oral anticoagulants

Labs

• *Increase:* Alk phosphatase, creatinine (due to interference with assay), bilirubin
• *False positive:* Urinary glucose test

SPECIAL CONSIDERATIONS

PATIENT/FAMILY EDUCATION

• Complete full course of therapy
• Take each dose with a full glass of water
• Maintain adequate fluid intake

* = non-FDA-approved use + = major clinical significance

- Notify physician of skin rash, sore throat, mouth sores, fever, or unusual bruising or bleeding
- Avoid sunlight or use sunscreen to prevent burns

MONITORING PARAMETERS

- Baseline and periodic CBC for patients on long-term or high-dose therapy

---

codeine

(koe'deen)

Chemical Class: Opiate, phenanthrene derivative
Therapeutic Class: Narcotic analgesic; antitussive
DEA Class: Schedule II

CLINICAL PHARMACOLOGY

Mechanism of Action: Binds to opiate receptors in the CNS causing inhibition of ascending pain pathways, altering the perception of and response to pain; suppresses cough by direct central action in the medulla

Pharmacokinetics

IM: Onset 10-30 min, peak 30-60 min

PO: Onset 30-60 min, peak 60-90 min

Metabolized in liver to morphine, excreted in urine (unchanged and metabolites), $t_{1/2}$ 2½-3½ hr

INDICATIONS AND USES: Mild to moderate pain, antitussive

DOSAGE

Adult

- *Analgesia:* PO/IM/SC 15-60 mg q4h prn
- *Antitussive:* PO 10-20 mg q4-6h, not to exceed 120 mg/d

Child

- *Analgesia:* PO/IM/SC 0.5-1 mg/kg/dose q4-6h prn, max 60 mg/dose
- *Antitussive:* PO 1-1.5 mg/kg/d in divided doses q4-6h prn, max 60 mg/dose

$ **AVAILABLE FORMS/COST OF THERAPY**

- Inj, Sol—IM; SC: 15 mg/ml, 2 ml × 10: **$8.21-$12.80;** 30, 60 mg/ml, 1 ml × 10: **$8.24-$12.89**
- Sol—Oral: 15 mg/5ml, 500 ml: **$30.08**
- Tab, Hypodermic—IM: 30 mg, 100's: **$50.34;** 60 mg, 100's: **$96.20**
- Tab, Uncoated—Oral: 15, 30, 60 mg, 100's: **$21.35-$87.78**

CONTRAINDICATIONS: Hypersensitivity

PRECAUTIONS: Head injury, increased intracranial pressure, acute abdominal conditions, elderly, severe impairment of hepatic or renal function, hypothyroidism, Addison's disease, prostatic hypertrophy, urethral stricture, history of drug abuse

PREGNANCY AND LACTATION: Pregnancy category C (category D if used for prolonged periods or in high doses at term); use during labor produces neonatal respiratory depression; passes into breast milk in very small amounts, compatible with breast feeding

SIDE EFFECTS/ADVERSE REACTIONS

CNS: Drowsiness, sedation, dizziness, agitation, dependency, lethargy, restlessness

CV: Bradycardia, palpitations, orthostatic hypotension, tachycardia

GI: Nausea, vomiting, anorexia, constipation

GU: Urinary retention

RESP: ***Respiratory depression, respiratory paralysis***

SKIN: Flushing, rash, urticaria

▼ **DRUG INTERACTIONS**

Drugs

- *Barbiturates:* Additive CNS depression
- *Cimetidine:* Increased effect of narcotic analgesics
- *Ethanol:* Additive CNS effects

• *Neuroleptics:* Hypotension and excessive CNS depression

SPECIAL CONSIDERATIONS

PATIENT/FAMILY EDUCATION

• Report any symptoms of CNS changes, allergic reactions
• Physical dependency may result when used for extended periods
• Change position slowly, orthostatic hypotension may occur
• Avoid hazardous activities if drowsiness or dizziness occurs
• Avoid alcohol, other CNS depressants unless directed by physician
• Minimize nausea by administering with food and remain lying down following dose

---

colchicine

(kol'chi-seen)

Colchicine, Colsalide improved

Chemical Class: Colchicum autumnale alkaloid

Therapeutic Class: Antigout agent

CLINICAL PHARMACOLOGY

Mechanism of Action: Inhibits microtubule formation in leukocytes, decreasing joint inflammation; has no direct analgesic effect

Pharmacokinetics

PO: Peak ½-2 hr, $t_{1/2}$ 20 min; deacetylated in liver; excreted in feces

INDICATIONS AND USES: Gouty arthritis (prevention, treatment), pseudogout,* Behçet's syndrome,* familial Mediterranean fever,* alcoholic cirrhosis*

DOSAGE

Adult

• *Prevention of gouty arthritis:* PO 0.5-1.8 mg qd depending on severity; IV 0.5-1 mg qd-bid
• *Treatment of gouty arthritis:* PO 0.5-1.2 mg, then 0.5-1.2 mg q1h, until pain decreases or side effects occur; IV 2 mg over 2-5 min, then 0.5 mg q6h, not to exceed 4 mg/24 hr; no colchicine should be given by any route for at least 7 days after a full course of IV therapy (4 mg)

$ AVAILABLE FORMS/COST OF THERAPY

• Inj, Sol—IV: 1 mg/2 ml, 2 ml × 6: **$19.55**
• Tab, Uncoated—Oral: 0.5, 0.6, 1 mg, 100's: **$3.80-$25.06**

CONTRAINDICATIONS: Hypersensitivity; serious GI, renal, hepatic, cardiac disorders; blood dyscrasias

PRECAUTIONS: Elderly, lactation, children; may induce ileal vitamin B_{12} malabsorption, extravasation may lead to shock

PREGNANCY AND LACTATION: Pregnancy category D (known teratogen)

SIDE EFFECTS/ADVERSE REACTIONS

CNS: Peripheral neuritis

GI: Nausea, vomiting, anorexia, malaise, diarrhea, metallic taste, cramps, peptic ulcer

GU: Hematuria, oliguria, azotemia, reversible azoospermia

HEME: ***Agranulocytosis, thrombocytopenia, aplastic anemia, pancytopenia***

MS: Myopathy (more common in persons with renal impairment)

SKIN: Dermatitis, pruritus, purpura, erythema, alopecia

▼ DRUG INTERACTIONS

Drugs

• *Cyclosporine:* Increased serum level of cyclosporine

Labs

• *Increase:* Alk phosphatase, AST/ALT
• *False positive:* Urine test for hemoglobin or RBCs; urinary 17-OHCS

SPECIAL CONSIDERATIONS

PATIENT/FAMILY EDUCATION

• Increase fluids to 3-4 L/day

• Avoid alcohol
• Take oral dose on empty stomach only

MONITORING PARAMETERS
• CBC, platelets, reticulocytes before and during therapy (q3mo)

colestipol
(koe-les'ti-pole)
Colestid
Chemical Class: Bile acid sequestrant
Therapeutic Class: Antihyperlipidemic

CLINICAL PHARMACOLOGY
Mechanism of Action: Combines with bile acids to form insoluble complex that is excreted through feces; increased fecal loss of bile acids leads to increased oxidation of cholesterol to bile acids, increased hepatic uptake of LDLs, and decreased serum LDL levels; serum triglyceride levels may increase or remain unchanged
Pharmacokinetics
PO: Not absorbed; excreted in feces
INDICATIONS AND USES: Primary hypercholesterolemia, xanthomas, pruritus due to biliary obstruction,* diarrhea due to bile acids*
DOSAGE
Adult
• PO 5-30 g qd in 2-4 divided doses, ac and hs; increase dose by 5 g at 1-2 mo intervals

$ **AVAILABLE FORMS/COST OF THERAPY**
• Granule—Oral: 5 g, 90's: **$105.00**
• Packet—Oral: 7.5 g, 60's: **$69.99**
• Tab, Uncoated—Oral: 1 g, 120's: **$34.40**

CONTRAINDICATIONS: Hypersensitivity, biliary obstruction
PRECAUTIONS: Lactation; children; bleeding disorders; may prevent absorption of fat-soluble vitamins such as A, D, E, and K; prolonged use may lead to the development of hyperchloremic acidosis; give all other medications 1 hr before colestipol or 4 hr after colestipol to avoid poor absorption
PREGNANCY AND LACTATION: Pregnancy category B
SIDE EFFECTS/ADVERSE REACTIONS
CNS: Headache, dizziness
GI: Constipation, abdominal pain, nausea, fecal impaction, hemorrhoids, flatulence, vomiting, steatorrhea, peptic ulcer
HEME: Bleeding
METAB: Decreased vitamin A, D, E, K absorption, hyperchloremic acidosis
SKIN: Rash; irritation of perianal area, tongue, skin

▼ **DRUG INTERACTIONS**
Drugs
• *Acetaminophen, digitoxin, digoxin, gemfibrozil, methotrexate, thiazides, thyroxine, triiodothyronine, warfarin:* Colestipol decreases absorption of these drugs
Labs
• *Increase:* Liver function studies, chloride, PO_4

SPECIAL CONSIDERATIONS
PATIENT/FAMILY EDUCATION
• Do not take colestipol in its dry form; it may be mixed with beverages, cereals, soups, and fruits

MONITORING PARAMETERS
• The decline in serum cholesterol levels usually occurs after one mo of treatment

colfosceril

(kohl-foss'sir-ill)
Exosurf Neonatal
Chemical Class: Phospholipid
Therapeutic Class: Synthetic lung surfactant

CLINICAL PHARMACOLOGY
Mechanism of Action: Maintains lung inflation by lowering surface tension. Each 10 ml vial contains 108 mg colfosceril palmitate, 12 mg cetyl alcohol, and 8 mg tyloxapol; cetyl alcohol acts as the spreading agent for colfosceril; tyloxapol acts as a dispersant
Pharmacokinetics
Administered intratracheally, distributed to all lobes, distal airways, and alveolar spaces; alveolar $t_{1/2}$ 12 hr

INDICATIONS AND USES: Prophylaxis for infants with birth weights of less than 1350 g who are at risk of developing respiratory distress syndrome (RDS); prophylaxis for infants with birth weights greater than 1350 g who have evidence of pulmonary immaturity; rescue treatment for infants who have developed RDS

DOSAGE
Child
• *Prophylaxis:* Intratracheal 5 ml/kg as soon as possible after birth and q12h for 2 doses to infants remaining on mechanical ventilation
• *Rescue treatment:* Intratracheal administer in two 5 ml/kg doses; give initial dose after diagnosis of RDS, then second dose in 12 hr
• Administered in two 2.5 ml/kg half-doses, instilled over 1 to 2 min in small bursts timed with inspiration; change body position between half-doses

$ AVAILABLE FORMS/COST OF THERAPY
• Inj, Lyphl-Susp—Intratracheal: 108 mg/10 ml vial: **$659.18**

CONTRAINDICATIONS: None

PRECAUTIONS: Colfosceril can rapidly affect po_2, pco_2, and lung compliance; pulmonary hemorrhage; mucous plugs; do not suction within 2 hr of dose

SIDE EFFECTS/ADVERSE REACTIONS
RESP: ***Apnea, pulmonary hemorrhage, pulmonary air leak, congenital pneumonia, pneumothorax, interstitial emphysema***

SPECIAL CONSIDERATIONS
MONITORING PARAMETERS
• Continuous ECG and transcutaneous O_2 saturation; pco_2; lung compliance; respiratory rate

colistin

(koe-lis'tin)
Coly-Mycin S Oral, Coly-Mycin S Otic (combination containing hydrocortisone [1%] and neomycin [4.71 mg/ml])
Chemical Class: Polymyxin B
Therapeutic Class: Antibiotic, miscellaneous; antidiarrheal

CLINICAL PHARMACOLOGY
Mechanism of Action: Bactericidal, surface-active basic polypeptide; binds to bacterial cytoplasmic membranes to allow leakage of intracellular contents
Pharmacokinetics
PO: Not significantly absorbed into systemic circulation

INDICATIONS AND USES: Treatment of diarrhea in infants and children caused by susceptible organisms; superficial bacterial infections of the external auditory canal

Antibacterial spectrum usually includes:
• Gram-negative organisms: *E. coli, Shigella*

DOSAGE

Adult

• TOP Instill in the ear canal, 4 gtt q6-8h

Child

• PO 5-15 mg/kg/d in 3 divided doses; TOP instill in the ear canal, up to 3 gtt q6-8h

$ AVAILABLE FORMS/COST OF THERAPY

• Powder: 66.7 g: **$381.25**
• Powder, Reconst—Oral: 25 mg/5 ml, 60 ml: **$27.07**
• Susp—Otic: 3 mg colistin, 1% hydrocortisone, 4.71 mg neomycin/ml, 10 ml: **$21.32**

CONTRAINDICATIONS: Hypersensitivity

PRECAUTIONS: Though not significantly absorbed, caution with decreased renal function

▼ DRUG INTERACTIONS

Drugs

• *Cephalosporins:* Additive nephrotoxicity

SPECIAL CONSIDERATIONS

PATIENT/FAMILY EDUCATION

• Shake well

corticotropin (ACTH)

(kor-ti-koe-troe'pin)

ACTH, ACTH Gel, Acthar, Acthar Gel H.P., Corticotropin

Chemical Class: Adrenocorticotropic hormone

Therapeutic Class: Pituitary hormone

CLINICAL PHARMACOLOGY

Mechanism of Action: Stimulates adrenal cortex to produce cortisol, corticosterone, several weakly androgenic steroids, and, to a limited extent, aldosterone

Pharmacokinetics

IV/IM/SC: Onset <1 hr; duration 2-4 hr, repository form has duration up to 3 days; plasma $t_{1/2}$ <20 min, excreted in urine; cortisol response dependent on total dose and total time of administration

INDICATIONS AND USES: Testing adrenocortical function; conditions in which the antiinflammatory effect of glucocorticoids is desired; ACTH has no advantage over glucocorticoids except perhaps in multiple sclerosis and dermatomyositis/polymyositis

DOSAGE

Adult

• *Testing of adrenocortical function:* IM/SC up to 80 U in divided doses qid; IV 10-25 U in 500 ml D_5W given over 8 hr
• *Antiinflammatory:* SC/IM 40 U in divided doses qid or 40 U q12-24h (gel/repository form)
• *Acute exacerbations of multiple sclerosis:* IM 80-120 U qd (gel/repository form) for up to 3 wk

Child

• *Antiinflammatory:* SC/IM 1.6 U/kg in divided doses qid or 0.8 U/kg q12-24h (gel/repository form)

$ AVAILABLE FORMS/COST OF THERAPY

• Inj, Lyphl-Sol—IM; SC: 25 U/vial, 1's: **$21.64;** 40 U/vial, 1's: **$31.84**
• Inj, Repos Gel—IM; SC: 80 U/ml, 5 ml: **$17.72-$39.85**
• Inj, Sol—IV: 40 U/ml, 5 ml: **$34.95;** 80 U/ml, 5 ml: **$55.35**

CONTRAINDICATIONS: Hypersensitivity, scleroderma, osteoporosis, CHF, peptic ulcer disease, hypertension, systemic fungal infections, smallpox vaccination, recent surgery, ocular herpes simplex, primary adrenocortical insufficiency/hyperfunction

PRECAUTIONS: Latent TB, hepatic disease, hyperthyroidism, childbearing-age women, psychiatric diagnosis, myasthenia gravis, acute gouty arthritis, posterior subcapsular cataracts, may mask some signs of infection; chronic administration of corticotropin may lead to adverse effects which are not reversible; in patients who receive prolonged corticotropin therapy the additional use of rapidly acting corticosteroids before, during, and after an unusual stressful situation is indicated

PREGNANCY AND LACTATION: Pregnancy category C

SIDE EFFECTS/ADVERSE REACTIONS

CNS: ***Convulsions,*** dizziness, euphoria, insomnia, headache, mood swings, behavioral changes, depression, psychosis, pseudotumor cerebri

CV: Hypertension, congestive heart failure

EENT: Posterior subcapsular cataracts, increased intraocular pressure

GI: Nausea, vomiting, ***peptic ulcer,*** pancreatitis, ulcerative esophagitis

METAB: Sodium retention, hypokalemic alkalosis, calcium loss, Cushingoid symptoms, hyperglycemia, growth retardation in children, menstrual irregularities, negative nitrogen balance due to protein catabolism

MS: Weakness, osteoporosis, compression fractures, muscle atrophy, steroid myopathy, myalgia, arthralgia, aseptic necrosis of femoral and humeral heads

SKIN: Impaired wound healing, rash, urticaria, hirsutism, petechiae, ecchymoses, sweating, acne, hyperpigmentation, suppression of skin test reactions

▼ **DRUG INTERACTIONS**

Drugs

• *Aminoglutethimide:* Decreased adrenal responsiveness to corticotropin
• *Barbiturates:* Increased cortisol clearance
• *Carbamazepine:* Increased cortisol clearance
• *Estrogens:* Decreased cortisol clearance
• *Isoniazid:* Decreased cortisol clearance
• *Oral contraceptives:* Decreased cortisol clearance
• *Phenytoin:* Increased cortisol clearance
• *Rifampin:* Increased cortisol clearance
• *Salicylates:* Decreased blood salicylate levels

Labs

• *Decrease:* Urinary estradiol, urinary estriol, ^{131}I uptake

SPECIAL CONSIDERATIONS

PATIENT/FAMILY EDUCATION

• Drug may mask infections
• Intercurrent illness may require increased corticosteroids
• Do not stop medication abruptly

cortisone

(kor′ti-sone)

Cortone

Chemical Class: Glucocorticoid, short-acting

Therapeutic Class: Corticosteroid, synthetic

CLINICAL PHARMACOLOGY

Mechanism of Action: Decreases inflammation by suppressing migration of polymorphonuclear leukocytes, macrophages, and fibroblasts, stabilizing leukocyte lysosomal membranes, and reversing increased capillary permeability

Pharmacokinetics

PO: Peak 2 hr, duration 1½ days

IM: Absorbed slowly over 24-48 hr

INDICATIONS AND USES: In replacement doses for primary or secondary adrenocortical insufficiency and congenital adrenal hyperplasia; in pharmacologic doses for hypercalcemia and localized or systemic inflammatory diseases responsive to corticosteroids

DOSAGE

Adult

• PO/IM 25-300 mg qd or q2d, titrated to patient response

$ **AVAILABLE FORMS/COST OF THERAPY**

• Inj, Sol—IM: 50 mg/ml, 10 ml: **$9.50-$25.38**

• Tab, Uncoated—Oral: 5 mg, 50's: **$6.23;** 10 mg, 100's: **$22.97;** 25 mg, 100's: **$8.50-$60.41**

CONTRAINDICATIONS: Psychosis, hypersensitivity, amebiasis, systemic fungal infections, child <2 yr, AIDS, live virus vaccines

PRECAUTIONS: Diabetes mellitus, glaucoma, osteoporosis, seizure disorders, ulcerative colitis, CHF, myasthenia gravis (if used with anticholinesterase agents), renal disease, esophagitis, peptic ulcer; in patients taking corticosteroids subjected to unusual stress, increased dosage of rapidly acting corticosteroids before, during, and after the stressful situation may be necessary

PREGNANCY AND LACTATION: Pregnancy category C; excreted in breast milk

SIDE EFFECTS/ADVERSE REACTIONS

CNS: ***Convulsions,*** dizziness, euphoria, insomnia, headache, mood swings, behavioral changes, depression, psychosis, pseudotumor cerebri

CV: Hypertension, congestive heart failure, thrombophlebitis, embolism

EENT: Posterior subcapsular cataracts, increased intraocular pressure, fungal infections

GI: Nausea, vomiting, ***peptic ulcer,*** pancreatitis, ulcerative esophagitis, intestinal perforation

HEME: ***Thrombocytopenia***

METAB: Sodium retention, hypokalemic alkalosis, calcium loss, Cushingoid symptoms, hyperglycemia, growth retardation in children, menstrual irregularities, negative nitrogen balance due to protein catabolism

MS: Weakness, osteoporosis, compression fractures, muscle atrophy, steroid myopathy, myalgia, arthralgia, aseptic necrosis of femoral and humeral heads, tendon rupture

SKIN: *Impaired wound healing,* rash, urticaria, hirsutism, petechiae, ecchymoses, sweating, acne, hyperpigmentation, suppression of skin test reactions

▼ **DRUG INTERACTIONS**

Drugs

• *Barbiturates, carbamazepine, phenytoin, rifampin:* Increased cortisone metabolism

• *Isoniazid:* Cortisone decreases isoniazid levels

• *Oral contraceptives, estrogens:* Increased cortisone effect

• *Salicylates:* Cortisone decreases salicylate level

Labs

• *Increase:* Cholesterol, Na, blood glucose, uric acid, Ca, urine glucose

• *Decrease:* Ca, K, T_4, T_3, thyroid ^{131}I uptake test, urine 17-OH CS, 17-KS, PBI

• *False negative:* Skin allergy tests

SPECIAL CONSIDERATIONS

PATIENT/FAMILY EDUCATION

• Drug may mask infections

• Intercurrent illness may require increased corticosteroids

• Affect, mood, or sleep may be affected

• Avoid salicylates and antiinflammatory drugs

• Do not stop medication abruptly

MONITORING PARAMETERS

• Serum K

cosyntropin

(koe-sin-troe'pin)
Cortrosyn
Chemical Class: Synthetic polypeptide
Therapeutic Class: Pituitary hormone

CLINICAL PHARMACOLOGY
Mechanism of Action: Stimulates adrenal cortex to produce cortisol; cosyntropin contains the first 24 of the 39 amino acids of natural ACTH; 0.25 mg of cosyntropin stimulates the adrenal cortex maximally and to the same extent as 25 units of natural ACTH
Pharmacokinetics
IV/IM: Onset 5 min, peak 1 hr, duration 2-4 hr
INDICATIONS AND USES: Testing adrenocortical function
DOSAGE
Adult
- IM/IV 0.25 mg

Child
- IM/IV age >2 yr 0.25 mg; age <2 yr 0.125 mg

$ AVAILABLE FORMS/COST OF THERAPY
- Inj, Dry-Sol—IM; IV: 0.25 mg, 10's: **$120.85**

CONTRAINDICATIONS: Hypersensitivity
PREGNANCY AND LACTATION: Pregnancy category C
SIDE EFFECTS/ADVERSE REACTIONS
SKIN: Rash, urticaria, pruritus, flushing
SPECIAL CONSIDERATIONS
MONITORING PARAMETERS
- Check plasma cortisol levels at baseline and 30-60 min after drug is administered

cromolyn

(kroe'moe-lin)
Crolom, Gastrocrom, Intal, Nasalcrom, Opticrom
Chemical Class: Mast cell stabilizer
Therapeutic Class: Antiasthmatic, topical antiinflammatory

CLINICAL PHARMACOLOGY
Mechanism of Action: Stabilizes membrane of the sensitized mast cell
Pharmacokinetics
Minimal oral absorption; 8% of total cromolyn dose absorbed after inhalation; after inhalation, peak level 15 min; elimination $t_{1/2}$ 80 min; excreted unchanged in feces
INDICATIONS AND USES: Allergic rhinitis, allergic conjunctivitis,* bronchial asthma, prevention of acute bronchospasm induced by environmental pollutants or exercise, systemic mastocytosis, prevention of food allergy
DOSAGE
Adult
- *Allergic conjunctivitis:* Ophthalmic sol 1-2 gtt OU 4-6 times/d
- *Allergic rhinitis:* Nasal sol 1 spray each nostril tid-qid
- *Bronchial asthma:* INH 2 puffs qid via inhaler or 20 mg qid by Spinhaler
- *Exercise-induced bronchospasm:* INH 2 puffs via inhaler or 20 mg via Spinhaler <1 hr before exercise
- *Systemic mastocytosis:* PO 200 mg qid

Child
- *Allergic conjunctivitis:* Age >2 yr ophthalmic sol 1-2 gtt OU 4-6 times/d
- *Allergic rhinitis:* Age >6 yr nasal sol 1 spray each nostril tid-qid
- *Exercise-induced bronchospasm:* Age 2-5 yr 20 mg qid via nebulized

solution; age >5 yr INH 2 puffs qid via inhaler or 20 mg qid by Spinhaler <1 hr before exercise

• *Bronchial asthma:* Age 2-5 yr 20 mg qid via nebulized solution; age >5 yr INH 2 puffs qid via inhaler or 20 mg qid by Spinhaler

• *Systemic mastocytosis:* Age <2 yr PO 5 mg/kg qid; age 2-12 yr PO 100 mg qid

$ **AVAILABLE FORMS/COST OF THERAPY**

• Sol—Inh: 10 mg/ml, 2 ml × 60: **$42.00-$48.25**

• Aer, Spray—Inh: 800 μg/spr, 112 spr's: **$37.98;** 200 spr's: **$60.43**

• Cap, Gel—Inh: 20 mg, 60's: **$35.44**

• Cap, Gel—Oral: 100 mg, 100's: **$94.10**

• Sol—Nasal: 5.2 mg/spr, 100 spr's: **$21.43**

• Sol—Ophth: 4%, 10 ml: **$17.30**

CONTRAINDICATIONS: Hypersensitivity to cromolyn, hypersensitivity to lactose (capsules for inhalation only)

PRECAUTIONS: Renal disease, hepatic disease, child <5 yr

PREGNANCY AND LACTATION: Pregnancy category B; avoid if lactating

SIDE EFFECTS/ADVERSE REACTIONS

CNS: Headache, dizziness, neuritis

EENT: Throat irritation, cough, nasal congestion, burning eyes, nasal stinging, nasal burning, *hoarseness*

GI: Nausea, vomiting, anorexia, dry mouth, *bitter taste,* diarrhea

GU: Frequency, dysuria

MS: Joint pain/swelling

RESP: Cough

SPECIAL CONSIDERATIONS

PATIENT/FAMILY EDUCATION

• Clear mucus before using

• Therapeutic effect may take up to 4 wk

• Empty contents of PO capsule into a half glass of hot water and stir until dissolved prior to administration

• Do not mix PO capsule with fruit juice, milk, or food

---

crotamiton

(kroe-tam'i-ton)

Eurax

Chemical Class: Synthetic chloroformate salt

Therapeutic Class: Scabicide

CLINICAL PHARMACOLOGY

Mechanism of Action: Toxic to *Sarcoptes scabiei*

Pharmacokinetics

Active topically, systemic absorption after topical use is unknown

INDICATIONS AND USES: Scabies in adults, scabies in children*

DOSAGE

Adult and Child

• TOP (cream, lotion), massage into skin of entire body from chin down; repeat application 24 hr later; reapply PRN for 48 hrs of exposure

$ **AVAILABLE FORMS/COST OF THERAPY**

• Lotion—Top: 10%, 60 g: **$10.57**

• Cre—Top: 10%, 60 g: **$9.91**

CONTRAINDICATIONS: Hypersensitivity, inflammation, abrasions, or breaks in skin, mucous membranes

PRECAUTIONS: Children

PREGNANCY AND LACTATION: Pregnancy category C

SIDE EFFECTS/ADVERSE REACTIONS

SKIN: Itching, rash, irritation, contact dermatitis

SPECIAL CONSIDERATIONS

PATIENT/FAMILY EDUCATION

• After patient bathes with soap and water, remove all crusts from chin down; massage crotamiton into skin

- From chin to toes including folds and creases
- 60 g is sufficient for two applications/adult
- Do not apply to face, lips, mouth, eyes, any mucous membrane, anus, or urethral meatus
- Clothing and bed linen should be changed the next morning
- A cleansing bath should be taken 48 hr after the last application
- Use topical corticosteroids to decrease contact dermatitis, antihistamines for pruritus; pruritus may continue for 4-6 wk

cyanide antidote

Therapeutic Class: Antidote, cyanide poisonings

CLINICAL PHARMACOLOGY

Mechanism of Action: Goals of therapy include decreased cyanide binding to cytochrome c and removal of cyanide from the blood; sodium nitrite reacts with hemoglobin to form methemoglobin, which competes with cytochrome oxidase for the cyanide ion; thiosulfate acts as a sulfur donor, and facilitates the conversion of cyanide to thiocyanate (relatively nontoxic)

INDICATIONS AND USES: Treatment of cyanide poisoning

DOSAGE

Adult

- Crush and inhale 0.3 ml ampul of amyl nitrite for 15-30 sec q1min until an IV sodium nitrite infusion is available; bolus 300 mg IV sodium nitrite; infuse 12 g sodium thiosulfate IV over 10 min; inj of both may be repeated at ½ the original dose

Child

- Crush and inhale 0.3 ml ampul of amyl nitrite for 15-30 sec q1min until an IV sodium nitrite infusion is available; bolus 300 mg IV sodium nitrite; infuse 7 g/m^2 (max 12.5 g) sodium thiosulfate IV over 10 min; injection of both may be repeated at ½ the original dose

$ **AVAILABLE FORMS/COST OF THERAPY**

- Kit—Inh; IV; Misc: 5 drop/300 mg/12.5 g: **$99.00-$144.49** (sodium nitrite 300 mg/10ml #2; sodium thiosulfate 12.5 g/50 ml #2; amyl nitrite 0.3 ml #12; syringes, stomach tube, tourniquet, and instructions)

PREGNANCY AND LACTATION: Pregnancy category C

cyanocobalamin (vitamin B_{12})

(sye-an-oh-koe-bal'a-min)

Bedoz, ✤ B_{12} Resin, Cobex, Crystamine, Crysti-12, Cyanabin, ✤ Cyanoject, Cyomin, Ener-B, Pernavite, Redisol, Rubesol-1000, Rubion, ✤ Rubramin PC, Sytobex

Chemical Class: Synthetic cobalt-containing B complex vitamin

Therapeutic Class: Vit B_{12}, water-soluble vitamin

CLINICAL PHARMACOLOGY

Mechanism of Action: Needed for adequate nerve functioning, protein and carbohydrate metabolism, normal growth, normal erythropoiesis

Pharmacokinetics

PO: Irregularly absorbed from the distal small gut; requires intrinsic factor but can be overcome with dosage increases (i.e., mean absorption rate of oral cyanocobalamin by patients with pernicious anemia is 1.2%; daily cobalamin turnover rate is about 2 μg/day, so oral doses of 100-250 μg are sufficient); peak 8-12 hr

IM: Sustained rise in serum concentration

Stored in liver, kidneys, stomach; 50%-90% excreted in urine; crosses placenta

INDICATIONS AND USES: Vit B_{12} deficiency, pernicious anemia, Vit B_{12} malabsorption syndrome, Schilling test; increased requirements with pregnancy, thyrotoxicosis, hemolytic anemia, hemorrhage, renal and hepatic disease, prevent and treat cyanide toxicity associated with nitroprusside*

DOSAGE

Adult

- *Deficiency:* PO 250 μg qd × 5-10 days, maintenance 250-500 μg qd; IM/SC 30-100 μg qd 5-10 days, maintenance 100-200 μg IM qmo
- *Pernicious anemia/malabsorption syndrome:* IM 100-1000 μg qd × 2 wk, then 100-1000 μg IM qmo
- *Schilling test:* IM 1000 μg in one dose

Child

- *Deficiency:* Total IM/SC dose is 1-5 mg given in single 100 μg doses qd over 2 or more wk; maintenance 60 μg IM qmo or more
- *Pernicious anemia/malabsorption syndrome:* IM 100-500 μg qd over 2 wk, then 60 μg IM/SC qmo
- *Schilling test:* IM 1000 μg in one dose

$ **AVAILABLE FORMS/COST OF THERAPY**

- Inj, Sol—IM; IV; SC: 0.1 mg/ml, 1 ml: **$1.71-$3.33;** 30 ml: **$1.95-$7.20;** 1 mg/ml, 1 ml: **$2.55;** 10 ml: **$1.10-$10.94**
- Tab—Oral: 500 μg, 100's: **$4.59**

CONTRAINDICATIONS: Hypersensitivity, optic nerve atrophy

PREGNANCY AND LACTATION: Pregnancy category A; excreted in breast milk in concentrations that approximate the mother's serum; compatible with breast feeding

SIDE EFFECTS/ADVERSE REACTIONS

CNS: Flushing, optic nerve atrophy

CV: ***CHF,*** peripheral vascular thrombosis, ***pulmonary edema***

GI: Diarrhea

METAB: Hypokalemia

SKIN: Itching, rash, pain at site

MISC: ***Anaphylactic shock***

▼ **DRUG INTERACTIONS**

Labs

- *False positive:* Intrinsic factor

SPECIAL CONSIDERATIONS

- Recommended Dietary Allowance: 0.5-2.6 μg/d depending on age and status, i.e., more during pregnancy and lactation
- Nutritional sources: egg yolks, fish, organ meats, dairy products, clams, oysters

MONITORING PARAMETERS

- CBC with reticulocyte count after 1st wk of therapy

---

cyclandelate

(sye-klan'da-late)

Cyclan, Cyclospasmol

Therapeutic Class: Peripheral vasodilator

CLINICAL PHARMACOLOGY

Mechanism of Action: Musculotropic; acts directly to relax vascular smooth muscle; no significant adrenergic stimulating or blocking actions

Pharmacokinetics

PO: Onset 15 min, peak 1½ hr, duration 4 hr

INDICATIONS AND USES: Possibly effective: Intermittent claudication, thrombophlebitis (to control associated vasospasm and muscular ischemia), Raynaud's phenomenon, ischemic cerebrovascular disease, arteriosclerosis obliterans, nocturnal leg cramps, dementia of cerebrovascular origin,* memory disorders,* migraine prophylaxis,* vertigo, tinnitus and visual disturbances attributable to chronic cerebrovascular insufficiency,* diabetic peripheral polyneuropathy*

DOSAGE

Adult

- PO 200 mg qid, not to exceed 400 mg qid; maintenance dose is 400-800 mg/d in 2-4 divided doses

$ AVAILABLE FORMS/COST OF THERAPY

- Cap, Gel—Oral: 200, 400 mg, 100's: **$5.66-$94.73**

CONTRAINDICATIONS: Hypersensitivity

PRECAUTIONS: Glaucoma, recent MI, hypertension, severe obliterative coronary artery or cerebrovascular disease ("steal" syndrome, diseased areas compromised by vasodilatory effects elsewhere)

PREGNANCY AND LACTATION: Pregnancy category C

SIDE EFFECTS/ADVERSE REACTIONS

CNS: Headache, paresthesias, dizziness, weakness

CV: ***Tachycardia***

GI: Heartburn, eructation, nausea, pyrosis

HEME: Increased bleeding time (rare)

SKIN: Sweating, flushing

SPECIAL CONSIDERATIONS

PATIENT/FAMILY EDUCATION

- Advise patient to quit smoking

---

cyclobenzaprine

(sye-kloe-ben'za-preen)

Flexeril

Chemical Class: Tricyclic amine

Therapeutic Class: Skeletal muscle relaxant, central acting

CLINICAL PHARMACOLOGY

Mechanism of Action: CNS (at brain stem) reduction of tonic somatic motor activity (both gamma [γ] and alpha [α] motor systems), producing skeletal muscle relaxant activity; effects similar to tricyclic antidepressants (including reserpine antagonism, norepinephrine potentiation, potent peripheral and central anticholinergic effects, and sedation)

Pharmacokinetics

PO: Onset 1 hr, peak 3-8 hr, duration 12-24 hr

$t_{1/2}$ 1-3 days; metabolized by liver; excreted in urine

INDICATIONS AND USES: Adjunct for relief of muscle spasm and pain in musculoskeletal conditions

DOSAGE

Adult

- PO 10 mg tid × 1 wk (range 20-40 mg/d), max 60 mg/d; use should not exceed 3 wk

$ AVAILABLE FORMS/COST OF THERAPY

- Tab, Coated—Oral: 10 mg, 100's: **$19.43-$87.10**

CONTRAINDICATIONS: Acute recovery phase of MI, dysrhythmias, heart block, CHF, hypersensitivity, child <12 yr, intermittent porphyria, thyroid disease

PRECAUTIONS: History of urinary retention, angle-closure glaucoma, increased intraocular pressure, and in patients taking anticholinergic medication, addictive personality, elderly; lowers seizure threshold

PREGNANCY AND LACTATION: Pregnancy category B; no data available, but closely related tricyclic antidepressants are excreted into breast milk

SIDE EFFECTS/ADVERSE REACTIONS

CNS: Dizziness, weakness, drowsiness, headache, tremor, depression, insomnia, confusion, paresthesia, nervousness, asthenia

CV: Postural hypotension, tachycardia, dysrhythmias
EENT: Diplopia, temporary loss of vision
GI: *Nausea,* vomiting, hiccups, *dry mouth,* constipation, dyspepsia, unpleasant taste
GU: Urinary retention, frequency, change in libido
SKIN: Rash, pruritus, fever, facial flushing, sweating

▼ DRUG INTERACTIONS

Drugs

• No drug interactions reported, however, consider MAOIs; hyperpyretic crisis, severe convulsions, and deaths have occurred in patients receiving closely related tricyclic antidepressants and MAOI drugs; separate use by 14 days

SPECIAL CONSIDERATIONS

PATIENT/FAMILY EDUCATION

• Caution with alcohol, other CNS depressants
• Caution with hazardous activities if drowsiness/dizziness occurs

---

cyclopentolate

(sye-kloe-pen′toe-late)
AK-Pentolate, Cyclogyl
Chemical Class: Anticholinergic
Therapeutic Class: Mydriatic, cycloplegic

CLINICAL PHARMACOLOGY

Mechanism of Action: Blocks response of iris sphincter muscle, muscle of accommodation of ciliary body to cholinergic stimulation, resulting in dilation, paralysis of accommodation

Pharmacokinetics

OPHTH: Peak 30-60 min (mydriasis), 25-74 min (cycloplegia), duration ¼-1 day

INDICATIONS AND USES: Cycloplegic refraction, mydriasis

DOSAGE

Adult

• OPHTH SOL 1 gtt of a 1%-2% sol, then 1 gtt in 5 min

Child >6 yr

• OPHTH SOL 1 gtt of a 0.5%-2% sol, then 1 gtt in 5 min of a 0.5%-1% sol

$ AVAILABLE FORMS/COST OF THERAPY

• Sol—Ophth: 0.5%, 2 ml: **$5.69;** 1%, 2 ml: **$1.04-$6.75;** 1%, 5 ml: **$2.60-$12.44**

CONTRAINDICATIONS: Hypersensitivity, infants <3 mo, open or narrow-angle glaucoma, conjunctivitis

PRECAUTIONS: Elderly (more risk of increased intraocular pressure), infants, children with spastic paralysis or brain damage

PREGNANCY AND LACTATION: Pregnancy category C

SIDE EFFECTS/ADVERSE REACTIONS

CV: Tachycardia
CNS: Psychotic reaction, behavior disturbances, ataxia, restlessness, hallucinations, somnolence, disorientation, confusion, failure to recognize people, ***grand mal seizures,*** irritability
EENT: Blurred vision, temporary burning sensation on instillation, eye dryness, photophobia, conjunctivitis, increased intraocular pressure
GI: Abdominal distention, vomiting, dry mouth, abdominal discomfort
MISC: Fever, flushing, dry skin, abdominal distension (in infants), bladder distension, irregular pulse, ***respiratory depression***

SPECIAL CONSIDERATIONS

PATIENT/FAMILY EDUCATION

• Review method of instillation: no more than one drop; pressure on lacrimal sac for 1 min
• Do not touch dropper to eye

cyclophosphamide

(sye-kloe-foss'fa-mide)

Cytoxan, Neosar, Procytox ♣

Chemical Class: Synthetic nitrogen mustard

Therapeutic Class: Antineoplastic alkylating agent

CLINICAL PHARMACOLOGY

Mechanism of Action: Active metabolites alkylate DNA, RNA, thus interfere with growth of susceptible rapidly proliferating malignant cells (mechanism is thought to involve cross-linking of tumor cell DNA); activity is not cell cycle phase specific

Pharmacokinetics

PO: Bioavailability >75%

IV: Peak, 2-3 hr (as metabolites) Metabolized by liver; excreted in urine (5%-25% unchanged); $t_{1/2}$ 3-12 hr; 60% bound to plasma proteins

INDICATIONS AND USES:

• Malignant Disease: Used concurrently or sequentially with other antineoplastic drugs for malignant lymphomas, Hodgkin's disease, lymphocytic lymphoma, Burkitt's lymphoma, multiple myeloma, chronic lymphocytic leukemia, chronic granulocytic leukemia, acute myelogenous and monocytic leukemia, acute lymphoblastic (stem cell) leukemia in children, mycosis fungoides (advanced disease), neuroblastoma (disseminated disease), adenocarcinoma of the ovary, retinoblastoma, carcinoma of the breast

• Nonmalignant Disease: Biopsy proven "minimal change" nephrotic syndrome in children; severe rheumatic conditions* (Wegener's granulomatosis, steroid-resistant vasculitides, progressive rheumatoid arthritis,* systemic lupus erythematosus,* polyarteritis nodosa,* polymyositis*), and multiple sclerosis*

DOSAGE

Adult

• *Malignant disease:* PO initially 1-5 mg/kg/day, maintenance is 1-5 mg/kg/day; IV initially 40-50 mg/kg in divided doses over 2-5 days, maintenance 10-15 mg/kg q7-10d, or 3-5 mg/kg q3d

Child

• *Malignant disease:* PO/IV 2-8 mg/kg or 60-250 mg/m^2 in divided doses for 6 or more days; maintenance 10-15 mg/kg q7-10d or 30 mg/kg q3-4wk; dose should be reduced by half when bone marrow depression occurs

• *Nephrotic syndrome:* PO 2.5 to 3 mg/kg/d × 60 to 90 days

$ **AVAILABLE FORMS/COST OF THERAPY**

• Inj, Lyphl-Sol—IV: 1, 2 g/vial: **$7.16-$86.00;** 100, 200, 500, 750 mg/vial: **$0.85-$49.37**

• Tab, Uncoated—Oral: 25 mg, 100's: **$152.31;** 50 mg, 100's: **$279.53**

CONTRAINDICATIONS: Hypersensitivity, suppressed bone marrow function

PRECAUTIONS: Radiation therapy

PREGNANCY AND LACTATION: Pregnancy category D; excreted in breast milk; contraindicated because of potential for adverse effects relating to immune suppression, growth, and carcinogenesis

SIDE EFFECTS/ADVERSE REACTIONS

CNS: Headache, dizziness

CV: ***Cardiotoxicity*** (high doses)

GI: Nausea, vomiting, diarrhea, weight loss, colitis, ***hepatotoxicity***

GU: ***Hemorrhagic cystitis, hematuria, neoplasms,*** *amenorrhea, azoospermia, sterility, ovarian fibrosis*

HEME: ***Thrombocytopenia, leukopenia, pancytopenia; myelosuppression***
METAB: Syndrome of inappropriate antidiuretic hormone (SIADH)
RESP: ***Fibrosis***
SKIN: *Alopecia,* dermatitis

▼ DRUG INTERACTIONS

Drugs

- *Allopurinol:* Increased cyclophosphamide toxicity
- *Digoxin:* Decreased digoxin absorption from tablets; Lanoxicaps and elixir not affected
- *Succinylcholine:* Prolonged neuromuscular blockade
- *Warfarin:* Inhibited hypoprothrombinemic response to warfarin

Labs

- *Increase:* Uric acid
- *False positive:* Pap test
- *False negative:* PPD, mumps, trichophytin, *Candida*
- *Decrease:* Pseudocholinesterase

SPECIAL CONSIDERATIONS

MONITORING PARAMETERS

- CBC, differential, platelet count qwk; withhold drug if WBC is <4000 or platelet count is <75,000
- Renal function studies: BUN, UA, serum uric acid, urine CrCl before, during therapy
- I&O ratio; report fall in urine output ≤30 ml/hr

---

cycloserine

(sye-kloe-ser′een)

Seromycin

Chemical Class: Streptomyces orchidaceus antibiotic; analog of D-alanine, R-enantiomer

Therapeutic Class: Antitubercular

CLINICAL PHARMACOLOGY

Mechanism of Action: Inhibits cell wall synthesis in susceptible strains of gram-positive and gram-negative bacteria and in *Mycobacterium tuberculosis*

Pharmacokinetics

PO: Peak 4-8 hr; therapeutic levels 25-30 μg/ml; blood levels <30 μg/ml minimizes toxicity; 65% excreted unchanged in urine; remaining metabolized to unknown substances; crosses placenta

INDICATIONS AND USES: Pulmonary and extrapulmonary tuberculosis, as adjunctive (like all antituberculosis drugs, cycloserine should be administered in conjunction with other effective chemotherapy and not as the sole therapeutic agent); acute UTIs caused by susceptible strains of gram-positive and gram-negative bacteria, especially *Enterobacter* sp and *E. coli* (when more conventional therapy has failed and when the organism has been demonstrated to be susceptible to the drug)

DOSAGE

Adult

- PO 250 mg q12h × 2 wk, then 250 mg q8h × 2 wk, then 250 mg q6h if there are no signs of toxicity; not to exceed 1 g/d

Child

- PO 10-20 mg/kg/d q12h (max 0.75-1 g) individualize doses

$ AVAILABLE FORMS/COST OF THERAPY

- Cap, Gel—Oral: 250 mg, 40's: **$131.21**

CONTRAINDICATIONS: Hypersensitivity, seizure disorders, renal disease, alcoholism (chronic), depression, severe anxiety, psychosis, anemia

PRECAUTIONS: Children

PREGNANCY AND LACTATION: Pregnancy category C; excreted into breast milk (72% of serum levels), 0.6% of mother's daily supply was estimated to be in the milk, compatible with breast feeding

SIDE EFFECTS/ADVERSE REACTIONS

CV: ***CHF***

CNS: Headache, anxiety, drowsiness, tremors, ***convulsions,*** lethargy, depression, confusion, psychosis, aggression

HEME: ***Megaloblastic anemia,*** Vit B_{12}, folic acid deficiency, leukocytosis

SKIN: Dermatitis, photosensitivity

▼ **DRUG INTERACTIONS**

Labs

- *Increase:* AST/ALT

SPECIAL CONSIDERATIONS

- L-enantiomer (l-cycloserine) in Gaucher's disease (Orphan Drug)
- Pyridoxine may prevent neurotoxicity

PATIENT/FAMILY EDUCATION

- Avoid concurrent alcohol

MONITORING PARAMETERS

- Mental status closely and liver function tests qwk

---

cyclosporine

(sye-kloe-spor'in)

Sandimmune, Neoral

Chemical Class: Fungus-derived *(Tolypocladium inflatun Gams),* cyclic peptide

Therapeutic Class: Immunosuppressant

CLINICAL PHARMACOLOGY

Mechanism of Action: Produces immunosuppression by inhibiting T-lymphocytes (mainly T-helper cells, but T-suppressor cells may also be suppressed); also inhibits lymphokine production and release including interleukin-2; does not cause bone marrow suppression

Pharmacokinetics

PO: Wide bioavailability (4%-89%), peak 3.5 hr

Blood level monitoring: maintenance of 24-hr trough levels of 250-800 ng/ml (whole blood, RIA) or 50-300 ng/ml (plasma, RIA) should minimize side effects and rejection events; 90% protein bound (lipoproteins), $t_{1/2}$ (biphasic) 1.2 hr, 25 hr; metabolized in liver (mixed function oxidase enzymes) to 17 metabolites, only 0.1% left unchanged; excretion primarily biliary-feces, 0.1% excreted in urine

INDICATIONS AND USES: PO/IV prophylaxis of organ rejection in kidney, liver, and heart allogeneic transplants in conjunction with adrenal corticosteroids; prophylaxis of organ rejection in pancreas,* bone marrow,* and heart/lung transplantation;* alopecia areata;* aplastic anemia;* atopic dermatitis;* Behçet's disease;* biliary cirrhosis;* Crohn's disease;* dermatomyositis;* Graves' ophthalmopathy;* insulin-dependent diabetes mellitus;* lupus nephritis;* multiple sclerosis;* myasthenia gravis,* nephrotic syndrome;* pemphigus and pemphigoid;* polymyositis;* psoriatic arthritis;* pulmonary sarcoidosis;* pyoderma gangrenosum;* rheumatoid arthritis;* severe psoriasis;* ulcerative colitis;* uveitis;* Orphan Drug Status: OPHTH keratoconjunctivitis sicca with Sjogren's syndrome; graft rejection following keratoplasty; corneal melting syndromes (i.e., Mooren's ulcer)

DOSAGE

Adult and Child

- PO 15 mg/kg several hr before surgery, daily for 2 wk, reduce dosage by 2.5 mg/kg/wk to 5-10 mg/kg/d; IV 5-6 mg/kg several hr before surgery, daily, switch to PO form as soon as possible

AVAILABLE FORMS/COST OF THERAPY

Sandimmune dosage forms:
- Cap, Elastic—Oral: 25 mg, 30's: **$37.50;** 50 mg, 30's: **$74.94**; 100 mg, 30's: **$149.88**
- Inj, Sol—IV: 250 mg/5 ml: **$22.28**
- Sol—Oral: 100 mg/5 ml, 50 ml: **$264.42**

Neoral dosage forms:
- Cap (soft gel) for micro emulsion: 25 mg, 30's: **$39.72;** 100 mg, 30's: **$158.76**
- Sol—Oral, for micro emulsion: 100 mg/5 ml, 50 ml: **$264.42**

CONTRAINDICATIONS: Hypersensitivity

PRECAUTIONS: Renal disease, hepatic disease, concurrent nephrotoxic drugs, anaphylaxis with first IV dose; malabsorption syndromes

PREGNANCY AND LACTATION: Pregnancy category C; excreted into breast milk; M:P ratios 0.17-0.4; contraindicated due to the potential for immune suppression and neutropenia, an unknown effect on growth, and possible association with carcinogenesis

SIDE EFFECTS/ADVERSE REACTIONS

CNS: Tremors, headache

CV: Hypertension (50% of renal transplants; most of cardiac transplants)

GI: Nausea, vomiting, diarrhea, *oral Candida, gum hyperplasia,* ***hepatotoxicity,*** pancreatitis

GU: ***Albuminuria, hematuria, proteinuria, renal failure***

METAB: Hypomagnesemia (related to neurotoxicity)

SKIN: Rash, acne, *hirsutism*

▼ DRUG INTERACTIONS

Drugs

- *Aminoglycosides, amphotericin B, co-trimoxazole, sulfonamides:* Additive nephrotoxicity with cyclosporine
- *Amiodarone, anabolic steroids, chloroquine, clarithromycin, oral contraceptives, erythromycin+, itraconazole, ketoconazole, miconazole:* Increased cyclosporine levels, potential for toxicity
- *Calcium channel blockers:* Diltiazem+, verapamil increase cyclosporine levels; isradipine, nifedipine, nitrendipine do not interact
- *Carbamazepine, co-trimoxazole, phenytoin, rifampin, sulfonamides:* Reduced cyclosporine levels, potential for therapeutic failure
- *Digitalis glycosides:* Cyclosporine in patients stabilized on digitalis leads to increased levels and potential toxicity
- *HMG-CoA reductase inhibitors:* Increased risk of reversible myopathy
- *Methotrexate:* Increased toxicity of both agents
- *Metoclopramide:* Increased bioavailability and serum levels of single dose cyclosporine
- *NSAIDs:* Increased risk of cyclosporine nephrotoxicity

SPECIAL CONSIDERATIONS

MONITORING PARAMETERS

- Renal function studies: BUN/creatinine qmo during treatment, 3 mo after treatment
- Liver function studies and serum levels during treatment

---

cyclothiazide

(cy-clo-thi'a-zide)

Anhydron, Fluidil

Chemical Class: Thiazide diuretic, sulfonamide derivative

Therapeutic Class: Diuretic antihypertensive

CLINICAL PHARMACOLOGY

Mechanism of Action: Alters renal tubular electrolyte reabsorption; acts on distal tubule by increasing excretion of water, sodium, chloride, potassium, magnesium; renal and extrarenal antihypertensive effects; decreased urinary calcium excretion

Pharmacokinetics

PO: Onset, <6 hr; peak effect, 7-12 hr; duration of effect, 18-24 hr; rapid absorption, eliminated unchanged via kidneys

INDICATIONS AND USES: Edema, hypertension, renal calculi,* diabetes insipidus*

DOSAGE

Adult

- 1-2 mg qd (max 6 mg qd)

Child

- 20-40 μg/kg/d

$ AVAILABLE FORMS/COST OF THERAPY

- Tab, Plain Coated—Oral: 2 mg, 100's: **$29.28**

CONTRAINDICATIONS: Anuria, hypersensitivity

PRECAUTIONS: Hypokalemia, renal disease (CrCl < 35 ml/min), hepatic disease, gout, diabetes mellitus, elderly

PREGNANCY AND LACTATION: Pregnancy category C; excreted into breast milk

SIDE EFFECTS/ADVERSE REACTIONS

CNS: Mood or mental changes

CV: Irregular heartbeat, weak pulse

GI: Dry mouth, increased thirst

GU: Decreased sexual ability

METAB: Hyperuricemia, gout

MS: Muscle cramps or pain, tiredness, weakness

SKIN: Skin rash, hives

▼ DRUG INTERACTIONS

Drugs

- *Antidiabetics:* Increased dosage requirements due to increased glucose levels
- *Carbenoxolone:* Additive potassium wasting, severe hypokalemia
- *Cholestyramine, colestipol:* Reduced absorption
- *Diazoxide:* Hyperglycemia
- *Digitalis glycosides:* Diuretic-induced hypokalemia increases risk of digitalis toxicity
- *Lithium+:* Increased lithium levels, potential toxicity

Labs

- *Increase:* Glucose, bilirubin, calcium, cholesterol (LDL), triglycerides, uric acid
- *Decrease:* Magnesium, potassium, sodium, protein-bound iodine, urinary calcium

SPECIAL CONSIDERATIONS

MONITORING PARAMETERS

- Ineffective with decreased renal function (CrCl<40 ml/min)
- Blood pressure, glucose, renal function tests, uric acid, and serum electrolytes

cyproheptadine

(si-proe-hep'ta-deen)

Periactin, Vimicon 🍁

Chemical Class: Piperidine

Therapeutic Class: H_1-receptor antagonist, antihistaminic and antiserotonergic agent

CLINICAL PHARMACOLOGY

Mechanism of Action: Serotonin and histamine antagonist with anticholinergic and sedative effects; competes with serotonin and histamine, respectively, for receptor sites

Pharmacokinetics

PO: Duration 4-6 hr; metabolized in liver; excreted by kidneys (40% unchanged)

INDICATIONS AND USES: Perennial and seasonal allergic rhinitis, vasomotor rhinitis, allergic conjunctivitis, allergic skin manifestations of urticaria and angioedema, cold urticaria, dermatographism, adjunctive with epinephrine and other standard measures for anaphylactic reactions, appetite stimulant,* cluster headaches,* SSRI induced sexual dysfunction*

DOSAGE

Adult

• PO 4 mg tid-qid, not to exceed 0.5 mg/kg/d

Child

• PO (0.25 mg/kg/d); 2-6 yr 2 mg bid-tid, not to exceed 12 mg/d; 7-14 yr 4 mg bid-tid, not to exceed 16 mg/d

$ AVAILABLE FORMS/COST OF THERAPY

• Syr—Oral: 2 mg/5 ml, 480 ml: **$6.38-$30.16**

• Tab, Uncoated—Oral: 4 mg, 100's: **$1.88-$39.43**

CONTRAINDICATIONS: Hypersensitivity to H_1-receptor antagonists, acute asthma attack, lower respiratory tract disease

PRECAUTIONS: Increased intraocular pressure due to closed-angle glaucoma, renal disease, cardiac disease, bronchial asthma, seizure disorder, stenosed peptic ulcers, prostatic hypertrophy, bladder neck obstruction, elderly

PREGNANCY AND LACTATION: Pregnancy category B; excreted in breast milk

SIDE EFFECTS/ADVERSE REACTIONS

CNS: Dizziness, drowsiness, poor coordination, fatigue, anxiety, euphoria, confusion, paresthesia, neuritis

CV: Hypotension, palpitations, tachycardia

EENT: Blurred vision, dilated pupils; tinnitus; nasal stuffiness; dry nose, throat, mouth

GI: Constipation, dry mouth, nausea, vomiting, anorexia, diarrhea, weight gain

GU: Retention, dysuria, frequency, increased appetite

RESP: Increased thick secretions, wheezing, chest tightness

SKIN: Rash, urticaria, photosensitivity

▼ DRUG INTERACTIONS

Labs

• *False negative:* Skin allergy tests

SPECIAL CONSIDERATIONS

PATIENT/FAMILY EDUCATION

• Avoid driving or other hazardous activity if drowsiness occurs, especially elderly

• Avoid concurrent use of alcohol or other CNS depressants

---

cytarabine

(sye-tare'a-been)

Cytosar, ♣Cytosar-U, Tarabine PFS

Chemical Class: Pyrimidine nucleoside

Therapeutic Class: Antineoplastic, antimetabolite

CLINICAL PHARMACOLOGY

Mechanism of Action: Competes with physiologic substrate of DNA synthesis, thus interfering with cell replication in the S phase of the cell cycle (before mitosis); potent immunosuppressant

Pharmacokinetics

SC or IM: Peak, 20-60 min (considerably lower than following IV)

IV: Peak, immeasurable in 30 min

INTRATHECAL: Level of cytarabine declines, with a first order $t_{1/2}$ of 2 hr

Distribution $t_{1/2}$ 10 min, elimination $t_{1/2}$ 2 hr; low protein binding (15%); deaminated in liver; excreted in urine (primarily inactive metabolite); crosses blood-brain barrier (moderate amounts)

INDICATIONS AND USES: Acute myelocytic leukemia, acute lymphocytic leukemia, chronic myelocytic leukemia, and in combination for non-Hodgkin's lymphomas in children

DOSAGE

Adult

• *Acute myelocytic leukemia:* IV INF 200 mg/m^2/day × 5 days; INTRATHECAL: 5-50 mg/m^2/d × 3 d/wk or 30 mg/m^2/d q4d, in combination

Child

• *Acute myelocytic leukemia:* IV INF 100 mg/m^2/day × 5-10 days

$ AVAILABLE FORMS/COST OF THERAPY

• Inj, Lyphl-Sol—Intrathecal; IV; SC: 1 g/vial: **$50.83;** 2 g: **$99.50;** 100 mg: **$6.07;** 500 mg: **$24.16**

CONTRAINDICATIONS: Hypersensitivity, infants

PRECAUTIONS: Renal disease, hepatic disease

PREGNANCY AND LACTATION: Pregnancy category C; contraindicated 1st trimester; breast feeding not recommended

SIDE EFFECTS/ADVERSE REACTIONS

CNS: Neuritis, dizziness, headache, personality changes, ataxia, mechanical dysphasia, ***coma***

CV: Chest pain, ***cardiopathy***

EENT: Sore throat, conjunctivitis

GI: Nausea, vomiting, anorexia, diarrhea, stomatitis, ***hepatotoxicity,*** abdominal pain, hematemesis, ***GI hemorrhage***

GU: Urinary retention, ***renal failure,*** uric acid nephropathy

HEME: Thrombophlebitis, bleeding, ***thrombocytopenia, leukopenia, myelosuppression, anemia***

METAB: ***Hyperuricemia***

SKIN: Rash, fever, freckling, cellulitis

RESP: ***Pneumonia,*** dyspnea

MISC: Cytarabine Syndrome—fever, myalgias, bone pain, chest pain, rash, conjunctivitis, malaise (6-12 hr after administration), *chills, infection*

▼ DRUG INTERACTIONS

Drugs

• *Bone marrow depressants:* Additive bone marrow depression

• *Cyclophosphamide:* Increased risk for cardiomyopathy and sudden death

• *Live viral vaccines:* Potentiation of viral replication, increased adverse effects, or decreased antibody response

Labs

• *Increase:* Uric acid (physiologic), alkaline phosphatase, AST, bilirubin

SPECIAL CONSIDERATIONS

PATIENT/FAMILY EDUCATION

• Avoid aspirin products and other NSAIDs

MONITORING PARAMETERS

• CBC (RBC, Hct, Hgb), differential, platelet count qwk

• Withhold drug if WBC is <4000/mm^3, platelet count is <75,000/mm^3, or RBC, Hct, Hgb are low

• Renal function studies, electrolytes, and uric acid before and during therapy

• Allopurinol may be necessary to control hyperuricemia and gout

• Liver function tests before and during therapy, as needed or qmo

• Bleeding

---

danazol

(da'na-zole)

Danocrine

Chemical Class: Ethisterone derivative

Therapeutic Class: Androgen

CLINICAL PHARMACOLOGY

Mechanism of Action: Suppresses the pituitary-ovarian axis by decreasing the hypothalamic-pituitary response to lowered estrogen production, altering sex steroid metabolism, and by competitively inhibiting the binding of steroids to their cytoplasmic receptors in target tissues; depresses the output of both follicle-stimulating hormone (FSH) and luteinizing hormone (LH); possesses weak androgenic activity

Pharmacokinetics

PO: Peak 2 hr, extensively metabolized in liver, excreted in urine, $t_{1/2}$ 4½ hr

INDICATIONS AND USES: Endometriosis amenable to hormonal management; reduction of nodularity, pain, and tenderness in fibrocystic breast disease; prevention of attacks of hereditary angioedema (cutaneous, abdominal, laryngeal); precocious puberty;* gynecomastia;* menorrhagia;* idiopathic immune thrombocytopenia;* lupus-associated thrombocytopenia;* autoimmune hemolytic anemia*

DOSAGE

Adult

- *Endometriosis:* PO initially 400 mg bid to achieve rapid response and amenorrhea, decrease to dose sufficient to maintain amenorrhea (100-200 mg bid) for 3-9 mo
- *Fibrocystic breast disease:* PO 100-400 mg/d in 2 divided doses
- *Hereditary angioedema:* PO initially 200 mg bid-tid, decrease dose by 50% or less at 1-3 mo intervals to lowest effective dose, if attack occurs, increase dose by up to 200 mg/d

$ AVAILABLE FORMS/COST OF THERAPY

- Cap, Gel—Oral: 50 mg, 100's: **$118.13;** 100 mg, 100's: **$177.26;** 200 mg, 100's: **$179.99-$295.38**

CONTRAINDICATIONS: Undiagnosed abnormal genital bleeding; markedly impaired hepatic, renal, or cardiac function; porphyria

PRECAUTIONS: Breast cancer, long-term use, epilepsy, migraine; cardiac, renal, or hepatic dysfunction

PREGNANCY AND LACTATION: Contraindicated in pregnancy, may result in androgenic effects in the fetus; initiate therapy during menstruation or rule out pregnancy prior to initiating therapy in women of child-bearing potential; contraindicated during breast feeding

SIDE EFFECTS/ADVERSE REACTIONS

CNS: Dizziness, headache, sleep disorders, fatigue, tremor, nervousness, emotional lability

CV: Elevated blood pressure

GI: Gastroenteritis, nausea, vomiting, constipation, hepatic dysfunction (doses >400 mg/d)

GU: Clitoral hypertrophy, testicular atrophy, hematuria, vaginitis (itching, dryness, burning, and vaginal bleeding), pelvic pain

MS: Muscle cramps, spasms, joint lock-up, joint swelling

SKIN: Acne, edema, *mild hirsutism, oily skin or hair,* flushing, sweating

MISC: Decrease in breast size, deepening of the voice, weight gain, changes in libido, glucose intolerance

▼ DRUG INTERACTIONS

Drugs

- *Carbamazepine:* Predictably increases serum carbamazepine concentrations; toxicity possible
- *Cyclosporine:* Increased serum cyclosporine concentrations; toxicity possible
- *Lovastatin:* Myositis with rhabdomyolysis has been reported
- *Oral anticoagulants+:* Enhanced hypoprothrombinemic response to warfarin

Labs

- *Increase:* Cholesterol
- *Decrease:* Cholesterol, T_4, T_3, thyroid ^{131}I uptake, 17-KS, PBI

• *Interference:* Glucose tolerance test

SPECIAL CONSIDERATIONS

PATIENT/FAMILY EDUCATION

• Notify physician if masculinizing effects occur (e.g., abnormal growth of facial or other fine body hair, deepening of the voice, etc.)

• Use nonhormonal contraceptive measures during therapy, discontinue use if pregnancy is suspected

• May administer with food if stomach upset occurs

MONITORING PARAMETERS

• Semen should be checked for volume, viscosity, sperm count, and motility q3-4mo, especially in adolescents

• Potassium, blood sugar, urine glucose during long-term therapy

• Daily weights, notify physician if weight gain >5 lbs

---

dantrolene

(dan'troe-leen)

Dantrium

Chemical Class: Hydantoin

Therapeutic Class: Skeletal muscle relaxant, direct acting

CLINICAL PHARMACOLOGY

Mechanism of Action: Reduces contraction of skeletal muscle by a direct action on excitation-contraction coupling, apparently by decreasing the amount of calcium released from the sarcoplasmic reticulum

Pharmacokinetics

PO: Peak 5 hr, highly protein bound, $t_{1/2}$ 8 hr, metabolized in liver, excreted in urine (metabolites and unchanged drug)

INDICATIONS AND USES: Control of spasticity resulting from upper motor neuron disorders such as spinal cord injury, stroke, cerebral palsy, or multiple sclerosis; malignant hyperthermia (prevention of initial and recurrent episodes, treatment of crises); exercise-induced muscle pain;* neuroleptic malignant syndrome;* heat stroke*

DOSAGE

Adult

• *Spasticity:* PO 25 mg qd initially, increase to tid-qid then increase dose by 25 mg q4-7d, max 400 mg/d

• *Malignant hyperthermia:* PO 4-8 mg/kg/d in 4 divided doses starting 1-2 hr before surgery, the same dose may be used for up to 3 days after a crisis to prevent further hyperthermia; IV 1 mg/kg, may repeat as needed to a cumulative dose of 10 mg/kg then switch to PO

Child

• *Spasticity:* PO 0.5 mg/kg/dose bid initially, increase to tid-qid at 4-7 day intervals then increase dose by 0.5 mg/kg to a max of 3 mg/kg/dose bid-qid, do not exceed 400 mg/d

• *Malignant hyperthermia:* Same as adult

$ AVAILABLE FORMS/COST OF THERAPY

• Cap, Gel—Oral: 25 mg, 100's: **$69.40;** 50 mg, 100's: **$103.96;** 100 mg, 100's: **$129.29**

• Inj, Sol—IV: 20 mg, 1's: **$55.21**

CONTRAINDICATIONS: (PO) Active hepatic disease; where spasticity is utilized to sustain upright posture and balance in locomotion or to obtain or maintain increased function; muscle spasm resulting from rheumatic disorders; (PO/IV) hypersensitivity

PRECAUTIONS: Age >35 yr (increased risk for hepatotoxicity), long-term use, impaired pulmonary function, severely impaired cardiac function, history of previous liver disease

PREGNANCY AND LACTATION: Pregnancy category C; do not use in nursing women

SIDE EFFECTS/ADVERSE REACTIONS

CNS: Dizziness, weakness, fatigue, drowsiness, headache, disorientation, insomnia, paresthesias, tremors, seizure, nervousness

CV: Erratic blood pressure, chest pain, palpitations

EENT: Nasal congestion, blurred vision, mydriasis

GI: Nausea, diarrhea, constipation, vomiting, increased AST and alk phosphatase, abdominal pain, dry mouth, anorexia, ***hepatitis, GI bleeding,*** dysphasia

GU: Urinary frequency, nocturia, impotence, crystalluria, hematuria, urinary incontinence, urinary retention

RESP: Pleural effusion, ***pulmonary edema***

SKIN: Rash, pruritus, photosensitivity, acne-like rash, urticaria, sweating

SPECIAL CONSIDERATIONS

PATIENT/FAMILY EDUCATION

- Use caution while driving or performing other tasks requiring alertness, coordination, or physical dexterity
- Take protective measures against exposure to UV light or sunlight until tolerance is determined (e.g. sunscreens, protective clothing)
- Avoid alcohol and other CNS depressants
- May cause weakness, malaise, fatigue, nausea, and diarrhea
- Notify physician if skin rash, itching, bloody or black tarry stools, or yellowish discoloration of skin or eyes occurs
- IV therapy may decrease the grip strength and increase weakness of leg muscles, especially walking down stairs; use caution
- Exercise caution at meals on the day of administration because difficulty swallowing and choking has been reported
- If improvement does not occur within 6 wk, physician may discontinue

MONITORING PARAMETERS

- Baseline and periodic LFTs (AST, ALT, alkaline phosphatase, total bilirubin)

---

dapiprazole

(da′pi-prah-zohl)

Rev-Eyes

Chemical Class: Pyridine derivative

Therapeutic Class: Ophthalmic α-adrenergic blocking agent

CLINICAL PHARMACOLOGY

Mechanism of Action: Blocks α-adrenergic receptors in smooth muscle producing miosis through an effect on the dilator muscle of the iris; no activity on ciliary muscle contraction or intraocular pressure

Pharmacokinetics

- Eye color affects the rate of pupillary constriction, individuals with brown irides may have a slightly slower rate of pupillary constriction than those with blue or green irides; eye color does not appear to affect the final pupil size

INDICATIONS AND USES: Iatrogenically induced mydriasis produced by adrenergic (phenylephrine) or parasympatholytic (tropicamide) agents

DOSAGE

Adult

- OPHTH instill 2 gtt, then 2 gtt 5 min later; do not use more than once/wk

$ AVAILABLE FORMS/COST OF THERAPY

- Sol—Ophth: 0.5%, 5 ml: **$32.74**

CONTRAINDICATIONS: Hypersensitivity, acute iritis

PRECAUTIONS: Children, severe cardiovascular disease

PREGNANCY AND LACTATION: Pregnancy category B; excretion into breast milk unknown, use caution in nursing mothers

SIDE EFFECTS/ADVERSE REACTIONS

EENT: Conjunctival injection, burning, ptosis, lid erythema, lid edema, itching, keratitis, corneal edema, browache, photophobia, headaches, eye dryness, tearing, blurring vision

SPECIAL CONSIDERATIONS

PATIENT/FAMILY EDUCATION

- May cause burning, itching, blurring, dryness of eye
- ***Preparation:*** Tear off aluminum seal, remove and discard rubber plugs from drug and diluent vials, pour diluent into drug vial, remove dropper and attach to vial, shake for several min

---

dapsone

(dap'sone)

Avlosulfan

Chemical Class: Sulfone

Therapeutic Class: Leprostatic

CLINICAL PHARMACOLOGY

Mechanism of Action: Similar to sulfonamides which are competitive antagonists of para-aminobenzoic acid (PABA) and prevent normal bacterial utilization of PABA for the synthesis of folic acid

Pharmacokinetics

PO: Rapid complete absorption, $t_{1/2}$ 25-31 hr, 73% bound to plasma proteins, metabolized in liver, excreted in urine and bile

INDICATIONS AND USES: All forms of leprosy (Hansen's disease) except for cases of proven dapsone resistance; dermatitis herpetiformis; *Pneumocystis carinii* pneumonia (PCP) in HIV+ patients (in combination with trimethoprim);* alternative to cotrimoxazole for PCP prophylaxis (alone or in combination with pyrimethamine);* prevention of the first episode of toxoplasmosis in HIV+ patients (in combination with pyrimethamine);* treatment of relapsing polychondritis;* prophylaxis of malaria;* brown recluse spider bites*

DOSAGE

Adult

- *Leprosy:* PO 50-100 mg qd for 3-10 yr (addition of rifampin 600 mg qd for the first 6 mo is recommended)
- *Dermatitis herpetiformis:* PO 50 mg qd initially, increase to 300 mg qd or higher to achieve full control, reduce dosage to min level as soon as possible
- *PCP prophylaxis:* PO 50 mg qd or 100 mg qod

Child

- *Leprosy:* PO 1-2 mg/kg/d, max 100 mg/d

$ **AVAILABLE FORMS/COST OF THERAPY**

- Tab, Uncoated—Oral: 25 mg, 100's: **$17.10;** 100 mg, 100's: **$18.20**

CONTRAINDICATIONS: Hypersensitivity to sulfones

PRECAUTIONS: Renal disease, hepatic disease, G-6-PD deficiency, anemia, severe cardiopulmonary disease, methemoglobin reductase deficiency

PREGNANCY AND LACTATION: Pregnancy category C; extensive, but uncontrolled, experience and two published surveys in pregnant women have not shown increases in the risk for fetal abnormalities if administered during all trimesters;

excreted in breast milk, hemolytic reactions can occur in neonates, discontinue nursing or discontinue drug; alternatively, some authors have suggested infants should be kept with mothers infected with leprosy, and breast feeding during drug therapy encouraged

SIDE EFFECTS/ADVERSE REACTIONS

CNS: Peripheral neuropathy, headache, insomnia, vertigo, paresthesia, psychosis

EENT: Blurred vision, optic neuritis, photophobia, tinnitus

GI: Nausea, vomiting, abdominal pain, anorexia

GU: Proteinuria, nephrotic syndrome, renal papillary necrosis

HEME: ***Hemolytic anemia*** (dose related), ***agranulocytosis, aplastic anemia***

SKIN: Drug-induced SLE, photosensitivity

▼ DRUG INTERACTIONS

Drugs

• *Didanosine:* Higher failure rate in pneumocystis infections, possibly due to inhibited dissolution of dapsone in stomach; administer dapsone 2-3 hr before didanosine

• *Probenecid:* Increased serum dapsone concentrations; clinical importance not established

• *Trimethoprim:* Increased serum dapsone concentrations; increased trimethoprim concentrations

SPECIAL CONSIDERATIONS

PATIENT/FAMILY EDUCATION

• Administer with meals to decrease GI symptoms

• Therapeutic effects may not occur for several mo, compliance with dosage schedule, duration is necessary

• Report sore throat, fever, pallor, yellowing of skin or eyes immediately

MONITORING PARAMETERS

• CBC weekly for the first mo, qmo for 6 mo and semiannually thereafter

• Periodic LFTs

D

deferoxamine

(de-fer-ox'a-meen)

Desferal

Chemical Class: Chelating agent

Therapeutic Class: Heavy metal antagonist

CLINICAL PHARMACOLOGY

Mechanism of Action: Chelates iron by forming a stable complex that prevents the iron from entering into further chemical reactions; readily chelates free serum iron, iron from ferritin and hemosiderin but not from transferrin; does not combine with the iron from cytochromes and hemoglobin

Pharmacokinetics

Rapidly metabolized by plasma enzymes, excreted in urine, $t_{1/2}$ 1 hr, iron chelate excreted renally giving urine a red color, some chelate also excreted in bile

INDICATIONS AND USES: Acute iron intoxication; promotion of iron excretion in patients who have secondary iron overload from multiple transfusions; aluminum accumulation in bone in renal failure patients,* aluminum-induced dialysis encephalopathy*

DOSAGE

Adult

• *Acute iron intoxication:* IM 1 g stat, then 0.5 g q4h for 2 doses, additional doses of 0.5 g q4-12h prn, max 6 g/d; IV 15 mg/kg/hr, max 6 g/d

• *Chronic iron overload:* IM 0.5-1 g/d; SC via portable pump infuse 1-2 g/d over 8-12 hr

Child

- *Acute iron intoxication:* IM 90 mg/kg/dose q8h, max 6 g/d; IV 15 mg/kg/hr, max 6 g/d
- *Chronic iron overload:* IV 15 mg/kg/hr, max 6 g/d; SC via portable pump infuse 20-40 mg/kg/d over 8-12 hr

$ **AVAILABLE FORMS/COST OF THERAPY**

- Inj, Sol—IM;IV; SC: 500 mg, 4's: **$39.81**

CONTRAINDICATIONS: Severe renal disease or anuria, hypersensitivity

PREGNANCY AND LACTATION: Pregnancy category C; excretion into breast milk unknown, use caution in nursing mothers

SIDE EFFECTS/ADVERSE REACTIONS

SKIN: Urticaria, erythema, pruritus, pain at inj site

CV: Hypotension (with rapid IV inj), tachycardia

GI: Diarrhea, abdominal cramps

EENT: Blurred vision, cataracts, ototoxicity

MS: Leg cramps

MISC: ***Anaphylaxis***

SPECIAL CONSIDERATIONS

PATIENT/FAMILY EDUCATION

- May turn urine red

MONITORING PARAMETERS

- Visual acuity tests, slit-lamp examinations, funduscopy, and audiometry are recommended periodically in patients treated for prolonged periods of time
- BUN, creatinine, CrC1
- Serum iron levels

demecarium bromide

(de-mi-kare'ee-um)

Humorsol

Chemical Class: Cholinesterase inhibitor, reversible

Therapeutic Class: Antiglaucoma agent, miotic

CLINICAL PHARMACOLOGY

Mechanism of Action: Produces intense miosis and ciliary muscle contraction due to inhibition of cholinesterase, allowing acetylcholine to accumulate at sites of cholinergic transmission; myopia may be induced or, if present, may be augmented by the increased refractive power of the lens

Pharmacokinetics

- Onset of miosis 15-60 min, duration 3-10 days, peak reduction of intraocular pressure 24 hr, duration 7-28 days

INDICATIONS AND USES: Open-angle glaucoma (should be used only when shorter-acting miotics have proved inadequate); conditions obstructing aqueous outflow, such as synechial formation, that are amenable to miotic therapy; following iridectomy; accommodative esotropia (accommodative convergent strabismus)

DOSAGE

Adult and Child

- *Glaucoma:* Initially instill 1 gtt of 0.125 or 0.25% sol (children) or 1-2 gtt (adults) in the glaucomatous eye, keep the patient under supervision and make tonometric examinations at least for 3 or 4 hr to be sure that no immediate rise in pressure occurs; usual dose 1-2 gtt bid to 1-2 gtt twice/wk, the 0.125% strength used bid usually results in smooth control of the physiologic diurnal variation in intraocular pressure

• *Strabismus:* Essentially equal visual acuity of both eyes is a prerequisite to successful treatment. Diagnosis: 1 gtt ou for 2 wk, then 1 gtt q2d for 2-3 wk, if the eyes become straighter, an accommodative factor is demonstrated. Therapy: In esotropia uncomplicated by amblyopia or anisometropia, instill not more than 1 gtt at a time OU qd for 2-3 wk (too severe a degree of miosis may interfere with vision), reduce to 1 gtt qod for 3-4 wk and reevaluate; may be continued in a dosage of 1 gtt q2d to 1 gtt twice/wk (the latter dosage may be maintained for several mo), evaluate the patient's condition every 4 to 12 wk, if improvement continues, change the schedule to 1 gtt qwk and eventually to a trial without medication; if after 4 mo control of the condition still requires 1 gtt q2d, therapy should be stopped

$ AVAILABLE FORMS/COST OF THERAPY

• Sol—Ophth: 0.125%, 5 ml: **$14.68;** 0.25%, 5 ml: **$15.74**

CONTRAINDICATIONS: Hypersensitivity, active uveal inflammation, glaucoma associated with iridocyclitis

PRECAUTIONS: Myasthenia gravis, narrow-angle glaucoma, asthma, spastic GI disturbances, peptic ulcer, bradycardia, hypotension, recent MI, epilepsy, parkinsonism, children (more frequent occurrence of iris cysts)

PREGNANCY AND LACTATION: Pregnancy category C; ionized at physiologic pH, transplacental passage in significant amounts would not be expected; excretion into breast milk unknown, but would be expected to be low due to ionization at physiologic pH

SIDE EFFECTS/ADVERSE REACTIONS

CNS: Headache, fainting, sweating

CV: Cardiac irregularities

EENT: Stinging, burning, lacrimation, eczematoid dermatitis, allergic follicular conjunctivitis, accommodative spasm, lid muscle twitching, conjunctival and ciliary redness, browache, myopia, blurred vision, iris cysts (more frequent in children), lens opacities, paradoxical increase in intraocular pressure

GI: Nausea, vomiting, abdominal cramps, diarrhea, salivation

GU: Urinary incontinence

RESP: Difficulty breathing

SPECIAL CONSIDERATIONS

PATIENT/FAMILY EDUCATION

• Local irritation and headache may occur at initiation of therapy

• Notify physician if abdominal cramps, diarrhea, or excessive salivation occurs

• Keep bottle tightly closed and out of the reach of children

• Avoid touching tip of container to any surface

• Wash hands immediately after use

• Use caution while driving at night or performing hazardous tasks in poor light

• Apply continuous gentle pressure on the lacrimal duct with the index finger for several seconds immediately following instillation of the drops to minimize systemic absorption

MONITORING PARAMETERS

• Frequent evaluations to detect iris cysts, especially in children

• Routine slit-lamp examination during prolonged administration

• Intraocular pressure

demeclocycline

(dem-e-kloe-sye'kleen)
Declomycin
Chemical Class: Tetracycline
Therapeutic Class: Antibiotic

CLINICAL PHARMACOLOGY
Mechanism of Action: Inhibits protein synthesis by binding with the 30S and possibly the 50S ribosomal subunit(s) of susceptible bacteria, may also cause alterations in the cytoplasmic membrane, bacteriostatic
Pharmacokinetics
PO: Peak 3-6 hr, $t_{1/2}$ 10-17 hr, excreted in urine, 65%-91% bound to serum protein
INDICATIONS AND USES: Chronic hyponatremia associated with the syndrome of inappropriate antidiuretic hormone (SIADH) secretion;* Rocky Mountain spotted fever, typhus fever, Q fever, rickettsialpox, tick fevers, *Mycoplasma pneumoniae,* psittacosis and ornithosis, lymphogranuloma venereum and granuloma inguinale, relapsing fever, chancroid, infections of the respiratory and urinary tract, syphilis and yaws, Vincent's infection, acute intestinal amebiasis (adjunct to amebicides), trachoma, inclusion conjunctivitis, severe acne.
Antibacterial spectrum usually includes:
• Gram-positive organisms: *Bacillus anthracis, Actinomyces israelii, Arachnia propionica, Clostridium perfringens, C. tetani, Listeria monocytogenes, Nocardia, Propionibacterium acnes*
• Gram-negative organisms: *Bartonella bacilliformis, Bordetella pertussis, Brucella, Calymmatobacterium granulomatis, Campylobacter fetus, Francisella tularensis, Haemophilus ducreyi, H. influenzae, Legionella pneumophilia, Leptotrichia buccalis, Neisseria gonorrhoeae, N. meningitidis, Pasteurella multocida, Pseudomonas pseudomallei, P. mallei, Shigella, Spirillum minus, Streptobacillus moniliformis, Vibrio cholerae, V. parahaemolyticus, Yersinia enterocolitica, Y. pestis*
• Other organisms: *Rickettsia akari, R. prowazeki, R. rickettsii, R. tsutsugamushi, R. typhi, Coxiella burnetii, Chlamydia trachomatis, C. psittaci, Mycoplasma hominis, M. pneumoniae, Ureaplasma urealyticum, Borrelia recurrentis, Leptospira, Treponema pallidum, T. pertenue*
DOSAGE
Adult
• PO 150 mg q6h or 300 mg q12h
• *Gonorrhea:* PO 600 mg, then 300 mg q12h for 4 days, total 3 g
• *SIADH:* PO 600-1200 mg/d in divided doses
Child >8 yr
• PO 6-12 mg/kg/d in divided doses q6-12h
$ AVAILABLE FORMS/COST OF THERAPY
• Cap, Elastic—Oral: 150 mg, 100's: **$285.30**
• Tab, Plain Coated—Oral: 150 mg, 100's: **$371.14;** 300 mg, 48's: **$324.15**
CONTRAINDICATIONS: Hypersensitivity to tetracyclines, children <8 yr
PRECAUTIONS: Renal disease, hepatic disease, nephrogenic diabetes insipidus, exposure to direct sunlight, outdated products
PREGNANCY AND LACTATION: Pregnancy category D; problems associated with use of the tetracyclines during or around pregnancy include adverse effects on fetal teeth and bones, maternal liver toxicity and congenital defects; excreted into

breast milk in low concentrations, use caution in nursing mothers

SIDE EFFECTS/ADVERSE REACTIONS

CNS: Fever, headache, paresthesia
CV: Pericarditis
GI: Dysphagia, oral candidiasis, *nausea,* vomiting, *diarrhea,* anorexia, glossitis, abdominal pain, enterocolitis, ***hepatotoxicity,*** flatulence, abdominal cramps, epigastric burning, stomatitis, ***pseudomembranous colitis***
GU: Increased BUN, polyuria, polydipsia, azotemia, nephrogenic diabetes insipidus
HEME: ***Eosinophilia, neutropenia, thrombocytopenia, hemolytic anemia***
SKIN: Rash, urticaria, *photosensitivity,* ***exfoliative dermatitis,*** pruritus
MISC: Decreased calcification of deciduous teeth, angioedema, pseudotumor cerebri (adults) and bulging fontanels (infants)

▼ DRUG INTERACTIONS

Drugs

• *Antacids+:* Reduced serum concentrations and efficacy of tetracyclines
• *Bismuth subsalicylate:* Significant reduction in tetracyline bioavailability; reduced antibacterial efficacy
• *Food+:* Food and dairy products containing high concentrations of cations may reduce serum concentrations of tetracyclines
• *Iron:* Oral iron products may reduce the serum concentrations of tetracyclines
• *Oral contraceptives:* Potential reduced effectiveness of oral contraceptives
• *Penicillin:* Impaired efficacy of penicillin therapy
• *Sodium bicarbonate+:* Reduced serum concentrations and efficacy of tetracyclines
• *Zinc:* May reduce serum concentrations of tetracyclines enough to reduce antibacterial efficacy

Labs

• *False negative:* Urine glucose with Clinistix or Tes-Tape
• *False increase:* Urinary catecholamines, AST, ALT, BUN

SPECIAL CONSIDERATIONS

PATIENT/FAMILY EDUCATION

• Avoid sun exposure, since burns may occur; sunscreen does not seem to decrease photosensitivity
• All prescribed medication must be taken to prevent superimposed infection
• Avoid milk products, take with full glass of water on an empty stomach 1 hr before meals or 2 hr after meals

MONITORING PARAMETERS

• LFTs during prolonged administration

desipramine

(dess-ip'ra-meen)
Norpramin, Pertofrane
Chemical Class: Dibenzazepine, secondary amine
Therapeutic Class: Antidepressant, tricyclic

CLINICAL PHARMACOLOGY

Mechanism of Action: Inhibits the reuptake of norepinephrine and serotonin at the presynaptic neuron prolonging neuronal activity; inhibits histamine and acetylcholine activity; mild peripheral vasodilator effects and possible "quinidine-like" actions

Pharmacokinetics

PO: Peak 2-4 hr, therapeutic response 2-4 wk, metabolized by liver, excreted by kidneys, $t_{1/2}$ 14-62 hr

INDICATIONS AND USES: Depression, facilitation of cocaine withdrawal,* eating disorders,* panic attacks*

DOSAGE

Adult

• PO 25 mg/d in single or divided doses initially, increase by 25 mg q3-5d to 100-200 mg/d, max 300 mg/d

Geriatric/Adolescent

• PO 25-100 mg/d, doses >150 mg/d not recommended

Child 6-12 yr

• PO 10-30 mg/d or 1-5 mg/kg/d in divided doses, max 5 mg/kg/d

$ AVAILABLE FORMS/COST OF THERAPY

• Tab, Plain Coated—Oral: 10, 25, 50, 75, 100 mg, 100's: **$10.43-$186.84;** 150 mg, 50's: **$109.50-$135.36**

CONTRAINDICATIONS: Hypersensitivity to tricyclic antidepressants, acute recovery phase of MI; concurrent use of MAOIs

PRECAUTIONS: Suicidal patients, convulsive disorders, prostatic hypertrophy, psychiatric disease, severe depression, increased intraocular pressure, narrow-angle glaucoma, urinary retention, cardiac disease, hepatic disease/renal disease, hyperthyroidism, electroshock therapy, elective surgery, elderly, abrupt discontinuation

PREGNANCY AND LACTATION: Pregnancy category C; excreted into breast milk, effect on the nursing infant unknown but may be of concern

SIDE EFFECTS/ADVERSE REACTIONS

CNS: Dizziness, confusion (especially in elderly), headache, anxiety, nervousness, panic, tremors, stimulation, weakness, fatigue, insomnia, nightmares, EPS (elderly), increased psychiatric symptoms, memory impairment

CV: Orthostatic hypotension, ***ECG changes, tachycardia, dysrhythmias,*** hypertension, palpitations, syncope, hypertensive episodes during surgery

EENT: Blurred vision, tinnitus, mydriasis, ophthalmoplegia, nasal congestion

GI: Constipation, dry mouth, nausea, vomiting, ***paralytic ileus,*** increased appetite, cramps, epigastric distress, jaundice, ***hepatitis,*** stomatitis, diarrhea

GU: Urinary retention

HEME: ***Agranulocytosis, thrombocytopenia, eosinophilia, leukopenia***

SKIN: Rash, urticaria, sweating, pruritus, photosensitivity

▼ DRUG INTERACTIONS

Drugs

• *Amphetamines:* Theoretical increase in effect of amphetamines, clinical evidence lacking

• *Anticholinergics:* Excessive anticholinergic effects

• *Barbiturates:* Reduced serum concentrations of cyclic antidepressants

• *Bethanidine:* Reduced antihypertensive effect of bethanidine

• *Carbamazepine:* Reduced cyclic antidepressant serum concentrations

• *Cimetidine:* Increased serum desipramine concentrations

• *Clonidine:* Reduced antihypertensive response to clonidine; enhanced hypertensive response with abrupt clonidine withdrawal

• *Debrisoquin:* Inhibited antihypertensive response of debrisoquin

• *Epinephrine+:* Markedly enhanced pressor response to IV epinephrine

• *Ethanol:* Additive impairment of motor skills; abstinent alcoholics may eliminate cyclic antidepressants more rapidly than non-alcoholics

• *Fluoxetine:* Marked increases in cyclic antidepressant plasma concentrations

• *Guanethidine:* Inhibited antihypertensive response to guanethidine
• *Moclobemide+:* Potential association with fatal or non-fatal serotonin syndrome
• *MAOIs:* Excessive sympathetic response, mania or hyperpyrexia possible
• *Neuroleptics:* Increased therapeutic and toxic effects of both drugs
• *Norepinephrine+:* Markedly enhanced pressor response to norepinephrine
• *Phenylephrine:* Enhanced pressor response to IV phenylephrine
• *Phenytoin:* Altered seizure control; decreased cyclic antidepressant serum concentrations
• *Propoxyphene:* Enhanced effect of cyclic antidepressants
• *Quinidine:* Increased cyclic antidepressant serum concentrations

Labs

• *Increase:* Serum bilirubin, blood glucose, alk phosphatase
• *Decrease:* VMA, 5-HIAA
• *False increase:* Urinary catecholamines

SPECIAL CONSIDERATIONS

PATIENT/FAMILY EDUCATION

• Therapeutic effects may take 2-3 wk
• Use caution in driving or other activities requiring alertness
• Avoid rising quickly from sitting to standing, especially elderly
• Avoid alcohol and other CNS depressants
• Do not discontinue abruptly after long-term use
• Wear sunscreen or large hat to prevent photosensitivity
• Increase fluids, bulk in diet if constipation occurs
• Gum, hard sugarless candy, or frequent sips of water for dry mouth

MONITORING PARAMETERS

• CBC, weight, ECG, mental status (mood, sensorium, affect, suicidal tendencies)
• Determination of desipramine plasma concentrations is not routinely recommended but may be useful in identifying toxicity, drug interactions, or noncompliance (adjustments in dosage should be made according to clinical response not plasma concentrations), therapeutic level is 50-200 nanogram/ml

desmopressin

(des-moe-press'in)

DDAVP, Stimute

Chemical Class: Synthetic antidiuretic hormone

Therapeutic Class: Pituitary hormone

CLINICAL PHARMACOLOGY

Mechanism of Action: Promotes reabsorption of water by action on renal tubular epithelium (antidiuretic hormone effect); causes vascular smooth muscle constriction (vasopressor effect); causes increase in plasma factor VIII levels, which increases platelet aggregation

Pharmacokinetics

NASAL: Onset 1 hr, peak 1-2 hr, duration 8-20 hr, terminal $t_{1/2}$ 76 min

INDICATIONS AND USES: Primary nocturnal enuresis (intranasal only); central diabetes insipidus; hemophilia A with factor VIII levels >5% (parenteral only); Von Willebrand's disease (Type I) (parenteral only); determination of the capacity of the kidneys to concentrate urine; chronic autonomic failure (e.g. nocturnal polyuria, overnight weight loss, morning postural hypotension);* intranasal treatment of hemophilia A and certain types of Von Willebrand's disease*

DOSAGE

Adult

• *Central diabetes insipidus:* NASAL (via rhinal tube) 0.1-0.4 ml qd, as a single or divided dose; most adults require 0.2 ml qd in 2 divided doses; the AM and PM doses should be separately adjusted for an adequate diurnal rhythm of water turnover; IV/SC 0.5-1 ml/d in 2 divided doses, adjusted separately for an adequate diurnal rhythm of water turnover; when switching from intranasal to IV the comparable antidiuretic dose is 1/10 the intranasal dose

• *Hemophilia A and von Willebrand's disease (Type I):* IV 0.3 mg/kg diluted in 50 ml NS infused slowly over 15-30 min

Child

• *Primary nocturnal enuresis: NASAL* (>6yr) initially 20 μg or 0.2 ml sol qhs, may increase up to 40 μg qhs prn, decrease to 10 μg qhs if the patient has shown a response to 20 μg

• *Central diabetes insipidus:* NASAL (via rhinal tube) (3 mo-12 yr) 0.05 to 0.3 ml qd, either as single dose or divided into 2 doses

• *Hemophilia A and von Willebrand's disease (Type I):* IV 0.3 mg/kg diluted in 50 ml NS (>10 kg) or 10 ml NS (≤10 kg) infused slowly over 15-30 min

$ AVAILABLE FORMS/COST OF THERAPY

• Aer, Spray—Nasal: 1.5 mg/ml, 2.5 ml: **$525.00**

• Inj, Sol—IV; SC: 4 μg/ml, 10 ml: **$238.89**

• Sol—Nasal: 0.1 mg/ml, 2.5 ml: **$56.19-$68.28**

CONTRAINDICATIONS: Hypersensitivity

PRECAUTIONS: Coronary artery disease, hypertensive cardiovascular disease

PREGNANCY AND LACTATION: Pregnancy category B; patients receiving desmopressin for diabetes insipidus have been reported to breast feed without apparent problems in the infant

SIDE EFFECTS/ADVERSE REACTIONS

CNS: Drowsiness, headache, lethargy, flushing

CV: Increased blood pressure

EENT: Nasal irritation, congestion, rhinitis

GI: Nausea, heartburn, cramps

GU: Vulvar pain

SPECIAL CONSIDERATIONS

PATIENT/FAMILY EDUCATION

• Nasal tube delivery system is supplied with a flexible calibrated plastic tube (rhinyle); draw solution into the rhinyle, insert one end of tube into nostril, blow on the other end to deposit solution deep into nasal cavity

• Notify physician if headache, shortness of breath, heartburn, nausea, abdominal cramps, or vulvar pain occurs

• Store in refrigerator or cool environment

MONITORING PARAMETERS

• Diabetes insipidus: Urine volume and osmolality, plasma osmolality

• Hemophilia A: Determine factor VIII coagulant activity before injecting desmopressin for hemostasis, if activity is <5% of normal do not rely on desmopressin

• Von Willebrand's disease: Assess levels of factor VIII coagulant, factor VIII antigen, and ristocetin cofactor; skin bleeding time may also be helpful

desonide

(dess'oh-nide)

DesOwen, Tridesilon

Chemical Class: Synthetic nonfluorinated agent, group IV (low) potency

Therapeutic Class: Topical corticosteroid

CLINICAL PHARMACOLOGY

Mechanism of Action: Depresses formation, release, and activity of endogenous mediators of inflammation such as prostaglandins, kinins, histamine, liposomal enzymes, and the complement system resulting in decreased edema, erythema, and pruritus

Pharmacokinetics

Absorbed through the skin (increased by inflammation and occlusive dressings), metabolized primarily in the liver

INDICATIONS AND USES: Psoriasis, eczema, contact dermatitis, pruritus; superficial bacterial infections of the external auditory canal (otic preparation)

DOSAGE

Adult and Child

• TOP apply to affected area bid-tid, rub completely into skin; OTIC instill 3-4 gtt tid-qid or insert wick saturated with solution and allow to remain *in situ*

$ **AVAILABLE FORMS/COST OF THERAPY**

• Cre—Top: 0.05%, 15, 60, 90 g: **$7.96-$54.81**

• Oint—Top: 0.05%, 15, 60 g: **$10.29-$31.88**

• Lotion—Top: 0.05%, 60, 120 ml: **$22.31-$32.50**

• Sol—Otic: 0.05% (with acetic acid 2%), 10 ml: **$16.18**

CONTRAINDICATIONS: Hypersensitivity to corticosteroids, fungal infections

PRECAUTIONS: Viral infections, bacterial infections, children; use on face, genitals, axilla

PREGNANCY AND LACTATION: Pregnancy category C; unknown whether topical application could result in sufficient systemic absorption to produce detectable amounts in breast milk (systemic corticosteroids are secreted into breast milk in quantities not likely to have detrimental effects on infant)

SIDE EFFECTS/ADVERSE REACTIONS

SKIN: Burning, dryness, itching, irritation, acne, folliculitis, hypertrichosis, perioral dermatitis, hypopigmentation, atrophy, striae, miliaria, allergic contact dermatitis, secondary infection

MISC: Systemic absorption of topical corticosteroids has produced reversible HPA axis suppression (more likely with occlusive dressings, prolonged administration, application to large surface areas, liver failure, and in children)

SPECIAL CONSIDERATIONS

PATIENT/FAMILY EDUCATION

• Apply sparingly only to affected area

• Avoid contact with the eyes

• Do not put bandages or dressings over treated area unless directed by physician

• Do not use on weeping, denuded, or infected areas

• Discontinue drug, notify physician if local irritation or fever develops

desoximetasone

(des-ox-i-met'a-sone)

Topicort, Topicort LP

Chemical Class: Group III (medium) potency: 0.05% (cream); Group II (high) potency: 0.25% (cream, ointment), 0.05% (gel)

Therapeutic Class: Topical corticosteroid

CLINICAL PHARMACOLOGY

Mechanism of Action: Depresses formation, release, and activity of endogenous mediators of inflammation such as prostaglandins, kinins, histamine, liposomal enzymes, and the complement system resulting in decreased edema, erythema, and pruritus

Pharmacokinetics

Absorbed through the skin (increased by inflammation and occlusive dressings), metabolized primarily in the liver

INDICATIONS AND USES: Psoriasis, eczema, contact dermatitis, pruritus

DOSAGE

Adult and Child

• Apply to affected area bid-tid, rub completely into skin

$ **AVAILABLE FORMS/COST OF THERAPY**

• Cre—Top: 0.05%, 15, 60 g: **$7.86-$31.44;** 0.25%, 15, 60, 120 g: **$10.25-$82.80**

• Gel—Top: 0.05%, 15, 60 g: **$14.25-$34.90**

• Oint—Top: 0.25%, 15, 60 g: **$16.30-$39.05**

CONTRAINDICATIONS: Hypersensitivity to corticosteroids, fungal infections; use on face, groin, or axilla

PRECAUTIONS: Viral infections, bacterial infections, children

PREGNANCY AND LACTATION: Pregnancy category C; unknown whether topical application could result in sufficient systemic absorption to produce detectable amounts in breast milk (systemic corticosteroids are secreted into breast milk in quantities not likely to have detrimental effects on infant)

SIDE EFFECTS/ADVERSE REACTIONS

SKIN: Burning, dryness, itching, irritation, acne, folliculitis, hypertrichosis, perioral dermatitis, hypopigmentation, atrophy, striae, miliaria, allergic contact dermatitis, secondary infection

MISC: Systemic absorption of topical corticosteroids has produced reversible HPA axis suppression (more likely with occlusive dressings, prolonged administration, application to large surface areas, liver failure, and in children)

SPECIAL CONSIDERATIONS

PATIENT/FAMILY EDUCATION

• Apply sparingly only to affected area

• Avoid contact with the eyes

• Do not put bandages or dressings over treated area unless directed by physician

• Do not use on weeping, denuded, or infected areas

• Discontinue drug, notify physician if local irritation or fever develops

desoxyribonuclease

(des-oxy-ribe-o-new'clee-ase)

Elase

Chemical Class: Lytic enzymes

Therapeutic Class: Topical enzyme preparation

CLINICAL PHARMACOLOGY

Mechanism of Action: Purulent exudates consist largely of fibrinous material and nucleoprotein; desoxyribonuclease attacks the DNA and fibrinolysin attacks principally the fibrin of blood clots and fibrinous exudates

INDICATIONS AND USES:
TOP—Debriding agent in general surgical wounds, ulcerative lesions (trophic, decubitus, stasis, arteriosclerotic), 2nd and 3rd degree burns, circumcision, episiotomy; Intravaginal—cervicitis (benign, postpartum, and postconization) and vaginitis; Irrigating agent—infected wounds (abscesses, fistulae, and sinus tracts), otorhinolaryngologic wounds, superficial hematomas (except when the hematoma is adjacent to or within adipose tissue)

DOSAGE

Adult

- *General topical use:* Apply thin layer of ointment and cover with petrolatum gauze or other nonadherant dressing, change qd-tid; sol may be applied topically as a liquid, wet dressing, or spray by using a conventional atomizer
- *Wet dressing:* Mix 1 vial of powder with 10-50 ml saline and saturate strips of fine-mesh gauze or unfolded sterile gauze sponge with sol; pack ulcerated area with gauze, allow to dry (approximately 6-8 hr) then remove dried gauze, repeat tid-qid
- *Intravaginal:* Apply 5 g of ointment deep into vagina qhs for 5 applications
- *Abscesses, empyema cavities, fistulae, sinus tracts, or SC hematomas:* Prepare sol by reconstituting contents of each vial of powder with 10 ml isotonic saline; drain and replace sol at 6-10 hr intervals

$ AVAILABLE FORMS/COST OF THERAPY

- Oint—Top: 10, 30 g: **$15.61-$24.22**
- Powder—Top: 15000 U desoxyribonuclease/25 U fibrinolysin, 10 ml: **$24.22**

CONTRAINDICATIONS: Hypersensitivity, parenteral use

PRECAUTIONS: History of sensitivity to bovine material

SIDE EFFECTS/ADVERSE REACTIONS

SKIN: Local hyperemia

SPECIAL CONSIDERATIONS

Successful enzymatic debridement depends on the following factors: surgical removal of any dense, dry eschar prior to administration; enzyme must be in constant contact with the substrate; periodic removal of accumulated necrotic debris; secondary closure or skin grafting as soon as possible after optimal debridement

PATIENT/FAMILY EDUCATION

- Frequency of application is more important than amount of ointment used
- Flush away necrotic debris with saline, peroxide, or warm water and dry gently prior to application
- Do not use sol ≥24 hr after reconstitution
- Refrigerate sol

dexamethasone

(dex-a-meth'a-sone)

Nasal: Decadron Phosphate Turbinaire

Ophthalmic: Ak-Dex Ophthalmic, Baldex, Decadron Phosphate Ophthalmic, Dexotic, I-methasone, Maxidex

Systemic: Dalalone D.P., Dalalone L.A., Decadron, Decaject, Dexacen LA-8, Dexasone L.A., Dexone LA, Solurex, Dalalone, Decadron Phosphate, Dexacen-4, Dexasone, Dexone, Hexadrol Phosphate, Solurex;

Topical: Aeroseb-Dex, Decaspray, Decaderm, Decadron Phosphate

Chemical Class: Glucocorticoid, long-acting; low-topical potency

Therapeutic Class: Corticosteroid

CLINICAL PHARMACOLOGY

Mechanism of Action: Controls the rate of protein synthesis, depresses the migrations of polymorphonuclear leukocytes and fibroblasts, reverses capillary permeability, and causes lysosomal stabilization at the cellular level to prevent or control inflammation

Pharmacokinetics

PO: Peak 1-2 hr

IM: Peak 8 hr

Metabolized in liver, excreted in urine and bile, biologic $t_{1/2}$ 36-54 hr

INDICATIONS AND USES:

Nasal: Allergic or inflammatory nasal conditions, nasal polyps (excluding polyps) originating within the sinuses)

Ophthalmic: Steroid-responsive inflammatory conditions of the palbebral and bulbar conjunctiva, lid, cornea, and anterior segment of the globe; corneal injury

Systemic: Anti-inflammatory or immunosuppressant agent in the treatment of a variety of diseases including those of hematologic, allergic, inflammatory, neoplastic, and autoimmune origin; acute mountain sickness;* antiemetic;* bacterial meningitis (to decrease incidence of hearing loss);* diagnosis of depression;* hirsutism;* prevention of neonatal respiratory distress syndrome (by administration to mother)*

Topical: Psoriasis, eczema, contact dermatitis, pruritis, steroid-responsive dermatoses

DOSAGE

Adult

- *Anti-inflammatory:* PO/IM/IV 0.75-9 mg/d in divided doses q6-12h; IM 8-16 mg q1-3 wk (acetate)
- *Cerebral edema:* IV 10 mg loading dose, then 4 mg IM/IV q6h
- *Shock:* IV 1-6 mg/kg or 40 mg q2-6h (phosphate)
- *Intralesional:* 0.8-1.6 mg (acetate)
- *Intra-articular and soft tissue:* 4-16 mg q1-3 wk (acetate); large joints 2-4 mg (phosphate); small joints 0.8-1 mg (phosphate); bursae 2-3 mg (phosphate); tendon sheaths 0.4-1 mg (phosphate); soft tissue infiltration 2-6 mg (phosphate); ganglia 1-2 mg (phosphate)
- *Nasal:* 2 sprays in each nostril bid-tid, max 12 sprays/day
- *Ophth:* INSTILL 1 gtt into conjunctival sac q1-4h depending on condition; apply ¼ inch ribbon of oint to lower conjunctival sac tid-qid; reduce frequency of administration once a favorable response is obtained
- *Top:* Apply to affected area bid-tid

Child 6-12 yr

- *Anti-inflammatory:* PO/IM/IV 0.08-0.3 mg/kg/d or 2.5-10 mg/m^2/d in divided doses q6-12h

• *Bacterial meningitis (>2 mo)*: IV 0.6 mg/kg/d divided q6h for 1st 4 days of antibiotic treatment, initiate with 1st dose of antibiotic
• *Cerebral edema:* PO/IM/IV 1-2 mg/kg loading dose, then 1-1.5 mg/kg/d (max 16 mg/d) in divided doses q4-6h
• *Physiologic replacement:* PO/IM/IV 0.03-0.15 mg/kg/d or 0.6-0.75 mg/m^2/d in divided doses q6-12h
• *Nasal:* 1-2 sprays into each nostril bid, max 8 sprays/day
• *Ophth:* Same as adult
• *Top:* Same ad adult

$ AVAILABLE FORMS/COST OF THERAPY

• Elixir—Oral: 0.5 mg/5ml, 100 ml: **$7.80-$16.96**
• Tab, Uncoated—Oral: 0.25, 0.5, 0.75, 1, 2 mg, 100's: **$3.56-$64.84;** 1.5, 4, 6 mg, 50's: **$10.40-$139.21**
• Inj, Sol (phosphate)—IM; IV: 4 mg/ml, 5 ml: **$1.05-$29.46;** 10 mg/ml, 10 ml: **$4.13-$25.25**
• Inj, Sol (phosphate)—IV: 20 mg/ml, 5 ml: **$8.22-$113.51;** 24 mg/ml, 5 ml: **$10.35**
• Inj, Sol (phosphate)—IM; IV: 40 mg/ml, 1 ml × 25: **$24.60**
• Inj, Susp—Intra-Articular; IM: (phosphate) 8 mg/ml, 5 ml: **$24.15;** (acetate) 8 mg/ml, 5 ml: **$11.71-$47.15;** 16 mg/ml, 5 ml: **$19.99**
• Aer, Spray—Inh, Nasal: 84 μg/spray, 12.6 g: **$24.79-$35.22**
• Oint—Ophth: 0.05%, 3.5 g: **$1.30-$6.34**
• Sol—Ophth: 0.1%, 5 ml: **$2.40-$15.56**
• Susp—Ophth: 0.1%, 5 ml: **$17.50**
• Aer—Top: 0.01%, 25, 58 g: **$14.86-$17.57**
• Gel—Top: 0.1%, 30 g: **$19.86**
• Cre—Top: 0.1%, 15, 30 g: **$11.75-$17.57**

CONTRAINDICATIONS: Systemic fungal infections, hypersensitivity, idiopathic thrombocytopenic purpura (IM); untreated localized infections of the nasal mucosa (nasal); acute superficial herpes simplex keratitis, fungal diseases of the ocular structures; most viral diseases of ocular structures, ocular TB, following uncomplicated removal of superficial corneal foreign body (ophth); fungal infections of the skin (top)

PRECAUTIONS: Psychosis, acute glomerulonephritis, amebiasis, cerebral malaria, child <2 yr, elderly, AIDS, tuberculosis, diabetes mellitus, glaucoma, osteoporosis, ulcerative colitis, CHF, myasthenia gravis, renal disease, esophagitis, peptic ulcer, ocular herpes simplex, live virus vaccines, hypertension; use on face, groin, and axilla (top)

PREGNANCY AND LACTATION: Pregnancy category C; used in patients with premature labor at about 24-36 wk gestation to stimulate fetal lung maturation; may appear in breast milk and could suppress growth, interfere with endogenous corticosteroid production, or cause unwanted effects in the nursing infant

SIDE EFFECTS/ADVERSE REACTIONS

CNS: Depression, vertigo, ***convulsions,*** headache, *mood changes*

CV: Hypertension, thrombophlebitis, ***thromboembolism,*** tachycardia, **CHF**

EENT: Increased intraocular pressure, blurred vision, cataracts; *nasal irritation, dryness, stinging,* rebound congestion, epistaxis, sneezing, nasal septum perforation, localized infections of nose and pharynx with *C. albicans,* sore throat (nasal); ***increased intraocular pressure,*** poor corneal wound healing, increased probability of corneal infection, glaucoma exacerbation, ***optic nerve***

damage, decreased acuity, cataracts, transient burning/stinging (ophth)
GI: Diarrhea, nausea, abdominal distention, ***GI hemorrhage,*** increased appetite, ***pancreatitis***
METAB: Cushingoid state, growth suppression in children, HPA suppression, decreased glucose tolerance
MS: Fractures, osteoporosis, aseptic necrosis of femoral and humeral heads, weakness, muscle mass loss
SKIN: Acne, poor wound healing, ecchymosis, bruising, petechiae, striae, thin fragile skin, suppression of skin test reactions

▼ **DRUG INTERACTIONS**

Drugs

• *Aminoglutethamide:* Enhanced elimination of dexamethasone; marked reduction in corticosteroid response
• *Antidiabetics:* Increased blood glucose in patients with diabetes
• *Barbiturates:* Reduced serum concentrations of corticosteroids
• *Carbamazepine:* Reduced serum concentrations of corticosteroids
• *Cholestyramine:* Possible reduced absorption of corticosteroids
• *Estrogens:* Enhanced effects of corticosteroids
• *Isoniazid:* Reduced plasma concentrations of isoniazid
• *Phenytoin:* Reduced therapeutic effect of corticosteroids
• *Rifampin:* Reduced therapeutic effect of corticosteroids
• *Salicylates:* Enhanced elimination of salicylates; subtherapeutic salicylate concentrations possible

Labs

• *Increase:* Cholesterol, blood glucose, urine glucose
• *Decrease:* Calcium, potassium, T_4, T_3, thyroid ^{131}I uptake test
• *False negative:* Skin allergy tests

SPECIAL CONSIDERATIONS

PATIENT/FAMILY EDUCATION

• May cause GI upset, take with meals or snacks; take single daily doses in AM
• Notify physician if unusual weight gain, swelling of lower extremities, muscle weakness, black tarry stools, vomiting of blood, puffing of the face, menstrual irregularities, prolonged sore throat, fever, cold, or infection occurs
• Signs of adrenal insufficiency include fatigue, anorexia, nausea, vomiting, diarrhea, weight loss, weakness, dizziness, and low blood sugar, notify physician if these signs and symptoms appear following dose reduction or withdrawal of therapy
• Avoid abrupt withdrawal of therapy following high dose or long-term therapy

MONITORING PARAMETERS

• Potassium and blood sugar during long-term therapy
• Edema, blood pressure, cardiac symptoms, mental status, weight
• Observe growth and development of infants and children on prolonged therapy
• Check lens and intraocular pressure frequently during prolonged use of ophthalmic preparations

dexchlorpheniramine

(dex'klor-fen-eer'a-meen)

Dex-Cpm; Dexchlor; Mylaramine; Polaramine, Poladex, Polargen

Chemical Class: Alkylamine, H_1 receptor antagonist
Therapeutic Class: Antihistamine

CLINICAL PHARMACOLOGY

Mechanism of Action: Acts on blood vessels, GI system, respiratory system, by competing with histamine for H_1-receptor site; decreases allergic response by blocking histamine

Pharmacokinetics

PO: Onset 20-60 min, peak 3 hr (7 ng/ml), duration 8-12 hr; protein binding 60%-70%; detoxified in liver; excreted by kidneys (metabolites/free drug); $t_{1/2}$, 20-24 hr

INDICATIONS AND USES: Allergy symptoms, rhinitis

DOSAGE

Adult

• PO 2-4 mg q6h prn

Child

• PO age 6-11 1 mg q6h; age 2-5 0.5 mg q6h

$ AVAILABLE FORMS/COST OF THERAPY

• Syr—Oral: 2 mg/5ml, 120 ml: **$3.19;** 480 ml: **$12.75-$39.70**

• Tab, Uncoated—Oral: 2 mg, 100's: **$37.43**

• Tab, Sust-Rel—Oral: 4 mg, 100's: **$31.67-$63.84;** 6 mg, 100's: **$44.23-$89.23**

CONTRAINDICATIONS: Hypersensitivity to H_1-receptor antagonists, acute asthma attack, lower respiratory tract disease

PRECAUTIONS: History of bronchial asthma; increased intraocular pressure; hyperthyroidism; cardiovascular disease; hypertension due to atropine-like actions; elderly

PREGNANCY AND LACTATION: Pregnancy category B

SIDE EFFECTS/ADVERSE REACTIONS

CNS: Dizziness, drowsiness, poor coordination, fatigue, anxiety, euphoria, confusion, paresthesia, neuritis

EENT: Blurred vision, dilated pupils, tinnitus, dry nose, throat

GI: Dry mouth, nausea, anorexia, diarrhea

GU: Retention, dysuria, frequency

HEME: ***Thrombocytopenia, agranulocytosis, hemolytic anemia***

RESP: Increased thick secretions, wheezing, chest tightness

SKIN: Photosensitivity

▼ DRUG INTERACTIONS

Labs

• *False negative:* Skin allergy tests

SPECIAL CONSIDERATIONS

PATIENT/FAMILY EDUCATION

• Caution in activities requiring mental alertness, i.e., driving or operating machinery due to slight to moderate drowsiness

• Alcohol or other sedative drugs may enhance the drowsiness

dexrazoxane

(dex-roz′ox-ane)

Zinecard

Chemical Class: EDTA derivative

Therapeutic Class: Cardioprotective chelating agent

CLINICAL PHARMACOLOGY

Mechanism of Action: Potent intracellular chelating agent; penetrates cell membranes; converted to a ring-opened chelating agent; interferes with iron-mediated free radical generation thought to be responsible for anthracycline-induced cardiomyopathy

Pharmacokinetics

IV: Peak 36.5 μg/ml at end of 15 min inf of 500 mg/m^2; rapid distribution, 42% excreted unchanged in urine, not protein bound, $t_{1/2}$ 2½ hr

INDICATIONS AND USES: Reduction of the incidence and severity of cardiomyopathy associated with doxorubicin in women with metastatic breast cancer who have received a cumulative doxorubicin dose of 300 mg/m^2

DOSAGE

Adult

• IV dosage ratio dexrazoxane: doxorubicin 10:1 (e.g., 500 mg/m^2

dexrazoxane:50 mg/m^2 doxorubicin); administer no more than 30 min of elapsed time before doxorubicin inj

$ AVAILABLE FORMS/COST OF THERAPY

• Lyphl-Powder, Inj—IV: 500 mg, 1's: **$221.45**

PRECAUTIONS: Additive myelosuppression, antitumor interference (reserve for patients with a cumulative doxorubicin dose of 300 mg/m^2)

PREGNANCY AND LACTATION: Pregnancy category C

SIDE EFFECTS/ADVERSE REACTIONS

GI: LFT abnormalities

GU: RFT abnormalities

HEME: ***Leukopenia, granulocytopenia, thrombocytopenia***

MISC: Pain on inj

SPECIAL CONSIDERATIONS

MONITORING PARAMETERS

• Does not eliminate the potential for anthracycline-induced cardiac toxicity; carefully monitor cardiac function

dextroamphetamine

(dex-troe-am-fet'a-meen)

Dexedrine, Dexedrine Spansules, Oxydess II, Spancap #1, Dextrostat

Chemical Class: Amphetamine

Therapeutic Class: Cerebral stimulant

DEA Class: Schedule II

CLINICAL PHARMACOLOGY

Mechanism of Action: Increases release of norepinephrine and dopamine in cerebral cortex and reticular activating system; promotes norepinephrine release from peripheral adrenergic nerve terminals

Pharmacokinetics

PO: Onset 30 min, peak 1-3 hr, duration 4-20 hr; metabolized by liver; urine excretion pH dependent (greater excretion with acidic urine); crosses placenta; $t_{1/2}$ 10-30 hr

INDICATIONS AND USES: Narcolepsy, attention deficit disorder with hyperactivity, exogenous obesity

DOSAGE

Adult

• *Narcolepsy:* PO 5-60 mg qd in divided doses

• *Obesity:* PO 10-15 mg qd (sus rel) in AM or 5-30 mg/day in divided doses of 5-10 mg, administer 30-60 min ac

Child

• *Narcolepsy:* Age >12 yr PO 10 mg qd increasing by 10 mg qd at weekly intervals; age 6-12 yr PO 5 mg qd increasing by 5 mg/wk (max 60 mg qd)

• *Obesity:* Age >12 yr PO same as adult

• *Attention deficit disorder:* Age >6 yr PO 5 mg qd-bid increasing by 5 mg qd at weekly intervals; age 3-6 yr PO 2.5 mg qd increasing by 2.5 mg qd at weekly intervals (max dose 40 mg/d)

$ AVAILABLE FORMS/COST OF THERAPY

• Tab, Uncoated—Oral: 5 mg, 100's: **$17.33-$19.86;** 10 mg, 100's: **$29.80**

• Cap, Gel, Sust Action—Oral: 5, 10, 15 mg, 50's: **$20.30-$32.30**

CONTRAINDICATIONS: Hypersensitivity, hyperthyroidism, hypertension, glaucoma, drug abuse, cardiovascular disease, anxiety, within 14 days of taking MAOIs

PRECAUTIONS: Tourette syndrome, child <3 yr; amphetamines have a high abuse potential

PREGNANCY AND LACTATION: Pregnancy category C; excreted in breast milk

SIDE EFFECTS/ADVERSE REACTIONS

CNS: Hyperactivity, insomnia, restlessness, talkativeness, dizziness, headache, chills, stimulation, dysphoria, irritability, aggressiveness, tremor, ***dependence, addiction***

CV: Palpitations, tachycardia, hypertension, decrease in heart rate, ***dysrhythmias, cardiomyopathy***

GI: Anorexia, dry mouth, diarrhea, constipation, weight loss, metallic taste

GU: Impotence, change in libido

SKIN: Urticaria

▼ **DRUG INTERACTIONS**

Drugs

- *Acetazolamide:* Reduced urinary excretion of dextroamphetamine
- *Antacids and sodium bicarbonate:* Increased GI absorption, decreased urinary excretion of dextroamphetamine
- *Tricyclic antidepressants:* Activity enhanced by dextroamphetamine
- *Furazolidone+, monoamine oxidase inhibitors+, phenelzine+, tranylcypromine+:* Hypertensive crisis due to dextroamphetamine
- *Guanadrel and guanethidine:* Inhibited by dextroamphetamine

Labs

- *Increase:* Elevation in plasma corticosteroid levels
- *Decrease:* Interfere with urinary steroid determinations

SPECIAL CONSIDERATIONS

PATIENT/FAMILY EDUCATION

- Tolerance or dependency is common
- Avoid OTC preparations unless approved by physician

dextromethorphan

(dex-troe-meth-or'fan)

Benylin DM, Bromfed DM, Children's Hold, Delsym, Dimetane DX, Hold DM, Naldecon DX, Pertussin, Pertussin ES, Robitussin Cough Calmers, Robitussin Pediatric, St. Joseph Cough Suppressant, Sucrets Cough Control, Suppress, TheraFlu, Triaminic DM, Trocal, Vicks Formula 44

Chemical Class: Levorphanol derivative

Therapeutic Class: Antitussive, nonnarcotic

CLINICAL PHARMACOLOGY

Mechanism of Action: Depresses cough center in medulla

Pharmacokinetics

PO: Onset 15-30 min, duration 3-6 hr

INDICATIONS AND USES: Nonproductive cough

DOSAGE

Adult

- PO 10-20 mg q4h, or 30 mg q6-8h, not to exceed 120 mg/d
- PO EXT-REL LIQ 60 mg bid, not to exceed 120 mg/d

Child

- PO: Age 6-12 yr 5-10 mg q4h, not to exceed 60 mg/d; age 2-6 yr 2.5-5 mg q4h, not to exceed 30 mg/d; EXT-REL LIQ Age 6-12 yr 30 mg bid, not to exceed 60 mg/d; age 2-6 yr 7.5 mg q6-8h, not to exceed 30 mg/d

$ **AVAILABLE FORMS/COST OF THERAPY**

- Loz—Oral: 5 mg, 24's: **$3.39**
- Syr—Oral: 5, 7.5, 10, 15 mg/5 ml, 120 ml: **$3.00**
- Liq, Ext-Rel—Oral: 30 mg/5 ml, 90 ml: **$4.33**

CONTRAINDICATIONS: Hypersensitivity to any component

PRECAUTIONS: Chronic, persistent, or productive cough; nausea/vomiting; fever; persistent headache

PREGNANCY AND LACTATION: Pregnancy category C

SIDE EFFECTS/ADVERSE REACTIONS

CNS: Dizziness

GI: Nausea

▼ **DRUG INTERACTIONS**

Drugs

- *Isocarboxazid, MAOIs, phenelzine:* Increased risk of toxicity due to dextromethorphan
- *Quinidine:* Reduced hepatic metabolism of dextromethorphan

---

dezocine

Dalgan

Chemical Class: Opioid, synthetic, aminotetralin series

Therapeutic Class: Narcotic agonist-antagonist analgesic

CLINICAL PHARMACOLOGY

Mechanism of Action: Depresses pain impulse transmission at the spinal cord level by interacting with opioid receptors

Pharmacokinetics

IM: Onset 30 min, peak 50-90 min, duration 2-4 hr

IV: Onset 10 min, peak 30 min, duration 2-4 hr

Metabolized by liver; excreted by kidneys; may cross placenta

INDICATIONS AND USES: Severe pain

DOSAGE

Adult

- IM 5-20 mg q3-6h, not to exceed 120 mg/d; IV 2.5-10 mg q2-4h

$ **AVAILABLE FORMS/COST OF THERAPY**

- Inj, Sol—IM; IV: 5 mg/ml: **$6.85-$7.28**

CONTRAINDICATIONS: Hypersensitivity

PRECAUTIONS: Patients physically dependent on narcotics (may precipitate withdrawal), addictive personality, increased intracranial pressure, respiratory depression, hepatic disease, renal disease, child <18 yr, elderly, biliary surgery, COPD, sulfite sensitivity

PREGNANCY AND LACTATION: Pregnancy category C

SIDE EFFECTS/ADVERSE REACTIONS

CNS: Drowsiness, dizziness, confusion, sedation, anxiety, headache, depression, delirium, sleep disturbances, dependency

CV: Hypotension, pulse irregularity, hypertension, chest pain, pallor, edema, thrombophlebitis

EENT: Blurred vision, slurred speech, diplopia

GI: Nausea, vomiting, anorexia, constipation, cramps, abdominal pain, dry mouth, diarrhea

GU: Urinary frequency, hesitancy, retention

RESP: ***Respiratory depression,*** hiccoughs

SKIN: Inj site reactions, pruritus, rash, sweating, chills

---

diazepam

(dye-az'e-pam)

Apo-Diazepam, ✤ E-Pam, ✤ Meval, ✤ Neo-calme, ✤ Novodipam, ✤ Q-Pam, Rival, ✤ Valium, Valrelease, Vivol ✤

Chemical Class: Benzodiazepine

Therapeutic Class: Antianxiety, amnestic, anticonvulsant, skeletal muscle relaxant, antitremor

DEA Class: Schedule IV

CLINICAL PHARMACOLOGY

Mechanism of Action: CNS depressant; potentiates the actions of

GABA, which mediates both pre- and post-synaptic inhibition in all regions of the CNS

Pharmacokinetics

PO: Rapidly absorbed; onset 15-45 min; peak, 0.5-1½ hr; duration 2-3 hr

IM: Absorption slow and erratic (deltoid muscle optimal site); onset 15-30 min; peak, 0.5-1½ hr; duration 1-1½ hr

IV: Onset 1-3 min, duration 15 min

Metabolized by liver, excreted by kidneys, crosses the blood-brain barrier; $t_{1/2}$ 20-50 hr

INDICATIONS AND USES: Anxiety, acute alcohol withdrawal, adjunctive anesthesia, amnesia in cardioversion, endoscopic procedures, etc., conscious sedation, insomnia, status epilepticus, adjunct in seizure disorders, skeletal muscle spasm relaxation, tremor,* tension headache,* panic disorder*

DOSAGE

Adult

- *Anxiety/convulsive disorders:* PO 2-10 mg tid-qid; EXT REL 15-30 mg qd
- *Sedative-hypnotic, alcohol withdrawal:* PO 10 mg tid-qid, tapered prn
- *Skeletal muscle relaxant:* PO 2-10 mg tid-qid
- *Status epilepticus:* IV BOL 5-20 mg, 2 mg/min, may repeat q5-10 min, not to exceed 60 mg; may repeat in 30 min if seizures reappear

Geriatric

- 2-2.5 mg qd-bid; titrated prn

Child

- IV BOL 0.1-0.3 mg/kg (over 3 min); may repeat q15 min × 2 doses
- *Tetanic muscle spasms:* Infants >30 days to <5 yr IM/IV 1-2 mg to 5-10 mg q3-4h prn
- *Anxiety/convulsive disorders:* >6 mo PO 1-2.5 mg tid-qid (0.04-0.2 mg/kg tid-qid prn)

$ **AVAILABLE FORMS/COST OF THERAPY**

- Inj, Sol—IM;IV: 5 mg/ml, 2 ml: **$2.59-$5.18**
- Tab, Uncoated—Oral: 2, 5, 10 mg, 100's: **$1.85-$102.64**
- Cap, Gel, Sust Action—Oral: 15 mg, 100's: **$172.10**
- Sol—Oral: 5 mg/5ml, 500 ml: **$38.79**

CONTRAINDICATIONS: Hypersensitivity to benzodiazepines, narrow angle glaucoma, psychosis

PRECAUTIONS: Elderly, debilitated, hepatic disease, renal disease, children, low serum albumin

PREGNANCY AND LACTATION: Pregnancy category D; drug and metabolite enter breast milk; M:P ratio 0.2:2.7; lethargy and loss of weight reported

SIDE EFFECTS/ADVERSE REACTIONS

CNS: Dizziness, drowsiness, confusion, headache, anxiety, tremors, stimulation, fatigue, depression, insomnia, hallucinations, withdrawal syndrome

CV: Orthostatic hypotension, ***ECG changes, tachycardia,*** hypotension; venous thrombosis, phlebitis, local irritation, swelling, and vascular impairment following IV inj into small veins on hand

EENT: Blurred vision, tinnitus, mydriasis

GI: Constipation, dry mouth, nausea, vomiting, anorexia, diarrhea

SKIN: Rash, dermatitis, itching

▼ **DRUG INTERACTIONS**

Drugs

- *Cimetidine:* Inhibits metabolism of diazepam with increased diazepam levels and adverse effects
- *Clozapine:* Several reports of cardiorespiratory collapse, causal relationship not established

D

• *Disulfiram:* Increased diazepam concentration via inhibiting oxidative metabolism
• *Ethanol:* Enhanced adverse psychomotor effects of diazepam; combined use dangerous in patients performing tasks requiring alertness
• *Oral contraceptives:* Increased diazepam concentration via inhibiting oxidative metabolism
• *Rifampin:* Reduced diazepam concentration

Labs

• *Increase:* AST/ALT, serum bilirubin
• *False increase:* 17-OHCS
• *Decrease:* RAIU

SPECIAL CONSIDERATIONS

• Flumazenil (Mazicon), a benzodiazepine receptor antagonist is indicated for complete or partial reversal of the sedative effects of benzodiazepines

PATIENT/FAMILY EDUCATION

• Avoid driving, activities that require alertness; drowsiness may occur
• Avoid alcohol, other psychotropic medications unless prescribed by physician

diazoxide

(dye-az-ox'ide)

Hyperstat, Proglycem

Chemical Class: Benzothiadiazine

Therapeutic Class: Antihypertensive, hyperglycemic

CLINICAL PHARMACOLOGY

Mechanism of Action: Vasodilates arteriolar smooth muscle by direct relaxation; reduction in blood pressure with concomitant increases in heart rate, cardiac output; decreases release of insulin from β-cells in pancreas, resulting in an increase in blood glucose

Pharmacokinetics

PO: Onset 1 hr, duration 8 hr

IV: Onset 1-2 min, peak 5 min, duration 3-12 hr

$t_{1/2}$ 20-36 hr, excreted slowly in urine, crosses blood-brain barrier, placenta

INDICATIONS AND USES: Hypertensive crisis when urgent decrease of diastolic pressure required; increase blood glucose levels in hyperinsulinism

DOSAGE

Adult

• *Hypertension:* IV BOL 1-3 mg/kg rapidly up to a max of 150 mg in a single inj; dose may be repeated at 5-15 min intervals until desired response is achieved; give IV in 30 sec or less
• *Hypoglycemia:* PO initial 1 mg/kg q8h, adjusted prn according to response; maintenance 3-8 mg/kg/d given bid-tid (max 15 mg/kg/d)

Child

• *Hypertension:* IV BOL 1-2 mg/kg rapidly; administration same as adult, not to exceed 150 mg
• *Hypoglycemia:* PO initial 3.3 mg/kg q8h, adjusted prn; maintenance 8-15 mg/kg/d given bid-tid

$ AVAILABLE FORMS/COST OF THERAPY

• Inj, Sol—IV: 15 mg/ml, 20 ml: **$42.41-$88.47**
• Cap—Oral: 50 mg, 100's: **$152.69**
• Susp—Oral: 50 mg/ml, 30 ml: **$105.88**

CONTRAINDICATIONS: Hypersensitivity to thiazides, sulfonamides; hypertension associated with aortic coarctation or AV shunt; pheochromocytoma; dissecting aortic aneurysm; functional hypoglycemia

PRECAUTIONS: Tachycardia; fluid, electrolyte imbalances; lactation; impaired cerebral or cardiac circulation; gout; diabetes mellitus

PREGNANCY AND LACTATION: Pregnancy category C

SIDE EFFECTS/ADVERSE REACTIONS

CNS: ***TIAs,*** sleepiness, euphoria, anxiety, EPS, confusion, tinnitus, blurred vision, dizziness, weakness, headache, malaise, insomnia, paresthesia

CV: ***Hypotension,*** T-wave changes, angina pectoris, palpitations, ***supraventricular tachycardia, edema,*** rebound hypertension

EENT: Diplopia, cataracts, ring scotoma, subconjunctival hemorrhage, lacrimation

GI: Changes in ability to taste, nausea, vomiting, dry mouth

GU: Reversible nephrotic syndrome, increased BUN, decreased urinary output, hematuria

HEME: Decreased hemoglobin/hematocrit, ***thrombocytopenia***

METAB: Hyperglycemia, hyperuricemia

SKIN: Rash, hypertrichosis

MISC: Allergic reactions, breast tenderness

▼ DRUG INTERACTIONS

Drugs

- *Hydralazine:* Severe hypotensive reactions
- *Phenytoin:* Decreased phenytoin levels in children, probably enhanced metabolism
- *Thiazide diuretics:* Hyperglycemia

SPECIAL CONSIDERATIONS

- Often administered concurrently with a diuretic to prevent congestive heart failure due to fluid retention
- Oral susp dosage form produces higher concentration than cap form
- Hyperglycemia transient (24-48 hr) after IV administration
- If not effective within 2-3 wk of treatment of hypoglycemia, reevaluate

dibucaine

(dye'byoo-kane)

Nupercainal

Chemical Class: Amide

Therapeutic Class: Topical anesthetic

CLINICAL PHARMACOLOGY

Mechanism of Action: Inhibits nerve impulses from sensory nerves

Pharmacokinetics

TOP: Onset up to 15 min; duration 3-4 hr; readily systemically absorbed through traumatized or abraded skin; hepatic and some renal biotransformation; renally excreted as metabolites

INDICATIONS AND USES: Pruritus, pain, sunburn, toothache, rectal pain and irritation, dermatitis (e.g., poison ivy), minor wounds

DOSAGE

Adult and Child

- TOP apply qid as needed

$ AVAILABLE FORMS/COST OF THERAPY

- Oint—Top: 1%, 30 g: **$1.80**
- Cre—Top: 0.5%, 45 g: **$1.00**

CONTRAINIDCATIONS: Hypersensitivity, infants <1 yr, application to large areas

PRECAUTIONS: Child <6 yr, sepsis, denuded skin

PREGNANCY AND LACTATION: Pregnancy category C

SIDE EFFECTS/ADVERSE REACTIONS

SKIN: Rash, irritation, sensitization

SPECIAL CONSIDERATIONS

Cross-sensitivity between amide derivatives and ester anesthetics or pramoxine has not been reported

dichlorphenamide

(die-klor-fen'a-mide)
Daranide
Chemical Class: Non-bacteriostatic sulfonamide
Therapeutic Class: Carbonic anhydrase inhibitor

CLINICAL PHARMACOLOGY
Mechanism of Action: Carbonic anhydrase inhibition reduces rate of aqueous humor formation, decreased intraocular pressure; inhibits hydrogen ion secretion in renal tubule with increased secretion of sodium, potassium, bicarbonate, and water
Pharmacokinetics
PO: Onset, 1 hr; peak effect, 2-4 hr; duration, 6-12 hr
INDICATIONS AND USES: Glaucoma, open-angle and angle-closure
DOSAGE
Adult
• 100-200 mg initially; then 100 mg q12h to response; maintenance 25-50 mg qd-tid
$ AVAILABLE FORMS/COST OF THERAPY
• Tab, Uncoated—Oral: 50 mg, 100's: **$50.11**
CONTRAINDICATIONS: Hepatic insufficiency, renal failure, adrenocortical insufficiency, hyperchloremic acidosis, hypokalemia, hyponatremia, impaired alveolar ventilation (pulmonary disease, edema, infection, or obstruction), and hypersensitivity
PRECAUTIONS: Hypokalemia when cirrhosis is present, or during concomitant use of steroids or ACTH; respiratory acidosis
PREGNANCY AND LACTATION: Pregnancy category C; safety in lactation not established
SIDE EFFECTS/ADVERSE REACTIONS
CNS: Convulsions, *weakness, malaise, fatigue,* nervousness, drowsiness, depression, dizziness, disorientation, confusion, ataxia, tremor, headache, lassitude, *paresthesias of the extremities*
EENT: Myopia, tinnitus,
GI: Melena, *anorexia, nausea, vomiting,* constipation, *taste alteration, diarrhea,* hepatic insufficiency
GU: Hematuria, glycosuria, *urinary frequency,* renal colic, renal calculi, phosphaturia, decreased libido, impotence
HEME: ***Blood dyscrasias***
METAB: Hypokalemia
MS: Flaccid paralysis
RESP: ***Acidosis*** (shortness of breath, troubled breathing)
SKIN: Urticaria, pruritus, skin eruptions, rash, ***Stevens-Johnson syndrome,*** photosensitivity
MISC: Weight loss, fever, hypersensitivity
▼ DRUG INTERACTIONS
Drugs
• *Amphetamines:* Increased amphetamine serum levels
• *Ephedrine:* Increased ephedrine serum levels
• *Methenamine compounds:* Alkalinization of urine decreases antibacterial effects
• *Phenytoin:* Increased risk of osteomalacia
• *Quinidine:* Alkalinization of urine increases quinidine serum levels
• *Salicylates:* Increased serum levels of carbonic anhydrase inhibitors, CNS toxicity
Labs
• *Increase:* Blood glucose levels, bilirubin, blood ammonia, calcium, chloride
• *Decrease:* Urine citrate, potassium
• *False positive:* Urinary protein, 17 OHCS

SPECIAL CONSIDERATIONS
PATIENT/FAMILY EDUCATION
- May cause drowsiness

diclofenac

(dye-kloe'fen-ac)
Voltaren, Voltaren SR (sodium), Cataflam (potassium)
Chemical Class: Phenylacetic acid
Therapeutic Class: Nonsteroidal antiinflammatory

CLINICAL PHARMACOLOGY
Mechanism of Action: Inhibits prostaglandin synthesis by decreasing enzyme needed for biosynthesis; analgesic, antiinflammatory, antipyretic properties
Pharmacokinetics
PO: Time to peak, sodium salt 2-3 hr, potassium salt 30 min; peak 0.28 g/ml; $t_{1/2}$, 2 hr, synovial $t_{1/2}$ 3 times longer. Completely absorbed, 99.7% bound to plasma proteins; metabolized in liver, 50% bioavailable after 1st pass, excreted in urine and bile
OPHTH: Limited systemic absorption
INDICATIONS AND USES: Acute, chronic rheumatoid arthritis, osteoarthritis, ankylosing spondylitis; acute pain; dysmenorrhea; management of postoperative inflammation following cataract extraction
DOSAGE
Adult
- *Osteoarthritis:* PO 100-150 mg/d in divided doses
- *Rheumatoid arthritis:* PO 150-200 mg/d in divided doses
- *Ankylosing spondylitis:* PO 100-125 mg/d; give 25 mg qid and 25 mg hs if needed
- *Pain, dysmenorrhea:* PO 50 mg tid; loading dose (100 mg) useful in some patients
- *Postoperative/cataracts:* TOP 1 gtt qid, starting 24 hr after surgery for 2 wk

$ AVAILABLE FORMS/COST OF THERAPY
Sodium
- Tab, Enteric Coated, Sust Action—Oral: 25 mg, 100's: **$49.23;** 50 mg, 100's: **$95.70;** 75 mg, 100's: **$115.90**
- Sol—Ophth: 0.1%, 5 ml: **$28.26**

Potassium
- Tab, Uncoated—Oral: 50 mg, 100's: **$135.20**

CONTRAINDICATIONS: Hypersensitivity to aspirin, iodides, other NSAIDs
PRECAUTIONS: Geriatric patients, bleeding disorders, GI disorders, cardiac disorders, hypersensitivity to other antiinflammatory agents, asthma
PREGNANCY AND LACTATION: Pregnancy category B; excreted in breast milk
SIDE EFFECTS/ADVERSE REACTIONS
CNS: Dizziness, drowsiness, fatigue, tremors, confusion, insomnia, anxiety, depression, nervousness, paresthesia, muscle weakness
CV: ***CHF,*** tachycardia, peripheral edema, palpitations, ***dysrhythmias, hypotension,*** hypertension, fluid retention
EENT: Tinnitus, hearing loss, blurred vision; OPHTH: burning, irritation, keratitis, elevated IOP, anterior chamber reaction, ocular allergy
GI: Nausea, anorexia, vomiting, diarrhea, ***jaundice, cholestatic hepatitis,*** constipation, flatulence, cramps, dry mouth, peptic ulcer, ***GI bleeding***
GU: ***Nephrotoxicity,*** dysuria, hematuria, ***oliguria, azotemia,*** cystitis, UTI
HEME: ***Blood dyscrasias,*** epistaxis, bruising

RESP: Dyspnea, hemoptysis, pharyngitis, ***bronchospasm, laryngeal edema,*** rhinitis, shortness of breath
SKIN: Purpura, rash, pruritus, sweating, erythema, petechiae, photosensitivity, alopecia

▼ DRUG INTERACTIONS

Drugs

- *ACE inhibitors, β-blockers, hydralazine:* Decreased antihypertensive effect
- *Diuretics:* Decreased diuretic and antihypertensive effect
- *Aminoglycosides, cyclosporine, lithium, methotrexate:* Increased serum levels and potential for toxicity
- *Cholestyramine, colestipol:* Decreased diclofenac levels with reduced therapeutic effect
- *Potassium sparing diuretics:* Some patients develop acute renal failure when NSAIDs and K-sparing diuretics are co-administered

SPECIAL CONSIDERATIONS

MONITORING PARAMETERS

- RFTs, serum potassium, CBC, stool tests for occult blood
- LFTs with chronic use

diclonine

(dye'clo-neen)
Dyclone
Chemical Class: Pramoxine derivative
Therapeutic Class: Topical anesthetic

CLINICAL PHARMACOLOGY

Mechanism of Action: Blocks nerve impulses at sensory nerve endings in the skin and mucous membranes

Pharmacokinetics

TOP: Onset 2-10 min, duration 30 min

INDICATIONS AND USES: Anesthetizing accessible mucous membranes (e.g., the mouth, pharynx, larynx, trachea, esophagus, and urethra) prior to endoscopic procedures; blocking the gag reflex; relieving pain associated with oral ulcers of stomatitis, postoperative wounds, and ano-genital lesions

DOSAGE

Adult

- Apply to desired area as a rinse, gargle, mouthwash, spray, wet compress, or swab prn; do not exceed 30 ml of 1% sol (300 mg)

$ AVAILABLE FORMS/COST OF THERAPY

- Sol—Top: 0.5%, 30 ml: **$27.60;** 1%, 30 ml: **$37.19**

CONTRAINDICATIONS: Hypersensitivity

PRECAUTIONS: Traumatized mucosa, sepsis in region intended for application, shock, heart block, child <12 yr

PREGNANCY AND LACTATION: Pregnancy category C; excretion into breast milk unknown

SIDE EFFECTS/ADVERSE REACTIONS

CNS: Excitation, depression, nervousness, dizziness, tremors, ***seizures,*** unconsciousness, drowsiness
CV: ***Myocardial depression, hypotension,*** bradycardia, ***cardiac arrest***
EENT: Blurred vision
GU: Urethritis (when used for urethral anesthesia)
RESP: ***Respiratory arrest***
SKIN: Slight irritation, stinging, urticaria, swelling, edema

SPECIAL CONSIDERATIONS

PATIENT/FAMILY EDUCATION

- Do not ingest food for 1 hr following use in the mouth or throat (increased risk of aspiration)
- Do not chew food or gum while mouth or throat area is anesthetized
- Avoid too frequent dosing to prevent accumulation and systemic side effects

dicloxacillin

(dye-klox'a-sill-in)

Dycill, Dynapen, Pathocil

Chemical Class: Penicillinase-resistant penicillin

Therapeutic Class: Broad-spectrum antibiotic

CLINICAL PHARMACOLOGY

Mechanism of Action: Bactericidal via cell wall synthesis inhibition

Pharmacokinetics

PO: Peak 1 hr, duration 4-6 hr; $t_{1/2}$, 30-60 min; absorption stable to acid; concurrent food decreases absorption; 98% plasma protein bound, excreted unchanged in urine

INDICATIONS AND USES: Infections of the upper respiratory tract, bone, and localized skin and skin structure caused by susceptible organisms. Antibacterial spectrum usually includes: gram-positive organisms: *Staphylococcus aureus, Streptococcus pyogenes, S. viridans, S. faecalis, S. bovis, S. pneumoniae,* including those producing penicillinase

DOSAGE

Adult

- PO 0.5-4 g/d in divided doses q6h

Child

- PO 12.5-25 mg/kg in divided doses q6h, max 4 g/d

$ AVAILABLE FORMS/COST OF THERAPY

- Cap, Gel—Oral: 250 mg, 100's: **$19.43-$93.96;** 500 mg, 100's: **$37.43-$76.85**
- Powder, Reconstitution—Oral: 62.5 mg/5 ml, 200 ml: **$15.53**

CONTRAINDICATIONS: Hypersensitivity to penicillins

PRECAUTIONS: Hypersensitivity to cephalosporins; asthma, eczema, mononucleosis

PREGNANCY AND LACTATION: Pregnancy category B; penicillins are excreted into breast milk in low concentrations, compatible with breast feeding

SIDE EFFECTS/ADVERSE REACTIONS

CNS: Lethargy, hallucinations, anxiety, depression, twitching, ***coma, convulsions***

GI: Nausea, vomiting, diarrhea, increased AST, ALT, abdominal pain, glossitis, colitis

GU: ***Oliguria, proteinuria, hematuria,*** *vaginitis, moniliasis,* ***glomerulonephritis***

HEME: Anemia, increased bleeding time, ***bone marrow depression, granulocytopenia***

▼ DRUG INTERACTIONS

Drugs

- *Aspirin, probenecid:* Increased dicloxacillin concentrations
- *Methotrexate:* Increased concentrations, increased potential for toxicity
- *Oral anticoagulants:* Reduced hypoprothrombinemic effects
- *Oral contraceptives:* Impaired contraceptive efficacy
- *Tetracyclines, chloramphenicol:* Decreased antimicrobial effectiveness of dicloxacillin

Labs

- *False positive:* Urine glucose, urine protein

SPECIAL CONSIDERATIONS

PATIENT/FAMILY EDUCATION

- Should be taken with water, 1 hr before or 2 hr after meals on an empty stomach

MONITORING PARAMETERS

- CBC, UA, RFTs, LFT periodically during prolonged therapy

dicumarol

(die-coom'er-all)

Chemical Class: Coumarin derivative

Therapeutic Class: Anticoagulant

CLINICAL PHARMACOLOGY

Mechanism of Action: Interferes with hepatic synthesis of vitamin-K dependent clotting factors (factors VII, IX, X, II); anticoagulant effects are dependent on the $t_{1/2}$, which are 6, 24, 36, and 50 hr, respectively

Pharmacokinetics

PO: $t_{1/2}$ 1-4 days; onset of action 1-5 days; duration of action, 2-10 days; onset and duration of effect dependent on depletion of clotting factors and varies in relation to factor half-lives; slow and incomplete absorption; >99% plasma protein bound, metabolized by hepatic microsomal enzymes; excreted as inactive metabolites in the urine and feces

INDICATIONS AND USES: Prophylaxis and treatment of deep venous thrombosis and pulmonary thromboembolism; prophylaxis of embolism associated with atrial fibrillation, MI, cardioversion of chronic atrial fibrillation, prosthetic heart valves, cerebral embolism

DOSAGE

Adult

- PO 25-200 mg/d, as indicated by prothrombin-time determinations

$ AVAILABLE FORMS/COST OF THERAPY

- Tab, Uncoated—Oral: 25 mg, 100's: **$9.94**

CONTRAINDICATIONS: Pregnancy; hemorrhagic tendencies; hemophilia; thrombocytopenic purpura; leukemia; recent or contemplated surgery of the eye or CNS; major regional lumbar block anesthesia, or surgery resulting in large, open surfaces; patients bleeding from the GI, respiratory, or GU tract; threatened abortion; aneurysm; ascorbic acid deficiency; history of bleeding diathesis; prostatectomy; continuous tube drainage of the small intestine; polyarthritis; diverticulitis; emaciation; malnutrition; cerebrovascular hemorrhage; eclampsia and preeclampsia; blood dyscrasias; severe uncontrolled or malignant hypertension; severe renal or hepatic disease; pericarditis and pericardial effusion; subacute bacterial endocarditis; visceral carcinoma; following spinal puncture and other diagnostic or therapeutic procedures with potential for uncontrollable bleeding; history of warfarin-induced necrosis

PRECAUTIONS: Patient selection (ensure cooperation, alcoholics, senile, psychotic); enhanced anticoagulant effects (carcinoma, hepatic disorders, vitamin K deficiency, steatorrhea, CHF, diarrhea, renal insufficiency, hyperthyroidism); decreased anticoagulant effects (edema, hyperlipidemia, diabetes mellitus, hypothyroidism, hereditary resistance to oral anticoagulants)

PREGNANCY AND LACTATION: Pregnancy category D; no adverse effect or any change in PT times have been noted in nursing infants; compatible with breast feeding

SIDE EFFECTS/ADVERSE REACTIONS

CV: Systemic cholesterol microembolization (purple toes syndrome)

GI: Nausea, diarrhea, sore mouth, mouth ulcers, paralytic ileus, intestinal obstruction from submucosal or intramural hemorrhage

GU: Red-orange urine

HEME: ***Hemorrhage***

METAB: Pyrexia, adrenal insufficiency
SKIN: ***Skin necrosis,*** dermatitis, exfoliative dermatitis, urticaria, alopecia
MISC: Hypersensitivity reactions

▼ **DRUG INTERACTIONS**

Drugs

• *Antithyroid drugs+, danazole+, salicylates+:* Increased anticoagulant effect via decreased hepatic synthesis of procoagulant factors
• *Allopurinol, amiodarone+, chloramphenicol, cimetidine, cotrimoxazole+, erythromycin, ethanol (acute ingestion), azoles (fluconazole, itraconazole, ketoconazole, miconazole), metronidazole+, phenylbutazone+, phenylramidol+, propafenone, quinolones (ciprafloxacin, norfloxacin, ofloxacin), sulfinpyrazone+:* Increased anticoagulant effect via inhibition of enzymatic metabolism of anticoagulant
• *Anabolic steroids+, cephalosporins (cefamandole, cefmetazole, cefoperazone, cefotetan, moxalactam), clofibrate+, thyroid hormones+:* Increased anticoagulant effect via alteration of procoagulant factor synthesis or catabolism
• *Anabolic steroids+, thyroid hormones+:* Increased anticoagulant effect via increased receptor affinity for anticoagulant
• *Aminoglycosides, binding resins:* Increase in anticoagulant effect via decreased vitamin K synthesis secondary to alterations in intestinal flora
• *Antidiabetics (initially), chloral hydrate (initially), clofibrate+, cotrimoxazole+, HMG-CoA reductase inhibitors, nalidixic acid, phenylbutasone+, phenytoin, salicylates+, sulfonamides, sulfinpyrazone+, triclofos:* Increase in anticoagulant effect via displacement of anitcoagulant from protein-binding sites
• *Glucagon, vitamin E:* Increased anticoagulant effect, mechanism unknown
• *Heparin:* Increased anticoagulant effect via severe factor IX deficiency
• *NSAIDs, salicylates+:* Inhibition of platelet aggregation, potential for GI ulceration or hemorrhage during therapy
• *Aminoglutethimide, barbiturates+, carbamazepine, ethanol (chronic), glutethimide, griseofulvin, nafcillin, phenytoin, pyrimidone+, rifampin+:* Decreased anticoagulant effect via accelerated metabolism of anticoagulant secondary to stimulation of hepatic microsomal enzyme activity
• *Binding resins:* Decreased anticoagulant effect via decreased absorption of anticoagulant from GI tract
• *Antidiabetics (with continued use):* Decreased anticoagulant effect via increased metabolism of anticoagulant
• *Vitamin K:* Decreased anticoagulant effect via increased hepatic synthesis of procoagulant factors

SPECIAL CONSIDERATIONS

• Warfarin is the coumarin anticoagulant of choice

MONITORING PARAMETERS:

• Dosage of anticoagulants must be individualized and adjusted according to PT determinations; it is recommended that PT determinations be performed prior to initiation of therapy, at 24-hr intervals while maintenance dosage is being established, then once or twice weekly for the following 3-4 wks, then at 1-4 wk intervals for the duration of treatment

dicyclomine

(dye-sye'kloe-meen)
Antispas, Bentyl, Bentylol, ✤ Byclomine, Dibent, Di-Spaz, Formulex, ✤ Neoquess, OR-Tyl, Spasmoject, Viserol
Chemical Class: Synthetic tertiary amine
Therapeutic Class: Gastrointestinal anticholinergic

CLINICAL PHARMACOLOGY
Mechanism of Action: Inhibits muscarinic actions of acetylcholine at postganglionic parasympathetic neuroeffector sites
Pharmacokinetics
PO: Onset 1-2 hr, duration 3-4 hr; metabolized by liver; $t_{1/2}$ (initial phase, 1.8 hr, secondary phase, 9-10 hr), excreted in urine
INDICATIONS AND USES: Irritable bowel syndrome, adjunctive treatment of peptic ulcer disease, infant colic
DOSAGE
Adult
• PO 10-20 mg tid-qid prn; IM 20 mg q4-6h prn
Child >2 yr
• PO 10 mg tid-qid prn
Child 6 mo-2 yr
• PO 5 mg tid-qid prn
$ AVAILABLE FORMS/COST OF THERAPY
• Cap, Gel—Oral: 10 mg, 100's: **$3.30-$24.36**
• Inj, Sol—IM: 10 mg/ml, 2 ml × 5: **$62.46;** 10 mg/ml, 10 ml: **$8.75-$39.90**
• Syr—Oral: 10 mg/5 ml, 480 ml: **$7.00-$27.12**
• Tab, Uncoated—Oral: 20 mg, 100's: **$2.85-$34.80**
CONTRAINDICATIONS: Hypersensitivity to anticholinergics, narrow angle glaucoma, GI obstruction, myasthenia gravis, paralytic ileus, GI atony, toxic megacolon
PRECAUTIONS: Hyperthyroidism, coronary artery disease, dysrhythmias, CHF, ulcerative colitis, hypertension, hiatal hernia, hepatic disease, renal disease, urinary retention, prostatic hypertrophy
PREGNANCY AND LACTATION: Pregnancy category B; (single case report of infant apnea) avoid in nursing women
SIDE EFFECTS/ADVERSE REACTIONS
CNS: Confusion, stimulation in elderly, headache, insomnia, dizziness, drowsiness, anxiety, weakness, hallucination; ***seizures, coma*** (child <3 mo)
CV: Palpitations, tachycardia
EENT: Blurred vision, photophobia, mydriasis, cycloplegia, increased ocular tension
GI: Dry mouth, constipation, ***paralytic ileus,*** heartburn, nausea, vomiting, dysphagia, absence of taste
GU: Hesitancy, rentention, impotence
SKIN: Urticaria, rash, pruritus, anhidrosis, fever, allergic reactions
▼ DRUG INTERACTIONS
Drugs
• *Amantadine, tricyclic antidepressants, MAOIs, H_1 antihistamines:* Increased anticholinergic effects
• *Phenothiazines, levodopa, ketoconazole:* Decreased therapeutic effects
• *Potassium chloride, wax matrix preparations:* Increased risk of KCl-induced gastrointestinal lesions
Labs
• *False negative:* Gastric acid secretion test

SPECIAL CONSIDERATIONS
PATIENT/FAMILY EDUCATION
• Suggest gum, hard candy, frequent rinsing of mouth for dryness of oral cavity

didanosine

(dye-dan'o-seen)

Videx, ddI, Dideoxyinosine

Chemical Class: Synthetic purine nucleoside of deoxyadenosine

Therapeutic Class: Anti-retroviral

CLINICAL PHARMACOLOGY

Mechanism of Action: Nucleoside analog, incorporates into viral DNA, leading to chain termination. Interferes with viral replication by inhibiting reverse transcriptase

Pharmacokinetics

PO: Peak, 0.5-1 hr; $t_{1/2}$, 1.6 hr; acid labile (administration with meal decreases peak concentrations and AUC); bioavailability variable, average 30%; extensive metabolism; renal elimination accounts for 50%, no accumulation reported

INDICATIONS AND USES: Advanced HIV infections in adults and children who have been unable to use zidovudine or who have not responded to treatment

DOSAGE

Adult

• PO >75 kg, 300 mg tab bid, or 375 mg buffered powder bid; 50-74 kg, 200 mg bid tab, or 250 mg bid buffered powder; 35-49 kg, 125 mg bid tab, or 167 mg bid buffered powder

Child

• PO 1.1-1.4 m^2, 100 mg bid tab, or 125 mg bid pedi powder; 0.8-1 m^2, 75 mg bid tabs, or 94 mg bid pedi powder; 0.5-0.7 m^2, 50 mg bid tabs, or 62 mg bid pedi powder; <0.4 m^2, 25 mg bid tabs, or 31 mg bid pedi powder

$ AVAILABLE FORMS/COST OF THERAPY

• Packet—Oral: 100, 167, 250 mg, 30's: **$44.51, $74.33, $111.26**

• Sol—Oral: 20 mg/ml, 100 ml: **$29.66;** 200 ml: **$59.32**

• Tab, Chewable—Oral: 25, 50, 100, 150 mg, 60's: **$22.25-$133.51**

CONTRAINDICATIONS: Hypersensitivity

PRECAUTIONS: Renal, hepatic disease, children, sodium-restricted diets, elevated amylase, preexisting peripheral neuropathy

PREGNANCY AND LACTATION: Pregnancy category B; unknown if excreted in breast milk, discontinuation of breast feeding recommended

SIDE EFFECTS/ADVERSE REACTIONS

CNS: ***Peripheral neuropathy, seizures,*** confusion, anxiety, hypertonia, abnormal thinking, asthenia, insomnia, ***CNS depression,*** pain, dizziness, chills, fever

CV: Hypertension, vasodilation, ***dysrhythmia,*** syncope, ***CHF,*** palpitation

EENT: Ear pain, otitis, photophobia, visual impairment, retinal depigmentation

GI: ***Pancreatitis,*** diarrhea, nausea, vomiting, abdominal pain, constipation, stomatitis, dyspepsia, liver abnormalities, flatulence, taste perversion, dry mouth, oral thrush, melena

HEME: ***Leukopenia, granulocytopenia, thrombocytopenia, anemia***

MS: Myalgia, arthritis, myopathy, muscular atrophy

RESP: Cough, pneumonia, dyspnea, ***bronchospasm,*** epistaxis, hypoventilation, sinusitis

SKIN: Rash, pruritus, alopecia, ecchymosis, hemorrhage, petechiae, sweating

MISC: Hypersensitivity

▼ DRUG INTERACTIONS

Drugs

• *Dapsone:* Buffering compound may inhibit dissolution of dapsone in the stomach

• *Food:* Reduced bioavailability
• *Itraconazole:* Alkalinization of stomach by didanosine reduces the solubility and absorption of itraconazole
• *Quinolones:* Decreased concentrations after binding to the aluminum and magnesium ions in the didanosine buffering compound

Labs

• *Increase:* Amylase, lipase, triglycerides, uric acid, ALT, AST, bilirubin, alk phosphatase, uric acid
• *Decrease:* Potassium

SPECIAL CONSIDERATIONS

MONITORING PARAMETERS

• Amylase, lipase, ophthalmologic examinations

---

dienestrol

(dye-en-ess'trole)

DV, Ortho Dienestrol

Chemical Class: Nonsteroidal synthetic estrogen

Therapeutic Class: Estrogen

CLINICAL PHARMACOLOGY

Mechanism of Action: Synthetic estrogen substitute. Acts on female GU tract and reproductive system

Pharmacokinetics

TOP: 50% systemic absorption (better than non-vaginal estrogen products); distributed mainly to adipose tissue; primarily hepatic degradation; excreted in urine

INDICATIONS AND USES: Atrophic vaginitis, kraurosis vulvae

DOSAGE

Adult

• VAG CREAM 1 applicatorful 1-2×/day qd × 2 wk, then ½ dose or every other day × 2 wk, then 1 application 2-3 × weekly as maintenance

$ AVAILABLE FORMS/COST OF THERAPY

• Cre—Vag: 0.01%, 78 g: **$22.98; $24.48** w/applicator

CONTRAINDICATIONS: Breast cancer, estrogen dependent neoplasia, thromboembolic disorders, reproductive cancer, genital bleeding (abnormal, undiagnosed)

PRECAUTIONS: Hypertension, asthma, blood dyscrasias, gallbladder disease, CHF, diabetes mellitus, bone disease, depression, migraine headache, convulsive disorders, hepatic disease, renal disease, family history of cancer of the breast or reproductive tract

PREGNANCY AND LACTATION: Pregnancy category X; no reports of adverse effects on nursing infant, may reduce milk volume and decreases in nitrogen and protein content

SIDE EFFECTS/ADVERSE REACTIONS

CNS: Dizziness, headache, migraines, depression

CV: ***Hypotension,*** thrombophlebitis, edema, ***thromboembolism, stroke, pulmonary embolism, MI***

GI: Nausea, vomiting, diarrhea, anorexia, ***pancreatitis,*** cramps, constipation, increased appetite, increased weight, ***cholestatic jaundice***

EENT: Contact lens intolerance, increased myopia, astigmatism

GU: Amenorrhea, cervical erosion, breakthrough bleeding, dysmenorrhea, vaginal candidiasis, breast changes, gynecomastia, testicular atrophy, impotence

METAB: Folic acid deficiency, hypercalcemia, hyperglycemia

SKIN: Rash, urticaria, acne, hirsutism, alopecia, oily skin, seborrhea, purpura, melasma

▼ **DRUG INTERACTIONS**

Drugs

- *Bromocriptine:* Estrogen may induce amenorrhea
- *Corticosteroids:* Estrogen can decrease clearance, increase elimination, and increase therapeutic and toxic effects
- *Cyclosporine:* Increased risk of toxicity
- *Dantrolene:* Increased risk of hepatotoxicity

Labs

- *Decrease:* Metyrapone test, T_3 resin uptake, antithrombin III, total cholesterol, folate, LDL lipoproteins, pregnanediol, pyridoxine
- *Increase:* Norepinephrine-induced platelet aggregability, protein-bound T_4, T_3 determination, calcium, clotting factors VII, VIII, IX, X, cortisol, glucose, HDL lipoproteins, phospholipids, prolactin, prothrombin, renin substrate, sodium, and triglycerides

---

diethylpropion

(die-ethyl-prop'ion)

Tenuate, Tenuate Dospan, Tepanil, Tepanil Ten-Tab, Nobesine, ✤ Regibon ✤

Chemical Class: Phenethylamine (amphetamine-like analog)

Therapeutic Class: Appetite suppressant

DEA Class: Schedule IV

CLINICAL PHARMACOLOGY

Mechanism of Action: Not completely established, may alter chemical control of nerve impulse transmission in the appetite control center of the hypothalamus, decreases hunger

Pharmacokinetics

PO: Duration 4 hr

PO-CONT REL: Duration 10-14 hr

Metabolized by liver; excreted by kidneys; $t_{1/2}$ 1-3½ hr

INDICATIONS AND USES: Treatment adjunct in exogenous obesity

DOSAGE

Adult

- PO 25 mg tid 1 hr ac, or 75 mg controlled release qd midmorning

$ **AVAILABLE FORMS/COST OF THERAPY**

- Tab, Uncoated—Oral: 25 mg, 100's: **$5.37-$37.86**
- Tab, Uncoated, Sust Action—Oral: 75 mg, 100's: **$48.45-$94.92**

CONTRAINDICATIONS: Hypersensitivity, hyperthyroidism, hypertension, glaucoma, angina pectoris, drug abuse, cardiovascular disease, children <12 yr, severe arteriosclerosis, agitated states

PRECAUTIONS: Convulsive disorders

PREGNANCY AND LACTATION: Pregnancy category B; excreted in breast milk, no reports of adverse effects

SIDE EFFECTS/ADVERSE REACTIONS

CNS: Hyperactivity, restlessness, anxiety, insomnia, dizziness, dysphoria, depression, tremors, headache, incoordination, fatigue, malaise, euphoria, depression, tremor, confusion

CV: Palpitations, tachycardia, hypertension, ***dysrhythmias,*** pulmonary hypertension, ECG changes

EENT: Mydriasis, blurred vision, eye irritation

GI: Nausea, vomiting, anorexia, unpleasant taste, pain, dry mouth, diarrhea, constipation

GU: Impotence, change in libido, menstrual irregularities, dysuria, polyuria, urinary frequency

HEME: ***Bone marrow depression***

SKIN: Urticaria, rash, erythema

MISC: Hair loss, ecchymosis, muscle/chest pain, excessive sweating, chills, flushing, fever

▼ **DRUG INTERACTIONS**

Drugs

- *MAOIs or within 14 days of MAOIs:* Hypertensive crisis

diethylstilbestrol

(dye-eth-il-stil-bess'trole)

DES, Honvol, ✤ Stilboestrol, ✤ Stilphostrol

Chemical Class: Nonsteroidal synthetic estrogen

Therapeutic Class: Antineoplastic estrogen

CLINICAL PHARMACOLOGY

Mechanism of Action: Increases cellular synthesis of DNA, RNA, and various proteins in responsive tissues of the female reproductive tract; reduces the release of gonadotropin-releasing hormone (GnRH) from the hypothalamus, leading to a reduction in release of FSH and LH from the pituitary

Pharmacokinetics

Primarily hepatic metabolism and renal excretion

INDICATIONS AND USES: Postcoital contraception;* inoperable breast and prostatic cancer

DOSAGE

Adult

- *Post-coital contraception:* PO 25 mg bid × 5 days, starting within 72 hr of intercourse
- *Prostatic cancer:* PO 1-3 mg qd, then 1 mg qd; IM 5 mg 2×/wk, then 4 mg 2×/wk; IV 0.25-1 g qd × 5 days, then 1-2 ×/wk; (diphosphate form) PO 50-200 mg tid
- *Breast cancer:* PO 15 mg qd

$ **AVAILABLE FORMS/COST OF THERAPY**

- Tab, Uncoated—Oral: 1 mg, 100's: **$9.14;** 5 mg, 100's: **$24.35**

Diphosphonate Salt:

- Inj, Sol—IV: 250 mg/5 ml, 1's: **$1.85**
- Tab, Uncoated—Oral: 50 mg, 50's: **$87.61**

CONTRAINDICATIONS: Thromboembolic disorders, reproductive cancer, genital bleeding (abnormal, undiagnosed)

PRECAUTIONS: Hypertension, asthma, blood dyscrasias, gallbladder disease, CHF, diabetes mellitus, bone disease blocking agents, hypercalcemia associated with metastatic breast disease

PREGNANCY AND LACTATION: Pregnancy category X; (increased incidence of vaginal and cervical carcinoma in female offspring exposed in-utero); may reduce quantity and quality of milk

SIDE EFFECTS/ADVERSE REACTIONS

CNS: Dizziness, headache, migraines, depression

CV: Hypotension, thrombophlebitis, edema, ***thromboembolism, stroke, pulmonary embolism, MI***

EENT: Contact lens intolerance, increased myopia, astigmatism

GI: Nausea, vomiting, diarrhea, anorexia, ***pancreatitis,*** cramps, constipation, increased appetite, increased weight, ***cholestatic jaundice***

GU: Amenorrhea, cervical erosion, breakthrough bleeding, dysmenorrhea, vaginal candidiasis, breast changes, *gynecomastia, testicular atrophy, impotence*

METAB: Folic acid deficiency, hypercalcemia, hyperglycemia

SKIN: Rash, urticaria, acne, hirsutism, alopecia, oily skin, seborrhea, purpura, melasma

▼ **DRUG INTERACTIONS**

Drugs

- *Anticonvulsants, barbiturates,*

phenylbutazone, rifampin: Decreased action of diethylstilbestrol
- *Corticosteroids:* Increased action

Labs
- *Increase:* BSP retention test, PBI, T_4, serum sodium, platelet aggregability, thyroxine-binding globulin (TBG), prothrombin, factors VII, VIII, IX, X, triglycerides
- *Decrease:* Serum folate, serum triglyceride, T_3 resin uptake test, glucose tolerance test, antithrombin III, pregnanediol, metyrapone test
- *False positive:* LE prep, antinuclear antibodies

SPECIAL CONSIDERATIONS

PATIENT/FAMILY EDUCATION
- Nausea, especially in the morning is primarily central in origin, but solid food often provides some relief

---

difenoxin

(dye-fen-ox'in)

Motofen

Chemical Class: Phenylpiperidine derivative; opiate agonist
Therapeutic Class: Antidiarrheal
DEA Class: Schedule IV

CLINICAL PHARMACOLOGY

Mechanism of Action: Slows intestinal motility through a local effect on the gastrointestinal wall; atropine is present to discourage deliberate overdosage

Pharmacokinetics

PO: Peak 40-60 min, duration 3-4 hr, terminal $t_{1/2}$ 12-14 hr, metabolized in liver to inactive metabolite, excreted in urine and feces

INDICATIONS AND USES: Acute nonspecific diarrhea, acute exacerbations of chronic functional diarrhea

DOSAGE

Adult
- PO 2 mg stat, then 1 mg after each loose stool or 1 mg q3-4h as needed, not to exceed 8 mg/24 hr

$ AVAILABLE FORMS/COST OF THERAPY
- Tab, Uncoated—Oral: 0.025 mg atropine/1 mg difenoxin, 100's: **$42.80**

CONTRAINDICATIONS: Hypersensitivity; diarrhea associated with organisms that penetrate the intestinal mucosa (toxigenic *E. coli, Salmonella* sp, *Shigella;*) pseudomembranous colitis; children <2 yr; jaundice

PRECAUTIONS: Hepatic disease, renal disease, ulcerative colitis, children, fluid and electrolyte imbalances, Down syndrome

PREGNANCY AND LACTATION: Pregnancy category C; excretion into breast milk unknown

SIDE EFFECTS/ADVERSE REACTIONS

CNS: Dizziness, drowsiness, lightheadedness, headache, fatigue, nervousness, insomnia, confusion
EENT: Burning eyes, blurred vision
GI: Nausea, vomiting, dry mouth, epigastric distress, constipation

▼ DRUG INTERACTIONS

Drugs
- *MAOIs:* May cause hypertensive crisis

SPECIAL CONSIDERATIONS

PATIENT/FAMILY EDUCATION
- Do not use for longer than 48 hr unless directed by physician
- Adhere strictly to recommended dosage
- Drowsiness or dizziness may occur, use caution when driving or operating dangerous machinery

MONITORING PARAMETERS
- Serum electrolytes if on long-term therapy

diflorasone

(die-floor'a-sone)

Florone, Florone E, Maxiflor, Psorcon

Chemical Class: Synthetic fluorinated agent, group II (high) potency

Therapeutic Class: Topical corticosteroid

CLINICAL PHARMACOLOGY

Mechanism of Action: Depresses formation, release, and activity of endogenous mediators of inflammation such as prostaglandins, kinins, histamine, liposomal enzymes, and the complement system resulting in decreased edema, erythema, and pruritus

Pharmacokinetics

Absorbed through the skin (increased by inflammation and occlusive dressings), metabolized primarily in the liver

INDICATIONS AND USES: Psoriasis, eczema, contact dermatitis, pruritus

DOSAGE

Adult and child

• Apply to affected area bid; rub completely into skin

$ AVAILABLE FORMS/COST OF THERAPY

• Cre—Top: 0.05%, 15, 30, 60 g: **$17.52-$54.96**

• Oint—Top: 0.05%, 15, 30, 60 g: **$22.30-$60.15**

CONTRAINDICATIONS: Hypersensitivity to corticosteroids, fungal infections; use on face, groin, or axilla

PRECAUTIONS: Viral infections, bacterial infections, children

PREGNANCY AND LACTATION: Pregnancy category C; unknown whether topical application could result in sufficient systemic absorption to produce detectable amounts in breast milk (systemic corticosteroids are secreted into breast milk in quantities not likely to have detrimental effects on infant)

SIDE EFFECTS/ADVERSE REACTIONS

SKIN: Burning, dryness, itching, irritation, acne, folliculitis, hypertrichosis, perioral dermatitis, hypopigmentation, atrophy, striae, miliaria, allergic contact dermatitis, secondary infection

MISC: Systemic absorption of topical corticosteroids has produced reversible HPA axis suppression (more likely with occlusive dressings, prolonged administration, application to large surface areas, liver failure, and in children)

SPECIAL CONSIDERATIONS

PATIENT/FAMILY EDUCATION

• Apply sparingly only to affected area

• Avoid contact with the eyes

• Do not put bandages or dressings over treated area unless directed by physician

• Do not use on weeping, denuded, or infected areas

• Discontinue drug, notify physician if local irritation or fever develops

diflunisal

(dye-floo'ni-sal)

Dolobid

Chemical Class: Salicylic acid derivative

Therapeutic Class: Nonsteroidal anti-inflammatory; nonnarcotic analgesic

CLINICAL PHARMACOLOGY

Mechanism of Action: Inhibits prostaglandin synthesis by decreasing activity of the enzyme cyclooxygenase, which results in decreased formation of prostaglandin precursors

Pharmacokinetics

PO: Peak 2-3 hr, onset 1 hr, >99% bound to plasma proteins, $t_{1/2}$ 8-12 hr (dose dependent), excreted mainly in urine as glucuronide conjugates

INDICATIONS AND USES: Mild to moderate pain, rheumatoid arthritis, osteoarthritis

DOSAGE

Adult

- *Mild to moderate pain:* PO 500-1000 mg initially, then 250-500 mg q8-12h
- *Osteoarthritis/rheumatoid arthritis:* PO 500-1000 mg/d in 2 divided doses, max 1500 mg/d

$ AVAILABLE FORMS/COST OF THERAPY

- Tab, Plain Coated—Oral: 250 mg, 60's: **$46.44-$57.06;** 500 mg, 60's: **$53.65-$71.34**

CONTRAINDICATIONS: Hypersensitivity or intolerance to NSAIDs

PRECAUTIONS: GI bleeding, peptic ulcer, history of GI disease, impaired renal function, compromised cardiac function, hypertension, children (potential association with Reye's syndrome), hepatic dysfunction

PREGNANCY AND LACTATION: Pregnancy category C; use during 3rd trimester not recommended due to effects on fetal cardiovascular system (closure of ductus arteriosus); excreted into breast milk in concentrations 2%-7% those in maternal plasma, use caution in nursing mothers

SIDE EFFECTS/ADVERSE REACTIONS

CNS: Stimulation, dizziness, somnolence, insomnia, confusion, *headache,* flushing, hallucinations, vertigo, paresthesias

CV: Palpitations, chest pain

EENT: Blurred vision, decreased acuity, corneal deposits

GI: Nausea, GI pain, diarrhea, vomiting, constipation, flatulance, GI bleeding, heartburn, anorexia, ***hepatitis,*** abnormal LFTs

HEME: ***Thrombocytopenia, agranulocytosis***

RESP: Dyspnea

SKIN: Rash, pruritus, sweating, dry mucous membranes, stomatitis, erythema multiforme, ***Stevens-Johnson syndrome, toxic epidermal necrolysis, exfoliative dermatitis,*** photosensitivity, urticaria

▼ DRUG INTERACTIONS

Drugs

- *Aminoglycosides:* Reduction of aminoglycoside clearance in premature infants
- *ACE inhibitors:* Inhibition of antihypertensive response
- *Beta blockers:* Reduced hypotensive effects of beta blockers
- *Furosemide:* Reduced diuretic and antihypertensive response to furosemide
- *Hydralazine:* Reduced antihypertensive response to hydralazine
- *Lithium:* Increased plasma lithium concentrations, toxicity
- *Methotrexate:* Reduced renal clearance of methotrexate, increased toxicity
- *Oral anticoagulants:* Increased risk of bleeding due to adverse effects on GI mucosa and platelet function
- *Potassium sparing diuretics:* Acute renal failure

Labs

- *Increase:* Coagulation studies, liver function studies, serum uric acid, amylase, CO_2, urinary protein
- *Decrease:* Serum potassium, PBI, cholesterol
- *Interference:* Urine catecholamines, pregnancy test

SPECIAL CONSIDERATIONS
PATIENT/FAMILY EDUCATION
• May cause GI upset, take with food
• Do not take aspirin or other NSAIDs while taking this medication
• Therapeutic response may take 2 wk
• Avoid alcohol
MONITORING PARAMETERS
• AST, ALT, bilirubin, creatinine, BUN, urine creatinine, CBC, hematocrit, if on long-term therapy

digitoxin

(di-ji-tox′in)
Crystodigin
Chemical Class: Digitalis preparation
Therapeutic Class: Antidysrhythmic; cardiac glycoside

CLINICAL PHARMACOLOGY
Mechanism of Action: Increases influx of calcium ions into intracellular cytoplasm by inhibiting sodium and potassium ion movement across the myocardial membranes, which results in a potentiation of the activity of contractile heart muscle fibers and an increase in the force of myocardial contraction (positive inotropic effect); inhibits adenosine triphosphatase (ATPase); decreases conduction through the SA and AV nodes (negative chronotropic effect)
Pharmacokinetics
PO: Onset 1-4 hr, peak 8-12 hr, $t_{1/2}$ 168-192 hr, 90%-97% bound to plasma proteins, metabolized by the liver, excreted via the kidneys (metabolites)
INDICATIONS AND USES: Congestive heart failure (CHF), atrial fibrillation, atrial flutter, paroxysmal atrial tachycardia (PAT), cardiogenic shock
DOSAGE
Adult
• Loading dose PO (rapid) 0.6 mg, followed by 0.4 mg, then 0.2 mg at q4-6h intervals; (slow) 0.2 mg bid for 4 days; maintenance dose PO 0.05-0.3 mg qd
Child
• Loading dose PO <1 yr 0.045 mg/kg, 1-2 yr 0.04 mg/kg, >2 yr 0.03 mg/kg divided into 3, 4 or more portions with >6 hr between doses; maintenance dose: PO 1/10 loading dose
$ **AVAILABLE FORMS/COST OF THERAPY**
• Tab, Uncoated—Oral: 0.05 mg, 100's: **$2.92;** 0.1 mg, 100's: **$5.14**
CONTRAINDICATIONS: Ventricular tachycardia, ventricular fibrillation, hypersensitivity to digitoxin
PRECAUTIONS: Hypokalemia, hypomagnesemia, hypercalcemia, hypothyroidism, severe pulmonary disease, sick sinus syndrome, hepatic disease, acute MI, AV block, elderly, Wolff-Parkinson-White syndrome
PREGNANCY AND LACTATION: Pregnancy category C; excretion into breast milk unknown, digoxin, a related cardiac glycoside is considered compatible with breast feeding
SIDE EFFECTS/ADVERSE REACTIONS
CNS: Anorexia, headache, weakness, apathy, drowsiness, mental depression, confusion, restlessness, disorientation, ***seizures,*** EEG abnormalities, delirium, hallucinations, neuralgia, psychosis
CV: ***Ventricular tachycardia, ventricular fibrillation,*** premature ventricular contractions (PVCs), ECG abnormalities, ***bradycardia,*** AV block, atrial fibrillation

EENT: Visual disturbances (blurred, yellow or green vision, halo effect)
GI: Nausea, vomiting, diarrhea, abdominal discomfort, ***hemorrhagic necrosis of the intestines***
HEME: Eosinophilia, thrombocytopenia
METAB: Gynecomastia
SKIN: Rash

▼ **DRUG INTERACTIONS**

Drugs

- *Aminoglutethamide:* Reduced serum concentrations of digitoxin
- *Calcium:* Elevated serum calcium concentrations following parenteral administration have been associated with acute digitalis toxicity
- *Charcoal:* Reduced serum digitoxin concentrations
- *Cholestyramine:* Reduced serum digitoxin concentrations
- *Diuretics:* Diuretic-induced hypokalemia may increase the risk of digitalis toxicity
- *Phenytoin:* Reduced serum digitoxin concentrations
- *Quinidine:* Increased digitalis concentrations, toxicity possible
- *Rifampin:* Reduced serum concentrations of digitoxin

Labs

- *Increase:* CPK

SPECIAL CONSIDERATIONS

PATIENT/FAMILY EDUCATION

- Do not discontinue medication without checking with physician
- Notify physician of loss of appetite, lower stomach pain, nausea, vomiting, diarrhea, unusual tiredness or weakness, drowsiness, headache, blurred or yellow vision, skin rash or hives, mental depression
- Avoid OTC medications unless directed by physician

MONITORING PARAMETERS

- Heart rate and rhythm, periodic ECGs
- Serum potassium, magnesium, calcium, CrCl
- Serum digitoxin levels when compliance, effectiveness, or systemic availability is questioned or toxicity suspected

digoxin

(di-jox'in)
Lanoxin, Lanoxicaps
Chemical Class: Digitalis preparation
Therapeutic Class: Antidysrhythmic; cardiac glycoside

CLINICAL PHARMACOLOGY

Mechanism of Action: Increases influx of calcium ions into intracellular cytoplasm by inhibiting sodium and potassium ion movement across the myocardial membranes, which results in a potentiation of the activity of contractile heart muscle fibers and an increase in the force of myocardial contraction (positive inotropic effect); inhibits adenosine triphosphatase (ATPase); decreases conduction through the SA and AV nodes (negative chronotropic effect)

Pharmacokinetics

IV: Onset 5-30 min, peak 1-5 hr
PO: Onset 30-120 min, peak 2-6 hr
$t_{1/2}$ 30-40 hr, 20%-25% bound to plasma proteins, excreted mainly by kidneys

INDICATIONS AND USES: Congestive heart failure (CHF), atrial fibrillation, atrial flutter, paroxysmal atrial tachycardia (PAT), cardiogenic shock

DOSAGE

Administer IV slowly over 5 min, IM route not recommended due to local irritation, pain, and tissue damage

Adult

- Loading dose (give ½ total dose initially, then ¼ total dose in each of 2 subsequent doses at 8-12 hr intervals); IV 0.5-1 mg; PO 0.75-1.5 mg; maintenance dose IV 0.1-0.4 mg qd; PO 0.125-0.5 mg qd

Child >10 yr

• Loading dose (administered as for adult) IV 8-12 μg/kg; PO 10-15 μg/kg; maintenance dose IV 2-3 μg/kg qd; PO 2.5-5 μg/kg qd

Child 5-10 yr

• Loading dose (administered as for adult) IV 15-30 μg/kg; PO 20-35 μg/kg; maintenance dose IV 4-8 μg/kg divided q12h; PO 5-10 μg/kg divided q12h

Child 2-5 yr

• Loading dose (administered as for adult) IV 25-35 μg/kg; IV 30-40 μg/kg; maintenance dose IV 6-9 μg/kg divided q12h; PO 7.5-10 μg/kg divided q12h

Child 1-24 months

• Loading dose (administered as for adult) IV 30-50 μg/kg; PO 35-60 μg/kg; maintenance dose IV 7.5-12 μg/kg divided q12h; PO 10-15 μg/kg divided q12h

Full term infant

• Loading dose (administered as for adult) IV 20-30 μg/kg; PO 25-35 μg/kg; maintenance dose IV 5-8 μg/kg divided q12h; PO 6-10 μg/kg divided q12h

Preterm infant

• Loading dose (administered as for adult) IV 15-25 μg/kg; PO 20-30 μg/kg; maintenance dose: IV 4-6 μg/kg divided q12h; PO 5-7.5 μg/kg divided q12h

$ AVAILABLE FORMS/COST OF THERAPY

• Inj, Sol—IM, IV: 0.1 mg/ml, 1 ml × 10: **$51.66;** 0.25 mg/ml, 2 ml × 10: **$21.50-$23.29**

• Elixir—Oral: 0.05 mg/ml, 60 ml: **$6.96-$17.06**

• Cap, Elastic—Oral: 0.05 mg, 100's: **$13.67;** 0.1 mg, 100's: **$14.93;** 0.2 mg, 100's: **$17.36**

• Tab, Uncoated—Oral: 0.125, 0.25, 0.5 mg, 100's: **$7.54-$20.05**

CONTRAINDICATIONS: Ventricular tachycardia, ventricular fibrillation, hypersensitivity to digoxin

PRECAUTIONS: Hypokalemia, hypomagnesemia, hypercalcemia, hypothyroidism, severe pulmonary disease, sick sinus syndrome, hepatic disease, acute MI, AV block, elderly, Wolff-Parkinson-White syndrome

PREGNANCY AND LACTATION: Pregnancy category C; excreted into breast milk, considered compatible with breast feeding

SIDE EFFECTS/ADVERSE REACTIONS

CNS: Anorexia, headache, weakness, apathy, drowsiness, mental depression, confusion, restlessness, disorientation, ***seizures,*** EEG abnormalities, delirium, hallucinations, neuralgia, psychosis

CV: ***Ventricular tachycardia, ventricular fibrillation,*** premature ventricular contractions (PVCs), ECG abnormalities, ***bradycardia,*** AV block, atrial fibrillation

EENT: Visual disturbances (blurred, yellow or green vision, halo effect)

GI: Nausea, vomiting, diarrhea, abdominal discomfort, ***hemorrhagic necrosis of the intestines***

HEME: Eosinophilia, thrombocytopenia

METAB: Gynecomastia

SKIN: Rash

▼ DRUG INTERACTIONS

Drugs

• *Aminoglycosides:* Neomycin reduces digoxin serum concentrations

• *Aminosalicylic acid:* Small reduction in digoxin serum concentrations

• *Amiodarone:* Accumulation of digoxin to concentrations which may result in toxicity

• *Calcium:* Elevated serum calcium concentrations following parenteral administration have been associated with acute digoxin toxicity
• *Calcium channel blockers:* Increased serum digoxin concentrations with verapamil, diltiazem, bepridil, nitrendipine
• *Charcoal:* Reduced serum digoxin concentrations
• *Cholestyramine:* Reduced serum digoxin concentrations
• *Cyclosporine:* Increased serum digoxin concentrations
• *Diuretics:* Diuretic-induced hypokalemia may increase the risk of digitalis toxicity
• *Hydroxychloroquine:* Increased serum digoxin concentrations
• *Metoclopramide:* Reduced serum digoxin concentrations when coadministered with slowly dissolving digoxin tablets
• *Phenytoin:* Small decreases in serum digoxin concentrations
• *Pirmenol:* Increased serum digoxin concentrations
• *Propafenone:* Increased serum digoxin concentrations
• *Propantheline:* Reduced serum digoxin concentrations when coadministered with slowly dissolving digoxin tablets
• *Quinidine+:* Increased digitalis concentrations, toxicity possible
• *Rifampin:* Reduced serum concentrations of digoxin
• *Spironolactone:* Interference with serum digoxin assays; possible true increases in serum digoxin concentrations
• *Sulfasalazine:* Reduced serum digoxin concentrations

Labs

• *Increase:* CPK

SPECIAL CONSIDERATIONS

PATIENT/FAMILY EDUCATION

• Do not discontinue medication without checking with physician
• Notify physician of loss of appetite, lower stomach pain, nausea, vomiting, diarrhea, unusual tiredness or weakness, drowsiness, headache, blurred or yellow vision, skin rash or hives, mental depression
• Avoid OTC medications unless directed by physician

MONITORING PARAMETERS

• Heart rate and rhythm, periodic ECGs
• Serum potassium, magnesium, calcium, CrCl
• Serum digoxin levels when compliance, effectiveness, or systemic availability is questioned or toxicity suspected
• Obtain serum drug concentrations at least 8-12 hr after a dose (preferably prior to next scheduled dose); therapeutic range 0.5-2.0 ng/ml

digoxin immune FAB

Digibind

Therapeutic Class: Antidote, digoxin specific

CLINICAL PHARMACOLOGY

Mechanism of Action: Antibody fragments bind to free digoxin to reverse digoxin toxicity by not allowing digoxin to bind to sites of action

Pharmacokinetics

IV: Onset of improvement in signs and symptoms of digoxin toxicity 30 min, $t_{1/2}$ 15-20 hr, fab fragment–digoxin complex accumulates in the blood and is excreted by the kidneys

INDICATIONS AND USES: Potentially life-threatening digoxin intoxication (has also been used successfully to treat life-threatening digitoxin overdose)

DOSAGE

Adult

• IV dose (mg) = dose ingested (mg) × 0.8 × 66.7; if digoxin liquid caps or digitoxin used, do not multiply ingested dose by 0.8; if ingested amount is unknown, give 800 mg IV. Alternatively, calculate the equimolar dose required from the total amount of digoxin (or digitoxin) in the patient's body. An estimate of the total body load can be made from a serum level: For digoxin body load in mg = serum digoxin concentration × 0.56 × weight in kg/1000. Each 40 mg vial will bind 0.6 mg of digoxin or digitoxin; calculate the number of vials required by dividing body load in mg by 0.6 mg/vial; dose (in number of vials) = body load (mg)/0.6 mg/vial

$ AVAILABLE FORMS/COST OF THERAPY

- Inj, Conc-Sol—IV: 40 mg/vial, 1's: **$401.99**

CONTRAINDICATIONS: Mild digoxin toxicity

PRECAUTIONS: Children, cardiac disease, renal disease, allergy to ovine products

PREGNANCY AND LACTATION: Pregnancy category C; excretion into breast milk unknown, use caution in nursing mothers

SIDE EFFECTS/ADVERSE REACTIONS

METAB: Hypokalemia

SKIN: Hypersensitivity, allergic reactions

▼ DRUG INTERACTIONS

Labs

- *Interference:* Immunoassay digoxin

SPECIAL CONSIDERATIONS

MONITORING PARAMETERS

- Potassium, serum digoxin level **prior** to therapy
- Continuous ECG monitoring

dihydroergotamine

(dye-hye-droe-er-got'a-meen)

D.H.E. 45

Chemical Class: Ergot alkaloid
Therapeutic Class: Antimigraine agent

CLINICAL PHARMACOLOGY

Mechanism of Action: Causes vasoconstriction of dilated cranial blood vessels associated with vascular headaches, with a concomitant decrease in the amplitude of pulsations

Pharmacokinetics

IM: Onset 15-30 min

IV: Onset within a few min

90% bound to plasma proteins, $t_{1/2}$ (terminal) 21-32 hr, metabolized by liver, excreted in urine and bile

INDICATIONS AND USES: Prevent or abort vascular headaches including migraine and cluster headaches; *Prevention of postoperative deep-vein thrombosis and pulmonary embolism in patients undergoing major abdominal, pelvic, thoracic, or hip-replacement surgery (in combination with heparin)

DOSAGE

Adult

- IM 1 mg at first sign of headache, repeat at 1 hr intervals prn, do not exceed 3 mg/attack or 6 mg/wk; IV 1 mg at first sign of headache, repeat in 1 hr prn, do not exceed 2 mg/attack or 6 mg/wk

$ AVAILABLE FORMS/COSTS OF THERAPY

- Inj, Sol—IM;IV: 1 mg/ml, 1 ml: **$10.27**

CONTRAINDICATIONS: Pregnancy, hypersensitivity, peripheral vascular disease, hepatic or renal impairment, coronary artery disease, uncontrolled hypertension, sepsis

PRECAUTIONS: Prolonged administration, excessive dosage

PREGNANCY AND LACTATION: Pregnancy category X; likely excreted into breast milk, ergotamine has caused symptoms of ergotism (e.g., vomiting, diarrhea) in the infant; excessive dosage or prolonged administration may inhibit lactation

SIDE EFFECTS/ADVERSE REACTIONS

CNS: Transient tachycardia or bradycardia, coronary vasoconstriction (large doses), chest pain, increase or decrease in blood pressure

GI: Nausea, vomiting

MISC: Numbness and tingling of fingers and toes, muscle pain in the extremities, weakness in the legs, itching, localized edema

▼ DRUG INTERACTIONS

Drugs

- *Dopamine:* Increased risk of vasoconstriction
- *Nitroglycerin:* Enhanced ergot effect, decreased antianginal effects

SPECIAL CONSIDERATIONS

PATIENT/FAMILY EDUCATION

- Initiate therapy at first sign of attack
- DO NOT exceed recommended dosage
- Notify physician of irregular heart beat, nausea, vomiting, numbness or tingling of fingers or toes, pain or weakness of extremities
- Prolonged use may lead to withdrawal headaches

dihydrotachysterol

(dye-hye-droe-tak-iss'ter-ole)

DHT Intensol, DHT, Hytakerol

Chemical Class: Vitamin D analog

Therapeutic Class: Fat-soluble vitamin

CLINICAL PHARMACOLOGY

Mechanism of Action: Stimulates intestinal calcium absorption and mobilization of bone calcium in the absence of parathyroid hormone and of functioning renal tissue; also increases renal phosphate excretion

Pharmacokinetics

PO: Onset 2 wk; hydroxylated in the liver to 25-hydroxydihydrotachysterol, which is the major circulating active form of the drug; excreted in feces

INDICATIONS AND USES: Treatment of acute, chronic, and latent forms of postoperative tetany, idiopathic tetany, hypoparathyroidism, pseudohypoparathyroidism; *familial hypophosphatemia, renal osteodystrophy in chronic renal failure, osteoporosis (with calcium and flouride)

DOSAGE

Adult

- PO 0.75-2.5 mg/d for 4 days initially, then 0.2-1 mg/d as required for normal serum calcium levels, max 1.5 mg/d

Child

- PO 1-5 mg/d for 4 days initially, then 0.5-1.5 mg/d as required for normal serum calcium levels

Neonate

- PO 0.05-0.1 mg/d

$ AVAILABLE FORMS/COST OF THERAPY

- Sol—Oral: 0.2 mg/ml, 30 ml: **$32.75**
- Tab, Uncoated—Oral: 0.125 mg,

50's: **$43.88;** 0.2 mg, 100's: **$88.64;** 0.4 mg, 50's: **$78.65**

• Cap, Gel—Oral: 0.125 mg, 50's: **$112.69**

CONTRAINDICATIONS: Hypercalcemia, hypersensitivity, and hypervitaminosis D

PRECAUTIONS: Renal stones, renal failure, heart disease

PREGNANCY AND LACTATION: Pregnancy category A (category D if used in doses above the recommended daily allowance); excretion into breast milk unknown; vit D is excreted into breast milk in limited amounts, considered compatible with breast feeding, however, serum calcium levels of the infant should be monitored if the mother is receiving pharmacologic doses

SIDE EFFECTS/ADVERSE REACTIONS

CNS: Drowsiness, headache, vertigo, fever, lethargy

EENT: Tinnitus

GI: Nausea, diarrhea, vomiting, jaundice, anorexia, dry mouth, constipation, cramps, metallic taste

GU: Polyuria, hypercalciuria, hyperphosphatemia, hematuria

MS: Myalgia, arthralgia, decreased bone development

▼ **DRUG INTERACTIONS**

Drugs

• *Cholestyramine, colestipol, mineral oil:* Decreased absorption of dihydrotachysterol

• *Thiazide diuretics, calcium supplements:* Hypercalcemia

• *Cardiac glycosides, verapamil:* Cardiac dysrhythmias

• *Corticosteroids, phenytoin, barbiturates:* Decreased effect of dihydrotachysterol

Labs

• *False increase:* Cholesterol

SPECIAL CONSIDERATIONS

PATIENT/FAMILY EDUCATION

• Notify physician of weakness, lethargy, headache, anorexia, weight loss, nausea, vomiting, abdominal cramps, diarrhea, constipation, vertigo, excessive thirst, excessive urine output, dry mouth, muscle or bone pain

• Compliance with dosage instructions, diet, and calcium supplementation are essential

MONITORING PARAMETERS

• Serum Ca^{++} and phosphate

• BUN, urinary Ca^{++}, AST, ALT, cholesterol, Cr, uric acid, urine pH, electrolytes may also be useful

---

dihydroxyaluminum sodium carbonate

(dye-hye-drox'ee-a-loom'-a-nim)

Rolaids

Chemical Class: Aluminum product

Therapeutic Class: Antacid

CLINICAL PHARMACOLOGY

Mechanism of Action: Neutralizes gastric acidity, reduces pepsin

Pharmacokinetics

PO: Onset 20-40 min, excreted in feces

INDICATIONS AND USES: Symptomatic relief of upset stomach associated with hyperacidity (heartburn, gastroesophageal reflux, acid indigestion, and sour stomach); hyperacidity associated with peptic ulcer, gastritis, peptic esophagitis, gastric hyperacidity, hiatal hernia

DOSAGE

Adult

• PO chew 1-2 tablets prn

$ **AVAILABLE FORMS/COST OF THERAPY**

• Tab, Chewable—Oral: 334 mg, 75's: **$4.33**

CONTRAINDICATIONS: Hypersensitivity to this drug or aluminum products

PRECAUTIONS: Elderly, fluid restriction, decreased GI motility, GI obstruction, dehydration, renal disease, sodium-restricted diets

PREGNANCY AND LACTATION: Pregnancy category C

SIDE EFFECTS/ADVERSE REACTIONS

GI: Constipation, anorexia, ***obstruction,*** fecal impaction

METAB: Hypophosphatemia, hypercalciuria

MISC: Aluminum intoxication, osteomalacia

▼ DRUG INTERACTIONS

Drugs

• *Tetracyclines, anticholinergics, phenothiazines, isoniazid, quinidine, phenytoin, digitalis, iron salts, ketoconazole:* Decreased effectiveness of these drugs

• May cause premature dissolution of enteric-coated tablets

SPECIAL CONSIDERATIONS

PATIENT/FAMILY EDUCATION

• Thoroughly chew chewable tablets before swallowing, follow with a glass of water

• May impair absorption of many drugs, do not take other drugs within 1-2 hr of administration

• Stools may appear white or speckled

diltiazem

(dil-tye'a-zem)

APO-Diltiaz, ♣ Cardizem, Cardizem SR, Cardizem CD, Dilacor XR

Chemical Class: Benzothiazepine, calcium channel blocker

Therapeutic Class: Antianginal, antihypertensive, antiarrhythmic

CLINICAL PHARMACOLOGY

Mechanism of Action: Inhibits calcium ion influx across cell membrane during cardiac depolarization; produces relaxation of coronary vascular smooth muscle, dilates coronary arteries, slows SA/AV node conduction times, dilates peripheral arteries

Pharmacokinetics

PO: Peak 2-3 hr

PO-SUS REL: Peak 6-11 hr

PO-QD CAPS: Peak 10-14 hr

$t_{1/2}$ 3.5-8 hr, 70%-80% bound to plasma proteins, metabolized by liver, excreted in urine (96% as metabolites)

INDICATIONS AND USES: Angina pectoris due to coronary artery spasm, chronic stable angina, essential hypertension, atrial fibrillation or flutter (IV), paroxysmal supraventricular tachycardia (IV); *prevention of reinfarction of non-Q-wave MI, tardive dyskinesia, Raynaud's syndrome, migraine headache prophylaxis

DOSAGE

Adult

• Immediate release PO 30 mg qid, gradually increase to 180-360 mg/d divided tid-qid until optimal response is obtained; sustained release PO 60-120 mg bid, adjust at 14 day intervals until optimal response obtained, optimum range 240-350 mg/d; once daily cap PO 180-240 mg qd, max 540 mg/d; parenteral, IV 0.25 mg/kg as a bolus over 2 min (a second 0.35 mg/kg bolus dose may be administered after 15 min if response is inadequate), then continuous infusion of 5-15 mg/hr for up to 24 hr; conversion from IV to PO, start PO approximately 3 hr after bolus dose; PO (mg/d) = [rate (mg/hr) × 3 + 3] × 10; 3 mg/hr = 120 mg/day; 5 mg/hr = 180 mg/day; 7 mg/hr = 240 mg/day; 11 mg/hr = 360 mg/day

$ AVAILABLE FORMS/COST OF THERAPY

• Cap, Gel, Sust Action—Oral:

60, 90, 120, 180, 240, 300 mg, 100's: **$70.77-$218.16**

• Tab, Plain Coated—Oral: 30, 60, 90, 120 mg, 100's: **$11.70-$125.50**

• Inj, Sol—IV: 5 mg/ml, 5 ml: **$12.98**

CONTRAINDICATIONS: Hypersensitivity, sick sinus syndrome or 2nd or 3rd degree heart block (except with a functioning pacemaker), hypotension <90 mm Hg systolic, acute MI with pulmonary congestion, atrial fibrillation or atrial flutter associated with an accessory bypass tract such as in WPW syndrome or short PR syndrome (IV), ventricular tachycardia (IV)

PRECAUTIONS: CHF, hypotension, hepatic injury, children, impaired renal or hepatic function

PREGNANCY AND LACTATION: Pregnancy category C; excreted into breast milk in concentrations which may approximate those in maternal serum, use caution in nursing mothers

SIDE EFFECTS/ADVERSE REACTIONS

CNS: Abnormal dreams, amnesia, depression, *dizziness,* gait abnormality, hallucinations, *headache,* insomnia, nervousness, paresthesia, personality change, somnolence, tremor

CV: Angina, arrhythmia, AV block (first degree), AV block (second or third degree), bradycardia, bundle branch block, ***congestive heart failure,*** ECG abnormality, *edema,* flushing, hypotension, palpitations, syncope, tachycardia, ventricular extrasystoles

GI: Anorexia, constipation, diarrhea, dysgeusia, dyspepsia, GERD, mild elevations of alkaline phosphatase, SGOT, SGPT, and LDH, *nausea,* thirst, vomiting, weight increase

SKIN: Petechiae, photosensitivity, pruritus, rash, urticaria

▼ **DRUG INTERACTIONS**

Drugs

• *Amiodarone:* Cardiotoxicity with bradycardia and decreased cardiac output

• *Benzodiazepines:* Marked increase in midazolam plasma concentrations, increased sedation likely

• *Beta-blockers:* Inhibition of metabolism of some beta-blockers, additive effects on cardiac conduction and hypotension

• *Carbamazepine:* Increase in carbamazepine toxicity, reduced diltiazem concentrations

• *Calcium channel blockers:* Increased nifedipine concentrations

• *Cyclosporine:* Increased cyclosporine blood concentrations, renal toxicity

• *H_2-receptor antagonists:* Serum diltiazem concentrations increased by cimetidine to a variable extent

SPECIAL CONSIDERATIONS

PATIENT/FAMILY EDUCATION

• Notify physician of irregular heart beat, pulse <50 bpm, shortness of breath, swelling of the hands and feet, pronounced dizziness, constipation, hypotension

• Swallow sustained release capsules whole, do not open, crush, or chew

dimenhydrinate

(dye-men-hye'dri-nate)

Calm-X, Dimetabs, Dinate, Dommanate, Dramamine, Dramanate, Dramocen, Dramoject, Dymenate, Gravol, ♣ Hydrate, Marmine, Nico-Vert, Triptone Caplets, Vertab

Chemical Class: H_1-receptor antagonist, ethanolamine derivative

Therapeutic Class: Antiemetic, antihistamine, anticholinergic

CLINICAL PHARMACOLOGY

Mechanism of Action: Has a depressant action on hyperstimulated labyrinthine function; antiemetic effects may be due to diphenhydramine moiety (dimenhydrinate is a mixture of diphenhydramine and 8-chlorotheophylline)

Pharmacokinetics

PO: Onset 15-30 min

IM: Onset 20-30 min

Duration 3-6 hr, metabolized in liver, excreted in urine

INDICATIONS AND USES: Prevention and treatment of motion sickness; Meniere's disease,* other vestibular disturbances*

DOSAGE

Adult

- PO 50-100 mg q4-6h, do not exceed 400 mg/d; IM/IV 50 mg prn

Child 6-12 yr

- PO 25-50 mg/q6-8h, do not exceed 150 mg/d; IM 1.25 mg/kg or 37.5 mg/m^2 qid, do not exceed 300 mg/d

Child 2-6 yr

- PO 12.5-25 mg q6-8h, do not exceed 75 mg/d

$ AVAILABLE FORMS/COST OF THERAPY

- Inj, Sol—IM; IV: 50 mg/ml, 10 ml: **$1.50-$15.60**
- Tab, Uncoated—Oral: 50 mg, 100's: **$1.92-$4.20**
- Tab, Chewable—Oral: 50 mg, 24's: **$5.43**
- Liq—Oral: 12.5 mg/4 ml, 120 ml: **$4.38**

CONTRAINDICATIONS: Neonates (IV products may contain benzyl alcohol), hypersensitivity

PRECAUTIONS: Children, prostatic hypertrophy, stenosing peptic ulcer, pyloroduodenal obstruction, bladder neck obstruction, narrow angle glaucoma, cardiac dysrhythmias, elderly

PREGNANCY AND LACTATION: Pregnancy category B; has been used for the treatment of hyperemesis gravidarum; small amounts are excreted into breast milk, use caution in nursing mothers

SIDE EFFECTS/ADVERSE REACTIONS

CNS: Drowsiness, confusion, nervousness, restlessness, headache, insomnia (especially in children), tingling, heaviness and weakness of hands, vertigo, dizziness, lassitude, excitation

CV: Palpitations, hypotension, tachycardia

EENT: Blurring of vision, diplopia, nasal stuffiness

GI: Nausea, vomiting, diarrhea, epigastric distress, constipation, anorexia, *dry mouth*

GU: Difficult or painful urination

HEME: ***Hemolytic anemia***

SKIN: Photosensitivity, urticaria, drug rash

▼ DRUG INTERACTIONS

Labs

- *False negative:* Allergy skin testing

SPECIAL CONSIDERATIONS

PATIENT/FAMILY EDUCATION

- May cause drowsiness, use caution driving or operating hazardous machinery

• For prevention of motion sickness administer 30 min before exposure to motion

dimercaprol

(dye-mer-kap'role)

BAL in Oil, British Anti-Lewisite*

Chemical Class: Dithiol compound, chelating agent

Therapeutic Class: Heavy metal antagonist, antidote

CLINICAL PHARMACOLOGY

Mechanism of Action: Promotes excretion of arsenic, gold, and mercury by chelation, increasing urinary and fecal elimination of the metals

Pharmacokinetics

IM: Peak 30-60 min, metabolism and excretion are complete within 4 hr, excretion via urine and feces

INDICATIONS AND USES: Treatment of arsenic, gold, and mercury poisoning; acute lead poisoning (in conjunction with calcium edetate disodium)

DOSAGE

Adult and Child

• *Mild arsenic and gold poisoning:* IM 2.5 mg/kg/dose q6h for 2 days, then q12h on 3rd day, then qd thereafter for 10 days

• *Severe arsenic and gold poisoning:* IM 3 mg/kg/dose q4h for 2 days, then q6h on 3rd day, then q12h thereafter for 10 days

• *Mercury poisoning:* IM 5 mg/kg initially followed by 2.5 mg/kg/dose qd-bid for 10 days

• *Lead poisoning:* IM 4 mg/kg alone for first dose, then 3-4 mg/kg/dose with calcium edetate disodium administered at a separate site q4h for 5-7 days

$ AVAILABLE FORMS/COST OF THERAPY

• Inj, Sol—IM: 100 mg/ml, 3 ml: **$33.00**

CONTRAINDICATIONS: Hepatic insufficiency (except postarsenical jaundice); iron, cadmium, or selenium poisoning; severe renal disease, hypersensitivity

PRECAUTIONS: Acute renal insufficiency, G-6-PD deficiency, acidic urine, hypertension

PREGNANCY AND LACTATION: Pregnancy category D; use only in life-threatening poisoning

SIDE EFFECTS/ADVERSE REACTIONS

CNS: Headache, anxiety

CV: Rise in blood pressure, tachycardia

EENT: Burning sensation in the lips, mouth and throat; feeling of constriction in the throat; conjunctivitis, lacrimation, blepharal spasm; rhinorrhea

GI: Nausea, vomiting, salivation, abdominal pain

GU: Burning sensation in the penis

SKIN: Sweating

▼ DRUG INTERACTIONS

Labs

• *Decrease:* RAIU test

SPECIAL CONSIDERATIONS

Administer by deep IM injection only

MONITORING PARAMETERS

• Blood pressure, pulse

• BUN, Cr, urine pH (alkaline urinary pH decreases renal damage)

• Specific heavy metal levels

dinoprostone

(dye-noe-prost'one)

Prepidil Gel, Prostin E_2

Chemical Class: Prostaglandin

Therapeutic Class: Abortifacient, oxytocic

D

CLINICAL PHARMACOLOGY

Mechanism of Action: Stimulates the myometrium of the gravid uterus to contract in a manner similar to contractions seen in the term uterus during labor

Pharmacokinetics

SUPP: Onset 10 min; duration 2-3 hr; metabolized in spleen, kidney, lungs; excreted in urine

INDICATIONS AND USES: Abortion during 2nd trimester, benign hydatidiform mole, expulsion of uterine contents in fetal deaths to 28 wk, missed abortion, cervical ripening, labor induction

DOSAGE

Adult

• *Abortifacient:* VAG SUPP 20 mg high into vagina, repeat q3-5h until abortion occurs, max 240 mg

• *Cervical ripening:* VAG GEL administer contents of 1 syringe (0.5 mg) into cervical canal just below the level of the internal os, repeat in 6 hr prn, max 1.5 mg/24 hr

$ AVAILABLE FORMS/COST OF THERAPY

• Inj, Sol—Vag: 0.5 mg/3 g, 1's: **$98.04**

• Supp—Vag: 20 mg/supp, 5's: **$111.91**

CONTRAINDICATIONS: SUPP: Hypersensitivity, acute PID, cardiac disease, pulmonary disease, renal disease, hepatic disease, viable fetus; GEL: History of cesarean section or major uterine surgery; cephalopelvic disproportion; history of difficult labor or traumatic delivery; grand multiparae with six or more previous term pregnancies; nonvertex presentation; hyperactive or hypertonic uterine patterns; fetal distress where delivery is not imminent; obstetric emergencies favoring surgical intervention; ruptured membranes; hypersensitivity; placenta previa or unexplained vaginal bleeding; vasa previa; active herpes genitalia

PRECAUTIONS: Asthma, glaucoma, hepatic/renal function impairment, hypotension, hypertension, cardiovascular disease, anemia, jaundice, diabetes, epilepsy, chorioamnionitis, cervicitis, infected endocervical lesions, acute vaginitis

PREGNANCY AND LACTATION: Pregnancy category C; complete any failed attempts at pregnancy termination by some other means

SIDE EFFECTS/ADVERSE REACTIONS

CNS: Headache, dizziness, chills, fever

CV: Hypotension, hypertension

EENT: Blurred vision

GI: Nausea, vomiting, diarrhea

GU: Vaginitis, vaginal pain, vulvitis, vaginismus

HEME: Transient leukocytosis

MS: Leg cramps, joint swelling, weakness

SKIN: Rash, skin color changes

SPECIAL CONSIDERATIONS

PATIENT/FAMILY EDUCATION

• Remain supine for 10-15 min (VAG SUPP), 15-30 min (GEL) after insertion

• Report excessive cramping, bleeding, chills, fever

MONITORING PARAMETERS

• Blood pressure

diphenhydramine

(dye-fen-hye'dra-meen)

Allerdryl, ✦ Allerdryl 50, Allergia-C, Banophen, Beldin, Belix, Ben-A-Vance, Ben-Rex, Bena-D-10, Benadryl, Benadryl Steri-Dose, Benahist, Bendramine, Benoject, Bydramine, Dibenil, Diphen, Diphenacen-50, Diphenhist, Dytuss, Fynex, Genahist, Hydramine, Hydril, Hyrexin, Noradryl, Norafed, Nordryl, Pharm-A-Dry, Shodryl, Tega Dryl, Truxadryl, Tusstat, Uad Dryl, Wehdryl

Chemical Class: Ethanolamine derivative

Therapeutic Class: Antihistamine, antiparkinson agent, antitussive, antiemetic, sleep aid

CLINICAL PHARMACOLOGY

Mechanism of Action: Competes with histamine for H_1-receptor sites on effector cells in the GI tract, blood vessels, and respiratory tract; also has anticholinergic and sedative effects

Pharmacokinetics

PO: Peak 2-4 hr, 78% bound to plasma proteins, metabolized in the liver, $t_{1/2}$ 2-8 hr

INDICATIONS AND USES: Perennial and seasonal allergic rhinitis; vasomotor rhinitis; allergic conjunctivitis; symptomatic relief of common cold; allergic and non-allergic pruritic symptoms; mild, uncomplicated urticaria and angioedema; adjunctive therapy of anaphylactic reactions, motion sickness, sleep aid, parkinsonism (including drug-induced), cough suppressant; *Acute dystonic reactions

DOSAGE

Adult

- PO/IM/IV 15-50 mg q4h, do not exceed 400 mg/d

Child

- PO/IM/IV 5 mg/kg/d or 150 mg/m^2/d divided q6-8h, do not exceed 300 mg/d

$ AVAILABLE FORMS/COST OF THERAPY

- Cap, Gel—Oral: 25, 50 mg, 100's: **$1.69-$29.24**
- Elixir—Oral: 12.5 mg/5ml, 480 ml: **$2.93-$15.48**
- Inj, Sol—IM, IV: 10 mg/ml, 30 ml: **$1.48-$8.85;** 50 mg/ml, 10 ml: **$4.49-$17.50**

CONTRAINDICATIONS: Hypersensitivity, narrow-angle glaucoma, bladder neck obstruction

PRECAUTIONS: Liver disease, elderly, increased intraocular pressure, hyperthyroidism, cardiovascular disease, hypertension, urinary retention, renal disease, stenosed peptic ulcers

PREGNANCY AND LACTATION: Pregnancy category C; excreted into breast milk; although levels are not thought to be sufficiently high after therapeutic doses to affect the infant, the manufacturer considers the drug contraindicated in nursing mothers due to the increased sensitivity of newborn or premature infants to antihistamines

SIDE EFFECTS/ADVERSE REACTIONS

CNS: Dizziness, drowsiness, poor coordination, fatigue, anxiety, euphoria, confusion, paresthesia, neuritis

CV: Hypotension, palpitations, tachycardia

EENT: Blurred vision, dilated pupils, tinnitus, nasal stuffiness, dry nose, throat

GI: Dry mouth, nausea, vomiting, anorexia, *constipation,* diarrhea

GU: Retention, dysuria, frequency, impotence

HEME: ***Thrombocytopenia, agranulocytosis, hemolytic anemia***

RESP: Increased thick secretions, wheezing, chest tightness
SKIN: Photosensitivity, rash, urticaria

▼ **DRUG INTERACTIONS**

Drugs
- *Barbiturates:* Excessive CNS depression

Labs
- *False negative:* Skin allergy tests

SPECIAL CONSIDERATIONS

PATIENT/FAMILY EDUCATION
- Notify physician if confusion, sedation, hypotension occurs
- Avoid driving or other hazardous activities if drowsiness occurs
- Avoid use of alcohol or other CNS or depressants while taking drug
- Use hard candy or gum (sugarless), frequent rinsing of mouth for dryness

---

diphenidol

(dye-fen'i-dole)
Vontrol
Chemical Class: Trihexyphenidyl derivative
Therapeutic Class: Antiemetic

CLINICAL PHARMACOLOGY
Mechanism of Action: Exerts a specific antivertigo effect on the vestibular apparatus to control vertigo and inhibits the chemoreceptor trigger zone to control nausea and vomiting
Pharmacokinetics
PO: Peak 1.5-3 hr, excreted in urine and feces
INDICATIONS AND USES: Nausea, vomiting, vertigo, Meniere's disease, labyrinthitis
DOSAGE
Adult
- PO 25-50 mg q4h

Child
- PO 0.4 mg/lb (0.88 mg/kg) q4h, do not exceed 2.5 mg/lb/d (5.5 mg/kg/d)

$ **AVAILABLE FORMS/COST OF THERAPY**
- Tab, Uncoated—Oral: 25 mg, 100's: **$50.40**

CONTRAINDICATIONS: Hypersensitivity, anuria, pregnancy
PRECAUTIONS: Child <50 lb, glaucoma, obstructive lesions of the GI and GU tracts, prostatic hypertrophy, pyloric and duodenal obstruction, organic cardiospasm
PREGNANCY AND LACTATION: Do not use in nausea and vomiting of pregnancy
SIDE EFFECTS/ADVERSE REACTIONS
CNS: Auditory and visual hallucinations, disorientation, confusion, *drowsiness,* overstimulation, depression, sleep disturbance, headache
CV: Transient lowering of blood pressure
EENT: Blurred vision
GI: Dry mouth, nausea, indigestion, heartburn, mild jaundice
SKIN: Rash

SPECIAL CONSIDERATIONS

Due to potential for hallucinations, disorientation, or confusion use should be limited to patients who are hospitalized or under comparable continuous, professional supervision

D

diphenoxylate

(dye-fen-ox'i-late)

Colonaid, Di-Atro, Dimotal, Diphenatol, Diphenoxylate W/Atropine, Lo-Rex, Lo-Trol, Lofene, Logen, Lomanate, Lomocot, Lomodix, Lomotil, Lomoxate, Lonox, Lotabs, Low-Quel; Nor-Mil, Romotil, Uni-Lom, Vi-Atro

Chemical Class: Meperidine analog
Therapeutic Class: Antidiarrheal
DEA Class: Schedule V

CLINICAL PHARMACOLOGY

Mechanism of Action: Direct effect on circular smooth muscle of the bowel that prolongs GI transit time; available only in combination with atropine sulfate

Pharmacokinetics

PO: Onset 1 hr, peak 2 hr, duration 3-4 hr; metabolized in liver, excreted in bile and urine

INDICATIONS AND USES: Diarrhea

DOSAGE

Adult

• PO 5 mg qid, then taper dose as tolerated

Child

• PO 0.3-0.4 mg/kg qd in four divided doses

$ **AVAILABLE FORMS/COST OF THERAPY**

• Sol—Oral: 2.5 mg diphenoxylate/0.025 mg atropine/5 ml, 60 ml: **$2.86-$12.50**

• Tab, Uncoated—Oral: 2.5 mg diphenoxylate/0.025 mg atropine, 100's: **$2.40-$44.80**

CONTRAINDICATIONS: Hypersensitivity to diphenoxylate or atropine, obstructive jaundice, diarrhea associated with pseudomembranous enterocolitis or enterotoxin-producing bacteria

PRECAUTIONS: Age <2 yr; acute ulcerative colitis (may induce toxic megacolon), severe hepatorenal disease

PREGNANCY AND LACTATION: Pregnancy category C; excreted in breast milk

SIDE EFFECTS/ADVERSE REACTIONS

CNS: Euphoria, depression, malaise/lethargy, confusion, *sedation/drowsiness, dizziness,* restlessness, headache, hyperthermia

CV: Tachycardia

EENT: Swelling of gums, *dry mouth, blurred vision*

GI: ***Toxic megacolon,*** *paralytic ileus,* pancreatitis, vomiting, nausea, anorexia, abdominal discomfort

GU: Urinary retention

MS: Muscle cramps

SKIN: Dry skin, urticaria

SPECIAL CONSIDERATIONS

PATIENT/FAMILY EDUCATION

• Avoid CNS depressants

dipivefrin

(dye-pi've-frin)

Propine

Chemical Class: Diesterified epinephrine
Therapeutic Class: Adrenergic agonist

CLINICAL PHARMACOLOGY

Mechanism of Action: Converted to epinephrine, which decreases aqueous production and increases outflow

Pharmacokinetics

Onset 30 min, peak 1 hr, duration 12 hr

INDICATIONS AND USES: Open-angle glaucoma

DOSAGE

Adult

• 1 gtt OU q12h

$ AVAILABLE FORMS/COST OF THERAPY

- Sol, Top—Ophth: 0.1%, 5 ml: **$9.31-$12.25;** 10 ml: **$17.16-$26.31**

CONTRAINDICATIONS: Hypersensitivity, narrow-angle glaucoma

PRECAUTIONS: Children, aphakia (may cause reversible macular edema)

PREGNANCY AND LACTATION: Pregnancy category B

SIDE EFFECTS/ADVERSE REACTIONS

CV: Hypertension, tachycardia, dysrhythmias

EENT: Burning, stinging, mydriasis, photophobia

SPECIAL CONSIDERATIONS

PATIENT/FAMILY EDUCATION

- May cause transient eye burning or stinging

---

dipyridamole

(dye-peer-id'a-mole)

Persantine

Chemical Class: Substituted pyrimidine

Therapeutic Class: Coronary vasodilator, antiplatelet

CLINICAL PHARMACOLOGY

Mechanism of Action: Inhibits adenosine deaminase and phosphodiesterase; increases adenosine and cyclic-3', 5'-adenosine monophosphate within platelets and inhibits thromboxane A_2 formation; this reduces platelet adhesion and causes coronary vasodilation that is abolished by theophylline

Pharmacokinetics

PO: Onset 30 min, peak 2-2½ hr, duration 6 hr

IV: Onset 1 min, peak 7 min, duration 30 min

Protein binding 91%-99%, conjugated in liver to glucuronide, excreted in bile, undergoes enterohepatic recirculation

INDICATIONS AND USES: With warfarin to prevent thromboembolic complications of cardiac valve replacement, with aspirin to prevent coronary bypass graft occlusion* or transient ischemic attack,* as diagnostic aid in thallium myocardial perfusion imaging for the evaluation of CAD

DOSAGE

Adult

- *Transient ischemic attack:* PO 50 mg tid, 1 hr ac, not to exceed 400 mg qd
- *Inhibition of platelet adhesion:* PO 50-75 mg qid in combination with aspirin or warfarin
- *Diagnostic aid in myocardial perfusion studies:* IV 0.14 mg/kg/min for 4 min, max dose 60 mg

Child

- *Inhibition of platelet adhesion:* PO 3-6 mg/kg/d in 3 divided doses

$ AVAILABLE FORMS/COST OF THERAPY

- Tab, Coated—Oral: 25, 50, 75 mg, 100's: **$2.16-$72.86**
- Inj, Sol—IV: 5 mg/ml, 10 ml × 5: **$720.00**

CONTRAINDICATIONS: Hypersensitivity, hypotension

PRECAUTIONS: Ischemic heart disease, bleeding disorders

PREGNANCY AND LACTATION: Pregnancy category C; excreted in breast milk

SIDE EFFECTS/ADVERSE REACTIONS

CNS: Headache, dizziness, weakness, fainting, syncope

CV: ***Angina pectoris, MI,*** *hypotension (5%),* hypertension, tachycardia, dysrhythmia

GI: Nausea, vomiting, anorexia, diarrhea

MS: Weakness, hypertonia

RESP: Dyspnea (3%)
SKIN: Rash, flushing

▼ **DRUG INTERACTIONS**

Drugs

• *Adenosine:* Dipyridamole reduces adenosine metabolism

• *Beta blockers:* Dipyridamole promotes bradycardia due to beta blockers

SPECIAL CONSIDERATIONS

• Contributes little to the antithrombotic effect of asprin

---

dirithromycin

(die-rith'ro-my-sin)
Dynabac

Chemical Class: Semi-synthetic, erythromycin analog (pro-drug for erythromycylamine)
Therapeutic Class: Macrolide antibiotic

CLINICAL PHARMACOLOGY

Mechanism of Action: Bacteriostatic via reversible binding to 23S component of 40S ribosomal unit, thereby impairing transpeptidation or translocation

Pharmacokinetics

PO: Peak, 0.48 mg/L at 4 hr after 500 mg dose; greater acid stability; 15%-32% protein bound; good tissue penetration into upper and lower respiratory tract and prostate; nonenzymatic hydrolysis to inactive metabolites; fecal and renal elimination; $t_{1/2}$, 44 hr

INDICATIONS AND USES: Infections of upper (including otitis media, pharyngitis, tonsillitis) and lower respiratory tract, skin and skin structure caused by susceptible organisms. Antibacterial spectrum usually includes: gram-positive organisms: *Streptococcus pneumonia, Staphylococcus aureus, Str. pyogenes;* gram-negative aerobes: *Legionella, Moraxella catarrhalis, Mycoplasma pneumonia, Chlamydia trachomatis*

DOSAGE

Adult

• PO 500 mg qd

$ **AVAILABLE FORMS/COST OF THERAPY**

• Cap—Oral: 250 mg, 60's: **$112.50**

CONTRAINDICATIONS: Hypersensitivity

PRECAUTIONS: Hepatic insufficiency

PREGNANCY AND LACTATION: Pregnancy category C; excreted into rodent breast milk, no human data

SIDE EFFECTS/ADVERSE REACTIONS

CNS: Headache, dizziness, vertigo
GI: Abdominal pain, diarrhea, nausea, vomiting

---

disopyramide

(dye-soe-peer'a-mide)
Disopyramide, Norpace, Norpace CR

Chemical Class: Substituted pyramide
Therapeutic Class: Antidysrhythmic (Class IA)

CLINICAL PHARMACOLOGY

Mechanism of Action: A type 1 antidysrhythmic drug; lengthens effective refractory period of the atrium and ventricle; decreases conduction velocity; has minimal effect on effective refractory period of the AV node; decreases the disparity in refractoriness between infarcted and adjacent normal myocardium

Pharmacokinetics

PO: Peak 30 min-3 hr, duration 6-12 hr; $t_{1/2}$ 4-10 hr; metabolized in liver; excreted unchanged in urine (50%) and feces (10%); crosses placenta; protein binding concentration dependent (50%-65% at plasma levels of 2-4 μg/ml)

INDICATIONS AND USES: PVCs, ventricular tachycardia, supraventricular tachycardia, atrial flutter, atrial fibrillation

DOSAGE

Adult

• PO 100-200 mg q6h; in renal dysfunction, if CrCl 30-40 ml/min, dose should be 100 mg q8h, if CrCl 15-30 ml/min, dose should be 100 mg q12h, if CrCl <15 ml/min, dose should be 100 mg q24h; may give loading dose of 300 mg for rapid effect; PO (SUS REL CAPS) 200-300 mg q12h; not recommended in renal dysfunction

Child

• PO age 12-18 yr: 6-15 mg/kg/d in divided doses q6h; age 4-12 yr: 10-15 mg/kg/d in divided doses q6h; age 1-4 yr: 10-20 mg/kg/d in divided doses q6h; age <1 yr: 10-30 mg/kg/d in divided doses q6h

$ AVAILABLE FORMS/COST OF THERAPY

• Cap, Gel—Oral: 100, 150 mg, 100's: **$9.75-$64.53**

• Cap, Gel, Sust Action—Oral: 100, 150 mg, 100's: **$28.43-$77.74**

CONTRAINDICATIONS: Hypersensitivity, 2nd or 3rd degree block, cardiogenic shock, CHF (uncompensated), sick sinus syndrome, QT prolongation

PRECAUTIONS: Children, diabetes mellitus, renal disease, hepatic disease, myasthenia gravis, narrow-angle glaucoma, cardiomyopathy, conduction abnormalities (including accessory pathways)

PREGNANCY AND LACTATION: Pregnancy category C; excreted in breast milk

SIDE EFFECTS/ADVERSE REACTIONS

CNS: Headache, dizziness, psychosis, fatigue, depression, paresthesias, anxiety, insomnia

CV: Hypotension, bradycardia, angina, PVCs, tachycardia, increased QRS or QT duration, ***cardiac arrest,*** edema, AV block, ***CHF,*** syncope, chest pain

EENT: Blurred vision, dry nose, throat, eyes, narrow-angle glaucoma

GI: Dry mouth (32%), *constipation* (11%), nausea, anorexia, flatulence, diarrhea, vomiting

GU: Retention, hesitancy (14%), impotence, urinary frequency, urgency

HEME: ***Thrombocytopenia, agranulocytosis,*** anemia (rare)

METAB: Hypoglycemia

MS: Weakness, pain in extremities

SKIN: Rash, pruritus, urticaria

▼ DRUG INTERACTIONS

Drugs

• *Beta blockers:* Enhanced negative inotropy

• *Barbiturates, phenobarbital, phenytoin, and rifampin:* Reduced disopyramide level

Labs

• *Increase:* Liver enzymes, lipids, BUN, creatinine

• *Decrease:* Hgb/Hct, blood glucose

SPECIAL CONSIDERATIONS

MONITORING PARAMETERS

• Monitor ECG closely; if PR, QRS, or QT interval increase by 25%, stop drug

---

disulfiram

(dye-sul'fi-ram)

Antabuse, Disulfiram

Chemical Class: Aldehyde dehydrogenase inhibitor; thiuram derivative

Therapeutic Class: Alcohol deterrent

CLINICAL PHARMACOLOGY

Mechanism of Action: Blocks oxidation of alcohol at acetaldehyde stage; accumulation of acetaldehyde produces disulfiram–alcohol reaction

Pharmacokinetics

PO: Onset 12 hr; effect lasts up to 2 wk; oxidized by liver; metabolites excreted by kidney, 20% excreted unchanged in feces

INDICATIONS AND USES: Adjunctive treatment of chronic alcoholism

DOSAGE

Adult

• PO 250-500 mg qd for 1-2 wk, then 125-500 mg qd until fully socially recovered

$ AVAILABLE FORMS/COST OF THERAPY

• Tab, Uncoated—Oral: 250, 500 mg, 100's: **$7.43-$66.11**

CONTRAINDICATIONS: Hypersensitivity, alcohol intoxication, psychoses, cardiovascular disease, recent use of metronidazole, isoniazid, paraldehyde, alcohol, or alcohol-containing preparations; patients with history of rubber contact dermatitis should be evaluated for hypersensitivity to thiuram derivatives before receiving

PRECAUTIONS: Hypothyroidism, hepatic disease, diabetes mellitus, seizure disorders, nephritis, stroke

PREGNANCY AND LACTATION: Pregnancy category X; excreted in breast milk

SIDE EFFECTS/ADVERSE REACTIONS

CNS: Headache, drowsiness, restlessness, dizziness, fatigue, tremors, psychosis, neuritis, sweating, ***convulsions,*** peripheral neuropathy

GI: Nausea, vomiting, anorexia, severe thirst, ***hepatotoxicity,*** metallic or garlic-like taste

SKIN: Rash, dermatitis, urticaria

MISC: ***Disulfiram–alcohol reaction: flushing, sweating, headache, nausea, vomiting, chest pain, palpitations, dyspnea, tachycardia, confusion, and hypotension. Reactions may occur with blood ethanol level as low as 5-10 mg per 100 ml.***

▼ DRUG INTERACTIONS

Drugs

• *Benzodiazepines, chlordiazepoxide, diazepam:* Disulfiram increases effect

• *Ethanol+, oral anticoagulants+, phenytoin+:* Disulfiram inhibits metabolism

• *Isoniazid, metronidazole:* Disulfiram promotes encephalopathy due to these

• *Theophylline:* Disulfiram increases level

Labs

• *Increase:* Cholesterol

• *Decrease:* ^{131}I uptake, VMA

SPECIAL CONSIDERATIONS

PATIENT/FAMILY EDUCATION

• Disulfiram–alcohol reaction may occur for 2 wk after last dose

• May occur with external use of alcohol-containing products (i.e., liniments)

---

dobutamine

(doe-byoo'ta-meen)

Dobutrex

Chemical Class: Catecholamine

Therapeutic Class: Adrenergic direct-acting β_1-agonist

CLINICAL PHARMACOLOGY

Mechanism of Action: Causes increased contractility, increased coronary blood flow and heart rate by direct action on β_1 receptors in heart; reduces systemic vascular resistance

Pharmacokinetics

IV: Onset 1-2 min, peak 10 min, $t_{1/2}$ 2 min; metabolized in liver (inactive metabolites); metabolites excreted in urine

INDICATIONS AND USES: Short-term treatment of adults with cardiac decompensation due to depressed myocardial contractility, diagnostic aid for ischemic heart disease*

DOSAGE

Adult

• IV INF 2.5-15 μg/kg/min; max dose 40 μg/kg/min

$ AVAILABLE FORMS/COST OF THERAPY

• Inj, Dry-Sol—IV: 12.5 mg/ml, 20 ml: **$42.81-$50.77**

CONTRAINDICATIONS: Hypersensitivity, hypertrophic cardiomyopathy, uncontrolled atrial fibrillation or flutter

PRECAUTIONS Children, hypertension, sulfite sensitivity (preparation contains sulfite)

PREGNANCY AND LACTATION: Pregnancy category C; excreted in breast milk

SIDE EFFECTS/ADVERSE REACTIONS

CNS: *Anxiety,* headache, dizziness, paresthesia

CV: Palpitations, *tachycardia,* hypertension, *PVCs*, angina, ***dysrhythmia***

GI: Heartburn, nausea, vomiting

METAB: Hypokalemia

MS: Leg cramps

SPECIAL CONSIDERATIONS

MONITORING PARAMETERS

• Continuously monitor ECG, BP, and PCWP

docusate

(dok'yoo-sate)

Colace, DC Softgels, Pro-Cal-Sof, Pro-Sof, Sulfalax Calcium, Surfak, Dialose, Diocto-K, Correctol Extra Gentle, Diocto, Dioeze, Disonate, DOK, DOS Softgel, Doxinate, D-S-S, Kasof, Modane Soft, Regulex SS, Regutol

Chemical Class: Anionic surfactant

Therapeutic Class: Laxative; stool softener

CLINICAL PHARMACOLOGY

Mechanism of Action: Detergent activity; facilitates admixture of fat and water to soften stool

Pharmacokinetics

PO: Onset 24-72 hr, absorbed to some extent in duodenum and jejunum, excreted in bile

INDICATIONS AND USES: Constipation associated with hard, dry stools; stool softener in patients who should avoid straining during defecation; cerumenolytic*

DOSAGE

Adult

• *Laxative:* PO 50-400 mg/d in 1-4 divided doses

• *Cerumenolytic:* Fill ear canal with liquid; produces substantial ear wax disintegration in 15 min, complete disintegration after 24 hr

Child <3 yr

• PO 10-40 mg/d in 1-4 divided doses

Child 3-6 yr

• PO 20-60 mg/d in 1-4 divided doses

Child 6-12 yr

• PO 40-150 mg/d in 1-4 divided doses

$ **AVAILABLE FORMS/COST OF THERAPY**

- Cap, Softgel—Oral: 50, 100, 250 mg, 100's: **$1.40-$22.88**
- Liq—Oral: 150 mg/15 ml, 480 ml: **$12.00-$87.25**
- Syr—Oral: 60 mg/15 ml, 480 ml: **$3.30-$18.41**

CONTRAINDICATIONS: Hypersensitivity, obstruction, fecal impaction, nausea/vomiting, acute abdominal pain, concomitant use of mineral oil

PREGNANCY AND LACTATION: Pregnancy category C; no reports linking use of docusate with congenital defects have been located; diarrhea has been reported in one infant exposed to docusate while breast feeding but relationship between symptom and drug is unknown

SIDE EFFECTS/ADVERSE REACTIONS

EENT: Throat irritation

GI: Nausea, anorexia, cramps, diarrhea, bitter taste

SKIN: Rash

SPECIAL CONSIDERATIONS

PATIENT/FAMILY EDUCATION

- Drink plenty of water during administration

---

dopamine

(doe'pa-meen)

Dopastat, Intropin, Revimine ♣

Chemical Class: Catecholamine

Therapeutic Class: Vasopressor; sympathomimetic

CLINICAL PHARMACOLOGY

Mechanism of Action: Stimulates both adrenergic and dopaminergic receptors in a dose-dependent manner; low doses (1-5 μg/kg/min) stimulate mainly dopaminergic receptors producing renal and mesenteric vasodilation; intermediate doses (5-15 μg/kg/min) stimulate both dopaminergic and β_1-adrenergic receptors producing cardiac stimulation and renal vasodilation; large doses (>15 μg/kg/min) stimulate α-adrenergic receptors producing vasoconstriction, increases in peripheral vascular resistance and blood pressure

Pharmacokinetics

IV: Onset 5 min, duration <10 min, metabolized in plasma, kidneys, and liver by MAO (75% to inactive metabolites, 25% to norepinephrine); $t_{1/2}$ 2 min

INDICATIONS AND USES: Shock, increase organ perfusion, CHF refractory to digitalis and diuretics, hepatorenal syndrome,* cirrhosis,* acute renal failure*

DOSAGE

Adult and child

- IV INF 1-20 μg/kg/min, titrated to desired response; do not exceed 50 μg/kg/min

$ **AVAILABLE FORMS/COST OF THERAPY**

- Inj, Conc-Sol—IV: 40, 80, 160 mg/ml, 5 ml: **$9.42-$378.44;** 80, 160, 320 mg/100 ml, 250 ml: **$19.30-$45.73**

CONTRAINDICATIONS: Pheochromocytoma, uncorrected tachydysrhythmia or ventricular fibrillation, hypersensitivity

PRECAUTIONS: Hypovolemia, arterial embolism, occlusive vascular disease, abrupt discontinuation, sulfite sensitivity, MAOIs

PREGNANCY AND LACTATION: Pregnancy category C; because dopamine is indicated only in life-threatening situations, chronic use would not be expected; no data available regarding use in breast feeding

SIDE EFFECTS/ADVERSE REACTIONS

CNS: Headache

CV: Ectopic beats, tachycardia, an-

ginal pain, palpitation, hypotension, vasoconstriction, aberrant conduction, bradycardia, widened QRS complex, hypertension
EENT: Dilated pupils (high doses)
GI: Nausea, vomiting
GU: Azotemia
RESP: Dyspnea
SKIN: Piloerection; necrosis, tissue sloughing with extravasation, ***gangrene*** (high doses for prolonged periods of time)

▼ **DRUG INTERACTIONS**

Drugs

- *Ergot alkaloids:* Gangrene has been reported

SPECIAL CONSIDERATIONS

Dilute before use if not prediluted; antidote for extravasation—infiltrate area as soon as possible with 10-15 ml NS containing 5-10 mg phentolamine

MONITORING PARAMETERS

- Urine flow, cardiac output, blood pressure

dornase alfa

(door'nace al'fa)
Pulmozyme
Chemical Class: Recombinant human deoxyribonuclease I
Therapeutic Class: Mucolytic; respiratory inhalant

CLINICAL PHARMACOLOGY

Mechanism of Action: Hydrolyzes DNA in sputum of CF patients and reduces sputum viscoelasticity

Pharmacokinetics

Does not produce significant elevations in serum DNase concentrations; no accumulation of serum DNase has been noted; following nebulization, enzyme levels are measurable in sputum within 15 min and decline rapidly thereafter

INDICATIONS AND USES: Cystic fibrosis (as an adjunct to standard therapies to reduce the frequency of respiratory infections requiring parenteral antibiotics and to improve pulmonary function)

DOSAGE

Adult and child ≥5

- NEB 2.5 mg qd; some patients (age >21, FVC >70%) may benefit from bid administration

$ **AVAILABLE FORMS/COST OF THERAPY**

- Sol—Inh: 1 mg/ml, 2.5 ml × 30: **$972.00**

CONTRAINDICATIONS: Hypersensitivity to dornase alfa, Chinese Hamster Ovary cell products, or any component of the product

PRECAUTIONS: Safety and efficacy have not been demonstrated in children <5 yr or patients with FVC <40% of predicted

PREGNANCY AND LACTATION: Pregnancy category B; excretion into breast milk unknown, however, since serum levels of DNase have not been shown to increase above endogenous levels, little drug would be expected to be excreted into breast milk

SIDE EFFECTS/ADVERSE REACTIONS

Most events likely reflected sequelae of the underlying lung disease
CNS: Fever, asthenia
CV: Chest pain
EENT: Voice alteration, pharyngitis, laryngitis, conjunctivitis
GI: Intestinal obstruction, gallbladder disease, liver disease, pancreatic disease, abdominal pain
METAB: Diabetes mellitus, weight loss
MS: Flu-like syndrome
RESP: Hypoxia, apnea, bronchiectasis, change in sputum, cough increase, dyspnea, hemoptysis, lung function decrease, nasal polyps, rhi-

nitis, sinusitis, sputum increase, wheeze

SKIN: Rash

SPECIAL CONSIDERATIONS

Safety and efficacy have been demonstrated only with the following nebulizers and compressors: disposable jet nebulizer *Hudson T Updraft II,* disposable jet nebulizer *Marquest Acorn II* in conjunction with a *Pulmo-Aide* compressor, and reusable *PARI LC Jet+* nebulizer in conjunction with the *PARI PRONEB* compressor

PATIENT/FAMILY EDUCATION

- Must be stored in refrigerator at 2-8°C and protected from strong light (keep refrigerated when transporting and do not leave at room temp for >24 hr)
- Do not dilute or mix with other drugs in nebulizer
- Not a cure for cystic fibrosis
- Proper use of nebulizer and compressor system used in the delivery of the drug

dorzolamide

(door-zol'a-mide)

Trusopt

Chemical Class: Sulfonamide derivative

Therapeutic Class: Carbonic anhydrase inhibitor

CLINICAL PHARMACOLOGY

Mechanism of Action: Inhibition of carbonic anhydrase in ciliary processes of the eye decreases aqueous humor secretion, reducing intraocular pressure

Pharmacokinetics

OPHTH: Systemically absorbed, amounts below the degree of inhibition anticipated to be necessary for pharmacological effect on renal function and respiration; 33% plasma protein bound; excreted as *N*-desethyl metabolite and unchanged in urine; $t_{1/2}$ in RBCs, 4 mo

INDICATIONS AND USES: Treatment of elevated intraocular pressure in patients with ocular hypertension or open-angle glaucoma

DOSAGE

Adult

- OPHTH 1 gtt in affected eye(s) tid

$ AVAILABLE FORMS/COST OF THERAPY

- Sol—Ophth: 2%, 5 ml: **$21.00;** 10 ml: **$42.00**

CONTRAINDICATIONS: Hypersensitivity

PRECAUTIONS: Renal/hepatic impairment (severe)

PREGNANCY AND LACTATION: Pregnancy category C

SIDE EFFECTS/ADVERSE REACTIONS

EENT: Ocular burning, stinging, or discomfort (25%); superficial punctate keratitis (12.5%); ocular allergic reactions, blurred vision, tearing, dryness, photophobia (1-5%)

GI: Bitter taste following administration (25%)

SPECIAL CONSIDERATIONS

PATIENT/FAMILY EDUCATION

- Can be administered concomitantly with other topical ophth products, separate administration by 10 min
- The preservative in dorzolamide sol, benzalkonium chloride, may be absorbed by soft contact lenses

doxapram

(dox'a-pram)

Dopram

Chemical Class: Monohydrated pyrrolidinone derivative

Therapeutic Class: Analeptic

CLINICAL PHARMACOLOGY

Mechanism of Action: Respiratory stimulation through activation of peripheral carotid chemoreceptors; with higher doses medullary respiratory centers are stimulated

Pharmacokinetics

IV: Onset 20-40 sec, peak 1-2 min, duration 5-10 min; metabolized by liver, metabolites excreted by kidneys; $t_{1/2}$ 2.4-4.1 hr

INDICATIONS AND USES: Chronic obstructive pulmonary disease (COPD) associated with acute hypercapnia (temporary measure in hospitalized patients); postanesthesia respiratory stimulation; drug-induced CNS depression; apnea of prematurity resistant to methylxanthines*

DOSAGE

Adult

- *Postanesthetic respiratory stimulation:* IV INJ 0.5-1 mg/kg, not to exceed 1.5 mg/kg total as a single inj, or 2 mg/kg total when given as multiple inj at 5 min intervals; IV INF 250 mg in 250 ml sol, initiate at 5 mg/min until response satisfactory, then maintain at 1-3 mg/min to sustain desired effect; recommended total dose 4 mg/kg
- *Drug-induced CNS depression:* IV INJ priming dose of 2 mg/kg, repeated in 5 min; repeat q1-2h till patient awakes; IV INF priming dose of 2 mg/kg, if no response continue supportive measures and repeat priming dose in 1-2 hr; if some respiratory stimulation occurs infuse 1 mg/ml sol at 1-3 mg/min, not to exceed 3 g/d
- *COPD:* IV INF 1-2 mg/min, not to exceed 3 mg/min; do not infuse for longer than 2 hr

Child

- *Apnea of prematurity:* IV 2.5-3 mg/kg loading dose, followed by continuous inf of 1 mg/kg/hr; titrate to lowest rate at which apnea is controlled; do not exceed 2.5 mg/kg/hr

$ **AVAILABLE FORMS/COST OF THERAPY**

- Inj, Sol—IV: 20 mg/ml, 20 ml: **$40.85-$42.75**

CONTRAINDICATIONS: Hypersensitivity; seizure disorders; severe hypertension; severe bronchial asthma; severe dyspnea; severe cardiac disorders; pneumothorax; pulmonary embolism; pulmonary fibrosis, conditions resulting in constriction of chest wall, muscles of respiration, or alveolar expansion; head injury; incompetence of ventilatory mechanism due to muscle paresis; flail chest

PRECAUTIONS: Bronchial asthma, pheochromocytoma, severe tachycardia, dysrhythmias, hypertension, children

PREGNANCY AND LACTATION: Pregnancy category B; excretion into breast milk unknown

SIDE EFFECTS/ADVERSE REACTIONS

CNS: Headache, dizziness, apprehension, disorientation, hyperactivity, ***convulsions,*** bilateral Babinski, involuntary movements, increased DTRs clonus, pyrexia

CV: Flushing, phlebitis, *variations in heart rate,* lowered T waves, dysrhythmias, *chest pain,* tightness in chest, *mild to moderate increase in BP*

EENT: ***Laryngospasm,*** pupillary dilation

GI: Nausea, vomiting, diarrhea, desire to defecate

GU: Urinary retention, spontaneous voiding, proteinuria

HEME: Decreased Hgb, Hct, or RBC; decreased WBC in patients with preexisting leukopenia; hemolysis (with rapid infusion)

RESP: Cough, dyspnea, tachypnea, ***bronchospasm,*** hiccoughs, rebound hypoventilation
SKIN: Local skin irritation with extravasation

SPECIAL CONSIDERATIONS

MONITORING PARAMETERS

• Baseline ABG then q30min (for use in COPD)

---

doxazosin

(dox-ay′zoe-sin)
Cardura
Chemical Class: Quinazoline derivative
Therapeutic Class: Peripheral α_1-adrenergic blocker

CLINICAL PHARMACOLOGY

Mechanism of Action: Selectively blocks postsynaptic α_1-adrenergic receptors; dilates both arterioles and veins; relaxes smooth muscle in bladder neck and prostate

Pharmacokinetics

PO: Onset 2 hr, peak 2-3 hr, $t_{1/2}$ 22 hr, extensively metabolized in liver, excreted via bile, feces, and urine, 98% bound to plasma proteins

INDICATIONS AND USES: Hypertension, benign prostatic hyperplasia (BPH), CHF*

DOSAGE

Adult

• PO 1 mg qd, increasing to 16 mg qd if required; usual range 4-16 mg/d

$ **AVAILABLE FORMS/COST OF THERAPY**

• Tab, Uncoated—Oral: 1, 2 mg, 100's: **$88.67;** 4 mg, 100's: **$93.10**; 8 mg, 100's: **$97.76**

CONTRAINDICATIONS: Hypersensitivity to quinazolines

PRECAUTIONS: Children, hepatic disease

PREGNANCY AND LACTATION: Pregnancy category C; may accumulate in breast milk, use caution in nursing mothers

SIDE EFFECTS/ADVERSE REACTIONS

CNS: Depression, *dizziness,* nervousness, paresthesia, somnolence, anxiety, insomnia, asthenia, ataxia, hypertonia, *headache,* fever
CV: Palpitations, postural hypotension, tachycardia, dysrhythmia, chest pain, edema, flushing
EENT: Abnormal vision, tinnitus, vertigo
GI: Nausea, vomiting, dry mouth, diarrhea, constipation, abdominal discomfort, flatulence
GU: Incontinence, polyuria
MS: Arthralgia, myalgia
RESP: Dyspnea
SKIN: Rash, pruritus

SPECIAL CONSIDERATIONS

PATIENT/FAMILY EDUCATION

• Alert patient to the possibility of syncopal and orthostatic symptoms, especially with first dose ("first-dose syncope")
• Take initial dose at bedtime, arise slowly from reclining position
• Report dizziness or palpitations to physician
• Use caution when driving or operating heavy machinery

---

doxepin

(dox′eh-pin)
Adapin, Sinequan, Triadapin, ✦ Zonalon
Chemical Class: Tertiary amine
Therapeutic Class: Antidepressant, tricyclic

CLINICAL PHARMACOLOGY

Mechanism of Action: Inhibits reuptake of norepinephrine and serotonin at the presynaptic neuron prolonging neuronal activity; inhibits histamine and acetylcholine activity; mild peripheral vasodilator effects and possible "quinidine-like" actions

Pharmacokinetics

PO: Metabolized by liver to desmethyldoxepin (active); excreted by kidneys, $t_{1/2}$ 8-24 hr, 80%-85% bound to plasma proteins

INDICATIONS AND USES: Depression, anxiety, chronic pain,* peptic ulcer disease,* panic disorder,* dermatologic disorders,* pruritus associated with atopic dermatitis and lichen simplex chronicus (TOP formulation)

DOSAGE

Adult

• PO 50-75 mg/d in divided doses; may increase to 300 mg/d or may give daily dose hs; TOP apply thin film of cream qid for up to 8 d

Adolescents

• PO 25-50 mg/d in single or divided doses; gradually increase to 100 mg/d

$ AVAILABLE FORMS/COST OF THERAPY

• Cre—Top: 5%, 30 g: **$19.80**

• Cap, Gel—Oral: 10, 25, 50, 75, 100, 150 mg, 100's: **$4.43-$184.60**

• Conc—Oral: 10 mg/ml, 120 ml: **$12.50-$26.13**

CONTRAINDICATIONS: Hypersensitivity to tricyclic antidepressants, urinary retention, narrow-angle glaucoma, acute recovery phase of MI, concurrent use of MAOIs

PRECAUTIONS: Suicidal patients, convulsive disorders, prostatic hypertrophy, psychiatric disease, severe depression, increased intraocular pressure, cardiac disease, hepatic disease/renal disease, hyperthyroidism, electroshock therapy, elective surgery, elderly, abrupt discontinuation, children

PREGNANCY AND LACTATION: Pregnancy category C (TOP formulation is category B); paralytic ileus has been observed in an infant exposed to doxepin and chlorpromazine at term; excreted into breast milk (as well as active metabolite), effect on nursing infant unknown but may be of concern

SIDE EFFECTS/ADVERSE REACTIONS

CNS: Dizziness, drowsiness, confusion (especially in elderly), headache, anxiety, nervousness, panic, tremors, stimulation, weakness, fatigue, insomnia, nightmares, EPS (elderly), increased psychiatric symptoms, memory impairment,

CV: Orthostatic hypotension, ***ECG changes, tachycardia, dysrhythmias,*** hypertension, palpitations, syncope

EENT: Blurred vision, tinnitus, mydriasis, ophthalmoplegia, nasal congestion

GI: Constipation, dry mouth, nausea, vomiting, ***paralytic ileus,*** increased appetite, cramps, epigastric distress, jaundice, ***hepatitis,*** stomatitis, diarrhea

GU: Urinary retention

HEME: ***Agranulocytosis, thrombocytopenia, eosinophilia, leukopenia***

SKIN: Rash, urticaria, sweating, pruritus, photosensitivity; *burning or stinging at application site, pruritus or eczema exacerbation, dryness/tightness of skin,* paresthesias, edema, irritation, tingling, scaling, crackling (TOP)

▼ DRUG INTERACTIONS

Drugs

• *Amphetamines:* Theoretical increase in effect of amphetamines, clinical evidence lacking

• *Anticholinergics:* Excessive anticholinergic effects

• *Barbiturates:* Reduced serum concentrations of cyclic antidepressants

• *Bethanidine:* Reduced antihypertensive effect of bethanidine

• *Carbamazepine:* Reduced cyclic antidepressant serum concentrations
• *Clonidine:* Reduced antihypertensive response to clonidine; enhanced hypertensive response with abrupt clonidine withdrawal
• *Debrisoquin:* Inhibited antihypertensive response of debrisoquin
• *Epinephrine+:* Markedly enhanced pressor response to IV epinephrine
• *Ethanol:* Additive impairment of motor skills; abstinent alcoholics may eliminate cyclic antidepressants more rapidly than non-alcoholics
• *Fluoxetine:* Marked increases in cyclic antidepressant plasma concentrations
• *Guanethidine:* Inhibited antihypertensive response to guanethidine
• *Moclobemide+:* Potential association with fatal or non-fatal serotonin syndrome
• *MAOIs:* Excessive sympathetic response, mania or hyperpyrexia possible
• *Neuroleptics:* Increased therapeutic and toxic effects of both drugs
• *Norepinephrine+:* Markedly enhanced pressor response to norepinephrine
• *Phenylephrine:* Enhanced pressor response to IV phenylephrine
• *Phenytoin:* Altered seizure control; decreased cyclic antidepressant serum concentrations
• *Propoxyphene:* Enhanced effect of cyclic antidepressants
• *Quinidine:* Increased cyclic antidepressant serum concentrations

Labs

• *Increase:* Serum bilirubin, blood glucose, alk phosphatase
• *Decrease:* VMA, 5-HIAA
• *False increase:* Urinary catecholamines

SPECIAL CONSIDERATIONS

PATIENT/FAMILY EDUCATION

• Therapeutic effects may take 2-3 wk
• Use caution in driving or other activities requiring alertness
• Avoid rising quickly from sitting to standing, especially elderly
• Avoid alcohol ingestion, other CNS depressants
• Do not discontinue abruptly after long-term use
• Wear sunscreen or large hat to prevent photosensitivity
• Increase fluids, bulk in diet if constipation occurs
• Sugarless gum, hard sugarless candy, or frequent sips of water for dry mouth
• Do not use occlusive dressings with TOP preparation
• If drowsiness occurs with TOP application, decrease surface area being treated or number of daily applications

MONITORING PARAMETERS

• CBC; weight; ECG; mental status: mood, sensorium, affect, suicidal tendencies

doxycycline

(dox-i-sye'kleen)

Apo-Doxy, ♣ Bio-Tab, Doryx, Doxy 100, Doxy 200, Doxy Caps, Doxychel Hyclate, Doxycin, ♣ Monodox, Vibramycin, Vibramycin IV, Vibra-Tabs

Chemical Class: Tetracycline
Therapeutic Class: Antibiotic; antimalarial

CLINICAL PHARMACOLOGY

Mechanism of Action: Inhibits protein synthesis by binding with the 30S and possibly the 50S ribosomal subunit(s) of susceptible organisms; may also cause alterations in cytoplasmic membrane

Pharmacokinetics

PO: Peak 1.5-4 hr; food decreases absorption approximately 20%; 90% bound to plasma proteins; not metabolized in liver, partially inactivated in the GI tract by chelate formation; $t_{1/2}$ 15-26 hr; excreted in urine (23%) and feces (30%)

INDICATIONS AND USES: Rocky mountain spotted fever, typhus fever and the typhus group, Q fever, rickettsialpox, tick fevers caused by Rickettsiae, respiratory tract infections, lymphogranuloma venereum, psittacosis (ornithosis), trachoma, inclusion conjunctivitis, uncomplicated urethral, endocervical, or rectal infections in adults, nongonococcal urethritis, relapsing fever, chancroid, plague, tularemia, cholera, *campylobacter fetus* infections, brucellosis, bartonellosis, granuloma inguinale, malaria prophylaxis.

Antibacterial spectrum usually includes:

• Gram-positive organisms: *Streptococcus pyogenes* (44% of strains found to be resistant), *Str. pneumoniae* (74% of strains found to be resistant), Enterococcus group (*Str. faecalis* and *Str. faecium*), α-hemolytic streptococci (viridans-group)

Gram-negative organisms: *Neisseria gonorrhoeae, Calymmatobacterium granulomatis, Haemophilus ducreyi, H. influenzae, Yersinia pestis, Francisella tularensis, Vibrio cholera, Bartonella bacilliformis, Brucella* sp

• Other organisms: Rickettsiae, *Clostridium* sp, *Chlamydia psittaci, C. trachomatis, Fusobacterium fusiforme, Actinomyces* sp, *Mycoplasma pneumoniae, Bacillus anthracis, Ureaplasma urealyticum, Propionibacterium acnes, Borrelia recurrentis, Entamoeba* sp, *Treponema pallidum, T. pertenue, Balantidium coli, Plasmodium falciparum*

DOSAGE

Adult

• PO/IV 100-200 mg/d in 1-2 divided doses

Child ≥ 8 yr

• PO/IV 2-5 mg/kg/d in 1-2 divided doses; do not exceed 200 mg/d

D

$ AVAILABLE FORMS/COST OF THERAPY

• Cap, Gel—Oral: 50, 100 mg, 50's: **$2.88-$176.65**

• Cap, Gel, Coated Pellets—Oral: 100 mg, 50's: **$88.49-$121.94**

• Tab, Plain Coated—Oral: 100 mg, 50's: **$6.38-$176.65**

• Powder, Reconst—Oral: 25 mg/5 ml, 60 ml: **$10.77**

• Syr—Oral: 50 mg/5ml, 480 ml: **$163.47**

• Inj, Sol—IV: 100 mg/vial: **$16.70-$21.07;** 200 mg/vial: **$33.69**

CONTRAINDICATIONS: Hypersensitivity to tetracyclines, children <8 yr

PRECAUTIONS: Hepatic disease, prolonged or repeated therapy

PREGNANCY AND LACTATION: Pregnancy category D; excreted into breast milk, theoretical possibility for dental staining seems remote because serum levels in infant undetectable; may modify bowel flora, have direct effects on infant, or interfere with interpretation of culture results if fever workup required

SIDE EFFECTS/ADVERSE REACTIONS

CNS: Fever, headache, paresthesia

CV: Pericarditis

GI: Nausea, vomiting, *diarrhea,* anorexia, glossitis, abdominal pain, enterocolitis, ***hepatotoxicity,*** flatulence, abdominal cramps, epigastric burning, stomatitis, ***psuedomembranous colitis***

GU: Increased BUN, polyuria, polydipsia, azotemia

HEME: ***Eosinophilia, neutropenia, thrombocytopenia, hemolytic anemia***

SKIN: Rash, urticaria, *photosensitivity,* ***exfoliative dermatitis,*** pruritus, highly irritating (avoid extravasation)

MISC: Decreased calcification of deciduous teeth, angioedema, pseudotumor cerebri (adults) and bulging fontanels (infants)

▼ DRUG INTERACTIONS

Drugs

- *Antacids+:* Reduced serum concentration and efficacy of doxycycline
- *Barbiturates:* Reduced serum doxycycline concentrations
- *Bismuth subsalicylate:* Reduced bioavailability of doxycycline
- *Carbamazepine:* Reduced serum doxycycline concentrations
- *Iron:* Reduced serum concentration and efficacy of doxycycline
- *Phenytoin:* Reduced serum doxycycline concentrations

Labs:

- *False negative:* Urine glucose with Clinistix or Tes-Tape
- *False increase:* Urinary catecholamines; ALT, AST

SPECIAL CONSIDERATIONS

PATIENT/FAMILY EDUCATION

- Avoid unnecessary exposure to sunlight
- Do not take with antacids, iron products
- Take with food

MONITORING PARAMETERS

- Periodic monitoring of renal, hepatic, and hematologic function tests during prolonged therapy

dronabinol

(droe-nab′i-nol)

Marinol

Chemical Class: Synthetic cannabinoid

Therapeutic Class: Antiemetic, appetite stimulant

DEA Class: Schedule II

CLINICAL PHARMACOLOGY

Mechanism of Action: Central sympathomimetic and neural cannabinoid receptor activity mediate effect; tachyphylaxis and tolerance develop to psychological effects but not appetite stimulant effect

Pharmacokinetics

PO: Onset 30-60 min; peak effect 2-4 hr; duration of psychoactive effect 4-6 hr, appetite stimulant effect 24 hr; absorption 90%; highly lipid soluble, 97% protein bound; metabolized in liver; metabolites and drug excreted in bile (85%) and urine (15%); metabolites detected in urine for 5 wk after single dose

INDICATIONS AND USES: Nausea related to cancer chemotherapy not responsive to conventional agents, AIDS-related anorexia

DOSAGE

Adult

- *Antiemetic:* PO 5 mg/m^2 1-3 hr before chemotherapy, then q2-4h up to 6 doses qd; max dose 15 mg/m^2
- *Appetite stimulant:* PO 2.5 mg bid, 1 hr ac, max dose 20 mg qd

$ AVAILABLE FORMS/COST OF THERAPY

- Cap, Elastic—Oral: 2.5, 5, 10 mg, 25's: **$48.51-$309.40**

CONTRAINDICATIONS: Hypersensitivity to any cannabinoid or sesame oil

PRECAUTIONS: Children, abuse or dependence

PREGNANCY AND LACTATION: Pregnancy category C; excreted in breast milk

SIDE EFFECTS/ADVERSE REACTIONS

CNS: Euphoria (24%), dizziness, difficulty concentrating, anxiety, mood change, confusion, depersonalization, hallucination, somnolence, abnormal thinking, ataxia

CV: Palpitations, tachycardia, vasodilation, orthostatic hypotension

EENT: Tinnitus, dry mouth, change in vision

GI: Nausea, vomiting, diarrhea

MS: Myalgias

RESP: Cough, rhinitis, sinusitis

SKIN: Sweating

▼ **DRUG INTERACTIONS**

Labs

• *Decrease:* FSH, LH, growth hormone, testosterone

SPECIAL CONSIDERATIONS

• May have additive sedative or behavioral effects with CNS depressants

---

droperidol

(droe-per′i-dole)

Inapsine

Chemical Class: Butyrophenone derivative

Therapeutic Class: Sedative; antiemetic

CLINICAL PHARMACOLOGY

Mechanism of Action: Alters the action of dopamine at subcortical levels in CNS to produce sedation; produces mild α-adrenergic blockade, peripheral vascular dilation and reduction of pressor effect of epinephrine

Pharmacokinetics

IV/IM: Onset 3-10 min (full effect may not be apparent for 30 min), duration 2-4 hr, metabolized in liver, excreted in urine and feces, $t_{1/2}$ 2.2 hr

INDICATIONS AND USES: Premedication for surgery; induction, maintenance in general anesthesia; antiemetic in cancer chemotherapy*

DOSAGE

Adult

• *Adjunct to general anesthesia:* IV 2.5 mg/10 kg given with analgesic or general anesthetic

• *Premedication for surgery:* IM 2.5-10 mg 30-60 min preoperatively

• *Maintaining general anesthesia:* IV 1.25-2.5 mg

Child 2-12 yr

• *Adjunct to general anesthesia:* IV 1-1.5 mg/10 kg, titrated to response needed

• *Premedication for surgery:* IM 1-1.5 mg/10 kg 30-60 min preoperatively

$ **AVAILABLE FORMS/COST OF THERAPY**

• Inj, Sol—IM; IV: 2.5 mg/ml, 2 ml: **$3.56-$5.31**

CONTRAINDICATIONS: Hypersensitivity

PRECAUTIONS: Elderly, cardiovascular disease (hypotension, bradydysrhythmias), renal disease, liver disease, Parkinson's disease, child <2 yr

PREGNANCY AND LACTATION: Pregnancy category C; has been used to promote analgesia for cesarean section patients without affecting respiration of the newborn; excretion into breast milk unknown, use caution in nursing mothers

SIDE EFFECTS/ADVERSE REACTIONS

CNS: Drowsiness, dystonia, akathisia, dizziness, chills, shivering, hallucinations

CV: Hypotension, tachycardia, hypertension

EENT: Oculogyric crisis

MS: Muscular rigidity

RESP: Respiratory depression, apnea, ***respiratory arrest, bronchospasm***

SPECIAL CONSIDERATIONS

MONITORING PARAMETERS

• Blood pressure, heart rate, respiratory rate

dyphylline

(dye'fi-lin)

Dilor, Dyflex-200, Dyflex-400, Dylline, Dyphylline, Lufyllin, Lufyllin-400, Neothylline, Protophylline ♣

Chemical Class: Xanthine derivative

Therapeutic Class: Bronchodilator

CLINICAL PHARMACOLOGY

Mechanism of Action: Possesses the peripheral vasodilator and bronchodilator actions characteristic of theophylline (approximately 1/10th as potent as theophylline); has diuretic and myocardial stimulant effects

Pharmacokinetics

PO: Bioavailability 68%-82%, peak 1 hr, $t_{1/2}$ 2 hr, not metabolized to theophylline, 83% excreted unchanged in urine

INDICATIONS AND USES: Bronchial asthma, bronchospasm in chronic bronchitis and emphysema

DOSAGE

Adult

• PO up to 15 mg/kg q6h; IM 250-500 mg q6h (administer by slow IM inj; do not administer IV), not to exceed 15 mg/kg/dose

$ **AVAILABLE FORMS/COST OF THERAPY**

• Elixir—Oral: 100 mg/15 ml, 480 ml: **$56.53;** 160 mg/5 ml, 480 ml: **$25.99**

• Inj, Sol—IM: 250 mg/ml, 2 ml: **$3.60-$14.75**

• Tab, Uncoated—Oral: 200, 400 mg, 100's: **$11.95-$132.55**

CONTRAINDICATIONS: Hypersensitivity, concurrent use with other xanthine preparations

PRECAUTIONS: Severe cardiac disease, hypertension, hyperthyroidism, acute myocardial injury, peptic ulcer, CHF, children

PREGNANCY AND LACTATION: Pregnancy category C; excreted into breast milk, compatible with breast feeding

SIDE EFFECTS/ADVERSE REACTIONS

CNS: Anxiety, restlessness, insomnia, dizziness, ***convulsions,*** headache, light-headedness, muscle twitching

CV: Palpitations, sinus tachycardia, hypotension, flushing, dysrhythmias

GI: Nausea, vomiting, anorexia, dyspepsia, epigastric pain

RESP: Tachypnea

SKIN: Flushing, urticaria

MISC: Fever, dehydration, ***albuminuria,*** hyperglycemia

▼ **DRUG INTERACTIONS**

Drugs

• *Probenecid:* Increased serum dyphylline concentrations

SPECIAL CONSIDERATIONS

PATIENT/FAMILY EDUCATION

• Administer with 8 oz of fluid to decrease GI upset

MONITORING PARAMETERS

• Minimal effective serum concentration 12 μg/ml

echothiophate iodide

(ek-oh-thye'oh-fate)

Phospholine Iodide

Chemical Class: Cholinesterase inhibitor, irreversible

Therapeutic Class: Miotic

CLINICAL PHARMACOLOGY

Mechanism of Action: Enhances

effect of endogenously liberated acetylcholine in iris, ciliary muscle, and other parasympathetically innervated structures of the eye; causes miosis, increase in facility of outflow of aqueous humor, fall in intraocular pressure, and potentiation of accommodation

Pharmacokinetics

OPHTH: Onset of miosis 10-30 min, duration of miosis 1-4 wk; onset of IOP reduction 4-8 hr, peak 24 hr, duration 7-28 days

INDICATIONS AND USES: Glaucoma (open-angle), accommodative esotropia

DOSAGE

Adult and Child

- OPHTH instill 1 gtt in conjunctival sac, not to exceed 1 gtt qd (accommodative estropia), or 1 gtt bid (glaucoma)

$ **AVAILABLE FORMS/COST OF THERAPY**

- Sol—Ophth: 0.03%, 0.06%, 0.125%, 0.25%, 5 ml: **$22.48-$29.76**

CONTRAINDICATIONS: Hypersensitivity, active uveal inflammation, most cases of angle-closure glaucoma (due to the possibility of increasing angle block)

PRECAUTIONS: Asthma, bradycardia, parkinsonism, peptic ulcer, myasthenia gravis, spastic GI disease, recent MI, epilepsy, history of quiescent uveitis

PREGNANCY AND LACTATION: Pregnancy category C; as a quaternary ammonium compound, is ionized at physiologic pH and transplacental passage in significant amounts would not be expected; excretion into breast milk unknown, use caution in nursing mothers

SIDE EFFECTS/ADVERSE REACTIONS

CNS: Headache

CV: Cardiac irregularities

EENT: Iris cysts, *burning, lacrimation,* lid muscle twitching, conjunctival and ciliary redness, browache, activation of latent iritis or uveitis, *visual blurring,* myopia, retinal detachment, lens opacities, conjunctival thickening, destruction of nasolacrimal canals

GI: Nausea, vomiting, abdominal cramps, diarrhea, salivation

GU: Urinary incontinence

RESP: Difficulty breathing

SKIN: Sweating

MISC: Fainting

▼ **DRUG INTERACTIONS**

Drugs

- *Neuromuscular blocking agents+:* Prolonged neuromuscular blocking effects of succinylcholine
- *Procaine:* Increased effect of procaine, clinical importance unknown

SPECIAL CONSIDERATIONS

PATIENT/FAMILY EDUCATION

- Local irritation and headache may occur at initiation of therapy
- Notify physician if abdominal cramps, diarrhea, or excessive salivation occur
- Wash hands immediately after administration
- Use caution while driving at night or performing hazardous tasks in poor light
- Minimize systemic absorption by applying gentle pressure to the inside corner of the eye for 3-5 min following administration

econazole

(e-kone'a-zole)

Spectazole

Chemical Class: Imidazole derivative

Therapeutic Class: Topical antifungal

CLINICAL PHARMACOLOGY

Mechanism of Action: Interferes

with fungal cell membrane, which increases permeability, leaking of cell nutrients

Pharmacokinetics

TOP: Systemic absorption extremely low, inhibitory concentrations have been found as deep as the middle region of the dermis, <1% of applied dose recovered in urine and feces

INDICATIONS AND USES: Tinea pedis (athlete's foot), tinea cruris (jock itch), tinea corporis (ringworm), cutaneous candidiasis, tinea versicolor. Antifungal spectrum usually includes: *Trichophyton rubrum, T. mentagrophytes, T. tonsurans, Microsporum canis, M. audouini, M. gypseum, Epidermophyton floccosum,* the yeasts, *Candida albicans, Pityrosporum orbiculare*

DOSAGE

Adult and Child

• TOP apply to affected area qd-bid depending on condition

$ AVAILABLE FORMS/COST OF THERAPY

• Cre—Top: 1%, 15, 30, 85 g: **$11.46-$37.56**

CONTRAINDICATIONS: Hypersensitivity

PREGNANCY AND LACTATION: Pregnancy category C; excretion into breast milk unknown, limited systemic absorption would minimize possibility of exposure to nursing infant

SIDE EFFECTS/ADVERSE REACTIONS

SKIN: Burning, itching, stinging, erythema, pruritic rash

SPECIAL CONSIDERATIONS

PATIENT/FAMILY EDUCATION

• For external use only, avoid contact with eyes, cleanse skin with soap and water and dry thoroughly prior to application

• Use medication for full treatment time outlined by physician, even though symptoms may have improved

• Notify physician if no improvement after 2 wk (jock itch, ringworm) or 4 wk (athlete's foot)

edetate calcium disodium

(ed'e-tate)

Calcium Disodium Versenate

Chemical Class: Chelating agent

Therapeutic Class: Heavy metal antagonist; antidote

CLINICAL PHARMACOLOGY

Mechanism of Action: The calcium in edetate calcium disodium is readily displaced by heavy metals, such as lead, to form stable complexes which are excreted in urine

Pharmacokinetics

IV/IM/SC: Not metabolized; distributed primarily in extracellular fluid; excreted in urine; $t_{1/2}$ 20-60 min

INDICATIONS AND USES: Acute and chronic lead poisoning, lead encephalopathy

DOSAGE

Adult

• *Acute lead encephalopathy:* IV 1.5 g/m^2/d as either an 8-24 hr inf or divided into 2 doses q12h for 3-5 days, with dimercaprol; may be given again after 4 days off drug; IM (preferred route) 250 mg/m^2/dose q4h for 3-5 days, with dimercaprol; may be given again after 4 days off drug

• *Lead poisoning:* IV 1 g/250-500 ml D_5W or 0.9% NaC1 over 1-2 hr q12h for 3-5 days; may repeat after 2 days; do not exceed 50 mg/kg/d in mildly affected or asymptomatic individuals; IM 35 mg/kg bid, do not exceed 50 mg/kg/d in mildly affected or asymptomatic individuals

Child

- *Acute lead encephalopathy:* Same as adult
- *Lead poisoning:* IM 35 mg/kg/d in divided doses q8-12h for 3-5 days; off 4 days before next course

$ AVAILABLE FORMS/COST OF THERAPY

- Inj, Sol—IV: 200 mg/ml, 5 ml: **$31.63**

CONTRAINDICATIONS: Anuria, hypersensitivity, active renal disease, hepatitis

PRECAUTIONS: Vomiting (may lead to dehydration and decreased urine flow), rapid IV inf (especially in lead encephalopathy)

PREGNANCY AND LACTATION: Pregnancy category B; excretion into breast milk unknown, use caution in nursing mothers

SIDE EFFECTS/ADVERSE REACTIONS

CNS: Fever, chills, tremors, *headache,* numbness, tingling

CV: Hypotension, cardiac rhythm irregularities

EENT: Sneezing, nasal congestion, lacrimation

GI: Cheilosis, nausea, vomiting, anorexia, excessive thirst, *mild increases in SGOT and SGPT*

GU: ***Acute necrosis of proximal tubules,*** infrequent changes in distal tubules and glomeruli, glycosuria, proteinuria, microscopic hematuria and large epithelial cells in urinary sediment

HEME: Transient bone marrow suppression, anemia

METAB: Zinc deficiency, hypercalcemia

MS: Myalgia, arthralgia, fatigue

SKIN: Rash

MISC: Malaise, pain at inj site

▼ DRUG INTERACTIONS

Labs

- *Decrease:* Cholesterol/triglycerides, potassium

SPECIAL CONSIDERATIONS

PATIENT/FAMILY EDUCATION

- Notify physician immediately if no urine output in a 12 hr period

MONITORING PARAMETERS

- Urinalysis and urine sediment daily during therapy to detect signs of progressive renal tubular damage
- Renal function tests, liver function tests, and serum electrolytes before and periodically during therapy
- ECG during IV therapy

---

edetate disodium

(ed'e-tate)

Chealamide, Disodium EDTA, Disotate, Endrate

Chemical Class: Chelating agent

Therapeutic Class: Heavy metal antagonist; antidote

CLINICAL PHARMACOLOGY

Mechanism of Action: Forms chelates with many divalent and trivalent metals which are then excreted in urine

Pharmacokinetics

IV: Not metabolized, $t_{1/2}$ 20-60 min, following chelation 95% excreted in urine as chelates within 24-48 hr

INDICATIONS AND USES: Emergency treatment of hypercalcemia; ventricular dysrhythmias associated with digitalis toxicity

DOSAGE

Adult

- IV INF 50 mg/kg/d (not to exceed 3 g/d), diluted in 500 ml of D_5W or 0.9% NaCl and infused over 3-4 hr for 5 consecutive days followed by 2 days without medication

Child

- IV INF 15-50 mg/kg/d (not to exceed 3 g/d), diluted in 500 ml of D_5W or 0.9% NaCl and infused over 3-4 hr for 5 consecutive days followed by 5 days without medication

$ AVAILABLE FORMS/COST OF THERAPY

• Inj, Sol—IV: 150 mg/ml, 20 ml: **$3.05-$26.70**

CONTRAINDICATIONS: Hypersensitivity, anuria

PRECAUTIONS: Intracranial lesions, seizure disorder, CAD, peripheral vascular disease, tuberculosis, CHF, diabetes

PREGNANCY AND LACTATION: Pregnancy category C; excretion into breast milk unknown, use caution in nursing mothers

SIDE EFFECTS/ADVERSE REACTIONS

CNS: Transient circumoral paresthesia, numbness, *headache,* febrile reactions, ***seizures***

CV: Transient drop in blood pressure, thrombophlebitis, dysrhythmias

GI: Nausea, vomiting, diarrhea

GU: ***Nephrotoxicity, acute tubular necrosis***

HEME: Anemia

METAB: Hyperuricemia, hypokalemia, hypomagnesemia, hypocalcemia

MS: Back pain, muscle cramps

RESP: ***Respiratory arrest***

SKIN: ***Exfoliative dermatitis,*** skin and mucous membrane reactions

▼ DRUG INTERACTIONS

Labs

• *Decrease:* Magnesium, alk phosphatase, potassium

• *False decrease:* Calcium via oxalate method

SPECIAL CONSIDERATIONS

Have patient remain supine for a short time after inf due to the possibility of orthostatic hypotension

MONITORING PARAMETERS

• ECG, blood pressure during inf

• Renal function before and during therapy

• Serum calcium, magnesium, potassium levels

edrophonium

(ed-roe-foe'nee-um)

Enlon, Reversol, Tensilon

Chemical Class: Quaternary ammonium compound

Therapeutic Class: Cholinergic; anticholinesterase

CLINICAL PHARMACOLOGY

Mechanism of Action: Facilitates transmission of impulses across myoneural junction by inhibiting destruction of acetylcholine by cholinesterase

Pharmacokinetics

IM: Onset 2-10 min, duration 12-45 min

IV: Onset <1 min, duration 6-24 min

Hydrolyzed by cholinesterase and metabolized by microsomal enzymes of liver, excreted by kidneys, $t_{1/2}$ 1.8 hr

INDICATIONS AND USES: Diagnosis of myasthenia gravis; curare antagonist; differentiation of myasthenic crisis from cholinergic crisis; evaluation of treatment requirements in myasthenia gravis

DOSAGE

Adult

• *Diagnosis of myasthenia gravis:* IV 1-2 mg over 15-30 sec, then 8 mg if no response; IM 10 mg; if cholinergic reaction occurs, retest after ½ hr with 2 mg IM

• *Evaluation of treatment requirements in myasthenia gravis:* IV 1-2 mg 1 hr after PO dose of anticholinesterase; if strength improves, an increase in neostigmine or pyridostigmine dose is indicated

• *Differentiation of myasthenic crisis from cholinergic crisis:* IV 1 mg, if no response in 1 min, may repeat; *myasthenic crisis* clear improvement in respiration, *cholinergic cri-*

sis increased oropharyngeal secretions and further weakening of respiratory muscles (intubation and controlled ventilation may be required)

• *Curare antagonist:* IV 10 mg over 30-45 sec, may repeat, not to exceed 40 mg

Child

• *Diagnosis of myasthenia gravis:* IV 0.04 mg/kg given over 1 min followed by 0.16 mg/kg given within 45 sec if no response; >34 kg IM 2 mg; <34 kg IM 1 mg; infant IV 0.1 mg, followed by 0.4 mg if no response, not to exceed 0.5 mg

• *Evaluation of treatment requirements in myasthenia gravis:* IV 0.04 mg/kg given 1 hr after PO intake of drug being used in treatment; if strength improves, an increase in neostigmine or pyridostigmine is indicated

$ AVAILABLE FORMS/COST OF THERAPY

• Inj, Sol—IM; IV: 10 mg/ml, 1 ml: **$0.69-$42.50**

CONTRAINDICATIONS: Mechanical intestinal and urinary obstructions, hypersensitivity

PRECAUTIONS: Seizure disorders, bronchial asthma, recent coronary occlusion, hyperthyroidism, dysrhythmias, peptic ulcer, megacolon, poor GI motility, bradycardia, hypotension

PREGNANCY AND LACTATION: Pregnancy category C; because it is ionized at physiologic pH, would not be expected to cross placenta in significant amounts; may cause premature labor; because it is ionized at physiologic pH, would not be expected to be excreted into breast milk

SIDE EFFECTS/ADVERSE REACTIONS

CNS: Dizziness, headache, sweating, weakness, ***convulsions,*** incoordination, ***paralysis,*** drowsiness, ***loss of consciousness***

CV: Tachycardia, dysrhythmias, bradycardia, hypotension, AV block, ECG changes, ***cardiac arrest,*** syncope

EENT: Miosis, blurred vision, lacrimation, visual changes

GI: Nausea, diarrhea, vomiting, cramps, increased salivary and gastric secretions, dysphagia, increased peristalsis

GU: Frequency, incontinence, urgency

MS: Weakness, fasciculations, muscle cramps and spasms; arthralgia

RESP: ***Respiratory depression, bronchospasm, constriction, laryngospasm, respiratory arrest,*** dyspnea, increased tracheobronchial secretions

SKIN: Rash, urticaria

▼ DRUG INTERACTIONS

Drugs

• *Quinidine:* Therapeutic effects of cholinergic drugs blocked by quinidine

SPECIAL CONSIDERATIONS

MONITORING PARAMETERS

• Pre- and postinjection strength

• Heart rate, respiratory rate, blood pressure

eflornithine

(eh-floor′ni-theen)

Ornidyl

Chemical Class: Ornithine decarboxylase inhibitor

Therapeutic Class: Antiprotozoal

CLINICAL PHARMACOLOGY

Mechanism of Action: Irreversibly inhibits ornithine decarboxylase; decarboxylation of ornithine by ornithine decarboxylase is an obligatory step in the biosynthesis of polyamines such as putrescine, spermidine, and spermine, which are ubiquitous in living cells and thought to play important roles in cell division and differentiation in all mammalian and many non-mammalian cells

Pharmacokinetics

IV: Not significantly bound to plasma proteins, crosses the blood-brain barrier, 80% excreted unchanged in urine within 24 hr, $t_{1/2}$ 3 hr

INDICATIONS AND USES: Treatment of meningoencephalitic stage of *Trypanosoma brucei gambiense* infection (sleeping sickness); *Pneumocystis carinii* pneumonia*

DOSAGE

Adult

• IV INF 100 mg/kg/dose infused over a minimum of 45 min q6h for 14 days

• **Note:** Eflornithine for inj concentrate is hypertonic and must be diluted with Sterile Water for Injection, USP, before inf

$ AVAILABLE FORMS/COST OF THERAPY

• Inj, Sol—IV: 200 mg/ml, 100 ml: Compassionate use through World Health Organization (WHO)

PRECAUTIONS: Seizure disorder, renal function impairment (reduced doses recommended)

PREGNANCY AND LACTATION: Pregnancy category C; excretion into breast milk unknown, use caution in nursing mothers

SIDE EFFECTS/ADVERSE REACTIONS

CNS: ***Seizures,*** headache, asthenia, dizziness

EENT: Hearing impairment

GI: Diarrhea, abdominal pain, anorexia

HEME: ***Myelosuppression, anemia, leukopenia, thrombocytopenia, eosinophilia***

SKIN: Alopecia

MISC: Facial edema

SPECIAL CONSIDERATIONS

The most frequent, serious, toxic effect of eflornithine is myelosuppression, which may be unavoidable if successful treatment is to be completed; decisions to modify dosage or to interrupt or cease treatment, depends on the severity of the observed adverse event(s), and the availability of support facilities

MONITORING PARAMETERS

• Serial audiograms if feasible

• CBC with platelets before and twice weekly during therapy and qwk after completion of therapy until hematologic values return to baseline levels

• Follow-up for at least 24 mo is advised to assure further therapy should relapses occur

---

emetine

(eh'mi-teen)

Chemical Class: Alkaloid related to ipecac

Therapeutic Class: Amebicide

CLINICAL PHARMACOLOGY

Mechanism of Action: Acts primarily in the bowel wall and liver; inhibits polypeptide chain elongation, thereby blocking protein synthesis in parasitic and mammalian cells, but not in bacteria

Pharmacokinetics

SC/IM: Concentrated primarily in the liver; appreciable levels also achieved in kidney, spleen, and lungs, which persist for several months; eliminated in urine for 40-60 days after administration

INDICATIONS AND USES: Intestinal amebiasis, extraintestinal amebiasis, balantidiasis, fascioliasis, paragonimiasis

DOSAGE

Adult

SC (preferred)/IM 1 mg/kg/d divided qd-bid, do not exceed 65 mg/d or 10 days of therapy; do not repeat course of therapy in <6 wk

• *Acute fulminating dysentery:* Administer only long enough to control diarrhea or dysenteric symptoms; usually 3-5 days
• *Amebic hepatitis or abscess:* Administer for 10 days

Child

• SC/IM (<8 yr) do not exceed 10 mg/d; (>8 yr) do not exceed 20 mg/d; 1 mg/kg/d in 2 doses for no more than 5 days has also been suggested

$ **AVAILABLE FORMS/COST OF THERAPY**

• Inj—SC; IM: 65 mg/ml, 1 ml: Drug not available

CONTRAINDICATIONS: Organic diseases of heart or kidney (except amebic hepatitis unresponsive to chloroquine); previous course of emetine within past 6 wk; pregnancy; children (except those with severe dysentery not controlled by other amebicides)

PRECAUTIONS: Elderly

PREGNANCY AND LACTATION: Pregnancy category X; safety for use has not been established in nursing mothers

SIDE EFFECTS/ADVERSE REACTIONS

CNS: Dizziness, headache
CV: Hypotension, tachycardia, precordial pain, ECG abnormalities, gallop rhythm, cardiac dilation, ***CHF***
GI: Nausea, vomiting
MS: Weakness, aching, tenderness, skeletal muscle stiffness (generally precedes more serious symptoms)
RESP: Dyspnea
SKIN: Aching, tenderness, and muscle weakness at inj site; eczematous, urticarial, or purpuric lesions

SPECIAL CONSIDERATIONS

Do NOT give IV

MONITORING PARAMETERS

• Blood pressure and pulse bid-tid
• ECG before, after the 5th dose, at the completion of therapy, and 1 wk later

enalapril/enalaprilat

(en-al'a-pril)
Vasotec, Vasotec IV
Chemical Class: Angiotensin-converting enzyme (ACE) inhibitor
Therapeutic Class: Antihypertensive

CLINICAL PHARMACOLOGY

Mechanism of Action: Selectively suppresses renin-angiotensin-aldosterone system; inhibits ACE, preventing conversion of angiotensin I to angiotensin II; results in dilation of arterial, venous vessels

Pharmacokinetics

PO: Peak ½-1½ hr (enalaprilat 3-4 hr); $t_{½}$ 1½ hr (enalaprilat 11 hr); metabolized by liver to active metabolite (enalaprilat), excreted in urine and feces
IV (enalaprilat): Onset 5-15 min

INDICATIONS AND USES: Hypertension, heart failure, left ventricular dysfunction (clinically stable asymptomatic patients, decreases rate of overt heart failure), diabetic nephropathy,* hypertensive emergencies (enalaprilat)*

DOSAGE

Adult

• PO 2.5-5 mg qd, increase prn, usually 10-40 mg/d divided qd-bid; IV (enalaprilat) 0.625-1.25 mg/dose given over 5 min q6h; Dosing adjustment in renal impairment: CrCl 10-50 ml/min, 75%-100% of normal dose; CrCl <10 ml/min, 50% of normal dose

Child

• PO 0.1 mg/kg/d initially, increase prn over 2 wk to max of 0.5 mg/

kg/d; IV (enalaprilat) 5-10 μg/kg/dose q8-24 hr

$ AVAILABLE FORMS/COST OF THERAPY

• Tab, Uncoated—Oral: 2.5 mg, 100's: **$71.76;** 5 mg, 100's: **$91.18;** 10 mg, 100's: **$95.74;** 20 mg, 100's: **$136.19**

• Inj, Sol—IV: 1.25 mg/ml, 1 ml: **$12.80**

CONTRAINDICATIONS: Hypersensitivity to ACE inhibitors

PRECAUTIONS: Impaired renal and liver function, dialysis patients, hypovolemia, diuretic therapy, collagen-vascular diseases, CHF, elderly, bilateral renal artery stenosis

PREGNANCY AND LACTATION: Pregnancy category C (first trimester), category D (second and third trimesters); ACE inhibitors can cause fetal and neonatal morbidity and death when administered to pregnant women; when pregnancy is detected, discontinue ACE inhibitors as soon as possible; detectable in breast milk in trace amounts; effect on nursing infant has not been determined, use with caution in nursing mothers

SIDE EFFECTS/ADVERSE REACTIONS

CNS: Anxiety, insomnia, paresthesia, *headache, dizziness, fatigue*

CV: Hypotension, postural hypotension, syncope (especially with first dose), palpitations, angina

GI: Nausea, constipation, vomiting, melena, abdominal pain

GU: Increased BUN/creatinine, decreased libido, impotence, UTI

HEME: ***Neutropenia, agranulocytosis***

METAB: Hyperkalemia, hyponatremia

MS: Arthralgia, arthritis, myalgia

RESP: *Cough,* asthma, bronchitis, dyspnea, sinusitis

SKIN: ***Angioedema,*** rash, flushing, sweating

▼ DRUG INTERACTIONS

Drugs

• *Lithium:* Increased risk of serious lithium toxicity

• *Loop diuretics:* Initiation of ACE inhibitor therapy in the presence of intensive diuretic therapy results in a precipitous fall in blood pressure in some patients; ACE inhibitors may induce renal insufficiency in the presence of diuretic-induced sodium depletion

• *NSAIDs:* Inhibition of the antihypertensive response to ACE inhibitors

• *Potassium:* Increased risk for hyperkalemia

• *Potassium sparing diuretics:* Increased risk for hyperkalemia

SPECIAL CONSIDERATIONS

PATIENT/FAMILY EDUCATION

• Do not use salt substitutes containing potassium without consulting physician

• Rise slowly to sitting or standing position to minimize orthostatic hypotension

• Notify physician of mouth sores, sore throat, fever, swelling of hands or feet, irregular heartbeat, chest pain

• Dizziness, fainting, light-headedness may occur during 1st few days of therapy

MONITORING PARAMETERS

• BUN, creatinine (watch for increased levels that may indicate acute renal failure)

• Potassium levels, although hyperkalemia rarely occurs

encainide

(en-kay′nide)

Enkaid

Chemical Class: Benzamide derivative

Therapeutic Class: Antiarrhythmic, Class IC

CLINICAL PHARMACOLOGY

Mechanism of Action: Blocks the sodium channel of Purkinje fibers and the myocardium; slows conduction, reduces membrane responsiveness, inhibits automaticity, and increases the ratio of effective refractory period to action potential duration

Pharmacokinetics

PO: Peak 30-90 min; metabolized in the liver to two active metabolites, O-demethyl encainide (ODE) and 3-methoxy-O-demethyl encainide (MODE) by >90% of patients; <10% of patients renal excretion is major route of elimination; $t_{1/2}$ 1-2 hr (rapid metabolizers), 6-11 hr (slow metabolizers); ODE $t_{1/2}$ 3-4 hr, MODE $t_{1/2}$ 6-12 hr

INDICATIONS AND USES: Documented life-threatening dysrhythmias (e.g., sustained ventricular tachycardia)

Encainide has been voluntarily withdrawn from the market because of continuing uncertainty about the implications of the Cardiac Arrhythmia Suppression Trial (CAST). The drug is still available on a limited basis through the Enkaid Continuing Patient Access Program. For further information contact Bristol-Myers Squibb at (800) 527-6741.

DOSAGE

Adult

- PO 25 mg q8h initially, increase gradually at 3-5 day intervals to 50 mg q8h if necessary

$ AVAILABLE FORMS/COST OF THERAPY

- Cap, Gel—Oral: 25 mg, 100's: **$63.79;** 35 mg, 100's: **$95.71;** 50 mg, 100's: **$127.60**

CONTRAINDICATIONS: Symptomatic nonsustained ventricular dysrhythmias, frequent premature ventricular complexes, 2nd or 3rd degree AV block, right bundle branch block when associated with a left hemiblock (unless pacemaker present), cardiogenic shock, hypersensitivity

PRECAUTIONS: Can cause new or worsened dysrhythmias; CHF; electrolyte disturbances; sick sinus syndrome; hepatic function impairment; renal function impairment; children

PREGNANCY AND LACTATION: Pregnancy category B; human experience very limited; excreted into breast milk along with active metabolites, use caution in nursing mothers

SIDE EFFECTS/ADVERSE REACTIONS

CNS: Dizziness, headache, anorexia, insomnia, nervousness, somnolence, tremor

*CV: **Ventricular tachycardia,*** CHF, 2nd or 3rd degree AV block, sinus bradycardia, sinus pause, sinus arrest, chest pain, palpitations, peripheral edema, PVCs, syncope

EENT: Blurred vision

GI: Elevated liver enzymes, ***hepatitis, jaundice,*** abdominal pain, constipation, diarrhea, dry mouth, dyspepsia, nausea, vomiting

METAB: Elevated blood glucose, increased insulin requirement

RESP: Dyspnea, increased cough

SKIN: Rash

▼ DRUG INTERACTIONS

Drugs

• *Quinidine:* Substantially increased encainide serum concentrations in rapid metabolizers

SPECIAL CONSIDERATIONS

MONITORING PARAMETERS

• Continuous ECG monitoring during initiation, baseline evaluation of left ventricular function

• The value of monitoring plasma concentrations of encainide and its metabolites has not been established

enoxacin

(en-ox'aa-sin)

Penetrex

Chemical Class: Fluoroquinolone

Therapeutic Class: Antiinfective

CLINICAL PHARMACOLOGY

Mechanism of Action: Interferes with the enzyme DNA gyrase needed for the synthesis of bacterial DNA; bactericidal

Pharmacokinetics

PO: Peak 1-3 hr, $t_{1/2}$ 3-6 hr, execreted in urine as unchanged drug and metabolites

INDICATIONS AND USES: Uncomplicated urethral or cervical gonorrhea due to *Neisseria gonorrhoeae;* uncomplicated UTI due to *E. coli, Staphylococcus epidermidis* or *S. saprophyticus;* complicated UTI due to *E. coli, Klebsiella pneumoniae, Proteus mirabilis, Pseudomonas aeruginosa, S. epidermidis* or *Enterobacter cloacae*

DOSAGE

Adult

• *Uncomplicated UTI:* PO 200 mg q12h for 3-7 days

• *Complicated UTI:* PO 400 mg q12h for 14 days

• *Uncomplicated gonorrhea:* PO 400 mg as a single dose

• Renal function impairment (CrCl <30 ml/min/1.73 m^2): PO after a normal initial dose, use 50% recommended dose q12h

$ AVAILABLE FORMS/COST OF THERAPY

• Tab, Uncoated—Oral: 200, 400 mg, 50's: **$142.19**

CONTRAINDICATIONS: Hypersensitivity to quinolones

PRECAUTIONS: Children (potential for arthropathy and osteochondrosis), elderly, renal disease, seizure disorders

PREGNANCY AND LACTATION: Pregnancy category C; excretion into breast milk unknown, due to the potential for arthropathy and osteochondrosis use extreme caution in nursing mothers

SIDE EFFECTS/ADVERSE REACTIONS

CNS: Dizziness, headache, fatigue, somnolence, depression, insomnia, anxiety, ***seizures***

EENT: Visual disturbances, dizziness

GI: Diarrhea, *nausea,* vomiting, anorexia, flatulence, heartburn, abdominal pain, dry mouth, increased AST/ALT, ***pseudomembranous colitis***

SKIN: Rash, pruritus, photosensitivity

▼ DRUG INTERACTIONS

Drugs

• *Antacids, food, iron, ranitidine, zinc:* Reduced serum enoxacin concentrations

• *Caffeine:* Large increases in serum caffeine concentrations

• *Tacrine:* increased serum tacrine concentrations

• *Theophylline:* Increased serum theophylline concentrations, potential toxicity

SPECIAL CONSIDERATIONS
PATIENT/FAMILY EDUCATION
- Administer on an empty stomach (1 hr before or 2 hr after meals)
- Drink fluids liberally
- Do not take antacids containing magnesium or aluminum or products containing iron or zinc within 4 hr before or 2 hr after dosing
- Observe caution while driving or performing other tasks requiring alertness
- Avoid excessive exposure to sunlight

---

enoxaparin
(e-nox-ah-pair′in)
Lovenox

Chemical Class: Low molecular weight heparin (fragments of 2000-8000 daltons)
Therapeutic Class: Anticoagulant/antithrombotic

CLINICAL PHARMACOLOGY
Mechanism of Action: Inhibits thrombosis by inactivating factor Xa and inhibiting the conversion of prothrombin to thrombin; has a higher ratio of anti-Factor Xa to antithrombin activity (3.35) than unfractionated heparin (1.22); does not significantly influence bleeding time, platelet function, prothrombin time (PT), or activated partial thromboplastin time (APTT) at recommended doses

Pharmacokinetics

SC: Peak activity 3-5 hr, $t_{1/2}$ 4½ hr

INDICATIONS AND USES: Prevention of deep vein thrombosis (DVT) following hip replacement surgery; Prevention of DVT following knee replacement surgery; treatment of DVT (1 mg/kg bid until warfarin therapy is therapeutic)

DOSAGE
Adult
- SC 30 mg bid beginning as soon as possible following surgery for 7-10 days

$ AVAILABLE FORMS/COST OF THERAPY
- Inj, Sol—SC: 30 mg/0.3 ml, 0.3 ml × 10: **$155.34**

CONTRAINDICATIONS: Active major bleeding, drug-induced thrombocytopenia, hypersensitivity to heparins or pork products

PRECAUTIONS: Bacterial endocarditis, bleeding disorder, active ulceration, angiodysplastic GI disease, hemorrhagic stroke; recent brain, spinal, or ophthalmological surgery; history of heparin-induced thrombocytopenia; renal function impairment; elderly; children

PREGNANCY AND LACTATION: Pregnancy category B; excretion into breast milk unknown, use caution in nursing mothers

SIDE EFFECTS/ADVERSE REACTIONS
CNS: Fever, confusion

CV: Edema

GI: Nausea

HEME: Hemorrhage, ***thrombocytopenia,*** hypochromic anemia

SKIN: Local irritation, pain, hematoma, erythema at inj site; ecchymosis

▼ DRUG INTERACTIONS
Labs
- *Increase:* AST, ALT

SPECIAL CONSIDERATIONS
PATIENT/FAMILY EDUCATION
- Administer lying down by deep SC inj into abdominal wall; alternate inj sites; introduce the whole length of the needle into a skin fold between the thumb and forefinger; hold the skin fold throughout the injection

• Report any unusual bruising or bleeding to physician

MONITORING PARAMETERS

• Platelets, occult blood, Hgb, Hct

ephedrine

(e-fed'rin)

Kondon's Nasal, Pretz-D, Vicks Vatronol

Chemical Class: Sympathomimetic alkaloid

Therapeutic Class: Bronchodilator; vasopressor; decongestant

CLINICAL PHARMACOLOGY

Mechanism of Action: Releases tissue stores of epinephrine and thereby produces α- and β-adrenergic stimulation

Pharmacokinetics

PO: Onset 15-60 min, duration 3-6 hr

IM: Onset 10-20 min 60%-77% of dose excreted as unchanged drug in urine, $t_{1/2}$ 2.5-3.6 hr

INDICATIONS AND USES: Bronchial asthma, nasal congestion (local treatment), vasopressor in shock, narcolepsy; enuresis,* myasthenia gravis*

DOSAGE

Adult

• IM/SC 25-50 mg, not to exceed 150 mg/24 hr; IV 10-25 mg, not to exceed 150 mg/24 hr; PO 25-50 mg bid-tid

• *Nasal congestion:* TOP Instill 3-4 gtt, q4h or small amount of gel in each nostril q4h

Child

• PO/SC/IV 3 mg/kg/d in divided doses q4-6h

• *Nasal congestion:* TOP Instill 3-4 gtt, q4h or small amount of gel in each nostril q4h

$ AVAILABLE FORMS/COST OF THERAPY

• Cap, Gel—Oral: 25 mg, 1000's: **$19.50-$23.70;** 50 mg, 1000's: **$29.70-$42.50**

• Inj, Sol—IM; IV; SC: 5 mg/ml, 10 ml × 10: **$121.25;** 25 mg/ml, 1 ml × 6: **$10.15;** 50 mg/ml, 1 ml × 6: **$11.17**

• Jelly—Nasal: 1%, 20 g: **$1.75**

• Spray—Nasal: 0.25%, 15 ml: **$5.00**

• Drops—Nasal: 0.5%, 30 ml: **$3.00**

CONTRAINDICATIONS: Hypersensitivity to sympathomimetics, narrow-angle glaucoma

PRECAUTIONS: Heart disease, coronary insufficiency, dysrhythmias, angina, hyperthyroidism, diabetes mellitus, prostatic hypertrophy, increased ICP, hypovolemia

PREGNANCY AND LACTATION: Pregnancy category C; routinely used to treat or prevent maternal hypotension following spinal anesthesia, may cause fetal heart rate changes; excretion into breast milk unknown, one case report of adverse effects (excessive crying, irritability, and disturbed sleeping patterns) in a 3-mo-old nursing infant whose mother consumed d-isoephedrine

SIDE EFFECTS/ADVERSE REACTIONS

CNS: Tremors, anxiety, insomnia, headache, dizziness, confusion, hallucinations, ***convulsions,*** CNS depression

CV: Palpitations, tachycardia, hypertension, chest pain, ***dysrhythmias***

EENT: Irritation, burning, sneezing, stinging, dryness, rebound congestion

GI: Anorexia, nausea, vomiting

GU: Dysuria, urinary retention

METAB: Hyperglycemia

RESP: Respiratory difficulty

SKIN: Contact dermatitis, pallor

▼ **DRUG INTERACTIONS**

Drugs

- *Acetazolamide:* Increased ephedrine serum concentrations, possible toxicity
- *Antacids:* Increased ephedrine serum concentrations
- *Guanadrel:* Inhibits antihypertensive response
- *Guanethidine:* Inhibits antihypertensive response
- *Moclobemide+:* Substantially enhanced pressor response to ephedrine, severe hypertension
- *MAOIs+:* Substantially enhanced pressor response to ephedrine, severe hypertension
- *Sodium bicarbonate:* Increased ephedrine serum concentrations

SPECIAL CONSIDERATIONS

PATIENT/FAMILY EDUCATION

- May cause wakefulness or nervousness, take last dose 4-6 hr prior to bedtime
- Notify physician of insomnia, dizziness, weakness, tremor, or irregular heart beat
- Do not use nasal products for >3-5 days

MONITORING PARAMETERS

- Heart rate, ECG, blood pressure (when using for vasopressor effect)

epinephrine

(ep-i-nef'rin)

Vasopressor: Adrenalin Chloride; Bronchodilator: Adrenalin Chloride, AsthmaHaler Mist, AsthmaNefrin, Bronitin Mist, Bronkaid Mist, Medihaler-Epi, microNefrin, Nephron Inhalant, Primatene Mist, S-2, Sus-Phrine, Vaponefrin, Racepinephrine; Decongestant: Adrenalin Chloride; Antiglaucoma agent: Epifrin, Glaucon; Emergency Kit: EpiPen, EpiPen Jr.

Chemical Class: Sympathomimetic amine

Therapeutic Class: Vasopressor, antiglaucoma agent, bronchodilator, decongestant

CLINICAL PHARMACOLOGY

Mechanism of Action: Stimulates α, β_1- and β_2- adrenergic receptors resulting in bronchodilation, cardiac stimulation, nasal decongestion, and dilation of skeletal muscle vasculature; effects on vasculature are dose dependent, small doses produce vasodilation while large doses produce vasoconstriction; decreases production of aqueous humor and increases aqueous outflow; dilates the pupil by contracting the dilator muscle

Pharmacokinetics

SC: Onset 3-5 min

INH: Onset 1 min

OPHTH: Onset 1 hr

Taken up into the adrenergic neuron and metabolized by monoamine oxidase and catechol-o-methyltransferase, circulating drug metabolized by liver, inactive metabolites excreted in urine

INDICATIONS AND USES: Cardiac arrest, acute asthmatic attacks, nasal congestion, open-angle glaucoma, anaphylactic reactions

DOSAGE

Adult

- *Bronchodilator:* IM/SC (1:1000) 0.1-0.5 mg q12-15 min-4 hr; IV 0.1-0.25 mg (single dose max 1 mg); SC suspension (1:200) 0.5-1.5 mg (0.1-0.3 ml); NEB instill 8-15 gtt into nebulizer reservoir, administer 1-3 inhalations 4-6 times/day; MDI 1-2 puffs at first sign of bronchospasm
- *Cardiac arrest:* IV/INTRACARDIAC 0.1-1 mg (1-10 ml of 1:10,000 dilution) q3-5 min prn; IV intermediate dose 2-5 mg q3-5 min; escalating dose 1 mg-3 mg-5 mg 3 min apart; high dose 0.1 mg/kg q3-5 min; INTRATRACHEAL 1 mg q3-5 min (higher doses, e.g., 0.1 mg/kg, should be considered only after 1 mg doses have failed)
- *Hypotension:* IV INF 1-4 μg/min
- *Anaphylactic reaction:* IM/SC 0.2-0.5 mg q20 min-4 hr (single dose max 1 mg)
- *Glaucoma:* OPHTH 1 gtt qd-bid
- *Nasal congestion:* INTRANASAL apply prn, do not use for >3-5 days

Child

- *Bronchodilator:* SC 10 μg/kg (0.01 ml/kg of 1:1000), max single dose 0.5 mg; susp (1:200) 0.005 ml/kg/dose (0.025 mg/kg/dose) q6h, max 0.15 ml (0.75 mg)/dose; NEB 0.25-0.5 ml of 2.25% racemic epinephrine solution diluted in 3 ml NS q1-4h
- *Cardiac arrest:* IV/INTRATRACHEAL 0.01 mg/kg (0.1 ml/kg) of 1:10,000 sol q3-5 min prn, max 5 ml
- *Refractory hypotension:* IV INF 0.1-4 μg/kg/min
- *Anaphylactic reaction:* SC 0.01 mg/kg q15 min for 2 doses then q4h prn, max 0.5 mg/dose
- *Nasal congestion* (>6 yr): INTRANASAL apply prn

Neonate

- *Cardiac arrest:* IV/INTRATRACHEAL 0.01-0.03 mg/kg (0.1-0.3 ml/kg) of 1:10,000 sol q3-5 min prn

$ **AVAILABLE FORMS/COST OF THERAPY**

- Inj, Sol—IM: 0.15, 0.3 mg/0.3 ml, 1's: **$24.60**
- Inj, Sol—IM; IV; SC: 0.1 mg/ml, 10 ml: **$5.25-$13.78;** 1 mg/ml, 1 ml: **$0.91-$15.00**
- Inj, Sol—IV: 5 mg/ml, 0.3 ml × 12: **$33.86**
- Inj, Susp—SC: 0.5%, 5.0 ml: **$35.68**
- Sol—Inh: 1%, 7.5 ml: **$13.19**
- Aer—Inh: 0.22 mg/inh, 15 ml: **$9.28;** 0.3 mg/inh, 15 ml: **$8.65**
- Sol—Ophth: 0.5%, 15ml: **$27.66**
- Sol—Ophth; Top: 1%, 2%, 10, 15 ml: **$16.88-$32.46**
- Sol—Nasal: 1 mg/ml, 1 oz: **$9.82**

CONTRAINDICATIONS: Hypersensitivity, cardiac dysrhythmias, angle-closure glaucoma, shock, local anesthesia of fingers and toes, general anesthesia with halogenated hydrocarbons or cyclopropane, organic brain damage, labor, coronary insufficiency

PRECAUTIONS: Elderly, cardiovascular disease, hypertension, diabetes, hyperthyroidism, psychoneurotic individuals, thyrotoxicosis, parkinsonism

PREGNANCY AND LACTATION: Pregnancy category C; excreted into breast milk, use caution in nursing mothers

SIDE EFFECTS/ADVERSE REACTIONS

CNS: Anxiety, headache, fear, hemiplegia, ***subarachnoid hemorrhage,*** restlessness, tremor, weakness, dizziness

CV: Palpitations, hypertension, ***dysrhythmias,*** anginal pain

GI: Nausea, vomiting
GU: Urinary retention
RESP: Respiratory difficulty
SKIN: Urticaria, wheal, hemorrhage at inj site, pallor

▼ **DRUG INTERACTIONS**

Drugs

• *Beta blockers+:* Noncardioselective beta blockers enhance pressor response to epinephrine resulting in hypertension and bradycardia
• *Chlorpromazine:* Reversal of epinephrine pressor response
• *Cyclic antidepressants+:* Pressor response to IV epinephrine markedly enhanced

SPECIAL CONSIDERATIONS

PATIENT/FAMILY EDUCATION

• Do not exceed recommended doses
• Wait at least 3-5 min between inhalations with MDI
• Notify physician of dizziness or chest pain
• Do not use nasal preparations for >3-5 days to prevent rebound congestion
• To avoid contamination of ophthal preparations do not touch tip of container to any surface
• Do not use ophthal preparations while wearing soft contact lenses
• Transitory stinging may occur on instillation of ophthal preparations
• Report any decrease in visual acuity immediately

MONITORING PARAMETERS

• Blood pressure, heart rate
• Intraocular pressure

ergocalciferol

(er-goe-kal-sif′e-role)
Calciferol, Drisdol, Deltalin
Chemical Class: Ergosterol derivative
Therapeutic Class: Vitamin, fat soluble

E

CLINICAL PHARMACOLOGY

Mechanism of Action: Regulates calcium homeostasis; promotes active absorption of calcium and phosphorus by the small intestine; increases rate of accretion and resorption of minerals in bone; promotes resorption of phosphate by renal tubules; also involved in magnesium metabolism

Pharmacokinetics

PO: Peak effect in approximately 1 mo following daily dosing; readily absorbed from GI tract; absorption requires intestinal presence of bile; inactive until hydroxylated in the liver and kidney to calcifediol and then to calcitriol (most active form)

INDICATIONS AND USES: Refractory rickets, familial hypophosphatemia and hypoparathyroidism

DOSAGE

Adult

• *Dietary supplementation:* PO 400 IU qd
• *Hypoparathyroidism:* PO 25,000-200,000 IU qd (with calcium supplements)
• *Refractory rickets:* PO 12,000-500,000 IU qd (with phosphate supplements)
• *Familial hypophosphatemia:* PO 10,000-80,000 IU qd (with 1-2 g/d elemental phosphorus)
• IM therapy reserved for patients with GI, liver, or biliary disease associated with vitamin D malabsorption

Child

• *Dietary supplementation:* PO 400 IU qd

• *Hypoparathyroidism:* PO 50,000-200,000 IU qd (with calcium supplements)

• *Refractory rickets:* PO 400,000-800,000 IU qd (with phosphate supplements)

$ AVAILABLE FORMS/COST OF THERAPY

• Sol—Oral: 8000 IU/ml, 60 ml: **$24.96-$64.98**

• Cap, Elastic—Oral: 50,000 IU, 100's: **$4.64-$12.00**

• Tab, Plain Coated—Oral: 50,000 IU, 100's: **$36.49**

• Inj, Sol—IM: 12.5 mg/ml, 1 ml × 5: **$74.00**

CONTRAINDICATIONS: Hypercalcemia, malabsorption syndrome, hypervitaminosis D, hypersensitivity, decreased renal function

PRECAUTIONS: Renal stones, coronary disease, arteriosclerosis, elderly

PREGNANCY AND LACTATION: Pregnancy category A (category D if used in doses above the recommended daily allowance); excreted into breast milk in limited amounts, compatible with breast feeding, however, serum calcium levels of the infant should be monitored if mother is receiving pharmacologic doses

SIDE EFFECTS/ADVERSE REACTIONS

CNS: Headache, somnolence, anorexia, irritability, hyperthermia, overt psychosis

CV: Generalized vascular calcification, hypertension, ***dysrhythmia***

EENT: Conjunctivitis (calcific), rhinorrhea

GI: Nausea, vomiting, dry mouth, constipation, metallic taste, polydipsia, ***pancreatitis,*** elevated AST and ALT

GU: Polyuria, nocturia, reversible azotemia, nephrocalcinosis, decreased libido, elevated BUN, albuminuria

METAB: Mild acidosis, hypercholesterolemia

MS: Weakness, muscle pain, bone pain

SKIN: Photophobia, pruritis

MISC: Weight loss

SPECIAL CONSIDERATIONS

PATIENT/FAMILY EDUCATION

• Compliance with dosage instructions, diet, and calcium supplementation are essential

• Notify physician of weakness, lethargy, headache, anorexia, weight loss, nausea, vomiting, abdominal cramps, diarrhea, constipation, vertigo, excessive thirst, excessive urine output, dry mouth, or muscle or bone pain

MONITORING PARAMETERS

• Serum and urinary calcium, phosphorus, and BUN q2wk

• X-ray bones monthly until condition is corrected and stabilized

• Ensure adequate calcium intake; maintain serum calcium concentration between 9-10 mg/dl

• Periodically determine magnesium and alk phosphatase

• 24 hr urinary calcium and phosphate (hypoparathyroid patients)

• Serum calcium times phosphorus should not exceed 70 mg/dl to avoid ectopic calcification

ergoloid

(er′goe-loid)

Gerimal, Hydergine, Hydergine LC, Niloric

Chemical Class: Dihydrogenated ergot alkaloids

Therapeutic Class: Cerebral metabolic enhancer

CLINICAL PHARMACOLOGY

Mechanism of Action: May increase brain metabolism, possibly increasing cerebral blood flow

Pharmacokinetics

PO: Rapidly absorbed, peak 0.6-3 hr, extensive first-pass metabolism by the liver, $t_{1/2}$ 2.6-5.1 hr

INDICATIONS AND USES: Age-related mental capacity decline

DOSAGE

Adult

• PO 1 mg tid initially, increase to 4.5-12 mg/d in divided doses

$ AVAILABLE FORMS/COST OF THERAPY

• Tab—SL: 0.5 mg, 100's: **$4.91-$15.75;** 1 mg, 100's: **$6.86-$54.87**

• Tab, Uncoated—Oral: 1 mg, 100's: **$13.88-$68.82**

• Cap, Elastic—Oral: 1 mg, 100's: **$72.36**

• Liq—Oral: 1 mg/ml, 100 ml: **$56.64**

CONTRAINDICATIONS: Hypersensitivity, acute or chronic psychosis

PRECAUTIONS: Acute intermittent porphyria

SIDE EFFECTS/ADVERSE REACTIONS

GI: Nausea, vomiting, sublingual irritation

SPECIAL CONSIDERATIONS

PATIENT/FAMILY EDUCATION

• Results may not be observed for 3-4 wk

• May cause transient GI disturbances, allow sublingual tablets to completely dissolve under tongue, do not chew or crush sublingual tablets

MONITORING PARAMETERS

• Before prescribing exclude the possibility that the patient's signs and symptoms arise from a potentially reversible and treatable condition

• Periodically reassess the diagnosis and the benefit of current therapy to the patient

ergonovine

(er-gone-o'veen)

Ergotrate Maleate

Chemical Class: Ergot alkaloid

Therapeutic Class: Oxytocic

CLINICAL PHARMACOLOGY

Mechanism of Action: Partial agonist or antagonist at α-adrenergic, dopaminergic, and tryptaminergic receptors; increases the strength, duration, and frequency of uterine contractions and decreases uterine bleeding when used after placental delivery

Pharmacokinetics

IM: Onset 7-8 min, duration 45 min

IV: Onset 40 sec, duration 3 hr

$t_{1/2}$ ½-2 hr, principally eliminated by nonrenal mechanisms (metabolism in liver, excretion in feces)

INDICATIONS AND USES: Postpartum/postabortal hemorrhage due to uterine atony; adjunct to coronary ateriography to diagnose coronary artery spasm;* migraine headache*

DOSAGE

Adult

• IM/IV 0.2 mg, severe uterine bleeding may require repeated doses, but rarely more than 0.2 mg per 2-4 hr (confine IV route to emergencies)

$ AVAILABLE FORMS/COST OF THERAPY

• Inj, Sol—IV: 0.2 mg/ml, 1 ml: **$4.74**

CONTRAINDICATIONS: Hypersensitivity to ergots, augmentation of labor, before delivery of placenta, threatened spontaneous abortion

PRECAUTIONS: Calcium deficiency, prolonged use, hypertension, heart disease, venoarterial shunts, mitral-valve stenosis, obliterative vascular disease, sepsis, hepatic or renal impairment

PREGNANCY AND LACTATION: Not recommended for routine use prior to delivery of the placenta; may lower prolactin levels, which may decrease lactation

SIDE EFFECTS/ADVERSE REACTIONS

CNS: Headache, dizziness, fainting
CV: Hypertension, chest pain
EENT: Tinnitus
GI: Nausea, vomiting
GU: Cramping
RESP: Dyspnea
SKIN: Sweating

SPECIAL CONSIDERATIONS

PATIENT/FAMILY EDUCATION

- May cause nausea, vomiting, dizziness, increased blood pressure, headache, chest pain, or shortness of breath

MONITORING PARAMETERS

- Blood pressure, pulse, and uterine response

---

ergotamine

(er-got'a-meen)

Ergostat, Gynergen, ✤ Medihaler Ergotamine ✤

Chemical Class: Ergot alkaloid
Therapeutic Class: Antimigraine agent

CLINICAL PHARMACOLOGY

Mechanism of Action: Partial agonist and/or antagonist activity against tryptaminergic, dopaminergic, and α-adrenergic receptors depending upon their site; uterine stimulant; causes constriction of peripheral and cranial blood vessels and produces depression of central vasomotor centers; reduces extracranial blood flow, causes a decline in the amplitude of pulsation in the cranial arteries

Pharmacokinetics

PO: Peak 2 hr, metabolized in liver, excreted as metabolites in bile, plasma $t_{1/2}$ 2 hr

INDICATIONS AND USES: Abortive therapy for vascular headaches including migraine and cluster headaches

DOSAGE

Adult

- SL 2 mg stat, then 1-2 mg q½h prn until relief, not to exceed 6 mg/d or 10 mg/wk

Older Child and Adolescent

- SL 1 mg stat, then 1 mg q½h prn until relief, not to exceed 3 mg/attack

$ AVAILABLE FORMS/COST OF THERAPY

- Tab—SL: 2 mg, 24's: **$17.72**

CONTRAINDICATIONS: Pregnancy, hypersensitivity, peripheral vascular disease, hepatic or renal impairment, CAD, uncontrolled hypertension, sepsis

PRECAUTIONS: Prolonged administration, excessive dosage

PREGNANCY AND LACTATION: Pregnancy category X; excreted into breast milk, has caused symptoms of ergotism (e.g. vomiting, diarrhea) in the infant; excessive dosage or prolonged administration may inhibit lactation

SIDE EFFECTS/ADVERSE REACTIONS

CV: Transient tachycardia or bradycardia, coronary vasoconstriction (large doses), chest pain, increase or decrease in blood pressure
GI: Nausea, vomiting
MISC: Numbness and tingling of fingers and toes, muscle pain in extremities, weakness in legs, itching, localized edema

▼ DRUG INTERACTIONS

Drugs

- *Dopamine:* Increased risk of vasoconstriction

• *Nitroglycerin:* Enhanced ergot effect, decreased antianginal effects

SPECIAL CONSIDERATIONS

PATIENT/FAMILY EDUCATION

• Initiate therapy at first sign of attack
• DO NOT exceed recommended dosage
• Notify physician of irregular heart beat, nausea, vomiting, numbness or tingling of fingers or toes, pain or weakness of extremities
• Prolonged use may lead to withdrawal headaches

erythrityl tetranitrate

(e-ri'thri-till)
Cardilate
Chemical Class: Nitrate
Therapeutic Class: Antianginal

CLINICAL PHARMACOLOGY

Mechanism of Action: Relaxes vascular smooth muscle resulting in generalized vasodilation; decreases peripheral venous resistance and venous filling pressure via selective action on venous capacitance vessels (preload reduction); reduces arteriolar resistance to a lesser extent (afterload reduction); may cause a beneficial redistribution of coronary blood flow resulting in decreased myocardial ischemia

Pharmacokinetics

PO: Onset 30 min, peak 1-1½ hr, duration 6 hr
SL: Onset 5-10 min, peak 30-45 min, duration 3 hr
Metabolized by liver, excreted in urine

INDICATIONS AND USES: Prophylaxis and long-term treatment of angina pectoris (not for acute relief of angina attacks); esophageal spasm*

DOSAGE

Adult

• PO 10 mg ac, max 100 mg/d; PO/SL 5-10 mg prn prior to situations likely to provoke angina attack or qhs for nocturnal angina

$ AVAILABLE FORMS/COST OF THERAPY

• Tab, Scored—Oral; SL: 5 mg, 100's: **$18.89;** 10 mg, 100's: **$54.77**

CONTRAINDICATIONS: Hypersensitivity to nitrates, severe anemia

PRECAUTIONS: Acute MI, CHF, severe liver or renal disease, hypotension, uncorrected hypovolemia, increased intracranial pressure

PREGNANCY AND LACTATION: Pregnancy category C; excretion into breast milk unknown, use caution in nursing mothers

SIDE EFFECTS/ADVERSE REACTIONS

CNS: Headache, dizziness, weakness, restlessness, twitching
CV: Postural hypotension, tachycardia, ***collapse,*** syncope, edema
EENT: Blurred vision
GI: Nausea, vomiting, dry mouth
HEME: Hemolytic anemia, ***methemoglobinemia***
SKIN: Pallor, sweating, rash

▼ DRUG INTERACTIONS

Labs

• *Decrease:* Cholesterol

SPECIAL CONSIDERATIONS

PATIENT/FAMILY EDUCATION

• Avoid alcohol products
• May cause headache, tolerance occurs over time
• May be taken before stressful activity, e.g., exercise, sexual intercourse
• Avoid hazardous activities if dizziness occurs
• Make position changes slowly to prevent fainting

MONITORING PARAMETERS

• Blood pressure, pulse

erythromycin

(er-ith-roe-mye'sin)

Systemic: E-Base, E-Mycin, Eryc, Ery-Tab, PCE Dispertab, Ilosone, E.E.S., Eryped, Eramycin, Ilotycin, Novorythro, ✦ Robimycin Robitabs, Wyamycin S; Topical: A/T/S, Akne-Mycin, C-Solve 2, Erycette, Eryderm, Erygel, Erymax, E-Solve 2, ETS-2%, Staticin, Theramycin Z, T-Stat

Ophth: AK-Mycin, Ilotycin

Chemical Class: Macrolide antibiotic

Therapeutic Class: Antibacterial

CLINICAL PHARMACOLOGY

Mechanism of Action: Binds to 50S ribosomal subunits of susceptible bacteria and suppresses protein synthesis

Pharmacokinetics

PO: Peak 4 hr, duration 6 hr, 70% bound to plasma proteins, $t_{1/2}$ 1-3 hr, metabolized in liver, excreted in bile, feces

INDICATIONS AND USES: Systemic: treatment of infections caused by susceptible strains of the designated microorganisms; Upper and lower respiratory tract infections caused by *Streptococcus pyogenes* and *Str. pneumoniae;* respiratory tract infections due to *Mycoplasma pneumoniae;* pertussis (whooping cough) caused by *Bordatella pertussis;* diphtheria, as an adjunct to antitoxin in infections due to *Corynebacterium diphtheriae;* erythrasma due to *Corynebacterium minutissimum;* intestinal amebiasis caused by *Entamoeba histolytica* (PO only); acute PID caused by *Neisseria gonorrhoeae;* infections due to *Listeria monocytogenes;* skin and soft tissue infections caused by *Str. pyogenes* and *Staphylococcus aureus;* primary syphilis caused by *Treponema pallidum;* infections caused by *Chlamydia trachomatis* (conjunctivitis of the newborn, pneumonia of infancy, urogenital infections during pregnancy, uncomplicated urethral, endocervical, or rectal infections in adults); nongonococcal urethritis caused by *Ureaplasma urealyticum;* Legionnaires' disease caused by *Legionella pneumophila;* prevention of initial/recurrent attacks of rheumatic fever; prevention of bacterial endocarditis; Topical: acne vulgaris; Ophthalmic: superficial ocular infections involving the conjunctiva or cornea; prophylaxis of ophthalmia neonatorum due to *Neisseria gonorrhoeae* or *Chlamydia trachomatis;* diabetic gastroparesis;* as an alternative to penicillins in anthrax;* Vincent's gingivitis;* erysipeloid;* tetanus, actinomycosis;* *Nocardia* infections (with a sulfonamide);* *Eikenella corrodens* infections;* *Borrelia* infections (including early Lyme disease);* campylobacter enteritis;* *Lymphogranuloma venereum;** chancroid*

DOSAGE

Adult

- PO base 333 mg q8h; estolate, stearate, or base 250-500 mg q6-12h; ethylsuccinate 400-800 mg q6-12h; IV 15-20 mg/kg/d divided q6h; TOP apply to affected area bid; OPHTH Apply ¼" ribbon of ointment qd-qid as needed
- *Endocarditis prophylaxis:* PO ethylsuccinate 800 mg 1 hr prior to procedure and 400 mg 6 hr after

Child

- PO base, ethylsuccinate 30-50 mg/kg/d divided q6-8h; estolate: 30-50 mg/kg/d divided q8-12h; stearate 20-40 mg/kg/d divided q6h; IV lactobionate 20-40 mg/kg/d divided q6h, do not exceed 4 g/d; gluceptate:

20-50 mg/kg/d divided q6h; TOP apply to affected area bid; OPHTH apply ¼″ ribbon of ointment qd-qid as needed

$ AVAILABLE FORMS/COST OF THERAPY

• Oint—Ophth: 5 mg/g, 3.5 g: **$1.87-$5.00**
• Gel—Top: 2%, 30, 50, 60 g: **$14.84-$34.51**
• Sol—Top: 1.5%, 60 ml: **$5.25-$21.41;** 2%, 60, 120 ml: **$3.90-$31.56**
• Swab, Medicated—Top: 2%, 60's: **$18.59-$19.68**
• Oint—Top: 2%, 25 g: **$18.00**
• Cap, Gel, Sust Action (base)—Oral: 250 mg, 100's: **$26.93-$40.82**
• Cap, Gel (estolate)—Oral: 250 mg, 100's: **$22.92-$50.97**
• Tab, Chewable (ethylsuccinate)—Oral: 200 mg, 40's: **$19.64**
• Tab, Plain Coated (base)—Oral: 250 mg, 100's: **$13.95-$16.33;** 333 mg, 60's: **$67.57;** 500 mg, 100's: **$25.60-$148.50**
• Tab, Plain Coated (stearate)—Oral: 250 mg, 100's: **$13.50-$18.16;** 500 mg, 100's: **$21.75-$40.84**
• Tab, Plain Coated (ethylsuccinate)—Oral: 400 mg, 100's: **$21.60-$30.87**
• Tab, Coated (estolate)—Oral: 500 mg, 50's: **$44.39**
• Tab, Enteric Coated, Sust Action (base)—Oral: 250 mg, 100's: **$12.12-$25.05;** 333 mg, 100's: **$34.49-$43.25;** 500 mg, 100's: **$17.95-$40.10**
• Susp (estolate)—Oral: 125 mg/5 ml, 480 ml: **$22.42-$42.09;** 250 mg/5 ml: 480 ml: **$36.77-$75.76**
• Susp (ethylsuccinate)—Oral: 200 mg/5 ml, 100, 480 ml: **$3.95-$27.31;** 400 mg/5 ml, 100, 480 ml: **$8.09-$49.06**
• Powder, Granules, Reconst (ethylsuccinate)—Oral: 200 mg/5 ml, 100, 200 ml: **$5.69-$14.80;** 400 mg/5 ml, 60, 100, 200 ml: **$7.78-$21.62**
• Drops (ethylsuccinate)—Oral: 200 mg/5 ml, 50 ml: **$6.21**
• Inj, Lyphl-Sol (lactobionate)—IV: 500 mg/vial, 1's: **$10.07-$11.15;** 1 g/vial, 1's: **$18.20-$18.94**
• Inj, Dry Sol (gluceptate)—IV: 1 g/ampul, 50 ml: **$22.45**

CONTRAINDICATIONS: Systemic: hypersensitivity, preexisting liver disease (estolate); Ophthalmic: hypersensitivity, epitheleal herpes simplex keratitis, vaccinia, varicella, mycobacterial, fungal infections, Topical: hypersensitivity

PRECAUTIONS: Systemic: hepatic disease, prolonged or repeated therapy; Ophthalmic: antibiotic hypersensitivity; Topical: child <12 yr

PREGNANCY AND LACTATION: Pregnancy category B; excreted into breast milk, may modify bowel flora, have direct effects on infant, or interfere with interpretation of culture results if fever workup is required; compatible with breast feeding

SIDE EFFECTS/ADVERSE REACTIONS

CV: ***Ventricular dysrhythmias*** (rare)
EENT: Hearing loss, tinnitus; poor corneal wound healing, temporary visual haze, overgrowth of nonsusceptible organisms (OPHTH)
GI: Nausea, vomiting, diarrhea, abdominal cramping and discomfort, anorexia, ***cholestatic hepatitis*** (most common with estolate), stomatitis, heartburn, pruritus ani
GU: Vaginitis, moniliasis
SKIN: Rash, urticaria, pruritus, thrombophlebitis (IV site); rash, urticaria, stinging, burning, pruritus, dry, scaly, oily skin (TOP)

▼ DRUG INTERACTIONS

Drugs

• *Astemizole+:* QT prolongation and dysrhythmia

- *Carbamazepine+:* Markedly increased carbamazepine concentrations, potential toxicity
- *Clozapine:* Elevated plasma clozapine concentrations, seizures
- *Cyclosporine+:* Elevated cyclosporine concentrations, nephrotoxicity
- *Lovastatin:* Rhabdomyloysis
- *Midazolam:* Increased plasma midazolam concentrations
- *Tacrolimus:* Increased tacrolimus concentrations, nephrotoxicity
- *Terfenadine+:* QT prolongation and dysrhythmia
- *Theophylline:* Increased theophylline concentrations, toxicity
- *Triazolam:* Increased triazolam concentrations
- *Warfarin+:* Markedly increased hypoprothrombinemic response to warfarin in some patients
- *Zopiclone:* Increased plasma concentrations and pharmacodynamic effects of zopiclone

Labs

- *Decrease:* Folate assay
- *False increase:* 17-OHCS/17-KS, AST/ALT

SPECIAL CONSIDERATIONS

PATIENT/FAMILY EDUCATION

- Take with food to minimize GI discomfort
- Complete full course of therapy
- Take each dose with 180-240 ml of water
- Notify physician of vomiting, diarrhea or stomach cramps, severe abdominal pain, yellow discoloration of the skin or eyes, darkened urine, pale stools, or unusual tiredness
- Wash, rinse, and dry affected area prior to TOP application
- Keep top preparations away from eyes, nose, and mouth
- Ophthal ointments may cause temporary blurring of vision following administration
- Do not touch tip of tube to any surface
- Notify physician if stinging, burning, or itching become profound or if redness, irritation, swelling, decreasing vision, or pain persists or worsens

MONITORING PARAMETERS

- LFTs if hepatotoxicity suspected
- Check daily for vein irritation and phlebitis in patients receiving IV forms

erythropoietin recombinant

(er-ith-row-poe'ee-tin)

Epogen, Procrit

Chemical Class: Amino acid glycoprotein

Therapeutic Class: Hematopoietic agent

CLINICAL PHARMACOLOGY

Mechanism of Action: Induces red blood cell production by stimulating the division and differentiation of committed erythroid progenitor cells; induces release of reticulocytes from bone marrow into the blood stream, where they mature to erythrocytes

Pharmacokinetics

SC: Peak 5-24 hr, onset takes several days, $t_{1/2}$ 4-13 hr in patients with chronic renal failure (20% shorter in patients with normal renal function), elimination poorly understood, some metabolism in liver and bone marrow, 10% excreted unchanged in urine

INDICATIONS AND USES: Anemia in patients with chronic renal failure, anemia related to zidovudine therapy in HIV-infected patients, anemia in cancer patients on chemotherapy increasing the procurement of autologous blood in patients about to undergo elective surgery,* anemia of prematurity*

DOSAGE

Adult

- *Chronic renal failure:* IV (dialysis patients)/IV or SC (nondialysis CRF patients) 50-100 U/kg 3 times/wk initially; increase dose if Hct increases by <5-6 points after 8 wk and is below target range; decrease dose when target Hct is reached, or Hct increases >4 points in any 2 wk period; maintenance dose should be individualized, but is generally about 25 U/kg 3 times/wk
- *Zidovudine-treated HIV-infected patients:* IV/SC 100 U/kg 3 times/wk initially; after 8 wk adjust dose by 50-100 U/kg to a max of 300 U/kg 3 times/wk
- *Cancer patients on chemotherapy:* SC 150 U/kg 3 times/wk initially; after 8 wk adjust dose by 50-100 U/kg to a max of 300 U/kg 3 times/wk

Neonate

- *Anemia of prematurity:* SC 150-250 U/kg 3 times/wk

$ **AVAILABLE FORMS/COST OF THERAPY**

- Inj, Sol—IV;SC: 2000 U/ml, 1 ml: **$24.00;** 3000 U/ml, 1 ml: **$36.00;** 4000 U/ml, 1 ml: **$48.00;** 10,000 U/ml, 1 ml: **$114-$120**

CONTRAINDICATIONS: Uncontrolled hypertension, hypersensitivity to mammalian cell-derived products or to human albumin

PRECAUTIONS: Severe anemia, seizure disorder, vascular disease, history of thrombosis, children, porphyria

PREGNANCY AND LACTATION: Pregnancy category C; excretion into breast milk unknown, use caution in nursing mothers

SIDE EFFECTS/ADVERSE REACTIONS

CNS: Headache, ***seizures***

CV: ***Hypertension,*** tachycardia

GI: Nausea, vomiting, diarrhea

HEME: Clotted vascular access

METAB: Hyperkalemia

MS: Arthralgia, myalgia

RESP: Shortness of breath

SKIN: Inj site stinging

SPECIAL CONSIDERATIONS

Iron supplementation (325 mg bid-tid) should be given during therapy to provide for increased requirements during expansion of red cell mass secondary to marrow stimulation by erythropoietin

PATIENT/FAMILY EDUCATION

- Do not shake vials as this may denature the glycoprotein rendering the drug inactive
- Notify physician if severe headache develops
- Frequent blood tests required to determine optimal dose

MONITORING PARAMETERS

- Hct (target range 30%-33%, max 36%), serum iron, ferritin (keep >100 ng/dl)
- Baseline erythropoietin level (treatment of patients with erythropoietin levels >200 mU/ml is not recommended)
- Blood pressure
- BUN, uric acid, creatinine, phosphorus, potassium on a regular basis

esmolol

(ess'moe-lol)

Brevibloc

Chemical Class: β_1-selective (cardioselective) adrenoceptor blocking agent

Therapeutic Class: Antidysrhythmic

CLINICAL PHARMACOLOGY

Mechanism of Action: Preferentially competes with β-adrenergic agonists for available β_1-receptor sites inhibiting the chronotropic and inotropic responses to β_1-adrenergic stimulation (cardioselective); slows conduction of AV node, decreases heart rate, decreases O_2 consumption in myocardium, also decreases renin-aldosterone-angiotensin system at higher doses; blocks β_2-receptors in bronchial system at higher doses; lacks membrane stabilizing or intrinsic sympathomimetic (partial agonist) activities

Pharmacokinetics

IV: Onset very rapid, duration short, 55% bound to plasma proteins, $t_{1/2}$ 9 min, metabolized by hydrolysis of the ester linkage by esterases in the cytosol of red blood cells, excreted via kidneys

INDICATIONS AND USES: Supraventricular tachycardia, noncompensatory sinus tachycardia, angina pectoris*

DOSAGE

Adult

- IV 500 μg/kg loading dose over 1 min; follow with 50 μg/kg/min inf for 4 min; if therapeutic response inadequate rebolus with 500 μg/kg over 1 min and increase inf by 50 μg/kg/min for 4 min; repeat this process until therapeutic effect achieved or max dose of 200 μg/kg/min

$ AVAILABLE FORMS/COST OF THERAPY

- Inj, Sol—IV: 250 mg/ml, 10 ml: **$56.40;** 10 mg/ml, 10 ml: **$11.90**

CONTRAINDICATIONS: Sinus bradycardia, heart block greater than first degree, cardiogenic shock or overt heart failure, hypersensitivity

PRECAUTIONS: Hypotension, peripheral vascular disease, diabetes, hypoglycemia, thyrotoxicosis, renal disease, asthma, children

PREGNANCY AND LACTATION: Pregnancy category C; potential for hypotension and subsequent decreased uterine blood flow and fetal hypoxia should be considered; excretion into breast milk unknown, use caution in nursing mothers

SIDE EFFECTS/ADVERSE REACTIONS

CNS: Insomnia, *fatigue, dizziness,* mental changes, memory loss, hallucinations, depression, *lethargy,* drowsiness, strange dreams

CV: Hypotension, ***bradycardia,*** CHF, cold extremities, ***2nd or 3rd degree heart block***

EENT: Sore throat, dry burning eyes, visual disturbances

GI: Nausea, diarrhea, vomiting, dry mouth, ***mesenteric arterial thrombosis, ischemic colitis***

GU: Impotence, sexual dysfunction

HEME: ***Agranulocytosis, thrombocytopenia***

METAB: Masked hypoglycemic response to insulin (sweating excepted)

RESP: ***Bronchospasm,*** dyspnea, wheezing

SKIN: Rash, pruritis, alopecia

▼ DRUG INTERACTIONS

Labs

- *Interference:* Glucose/insulin tolerance test

SPECIAL CONSIDERATIONS

Transfer to alternative agent (e.g., propranolol, digoxin, verapamil): ½ hr after 1st dose of alternative agent, reduce esmolol inf rate by 50%; following 2nd dose of alternative agent, monitor patient's response and, if satisfactory control is maintained for the 1st hr, discontinue esmolol inf

MONITORING PARAMETERS

- Blood pressure, ECG, heart rate, respiratory rate, IV site

estazolam

(ess-ta'zoe-lam)

ProSom

Chemical Class: Benzodiazepine
Therapeutic Class: Sedative-hypnotic
DEA Class: Schedule IV

CLINICAL PHARMACOLOGY

Mechanism of Action: Facilitates inhibitory effect of γ-aminobutyric acid (GABA) on neuronal excitability by increasing membrane permeability to chloride ions

Pharmacokinetics

PO: Onset 15-45 min, peak 2 hr, duration 7-8 hr, 93% bound to plasma proteins, metabolized by liver, excreted by kidneys (inactive/active metabolites)

INDICATIONS AND USES: Insomnia

DOSAGE

Adult

• PO 1-2 mg qhs

Elderly

• PO 0.5-1 mg qhs

$ **AVAILABLE FORMS/COST OF THERAPY**

• Tab, Uncoated—Oral: 1 mg, 100's: **$85.22;** 2 mg, 100's: **$94.93**

CONTRAINDICATIONS: Hypersensitivity to benzodiazepines, pregnancy

PRECAUTIONS: Renal or hepatic function impairment, elderly, depression, history of drug abuse, abrupt withdrawal, respiratory depression, sleep apnea

PREGNANCY AND LACTATION: Pregnancy category X; may cause fetal damage when administered during pregnancy; excreted into breast milk, may accumulate in breast-fed infants and is therefore not recommended

SIDE EFFECTS/ADVERSE REACTIONS

CNS: Somnolence, asthenia, hypokinesia, hangover, abnormal thinking, anxiety, agitation, amnesia, apathy, emotional lability, hostility, seizure, sleep disorder, stupor, twitch, ataxia, decreased libido, decreased reflexes, neuritis

CV: Dysrhythmia, syncope

EENT: Ear pain, eye irritation/pain/swelling, photophobia, pharyngitis, rhinitis, sinusitis, epistaxis,

GI: Dyspepsia, decreased/increased appetite, flatulence, gastritis, enterocolitis, melena, mouth ulceration, abdominal pain, increased AST

GU: Frequent urination, menstrual cramps, urinary hesitancy/urgency, vaginal discharge/itching, hematuria, nocturia, oliguria, penile discharge, urinary incontinence

HEME: ***Agranulocytosis***

MS: Lower extremity pain, back pain

RESP: Cold symptoms, asthma, cough, dyspnea, hyperventilation

SKIN: Urticaria, acne, dry skin, photosensitivity

▼ **DRUG INTERACTIONS**

Drugs

• *Cimetidine:* Increased serum benzodiazepine concentrations
• *Clozapine:* Isolated cases of cardiorespiratory collapse
• *Disulfiram:* May increase benzodiazepine serum concentrations
• *Ethanol:* Enhanced adverse psychomotor effects of benzodiazepines
• *Rifampin:* Reduced serum benzodiazepine concentrations

SPECIAL CONSIDERATIONS

PATIENT/FAMILY EDUCATION

• Avoid alcohol and other CNS depressants
• Do not discontinue abruptly after prolonged therapy
• May experience disturbed sleep for the first or second night after discontinuing the drug

• May cause drowsiness or dizziness, use caution while driving or performing other tasks requiring alertness
• Inform physician if you are planning to become pregnant, are pregnant, or if you become pregnant while taking this medicine

MONITORING PARAMETERS
• Periodic CBC, U/A, blood chemistry analyses during prolonged therapy

---

esterified estrogens

Climestrone, ✤ Estratab, Menest, Neo-Estrone ✤

Chemical Class: Estrogen derivative
Therapeutic Class: Estrogen

CLINICAL PHARMACOLOGY
Mechanism of Action: Needed for adequate functioning of female reproductive system; affects release of pituitary gonadotropins, inhibits ovulation, conserves calcium and phosphorus, and encourages bone formation
Pharmacokinetics
PO: Well absorbed, metabolized and inactivated in the liver, excreted in urine

INDICATIONS AND USES: Symptoms associated with menopause, female hypogonadism, female castration, primary ovarian failure, breast cancer (palliation), prostatic carcinoma (palliation), postpartum breast engorgement, osteoporosis

DOSAGE
Adult
• *Menopause:* PO 0.3-1.25 mg qd or days 1-25 of mo (combined with progestin in women with intact uterus)
• *Female hypogonadism:* PO 2.5 to 7.5 mg/d in divided doses for 20 days, followed by 10 day rest period, repeat if bleeding does not occur by the end of this period; if bleeding occurs before the end of the 10 day period, begin 2.5-7.5 mg/d in divided doses days 1-20 of month (administer oral progestin during last 5 days of estrogen cycle)
• *Female castration and primary ovarian failure:* PO 1.25 mg 3 wk on, 1 wk off
• *Prostate cancer (inoperable, progressing):* 1.25-2.5 mg tid
• *Breast cancer (inoperable, progressing):* 10 mg tid for 3 mo or longer

$ **AVAILABLE FORMS/COST OF THERAPY**
• Tab, Sugar Coated—Oral: 0.3 mg, 100's: **$12.20-$20.80;** 0.625 mg, 100's: **$17.25-$28.97;** 1.25 mg, 100's: **$29.05-$39.64;** Oral 2.5 mg, 100's: **$68.65**

CONTRAINDICATIONS: Breast cancer (except in appropriately selected patients being treated for metastatic disease), estrogen-dependent neoplasia, pregnancy, undiagnosed abnormal genital bleeding, active thrombophlebitis or thromboembolic disorders, past history of thrombophlebitis, thrombosis, or thromboembolic disorders associated with previous estrogen use

PRECAUTIONS: Hypertension, asthma, blood dyscrasias, gallbladder disease, CHF, diabetes mellitus, bone disease, depression, migraine headache, convulsive disorders, hepatic disease, renal disease, family history of cancer of breast or reproductive tract

PREGNANCY AND LACTATION: Pregnancy category X; no reports of adverse effects from estrogens in the nursing infant have been located; potential exists for decreased milk volume and decreased nitrogen and protein content

SIDE EFFECTS/ADVERSE REACTIONS

CNS: Headache, migraine, dizziness, mental depression, chorea, convulsions

CV: Edema, ***thromboembolism, stroke, pulmonary embolism, MI***

EENT: Steepening of corneal curvature, intolerance to contact lenses

GI: Nausea, vomiting, abdominal cramps, bloating, ***cholestatic jaundice,*** colitis, acute pancreatitis

GU: Breakthrough bleeding, spotting, change in menstrual flow, dysmenorrhea, premenstrual-like syndrome, amenorrhea, increase in size of uterine fibromyomata, vaginal candidiasis, change in cervical erosion and degree of cervical secretion, cystitis-like syndrome, hemolytic uremic syndrome, endometrial cystic hyperplasia, gynecomastia, testicular atrophy, impotence

HEME: Aggravation of prophyria

METAB: Reduced carbohydrate tolerance, increased triglycerides

SKIN: Chloasma or melasma, erythema nodosum/multiforme, hemorrhagic eruption, scalp hair loss, hirsutism, urticaria, dermatitis

MISC: Changes in libido, *breast tenderness, enlargement*

▼ **DRUG INTERACTIONS**

Drugs

- *Corticosteroids:* Excessive corticosteroid effects

SPECIAL CONSIDERATIONS

PATIENT/FAMILY EDUCATION

- Notify physician of pain in groin or calves, sharp chest pain or sudden shortness of breath, abnormal vaginal bleeding, missed menstrual period, lumps in breast, sudden severe headache, dizziness or fainting, vision or speech disturbance, weakness or numbness in an arm or leg, severe abdominal pain, yellowing of the skin or eyes, severe depression
- Take with food or milk to decrease GI symptoms

MONITORING PARAMETERS

- Pretreatment physical exam with reference to blood pressure, breasts, pelvic, and Pap smear
- Baseline glucose, triglycerides, cholesterol, liver function tests, calcium; repeat yearly

estradiol

(ess-tra-dye'ole)

Oral: Estrace

Estradiol Cypionate Inj: depGynogen, Depo-Estradiol, Depogen, Dura-Estrin, E-Cypionate, Estra-D, Estro-Cyp, Estrofem, Estroject-LA, Estronol-LA, Hormogen Depot

Estradiol Valerate Inj: Deladiol-40, Deoestrogen, Dioval, Dioval 40, Dioval XX, Duragen-20, Duragen-40, Estradiol LA, Estradiol LA 20, Estradiol LA 40, Estra-L 20, Estra-L 40, Estraval, Gynogen LA 10, Gynogen LA 20, Gynogen LA 40, LAE 20, Valergen-10, Valergen-20, Valeragen-40

Transdermal: Estraderm

Chemical Class: Synthetic estrogen

Therapeutic Class: Estrogen

CLINICAL PHARMACOLOGY

Mechanism of Action: Needed for adequate functioning of female reproductive system; affects release of pituitary gonadotropins (inhibits ovulation, decreases serum testosterone), inhibits bone resorption

Pharmacokinetics

PO/IM/TRANSDERM: Degraded in liver; excreted in urine; crosses placenta; excreted in breast milk

INDICATIONS AND USES: Menopause, breast cancer,* prostatic cancer, atrophic vaginitis, hypogonadism, castration, primary ovarian failure, prevention of osteoporosis, prevention of atherosclerotic disease*

DOSAGE

Adult

- *Menopause/hypogonadism/castration/ovarian failure:* PO 1-2 mg qd 3wk on, 1 wk off or 5 days on, 2 days off; IM 1-5 mg q3-4wk (cypionate); 10-20 mg q4wk (valerate); TRANSDERM .05-0.1 mg worn continuously, change twice/week
- *Prostatic cancer:* IM 30 mg q1-2 wk (valerate); PO 1-2 mg tid (oral estradiol)
- *Breast cancer:* PO 10 mg tid for 3 mo or longer
- *Atrophic vaginitis:* VAG CREAM 2-4 g (marked on applicator) qd for 1-2 wk, then 1 g 1-3 times/wk

$ **AVAILABLE FORMS/COST OF THERAPY**

- Tab, Uncoated—Oral: 0.5 mg, 100's: **$24.64;** 1 mg, 100's: **$32.83;** 2 mg, 100's: **$47.94**
- Cre—Vag: 0.01%, 42.5 g: **$25.68**
- Film, Cont Release—Percutaneous: 0.05 mg/day, 24's: **$50.96;** 0.1 mg/day, 24's: **$55.54**
- Inj (Valerate)—IM: 10, 20, 40 mg/ml, 10 ml: **$4.17-$24.20**
- Inj (Cypionate)—IM: 5 mg/ml, 10 ml: **$4.99-$11.25**

CONTRAINDICATIONS: Breast cancer, thromboembolic disorders, endometrial cancer, genital bleeding (abnormal, undiagnosed)

PRECAUTIONS: Hypertension, asthma, blood dyscrasias, gallbladder disease, CHF, diabetes mellitus, bone disease, depression, migraine headache, convulsive disorders, hepatic disease, renal disease, family history of cancer of breast or reproductive tract, children (accelerated epiphyseal closure)

PREGNANCY AND LACTATION: Pregnancy category X; compatible with breast feeding but may decrease quantity and quality of breast milk

SIDE EFFECTS/ADVERSE REACTIONS

CNS: Dizziness, headache, migraines, depression

CV: Hypotension, thrombophlebitis, edema, ***thromboembolism, stroke, pulmonary embolism, MI***

EENT: Contact lens intolerance, increased myopia, astigmatism

GI: Nausea, vomiting, diarrhea, anorexia, pancreatitis, cramps, constipation, increased appetite, increased weight, ***cholestatic jaundice***

GU: Amenorrhea, cervical erosion, breakthrough bleeding, dysmenorrhea, vaginal candidiasis, breast changes, *gynecomastia, testicular atrophy, impotence*

METAB: Folic acid deficiency, hypercalcemia, hyperglycemia

SKIN: Rash, urticaria, acne, hirsutism, alopecia, oily skin, seborrhea, purpura, melasma

▼ **DRUG INTERACTIONS**

Drugs

- *Anticoagulants, oral hypoglycemics:* Decreased action
- *Anticonvulsants, barbiturates, phenylbutazone, rifampin:* Decreased action of estrogens
- *Corticosteroids:* Increased action

Labs

- *Increase:* T_4, T_3 (because of increased TBG levels, free thryroid hormone levels unaffected), glucose, HDL, prolactin, factors II, VII, VIII, IX, and X, triglycerides
- *Decrease:* T_3U, antithrombin III, folate

estrogens, conjugated

C.E.S, 🍁 Conjugated Estrogens, Premarin, Premarin Intravenous, Combination products packaged with medroxyprogesterone acetate (MPA): Prempro (daily product), Premphase (cycled product)

Chemical Class: Equine estrogen product

Therapeutic Class: Estrogen

CLINICAL PHARMACOLOGY

Mechanism of Action: Needed for adequate functioning of female reproductive system; affects release of pituitary gonadotropins, inhibits bone resorption

Pharmacokinetics

PO/IV/IM: Degraded in liver, excreted in urine, crosses placenta, excreted in breast milk

INDICATIONS AND USES: Menopause, breast cancer (inoperable, in post-menopausal women and men), prostatic cancer, dysfunctional uterine bleeding, hypogonadism, castration, primary ovarian failure, prevention of osteoporosis, prevention of cardiovascular disease*

DOSAGE

Adult

- *Menopause/atrophic vaginitis:* PO 0.3-1.25 mg qd cyclically or continuously
- *Atrophic vaginitis:* VAG CREAM 2-4 g qd cyclically, reduce dosage as tolerated
- *Osteoporosis prevention:* PO 0.625 mg qd cyclically or continuously
- *Prostatic cancer:* PO 1.25-2.5 mg tid
- *Breast cancer:* PO 10 mg tid for 3 mo or longer
- *Dysfunctional uterine bleeding:* IV/IM 25 mg, repeat in 6-12 hr

Castration/primary ovarian failure: PO 1.25 mg qd cyclically or continuously, reduce as tolerated

- *Hypogonadism:* PO 2.5 mg qd-tid cyclically

$ AVAILABLE FORMS/COST OF THERAPY

- Cre, Top—Vag: 0.625 mg/g, 45 g: **$29.15-$32.46**
- Inj, Lyphl-Sol—IM;IV: 25 mg/5 ml, 5 ml: **$32.11;** 30 ml: **$3.00**
- Tab, Sugar Coated—Oral: 0.3 mg, 100's: **$28.31;** 0.625 mg, 100's: **$28.16-$42.41;** 0.9 mg, 100's: **$46.73;** 1.25 mg, 100's: **$53.99-$56.68;** 2.5 mg, 100's: **$93.49**

Combination Products (package contains separate pills of estrogen and MPA):

- Tab, Uncoated—Oral: 0.625 mg/2.5 mg MPA (both hormones dosed qd), 168's: **$50.40**
- Tab, Uncoated—Oral: 0.625 mg/5 mg MPA (estrogen dosed qd day 1-28, MPA dosed day 15-28), 126's: **$46.20**

CONTRAINDICATIONS: Breast cancer, thromboembolic disorders, endometrial cancer, genital bleeding (abnormal, undiagnosed)

PRECAUTIONS: Hypertension, asthma, blood dyscrasias, gallbladder disease, CHF, diabetes mellitus, bone disease, depression, migraine headache, convulsive disorders, hepatic disease, renal disease, family history of cancer of breast or reproductive tract

PREGNANCY AND LACTATION: Pregnancy category X; may decrease quantity and quality of breast milk

SIDE EFFECTS/ADVERSE REACTIONS

CNS: Dizziness, headache, migraine, depression

CV: Hypotension, thrombophlebitis, edema, ***thromboembolism, stroke, pulmonary embolism, MI***

EENT: Contact lens intolerance, increased myopia, astigmatism
GI: *Nausea,* vomiting, diarrhea, anorexia, pancreatitis, cramps, constipation, increased appetite, increased weight, ***cholestatic jaundice***
GU: Amenorrhea, cervical erosion, breakthrough bleeding, dysmenorrhea, vaginal candidiasis, breast changes, *gynecomastia, testicular atrophy, impotence*
METAB: Folic acid deficiency, hypercalcemia (in metastatic bone disease), hyperglycemia
SKIN: Rash, urticaria, acne, hirsutism, alopecia, oily skin, seborrhea, purpura, melasma

▼ DRUG INTERACTIONS

Drugs

• *Anticoagulants, oral hypoglycemics:* Decreased action
• *Anticonvulsants, barbiturates, phenylbutazone, rifampin:* Decreased action of estrogens
• *Corticosteroids:* Increased action

Labs

• *Increase:* T_4, T_3 (because of increased TBG levels, free thyroid hormone levels unaffected), glucose, HDL, prolactin, factors II, VII, VIII, IX, and X, triglycerides
• *Decrease:* T_3U, antithrombin III, folate

estrone

(ess′trone)

Aquest, Estrone Aqueous, Estrone-5, Estronol, Femogen Forte, ✦ Kestrone-5, Theelin Aqueous

Chemical Class: Estrogen derivative
Therapeutic Class: Estrogen

CLINICAL PHARMACOLOGY

Mechanism of Action: Needed for adequate functioning of female reproductive system; affects release of pituitary gonadotropins, inhibits ovulation, inhibits bone resorption

Pharmacokinetics

IM: Degraded in liver; excreted in urine; crosses placenta; excreted in breast milk

INDICATIONS AND USES: Menopause, inoperable prostatic cancer, atrophic vaginitis, hypogonadism, primary ovarian failure, dysfunctional uterine bleeding

DOSAGE

Adult

• *Dysfunctional uterine bleeding:* IM 2-5 mg qd for several days
• *Menopause/atrophic vaginitis:* IM 0.1-0.5 mg 2-3 times/wk, cyclically or continuously
• *Female hypogonadism/primary ovarian failure:* IM 0.1-2 mg qwk in one dose or divided doses, cyclically or continuously
• *Prostatic cancer:* IM 2-4 mg 2-3 times/wk

$ AVAILABLE FORMS/COST OF THERAPY

• Inj, Susp—IM: 2 mg/ml, 10 ml: **$4.95-$25.56;** 5 mg/ml, 10 ml: **$5.85-$12.75**

CONTRAINDICATIONS: Breast cancer, thromboembolic disorders, endometrial cancer, genital bleeding (abnormal, undiagnosed)

PRECAUTIONS: Hypertension, asthma, blood dyscrasias, gallbladder disease, CHF, diabetes mellitus, migraine headache, hepatic disease, renal disease, family history of breast or endometrial cancer, uterine fibroids, endometriosis

PREGNANCY AND LACTATION: Pregnancy category X; estradiol considered compatible with breast feeding, no data on estrone; may decrease quantity and quality of breast milk

SIDE EFFECTS/ADVERSE REACTIONS
CNS: Dizziness, headache, migraine, depression
CV: Hypotension, thrombophlebitis, edema, ***thromboembolism, stroke, pulmonary embolism, MI***
EENT: Contact lens intolerance, increased myopia, astigmatism
GI: Nausea, vomiting, diarrhea, anorexia, pancreatitis, cramps, constipation, increased appetite, increased weight, ***cholestatic jaundice***
GU: Amenorrhea, cervical erosion, breakthrough bleeding, dysmenorrhea, vaginal candidiasis, breast pain and enlargement, *gynecomastia, testicular atrophy, impotence*
METAB: Folic acid deficiency, hypercalcemia, hyperglycemia
SKIN: Rash, urticaria, acne, hirsutism, alopecia, oily skin, seborrhea, purpura, melasma

▼ **DRUG INTERACTIONS**

Drugs

• *Anticoagulants, oral hypoglycemics:* Decreased action
• *Anticonvulsants, barbiturates, phenylbutazone, rifampin:* Decreased action of estrogens
• *Corticosteroids:* Increased action

Labs

• *Increase:* T_4, T_3 (because of increased TBG levels, free thyroid hormone levels unaffected), glucose, HDLs, prolactin, factors II, VII, VIII, IX, and X, triglycerides
• *Decrease:* T_3U, antithrombin III, folate

estropipate

(es-tro-pip'ate)
Ogen
Chemical Class: Natural estrogen compound with piperazine
Therapeutic Class: Estrogen

CLINICAL PHARMACOLOGY
Mechanism of Action: Necessary for adequate functioning of female reproductive system and secondary sex characteristics; affects release of pituitary gonadotropins, promotes adequate calcium use in bone structures

Pharmacokinetics

PO: Metabolized in liver (significant first pass effect) primarily to estrone; excreted in urine

INDICATIONS AND USES: Vasomotor symptoms, atrophic vaginitis or kraurosis vulvae associated with menopause; female hypogonadism, female castration or primary ovarian failure; osteoporosis prevention, CAD prevention*

DOSAGE

Adult

• *Vasomotor symptoms, atrophic vaginitis:* PO 0.625 mg qd; VAG 2-4 g qd prn initially, then weekly or twice weekly
• *Female hypogonadism, female castration, or primary ovarian failure:* PO 1.25-7.5 mg/day × 3 wk, followed by a rest period of 8-10 days, repeated cyclically
• *Osteoporosis prevention:* PO 0.625 mg qd for 25-31 days monthly

$ **AVAILABLE FORMS/COST OF THERAPY**

• Tab, Uncoated—Oral: 0.625 mg, 100's: **$34.66-$53.22;** 1.25 mg, 100's: **$47.40-$74.35;** 2.5 mg, 100's: **$100.35-$129.40**
• Cre—Vag: 1.5 mg/g, 42.5-45 g: **$39.14**

CONTRAINDICATIONS: Breast cancer, reproductive cancer, genital bleeding (abnormal, undiagnosed), pregnancy

PRECAUTIONS: Hypertension, asthma, blood dyscrasias, gallbladder disease, CHF, diabetes mellitus, bone disease, depression, migraine headache, convulsive disorders, hepatic disease, renal disease, family history of cancer of breast or reproductive tract, thromboembolic disorders

PREGNANCY AND LACTATION: Pregnancy category X; small amounts excreted in breast milk, may influence quantity and quality (decreased composition of nitrogen and protein content) of milk

SIDE EFFECTS/ADVERSE REACTIONS

CNS: Dizziness, headache, migraine headaches, depression

CV: Hypotension, thrombophlebitis, edema, ***thromboembolism, stroke, pulmonary embolism, MI***

EENT: Contact lens intolerance, increased myopia, astigmatism

GI: Nausea, vomiting, diarrhea, anorexia, pancreatitis, cramps, constipation, increased appetite, increased weight, ***cholestatic jaundice,*** colitis, acute pancreatitis

GU: Amenorrhea, cervical erosion, breakthrough bleeding, dysmenorrhea, vaginal candidiasis, breast changes

METAB: Folic acid deficiency, hypercalcemia, hyperglycemia

SKIN: Rash, urticaria, acne, hirsutism, alopecia, oily skin, seborrhea, purpura, chloasma or melasma, erythema nodosum/multiforme, changes in libido

MISC: Weight gain

▼ **DRUG INTERACTIONS**

Drugs

- *Benzodiazepines:* Estrogens inhibit oxidative metabolism, increased levels of chlordiazepoxide, diazepam, alprazolam, triazolam
- *Corticosteroids:* Via increased serum cortisol-binding globulin, retards the metabolism of corticosteroids
- *Cyclosporine:* Increased cyclosporine levels
- *Dantrolene:* Increased hepatotoxic risk
- *Griseofulvin:* Griseofulvin enhances metabolism of estrogens, reduced efficacy
- *Smoking, tobacco+:* Increased cardiovascular risk; increased hepatic metabolism of estrogen resulting in lowered serum levels

Labs

- *Increase:* Norepinephrine-induced platelet aggregability, BSP retention, PBI, T_4, T_3, cortisol, glucose, phospholipids, prolactin, prothrombin, and clotting factors VII, VIII, IX, and X, Na, triglycerides, renin substrate, serum calcium
- *Decrease:* Metyrapone test, antithrombin III, pregnanediol excretion, pyridoxine, and folate concentrations

SPECIAL CONSIDERATIONS

Unopposed estrogen increases risk of endometrial cancer; recommended administration of concurrent progestational agents

ethacrynic acid

(eth-a-kri′nik)

Edecrin, Edecrin Sodium

Chemical Class: Ketone derivative

Therapeutic Class: Loop diuretic

CLINICAL PHARMACOLOGY

Mechanism of Action: Acts on loop of Henle to inhibit resorption of sodium and water

Pharmacokinetics

PO: Onset ½ hr, peak 2 hr, duration 6-8 hr

IV: Onset 5 min, peak 15-30 min, duration 2 hr

Excreted in urine and feces, crosses placenta; $t_{1/2}$ 30-70 min

INDICATIONS AND USES: Pulmonary edema; edema in CHF, liver disease, renal disease including nephrotic syndrome, ascites; glaucoma;* hypertension (in combination with other agents),* hypercalcemia*

DOSAGE

Adult

• PO 50-200 mg/d; may give up to 200 mg bid; adjust dose in 25-50 mg increments; IV 50 mg or 0.5-1.0 mg/kg given over several min

Child

• PO 25 mg, increased by 25 mg/d until desired effect occurs; not established for infants or parenterally

$ AVAILABLE FORMS/COST OF THERAPY

• Inj, Sol—IV: 50 mg/vial: **$19.05**

• Tab, Uncoated—Oral: 25 mg, 100's: **$29.86;** 50 mg, 100's: **$42.56**

CONTRAINDICATIONS: Anuria, hypovolemia, electrolyte depletion, infants

PRECAUTIONS: Dehydration, ascites, severe renal disease, hypoproteinemia, cirrhosis (may precipitate hepatic encephalopathy), concurrent administration of other ototoxic drugs, sulfa allergy

PREGNANCY AND LACTATION: Pregnancy category B; no data on nursing; contraindicated per manufacturer

SIDE EFFECTS/ADVERSE REACTIONS

CNS: Headache, fatigue, weakness, vertigo, encephalopathy in hepatic disease

CV: ***Chest pain,*** hypotension, ***circulatory collapse,*** ECG changes

EENT: Hearing loss, ear pain, tinnitus, blurred vision

ENDO: Decreased glucose tolerance, hyperglycemia

GI: Nausea, ***severe diarrhea,*** dry mouth, vomiting, anorexia, cramps, upset stomach, abdominal pain, ***acute pancreatitis,*** jaundice, ***GI bleeding;*** abdominal distension

GU: Polyuria, ***renal failure,*** glycosuria, sexual dysfunction

HEME: ***Thrombocytopenia, agranulocytosis, leukopenia, neutropenia***

METAB: Hypokalemia, hypochloremic alkalosis, hypomagnesemia, hyperuricemia, hypocalcemia, hyponatremia

MS: Cramps, arthritis, stiffness

SKIN: Rash, pruritis, purpura, ***Stevens-Johnson syndrome,*** sweating, photosensitivity

▼ DRUG INTERACTIONS

Drugs

• *Aminoglycosides:* Increased ototoxicity

• *ACE inhibitors:* Renal insufficiency, hypotension

• *Digitalis:* Hypokalemia induced digitalis toxicity

---

ethambutol

(e-tham'byoo-tole)

Etibi, ♣ Myambutol

Chemical Class: Diisopropylethylene diamide derivative

Therapeutic Class: Antitubercular

CLINICAL PHARMACOLOGY

Mechanism of Action: Inhibits RNA synthesis, decreases tubercle bacilli replication

Pharmacokinetics

PO: Peak 2-4 hr, $t_{1/2}$ 3-4 hr; metabolized in liver; excreted in urine (unchanged drug/inactive metabolites), and feces, crosses placenta

INDICATIONS AND USES: Adjunct in treatment of pulmonary tuberculosis

DOSAGE

Adult and Child >13 yr

• *Initial treatment:* PO 15 mg/kg/d as a single daily dose

• *Retreatment:* PO 25 mg/kg/d as single dose for 2 mo with at least 1 other drug, then decrease to 15 mg/kg/d as single daily dose

$ AVAILABLE FORMS/COST OF THERAPY

• Tab, Uncoated—Oral: 100 mg, 100's: **$47.45;** 400 mg, 100's: **$158.75**

CONTRAINDICATIONS: Hypersensitivity, optic neuritis, child <13 yrs

PRECAUTIONS: Renal disease, diabetic retinopathy, cataracts, ocular defects, hepatic and hematopoietic disorders, gout

PREGNANCY AND LACTATION: Pregnancy category B; compatible with breast feeding

SIDE EFFECTS/ADVERSE REACTIONS

CNS: Headache, confusion, fever, malaise, dizziness, disorientation, hallucinations

EENT: Blurred vision, optic neuritis, photophobia, decreased visual acuity, changes in color perception, bloody sputum

GI: Abdominal distress, anorexia, nausea, vomiting

HEME: Thrombocytopenia

METAB: Elevated uric acid, acute gout, liver function impairment

MS: Joint pain

SKIN: Dermatitis, pruritis

▼ DRUG INTERACTIONS

Drugs

• *Aluminum salts:* Delayed absorption of ethambutol

SPECIAL CONSIDERATIONS

PATIENT/FAMILY EDUCATION

• Administer with meals to decrease GI symptoms

MONITORING PARAMETERS

• Perform visual acuity testing before beginning therapy and periodically during drug administration (qmo if dose >15 mg/kg/d)

ethanolamine oleate

(eth-an-ole'a-meen ol'ee-ate)

Ethamolin

Therapeutic Class: Sclerosing agent

CLINICAL PHARMACOLOGY

Mechanism of Action: Following IV inj, irritates intimal endothelium of the vein and produces a sterile dose-related inflammatory response, leading to fibrosis and occlusion of the vein; oleic acid component of compound is responsible for the inflammatory response and may also activate coagulation

Pharmacokinetics

IV: Disappears from inj site within 5 min via portal vein; sclerosis of varices lasts 2½ mo

INDICATIONS AND USES: Esophageal varices to prevent rebleeding

DOSAGE

Adult

• IV 1.5-5 ml per varix; max total dose per treatment should not exceed 20 ml or 0.4 ml/kg for a 50 kg patient

Child

• IV 2-5 ml per varix to a max of 20 ml

$ AVAILABLE FORMS/COST OF THERAPY

• Inj, Sol—IV: 5%, 2 ml: **$24.00**

CONTRAINDICATIONS: Hypersensitivity

PRECAUTIONS: Severe inj necrosis; concomitant cardiorespiratory disease

PREGNANCY AND LACTATION: Pregnancy category C

SIDE EFFECTS/ADVERSE REACTIONS

GI: Esophageal ulcer, stricture

METAB: Pyrexia

RESP: Pleural effusion/infiltration, pneumonia

MISC: Retrosternal pain

ethchlorvynol

(eth-klor-vi'nole)

Placidyl

Chemical Class: Tertiary acetylenic alcohol

Therapeutic Class: Sedative-hypnotic

DEA Class: Schedule IV

CLINICAL PHARMACOLOGY

Mechanism of Action: Produces cerebral depression; mechanism unknown

Pharmacokinetics

PO: Onset 15-60 min; peak 2 hr; duration 5 hr; $t_{1/2}$, 10-20 hr; extensive distribution to adipose tissue; metabolized by liver (90%); renal elimination

INDICATIONS AND USES: Sedation, insomnia

DOSAGE

Adult

- *Sedation:* PO 200 mg bid or tid
- *Insomnia:* PO 500 mg-1 g ½ hr before hs; may repeat 100-200 mg if needed

Child

- PO 25 mg/kg in one dose not to exceed 1 g

$ **AVAILABLE FORMS/COST OF THERAPY**

- Cap, Gel—Oral: 200 mg, 100's: **$105.07;** 500 mg, 100's: **$129.44;** 750 mg, 100's: **$66.50-$171.78**

CONTRAINDICATIONS: Hypersensitivity, uncontrolled pain, porphyria, drug abuse/dependency

PRECAUTIONS: Depression, hepatic disease, renal disease, suicidal tendencies, elderly

PREGNANCY AND LACTATION: Pregnancy category C

SIDE EFFECTS/ADVERSE REACTIONS

CNS: Fatigue, drowsiness, dizziness, sedation, ataxia, nightmares, hangover, giddiness, weakness, hysteria

CV: Hypotension

EENT: Blurred vision, bitter aftertaste

GI: Nausea, vomiting

HEME: ***Thrombocytopenia***

SKIN: *Rash,* urticaria

SPECIAL CONSIDERATIONS

Geriatric patients may be more sensitive to usual adult dose

ethinyl estradiol

(eth-in'il ess-tra-dye'ole)

Estinyl, Feminone ✦

Chemical Class: Synthetic estrogen

Therapeutic Class: Estrogen

CLINICAL PHARMACOLOGY

Mechanism of Action: Needed for adequate functioning of female reproductive system and secondary sex characteristics; affects release of pituitary gonadotropins, inhibits ovulation, promotes adequate calcium use in bone structures

Pharmacokinetics

PO: Degraded in liver; excreted in urine

INDICATIONS AND USES: Vasomotor symptoms associated with menopause, atrophic vaginitis; kraurosis vulvae, breast engorgement, female hypogonadism, osteoporosis, contraceptive (combined with progestins), female breast cancer (inoperable, progressing), prostatic carcinoma (inoperable)

DOSAGE

Adult

- *Menopause:* PO 0.02-0.5 mg qd 3 wk on, 1 wk off
- *Prostatic cancer:* PO 0.15-2 mg qd
- *Hypogonadism:* PO 0.05 mg qd-tid × 2 wk/mo, then 2 wk proges-

terone, then 3-6 mo cycles, then 2 mo off

• *Breast cancer:* PO 1 mg tid

• *Breast engorgement:* PO 0.5-1 mg qd × 3 days, then tapered off over 7 days

• *Combined oral contraceptive:* Combined with progestins, 30-80 mcg cycled 21 days, off 7 days

$ AVAILABLE FORMS/COST OF THERAPY

• Tab, Coated—Oral: 0.02 mg, 100's: **$28.69;** 0.05 mg, 100's: **$48.35;** 0.5 mg, 100's: **$97.72**

See oral contraceptives monograph for combined oral contraceptives containing ethinyl estradiol

CONTRAINDICATIONS: Breast cancer (except for appropriately selected patients being treated for metastatic disease), thromboembolic disorders, reproductive cancer, genital bleeding (abnormal, undiagnosed), pregnancy

PRECAUTIONS: Hypertension, asthma, blood dyscrasias, gallbladder disease, CHF, diabetes mellitus, bone disease, depression, migraine headache, convulsive disorders, hepatic disease, renal disease, family history of cancer of breast or reproductive tract

PREGNANCY AND LACTATION: Pregnancy category X; small amounts excreted in breast milk, may influence quantity and quality (decreased composition of nitrogen and protein content) of milk

SIDE EFFECTS/ADVERSE REACTIONS

CNS: Dizziness, headache, migraine headaches, depression

CV: Hypotension, thrombophlebitis, edema, ***thromboembolism, stroke, pulmonary embolism, MI***

EENT: Contact lens intolerance, increased myopia, astigmatism

GI: Nausea, vomiting, diarrhea, anorexia, pancreatitis, cramps, constipation, increased appetite, increased weight, ***cholestatic jaundice,*** colitis, acute pancreatitis

GU: Amenorrhea, cervical erosion, breakthrough bleeding, dysmenorrhea, vaginal candidiasis, breast changes, *gynecomastia, testicular atrophy, impotence*

METAB: Folic acid deficiency, hypercalcemia, hyperglycemia

SKIN: Rash, urticaria, acne, hirsutism, alopecia, oily skin, seborrhea, purpura, chloasma or melasma, erythema nodosum/multiforme, changes in libido

MISC: Weight gain

▼ DRUG INTERACTIONS

Drugs

• *Antibiotics:* Impaired contraceptive efficacy via reducing bacterial hydrolysis in GI tract, interrupting enterohepatic circulation

• *Anticonvulsants:* Reduce contraceptive efficacy via enhanced metabolism

• *Benzodiazepines:* Estrogens inhibit oxidative metabolism, increased levels of chlordiazepoxide, diazepam, alprazolam, triazolam

• *Corticosteroids:* Via increased serum cortisol-binding globulin, retards the metabolism of corticosteroids

• *Cyclosporine:* Increased cyclosporine levels

• *Dantrolene:* Increased hepatotoxic risk

• *Griseofulvin:* Griseofulvin enhances metabolism of estrogens, reduced efficacy

• *Rifampin:* Enhanced metabolism of contraceptive steroids, reduced efficacy

• *Smoking, tobacco+:* Increased cardiovascular risk

Labs

• *Increase:* Norepinephrine-induced platelet aggregability, BSP retention, PBI, T_4, T_3, cortisol, glucose,

phospholipids, prolactin, prothrombin, and clotting factors VII, VIII, IX, and X, Na, triglycerides, renin substrate, serum calcium
• *Decrease:* Metyrapone test, antithrombin III, pregnanediol excretion, pyridoxine, and folate concentrations

ethionamide

(e-thye-on'am-ide)
Trecator-SC
Chemical Class: Thiomine derivative
Therapeutic Class: Antitubercular

CLINICAL PHARMACOLOGY
Mechanism of Action: Bacteriostatic against *Mycobacterium tuberculosis* via inhibition of peptide synthesis
Pharmacokinetics
PO: Peak 3 hr $t_{1/2}$, 3 hr; metabolized in liver; renal excretion (primarily inactive metabolites)
INDICATIONS AND USES: Pulmonary, extrapulmonary TB when other antitubercular drugs have failed
DOSAGE
Adult
• PO 500 mg-1 g qd in divided doses, with another antitubercular drug and pyridoxine
Child
• PO 15-20 mg/kg/d in 3-4 doses, not to exceed 1 g; concomitant pyridoxine recommended
$ AVAILABLE FORMS/COST OF THERAPY
• Tab, Sugar Coated—Oral: 250 mg, 100's: **$170.15**
CONTRAINDICATIONS Hypersensitivity, severe hepatic disease
PRECAUTIONS: Renal disease, diabetes, hepatic impairment
PREGNANCY AND LACTATION: Pregnancy category D
SIDE EFFECTS/ADVERSE REACTIONS
CNS: Headache, drowsiness, tremors, ***convulsions,*** depression, psychosis, dizziness, peripheral neuritis, olfactory disturbances
CV: Postural hypotension
EENT: Blurred vision, optic neuritis
GI: Anorexia, nausea, vomiting, diarrhea (50% can't tolerate >500 mg), metallic taste, jaundice
GU: Impotence, menorrhagia
HEME: ***Thrombocytopenia,*** purpura
METAB: Difficulty managing diabetes mellitus
SKIN: Dermatitis, alopecia, acne
MISC: Gynecomastia
▼ DRUG INTERACTIONS
Drugs
• *Cycloserine:* Increased neurotoxicity
Labs
• *Increase:* Serum transaminases
SPECIAL CONSIDERATIONS
Use only with at least one other effective antituberculous agent
MONITORING PARAMETERS
• Serum transaminases (AST, ALT) bi-weekly during therapy

ethosuximide

(eth-oh-sux'i-mide)
Zarontin
Chemical Class: Succinimide
Therapeutic Class: Anticonvulsant

CLINICAL PHARMACOLOGY
Mechanism of Action: Increases seizure threshold and inhibits spike-and-wave formation in absence (petit mal) seizures; decreases amplitude, frequency, duration, spread of discharge in minor motor seizures
Pharmacokinetics
PO: Peak 3-7 hr; steady state 4-7 days; therapeutic serum concentrations 40-100 μg/ml; rapid and com-

plete absorption; freely distributed, except to fat; insignificant protein binding; metabolized by liver; excreted in urine (20% unchanged); $t_{1/2}$ 56-60 hr (adults); 26-30 hr (children)

INDICATIONS AND USES: Absence seizures, partial seizures, tonic-clonic seizures

DOSAGE

Adult and Child >6 yr

• PO 250 mg bid initially; may increase by 250 mg q4-7d, not to exceed 1.5 g/d

Child 3-6 yr

• PO 250 mg/d or 125 mg bid; may increase by 250 mg q4-7d, not to exceed 1 g/d (20 mg/kg/d)

$ AVAILABLE FORMS/COST OF THERAPY

• Syr—Oral: 250 mg/5 ml, 480 ml: **$63.20-$75.44**

• Cap, Gel—Oral: 250 mg, 100's: **$71.72**

CONTRAINDICATIONS Hypersensitivity

PRECAUTIONS: Hepatic function impairment; renal dysfunction; blood dyscrasias

PREGNANCY AND LACTATION: Pregnancy category C; freely enters breast milk; no adverse effects on infants reported; compatible with breast feeding

SIDE EFFECTS/ADVERSE REACTIONS

CNS: Drowsiness, dizziness, fatigue, euphoria, lethargy, anxiety, aggressiveness, irritability, depression, headache, insomnia

EENT: Myopia, blurred vision

GI: Nausea, vomiting, heartburn, anorexia, diarrhea, abdominal pain, cramps, constipation, hiccoughs, weight loss, gum hypertrophy, tongue swelling

GU: Vaginal bleeding, ***hematuria, renal damage***

HEME: ***Agranulocytosis, aplastic anemia, thrombocytopenia, leukocytosis, eosinophilia, pancytopenia***

SKIN: Urticaria, pruritic erythema, hirsutism, ***Stevens-Johnson syndrome***

MISC: SLE

▼ DRUG INTERACTIONS

Drugs

• *CNS depression-producing medications:* Enhanced CNS depression

• *Haloperidol:* Change in pattern or frequency of seizures

Labs

• *False positive:* Direct Coombs' test

SPECIAL CONSIDERATIONS

PATIENT/FAMILY EDUCATION

• Take doses at regularly spaced intervals

• May cause drowsiness

• OK with food or milk

MONITORING PARAMETERS

• Blood counts, RFTs, LFTs, urinalysis periodically

---

ethotoin

(eth-oh-to'in)

Peganone

Chemical Class: Hydantoin derivative

Therapeutic Class: Anticonvulsant

CLINICAL PHARMACOLOGY

Mechanism of Action: Stabilizes neuronal membranes at the cell body, axon, and synapse and limit the spread of neuronal or seizure activity

Pharmacokinetics

PO: Therapeutic serum concentration 15-50 µg/ml; rapid absorption; metabolized by liver (substantial nonlinear kinetics); excreted in urine; $t_{1/2}$ 3-9 hr

INDICATIONS AND USES: Generalized tonic-clonic or complex-partial seizures (second line agent)

DOSAGE

Adult

• PO 250 mg qid initially; may increase over several days to 3 g/d in divided doses (<2 g/d ineffective in most adults)

Child

• PO 250 mg bid; may increase by 250 mg qid

$ **AVAILABLE FORMS/COST OF THERAPY**

• Tab, Uncoated—Oral: 250 mg, 100's: **$41.28;** 500 mg, 100's: **$77.47**

CONTRAINDICATIONS Hypersensitivity to hydantoins, blood dyscrasias, hematologic disease, hepatic disease

PRECAUTIONS: Geriatric patients metabolize hydantoins slowly

PREGNANCY AND LACTATION: Pregnancy category D (fetal hydantoin syndrome)

SIDE EFFECTS/ADVERSE REACTIONS

CNS: Fatigue, insomnia, numbness, fever, headache, dizziness, ataxia

CV: Chest pain

EENT: Nystagnus, diplopia

GI: Nausea, vomiting, diarrhea, gingival hypertrophy

HEME: ***Agranulocytosis, thrombocytopenia, leukopenia, pancytopenia, megaloblastic anemia,*** lymphadenopathy

SKIN: Rash

▼ **DRUG INTERACTIONS**

Drugs

• *Alcohol or CNS depression-producing drugs:* Enhanced CNS depression

• *Amiodarone:* Increased plasma concentration of ethotoin

• *Antacids:* Decrease bioavailability of ethotoin

• *Chloramphenicol, cimetidine, disulfiram, isoniazid, phenylbutazone, sulfonamides:* All inhibit metabolism and increase concentration of ethotoin

• *Estrogen contraceptives, corticosteroids, corticotropin, estrogens:* All may have effects decreased because of increased metabolism

• *Fluconazole:* Decreases the metabolism of ethotoin

• *Lidocaine:* Concurrent IV use may produce additive cardiac depressant effects

• *Methadone:* Increased methadone metabolism, decreased activity

• *Oral anticoagulants:* Increased serum concentration of ethotoin; increased anticoagulant effect initially, then decreased with continued use

• *Oral diazoxide:* Decreased efficacy of both agents

• *Rifampin:* Increased metabolism of ethotoin, decreased effect

• *Streptozocin:* Ethotoin may protect pancreatic beta cells from the toxic effects of streptozocin

• *Sucralfate:* Decreased ethotoin absorption

• *Valproic acid:* Displaces ethotoin from binding sites, inhibits ethotoin metabolism, increased or additive liver toxicity

• *Xanthines:* Increased hepatic xanthine metabolism, decreased serum concentration, xanthines inhibit ethotoin absorption with decreased serum ethotoin levels

Labs

• *Increase:* Serum glucose, urine glucose, BSP, alk phosphatase

• *Decrease:* Urinary steroids, PBI, dexamethasone/metyrapone tests, Schilling test, thyroid function tests

SPECIAL CONSIDERATIONS

PATIENT/FAMILY EDUCATION

• May cause drowsiness

• Avoid alcoholic beverages

• Strictly enforced program of teeth cleaning and plaque control to prevent gingival hyperplasia is necessary

• Take doses at regularly spaced intervals

ethylnorepinephrine

(eth'il-nor-ep-i-nef'rin)
Bronkephrine
Chemical Class: Catecholamine
Therapeutic Class: Adrenergic bronchodilator

CLINICAL PHARMACOLOGY
Mechanism of Action: α-Stimulation with vasoconstriction, pressor response, nasal decongestion; β_1 stimulation with increased myocardial contractility and β_2-stimulation with vasodilation and bronchial dilation
Pharmacokinetics
IM/SC: Onset 6-12 min, duration 1-2 hr
INDICATIONS AND USES: Bronchospasm
DOSAGE
Adult
• IM/SC 0.5-1 ml
Child
• IM/SC 0.1-0.5 ml
$ AVAILABLE FORMS/COST OF THERAPY
• Inj, Sol—SC; IM: 2 mg/ml, 1 ml: **$4.39**
CONTRAINDICATIONS: Hypersensitivity, narrow-angle glaucoma
PRECAUTIONS: Cardiac disorders, hyperthyroidism, diabetes mellitus, prostatic hypertrophy
PREGNANCY AND LACTATION: Pregnancy category C
SIDE EFFECTS/ADVERSE REACTIONS
CNS: Tremors, anxiety, insomnia, headache, dizziness, confusion
CV: Palpitations, tachycardia, hypertension, chest pain, ***dysrhythmias***
GI: Anorexia, nausea, vomiting

▼ DRUG INTERACTIONS
Drugs
• *Beta blockers+:* Enhanced pressor response—hypertension, bradycardia
• *MAOIs or tricyclic antidepressants+:* Enhanced pressor response
• *Chlorpromazine, neuroleptics:* Neuroleptics may reverse the pressor response of epinephrine

etidocaine

(eh-tee'doe-kane)
Duranest
Chemical Class: Amide
Therapeutic Class: Local anesthetic

CLINICAL PHARMACOLOGY
Mechanism of Action: Competes with calcium for sites in nerve membrane that control sodium transport across cell membrane; decreases rise of depolarization phase of action potential
Pharmacokinetics
Onset 2-8 min, duration 3-6 hr; metabolized by liver; high lipid solubility; $t_{1/2}$ 2.7 hr (adult), 4-8 hr (neonate); metabolites excreted in urine
INDICATIONS AND USES: Peripheral nerve block, caudal anesthesia, central neural block, vaginal block
DOSAGE
Amount varies with route and procedure
• Peripheral nerve block, central nerve block or lumbar peridural, caudal: 1%
• Intra-abdominal or pelvic surgery, lower limb surgery or cesarean section: 1% or 1.5%
• Maxillary infiltration or inferior alveolar nerve block: 1.5%
$ AVAILABLE FORMS/COST OF THERAPY
• Inj—Sol (w/epinephrine): 1%, 30 ml: **$19.52;** 1.5%, 20 ml: **$20.90**

• Inj—Sol: 1.5%, 1.8 ml × 100: **$62.50**

CONTRAINDICATIONS Hypersensitivity, child <12 yr, elderly, severe liver disease

PRECAUTIONS: Severe drug allergies

PREGNANCY AND LACTATION: Pregnancy category B; although no breast milk excretion data, problems in humans have not been documented

SIDE EFFECTS/ADVERSE REACTIONS

CNS: Anxiety, restlessness, ***convulsions, loss of consciousness,*** drowsiness, disorientation, tremors, shivering

CV: ***Myocardial depression, cardiac arrest, dysrhythmias,*** bradycardia, hypotension, hypertension, ***fetal bradycardia***

EENT: Blurred vision, tinnitus, pupil constriction

GI: Nausea, vomiting

RESP: ***Status asthmaticus, respiratory arrest, anaphylaxis***

SKIN: Rash, urticaria, allergic reactions, edema, burning, skin discoloration at inj site, tissue necrosis

▼ **DRUG INTERACTIONS**

Drugs

• *CNS depressants:* Additive depressant effects

---

etidronate

(ee-tid'roe-nate)

Didronel, Didronel IV

Chemical Class: Bisphosphate

Therapeutic Class: Bone resorption inhibitor, anti-hypercalcemic

CLINICAL PHARMACOLOGY

Mechanism of Action: Bone crystal poison; decreases bone resorption and new bone development (accretion)

Pharmacokinetics

Therapeutic response, Paget's Disease and osteoporosis 1-3 mo; hypercalcemia 24 hr; duration of effect, Paget's Disease 1 yr after discontinuing therapy; hypercalcemia 14 days of normocalcemia; poorly absorbed (1%-6%); chemically adsorbed to bone; not metabolized; excreted in urine/feces

INDICATIONS AND USES: Paget's disease, heterotopic ossification, hypercalcemia of malignancy, osteoporosis*

DOSAGE

Adult

• *Paget's disease:* PO 5-10 mg/kg/d 2 hr ac with H_2O, not to exceed 20 mg/kg/d, max course, 6 mo

• *Heterotropic ossification:* PO 20 mg/kg qd × 2 wk, then 10 mg/kg/d for 10 wk, total 12 wk

• *Hypercalcemia:* IV 7.5 mg/kg/d for 3 successive days (diluted in at least 250 ml normal saline) over at least 2 hr; pretreatment interval at least 7 days

• *Osteoporosis:* PO 400 mg 2 hr ac with H_2O × 2 wk, repeat every 3 mo

$ **AVAILABLE FORMS/COST OF THERAPY**

• Inj, Sol—IV: 300 mg/6ml, 6 ml: **$63.60**

• Tab, Uncoated—Oral: 200 mg, 60's: **$108.89;** 400 mg, 60's: **$217.78**

CONTRAINDICATIONS Pathologic fractures, children, colitis, severe renal disease

PRECAUTIONS: Renal disease, restricted Vit D and calcium intake

PREGNANCY AND LACTATION: Pregnancy category B; breast milk excretion not known, problems in humans have not been documented

SIDE EFFECTS/ADVERSE REACTIONS

GI: Nausea, diarrhea

MS: Bone pain, hypocalcemia, decreased mineralization of nonaffected bones

▼ **DRUG INTERACTIONS**

Drugs

- *Antacids containing calcium, magnesium, or aluminum:* Decreased absorption of oral etidronate

SPECIAL CONSIDERATIONS

PATIENT/FAMILY EDUCATION

- Administer on empty stomach with H_2O, 2 hours ac
- Exceeding the 2 wk treatment periods for osteoporosis may lead to bone demineralization and osteomalacia

etodolac

(e-toe'doe-lack)

Lodine

Chemical Class: Pyranoindoleacetic acid

Therapeutic Class: Nonsteroidal antiinflammatory drug (NSAID)

CLINICAL PHARMACOLOGY

Mechanism of Action: Decreases prostaglandin synthesis by inhibiting cyclooxygenase, an enzyme needed for biosynthesis; analgesic, antiinflammatory, and antipyretic activity

Pharmacokinetics

PO: Peak serum levels 1-2 hr; analgesic onset 30 min; analgesic duration 4-12 hr; $t_{1/2}$ 7.3 hr; rapidly and completely absorbed; serum protein binding >90%, metabolized by liver; metabolites excreted in urine

INDICATIONS AND USES: Mild to moderate pain, osteoarthritis; rheumatoid arthritis,* ankylosing spondylitis,* tendinitis,* bursitis,* acute painful shoulder,* acute gout*

DOSAGE

Adult

- *Osteoarthritis:* PO 800-1200 mg/d in divided doses initially, then adjust dose to 600-1200 mg/d in divided doses; do not exceed 1200 mg/d; patients <60 kg not to exceed 20 mg/kg
- *Analgesia:* PO 200-400 mg q6-8h prn for acute pain; do not exceed 1200 mg/d; patients <60 kg, not to exceed 20 mg/kg

$ AVAILABLE FORMS/COST OF THERAPY

- Cap, Gel—Oral: 200 mg, 100's: **$103.44;** 300 mg, 100's: **$117.15**
- Tab, Uncoated—Oral: 400 mg, 100's: **$123.83**

CONTRAINDICATIONS Hypersensitivity; patients in whom aspirin, iodides, or other NSAIDs have produced asthma, rhinitis, urticaria, nasal polyps, angioedema, bronchospasm

PRECAUTIONS: Children; bleeding; GI, cardiac disorders; elderly; renal, hepatic disorders

PREGNANCY AND LACTATION: Pregnancy category C (category D if used near term); breast milk excretion unknown, problems in humans have not been documented

SIDE EFFECTS/ADVERSE REACTIONS

CNS: Dizziness, headache, drowsiness, fatigue, tremors, confusion, insomnia, anxiety, depression, lightheadedness, vertigo

CV: Tachycardia, peripheral edema, fluid retention, palpitations, dysrhythmias, CHF

EENT: Tinnitus, hearing loss, blurred vision

GI: Nausea, anorexia, vomiting, diarrhea, jaundice, ***cholestatic hepatitis,*** constipation, flatulence, cramps, dry mouth, peptic ulcer, dyspepsia, ***GI bleeding***

GU: ***Nephrotoxicity: dysuria, hematuria, oliguria, azotemia,*** cystitis, UTI

HEME: ***Blood dyscrasias***

SKIN: Erythema, urticaria, purpura, rash, pruritus, sweating

▼ **DRUG INTERACTIONS**

Drugs

- *Anticoagulants:* Increased risk of bleeding
- *Cefamandole, cefoperazone, cefotetan, moxalactam:* Hypoprothrombinemia from antibiotics, increased risk of bleeding
- *Cyclosporine:* Additive nephrotoxicity
- *Lithium:* Decreased excretion of lithium, potential lithium toxicity
- *Methotrexate:* Increased risk of methotrexate toxicity
- *Plicamycin, valproic acid:* Additive inhibition of platelet aggregation, increased risk of bleeding

SPECIAL CONSIDERATIONS

PATIENT/FAMILY EDUCATION

- Administer with food to decrease GI symptoms, since extent of absorption is not affected by food

MONITORING PARAMETERS

- Hgb, stool for blood, renal and liver function tests quarterly in high risk and yearly in low risk patients

etretinate

(e-tret′in-ate)

Tegison

Chemical Class: Related to both retinoic acid and retinol (vitamin A)

Therapeutic Class: Systemic antipsoriatic

CLINICAL PHARMACOLOGY

Mechanism of Action: Unknown; might reduce cell proliferation by inhibiting ornithine decarboxylase, a rate limiting enzyme in regulation of cell growth, proliferation, and differentiation

Pharmacokinetics

Peak 102-389 ng/ml at 2-6 hr during chronic therapy; $t_{1/2}$ 120 days; absorbed in small intestine; accumulates in adipose tissue, especially the liver and subcutaneous fat; significant first pass hepatic metabolism to active acid form; primarily biliary excretion

INDICATIONS AND USES: Severe recalcitrant psoriasis, including erythrodermic and generalized pustular types; bronchial metaplasia,* mycosis fungoides,* actinic keratoses,* arsenical keratoses,* basal cell carcinomas, genodermatosis,* pustular bacterids,* hyperkeratotic eczema of palms/soles,* cutaneous lupus erythematosus*

DOSAGE

Adult

- Psoriasis: PO 0.75-1 mg/kg/d in divided doses, not to exceed 1.5 mg/kg/d; maintenance dose 0.5-0.75 mg/kg/d generally beginning after 8-16 wk of therapy

$ AVAILABLE FORMS/COST OF THERAPY

- Cap, Gel—Oral: 10 mg, 30's: **$59.66;** 25 mg, 30's: **$93.30**

CONTRAINDICATIONS: Pregnancy

PRECAUTIONS: Children, hepatic disease, diabetes, obesity, increased alcohol intake

PREGNANCY AND LACTATION: Pregnancy category X (effective contraception must be used at least 1 mo before, during, and following discontinuation of therapy for an indefinite period of time); excreted into milk of lactating rats, human breast milk data not available, not recommended during lactation

SIDE EFFECTS/ADVERSE REACTIONS

CNS: Fatigue, headache, dizziness, fever, pain, anxiety, amnesia, depression, pseudotumor cerebri

CV: Edema, ***CV obstruction, atrial fibrillation,*** chest pain, coagulation disorders

EENT: Eye irritation, pain, double vision, change in lacrimation, earache, otitis externa, dry nose, eyes, mouth, nosebleed, cheilitis, sore tongue

GI: Anorexia, abdominal pain, nausea, ***hepatitis,*** constipation, diarrhea, flatulence, weight loss

GU: WBC in urine, ***proteinuria,*** glycosuria, *increased BUN/creatinine,* ***hematuria, casts, acetonuria, hemoglobinuria, dysuria***

METAB: Increase or decrease K, Ca, P, Na, Cl; elevation of plasma triglycerides, total cholesterol; decrease in HDL cholesterol; increased or decreased fasting blood sugar

MS: Hyperostosis, bone pain, cramps, myalgia, gout, hypertonia

RESP: Dyspnea, cough

SKIN: Alopecia; peeling of palms, soles, fingertips; itching; rash; dryness; red scaling face; bruising; sunburn; pyogenic granuloma; paronychia; onycholysis; perspiration change, nail changes

▼ **DRUG INTERACTIONS**

Drugs

- *Alcohol:* Additive hypertriglyceridemia
- *Isotretinoin, tretinoin, vitamin A:* Additive toxic effects
- *Methotrexate:* Increased potential for hepatotoxicity
- *Tetracyclines:* Increased potential for pseudotumor cerebri

Labs

- *Increase:* Plasma triglycerides; cholesterol, SGPT, SGOT, LDH
- *Decrease:* HDL cholesterol

SPECIAL CONSIDERATIONS

PATIENT/FAMILY EDUCATION

- Take with food or milk
- Contact lens intolerance is common

MONITORING PARAMETERS

- Lipid levels

---

famotidine

(fam-o'tah-deen)

Pepcid, Pepcid IV, Pepcid AC

Chemical Class: Thiazole derivative

Therapeutic Class: H_2 histamine receptor antagonist

CLINICAL PHARMACOLOGY

Mechanism of Action: Competitively inhibits histamine at histamine H_2 receptor sites on parietal cells, decreasing basal and nocturnal gastric secretion while pepsin remains at stable levels

Pharmacokinetics

PO: Onset 30-60 min, duration 6-12 hr, peak 1-3 hr

IV: Onset immediate, peak 30-60 min, duration 6-12 hr

Oral absorption 50%; plasma protein-binding 15%-20%; metabolized in liver 30% (active metabolites); 70% excreted by kidneys unchanged; $t_{1/2}$ 2½-3½ hr (>20 hr with CrCl <10 ml/min)

INDICATIONS AND USES: Short-term treatment of active duodenal ulcer, maintenance therapy for duodenal ulcer, Zollinger-Ellison syndrome, multiple endocrine adenomas, gastric ulcers,* gastroesophageal reflux,* GI bleeding,* prophylaxis for aspiration pneumonitis*

DOSAGE

Adult

- *Duodenal ulcer:* PO 40 mg qd hs ×4-8 wk, then 20 mg qd hs if needed (maintenance); IV 20 mg q12h if unable to take PO
- *Hypersecretory conditions:* PO 20 mg q6h; may give 160 mg q6h if needed; IV 20 mg q12h if unable to take PO

$ **AVAILABLE FORMS/COST OF THERAPY**

- Granule, Reconst—Oral Susp: 40 mg/5 ml: **$76.25**

• Tab, Plain Coated—Oral (OTC): 10 mg, 18's: **$5.82**
• Tab, Plain Coated—Oral: 20 mg, 100's: **$154.13;** 40 mg, 100's: **$297.78**
• Inj, Sol—IV: 10 mg/ml, 2 ml: **$3.60;** 4 ml: **$7.19**

CONTRAINDICATIONS: Hypersensitivity

PRECAUTIONS: Severe renal disease, severe hepatic function, elderly

PREGNANCY AND LACTATION: Pregnancy category B; concentrated in breast milk (less than cimetidine or ranitidine), M:P ratio, 1.78 at 6 hr, no problems reported with other H_2 histamine receptor antagonists, compatible with breast feeding

SIDE EFFECTS/ADVERSE REACTIONS

CNS: Headache, dizziness, paresthesia, ***seizure,*** depression, anxiety, somnolence, insomnia, fever

EENT: Taste change, tinnitus, orbital edema

GI: Constipation, nausea, vomiting, anorexia, cramps, abnormal liver enzymes

HEME: ***Thrombocytopenia***

MS: Myalgia, arthralgia

RESP: ***Bronchospasm***

SKIN: Rash

▼ **DRUG INTERACTIONS**

Drugs

• *Enoxacin, ketoconazole:* Reduction in gastric acidity reduces absorption, decreased plasma levels, potential for therapeutic failure
• *Antacids:* Decreased absorption of famotidine

Labs

• *False negative:* Gastric acid secretion test, skin test using allergen extracts

felodipine

(fell-o'da-peen)

Plendil

Chemical Class: Dihydropyridine

Therapeutic Class: Calcium-channel blocker

CLINICAL PHARMACOLOGY

Mechanism of Action: Inhibits calcium ion influx across cell membrane, resulting in dilation of peripheral arteries; no effects on cardiac conduction system; generally associated with increased heart rate, myocardial contractility, cardiac output, and significantly decreased peripheral vascular resistance

Pharmacokinetics

Onset, 2-5 hr; peak ½-5 hr; elimination $t_{1/2}$ 11-16 hr; well absorbed; 99% protein bound; metabolized in liver; 0.5% excreted unchanged in urine

INDICATIONS AND USES Essential hypertension, vasospastic angina,* effort-associated angina,* primary pulmonary hypertension,* esophageal disorders,* biliary and renal colic,* Raynaud's syndrome*

DOSAGE

Adult

• *Hypertension:* PO 5 mg qd initially, usual range 5-10 mg qd; do not exceed 20 mg qd; do not adjust dosage at intervals of <2 wk

$ **AVAILABLE FORMS/COST OF THERAPY**

• Tab, Uncoated, Sust Action—Oral: 2.5, 5 mg, 100's: **$85.38;** 10 mg, 100's: **$153.42**

CONTRAINDICATIONS: Hypersensitivity

PRECAUTIONS: Hypotension <90 mm Hg systolic, hepatic injury, children, renal disease, elderly

PREGNANCY AND LACTATION: Pregnancy category C

SIDE EFFECTS/ADVERSE REACTIONS

CNS: Headache, fatigue, dizziness, anxiety, depression, insomnia, lightheadedness, tinnitus

CV: Edema, hypotension, palpitations, ***MI, pulmonary edema,*** tachycardia, syncope

EENT: Cough, nasal congestion, epistaxis

GI: Gastric upset, gingival hyperplasia

GU: Nocturia, polyuria

HEME: Anemia

RESP: Shortness of breath, wheezing

SKIN: Rash, pruritus

MISC: Flushing, sexual difficulties

▼ **DRUG INTERACTIONS**

Drugs

- *Beta-blockers:* Increased Beta-blocker serum levels, potential for hypotension
- *Cimetidine, ranitidine:* Increased felodipine level
- *Grapefruit juice:* Inhibits felodipine metabolism, 200% increase in AUC

SPECIAL CONSIDERATIONS

PATIENT/FAMILY EDUCATION

- Administer as whole tablet (do not crush or chew)
- Avoid grapefruit juice (see drug interactions)

fenfluramine

(fen-fluer′a-meen)

Pondimin

Chemical Class: Amphetamine derivative

Therapeutic Class: Anorexiant

DEA Class: Schedule IV

CLINICAL PHARMACOLOGY

Mechanism of Action: Influences serotonergic pathways in CNS to suppress appetite

Pharmacokinetics

PO: Onset 1-2 hr, duration 4-6 hr; lipid soluble, crosses placenta; metabolized by liver; excreted by kidneys; $t_{1/2}$ 20 hr (11 hr if urine pH <5)

INDICATIONS AND USES: Exogenous obesity

DOSAGE

Adult

- PO 20 mg tid ac, not to exceed 40 mg tid

$ **AVAILABLE FORMS/COST OF THERAPY**

- Tab, Uncoated—Oral: 20 mg, 100's: **$31.03**

CONTRAINDICATIONS: Hypersensitivity to sympathomimetic amine, glaucoma, drug abuse, CVD, alcoholism, age <12 yr, hypertension, hyperthyroidism, agitated states, within 14 days following MAOIs

PRECAUTIONS: Diabetes mellitus, depression

PREGNANCY AND LACTATION: Pregnancy category C; excreted in breast milk

SIDE EFFECTS/ADVERSE REACTIONS

CNS: Insomnia, euphoria, anxiety, drowsiness, depression, dizziness, headache, irritability, confusion, mood changes, weakness, vivid dreams, incoordination, tremor

CV: Palpitations, tachycardia, hypertension, dysrhythmias, pulmonary hypertension

EENT: Mydriasis, blurred vision, eye irritation

GI: Nausea, vomiting, *dry mouth, diarrhea,* constipation, abdominal pain

GU: Impotence, change in libido, dysuria, urinary frequency

HEME: ***Bone marrow depression, leukopenia, agranulocytosis***

MS: Myalgia

SKIN: Urticaria, rash, burning, sweating, chills, fever, erythema
MISC: Hair loss, flushing, fever

▼ **DRUG INTERACTIONS**

Drugs

• *Acetazolamide:* Reduced urinary excretion of fenfluramine
• *Antacids and sodium bicarbonate:* Increased GI absorption, decreased urinary excretion of fenfluramine
• *Furazolidone+, monoamine oxidase inhibitors+, phenelzine+,* and *tranylcypromine+:* Hypertensive crisis

SPECIAL CONSIDERATIONS

PATIENT/FAMILY EDUCATION

• Avoid OTC preparations unless approved by physician
• Do not stop drug abruptly

fenoprofen

(fen-oh-proe'fen)
Nalfon
Chemical Class: Propionic acid derivative
Therapeutic Class: Nonsteroidal antiinflammatory drug (NSAID)

CLINICAL PHARMACOLOGY

Mechanism of Action: Inhibits prostaglandin synthesis by decreasing cyclo-oxygenase activity

Pharmacokinetics

PO: Rapid absorption, peak level 2 hr, $t_{1/2}$ 3 hr; metabolized in liver; metabolites excreted in urine; 99% protein binding to albumin; does not cross placenta

INDICATIONS AND USES: Mild to moderate pain, osteoarthritis, rheumatoid arthritis, acute gouty arthritis,* ankylosing spondylitis,* migraine,* fever*

DOSAGE

Adult

• *Pain:* PO 200 mg q4-6h prn
• *Arthritis:* PO 300-600 mg qid, not to exceed 3.2 g/d

$ **AVAILABLE FORMS/COST OF THERAPY**

• Cap, Gel—Oral: 200 mg, 100's: **$23.60-$48.42;** 300 mg, 100's: **$30.57-$38.76**
• Tab, Uncoated—Oral: 600 mg, 100's: **$20.70-$62.80**

CONTRAINDICATIONS: Hypersensitivity, severe renal disease, severe hepatic disease, aspirin-induced asthma/rhinitis syndrome

PRECAUTIONS: Children, bleeding disorders, peptic ulcer disease, GI disorders, CHF, hypersensitivity to other antiinflammatory agents

PREGNANCY AND LACTATION: Pregnancy category B (D 3rd trimester); excreted in breast milk

SIDE EFFECTS/ADVERSE REACTIONS

CNS: Headache, anxiety, dizziness, drowsiness, fatigue, tremors, confusion, insomnia, depression
CV: Peripheral edema, tachycardia, palpitations, dysrhythmias
EENT: Tinnitus, hearing loss, blurred vision
GI: Dyspepsia, nausea, constipation, ***peptic ulcer*** after 1 yr of therapy), anorexia, vomiting, diarrhea, ***cholestatic hepatitis*** , cramps, dry mouth
GU: ***Interstitial nephritis,*** dysuria, hematuria, ***azotemia***
HEME: Thrombocytopenia, hemolytic anemia, aplastic anemia, agranulocytosis
METAB: Hyperkalemia
SKIN: Rash, pruritus, sweating, purpura

▼ **DRUG INTERACTIONS**

Drugs

• *ACE inhibitors, beta blockers, hydralazine:* Impaired antihypertensive effect
• *Bile acid binding resins:* Reduced absorption of fenoprofen

F

• *Cyclosporine:* Enhanced nephrotoxicity
• *Lithium:* Reduced excretion of lithium
• *Methotrexate:* Reduced excretion of methotrexate
• *Sulfonylureas+:* Increased hypoglycemic effect
• *Warfarin:* Increased bleeding risk

Labs

• *Increase:* Free and total triiodothyronine levels

SPECIAL CONSIDERATIONS

PATIENT/FAMILY EDUCATION

• Take with food to decrease GI symptoms; empty stomach facilitates absorption

fentanyl

(fen'ta-nill)

Sublimaze, Fentanyl Oralet, Duragesic-25, 50, 75, 100

Chemical Class: Opiate, synthetic phenylpiperidine derivative

Therapeutic Class: Narcotic analgesic

DEA Class: Schedule II

CLINICAL PHARMACOLOGY

Mechanism of Action: Inhibits ascending pain pathways primarily through interaction with opioid μ-receptors located in the brain, spinal cord, and smooth muscle; has less emetic activity than morphine

Pharmacokinetics

IM: Onset 7-15 min, peak 30 min, duration 1-2 hr

IV: Onset 1-2 min, peak 3-5 min, duration ½-1 hr

LOZ: Onset 5-15 min, peak 20-30 min; 50% bioavailability with rapid transmucosal and slower GI absorption

TRANSDERMAL: Steady state plasma level 24 hr after application, 6 days after change of dose; plasma level $t_{1/2}$ 17 hr after patch removal due to some continued absorption

Metabolized by liver; excreted by kidneys, excretion $t_{1/2}$ 2½-4 hr; highly lipophilic, 80% bound to plasma proteins, crosses placenta, stored in fat and muscle (may lead to prolonged effect with repeated administration)

INDICATIONS AND USES: Perioperative analgesia, adjunct to general anesthesia (alone or combined with droperidol), chronic pain (transdermal)

DOSAGE

Adult and Child >12 yr

• *Sedation for minor procedure:* IV/IM 0.5-1.5 μg/kg q30-60 min; buccal 5 μg/kg
• *Preoperatively:* IM 0.05-0.1 mg q30-60 min before surgery
• *Adjunct to anesthesia:* IV 2-50 μg/kg
• *Analgesia:* IV/IM 0.5-1.5 μg/kg q1-2h prn; TRANSDERMAL 25 μg/hr, increase at at least 6 day intervals until pain relief occurs: change system q72h

Child 1-12 yr

• *Sedation for minor procedure:* IV/IM 1-2 μg/kg q30-60 min; buccal 5-10 μg/kg (age >2 yr only)
• *Adjunct to anesthesia:* IV 2-50 μg/kg
• *Analgesia:* IV 1-2 μg/kg bolus, then 1-3 μg/kg qh prn

Notes:

1. IV/IM dose of 0.1 mg fentanyl equianalgesic to 10 mg of morphine, 75 mg of meperidine
2. Transdermal fentanyl dose of 100 μg/hr equianalgesic to 60 mg morphine IM or 360 mg morphine PO per 24 hr
3. Buccal dose of 5 μg fentanyl equianalgesic to 1 μg IM fentanyl

AVAILABLE FORMS/COST OF THERAPY

• Inj, Sol—IM; IV: 0.05 mg/ml, 2 ml × 10: **$9.35-$25.81**
• Loz, Top—Oral: 200, 300, 400 µg, 1's: **$27.99**
• Film, Cont Release—Percutaneous: 25 µg/hr, 5's: **$49.97;** 50 µg/hr, 5's: **$74.92;** 75 µg/hr, 5's: **$114.42;** 100 µg/hr, 5's: **$142.56**

CONTRAINDICATIONS: Hypersensitivity to opiates, myasthenia gravis, MAOI within 14 days, lozenge for child <15 kg, transdermal for child <12 yr

PRECAUTIONS: Elderly, respiratory depression, increased intracranial pressure, seizure disorders, severe respiratory disorders, cardiac dysrhythmias

PREGNANCY AND LACTATION: Pregnancy category C; excreted in breast milk

SIDE EFFECTS/ADVERSE REACTIONS

CNS: Dizziness, somnolence, confusion, asthenia, delirium, euphoria
CV: Bradycardia, hypotension or hypertension
EENT: Blurred vision, miosis, *dry mouth*
GI: Nausea, vomiting, constipation
GU: Urinary retention
MS: Muscle rigidity
RESP: ***Respiratory depression,*** laryngospasm
SKIN: Pruritis, sweating

SPECIAL CONSIDERATIONS

• Increased skin temperature increases absorption rate of transdermal preparation

ferrous salts

Femiron, Feostat, Ferrets, Fumasorb, Fumerin, Hemocyte, Ircon, Nephro-Fer, Span-FF, Fergon, Ferralet, Ferralet S.R., Simron, Feosol, Feratab, Fer-In-Sol, Fer-Iron, Fero-Gradumet, Ferospace, Ferralyn, Ferra-TD, Mol-Iron, Slow-Fe

Chemical Class: Iron preparation
Therapeutic Class: Hematinic

CLINICAL PHARMACOLOGY

Mechanism of Action: Replaces iron stores; hematologic response begins in 3 days

Pharmacokinetics

PO: Absorbed in duodenum and upper jejunum, absorption decreased by food and achlorhydria; bound to transferrin; crosses placenta; excreted in feces, urine

INDICATIONS AND USES: Prevention and treatment of iron deficiency anemia

DOSAGE (all expressed in elemental iron)

Adult

• *Iron deficiency:* 60-100 mg bid
• *Prophylaxis:* 60-100 mg qd

Child

• *Iron deficiency:* 3-6 mg/kg/d in 3 divided doses
• *Prophylaxis:* 1-2 mg/kg/d in 3 divided doses

Note: Ferrous fumarate is 33% elemental iron (325 mg has 106 mg); gluconate 12% elemental iron (325 mg has 38 mg); sulfate 20% elemental iron (325 mg has 65 mg)

AVAILABLE FORMS/COST OF THERAPY

Ferrous fumarate
• Tab—Oral: 325 mg, 100's: **$1.87-$7.43**
• Tab, Chewable—Oral: 100 mg, 100s: **$14.69**

• Cap—Oral: 325 mg, 100s: **$5.20-$8.67**
• Susp—Oral: 45 mg/0.6 ml, 60 ml: **$14.27;** 100 mg/5 ml, 240 ml: **$16.45**
Ferrous gluconate
• Tab—Oral: 325 mg, 100s: **$1.45-$9.00**
• Elixir—Oral: 300 mg/5 ml, 480 ml: **$11.20**
Ferrous sulfate
• Tab—Oral: 195 mg, 100's: **$7.86;** 325 mg, 100's: **$1.50-$4.83**
• Cap—Oral: 325 mg, 100's: **$3.90**
• Elixir—Oral: 90 mg/5 ml, 480 ml: **$14.76;** 125 mg/5 ml, 480 ml: **$4.80;** 220 mg/5 ml, 480 ml: **$108.66;** 300 mg/5 ml, 480 ml: **$5.10**

CONTRAINDICATIONS: Hypersensitivity, ulcerative colitis/regional enteritis, hemosiderosis/hemochromatosis, peptic ulcer disease, hemolytic anemia, cirrhosis

PREGNANCY AND LACTATION: Pregnancy category A; excreted in breast milk

SIDE EFFECTS/ADVERSE REACTIONS

GI: Nausea, constipation, epigastric pain, black stools, vomiting, diarrhea

SKIN: Temporarily discolored tooth enamel and eyes

▼ **DRUG INTERACTIONS**

Drugs

• *Antacids, bile acid binding resins:* Reduce iron absorption
• *Ascorbic acid:* Increases iron absorption
• *Ciprofloxacin, levothyroxine, methyldopa, norfloxacin, penicillamine, tetracyclines, vitamin E:* Absorption reduced by iron

Labs

• *False positive:* Occult blood by guaiac method

SPECIAL CONSIDERATIONS

Iron changes stools black or dark green

---

finasteride

(feen-as'ter-ide)
Proscar
Chemical Class: 5α-reductase inhibitor
Therapeutic Class: Androgen hormone inhibitor

CLINICAL PHARMACOLOGY

Mechanism of Action: Inhibits the enzyme responsible for converting testosterone to 5α-dihydrotestosterone (DHT) reducing the levels of DHT available for development of the prostate gland and other DHT-dependent organs

Pharmacokinetics

PO: Bioavailability 63%, peak 1-2 hr, plasma protein binding 90%, metabolized in the liver, 39% excreted in urine (metabolites), 57% in feces, $t_{1/2}$ 6 hr, crosses blood-brain barrier

INDICATIONS AND USES: Symptomatic benign prostatic hypertrophy (<50% of patients experience an increase in urinary flow and improvement in symptoms), prostate cancer*

DOSAGE

Adult

• PO 5 mg qd

$ **AVAILABLE FORMS/COST OF THERAPY**

• Tab, Plain Coated—Oral: 5 mg, 100's: **$195.46**

CONTRAINDICATIONS: Hypersensitivity, children, women

PRECAUTIONS: Hepatic function impairment, obstructive uropathy

PREGNANCY AND LACTATION: Pregnancy category X; not indicated for use in women

SIDE EFFECTS/ADVERSE REACTIONS

GU: Impotence, decreased libido, decreased volume of ejaculate

▼ **DRUG INTERACTIONS**

Labs

• *Decrease:* Prostate specific antigen (PSA) (does not suggest beneficial effect on prostate cancer)

SPECIAL CONSIDERATIONS

PATIENT/FAMILY EDUCATION

• Female partners of patients receiving finasteride should avoid exposure to semen

MONITORING PARAMETERS

• 6-12 mo of therapy may be necessary in some patients to assess effectiveness

---

flavoxate

(fla-vox'ate)

Urispas

Chemical Class: Flavone derivative

Therapeutic Class: Genitourinary muscle relaxant

CLINICAL PHARMACOLOGY

Mechanism of Action: Relaxes the detrusor and other smooth muscle by cholinergic blockade, also exerts a direct effect on the muscle

Pharmacokinetics

PO: Onset 55 min, peak 112 min, 57% excreted in urine within 24 hr

INDICATIONS AND USES: Relief of nocturia, incontinence, suprapubic pain, dysuria, frequency associated with urologic conditions (symptomatic only)

DOSAGE

Adult and Child >12 yr

• PO 100-200 mg tid-qid, reduce dose when symptoms improve

$ **AVAILABLE FORMS/COST OF THERAPY**

• Tab, Plain Coated—Oral: 100 mg, 100's: **$75.20**

CONTRAINDICATIONS: Pyloric or duodenal obstruction; obstructive intestinal lesions or ileus; achalasia; GI hemorrhage; obstructive uropathies of the lower urinary tract

PRECAUTIONS: Glaucoma, children <12 yr

PREGNANCY AND LACTATION: Pregnancy category B; excretion into breast milk unknown, use caution in nursing mothers

SIDE EFFECTS/ADVERSE REACTIONS

CNS: Vertigo, headache, mental confusion (especially in the elderly), *drowsiness,* nervousness

CV: Tachycardia and palpitation

EENT: Increased ocular tension, *blurred vision,* disturbance in eye accommodation

GI: Nausea, vomiting, dry mouth

GU: Dysuria

HEME: ***Leukopenia***

SKIN: Urticaria and other dermatoses

SPECIAL CONSIDERATIONS

PATIENT/FAMILY EDUCATION

• May cause drowsiness or blurred vision

---

flecainide

(fle'-kah-nide)

Tambocor

Chemical Class: Benzamide derivative

Therapeutic Class: Antidysrhythmic, Class IC

CLINICAL PHARMACOLOGY

Mechanism of Action: Produces a dose-related decrease in intracardiac conduction in all parts of the heart with the greatest effect on the His-Purkinje system; causes slight prolongation of refractory periods; decreases the rate of rise of the action potential without affecting its duration

Pharmacokinetics

PO: Peak 3 hr, 40%-50% bound to plasma proteins (α_1-glycoprotein),

$t_{1/2}$ 12-27 hr, metabolized by liver, excreted by kidneys

INDICATIONS AND USES: Paroxysmal atrial fibrillation (PAF) and paroxysmal supraventricular tachycardias (PSVT) associated with disabling symptoms; documented life-threatening ventricular dysrhythmias

DOSAGE

Adult

- *PSVT and PAF:* PO 50 mg q12h; may increase q4d by 50 mg q12h to desired response, not to exceed 300 mg/d
- *Sustained ventricular tahcycardia:* PO 100 mg q12h; may increase q4d by 50 mg q12h to desired response, not to exceed 400 mg/d

Child

- PO 3 mg/kg/d divided tid, may increase up to 11 mg/kg/d for uncontrolled patients with subtherapeutic levels

$ AVAILABLE FORMS/COST OF THERAPY

- Tab, Uncoated—Oral: 50 mg, 100's: **$63.42;** 100 mg, 100's: **$115.14;** 150 mg, 100's: **$158.46**

CONTRAINDICATIONS: Hypersensitivity, severe heart block, cardiogenic shock, nonsustained ventricular dysrhythmias, frequent PVCs, non-life-threatening dysrhythmias (due to proarrhythmic effects), recent MI

PRECAUTIONS: Children, renal disease, liver disease, CHF, respiratory depression, myasthenia gravis, sick sinus syndrome, electrolyte disturbances

PREGNANCY AND LACTATION: Pregnancy category C; excreted into breast milk with milk-plasma ratios 1.6:3.7, but considered compatible with breast feeding

SIDE EFFECTS/ADVERSE REACTIONS

CNS: Dizziness, lightheadedness, faintness, unsteadiness, headache, fatigue, tremor, hypoesthesia, paresthesia, paresis, ataxia, vertigo, syncope, somnolence, anxiety, insomnia, depression, malaise, twitching, weakness, ***convulsions,*** neuropathy, stupor, amnesia, confusion, euphoria

CV: Palpitation, chest pain, edema, ***dysrhythmia, CHF, AV block, bradycardia, sinus pause, sinus arrest, tachycardia, angina pectoris, hypertension, hypotension***

EENT: Visual disturbances, blurred vision, diplopia, eye pain/irritation, photophobia, nystagmus

GI: Nausea, constipation, abdominal pain, vomiting, dyspepsia, anorexia, flatulence, change in taste, dry mouth

GU: Impotence, decreased libido, polyuria, urinary retention

HEME: ***Leukopenia, thrombocytopenia***

MS: Arthralgia, myalgia

RESP: ***Bronchospasm***

SKIN: Rash, urticaria, ***exfoliative dermatitis,*** pruritus, alopecia

▼ DRUG INTERACTIONS

Drugs

- *Amiodarone:* Reduced flecainide dosage requirements

Labs

- *Increase:* CPK

SPECIAL CONSIDERATIONS

MONITORING PARAMETERS

- Monitor trough plasma levels periodically, especially in patients with moderate to severe chronic renal failure or severe hepatic disease and CHF; therapeutic range 0.2-1 μg/ml

fluconazole

(floo-con'a-zole)

Diflucan

Chemical Class: Bis-triazole

Therapeutic Class: Antifungal

CLINICAL PHARMACOLOGY

Mechanism of Action: Interferes with cytochrome P-450 activity, decreasing ergosterol synthesis (principal sterol in fungal cell membrane) and inhibiting cell membrane formation

Pharmacokinetics

IV/PO: Peak 1-2 hr (PO), 11%-12% bound to plasma proteins, extensive distribution into all studied body fluids, $t_{1/2}$ 20-50 hr, cleared primarily by renal excretion

INDICATIONS AND USES: Oropharyngeal and esophageal candidiasis; candidal UTI, peritonitis and systemic candidal infections; vaginal candidiasis; prophylaxis of candidiasis in patients undergoing bone marrow transplant who receive cytotoxic chemotherapy or radiation therapy; cryptococcal meningitis

DOSAGE

Adult

- *Cryptococcal meningitis:* PO/IV 400 mg on 1st day, then 200 mg qd for 10-12 wk after CSF becomes culture negative, increase up to 400 mg/d based on response
- *Esophageal candidiasis:* PO/IV 200 mg on 1st day, then 100 mg qd for at least 3 wk and for 2 wk following resolution of symptoms; doses up to 400 mg/d may be used based on response
- *Oropharyngeal candidiasis:* PO/IV 200 mg on 1st day, then 100 mg qd for at least 2 wk
- *Other candidiasis:* PO/IV 50-200 mg/d, doses up to 400 mg/d may be used based on response
- *Prevention of candidiasis in bone marrow transplant:* PO/IV 400 mg qd, initiate several days before anticipated onset of neutropenia, continue 7 days after neutrophil count rises above 1000 cells/mm^3
- *Renal function impairment:* PO/IV reduce dose by 50% in patients with CrCl <50 ml/min
- *Vaginal candidiasis:* PO 150 mg as a single dose

$ AVAILABLE FORMS/COST OF THERAPY

- Inj, Sol—IV: 2 mg/ml, 100 ml: **$487.49**
- Powder—Oral: 50 mg/5ml, 60 ml: **$28.12;** 200 mg/5ml, 60 ml: **$102.12**
- Tab, Plain Coated—Oral: 50 mg, 30's: **$131.25;** 100 mg, 30's: **$206.24;** 150 mg, 12's: **$127.50;** 200 mg, 30's: **$337.50**

CONTRAINDICATIONS: Hypersensitivity

PRECAUTIONS: Hypersensitivity to other azoles, children, renal disease

PREGNANCY AND LACTATION: Pregnancy category C; excreted into breast milk in concentrations similar to plasma; not recommended in nursing mothers

SIDE EFFECTS/ADVERSE REACTIONS

CNS: Headache, ***seizures***

GI: ***Hepatic injury,*** nausea, vomiting, diarrhea, cramping, flatus

HEME: ***Leukopenia, thrombocytopenia***

METAB: Hypercholesterolemia, hypertriglyceridemia, hyopkalemia

SKIN: ***Exfoliative skin disorders***

▼ DRUG INTERACTIONS

Drugs

- *Phenytoin:* Increases in plasma phenytoin concentrations, possible toxicity
- *Tacrolimus:* Increased tacrolimus concentrations which may result in nephrotoxicity

• *Warfarin:* Enhanced hypoprothrombinemic resonse to warfarin

Labs:

• *Increase:* AST

SPECIAL CONSIDERATIONS

MONITORING PARAMETERS

• Periodic renal and liver function tests

---

flucytosine

(floo-sye'toe-seen)

Ancobon, Ancotil ♣

Chemical Class: Pyrimidine (fluorinated)

Therapeutic Class: Antifungal

CLINICAL PHARMACOLOGY

Mechanism of Action: Acts directly on fungal organisms by competitive inhibition of purine and pyrimidine uptake and indirectly by metabolism within the fungal organism to 5-fluorouracil which inhibits synthesis of both DNA and RNA

Pharmacokinetics

PO: Peak 2 hr, $t_{1/2}$ 2-5 hr, excreted in urine (unchanged), well-distributed to peritoneal fluid, aqueous humor, joints, and other body fluids and tissues, CSF concentrations approximately 65%-90% of serum levels

INDICATIONS AND USES: Serious infections caused by susceptible strains of *Candida* (septicemia, endocarditis, UTIs) or *Cryptococcus* (meningitis, pulmonary, urinary tract infections, septicemia); treatment of chromomycosis*

DOSAGE

Adult and Child >50 kg

• PO 50-150 mg/kg/d divided q6h; initiate dose at the lower level if renal impairment is present

Adult and Child <50 kg

• PO 1.5-4.5 g/m^2/d in 4 divided doses

$ AVAILABLE FORMS/COST OF THERAPY

• Cap, Gel—Oral: 250 mg, 100's: **$103.35;** 500 mg, 100's: **$198.93**

CONTRAINDICATIONS: Hypersensitivity

PRECAUTIONS: Renal disease, impaired hepatic function, bone marrow depression, blood dyscrasias, radiation/chemotherapy

PREGNANCY AND LACTATION: Pregnancy category C; 4% of drug metabolized to 5-fluorouracil, an antineoplastic suspected of producing congenital defects in humans; excretion into breast milk unknown, use caution in nursing mothers

SIDE EFFECTS/ADVERSE REACTIONS

CNS: Ataxia, hearing loss, headache, paresthesia, parkinsonism, peripheral neuropathy, pyrexia, vertigo, sedation, confusion, hallucinations, psychosis

CV: Chest pain, ***cardiac arrest***

GI: Nausea, vomiting, abdominal pain, diarrhea, *anorexia,* dry mouth, duodenal ulcer, ***GI hemorrhage,*** hepatic dysfunction, jaundice, ulcerative colitis, bilirubin elevation, elevation of hepatic enzymes

GU: Azotemia, creatinine and BUN elevation, crystalluria, ***renal failure***

HEME: Anemia, ***agranulocytosis, aplastic anemia, eosinophilia, leukopenia, pancytopenia, thrombocytopenia***

METAB: Hypoglycemia, hypokalemia

RESP: ***Respiratory arrest,*** dyspnea

SKIN: Rash, pruritus, urticaria, photosensitivity

▼ DRUG INTERACTIONS

Labs

• *False increase:* Serum creatinine (when Ektachem analyzer is used)

SPECIAL CONSIDERATIONS

Rarely used as monotherapy; generally used in combination with amphotericin B

PATIENT/FAMILY EDUCATION

• Reduce or avoid GI upset by taking caps a few at a time over a 15 min period

MONITORING PARAMETERS

• Creatinine, BUN, alk phosphatase, AST, ALT, CBC

• Serum flucytosine concentrations (therapeutic range 25-100 μg/ml)

fludrocortisone

(floo-droe-kor′ti-sone)

Florinef Acetate

Chemical Class: Mineralocorticoid

Therapeutic Class: Adrenal corticosteroid

CLINICAL PHARMACOLOGY

Mechanism of Action: Acts on the distal tubules of the kidney to enhance reabsorption of sodium ions from tubular fluid into the plasma; increases urinary excretion of both potassium and hydrogen ions

Pharmacokinetics

PO: Peak 1.7 hr, plasma $t_{1/2}$ 3½ hr, biological $t_{1/2}$ 18-36 hr, metabolized by liver, excreted in urine

INDICATIONS AND USES: Adrenocortical insufficiency in Addison's disease; salt-losing adrenogenital syndrome; severe orthostatic hypotension*

DOSAGE

Adult

• PO 0.05-0.2 mg qd

Child

• PO 0.05-0.1 mg qd

$ **AVAILABLE FORMS/COST OF THERAPY**

• Tab, Uncoated—Oral: 0.1 mg, 100's: **$44.86**

CONTRAINDICATIONS: Hypersensitivity, systemic fungal infections

PRECAUTIONS: Trauma, surgery, severe illness (supportive dosage may be required); abrupt discontinuation

PREGNANCY AND LACTATION: Pregnancy category C; observe newborn for signs and symptoms of adrenocortical insufficiency; corticosteroids are found in breast milk, use caution in nursing mothers

SIDE EFFECTS/ADVERSE REACTIONS

CNS: Headache

CV: Edema, hypertension, ***CHF,*** enlargement of the heart, flushing

METAB: Hypokalemic alkalosis

MS: Fractures, osteoporosis, weakness

SKIN: Bruising, increased sweating, hives, allergic rash

▼ **DRUG INTERACTIONS**

Labs

• *Increase:* K, Na

• *Decrease:* Hematocrit

SPECIAL CONSIDERATIONS

PATIENT/FAMILY EDUCATION

• Notify physician of dizziness, severe headache, swelling of feet or lower legs, unusual weight gain

• Do not discontinue abruptly

MONITORING PARAMETERS

• Serum electrolytes, blood pressure, serum renin

flumazenil

(floo-maz′en-ill)

Romazicon

Chemical Class: Imidazobenzodiazepine derivative

Therapeutic Class: Benzodiazepine receptor antagonist

CLINICAL PHARMACOLOGY

Mechanism of Action: Antagonizes the actions of benzodiazepines in the CNS, competitively inhibits activity at the benzodiazepine recognition site on the GABA/benzodiazepine receptor

Pharmacokinetics

IV: 50% bound to plasma proteins, metabolized in the liver, primarily excreted in urine, terminal $t_{1/2}$ 41-79 min

INDICATIONS AND USES: Complete or partial reversal of sedative effects of benzodiazepines

DOSAGE

Adult

• *Reversal of conscious sedation*: IV 0.2 mg (2 ml) initially over 15 sec, repeat at 60 sec intervals prn to a max total dose of 1 mg (10 ml)

• *Suspected benzodiazepine overdose:* IV 0.2 mg (2 ml) given over 30 sec; wait 30 sec, then give 0.3 mg (3 ml) over 30 sec if consciousness does not occur; further doses of 0.5 mg (5 ml) can be given over 30 sec at intervals of 1 min up to cumulative dose of 3 mg; patients with a partial response at 3 mg may require additional titration up to a total dose of 5 mg (administered slowly in the same manner)

$ AVAILABLE FORMS/COST OF THERAPY

• Inj, Sol—IV: 0.1 mg/ml, 10 ml: **$44.77**

CONTRAINDICATIONS: Hypersensitivity to flumazenil or benzodiazepines, serious cyclic antidepressant overdose, patients given benzodiazepine for control of life-threatening condition

PRECAUTIONS: Children, elderly, renal disease, seizure disorders, head injury, labor and delivery, hepatic disease, hypoventilation, panic disorder, drug and alcohol dependency, ambulatory patients (sedation may occur)

PREGNANCY AND LACTATION: Pregnancy category C; excretion into breast milk unknown, use caution in nursing mothers

SIDE EFFECTS/ADVERSE REACTIONS

CNS: ***Seizures,*** headache, *dizziness,* agitation, emotional lability, confusion, somnolence

CV: ***Cardiac dysrhythmias,*** hypertension, palpitations, cutaneous vasodilation, bradycardia, tachycardia, chest pain

EENT: Abnormal vision, blurred vision, tinnitus

GI: Nausea, vomiting, hiccoughs

SKIN: Increased sweating

MISC: Inj site pain, fatigue

SPECIAL CONSIDERATIONS

PATIENT/FAMILY EDUCATION

• Sedation may occur; do not engage in any activities requiring complete alertness, operate hazardous machinery or a motor vehicle until at least 18 to 24 hr after discharge

• Do not use any alcohol or nonprescription drugs for 18 to 24 hr after flumazenil administration

MONITORING PARAMETERS

• Monitor for sedation, respiratory depression, or other residual benzodiazepine effects for an appropriate period (up to 120 min) based on dose and duration of effect of the benzodiazepine employed

flunisolide

(floo-niss'oh-lide)

AeroBid, Nasalide

Chemical Class: Glucocorticoid

Therapeutic Class: Anti-inflammatory agent; corticosteroid, inhalant; corticosteroid, topical

CLINICAL PHARMACOLOGY

Mechanism of Action: Decreases inflammation by suppression of migration of polymorphonuclear leukocytes, fibroblasts, reversal of increased capillary permeability, and lysosomal stabilization

Pharmacokinetics

INH: Systemic availability 40%

NASAL: 50% absorption after nasal inhalation

Rapidly metabolized in liver to inactive metabolites, $t_{1/2}$ 1.8 hr, excreted in urine and feces

INDICATIONS AND USES: Seasonal or perennial rhinitis, nasal polyps (nasal sol);* steroid-dependent asthma (oral inhaler)

DOSAGE

Adult

• Nasal sol 2 sprays (50 µg) in each nostril bid-tid, max 8 sprays/nostril/d (400 µg/day); Oral inhaler 2 inhalations (500 µg) bid, not to exceed 4 inhalations bid (2000 µg)

Child

• Nasal sol 1 spray (25 µg) in each nostril tid or 2 sprays (50 µg) in each nostril bid, max 4 sprays/nostril/d (200 µg/d); Oral inhaler (age 6-15 yr) 2 inhalations bid (1000 µg/d)

$ **AVAILABLE FORMS/COST OF THERAPY**

• Aer—Inh: 250 µg, 7 g: **$47.59**
• Sol—Nasal: 0.25 mg/ml, 25 ml: **$26.52**

CONTRAINDICATIONS: Hypersensitivity; fungal, bacterial infection of nose (nasal sol); status asthmaticus (oral inhaler)

PRECAUTIONS: Quiescent tuberculosis infections of the respiratory tract; nasal septal ulcers, recurrent epistaxis, nasal surgery or trauma; untreated fungal, bacterial, or viral infections

PREGNANCY AND LACTATION: Pregnancy category C; excretion into breast milk unknown, use caution in nursing mothers

SIDE EFFECTS/ADVERSE REACTIONS

CNS: Headache, nervousness, restlessness, dizziness

EENT: Hoarseness, *Candida* infection of oral cavity, *sore throat,* hoarseness/dysphonia (oral sol); nasal irritation and stinging, dryness, rebound congestion, epistaxis, sneezing (nasal sol)

GI: Nausea, vomiting, dry mouth

SKIN: Urticaria

SPECIAL CONSIDERATIONS

PATIENT/FAMILY EDUCATION

• To be used on a regular basis, not for acute symptoms
• Use bronchodilators before oral inhaler (for patients using both)
• Nasal sol may cause drying and irritation of nasal mucosa
• Clear nasal passages prior to use of nasal sol

MONITORING PARAMETERS

• Monitor children for growth as well as for effects on the HPA axis during chronic therapy
• Monitor patients switched from chronic systemic corticosteroids to avoid acute adrenal insufficiency in response to stress

fluocinolone

(floo-oh-sin'oh-lone)

Derma-Smoothe/FS, Fluonid, Flurosyn, FS Shampoo, Synalar, Synalar HP, Syncmol

Chemical Class: Synthetic fluorinated agent; Group IV (low) potency: 0.01% cream and lotion; Group III (medium) potency: 0.025% cream and ointment; Group II (high) potency: 0.2% cream

Therapeutic Class: Topical corticosteroid

CLINICAL PHARMACOLOGY

Mechanism of Action: Depresses

F

formation, release, and activity of endogenous mediators of inflammation such as prostaglandins, kinins, histamine, liposomal enzymes, and the complement system resulting in decreased edema, erythema, and pruritus

Pharmacokinetics

Absorbed through the skin (increased by inflammation and occlusive dressings), metabolized primarily in the liver

INDICATIONS AND USES: Psoriasis, eczema, contact dermatitis, pruritus

DOSAGE

Adult and Child

• Apply to affected area bid-tid; rub completely into skin

$ AVAILABLE FORMS/COST OF THERAPY

• Cre—Top: 0.01%, 15, 30, 60 g: **$1.26-$18.95;** 0.025%, 15, 30, 60 g: **$1.58-$33.86;** 0.2%, 12 g: **$26.27**

• Oint—Top: 0.025%, 15, 30, 60 g: **$2.04-$32.24**

• Sol—Top: 0.01%, 20, 60 ml: **$3.53-$34.03**

• Oil—Top: 0.01%, 120 ml: **$17.00**

• Shampoo—Top: 0.01%, 4 oz: **$12.35**

CONTRAINDICATIONS: Hypersensitivity to corticosteroids, fungal infections, use on face, groin, or axilla

PRECAUTIONS: Viral infections, bacterial infections, children

PREGNANCY AND LACTATION: Pregnancy category C; unknown whether topical application could result in sufficient systemic absorption to produce detectable amounts in breast milk (systemic corticosteroids are secreted into breast milk in quantities not likely to have detrimental effects on infant)

SIDE EFFECTS/ADVERSE REACTIONS

SKIN: Burning, dryness, itching, irritation, acne, folliculitis, hypertrichosis, perioral dermatitis, hypopigmentation, atrophy, striae, miliaria, allergic contact dermatitis, secondary infection

MISC: Systemic absorption of topical corticosteroids has produced reversible HPA axis suppression (more likely with occlusive dressings, prolonged administration, application to large surface areas, liver failure, and in children)

SPECIAL CONSIDERATIONS

PATIENT/FAMILY EDUCATION

• Apply sparingly only to affected area

• Avoid contact with eyes

• Do not put bandages or dressings over treated area unless directed by physician

• Do not use on weeping, denuded, or infected areas

• Discontinue drug, notify physician if local irritation or fever develops

fluocinonide

(floo-oh-sin′oh-nide)

Fluonex, Lidemol, ♣ Lidex, Lidex-E

Chemical Class: Synthetic fluorinated agent; Group II (high) potency

Therapeutic Class: Topical corticosteroid

CLINICAL PHARMACOLOGY

Mechanism of action: Depresses formation, release, and activity of endogenous mediators of inflammation such as prostaglandins, kinins, histamine, liposomal enzymes, and the complement system resulting in decreased edema, erythema, and pruritus

Pharmacokinetics

Absorbed through the skin (increased by inflammation and occlusive dressings), metabolized primarily in the liver

INDICATIONS AND USES: Psoriasis, eczema, contact dermatitis, pruritus

DOSAGE

Adult and Child

• Apply to affected area bid-tid; rub completely into skin

$ AVAILABLE FORMS/COST OF THERAPY

• Cre—Top: 0.05%, 15, 30, 60, 120 g: **$4.43-$60.54**

• Gel—Top: 0.05%, 15, 30, 60, 120 g: **$10.65-$85.16**

• Oint—Top: 0.05%, 15, 30, 60, 120 g: **$16.20-$129.60**

• Sol—Top: 0.05%, 20, 60 ml: **$5.67-$40.09**

CONTRAINDICATIONS: Hypersensitivity to corticosteroids, fungal infections, use on face, groin, or axilla

PRECAUTIONS: Viral infections, bacterial infections, children

PREGNANCY AND LACTATION: Pregnancy category C; unknown whether topical application could result in sufficient systemic absorption to produce detectable amounts in breast milk (systemic corticosteroids are secreted into breast milk in quantities not likely to have detrimental effects on infant)

SIDE EFFECTS/ADVERSE REACTIONS

SKIN: Burning, dryness, itching, irritation, acne, folliculitis, hypertrichosis, perioral dermatitis, hypopigmentation, atrophy, striae, miliaria, allergic contact dermatitis, secondary infection

MISC: Systemic absorption of topical corticosteroids has produced reversible HPA axis suppression (more likely with occlusive dressings, prolonged administration, application to large surface areas, liver failure, and in children)

SPECIAL CONSIDERATIONS

PATIENT/FAMILY EDUCATION

• Apply sparingly only to affected area

• Avoid contact with eyes

• Do not put bandages or dressings over treated area unless directed by physician

• Do not use on weeping, denuded, or infected areas

• Discontinue drug, notify physician if local irritation or fever develops

fluorescein

(flure'e-seen)

AK-Fluor, Fluorescite, Fluorets, Fluor-I-Strip, Fluor-I-Strip-A.T., Ful-Glo, Funduscein-10, Funduscein-25, Fluorets, Ophthifluor

Chemical Class: Xanthine dye

Therapeutic Class: Diagnostic agent, optic

CLINICAL PHARMACOLOGY

Mechanism of Action: Breaks in corneal tissue absorb dye and appear bright green under cobalt blue light

INDICATIONS AND USES: Diagnostic aid in identifying foreign bodies, fitting hard contact lenses, fundus photography, tonometry, identifying corneal abrasions, retinal angiography

DOSAGE

Adult

• *Detection of foreign bodies/corneal abrasions:* OPHTH 1 gtt 2% sol, allow a few sec for staining, wash out excess with sterile irrigating solution; STRIPS moisten strip with sterile water, place moistened strip at the fornix in lower cul-de-sac close to the punctum, have patient close lid tightly over strip until desired amount of staining obtained

• *Retinal angiography:* IV 500-750 mg inj rapidly in antecubital vein

Child

• *Retinal angiography:* IV 7.5 mg/kg inj rapidly in antecubital vein

$ AVAILABLE FORMS/COST OF THERAPY

• Inj, Sol—IV: 100 mg/ml, 12 × 5 ml: **$6.00**

• Inj, Sol—IV; Ophth: 25%, 12 × 5 ml: **$3.95-$90.72**

• Sol—Ophth: 2%, 15 ml: **$12.44**

• Strip—Ophth: 0.6 mg, 300's: **$36.88;** 1, 9 mg, 300's: **$62.18**

CONTRAINDICATIONS: Hypersensitivity, soft contact lenses (lenses may become discolored)

PRECAUTIONS: History of allergies, asthma

PREGNANCY AND LACTATION: Pregnancy category C; avoid parenteral use, especially in first trimester; excreted into breast milk, use caution in nursing mothers

SIDE EFFECTS/ADVERSE REACTIONS

CNS: Headache, dizziness, paresthesia, ***convulsions***

CV: Bradycardia, ***shock, cardiac arrest,*** hypotension, syncope

EENT: Stinging, burning, conjunctival redness, urticaria, pruritis

GI: Nausea, vomiting, GI distress, strong taste

GU: Bright yellow discoloration of urine

RESP: ***Dyspnea, acute pulmonary edema, bronchospasm***

SKIN: Severe local tissue damage with extravasation, yellowish discoloration of skin

SPECIAL CONSIDERATIONS

PATIENT/FAMILY EDUCATION

• May cause temporary yellowish discoloration of skin (fades in 6-12 hr)

• Urine will appear bright yellow (fades in 24-36 hr)

• Soft contact lenses may become stained, wait at least 1 hr after thorough rinsing of eye before replacing lenses

MONITORING PARAMETERS

• Luminescence appears in the retina and choroidal vessels 9-15 min following IV inj; can be observed by standard viewing equipment

fluorometholone

(flure-oh-meth'oh-lone)

Flarex, Fluor-Op, FML, FML Forte, FML S.O.P.

Chemical Class: Corticosteroid

Therapeutic Class: Ophthalmic antiinflammatory

CLINICAL PHARMACOLOGY

Mechanism of Action: Inhibits the edema, fibrin deposition, capillary dilation, leukocyte migration, capillary proliferation, fibroblast proliferation, deposition of collagen, and scar formation associated with inflammation

Pharmacokinetics

Absorbed into aqueous humor with slight systemic absorption

INDICATIONS AND USES: Steroid-responsive inflammatory conditions of the palpebral and bulbar conjunctiva, lid, cornea, and anterior segment of the globe; corneal injury; graft rejection after keratoplasty

DOSAGE

Adult and Child

• Susp instill 1 gtt in conjunctival sac q1h during the day and q2h during night, reduce to tid-qid when a favorable response is observed; ointment apply 1/4″ ribbon in lower conjunctival sac tid-qid, taper when favorable response is observed

AVAILABLE FORMS/COST OF THERAPY

• Oint, Top—Ophth: 0.1%, 3.5 g: **$18.01**
• Powder—Ophth: 0.1%, 10 ml: **$18.60**
• Sol—Ophth: 0.1%, 5 ml: **$12.50**
• Susp—Ophth: 0.25%, 10 ml: **$22.03**

CONTRAINDICATIONS: Hypersensitivity, acute superficial herpes simplex, fungal/viral diseases of the eye or conjunctiva, ocular TB

PRECAUTIONS: Corneal abrasions, glaucoma, children, eye infections

PREGNANCY AND LACTATION: Pregnancy category C

SIDE EFFECTS/ADVERSE REACTIONS

EENT: Poor corneal wound healing, increased possibility of corneal infections, glaucoma exacerbation, ***optic nerve damage,*** decreased acuity, visual field defects, cataracts, transient stinging or burning

SPECIAL CONSIDERATIONS

PATIENT/FAMILY EDUCATION

• Do not discontinue use without consulting physician
• Notify physician if condition worsens or persists or if pain, itching, or swelling of the eye occurs

fluoxetine

(floo-ox′e-teen)

Prozac

Chemical Class: Selective serotonin reuptake inhibitor (SSRI)

Therapeutic Class: Antidepressant

CLINICAL PHARMACOLOGY

Mechanism of Action: Selectively inhibits CNS neuronal uptake of serotonin (5HT)

Pharmacokinetics

PO: Peak 4-8 hr, 94.5% bound to plasma proteins, metabolized to norfluoxetine (active), $t_{1/2}$ 48-216 hr (including active metabolite)

INDICATIONS AND USES: Depression, obsessive-compulsive disorder, obesity,* bulimia nervosa*

DOSAGE

Adult

• PO 20 mg QAM, increase after 4-6 wks prn, max 80 mg/d; doses >20 mg can be divided into morning and noon doses

AVAILABLE FORMS/COST OF THERAPY

• Cap, Gel—Oral: 10 mg, 100's: **$214.62;** 20 mg, 100's: **$220.14**
• Sol—Oral: 20 mg/5 ml, 120 ml: **$97.75**

CONTRAINDICATIONS: Hypersensitivity to SSRIs, concurrent use with MAOI, or within 14 days of discontinuing MAOI

PRECAUTIONS: Renal or hepatic function impairment, elderly, children, bipolar affective disorder, seizure disorder, suicidal ideation, diabetes

PREGNANCY AND LACTATION: Pregnancy category B; excreted into breast milk, use caution in nursing mothers

SIDE EFFECTS/ADVERSE REACTIONS

CNS: Nervousness, insomnia, drowsiness, fatigue, tremor, dizziness, anxiety, headache, decreased libido, apathy, euphoria, hallucinations, delusions, psychosis, ***seizures,*** serotonergic syndrome (anxiety, hyperreflexia, confusion)

CV: Palpitations, hot flushes

EENT: Visual disturbance, blurred vision

GI: Anorexia, nausea, diarrhea/loose stools, dyspepsia, dry mouth, constipation, taste changes

GU: Sexual dysfunction, painful menstruation

METAB: Hypoglycemia, altered glycemic control

MS: Joint/muscle pain
SKIN: Sweating, rash, pruritus
MISC: Weight loss

▼ **DRUG INTERACTIONS**

Drugs

- *Alprazolam:* Increased alprazolam concentrations
- *Beta blockers:* Increased beta blocking effects of propranolol and metoprolol, cardiac toxicity may result
- *Carbamazepine:* Carbamazepine toxicity, parkinsonism, serotonin syndrome with concomitant use
- *Cyclic antidepressants:* Increased cyclic antidepressant concentrations, toxicity
- *Lithium:* Increased potential for neurotoxicity
- *MAOI+:* Severe or fatal reactions may occur, wait 5 wk after stopping fluoxetine before starting MAOI and 2 wk after stopping MAOI before starting fluoxetine
- *Moclobemide:* Reduced clearance of moclobemide
- *Phenytoin:* Increased phenytoin concentrations, toxicity
- *Selegiline+:* Mania, hypertension, vasoconstriction
- *Tryptophan:* Agitation, restlessness, poor concentration, nausea; reduced response to fluoxetine

Labs

- *Increase:* Serum bilirubin, blood glucose, alk phosphatase
- *Decrease:* VMA, 5-HIAA
- *False increase:* Urinary catecholamines

SPECIAL CONSIDERATIONS

PATIENT/FAMILY EDUCATION

- May cause dizziness or drowsiness, use caution while driving or performing tasks which require alertness
- Therapeutic response may take 4-6 wk
- May cause insomnia, administer in AM

fluoxymesterone

(floo-ox-ee-mess'te-rone)
Halotestin, Hysterone
Chemical Class: Halogenated derivative of 17-α-methyltestosterone
Therapeutic Class: Anabolic steroid; androgen
DEA Class: Schedule III

CLINICAL PHARMACOLOGY

Mechanism of Action: Promotes weight gain via retention of nitrogen, potassium, and phosphorus, increased protein anabolism, and decreased amino acid catabolism; endogenous androgens are essential for normal growth and development of male sex organs and maintenance of secondary sex characteristics

Pharmacokinetics

PO: Metabolized in liver, excreted in urine, $t_{1/2}$ 9.2 hr

INDICATIONS AND USES: Males: primary hypogonadism (congenital or acquired), hypogonadotropic hypogonadism (congenital or acquired), delayed puberty; Females: palliative therapy of metastatic breast cancer, postpartum breast pain/engorgement

DOSAGE

Adult Males

- *Hypogonadism:* PO 5-20 mg qd
- *Delayed puberty:* 2.5-20 mg qd for 4-6 mo

Adult Females

- *Breast cancer:* PO 10-40 mg/d in divided doses
- *Breast engorgement:* PO 2.5 mg after delivery, 5-10 mg/d in divided doses for 4-5 days

$ **AVAILABLE FORMS/COST OF THERAPY**

- Tab, Uncoated—Oral: 2 mg, 100's: **$44.82;** 5 mg, 100's: **$109.96;** 10 mg, 100's: **$65.00-$163.52**

CONTRAINDICATIONS: Hypersensitivity; serious cardiac, hepatic, or renal disease; carcinoma of breast or prostate (males); pregnancy, enhancement of athletic performance

PRECAUTIONS: Epilepsy, migraine headaches, children, BPH, acute intermittent porphyria, hypercholesterolemia

PREGNANCY AND LACTATION: Pregnancy category X; causes virilization of external genitalia of female fetus; excretion into breast milk unknown, use extreme caution in nursing mothers

SIDE EFFECTS/ADVERSE REACTIONS

CNS: Dizziness, headache, fatigue, tremors, paresthesias, flushing, sweating, anxiety, lability, insomnia, decreased or increased libido

CV: Increased blood pressure

EENT: Conjunctional edema, nasal congestion

GI: Nausea, vomiting, constipation, weight gain, ***cholestatic jaundice***

GU: ***Hematuria,*** *amenorrhea,* vaginitis, *clitoral hypertrophy,* testicular atrophy, excessive frequency and duration of erection, oligospermia

HEME: Suppression of clotting factors II, V, VII, and X; polycythemia

METAB: Abnormal GTT; hypercalcemia; sodium, chloride, water, potassium, calcium, and inorganic phosphate retention; increased serum cholesterol

MS: Cramps, spasms

SKIN: Rash, acneiform lesions, oily hair, skin, flushing, sweating, acne vulgaris, alopecia, hirsutism

MISC: *Virilization (females),* decreased breast size, gynecomastia

▼ **DRUG INTERACTIONS**

Drugs

- *Warfarin+:* Enhanced hypoprothrombinemic response to oral anticoagulants

Labs

- *Increase:* Serum cholesterol, blood glucose, urine glucose
- *Decrease:* Serum Ca, serum K, T_4, T_3, thyroid ^{131}I uptake test, urine 17-OHCS, 17-KS, PBI, BSP

SPECIAL CONSIDERATIONS

PATIENT/FAMILY EDUCATION

- May cause GI upset
- Notify physician if swelling of extremities, priapism, or jaundice occur (males)
- Notify physician if hoarseness, deepening of voice, male-pattern baldness, hirsutism, acne, or menstrual irregularities occur (females)

MONITORING PARAMETERS

- Frequent urine and serum calcium determinations (females)
- Periodic LFTs
- X-ray examinations of bone age q6mo during treatment of prepubertal males
- Hgb and Hct periodically to check for polycythemia

---

fluphenazine

(floo-fen'a-zeen)

Permitil, Prolixin, Prolixin Decanoate, Prolixin Enanthate

Chemical Class: Phenothiazine, piperazine

Therapeutic Class: Antipsychotic/neuroleptic

CLINICAL PHARMACOLOGY

Mechanism of Action: Blocks postsynaptic D_1 and D_2 receptors in the basal ganglia, hypothalamus, limbic system, brain stem, and medulla; depresses various components of the reticular activating system which is involved in the control of basal metabolism and body temperature, wakefulness, vasomotor tone, emesis, and hormonal balance; also exerts anticholinergic and α-adrenergic blocking effects

Pharmacokinetics

PO: Peak 2-4 hr, onset 1 hr, duration 6-8 hr

IM/SC: Peak 2-3 days, onset 1-3 days, duration 1-3 wk, $t_{1/2}$ 3½-4 hr (enanthate); 1-2 days, onset 1-3 days, duration ≥4 wk, 6.8-14.3 hr (decanoate) Widely distributed in tissues, 91%-99% bound to plasma proteins, metabolized in liver, excreted in urine and bile

INDICATIONS AND USES: Management of psychotic disorders, Huntington's chorea,* control of acute agitation,* dementia*

DOSAGE

Adult

• PO 0.5-10 mg/d divided q6-8h initially; reduce dosage gradually to daily maintenance doses of 1-5 mg (may give as single daily dose); IM 1.25-10 mg/d divided q6-8h; IM/SC (enanthate and decanoate) 12.5-25 mg q1-3wk based on patient response, do not exceed 100 mg

Child

• PO 0.25-3.5 mg/d in divided doses q 4-6 hr, max 10 mg/day

$ **AVAILABLE FORMS/COST OF THERAPY**

• Conc—Oral: 5 mg/ml, 120 ml: **$69.97-$113.71**

• Elixir—Oral: 2.5 mg/5ml, 60 ml: **$17.00-$18.08**

• Inj, Sol—IM: 2.5 mg/ml, 10 ml: **$26.50-$59.20**

• Tab, Plain Coated—Oral: 1, 2.5, 5, 10 mg, 100's: **$23.63-$190.08**

• Inj, Sol (decanoate)—IM; SC: 25 mg/ml, 5 ml: **$20.99-$103.75**

• Inj, Sol (enanthate)—SC: 25 mg/ml, 5 ml: **$110.53**

CONTRAINDICATIONS: Hypersensitivity to phenothiazines, liver damage, cerebral arteriosclerosis, CAD, severe hypertension/hypotension, blood dyscrasias, coma, subcortical brain damage, bone marrow depression

PRECAUTIONS: Depression, acute pulmonary infection, chronic respiratory disorders, cardiovascular disease, glaucoma, seizure disorder, impaired hepatic/renal function, elderly, children <12 yr, alcohol withdrawal, electroconvulsive therapy

PREGNANCY AND LACTATION: Pregnancy category C; EPS in the newborn have been attributed to *in utero* exposure; other reports have indicated that phenothiazines are relatively safe during pregnancy; excretion into breast milk unknown, use caution in nursing mothers

SIDE EFFECTS/ADVERSE REACTIONS

CNS: EPS: pseudoparkinsonism, akathisia, dystonia, ***tardive dyskinesia;*** drowsiness, headache, vertigo, fatigue, insomnia, ***seizures, neuroleptic malignant syndrome***

CV: Orthostatic hypotension, hypertension, ***cardiac arrest,*** ECG changes, ***tachycardia***

EENT: Blurred vision, glaucoma, dry eyes

GI: Dry mouth, nausea, vomiting, anorexia, constipation, diarrhea, jaundice, weight gain, ***paralytic ileus, hepatitis***

GU: Urinary retention, frequency or incontinence, bladder paralysis, polyuria, enuresis, priapism, ejaculation inhibition, male impotence

HEME: Anemia, ***leukopenia, leukocytosis, agranulocytosis, thrombocytopenia, aplastic anemia, hemolytic anemia***

METAB: Lactation, moderate breast engorgement (females), galactorrhea, SIADH, amenorrhea, menstrual irregularities, hyperglycemia or hypoglycemia, hyopnatremia

RESP: Laryngospasm, bronchospasm, dyspnea

* = non-FDA-approved use

+ = major clinical significance

SKIN: *Rash,* photosensitivity, dermatitis
MISC: Heat intolerance

▼ **DRUG INTERACTIONS**

Drugs

• *Anticholinergics:* Inhibition of therapeutic response to neuroleptics, additive anticholinergic effects
• *Barbiturates:* Reduced serum neuroleptic concentrations
• *Beta blockers:* Potential increases in serum concentrations of both drugs
• *Bromocriptine:* Reduced effects of both drugs
• *Cyclic antidepressants:* Increased serum concentrations of both drugs
• *Epinephrine:* Reversal of pressor response to epinephrine
• *Levodopa:* Inhibition of the antiparkinsonian effect of levodopa
• *Lithium:* Rare cases of severe neurotoxicity have been reported in acute manic patients
• *Meperidine:* Hypotension, excessive CNS depression
• *Orphenadrine:* Reduced serum neuroleptic concentrations

Labs

• *Increase:* Liver function tests, cardiac enzymes, cholesterol, blood glucose, prolactin, bilirubin, PBI, cholinesterase
• *Decrease:* Hormones (blood and urine)
• *False positive:* Pregnancy tests, PKU
• *False negative:* Urinary steroids, 17-OHCS, pregnancy tests

SPECIAL CONSIDERATIONS

Concentrate must be diluted prior to administration; use only the following diluents: water, saline, 7-Up, homogenized milk, carbonated orange beverage, and pineapple, apricot, prune, orange, V-8, tomato, and grapefruit juices; do not mix with beverages containing caffeine, tannics (tea), or pectinates (apple juice), as physical incompatibility may result

PATIENT/FAMILY EDUCATION

• May cause drowsiness, use caution while driving or performing other tasks requiring alertness
• Avoid contact with skin when using concentrates
• Avoid prolonged exposure to sunlight
• May discolor urine pink or reddish-brown
• Use caution in hot weather, heat stroke may result
• Notify physician if sore throat, fever, skin rash, weakness, tremors, impaired vision, or jaundice occur
• Arise slowly from a reclining position

MONITORING PARAMETERS

• Monitor closely for the appearance of tardive dyskinesia

flurandrenolide

(flure-an-dren′oh-lide)
Cordran, Cordran SP, Cordran Tape
Chemical Class: Synthetic fluorinated agent; Group III (medium) potency
Therapeutic Class: Topical corticosteroid

CLINICAL PHARMACOLOGY

Mechanism of Action: Depresses formation, release, and activity of endogenous mediators of inflammation such as prostaglandins, kinins, histamine, liposomal enzymes, and the complement system resulting in decreased edema, erythema, and pruritus

Pharmacokinetics

Absorbed through the skin (increased by inflammation and occlusive dressings), metabolized primarily in the liver

INDICATIONS AND USES: Psoriasis, eczema, contact dermatitis, pruritus

DOSAGE

Adult and Child

- Apply to affected area bid-tid; rub completely into skin; apply tape q12-24h

$ AVAILABLE FORMS/COST OF THERAPY

- Lotion—Top: 0.05%, 15, 60 ml: **$11.76-$30.90**
- Cre—Top: 0.025%, 30, 60 g: **$13.03-$18.41;** 0.05%, 15, 30, 60, 225 g: **$11.76-$86.45**
- Oint—Top: 0.025%, 30, 60, 225 g: **$13.03-$49.36;** 0.05%, 15, 30, 60 g: **$11.76-$30.90**
- Tape, Medicated—Top: 4 μg/sq cm, 12's: **$12.91**

CONTRAINDICATIONS: Hypersensitivity to corticosteroids, fungal infections, use on face, groin, or axilla

PRECAUTIONS: Viral infections, bacterial infections, children

PREGNANCY AND LACTATION: Pregnancy category C; unknown whether topical application could result in sufficient systemic absorption to produce detectable amounts in breast milk (systemic corticosteroids are secreted into breast milk in quantities not likely to have detrimental effects on infant)

SIDE EFFECTS/ADVERSE REACTIONS

SKIN: Burning, dryness, itching, irritation, acne, folliculitis, hypertrichosis, perioral dermatitis, hypopigmentation, atrophy, striae, miliaria, allergic contact dermatitis, secondary infection

MISC: Systemic absorption of topical corticosteroids has produced reversible HPA axis suppression (more likely with occlusive dressings, prolonged administration, application to large surface areas, liver failure, and in children)

SPECIAL CONSIDERATIONS

PATIENT/FAMILY EDUCATION

- Apply sparingly only to affected area
- Avoid contact with the eyes
- Do not put bandages or dressings over treated area unless directed by physician
- Do not use on weeping, denuded, or infected areas
- Discontinue drug, notify physician if local irritation or fever develops

---

flurazepam

(flure-az'e-pam)

Dalmane, Somnol ✤

Chemical Class: Benzodiazepine
Therapeutic Class: Sedative-hypnotic
DEA Class: Schedule IV

CLINICAL PHARMACOLOGY

Mechanism of Action: Facilitates the inhibitory effect of γ-aminobutyric acid (GABA) on neuronal excitability by increasing membrane permeability to chloride ions

Pharmacokinetics

PO: Onset 15-45 min, peak ½-1 hr, 97% bound to plasma proteins, metabolized by liver to an active metabolite (N-desalkylflurazepam), $t_{1/2}$ of active metabolite 47-100 hr

INDICATIONS AND USES: Insomnia

DOSAGE

Adult

- PO 15-30 mg qhs

Elderly and Child >15 yr

- PO 15 mg qhs

$ AVAILABLE FORMS/COST OF THERAPY

- Cap, Gel—Oral: 15, 30 mg, 100's: **$5.25-$58.43**

CONTRAINDICATIONS: Hypersensitivity to benzodiazepines, pregnancy

PRECAUTIONS: Renal or hepatic function impairment, elderly, depression, history of drug abuse, abrupt withdrawal, respiratory depression, sleep apnea

PREGNANCY AND LACTATION: Contraindicated in pregnancy; administration to nursing mothers is not recommended

SIDE EFFECTS/ADVERSE REACTIONS

CNS: Lethargy, drowsiness, daytime sedation, dizziness, confusion, lightheadedness, headache, anxiety, irritability

CV: Chest pain, pulse changes, palpitations, hypotension (rare)

GI: Nausea, vomiting, diarrhea, heartburn, abdominal pain, constipation

HEME: ***Leukopenia, granulocytopenia*** (rare)

SKIN: Dermatitis/allergy, sweating, flushes, pruritus, rash

▼ **DRUG INTERACTIONS**

Drugs

- *Cimetidine:* Increased serum benzodiazepine concentrations
- *Clozapine:* Isolated cases of cardiorespiratory collapse
- *Disulfiram:* May increase benzodiazepine serum concentrations
- *Ethanol:* Enhanced adverse psychomotor effects of benzodiazepines
- *Rifampin:* Reduced serum benzodiazepine concentrations

Labs

- *Increase:* AST/ALT, serum bilirubin
- *Decrease:* RAI uptake
- *False increase:* Urinary 17-OHCS

SPECIAL CONSIDERATIONS

PATIENT/FAMILY EDUCATION

- Avoid alcohol and other CNS depressants
- Do not discontinue abruptly after prolonged therapy
- May experience disturbed sleep for the first or second night after discontinuing the drug
- May cause drowsiness or dizziness, use caution while driving or performing other tasks requiring alertness
- Inform physician if you are planning to become pregnant, you are pregnant, or if you become pregnant while taking this medicine

flurbiprofen

(flure-bi'proe-fen)

Ansaid, Ocufen (ophthalmic), Froben ✤

Chemical Class: Phenylalkanoic acid

Therapeutic Class: Nonsteroidal antiinflammatory drug (NSAID)

CLINICAL PHARMACOLOGY

Mechanism of Action: Inhibits cyclooxygenase activity and prostaglandin synthesis; other mechanisms such as inhibition of lipoxygenase, leukotriene synthesis, lysosomal enzyme release, neutrophil aggregation, and various cell-membrane functions may exist as well

Pharmacokinetics

PO: Peak 1.5 hr, >99% bound to plasma proteins, extensively metabolized, excreted primarily in urine, $t_{1/2}$ 5.7 hr

INDICATIONS AND USES: Rheumatoid arthritis, osteoarthritis, ankylosing spondylitis,* mild to moderate pain,* primary dysmenorrhea,* tendinitis,* bursitis,* acute painful shoulder,* acute gout,* migraine,* inhibition of intraoperative miosis (ophth), cystoid macular edema* (ophth), inflammation after cataract or glaucoma laser surgery and uveitis syndromes* (ophth)

DOSAGE

Adult

• *Rheumatoid and osteoarthritis:* PO 200-300 mg/d divided bid-qid

• *Dysmenorrhea:* PO 50 mg qid

• *Inhibition of intraoperative miosis:* OPHTH 1 gtt q30 min beginning 2 hr before surgery (total 4 gtt)

$ AVAILABLE FORMS/COST OF THERAPY

• Tab, Coated—Oral: 50 mg, 100's: **$68.15-$80.09;** 100 mg, 100's: **$106.38-$125.00**

• Sol—Ophth: 0.03%, 2.5 ml: **$8.73-$14.49**

CONTRAINDICATIONS: Hypersensitivity to NSAIDs or ASA, dendritic keratitis (ophth)

PRECAUTIONS: Bleeding tendencies, peptic ulcer, renal/hepatic function impairment, elderly, CHF, hypertension

PREGNANCY AND LACTATION: Pregnancy category C; excreted into breast milk, use caution in nursing mothers

SIDE EFFECTS/ADVERSE REACTIONS

CNS: Dizziness, headache, lightheadedness

CV: ***CHF,*** hypotension, hypertension, palpitation, dysrhythmias, tachycardia, edema, chest pain

EENT: Visual disturbances, photophobia, dry eyes, hearing disturbances, tinnitus, *burning/stinging upon instillation*

GI: Nausea, vomiting, diarrhea, constipation, abdominal cramps, *dyspepsia,* flatulence, ***gastric or duodenal ulcer with bleeding or perforation,*** occult blood in stool, ***hepatitis,*** pancreatitis

HEME: ***Neutropenia, eosinophilia, leukopenia, pancytopenia, thrombocytopenia, agranulocytosis***

GU: ***Acute renal failure***

METAB: Hyperglycemia, hypoglycemia, hyperkalemia, hyponatremia

RESP: Dyspnea, bronchospasm

SKIN: Rash, urticaria, photosensitivity

▼ DRUG INTERACTIONS

Drugs

• *Aminoglycosides:* Reduction of aminoglycoside clearance in premature infants

• *ACE inhibitors:* Inhibition of antihypertensive response

• *Beta blockers:* Reduced hypotensive effects of beta blockers

• *Furosemide:* Reduced diuretic and antihypertensive response to furosemide

• *Hydralazine:* Reduced antihypertensive response to hydralazine

• *Lithium:* Increased plasma lithium concentrations, toxicity

• *Methotrexate:* Reduced renal clearance of methotrexate, increased toxicity

• *Potassium sparing diuretics:* Acute renal failure

Labs

• *Increase:* Bleeding time

SPECIAL CONSIDERATIONS

PATIENT/FAMILY EDUCATION

• Avoid aspirin and alcoholic beverages

• Take with food, milk, or antacids to decrease GI upset

• Notify physician if edema, black stools, or persistent headache occurs

MONITORING PARAMETERS

• CBC, BUN, serum creatinine, LFTs, occult blood loss, periodic eye exams

flutamide

(floo'ta-mide)
Eulexin

Chemical Class: Acetanilid
Therapeutic Class: Androgen inhibitor; antineoplastic

CLINICAL PHARMACOLOGY

Mechanism of Action: Inhibits androgen uptake or inhibits nuclear binding of androgen in target tissues; arrests tumor growth in androgen-sensitive tissue, i.e., prostate gland

Pharmacokinetics

PO: Rapidly and completely absorbed, 94% bound to plasma proteins, excreted in urine and feces as metabolites, $t_{1/2}$ 6 hr, geriatric $t_{1/2}$ 8 hr

INDICATIONS AND USES: Metastatic prostatic carcinoma (stage D_2) in combination with LHRH agonistic analogs (e.g., leuprolide)

DOSAGE

Adult

• PO 250 mg (125 mg × 2) q8h

$ AVAILABLE FORMS/COST OF THERAPY

• Cap, Gel—Oral: 125 mg, 180's: **$268.64**

CONTRAINDICATIONS: Hypersensitivity

PREGNANCY AND LACTATION: Pregnancy category D

SIDE EFFECTS/ADVERSE REACTIONS

CNS: Hot flashes, drowsiness, confusion, depression, anxiety
CV: Edema, hypertension
GI: Diarrhea, nausea, vomiting, increased liver function studies, anorexia, ***hepatitis***
GU: Decreased libido, impotence
HEME: ***Anemia, leukopenia, thrombocytopenia***
SKIN: Rash, photosensitivity
MISC: Gynecomastia

▼ DRUG INTERACTIONS

Drugs

• *Warfarin:* Increased hypoprothrombinemic effect

SPECIAL CONSIDERATIONS

PATIENT/FAMILY EDUCATION

• Feminization may occur during therapy
• Do not discontinue therapy without discussion with physician

MONITORING PARAMETERS

• Periodic LFTs during long-term treatment

F

fluvoxamine

(floo-vox'a-meen)
Luvox

Chemical Class: Selective serotonin reuptake inhibitor (SSRI)
Therapeutic Class: Antidepressant

CLINICAL PHARMACOLOGY

Mechanism of Action: Selectively inhibits CNS neuronal uptake of serotonin (5HT)

Pharmacokinetics

PO: Peak 3-8 hr, 77%-80% bound to plasma proteins, primarily eliminated by kidneys, $t_{1/2}$ 13.6-15.6 hr

INDICATIONS AND USES: Obsessive-compulsive disorder, depression*

DOSAGE

Adult

• PO 50 mg qhs initially, increase in 50 mg increments q4-7d, as tolerated, until max therapeutic benefit is achieved; do not exceed 300 mg/d; doses >100 mg should be divided bid

$ AVAILABLE FORMS/COST OF THERAPY

• Tab, Uncoated—Oral: 50 mg, 100's: **$183.68**; 100 mg, 100's: **$188.95**

CONTRAINDICATIONS: Hypersensitivity to SSRIs, coadministration with astemizole or terfenidine, concurrent use with MAOI, or within 14 days of discontinuing MAOI

PRECAUTIONS: History of mania, seizure disorder, liver dysfunction, suicidal ideation, children

PREGNANCY AND LACTATION: Pregnancy category C; excreted into breast milk, use caution in nursing mothers

SIDE EFFECTS/ADVERSE REACTIONS

CNS: Headache, insomnia, somnolence, nervousness, anxiety, dizziness, tremor, depression, decreased libido, agitation

CV: Palpitations, orthostatic hypotension, hypertension, syncope, tachycardia

EENT: Taste perversion/change, amblyopia

GI: Nausea, vomiting, *diarrhea, dyspepsia, dry mouth,* anorexia, constipation, flatulence

GU: Sexual dysfunction, urinary frequency, abnormal ejaculation

RESP: Dyspnea

SKIN: Sweating

▼ **DRUG INTERACTIONS**

Drugs

- *Alprazolam:* Increased alprazolam plasma concentrations
- *Astemizole:* Inhibition of enzyme that metabolizes astemizole, potential for cardiac dysrhythmias
- *Clozapine:* Increased clozapine plasma concentrations
- *Moclobemide:* Increased risk of headache and fatigue
- *Terfenadine:* Inhibition of enzyme that metabolizes terfenidine, potential for cardiac dysrhythmias
- *Theophylline:* Increased theophylline concentrations, toxicity

Labs

- *Increase:* Serum bilirubin, blood glucose, alk phosphatase
- *Decrease:* VMA, 5-HIAA
- *False increase:* Urinary catecholamines

SPECIAL CONSIDERATIONS

PATIENT/FAMILY EDUCATION

- May cause dizziness or drowsiness, use caution driving or performing tasks requiring alertness

---

folic acid

(foe'lik)

Folvite, Novofolacid ♣

Chemical Class: Vitamin, water soluble

Therapeutic Class: Hemostatic, nutrient

CLINICAL PHARMACOLOGY

Mechanism of Action: Required for nucleoprotein synthesis and maintenance of normal erythropoiesis; stimulates production of RBC, WBC, and platelets in certain megaloblastic anemias

Pharmacokinetics

PO: Peak 1 hr, metabolized in liver to 7,8-dihydrofolic acid and eventually to 5,6,7,8-tetrahydrofolic acid, excreted in urine (percentage dependent on dose)

INDICATIONS AND USES: Treatment of megaloblastic anemias due to folic acid deficiency; prophylaxis of fetal neural tube defects

DOSAGE

Adult and Child >11 yr

- *Folic acid deficiency:* PO/IV/IM/SC 1 mg/d initially; maintenance dose 0.5 mg/d
- *Prophylaxis of fetal neural tube defects:* PO at least 0.4 mg/d beginning at least 1 mo prior to conception and increasing to 0.8 mg/d during pregnancy

Child

- *Folic acid deficiency:* PO/IV/IM/SC 1 mg/d initially; maintenance dose 0.1-0.4 mg/d

Infants

- *Folic acid deficiency:* PO/IV/IM/SC 15 μg/kg/dose daily or 50 μg/day

$ **AVAILABLE FORMS/COST OF THERAPY**

- Inj, Sol—IM; IV; SC: 5 mg/ml, 10 ml: **$11.85-$14.33**
- Inj, Sol—IV: 10 mg/ml, 10 ml: **$3.10-$17.85**
- Tab, Uncoated—Oral: 0.4, 0.8 mg, 100's: **$1.08-$2.99**; 1 mg, 100's: **$0.89-$16.00**

CONTRAINDICATIONS: Hypersensitivity, anemias other than megaloblastic/macrocytic anemia, Vit B_{12} deficiency anemia

PREGNANCY AND LACTATION: Pregnancy category A; folic acid deficiency during pregnancy is a common problem in undernourished women and in women not receiving supplements; evidence has accumulated that folic acid deficiency, or abnormal folate metabolism, may be related to the occurence of neural tube defects; actively excreted in human breast milk; compatible with breast feeding; US RDA during lactation is 0.5 mg/d

SIDE EFFECTS/ADVERSE REACTIONS

RESP: Bronchospasm (rare)

SKIN: Allergic reactions have been reported, rash, itching

$ **DRUG INTERACTIONS**

Drugs

- *Phenytoin:* Decreased serum phenytoin concentrations; long-term phenytoin frequently leads to subnormal folate levels
- *Pyrimethamine:* Inhibition of antimicrobial effect of pyrimethamine

SPECIAL CONSIDERATIONS

PATIENT/FAMILY EDUCATION

- Take only under medical supervision

MONITORING PARAMETERS

- CBC; serum folate concentrations <0.005 μg/ml indicate folic acid deficiency and concentrations <0.002 μg/ml usually result in megaloblastic anemia

---

foscarnet

(foss-car′net)

Foscavir

Chemical Class: Organic analog of inorganic pyrophosphate
Therapeutic Class: Antiviral

CLINICAL PHARMACOLOGY

Mechanism of Action: Selective inhibition at the pyrophosphate binding site on virus-specific DNA polymerases and reverse transcriptases; does not require activation by thymidine kinase or other kinases

Pharmacokinetics

IV: 14%-17% bound to plasma proteins, 80%-90% excreted unchanged in urine, $t_{1/2}$ 2-8 hr in normal renal function

INDICATIONS AND USES: CMV retinitis in patients with AIDS; acyclovir-resistant HSV and herpes zoster infections*

DOSAGE

Adult and Adolescent

- *Induction:* IV INF 60 mg/kg via infusion pump over 1 hr q8h for 2-3 wk depending on clinical response
- *Maintenance:* IV INF 90-120 mg/kg/d via infusion pump over 2 hr
- *Dose adjustment in renal impairment (based on CrCl ml/min/kg):* Induction for CrCl ≥1.6, 60 mg/kg/8h; CrCl 1.3, 50 mg/kg/8h; CrCl 1.0, 40 mg/kg/8h; CrCl 0.7, 30 mg/kg/8h; CrCl 0.4, 20 mg/kg/8h; maintenance for CrCl ≥1.4, 100 mg/kg/d; CrCl 0.7, 70 mg/kg/d; CrCl 0.5, 60 mg/kg/d

$ **AVAILABLE FORMS/COST OF THERAPY**

- Sol—IV: 24 mg/ml, 250 ml: **$73.28**

CONTRAINDICATIONS: Hypersensitivity

PRECAUTIONS: Renal function impairment, electrolyte disturbances, neurologic abnormalities, cardiac abnormalities, seizure disorder, elderly, children, severe anemia

PREGNANCY AND LACTATION: Pregnancy category C; excretion into breast milk unknown, use caution in nursing mothers

SIDE EFFECTS/ADVERSE REACTIONS

CNS: Fever, headache, ***seizure***

CV: Hypertension, palpitations, ECG abnormalities (sinus tachycardia, 1st degree AV block, non-specific ST-T segment changes), hypotension, flushing, cardiomyopathy, ***cardiac failure/arrest,*** bradycardia, extrasystole, dysrhythmias, phlebitis

EENT: Vision abnormalities, taste perversions, eye abnormalities, eye pain, conjunctivitis

GI: Nausea, vomiting, anorexia, *diarrhea,* abdominal pain, constipation, dysphagia, dyspepsia, rectal hemorrhage, dry mouth, melena, flatulence, ulcerative stomatitis, ***pancreatitis***

GU: ***Abnormal renal function (acute renal failure, decreased CrCl and increased serum creatinine),*** albuminuria, dysuria, polyuria, urethral disorder, urinary retention, UTI, nocturia

HEME: ***Anemia, granulocytopenia, leukopenia, thrombocytopenia,*** platelet abnormalities, thrombosis, WBC abnormalities, lymphadenopathy

METAB: Hypokalemia, hypocalcemia, hypomagnesemia, hypo- or hyperphosphatemia, hyponatremia, decreased weight, increased alkaline phosphatase, acidosis, cachexia, thirst, hypercalcemia, increased LDH and BUN

MS: Back/chest pain, arthralgia, myalgia

RESP: Coughing, dyspnea, pneumonia, sinusitis, pharyngitis, rhinitis, respiratory disorders, pulmonary infiltration, stridor, pneumothorax, hemoptysis, bronchospasm

SKIN: Rash, sweating, pruritus, skin ulceration, seborrhea, erythematous rash, maculopapular rash, skin discoloration, facial edema

SPECIAL CONSIDERATIONS

- Hydration to establish diuresis both prior to and during administration is recommended to minimize renal toxicity; the standard 24 mg/ml sol may be used undiluted via a central venous catheter, dilute to 12 mg/ml with D_5W or NS when a peripheral vein catheter is used

PATIENT/FAMILY EDUCATION

- Foscarnet is not a cure for CMV retinitis
- Notify physician of perioral tingling, numbness in the extremities, or paresthesias (could signify electrolyte imbalances)

MONITORING PARAMETERS

- Serum creatinine, calcium, phosphorus, potassium, magnesium at baseline and 2-3 times/wk during induction and at least every 1-2 wk during maintenance
- Hemoglobin
- Regular ophthalmologic examinations

fosinopril

(foss-in-o'pril)

Monopril

Chemical Class: Angiotensin-converting enzyme (ACE) inhibitor

Therapeutic Class: Antihypertensive

CLINICAL PHARMACOLOGY

Mechanism of Action: Selectively

suppresses renin-angiotensin-aldosterone system; inhibits ACE preventing conversion of angiotensin I to angiotensin II; results in dilation of arterial, venous vessels

Pharmacokinetics

PO: Onset 1 hr, duration 24 hr, peak 3 hr, metabolized to active metabolite (fosinoprilat), t½ (fosinoprilat) 12 hr, excreted in urine (50%) and feces (50%)

INDICATIONS AND USES: Hypertension, CHF,* diabetic nephropathy*

DOSAGE

Adult

• PO 10 mg qd initially, then 20-40 mg/d divided bid or qd, max 80 mg/d

$ AVAILABLE FORMS/COST OF THERAPY

• Tab, Uncoated—Oral: 10 mg, 100's: **$70.86;** 20 mg, 100's: **$75.84**

CONTRAINDICATIONS: Hypersensitivity to ACE inhibitors

PRECAUTIONS: Impaired renal and liver function, dialysis patients, hypovolemia, diuretic therapy, collagen-vascular diseases, CHF, elderly, bilateral renal artery stenosis

PREGNANCY AND LACTATION: Pregnancy category C (first trimester), category D (second and third trimesters); ACE inhibitors can cause fetal and neonatal morbidity and death when administered to pregnant women; when pregnancy is detected, discontinue ACE inhibitors as soon as possible; detectable in breast milk in trace amounts, a newborn would receive <0.1% of the mg/kg maternal dose; effect on nursing infant has not been determined, use with caution in nursing mothers

SIDE EFFECTS/ADVERSE REACTIONS

CNS: Anxiety, insomnia, paresthesia, *headache, dizziness, fatigue*

CV: Hypotension, postural hypotension, syncope (especially with first dose), palpitations, angina

GI: Nausea, constipation, vomiting, melena, abdominal pain

GU: Increased BUN, creatinine, decreased libido, impotence, UTI

HEME: ***Neutropenia, agranulocytosis***

METAB: Hyperkalemia, hyponatremia

MS: Arthralgia, arthritis, myalgia

RESP: *Cough,* asthma, bronchitis, dyspnea, sinusitis

SKIN: ***Angioedema,*** rash, flushing, sweating

▼ DRUG INTERACTIONS

Drugs

• *Lithium:* Increased risk of serious lithium toxicity

• *Loop diuretics:* Initiation of ACE inhibitor therapy in the presence of intensive diuretic therapy results in a precipitous fall in blood pressure in some patients; ACE inhibitors may induce renal insufficiency in the presence of diuretic-induced sodium depletion

• *NSAIDs:* Inhibition of the antihypertensive response to ACE inhibitors

• *Potassium sparing diuretics:* Increased risk for hyperkalemia

SPECIAL CONSIDERATIONS

PATIENT/FAMILY EDUCATION

• Do not use salt substitutes containing potassium without consulting physician

• Rise slowly to sitting or standing position to minimize orthostatic hypotension

• Notify physician of mouth sores, sore throat, fever, swelling of hands or feet, irregular heartbeat, chest pain

• Dizziness, fainting, lightheadedness may occur during 1st few days of therapy

MONITORING PARAMETERS

• BUN, creatinine (watch for in-

creased levels that may indicate acute renal failure)
- Potassium levels, although hyperkalemia rarely occurs

---

furazolidone

(fyur-a-zoh′li-done)
Furoxone
Chemical Class: Synthetic nitrofuran derivative
Therapeutic Class: Antibacterial, antiprotozoal

CLINICAL PHARMACOLOGY
Mechanism of Action: Exerts bactericidal action via interference with several bacterial enzyme systems; inhibits the enzyme MAO
Pharmacokinetics
PO: Systemically absorbed, extensively metabolized (possibly in the intestine), colored metabolites excreted in urine
INDICATIONS AND USES: Bacterial or protozoal diarrhea and enteritis caused by susceptible organisms. Antibacterial spectrum usually includes: gram-positive organisms: staphylococci; gram-negative organisms: *E. coli, Salmonella, Shigella, Proteus, Enterobacter aerogenes, Vibrio cholerae;* protozoan organisms: *Giardia lamblia*
DOSAGE
Adult
- PO 100 mg qid

Child
- PO 25-50 mg qid (≥5 yr); 17-25 mg qid (1-4 yr); 8-17 mg qid (1 mo-1 yr)

$ AVAILABLE FORMS/COST OF THERAPY
- Liq—Oral: 50 mg/15 ml, 60 ml: **$11.19**
- Tab, Coated—Oral: 100 mg, 100's: **$190.98**

CONTRAINDICATIONS: Hypersensitivity, infants <1 mo
PRECAUTIONS: Hypertension, diabetes, G-6-PD deficiency
PREGNANCY AND LACTATION: Pregnancy category C; could theoretically produce hemolytic anemia in a G-6-PD deficient newborn if given at term; excretion into breast milk unknown, use caution in nursing mothers
SIDE EFFECTS/ADVERSE REACTIONS
CNS: Headache, malaise, fever
CV: Orthostatic hypotension, ***hypertensive crisis***
GI: Colitis, proctitis, anal pruritus, staphylococcic enteritis, nausea, vomiting
HEME: Hemolysis in G-6-PD deficiency
METAB: Hypoglycemia
MS: Arthralgia
SKIN: Vesicular morbilliform rash
$ DRUG INTERACTIONS
Drugs
- *Amphetamines:* Hypertensive crisis
- *Ethanol:* Disulfiram-like reaction

Food
- Foods high in amine content: Hypertensive crisis

Labs
- *False positive:* Urine glucose with Clinitest

SPECIAL CONSIDERATIONS

PATIENT/FAMILY EDUCATION
- Avoid ingestion of alcohol during and within 4 days after furazolidone therapy
- Avoid foods containing tyramine, especially if therapy extends beyond 5 days
- Avoid OTC drugs containing sympathomimetic drugs
- May color the urine brown

furosemide

(fur-oh'se-mide)

Detue, Furocot, Lasix, Luramide, Novosemide, ✦ Uritol ✦

Chemical Class: Sulfonamide derivative

Therapeutic Class: Loop diuretic

CLINICAL PHARMACOLOGY

Mechanism of Action: Inhibits the absorption of sodium and chloride not only in the proximal and distal tubules but also in the loop of Henle

Pharmacokinetics

PO: Onset 1 hr, peak 1-2 hr, duration 6-8 hr, absorbed 70%

IV/IM: Onset 5 min (slightly delayed with IM), peak ½ hr (IM), duration 2 hr; 98% bound to plasma proteins; 50% of PO dose and 80% of IV dose excreted in the urine within 24 hr; remainder eliminated by nonrenal pathways (liver metabolism, excreted unchanged in feces); $t_{1/2}$ 30 min (9 hr in renal failure)

INDICATIONS AND USES: Edema associated with CHF, hepatic cirrhosis, renal disease, nephrotic syndrome; hypertension; pulmonary edema, hypercalcemia*

DOSAGE

Adult

PO 20-80 mg/d in AM; may give another dose in 6 hr; increase in increments of 20-40 mg up to 600 mg/d if response is not satisfactory; IM/IV 20-40 mg, increased by 20 mg q2h until desired response (Rule of thumb: IV dose = ½ PO dose)

• *Pulmonary edema:* IV 40 mg given over several min, repeated in 1 hr; increase to 80 mg if needed

Child

• PO/IM/IV 1-2 mg/kg/dose up to 6 mg/kg/d in divided doses q6-12h

$ AVAILABLE FORMS/COST OF THERAPY

• Inj, Sol—IM; IV: 10 mg/ml, 10 ml: **$2.36-$78.13**

• Sol—Oral: 10 mg/ml, 60, 120 ml: **$6.60-$18.40;** 40 mg/5 ml, 500 ml: **$29.04**

• Tab, Uncoated—Oral: 20, 40, 80 mg, 100's: **$2.03-$24.95**

CONTRAINDICATIONS: Hypersensitivity to sulfonamides, anuria

PRECAUTIONS: Diabetes mellitus, dehydration, severe renal disease, hepatic cirrhosis, ascites, SLE, gout

PREGNANCY AND LACTATION: Pregnancy category C; cardiovascular disorders, such as pulmonary edema, severe hypertension, or CHF are probably the only valid indications for this drug during pregnancy; excreted into breast milk, no reports of adverse effects in nursing infants have been found; thiazide diuretics have been used to suppress lactation

SIDE EFFECTS/ADVERSE REACTIONS

CNS: Vertigo, headache, dizziness, paresthesia, restlessness, fever

CV: Orthostatic hypotension, chest pain, ECG changes, ***circulatory collapse***

EENT: Blurred vision, ototoxicity

GI: Anorexia, *nausea,* vomiting, dry mouth, diarrhea, oral and gastric irritation, cramping, constipation, pancreatitis, jaundice, ***ischemic hepatitis***

GU: Urinary bladder spasm, hyperuricemia, glycosuria

HEME: ***Anemia, leukopenia,*** purpura, ***aplastic anemia, thrombocytopenia, agranulocytosis***

METAB: Hyperglycemia

SKIN: Photosensitivity, urticaria, pruritus, necrotizing angiitis, interstitial nephritis, ***exfoliative dermatitis,*** erythema multiforme, *rash*

▼ **DRUG INTERACTIONS**

Drugs

• *ACE inhibitors:* Initiation of ACE inhibitor in the presence of intensive diuretic therapy may result in precipitous fall in blood pressure; ACE inhibitors may induce renal insufficiency in the presence of diuretic-induced sodium depletion

• *Bile acid binding resins:* Reduced bioavailability and diuretic response of furosemide

• *Clofibrate:* Enhanced effects of both drugs especially in patients with hypoalbuminemia

• *Digitalis glycosides:* Diuretic-induced hypokalemia may increase risk of digitalis toxicity

• *NSAIDs:* Reduced diuretic and antihypertensive efficacy of furosemide

• *Phenytoin:* Reduced diuretic response to furosemide

Labs

• *Interference:* GTT

SPECIAL CONSIDERATIONS

PATIENT/FAMILY EDUCATION

• May cause GI upset, take with food or milk

• Take early in the day

• Avoid prolonged exposure to sunlight

MONITORING PARAMETERS

• Frequent serum electrolyte, calcium, glucose, uric acid, creatinine, and BUN determinations during first months of therapy and periodically thereafter

gabapentin

(ga'ba-pen-tin)

Neurontin

Chemical Class: Substituted cyclohexanacetic acid

Therapeutic Class: Anticonvulsant

CLINICAL PHARMACOLOGY

Mechanism of Action: Structurally related to γ-aminobutyric acid (GABA) but does not interact with GABA receptors; may act via gabapentin binding sites in neocortex and hippocampus

Pharmacokinetics

PO: Over dosage range of 300 to 600 mg tid, bioavailability drops 60 percent; not protein bound; not metabolized; elimination $t_{1/2}$ 5-7 hr if CrCl normal, 52 hr if CrCl <30 ml/min; removed by hemodialysis.

INDICATIONS AND USES: Adjunctive therapy for partial seizures with or without secondary generalization

DOSAGE

Adult and Child >12 yr

• PO 900 to 2400 mg/d given in 3 divided doses; start with 300 mg on day 1, 300 mg bid on day 2, and 300 mg tid on day 3; adjustment for renal dysfunction: CrCl >60 ml/min, daily dose 1200 mg, CrCl 30-60 ml/min, daily dose 600 mg, CrCl 15-30 ml/min, daily dose 300 mg, CrCl <15 ml/min, daily dose 150 mg, hemodialysis, 200-300 mg after dialysis

$ **AVAILABLE FORMS/COST OF THERAPY**

• Cap, Gel—Oral: 100 mg, 100's: **$36.00;** 300 mg, 100's: **$90.00;** 400 mg, 100's: **$108.00**

CONTRAINDICATIONS: Hypersensitivity

PRECAUTIONS: Severe renal dysfunction, age <12 yr, tumorigenic in rats (pancreatic adenomas and carcinomas); significance to humans unknown

PREGNANCY AND LACTATION: Pregnancy category C; excretion into breast milk unknown

SIDE EFFECTS/ADVERSE REACTIONS

CNS: Somnolence (19%), dizziness (17%), ataxia (13%), fatigue (11%),

nystagmus (8%), tremor (7%), nervousness, dysarthria, amnesia, depression, abnormal thinking
EENT: Diplopia, rhinitis
GI: Dyspepsia, dry mouth
GU: Impotence
HEME: ***Leukopenia (1%)***
MS: Myalgia, twitching
SKIN: Flushing, pruritus

▼ **DRUG INTERACTIONS**

Drugs

- *Antacids:* Reduce bioavailability of gabapentin by 20%
- *Cimetidine:* Reduces renal clearance of gabapentin by 14%

Labs

- *False positive:* Urine protein by Multistix method

SPECIAL CONSIDERATIONS

PATIENT/FAMILY EDUCATION

Do not stop abruptly—taper over 1 wk

MONITORING PARAMETERS

- Drug level monitoring not necessary

---

gallium nitrate

(gal'ee-yum)
Ganite
Chemical Class: Hydrated nitrate salt of the group IIIa element, gallium
Therapeutic Class: Hypocalcemic agent

CLINICAL PHARMACOLOGY

Mechanism of Action: Inhibits calcium resorption from bone, reducing increased bone turnover; precise mechanism has not been determined

Pharmacokinetics

IV: Steady state achieved in 24-48 hr, not metabolized, excreted by the kidneys

INDICATIONS AND USES: Symptomatic cancer-related hypercalcemia unresponsive to adequate hydration

DOSAGE

Adult

- IV INF 200 mg/m^2/d for 5 consecutive days; dilute in 1 L NS or D_5W and infuse over 24 hr

$ **AVAILABLE FORMS/COST OF THERAPY**

- Inj, Sol—IV: 25 mg/ml, 20 ml: **$110.00**

CONTRAINDICATIONS: Hypersensitivity, severe renal disease (serum creatinine >2.5 mg/dl)

PRECAUTIONS: Children, mild renal disease

PREGNANCY AND LACTATION: Pregnancy category C; excretion into breast milk unknown, use caution in nursing mothers

SIDE EFFECTS/ADVERSE REACTIONS

CNS: Lethargy, confusion, hypothermia, fever, paresthesia
CV: Tachycardia, edema, hypotension
EENT: Acute optic neuritis, visual impairment, decreased hearing
GI: Nausea, vomiting, diarrhea, constipation
GU: ***Nephrotoxicity, acute renal failure***
HEME: ***Anemia*** (very high doses), ***leukopenia***
METAB: Hypocalcemia, *transient hypophosphatemia, decreased serum bicarbonate*
RESP: Dyspnea, rales, rhonchi, pleural effusion, pulmonary infiltrates
SKIN: Rash

▼ **DRUG INTERACTIONS**

Drugs

- *Aminoglycosides:* Increased risk of nephrotoxicity
- *Amphotericin B:* Increased risk of nephrotoxicity

SPECIAL CONSIDERATIONS

Maintain adequate hydration

throughout the treatment period; avoid overhydration in patients with compromised cardiovascular status

MONITORING PARAMETERS

- Serum creatinine daily (discontinue if exceeds 2.5 mg/dl)
- Urine output (≥2 L/day is recommended)
- Serum calcium and phosphorus

ganciclovir (DHPG)

(gan-sy'clo-ver)

Cytovene

Chemical Class: Synthetic nucleoside analog

Therapeutic Class: Antiviral

CLINICAL PHARMACOLOGY

Mechanism of Action: Preferentially phosphorylated in virus-infected cells to ganciclovir-triphosphate which inhibits viral DNA synthesis by: (1) competitive inhibition of viral DNA polymerases and (2) direct incorporation into viral DNA, resulting in eventual termination of viral DNA elongation

Pharmacokinetics

IV: $t_{1/2}$ 1.7-5.8 hr (prolonged in renal failure), excreted unchanged by the kidneys, crosses blood-brain barrier, 1%-2% bound to plasma proteins

INDICATIONS AND USES: CMV retinitis in immunocompromised patients; prevention of CMV disease in transplant patients at risk; other CMV disease (e.g., pneumonitis, gastroenteritis, hepatitis)*

DOSAGE

Adult and Child >3 mo

- *CMV retinitis:* Induction IV 5 mg/kg q12h as a 1-2 hr inf for 14-21 days; maintenance IV 5 mg/kg/d as a single daily dose for 7 days/wk or 6 mg/kg/d for 5 days/wk; PO 1 g tid with food
- *CMV prevention in transplant patients:* Induction IV 5 mg/kg q12h as a 1-2 hr inf for 7-14 days; maintenance IV 5 mg/kg/d as a single daily dose for 7 days/wk or 6 mg/kg/d for 5 days/wk
- *Dosage reduction in renal function impairment:* (CrCl measured in ml/min/1.73 m^2): Induction
- *Maintenance dose:* 50% of induction dose, monitor for disease progression

$ **AVAILABLE FORMS/COST OF THERAPY**

- Cap, Gel—Oral: 250 mg, 180's: **$702.00**
- Inj, Lyph-Sol—IV: 500 mg/vial, 25's: **$870.00**

CONTRAINDICATIONS: Hypersensitivity to acyclovir or ganciclovir

PRECAUTIONS: Preexisting cytopenias, renal function impairment, children <6 mo, elderly, platelet count <25,000/mm^3

PREGNANCY AND LACTATION: Pregnancy category C; excretion into breast milk unknown, not recommended in nursing mothers due to potential for serious adverse reactions in the nursing infant; do not resume nursing for at least 72 hr after last dose of ganciclovir

SIDE EFFECTS/ADVERSE REACTIONS

CNS: Headache, confusion, abnormal thoughts or dreams, ataxia, ***coma,*** dizziness, nervousness, paresthesia, psychosis, somnolence, tremor, fever, chills, malaise

CV: Dysrhythmia, hypertension, hypotension

EENT: Retinal detachment in CMV retinitis

GI: Nausea, vomiting, anorexia, diarrhea, ***hemorrhage,*** abdominal pain, abnormal LFTs

GU: Hematuria; increased serum creatinine, BUN

HEME: ***Granulocytopenia, thrombocytopenia, anemia, eosinophilia***
METAB: Decrease in blood glucose
RESP: Dyspnea
SKIN: Rash, alopecia, pruritus, urticaria
MISC: Sepsis, infections

▼ **DRUG INTERACTIONS**

Drugs

- *Zidovudine+:* Increased hematological toxicity

SPECIAL CONSIDERATIONS

PATIENT/FAMILY EDUCATION

- Ganciclovir is not a cure for CMV retinitis, progression may occur during or following therapy
- Compliance with laboratory monitoring is essential

MONITORING PARAMETERS

- CBC with differential and platelets q2d during induction and weekly thereafter
- Serum creatinine q2wk

---

gemfibrozil

(gem-fi'broe-zil)
Lopid
Chemical Class: Fibric acid derivative
Therapeutic Class: Antilipemic

CLINICAL PHARMACOLOGY

Mechanism of Action: Inhibits peripheral lipolysis and decreases hepatic extraction of free fatty acids, thus reducing hepatic triglyceride production; inhibits synthesis of VLDL carrier apolipoprotein B, leading to a decrease in VLDL production

Pharmacokinetics

PO: Peak 1-2 hr, >90% bound to plasma proteins, $t_{1/2}$ 1½ hr (biologic $t_{1/2}$ considerably longer due to enterohepatic recycling) metabolized in liver, excreted in urine (glucuronide conjugates)

INDICATIONS AND USES: Hypertriglyceridemia (Types IV and V hyperlipidemia); Type IIb hyperlipidemia

DOSAGE

Adult

- PO 600 mg bid, 30 min before morning and evening meals

$ **AVAILABLE FORMS/COST OF THERAPY**

- Tab, Plain Coated—Oral: 600 mg, 60's: **$40.87-$65.75**

CONTRAINDICATIONS: Severe hepatic disease, preexisting gallbladder disease, severe renal disease, primary biliary cirrhosis, hypersensitivity

PRECAUTIONS: Children, suspected cholelithiasis

PREGNANCY AND LACTATION: Pregnancy category B; excretion into breast milk unknown, use caution in nursing mothers

SIDE EFFECTS/ADVERSE REACTIONS

CNS: Fatigue, vertigo, headache, paresthesia, hypesthesia
CV: Atrial fibrillation
EENT: Blurred vision, retinal edema, cataracts
GI: *Dyspepsia, abdominal pain,* diarrhea, nausea, vomiting, constipation, taste perversion
GU: Impotence
HEME: ***Anemia, leukopenia, bone marrow hypoplasia, eosinophilia, thrombocytopenia***
METAB: Increased blood glucose
MS: Myopathy, myasthenia, myalgia, painful extremities, arthralgia, synovitis, ***rhabdomyolysis***
SKIN: ***Exfoliative dermatitis,*** dermatitis, pruritus, alopecia
MISC: Weight loss

▼ **DRUG INTERACTIONS**

Drugs

- *Binding resins:* Reduced bioavailability of gemfibrozil, separate doses by >2 hr

G

• *Lovastatin:* Increased likelihood of lovastatin-induced myopathy

Labs

• *Increase:* Liver function studies, CPK, BSP, thymol turbidity, glucose

• *Decrease:* Hgb, Hct, WBC

SPECIAL CONSIDERATIONS

PATIENT/FAMILY EDUCATION

• May cause dizziness or blurred vision, use caution while driving or performing other tasks requiring alertness

• Notify physician if GI side effects become pronounced

MONITORING PARAMETERS

• Serum CK level in patients complaining of muscle pain, tenderness, or weakness

• Periodic CBC during first 12 mo of therapy

• Periodic LFTs, discontinue therapy if abnormalities persist

• Blood glucose

---

gentamicin

(jen-ta-mye'sin)

Garamycin, Garamycin Intrathecal, Garamycin Pediatric, Jenamicin

Ophthalmic: Garamycin Ophthalmic, Genoptic Ophthalmic, Genoptic Gentacidin, Gent-AK, Gentak

Topical: G-Myticin, Garamycin

Chemical Class: Aminoglycoside

Therapeutic Class: Antibiotic

CLINICAL PHARMACOLOGY

Mechanism of Action: Interferes with protein synthesis in bacterial cell by binding to 30S ribosomal subunit, which causes misreading of genetic code, inaccurate peptide sequence forms in protein chain, causing bacterial death

Pharmacokinetics

IM: Onset rapid, peak 30-90 min

IV: Onset immediate, peak 30 min after a 30 min inf

<30% bound to plasma proteins, plasma $t_{1/2}$ 1-2 hr, duration 6-8 hr, not metabolized, eliminated unchanged in urine via glomerular filtration

INDICATIONS AND USES: Bacterial neonatal sepsis; bacterial septicemia; serious bacterial infections of the CNS (meningitis), urinary tract, respiratory tract, GI tract, skin, bone, and soft tissue; Superficial ocular infections involving the conjunctiva or cornea, infection prophylaxis in minor cuts, wounds, burns, and skin abrasions; superficial infections of the skin alternative regimen for PID (in combination with clindamycin)*

Antibacterial spectrum usually includes:

• Gram-positive organisms: *Staphylococcus* sp (including penicillin- and methicillin-resistant strains), *Streptococcus faecalis* (in combination with cell wall synthesis inhibitor)

• Gram-negative organisms: *Escherichia coli, Proteus* sp (indole-positive and indole-negative), *Pseudomonas aeruginosa, Klebsiella* sp, *Enterobacter* sp, *Serratia* sp, *Citrobacter* sp, *Providencia* sp, *Salmonella* sp and *Shigella* sp, *Yersinia pestis*

DOSAGE

• Use ideal body weight for dosage calculations

Adult

• *Severe systemic infections:* IV INF 3-5 mg/kg/d diluted in 50-100 ml NS or D_5 W and infused over 30-60 min in divided doses q8h, adjust dosage based on results of gentamicin peak and trough levels (once-daily dosage:* 7 mg/kg q24h; not for pediatrics, pregnant, burns, ascites, dialysis, enterococcal endocarditis); IM 3 mg/kg/d in divided doses q8h, adjust dosage based on results of gentamicin peak and trough levels; INTRATHECAL 4-8 mg/d

- INSTILL 1 gtt q2-4h; OPHTH apply 1/4″ ribbon of ointment to conjunctival sac bid-tid
- TOP rub into affected area qd-qid; cover with sterile bandage if needed

Infants and Children <5 yr

- IV/IM 2.5 mg/kg/dose q8h, adjust dosage based on results of gentamicin peak and trough levels; INTRATHECAL (>3 mo) 1-2 mg/d

Child ≥5 yr

- IV/IM 1.5-2.5 mg/kg/dose q8h, adjust dosage based on results of gentamicin peak and trough levels

$ AVAILABLE FORMS/COST OF THERAPY

- Inj, Sol—IM; IV: 2 mg/ml, 2 ml: **$2.70**; 10 mg/ml, 2 ml: **$0.60-$32.81**; 40 mg/ml, 2 ml: **$1.26-$51.56**
- Sol—Ophth: 3 mg/ml, 5, 15 ml: **$3.75-14.86**
- Oint—Ophth: 3 mg/g, 3.5 g: **$3.85-$14.86**
- Oint—Top: 1 mg/g, 15, 30, 45 g: **$2.03-$86.40**
- Cre—Top: 0.1%, 15, 30, 45 g: **$2.03-$86.40**

CONTRAINDICATIONS: Hypersensitivity to aminoglycosides

PRECAUTIONS: Neonates, renal disease, myasthenia gravis, hearing deficits, Parkinson's disease, elderly, dehydration, hypokalemia, prolonged use

PREGNANCY AND LACTATION: Pregnancy category C; ototoxicity has not been reported as an effect of *in utero* exposure; eighth cranial nerve toxicity in the fetus is well known following exposure to other aminoglycosides and could potentially occur with gentamicin; potentiation of $MgSO_4$-induced neuromuscular weakness in neonates has been reported, use caution during the last 32 hr of pregnancy; data on excretion into breast milk are lacking

SIDE EFFECTS/ADVERSE REACTIONS

CNS: Confusion, depression, numbness, tremors, ***convulsions,*** muscle twitching, ***neurotoxicity,*** dizziness, vertigo, myasthenia gravis-like syndrome

CV: Hypotension, hypertension, palpitations

EENT: ***Ototoxicity, deafness,*** visual disturbances, tinnitus; Ophth: Lid itching, lid swelling, conjunctival erythema, mydriasis, conjunctival paresthesia, poor corneal wound healing, temporary visual haze (ointment), overgrowth of nonsusceptible organisms, transient irritation, burning, stinging, itching, inflammation

GI: Nausea, vomiting, anorexia, increased ALT, AST, bilirubin, hepatomegaly, splenomegaly

GU: ***Oliguria, hematuria, renal damage, azotemia, renal failure, nephrotoxicity***

HEME: ***Agranulocytosis, thrombocytopenia, leukopenia, eosinophilia,*** anemia

METAB: Decreased serum calcium, sodium, potassium, magnesium

RESP: ***Respiratory depression***

SKIN: Rash, burning, urticaria, dermatitis, alopecia, photosensitivity, pruritis

▼ DRUG INTERACTIONS

Drugs

- *Amphotericin B:* Synergistic nephrotoxicity
- *Cephalosporins:* Increased potential for nephrotoxicity in patients with pre-existing renal disease

• *Cyclosporine:* Additive renal damage
• *Ethacrynic acid+:* Increased risk of ototoxicity
• *Extended spectrum penicillins:* Potential for inactivation of gentamicin in patients with renal failure
• *Methoxyflurane:* Enhanced renal toxicity
• *Neuromuscular blocking agents+:* Potentiation of respiratory suppression produced by neuromuscular blocking agents
• *NSAIDs:* Reduced renal clearance of aminoglycosides in premature infants

SPECIAL CONSIDERATIONS

PATIENT/FAMILY EDUCATION

• Report headache, dizziness, loss of hearing, ringing, roaring in ears, or feeling of fullness in head
• Tilt head back, place medication in conjunctival sac, and close eyes
• Apply light finger pressure on lacrimal sac for 1 min following instill (gtt)
• May cause temporary blurring of vision following administration
• Notify physician if stinging, burning, or itching becomes pronounced or if redness, irritation, swelling, decreasing vision, or pain persists or worsens
• Do not touch tip of container to any surface
• For external use only
• Cleanse affected area of skin prior to application
• Notify physician if condition worsens or if rash or irritation develops

MONITORING PARAMETERS

• Urinalysis for proteinuria, cells, casts
• Urine output
• Serum peak, drawn at 30-60 min after IV inf or 60 min after IM inj, trough level drawn just before next dose; adjust dosage per levels (usual therapeutic plasma levels, peak 4-8 µg/ml, trough ≤2 µg/ml)
• Serum creatinine for CrCl calculation
• Serum calcium, magnesium, sodium
• Audiometric testing, assess hearing before, during, after treatment

---

glipizide

(glip'i-zide)
Glucotrol, Glucotrol XL
Chemical Class: Sulfonylurea (2nd generation)
Therapeutic Class: Antidiabetic

CLINICAL PHARMACOLOGY

Mechanism of Action: Stimulates insulin release from β-cells in the pancreatic islets possibly as a result of increased intracellular cAMP; may improve the binding between insulin and insulin receptors or increase the number of receptors; extrapancreatic effects include suppression of glucagon release and hepatic glucose production

Pharmacokinetics

PO: Completely absorbed by GI route, onset 1-1½ hr, duration 10-24 hr, $t_{1/2}$ 2-4 hr, metabolized in liver to inactive metabolites, excreted in urine, 90%-95% bound to plasma proteins

INDICATIONS AND USES: Type II diabetes mellitus

DOSAGE

Adult

• PO 2.5-5 mg 30 min before breakfast; adjust dose in 2.5-5 mg increments; do not exceed 20 mg/dose, 40 mg/d (Note: Little if any benefit from daily doses >20 mg)

$ AVAILABLE FORMS/COST OF THERAPY

• Tab, Uncoated—Oral: 5 mg, 100's: **$27.30-$35.45;** 10 mg, 100's: **$50.12-$65.08**

---

* = non-FDA-approved use + = major clinical significance

• Tab, Coated, Sust Action—Oral: 5 mg, 100's: **$30.67;** 10 mg, 100's: **$60.69**

CONTRAINDICATIONS: Hypersensitivity to sulfonylureas; diabetes complicated by ketoacidosis

PRECAUTIONS: Elderly, cardiac disease, severe renal disease, severe hepatic disease, thyroid disease, adrenal or pituitary insufficiency, debilitated or malnourished patients

PREGNANCY AND LACTATION: Pregnancy category C; in general avoid the sulfonylurea agents in pregnancy since they will not provide adequate blood glucose control; excretion into breast milk unknown, because of the potential for hypoglycemia in nursing infants use with caution in nursing mothers

SIDE EFFECTS/ADVERSE REACTIONS

CNS: Dizziness, drowsiness, headache, paresthesia

EENT: Tinnitus, vertigo

GI: Nausea, diarrhea, constipation, gastralgia, cholestatic jaundice, elevated liver function tests

GU: Mild to moderate elevations in BUN and creatinine

HEME: ***Leukopenia, thrombocytopenia, aplastic anemia, agranulocytosis, hemolytic anemia, pancytopenia,*** hepatic porphyria

METAB: ***Hypoglycemia,*** SIADH

MS: Weakness, fatigue

SKIN: Erythema, morbilliform or maculopapular eruptions, urticaria, pruritus, eczema

▼ **DRUG INTERACTIONS**

Drugs

• *Anabolic steroids:* Enhanced hypoglycemic response
• *Beta blockers:* Altered response to hypoglycemia; prolonged recovery of normoglycemia, hypertension, blockade of tachycardia; may increase blood glucose concentration
• *Clofibrate:* Enhanced effects of oral hypoglycemic drugs
• *Corticosteroids:* Increased blood glucose in diabetic patients
• *Ethanol+:* Excessive intake may lead to altered glycemic control; "Antabuse"-like reaction may occur
• *Halofenate:* Increased serum concentration of sulfonylureas
• *MAOIs:* Excessive hyopglycemia may occur in patients with diabetes
• *Phenylbutazole+:* Increases serum concentrations of oral hypoglycemic drugs
• *Rifampin:* Reduced sulfonylurea concentrations
• *Salicylate:* Enhanced hypoglycemic response to sulfonylureas
• *Sulfonamides:* Enhanced hypoglycemic effects of oral antidiabetic agents
• *Thiazide diuretics:* Potential increased dosage requirement of antidiabetic drugs

SPECIAL CONSIDERATIONS

PATIENT/FAMILY EDUCATION

• Administer 30 min ac
• Avoid alcohol and salicylates
• Notify physician of fever, sore throat, rash, unusual bruising, or bleeding

MONITORING PARAMETERS

• Fasting blood glucose, glycosylated Hgb

glucagon

(gloo'ka-gon)

Chemical Class: Polypeptide hormone

Therapeutic Class: Antihypoglycemic agent

CLINICAL PHARMACOLOGY

Mechanism of Action: Accelerates liver glycogenolysis and inhibits glycogen synthetase resulting in blood glucose elevation; stimulates hepatic gluconeogenesis; relaxes smooth muscle of the GI tract

Pharmacokinetics

IV/IM/SC: Onset within 15 min; degraded in liver, kidney and plasma; $t_{1/2}$ 3-6 min

INDICATIONS AND USES: Hypoglycemia; diagnostic aid in radiologic examination of GI tract when hypotonic state is advantageous

DOSAGE

Adult

- *Hypoglycemia:* IV/IM/SC 0.5-1 mg, may repeat in 20 min prn
- *Diagnostic aid:* IV/IM/SC 0.25-2.0 mg 10 min prior to procedure

Child

- *Hypoglycemia:* IV/IM/SC 30 μg/kg/dose, not to exceed 1 mg/dose, repeat in 20 min prn

Neonate

- *Hypoglycemia:* IV/IM/SC 30 μg/kg/dose, max 1 mg/dose

$ **AVAILABLE FORMS/COST OF THERAPY**

- Inj, Dry-Sol—IM; IV; SC: 10 mg/10 ml, 10's: **$270.06**
- Inj, Sol—IM; IV; SC: 1 mg/vial, 1's: **$27.07-$34.55**

CONTRAINDICATIONS: Hypersensitivity

PRECAUTIONS: Insulinoma, pheochromocytoma

PREGNANCY AND LACTATION: Pregnancy category B; excretion into breast milk unknown, use caution in nursing mothers

SIDE EFFECTS/ADVERSE REACTIONS

CV: Hypotension

GI: Nausea, vomiting

RESP: ***Respiratory distress***

SKIN: Urticaria

▼ **DRUG INTERACTIONS**

Drugs

- *Oral anticoagulants:* Enhanced hypoprothrombinemic response to warfarin, and possibly other oral anticoagulants

SPECIAL CONSIDERATIONS

PATIENT/FAMILY EDUCATION

- Notify physician when hypoglycemic reactions occur so that antidiabetic therapy can be adjusted

---

glutethimide

(gloo-teth'i-mide)

Doriden, Doriglute, Dorimide

Chemical Class: Piperidine derivative

Therapeutic Class: Sedative-hypnotic

DEA Class: Schedule II

CLINICAL PHARMACOLOGY

Mechanism of Action: Depresses activity in brain cells primarily in reticular activating system in brain stem, also selectively depresses neurons in posterior hypothalamus, limbic structures; exhibits pronounced anticholinergic activity; suppresses REM sleep and is associated with REM rebound

Pharmacokinetics

PO: Erratically absorbed from GI tract, peak 1-6 hr, $t_{1/2}$ 10-12 hr, 50% bound to plasma proteins, metabolized in liver to an active metabolite; significant enterohepatic recirculation

INDICATIONS AND USES: Short-term relief of insomnia

DOSAGE

Adult

- PO 250-500 mg hs

$ **AVAILABLE FORMS/COST OF THERAPY**

- Tab, Uncoated—Oral: 500 mg, 100's: **$10.50-$17.93**

CONTRAINDICATIONS: Hypersensitivity, porphyria

PRECAUTIONS: History of drug abuse, children, elderly

PREGNANCY AND LACTATION: Pregnancy category C; newborn infants of mothers dependent on glutethimide may exhibit withdrawal symptoms; excretion into breast milk unknown, use caution in nursing mothers

SIDE EFFECTS/ADVERSE REACTIONS

CNS: Residual sedation, dizziness, ataxia, stimulation, headache, hangover

EENT: Blurred vision

GI: Nausea, vomiting, hiccups, diarrhea, jaundice, dry mouth

HEME: ***Thrombocytopenia, aplastic anemia, leukopenia, megaloblastic anemia,*** porphyria

SKIN: Rash, urticaria, purpura, ***exfoliative dermatitis (rare)***

▼ **DRUG INTERACTIONS**

Drugs

- *Ethanol:* Excessive CNS depression and impaired psychomotor performance
- *Oral anticoagulants+:* Decreased hypoprothrombinemic response to warfarin, and probably other oral anticoagulants

Labs

- *Interference:* 17-OHCS

SPECIAL CONSIDERATIONS

Has generally been replaced with safer and more effective agents

PATIENT/FAMILY EDUCATION

- Use caution when driving or performing tasks requiring alertness
- Avoid alcohol and other CNS depressants

MONITORING PARAMETERS

- Toxic serum glutethimide concentrations are >6 μg/ml

glyburide

(glye'byoor-ide)

DiaBeta, Glynase Prestab, Micronase

Chemical Class: Sulfonylurea (2nd generation)

Therapeutic Class: Antidiabetic

CLINICAL PHARMACOLOGY

Mechanism of Action: Stimulates insulin release from β-cells in the pancreatic islets possibly as a result of increased intracellular cAMP; may improve the binding between insulin and insulin receptors or increase the number of receptors; extrapancreatic effects include suppression of glucagon release and hepatic glucose production

Pharmacokinetics

PO: Completely absorbed by GI route, onset 2-4 hr, peak 2-8 hr, duration 24 hr, $t_{1/2}$ 10 hr (4 hr for micronized formulation), metabolized in liver to weakly active metabolites; excreted in urine, feces (metabolites); 90%-95% bound to plasma proteins

INDICATIONS AND USES: Type II diabetes mellitus

DOSAGE

Adult

- PO 1.25-5 mg qd (0.75-3 mg for micronized formulation) with breakfast or first main meal; not to exceed 20 mg/d (12 mg/d for micronized formulation); (Note: Daily doses >10 mg [6 mg for micronized] provide little added benefit)

$ AVAILABLE FORMS/COST OF THERAPY

- Tab, Uncoated—Oral: 1.25 mg, 100's: **$18.32-$21.52;** 2.5 mg, 100's: **$27.77-$35.87;** 5 mg, 100's: **$50.99-$60.62**
- Tab, Uncoated, Micronized—Oral: 1.5 mg, 100's: **$23.97-$32.50;** 3 mg,

100's: **$40.32-$54.93;** 6 mg, 100's: **$82.40**

CONTRAINDICATIONS: Hypersensitivity to sulfonylureas; diabetes complicated by ketoacidosis

PRECAUTIONS: Elderly, cardiac disease, severe renal disease, severe hepatic disease, thyroid disease, adrenal or pituitary insufficiency, debilitated or malnourished patients

PREGNANCY AND LACTATION: Pregnancy category B; in general avoid the sulfonylurea agents in pregnancy since they will not provide adequate blood glucose control; excretion into breast milk unknown; because of the potential for hypoglycemia in nursing infants, use with caution in nursing mothers

SIDE EFFECTS/ADVERSE REACTIONS

CNS: Dizziness, drowsiness, headache, paresthesia

EENT: Tinnitus, vertigo

GI: Nausea, diarrhea, constipation, gastralgia, cholestatic jaundice, elevated liver function tests

GU: Mild to moderate elevations in BUN and creatinine

HEME: ***Leukopenia, thrombocytopenia, aplastic anemia, agranulocytosis, hemolytic anemia, pancytopenia,*** hepatic porphyria

METAB: ***Hypoglycemia,*** SIADH

MS: Weakness, fatigue

SKIN: Erythema, morbilliform or maculopapular eruptions, urticaria, pruritus, eczema

▼ **DRUG INTERACTIONS**

Drugs

- *Anabolic steroids:* Enhanced hypoglycemic response
- *Beta blockers:* Altered response to hypoglycemia; prolonged recovery of normoglycemia, hypertension, blockade of tachycardia; may increase blood glucose concentration
- *Clofibrate:* Enhanced effects of oral hypoglycemic drugs
- *Corticosteroids:* Increased blood glucose in diabetic patients
- *Ethanol+:* Excessive intake may lead to altered glycemic control; "Antabuse"-like reaction may occur
- *Halofenate:* Increased serum concentration of sulfonylureas
- *MAOIs:* Excessive hypoglycemia may occur in patients with diabetes
- *Phenylbutazole+:* Increases serum concentrations of oral hypoglycemic drugs
- *Rifampin:* Reduced sulfonylurea concentrations
- *Salicylate:* Enhanced hypoglycemic response to sulfonylureas
- *Sulfonamides:* Enhanced hypoglycemic effects of oral antidiabetic agents
- *Thiazide diuretics:* Potential increased dosage requirement of antidiabetic drugs

SPECIAL CONSIDERATIONS

Micronized formulations do not provide bioequivalent serum concentrations to nonmicronized formulations, retitrate patients when transferring from any hypoglycemic to micronized glyburide

PATIENT/FAMILY EDUCATION

- Avoid alcohol and salicylates
- Notify physician of fever, sore throat, rash, unusual bruising, or bleeding

MONITORING PARAMETERS

- Fasting blood glucose, glycosylated Hgb

glycerin

(gli'ser-in)

(Laxative) Fleet Babylax, Glycerin USP, Glycerol, Sani-Supp; (Ophthal) Ophthalgan Ophthalmic; (Oral) Osmoglyn

Chemical Class: Trihydric alcohol

Therapeutic Class: Laxative, hyperosmotic; antiglaucoma agent; osmotic diuretic

CLINICAL PHARMACOLOGY

Mechanism of Action: (Laxative) draws fluid into the colon, stimulates defecation; (Ophthal) attracts water through the semipermeable corneal epithelium, reducing edema and corneal haze transiently; (Oral) adds to the tonicity of blood, reduces intraocular and intracranial pressure

Pharmacokinetics

PO: Well absorbed, onset 10-60 min, duration 2-3 hr

OPHTH: Onset 10 min, peak 20 min, duration 4-8 hr

PR: Poorly absorbed, onset 15-30 min

Metabolized and eliminated by kidney

INDICATIONS AND USES: (Rect) constipation; (Ophth) edematous cornea; (Oral) interruption of acute glaucoma attack, reduction of intraocular pressure pre- and post-ocular surgery, lowering intracranial pressure*

DOSAGE

Adult

- *Constipation:* PR 1 adult supp 1-2 times/d prn or 5-15 ml as an enema
- *Reduction of corneal edema:* OPHTH instill 1 gtt q3-4h
- *Reduction of intraocular pressure:* PO 1-1.8 g/kg 1-1½ hr preoperatively; additional doses may be administered at 5 hr intervals
- *Reduction of intracranial pressure:* PO 1.5 g/kg/d divided q4h or 1 g/kg/dose q6h

Child

- *Constipation:* PR (<6 yr) 1 infant supp 1-2 times/d prn or 2-5 ml as an enema; (>6 yr) same as adult
- *Reduction of corneal edema:* Same as adult
- *Reduction of intraocular pressure:* Same as adult
- *Reduction of intracranial pressure:* Same as adult

Neonate

- *Constipation:* PR 0.5 ml/kg/dose

$ AVAILABLE FORMS/COST OF THERAPY

- Sol—Ophth: 99.5%, 7.5 ml: **$21.25**
- Sol—Oral: 50%, 500 ml: **$3.97-$14.80**
- Supp—Rect: Ped 12's: **$0.76-$4.82;** Adult 12's: **$0.86-$4.82**
- Liq—Rect: Ped 4 ml, 6's: **$2.48**

CONTRAINDICATIONS: (Laxative) hypersensitivity, symptoms of appendicitis, acute surgical abdomen, fecal impaction, intestinal obstruction, undiagnosed abdominal pain; (Ophth) hypersensitivity; (Oral) well established anuria, severe dehydration, pulmonary edema, cardiac decompensation, hypersensitivity

PRECAUTIONS: (Laxative) fluid and electrolyte imbalance, chronic use, rectal bleeding; (Oral) hypervolemia, confused mental status, CHF, diabetes, severe dehydration, cardiac/renal/hepatic disease

PREGNANCY AND LACTATION: Pregnancy category C; data regarding use in breast feeding are unavailable

SIDE EFFECTS/ADVERSE REACTIONS

CNS: Headache, confusion, disorientation (oral); dizziness, fainting (laxative)

CV: ***Dysrhythmias*** (oral); palpitations (laxative)

EENT: Pain or irritation upon instillation (ophth)

GI: Nausea, vomiting (oral); excessive bowel activity, perianal irritation, abdominal pain, flatulence, bloating (laxative)

METAB: ***Hyperosmolar nonketotic coma***

SPECIAL CONSIDERATIONS

PATIENT/FAMILY EDUCATION

- Do not use laxative in the presence of abdominal pain, nausea, or vomiting
- Do not use longer than 1 wk, discontinue when regularity returns
- Prolonged or frequent use may result in dependency or electrolyte imbalance
- Notify physician if unrelieved constipation, rectal bleeding, muscle cramps, weakness, or dizziness occurs

MONITORING PARAMETERS

- Blood glucose, intraocular pressure

---

glycopyrrolate

(glye-koe-pye'roe-late)

Robinul, Robinul Forte

Chemical Class: Quaternary anticholinergic

Therapeutic Class: Anticholinergic; antispasmodic; gastrointestinal agent

CLINICAL PHARMACOLOGY

Mechanism of Action: Inhibits action of acetylcholine on structures innervated by postganglionic cholinergic nerves and on smooth muscles that respond to acetylcholine but lack cholinergic innervation; diminishes volume and free acidity of gastric secretions and controls excessive pharyngeal, tracheal, and bronchial secretions; antagonizes muscarinic symptoms (e.g., bronchorrhea, bronchospasm, bradycardia, and intestinal hypermotility) induced by cholinergic drugs such as the anticholinesterases

Pharmacokinetics

PO: Onset 1 hr, duration 6 hr

IM: Onset 15-30 min, duration 7 hr

IV: Onset 1-10 min, duration 7 hr

Does not penetrate CNS, excreted primarily unchanged via bile, feces

INDICATIONS AND USES: Peptic ulcer (adjunctive therapy); decreases secretions prior to induction of anesthesia, intubation, and surgery; protection against peripheral muscarinic effects of cholinergic agents such as neostigmine and pyridostigmine used to reverse neuromuscular blockade due to non-depolarizing muscle relaxants

DOSAGE

Adult

- *Preoperatively:* IM 0.004 mg/kg 0.5-1 hr before surgery
- *Peptic ulcer:* PO 1-2 mg bid-tid; IM/IV 0.1-0.2 mg tid-qid
- *Reversal of neuromuscular blockade:* IV 0.2 mg for each 1 mg of neostigmine or 5 mg of pyridostigmine administered

Child

- *Preoperatively:* IM (<2 yr) 4.4-8.8 μg/kg 0.5-1 hr before surgery; (>2 yr) 4.4 μg/kg 0.5-1 hr before surgery
- *Reversal of neuromuscular blockade:* same as adult

$ AVAILABLE FORMS/COST OF THERAPY

- Inj, Sol—IM; IV: 0.2 mg/ml, 20 ml:**$1.35-$4.59**
- Tab, Uncoated—Oral: 1 mg, 100's: **$17.55;** 2 mg, 100's: **$27.96**

CONTRAINDICATIONS: Narrow-angle glaucoma, obstructive uropathy, GI tract obstruction, paralytic ileus, intestinal atony, acute hemorrhage, severe ulcerative colitis, toxic megacolon, myasthenia gravis

PRECAUTIONS: Glaucoma, asthma, elderly, prostatic hypertrophy, renal disease, CHF, pulmonary disease, hyperthyroidism, CAD, hypertension

PREGNANCY AND LACTATION: Pregnancy category B; has been used prior to cesarean section to decrease gastric secretions; quaternary structure results in limited placental transfer; excretion into breast milk is unknown but should be minimal due to quaternary structure

SIDE EFFECTS/ADVERSE REACTIONS

CNS: Confusion, anxiety, restlessness, irritability, delusions, hallucinations, headache, sedation, depression, incoherence, dizziness, lethargy, flushing, weakness

CV: Palpitations, tachycardia, postural hypotension, paradoxical bradycardia

EENT: Blurred vision, photophobia, dilated pupils, difficulty swallowing, increased intraocular pressure, mydriasis, cycloplegia, nasal congestion

GI: Dry mouth, constipation, nausea, vomiting, abdominal distress, paralytic ileus, altered taste perception

GU: Hesitancy, retention, impotence

SKIN: Urticaria, allergic reactions, decreased sweating

SPECIAL CONSIDERATIONS

PATIENT/FAMILY EDUCATION

- May cause drowsiness, dizziness, or blurred vision; use caution driving or performing tasks requiring alertness
- Notify physician if skin rash, flushing, or eye pain occurs

gonadorelin

(goe-nad-oh-rell'in)

Lutrepulse (acetate), Factrel (HCl)

Chemical Class: Synthetic endogenous gonadotropin-releasing hormone (GnRH)

Therapeutic Class: Diagnostic agent; gonadotropic hormone

CLINICAL PHARMACOLOGY

Mechanism of Action: Stimulates release of lutenizing hormone (LH) from the anterior pituitary

Pharmacokinetics

IV: Rapidly metabolized to various biologically inactive peptide fragments which are readily excreted in urine; $t_{1/2}$ 2-10 min (initial), 10-40 min (terminal)

INDICATIONS AND USES: Induction of ovulation in primary hypothalamic amenorrhea (acetate); evaluating functional capacity and response of the gonadotropes of the anterior pituitary (suspected gonadotropin deficiency, evaluating residual gonadotropic function of the pituitary following removal of a pituitary tumor by surgery and/or irradiation)

DOSAGE

Adult

- *Primary hypothalamic amenorrhea:* IV (acetate) 5 μg q90 min delivered via the Lutrepulse pump (range 1-20 μg), recommended treatment interval is 21 days; when ovulation occurs with the Lutrepulse pump in place, continue therapy for another 2 wk to maintain the corpus luteum
- *Evaluating functional capacity and response of gonadotropes of the anterior pituitary:* IV/SC (HCl): 100 μg; in females, perform the test in

the early follicular phase (days 1-7) of menstrual cycle

Child

• *Evaluating functional capacity and response of gonadotropes of the anterior pituitary:* IV (HCl): 100 μg

$ AVAILABLE FORMS/COST OF THERAPY

Acetate:

• Inj, Sol—IV: 0.8 mg, 1's: **$144.94;** 3.2 mg, 1's: **$437.44**

• Kit—IV: 0.8 mg, 1's: **$282.44;** 3.2 mg, 1's: **$574.44**

HCl:

• Inj, Sol—IV; SC: 50 μg/ml, 2 ml: **$65.26;** 250 μg/ml, 2 ml:**$108.75**

CONTRAINDICATIONS: (Acetate and HCl) hypersensitivity; (Acetate) any condition that could be exacerbated by pregnancy; reproductive hormone-dependent tumor; ovarian cysts; anovulation not of hypothalamic origin

PRECAUTIONS: Ovarian hyperstimulation is possible; multiple pregnancy is possible

PREGNANCY AND LACTATION: Pregnancy category B; possibility of fetal harm appears remote if used during pregnancy

SIDE EFFECTS/ADVERSE REACTIONS

CNS: Headache, lightheadedness, flushing

GI: Nausea, abdominal discomfort

GU: Ovarian hyperstimulation (sudden ovarian enlargement, ascites, pleural effusion), multiple pregnancy

RESP: ***Anaphylaxis***

SKIN: Local reactions at inf pump catheter site (inflammation, infection, mild phlebitis, hematoma)

▼ DRUG INTERACTIONS

Drugs/Labs

• *Androgen, estrogen, glucocorticoid, and progestin-containing preparations:* directly affect pituitary secretion of gonadotropins

• Do not conduct diagnostic tests during administration of these agents

SPECIAL CONSIDERATIONS

Therapy with the acetate formulation should only be conducted by physicians familiar with pulsatile GnRH delivery and the clinical ramifications of ovulation induction

MONITORING PARAMETERS

• (Acetate) ovarian ultrasound at baseline, therapy day 7, therapy day 14

• Mid-luteal phase serum progesterone

• Clinical observation of inf site at each visit

• Physical exam including pelvic at regularly scheduled visits

---

goserelin

(go'seh-rel-in)

Zoladex

Chemical Class: Synthetic decapeptide analog of LHRH

Therapeutic Class: Gonadotropin-releasing hormone

CLINICAL PHARMACOLOGY

Mechanism of Action: Causes initial increase in serum luteinizing hormone (LH) and follicle stimulating hormone (FSH); chronic administration leads to sustained suppression of pituitary gonadotropins with subsequent reductions in serum testosterone (males) and estradiol (females)

Pharmacokinetics

SC: Peak 12-15 days; released from depot at slower rate for first 8 days, and then more rapidly during the remainder of the 28-day dosing period; $t_{1/2}$ 4.2 hr; cleared via a combination of hepatic metabolism and urinary excretion

INDICATIONS AND USES: Advanced prostate carcinoma, endometriosis, breast cancer*

DOSAGE

Adult

• SC 3.6 mg into upper abdominal wall q28d; recommended duration in endometriosis is 6 mo

$ AVAILABLE FORMS/COST OF THERAPY

• Implant, Cont Rel—SC: 3.6 mg, 1's: **$358.55**

CONTRAINDICATIONS: Hypersensitivity, pregnancy

PRECAUTIONS: Patients at risk for osteoporosis (alcoholism, tobacco abuse, family history, chronic anticonvulsant therapy, chronic corticosteroid use)

PREGNANCY AND LACTATION: Pregnancy category X; excretion into breast milk unknown, use caution in nursing mothers

SIDE EFFECTS/ADVERSE REACTIONS

CNS: Headaches, anxiety, *depression, emotional lability,* nervousness, insomnia, ***spinal cord compression***

CV: ***Dysrhythmia, cerebrovascular accident,*** hypertension, ***MI,*** chest pain, *hot flashes*

GI: Nausea, vomiting, constipation, diarrhea, ulcer

GU: Spotting, breakthrough bleeding, decreased libido, renal insufficiency, urinary obstruction, UTI, vaginal dryness

METAB: Gout, hyperglycemia

MS: Osteoneuralgia, decreased bone mineral density

SKIN: Rash, pain on inj, alopecia, dry skin, skin discoloration, *sweating*

MISC: Change in breast size, gynecomastia, breast tenderness

▼ DRUG INTERACTIONS

Labs

• *Increase:* Alk phosphatase, estradiol, FSH, LH, testosterone levels

• *Decrease:* Testosterone levels, progesterone

SPECIAL CONSIDERATIONS

PATIENT/FAMILY EDUCATION

• Notify physician if regular menstruation persists (females)

• An initial flare in bone pain may occur (prostate cancer therapy)

MONITORING PARAMETERS

• PSA, acid phosphatase, alk phosphatase

• Testosterone level (<25 ng/dl)

G

---

granisetron

(gra-ni'se-tron)

Kytril

Chemical Class: Serotonin antagonist

Therapeutic Class: Antiemetic

CLINICAL PHARMACOLOGY

Mechanism of Action: Selective serotonin-3 receptor antagonist; reduces vagal input and chemoreceptor trigger zone activity mediated by serotonin

Pharmacokinetics

PO: Onset 15-30 min

IV: Onset 1-3 min

Mean $t_{1/2}$ 9 hr in cancer patients (range 1-31 hr); mean 5 hr in normals (range 1-15 hr); 65% protein bound; metabolized by cytochrome P-450 3A, some metabolites active; 12% of drug excreted unchanged in urine; metabolites excreted in urine and feces

INDICATIONS AND USES: Prevention and treatment of emesis due to cancer chemotherapy

DOSAGE

Adult

• IV 10 μg/kg infused over 3-5 min, beginning 30 min before initiation of chemotherapy; no adjustment for renal or hepatic disease; PO 1 mg q12h; 1st dose given 1 hr before chemotherapy, only on the day(s) chemotherapy is given

Child (age 2-16 yr)

• IV 10 μg/kg inf over 3-5 min, beginning 30 min before initiation of chemotherapy; no adjustment for renal or hepatic disease

$ AVAILABLE FORMS/COST OF THERAPY

• Inj, Sol—IV: 1 mg/ml, 1 ml: **$166.00**

• Tab, Uncoated—Oral: 1 mg, 2's: **$78.75**

CONTRAINDICATIONS: Hypersensitivity

PRECAUTIONS: Child <2 yr

PREGNANCY AND LACTATION: Pregnancy category B; breast milk excretion unknown

SIDE EFFECTS/ADVERSE REACTIONS

CNS: Headache, weakness, somnolence, anxiety

CV: Hypertension, hypotension, atrioventricular block, ventricular ectopy

EENT: Dysgeusia

GI: Diarrhea, constipation, elevated transaminase

MISC: Fever

▼ DRUG INTERACTIONS

Drugs

• *Ketoconazole:* Inhibits granisetron metabolism

• *Cytochrome P-450 inducers or inhibitors:* May change granisetron metabolism

griseofulvin

(gri-see-oh-ful'vin)

Fulvicin-U/F, Grifulvin V, Grisactin, Grisactin 500, Fulvicin P/G, Grisactin-Ultra, Gris-PEG

Chemical Class: Penicillium griseofulvum derivative

Therapeutic Class: Antifungal

CLINICAL PHARMACOLOGY

Mechanism of Action: Deposited in the keratin precursor cells, which are gradually exfoliated and replaced by noninfected tissue; has a greater affinity for diseased tissue; tightly bound to the new keratin which becomes highly resistant to fungal invasions

Pharmacokinetics

PO: GI absorption exhibits high interindividual variability; absorption increased by meals with high fat content; ultramicrosize absorbed 1.5 times more efficiently than conventional microsized formulation; peak 4 hr; $t_{1/2}$ 9-24 hr, metabolized in liver; excreted in urine (inactive metabolites), feces, perspiration

INDICATIONS AND USES: Fungal infections of the skin, hair, and nails (i.e tinea corporis, tinea pedis, tinea cruris, tinea barbae, tinea capitis, and tinea unguium) caused by susceptible organisms. Antifungal spectrum usually includes: *Trichophyton rubrum, T. tonsurans, T. mentagrophytes, T. interdigitalis, T. verrucosum, T. megninii, T. gallinae, T. crateriform, T. sulphureum, T. schoenleinii, Microsporum audouinii, M. canis, M. gypseum, Epidermophyton floccosum*

DOSAGE

Adult

• PO (microsize) 500-1000 mg/d in single or divided doses; (ultramicrosize) 330-375 mg/d in single or divided doses, max 750 mg/d

Child ≥2 yr

• PO (microsize) 10-15 mg/kg/d in single or divided doses; (ultramicrosize) 5.5-7.3 mg/kg/d in single or divided doses

Duration

• *Tinea corporis:* 2-4 wk

• *Tinea capitis:* At least 4-6 wk

• *Tinea pedis:* 4-8 wk

• *Tinea unguium:* 3-6 mo

$ AVAILABLE FORMS/COST OF THERAPY

Microsize:

• Tab, Uncoated—Oral: 250 mg, 100's: **$67.04-$70.78;** 500 mg, 100's: **$107.04-$122.73**

• Cap, Gel—Oral: 125 mg, 100's: **$27.98;** 250 mg, 100's: **$69.70**

• Susp—Oral: 125 mg/5 ml, 120 ml: **$22.32**

Ultramicrosize:

• Tab, Uncoated—Oral: 125, 165, 250, 330 mg, 100's: **$33.11-$114.53**

CONTRAINDICATIONS: Hypersensitivity, porphyria, hepatocellular failure

PRECAUTIONS: Penicillin allergy (possible cross-sensitivity), lupus erythematosus

PREGNANCY AND LACTATION: Pregnancy category C; since the use of an antifungal is seldom essential during pregnancy, avoid use during this time; excretion into breast milk unknown, use caution in nursing mothers

SIDE EFFECTS/ADVERSE REACTIONS

CNS: Headache, fatigue, dizziness, insomnia, mental confusion, paresthesias (chronic use)

GI: Oral thrush, nausea, vomiting, epigastric distress, diarrhea, ***hepatic toxicity, GI bleeding***

GU: Proteinuria, menstrual irregularities

HEME: ***Leukopenia, granulocytopenia***

SKIN: Rash, urticaria, angioneurotic edema, photosensitivity

▼ DRUG INTERACTIONS

Drugs

• *Cyclosporine:* Decreased blood concentrations of cyclosporine

• *Oral anticoagulants:* Reduced hypoprothrombinemic response to warfarin and possibly other anticoagulants

• *Oral contraceptives:* Menstrual irregularities, increased risk of pregnancy possible

SPECIAL CONSIDERATIONS

Prior to therapy, the type of fungus responsible for the infection should be identified

PATIENT/FAMILY EDUCATION

• Response to therapy may not be apparent for some time, complete entire course of therapy

• Avoid prolonged exposure to sunlight or sunlamps

• Notify physician if sore throat or skin rash occurs

• Store oral suspensions at room temp in light resistant container

MONITORING PARAMETERS

• Periodic assessments of renal, hepatic, and hematopoietic function during prolonged therapy

G

guaifenesin

(gwye-fen'e-sin)

Amonidrin, Anti-tuss, Breonesin, Fenesin, Gee-Gee, Genatuss, GG-Cen, Glyate, Glycotuss, Glytuss, Guiatuss, Halotussin, Humibid, Humibid L.A., Hytuss, Hytuss 2X, Malotuss, Mytussin, Naldecon Senior EX, Robitussin, Scot-Tussin Expectorant, Sinumist-SR, Uni-Tussin

Chemical Class: Glyceryl derivative

Therapeutic Class: Expectorant; mucolytic

CLINICAL PHARMACOLOGY

Mechanism of Action: Increases the output of respiratory tract fluid by reducing adhesiveness and surface tension, promotes ciliary action and facilitates removal of viscous mucus

Pharmacokinetics

PO: Readily absorbed from GI tract;

rapidly metabolized; excreted in urine; $t_{1/2}$ 1 hr

INDICATIONS AND USES: Dry, nonproductive cough; sinusitis*

DOSAGE

Adult

- PO 100-400 mg q4-6h or 600 mg sustained release q12h; not to exceed 2.4 g/d

Child

- PO (6-12 yr) 100-200 mg q4h, not to exceed 1.2 g/d; (2-6 yr) 50-100 mg q4h, not to exceed 600 mg/d

$ **AVAILABLE FORMS/COST OF THERAPY**

- Cap, Sprinkle—Oral: 300 mg, 100's: **$41.48**
- Liq—Oral: 100 mg/5 ml, 480 ml: **$72.48**
- Tab, Coated, Sust Action—Oral: 600 mg, 100's: **$18.56-$41.99**
- Tab, Uncoated—Oral: 200 mg, 100's: **$23.95-$27.19**

CONTRAINDICATIONS: Hypersensitivity

PRECAUTIONS: Recurrent cough, cough associated with fever, rash, persistant headache, excessive secretions

PREGNANCY AND LACTATION: Pregnancy category C; excretion into breast milk unknown

SIDE EFFECTS/ADVERSE REACTIONS

CNS: Dizziness, headache, drowsiness

GI: Nausea, vomiting, stomach pain

SKIN: Rash

▼ **DRUG INTERACTIONS**

Labs

- *Interference:* 5-HIAA, VMA

SPECIAL CONSIDERATIONS

PATIENT/FAMILY EDUCATION

- Drink a full glass of water with each dose to help further loosen mucus
- Notify physician if cough persists after medication has been used for 7 days or cough is associated with headache, high fever, skin rash, or sore throat

---

guanabenz

(gwan'a-benz)

Wytensin

Chemical Class: Dichlorobenzene derivative

Therapeutic Class: Antihypertensive

CLINICAL PHARMACOLOGY

Mechanism of Action: Stimulates central α_2-adrenergic receptors resulting in decreased sympathetic outflow to the heart, kidneys, and peripheral vasculature; decreases systolic and diastolic blood pressure, systemic vascular resistance, and slightly slows pulse

Pharmacokinetics

PO: Extensive first-pass metabolism, peak 2-5 hr, onset 1 hr, duration 12 hr, 90% bound to plasma proteins, metabolized (site undetermined) and excreted in urine and feces, $t_{1/2}$ approximately 6 hr

INDICATIONS AND USES: Hypertension

DOSAGE

Adult

- PO 4 mg bid initially, increase in 4-8 mg/d increments q1-2 wk prn, not to exceed 32 mg bid

$ **AVAILABLE FORMS/COST OF THERAPY**

- Tab, Uncoated—Oral: 4 mg, 100's: **$52.76-$70.18;** 8 mg, 100's: **$79.20-$105.35**

CONTRAINDICATIONS: Hypersensitivity

PRECAUTIONS: Severe coronary insufficiency, recent MI, cerbrovascular disease, severe renal/hepatic failure, sudden discontinuation

PREGNANCY AND LACTATION: Pregnancy category C; excretion into breast milk unknown, use caution in nursing mothers

SIDE EFFECTS/ADVERSE REACTIONS

CNS: *Drowsiness/sedation, dizziness, weakness, headache,* anxiety, ataxia, depression, sleep disturbance

CV: Chest pain, edema, dysrhythmias, palpitations, ***rebound hypertension with abrupt cessation***

EENT: Nasal congestion, blurred vision

GI: *Dry mouth,* nausea, epigastric pain, diarrhea, vomiting, constipation, abdominal discomfort, taste disorder

GU: Urinary frequency, disturbances of sexual function

METAB: Gynecomastia

MS: Myalgias

RESP: Dyspnea

SKIN: Rash, pruritis

▼ **DRUG INTERACTIONS**

Drugs

• *Beta blockers:* Rebound hypertension from guanabenz withdrawal exacerbated by noncardioselective beta blockers

• *Piribedil:* Inhibited antiparkinsonian effect of piribedil

SPECIAL CONSIDERATIONS

PATIENT/FAMILY EDUCATION

• Avoid hazardous activities, since drug may cause drowsiness

• Do not discontinue oral drug abruptly, or withdrawal symptoms may occur (anxiety, increased BP, headache, insomnia, increased pulse, tremors, nausea, sweating

• Do not use OTC (cough, cold, or allergy) products unless directed by physician

• Rise slowly to sitting or standing position to minimize orthostatic hypotension, especially elderly

• May cause dizziness, fainting, light-headedness during 1st few days of therapy

• May cause dry mouth; use hard candy, saliva product, or frequent rinsing of mouth

guanadrel

(gwahn'a-drel)

Hylorel

Chemical Class: Guanidine derivative

Therapeutic Class: Antihypertensive

CLINICAL PHARMACOLOGY

Mechanism of Action: Slowly displaces norepinephrine from its storage in nerve endings and thereby blocks the release of norepinephrine normally produced by nerve stimulation; leads to reduced arteriolar vasoconstriction, especially the reflex increase in sympathetic tone that occurs with a change in position

Pharmacokinetics

PO: Peak 1½-2 hr, onset 2 hr, duration 4-14 hr, <20% bound to plasma proteins, metabolized in liver, excreted in urine (40% as unchanged drug), $t_{1/2}$ approximately 10 hr (high interindividual variation)

INDICATIONS AND USES: Hypertension (not first line)

DOSAGE

Adult

• PO 10 mg/d as a single dose or divided bid; usual range 20-75 mg/d generally divided bid-qid; renal function impairment, CrCl 30-60 ml/min, 5 mg qd; CrCl <30 ml/min, 5 mg qod

$ **AVAILABLE FORMS/COST OF THERAPY**

• Tab, Uncoated—Oral: 10 mg, 100's: **$71.99;** 25 mg, 100's: **$104.20**

CONTRAINDICATIONS: Pheochromocytoma, hypersensitivity, CHF, concurrent use with or within 1 wk of MAOI

PRECAUTIONS: Cerebral vascular disease, CAD, elective surgery, asthma, renal function impairment, children, peptic ulcer, elderly

PREGNANCY AND LACTATION: Pregnancy category B; excretion into breast milk unknown, use caution in nursing mothers

SIDE EFFECTS/ADVERSE REACTIONS

CNS: Fatigue, headache, faintness, drowsiness, paresthesias, confusion, psychological problems, *depression,* sleep disorder

CV: Palpitations, bradycardia, chest pain, syncope, *peripheral edema, orthostatic hypotension,* ***CHF***

EENT: Nasal stuffiness, tinnitus, visual changes, sore throat, double vision, dry burning eyes

GI: Increased bowel movements, abdominal pain, constipation, anorexia, glossitis, nausea, vomiting, dry mouth/throat

GU: Nocturia, urinary frequency/urgency, ejaculation disturbances, impotence, hematuria

MS: Leg cramps, joint pain, aching limbs

RESP: ***Bronchspasm***

SKIN: Rash, purpura, alopecia

MISC: Weight gain/loss

▼ **DRUG INTERACTIONS**

Drugs

- *Methylphenidate:* Inhibition of antihypertensive response to guanadrel
- *Norepinephrine:* Exaggerated pressor response to norepinephrine
- *Phenylephrine:* Enhanced pupillary response to phenylephrine eye drops
- *Phenothiazines:* Inhibition of antihypertensive response to guanadrel

SPECIAL CONSIDERATIONS

PATIENT/FAMILY EDUCATION

- Arise slowly from a reclining position, especially in the morning
- Avoid OTC medications except as directed by physician
- Avoid driving, hazardous activities if drowsiness occurs

MONITORING PARAMETERS

- Sitting and standing blood pressure, pulse

---

guanethidine

(gwahn-eth'i-deen)

Ismelin

Chemical Class: Guanidine derivative

Therapeutic Class: Antihypertensive

CLINICAL PHARMACOLOGY

Mechanism of Action: Slowly displaces norepinephrine from its storage in nerve endings and thereby blocks the release of norepinephrine normally produced by nerve stimulation; leads to reduced arteriolar vasoconstriction, especially the reflex increase in sympathetic tone that occurs with a change in position

Pharmacokinetics

PO: Oral absorption highly variable (3%-30%), full therapeutic effect can take 1-3 wk, metabolized in liver, excreted in urine (25%-50% as unchanged drug), $t_{1/2}$ 4-8 days

INDICATIONS AND USES: Hypertension (not first line)

DOSAGE

Adult

- *Ambulatory patients:* PO 10 mg qd, increase at 5-7 day intervals to a max of 25-50 mg/d
- *Hospitalized patients:* PO 25-50 mg qd, increase by 25-50 mg/d to desired therapeutic response

Child

- PO 0.2 mg/kg/d, increase by 0.2 mg/kg/d at 7-10 day intervals to a max of 3 mg/kg/d

AVAILABLE FORMS/COST OF THERAPY

• Tab, Uncoated—Oral: 10 mg, 100's: **$49.67;** 25 mg, 100's: **$81.17**

CONTRAINDICATIONS: Hypersensitivity, pheochromocytoma, CHF, concurrent use with or within 1 wk of MAOI

PRECAUTIONS: Elective surgery (discontinue 2 wk prior to procedure), fever (reduced dosage requirements), asthma, recent MI, CAD, peptic ulcer, elderly

PREGNANCY AND LACTATION: Pregnancy category C; excreted into breast milk in small quantities, problems in humans have not been documented

SIDE EFFECTS/ADVERSE REACTIONS

CNS: Dizziness, weakness, lassitude, fatigue, tremor, mental depression

CV: Bradycardia, fluid retention, edema, angina, *orthostatic hypotension,* syncope, ***CHF***

EENT: Blurred vision, ptosis of the lids, *nasal congestion*

GI: Nausea, vomiting, dry mouth, parotid tenderness, *diarrhea*

GU: Inhibition of ejaculation, rise in BUN, nocturia, urinary incontinence, priapism, impotence

HEME: Anemia, ***thrombocytopenia, leukopenia***

MS: Myalgia

RESP: Dyspnea, asthma

SKIN: Dermatitis, alopecia

▼ **DRUG INTERACTIONS**

Drugs

• *Amphetamines, cyclic antidepressants, ephedrine, haloperidol+, methylphenidate, phenothiazines:* Inhibition of antihypertensive response to guanethidine

• *Norepinephrine:* Exaggerated pressor response to norepinephrine

• *Phenylephrine:* Enhanced pupillary response to phenylephrine eye drops

Labs

• *Increase:* BUN

• *Decrease:* Blood glucose, VMA excretion, urinary norepinephrine

SPECIAL CONSIDERATIONS

PATIENT/FAMILY EDUCATION

• Arise slowly from a reclining position, especially in the morning

• Use alcohol with caution

• Use caution when standing for prolonged periods of time, exercising, and during hot weather (enhanced orthostatic hypotension)

• Avoid OTC medications unless discussed with physician

• Notify physician of fever, severe diarrhea

• Do not discontinue abruptly

MONITORING PARAMETERS

• Sitting and standing blood pressure, pulse

---

guanfacine

(gwahn'fa-seen)

Tenex

Chemical Class: Dichlorobenzene derivative

Therapeutic Class: Antihypertensive

CLINICAL PHARMACOLOGY

Mechanism of Action: Stimulates central α_2-adrenergic receptors resulting in decreased sympathetic outflow to the heart, kidneys, and peripheral vasculature; decreases systolic and diastolic blood pressure, systemic vascular resistance, and slightly slows pulse

Pharmacokinetics

PO: Peak 1-4 hr, onset (multiple doses) 1 wk, 70% bound to plasma proteins, 50% bound to erythrocytes, metabolized in liver, excreted in urine (40% as unchanged drug), $t_{1/2}$ 17 hr

G

INDICATIONS AND USES: Hypertension, heroin withdrawal syndrome,* migraine headache*

DOSAGE

Adult

• PO 1 mg qd, increase to 2 mg qd after 3-4 wk prn

$ **AVAILABLE FORMS/COST OF THERAPY**

• Tab, Uncoated—Oral: 1 mg, 100's: **$83.04;** 2 mg, 100's: **$113.85**

CONTRAINDICATIONS: Hypersensitivity

PRECAUTIONS: Chronic renal or hepatic failure, severe coronary insufficiency, recent MI, cerebrovascular disease, children

PREGNANCY AND LACTATION: Pregnancy category B; excretion into human breast milk unknown, excreted in the milk of lactating rats, use caution in nursing mothers

SIDE EFFECTS/ADVERSE REACTIONS

CNS: Somnolence, dizziness, headache, fatigue

CV: Bradycardia, chest pain, palpitations

EENT: Taste change, tinnitus, vision change, rhinitis, nasal congestion

GI: Dry mouth, constipation, cramps, nausea, diarrhea

GU: Impotence, urinary incontinence

MS: Leg cramps

RESP: Dyspnea

SKIN: Dermatitis, pruritus, purpura

▼ **DRUG INTERACTIONS**

Drugs

• *Beta blockers:* Rebound hypertension from halazepam withdrawal exacerbated by noncardioselective beta blockers

• *Piribedil:* Inhibited antiparkinsonian effect of piribedil

SPECIAL CONSIDERATIONS

PATIENT/FAMILY EDUCATION

• Avoid hazardous activities, since drug may cause drowsiness

• Do not discontinue oral drug abruptly, or withdrawal symptoms may occur after 3-4 days (anxiety, increased B/P, headache, insomnia, increased pulse, tremors, nausea, sweating)

• Do not use OTC (cough, cold, or allergy) products unless directed by physician

• Rise slowly to sitting or standing position to minimize orthostatic hypotension, especially elderly

• Dizziness, fainting, light-headedness may occur during 1st few days of therapy

• May cause dry mouth; use hard candy, saliva product, or frequent rinsing of mouth

---

halazepam

(hal-az'e-pam)

Paxipam

Chemical Class: Benzodiazepine

Therapeutic Class: Anxiolytic

DEA Class: Schedule IV

CLINICAL PHARMACOLOGY

Mechanism of Action: Facilitates the inhibitory effect of γ-aminobutyric acid (GABA) on neuronal excitability by increasing membrane permeability to chloride ions

Pharmacokinetics

PO: Peak 1-3 hr, metabolized by the liver to active metabolites, eliminated in the urine, $t_{1/2}$ 14 hr

INDICATIONS AND USES: Anxiety

DOSAGE

Adult

• PO 20-40 mg tid-qid

Geriatric

• PO 20 mg qd-bid

$ **AVAILABLE FORMS/COST OF THERAPY**

• Tab, Uncoated—Oral: 20 mg, 100's: **$44.74;** 40 mg, 100's: **$62.18**

CONTRAINDICATIONS: Hypersensitivity to benzodiazepines, narrow angle glaucoma, psychosis, pregnancy

PRECAUTIONS: Elderly, debilitated, hepatic disease, renal disease, history of drug abuse, abrupt withdrawal, respiratory depression

PREGNANCY AND LACTATION: Pregnancy category D; may cause fetal damage when administered during pregnancy; excreted into breast milk, may accumulate in breast-fed infants and is therefore not recommended

SIDE EFFECTS/ADVERSE REACTIONS

CNS: Somnolence, asthenia, hypokinesia, hangover, abnormal thinking, anxiety, agitation, amnesia, apathy, emotional lability, hostility, seizure, sleep disorder, stupor, twitch, ataxia, decreased libido, decreased reflexes, neuritis

CV: Dysrhythmia, syncope

EENT: Ear pain, eye irritation/pain/swelling, photophobia, pharyngitis, rhinitis, sinusitis, epistaxis

GI: Dyspepsia, decreased/increased appetite, flatulence, gastritis, enterocolitis, melena, mouth ulceration, abdominal pain, increased AST

GU: Frequent urination, menstrual cramps, urinary hesitancy/urgency, vaginal discharge/itching, hematuria, nocturia, oliguria, penile discharge, urinary incontinence

HEME: ***Agranulocytosis***

MS: Lower extremity pain, back pain,

RESP: Cold symptoms, asthma, cough, dyspnea, hyperventilation

SKIN: Urticaria, acne, dry skin, photosensitivity

▼ **DRUG INTERACTIONS**

Drugs

• *Cimetidine:* Increased plasma concentrations of halazepam

Labs

• *Increase:* AST/ALT, serum bilirubin

• *Decrease:* RAIU

• *False increase:* 17-OHCS

SPECIAL CONSIDERATIONS

PATIENT/FAMILY EDUCATION

• Avoid alcohol and other CNS depressants

• Do not discontinue abruptly after prolonged therapy

• May cause drowsiness or dizziness, use caution while driving or performing other tasks requiring alertness

• Inform physician if you are planning to become pregnant, you are pregnant, or if you become pregnant while taking this medicine

• May be habit forming

MONITORING PARAMETERS

• Periodic CBC, U/A, blood chemistry analyses during prolonged therapy

---

halcinonide

(hal-sin′o-nide)

Halog, Halog-E

Chemical Class: Synthetic fluorinated agent; Group II (high) potency

Therapeutic Class: Topical corticosteroid

CLINICAL PHARMACOLOGY

Mechanism of Action: Depresses formation, release, and activity of endogenous mediators of inflammation such as prostaglandins, kinins, histamine, liposomal enzymes, and the complement system resulting in decreased edema, erythema, and pruritus

Pharmacokinetics

Absorbed through the skin (increased by inflammation and occlusive dressings), metabolized primarily in the liver

INDICATIONS AND USES: Psoriasis, eczema, contact dermatitis, pruritus

DOSAGE

Adult and Child

• Apply to affected area bid-tid; rub completely into skin

AVAILABLE FORMS/COST OF THERAPY

• Cre, Oint—Top: 0.1%, 15, 30, 60, 240 g: **$17.84-$162.06**

• Sol—Top: 0.1%, 20, 60 ml: **$22.08-$49.45**

CONTRAINDICATIONS: Hypersensitivity to corticosteroids, fungal infections, use on face, groin, or axilla

PRECAUTIONS: Viral infections, bacterial infections, children

PREGNANCY AND LACTATION: Pregnancy category C; unknown whether top application could result in sufficient systemic absorption to produce detectable amounts in breast milk (systemic corticosteroids are secreted into breast milk in quantities not likely to have detrimental effects on infant)

SIDE EFFECTS/ADVERSE REACTIONS

SKIN: Burning, dryness, itching, irritation, acne, folliculitis, hypertrichosis, perioral dermatitis, hypopigmentation, atrophy, striae, miliaria, allergic contact dermatitis, secondary infection

MISC: Systemic absorption of topical corticosteroids has produced reversible HPA axis suppression (more likely with occlusive dressings, prolonged administration, application to large surface areas, liver failure, and in children)

SPECIAL CONSIDERATIONS

PATIENT/FAMILY EDUCATION

• Apply sparingly only to affected area

• Avoid contact with the eyes

• Do not put bandages or dressings over treated area unless directed by physician

• Do not use on weeping, denuded, or infected areas

• Discontinue drug, notify physician if local irritation or fever develops

halobetasol

(hal-oh-be'ta-sol)

Ultravate

Chemical Class: Synthetic fluorinated agent; Group I (very high) potency

Therapeutic Class: Topical corticosteroid

CLINICAL PHARMACOLOGY

Mechanism of Action: Depresses formation, release, and activity of endogenous mediators of inflammation such as prostaglandins, kinins, histamine, liposomal enzymes, and the complement system resulting in decreased edema, erythema, and pruritus

Pharmacokinetics

Absorbed through the skin (increased by inflammation and occlusive dressings), metabolized primarily in the liver

INDICATIONS AND USES: Psoriasis, eczema, contact dermatitis, pruritus

DOSAGE

Adult and Child

• Apply to affected area bid-tid; rub completely into skin; total dosage should not exceed 50 g/wk because of the drug's potential to suppress the hypothalamic-pituitary-adrenal (HPA) axis; treatment beyond 2 consecutive wk not recommended

AVAILABLE FORMS/COST OF THERAPY

• Cre, Oint—Top: 0.05%, 15, 50 g: **$20.90-$51.19**

CONTRAINDICATIONS: Hypersensitivity to corticosteroids, fungal infections, use on face, groin, or axilla, occlusive dressings

PRECAUTIONS: Viral infections, bacterial infections, children

PREGNANCY AND LACTATION: Pregnancy category C; unknown whether TOP application could result in sufficient systemic absorption to produce detectable amounts in breast milk (systemic corticosteroids are secreted into breast milk in quantities not likely to have detrimental effects on infant)

SIDE EFFECTS/ADVERSE REACTIONS

SKIN: Burning, dryness, itching, irritation, acne, folliculitis, hypertrichosis, perioral dermatitis, hypopigmentation, atrophy, striae, miliaria, allergic contact dermatitis, secondary infection

MISC: Systemic absorption of topical corticosteroids has produced reversible HPA axis suppression (more likely with occlusive dressings, prolonged administration, application to large surface areas, liver failure, and in children)

SPECIAL CONSIDERATIONS

PATIENT/FAMILY EDUCATION

- Apply sparingly only to affected area
- Avoid contact with the eyes
- Do not put bandages or dressings over treated area
- Do not use on weeping, denuded, or infected areas
- Discontinue drug, notify physician if local irritation or fever develops
- Treatment should be limited to two wk, and amounts greater than 50 g/wk should not be used

haloperidol

(ha-loe-per′idole)

Haldol, Haldol Decanoate

Chemical Class: Butyrophenone

Therapeutic Class: Antipsychotic/neuroleptic

CLINICAL PHARMACOLOGY

Mechanism of Action: Competitively blocks postsynaptic dopamine receptors in the mesolimbic dopaminergic system which increases turnover of brain dopamine producing an antipsychotic action; blockade of dopamine receptors in the nigrostriatal dopamine pathway produces extrapyramidal motor reactions; blockade of dopamine receptors in the tuberoinfundibular system decreases growth hormone release and increases prolactin release by the pituitary; also some blockade of α-adrenergic receptors of the autonomic nervous system

Pharmacokinetics

PO: Peak 3-6 hr, $t_{1/2}$ 17 hr

IM: Peak 10-20 min, $t_{1/2}$ 17 hr

IM (decanoate): Peak 3-9 days, $t_{1/2}$ approximately 3 wk

>90% bound to plasma proteins, metabolized by the liver, excreted in urine and feces

INDICATIONS AND USES: Psychosis, Gilles de la Tourette syndrome, severe behavioral problems, hyperactive children (short-term), prolonged parenteral neuroleptic therapy for chronic schizophrenia (decanoate), antiemetic* (small doses)

DOSAGE

Adult

- *Psychosis/Tourette's syndrome:* PO 0.5-5 mg bid or tid initially depending on severity of condition; dose is increased to desired dose, max 100 mg/d; IM 2-5 mg q1-8h

• *Chronic schizophrenia:* IM 10-15 times the individual patient's stabilized PO dose q4wk (decanoate)

Child 3-12 yr

• *Psychosis:* PO/IM 0.05-0.15 mg/kg/d in 2-3 divided doses

• *Tourette's syndrome:* PO 0.05-0.075 mg/kg/d in 2-3 divided doses

• *Hyperactivity:* PO 0.05-0.075 mg/kg/d in 2-3 divided doses

$ AVAILABLE FORMS/COST OF THERAPY

• Conc—Oral: 2 mg/ml, 120 ml: **$26.75-$96.23**

• Inj, Sol—IM: 5 mg/ml, 10 ml: **$16.68-$58.67**

• Tab, Uncoated—Oral: 0.5, 1, 2, 5, 10, 20 mg, 100's: **$1.88-$338.66**

CONTRAINDICATIONS: Severe toxic CNS depression, comatose states from any cause, hypersensitivity, Parkinson's disease

PRECAUTIONS: Elderly, severe cardiac disorders, seizure disorder, hepatic dysfunction, child <3 yr, alcohol withdrawal, electroconvulsive therapy, abrupt withdrawal, glaucoma

PREGNANCY AND LACTATION: Pregnancy category C; has been used for hyperemesis gravidarum, chorea gravidarum, and manic-depressive illness during pregnancy; excreted into breast milk, effect on nursing infant unknown but may be of concern

SIDE EFFECTS/ADVERSE REACTIONS

CNS: EPS (pseudoparkinsonism, akathisia, dystonia, tardive dyskinesia), drowsiness, headache, ***seizures, neuroleptic malignant syndrome,*** confusion, insomnia, restlessness, anxiety, euphoria, agitation, depression, lethargy, vertigo, exacerbation of psychotic symptoms including hallucinations, catatonic-like behavioral states

CV: ***Tachycardia,*** hypotension, hypertension, ECG changes

EENT: Blurred vision, glaucoma, dry eyes, cataracts, retinopathy

GI: Anorexia, constipation, diarrhea, hypersalivation, dyspepsia, *nausea,* vomiting, *dry mouth*

GU: Urinary retention, priapism

HEME: Transient leukopenia, leukocytosis, minimal decreases in red blood cell counts, anemia, ***agranulocytosis***

METAB: Lactation, breast engorgement, mastalgia, menstrual irregularities, gynecomastia, impotence, increased libido, hyperglycemia, hypoglycemia, hyponatremia

RESP: Laryngospasm, bronchospasm, increased depth of respiration

SKIN: Maculopapular and acneiform skin reactions, isolated cases of photosensitivity, loss of hair, diaphoresis

▼ DRUG INTERACTIONS

Drugs

• *Anticholinergics:* Inhibition of therapeutic effect of neuroleptics

• *Barbiturates:* Potential reduction of serum neuroleptic concentrations

• *Bromocriptine:* Inhibition of bromocriptine's ability to lower serum prolactin concentrations in patients with pituitary adenoma; theoretical inhibition of antipsychotic effects of neuroleptics

• *Carbamazepine:* Decreased serum haloperidol concentrations

• *Guanethidine+:* Inhibition of antihypertensive effect of guanethidine

• *Levodopa:* Inhibition of antiparkinsonian effects of levodopa

• *Lithium:* Rare reports of severe neurotoxicity in patients receiving lithium and neuroleptics

Labs

• *Increase:* Liver function tests, cardiac enzymes, cholesterol, blood glucose, prolactin, bilirubin, PBI, cholinesterase

• *Decrease:* Hormones (blood, urine)

• *False positive:* Pregnancy tests, PKU

• *False negative:* Urinary steroids

SPECIAL CONSIDERATIONS

PATIENT/FAMILY EDUCATION

• Do not mix liquid formulation with coffee or tea
• Use calibrated dropper
• Take with food or milk
• Arise slowly from reclining position
• Do not discontinue abruptly
• Use a sunscreen during sun exposure to prevent burns
• Take special precautions to stay cool in hot weather

MONITORING PARAMETERS

• Observe closely for signs of tardive dyskinesia

haloprogin

(ha-loe-proe′jin)

Halotex

Chemical Class: Iodinated phenolic ester

Therapeutic Class: Local anti-infective, antifungal

CLINICAL PHARMACOLOGY

Mechanism of Action: Interferes with fungal cell membrane permeability

Pharmacokinetics

TOP: Absorbed poorly through the skin

INDICATIONS AND USES: Tinea pedis (athlete's foot), tinea cruris (jock itch), tinea corporis (ringworm), tinea manuum, tinea versicolor. Antifungal spectrum usually includes: *Trichophyton rubrum, T. tonsurans, T. mentagrophytes, Microsporum canis, Epidermophyton floccosum, Malassezia furfur*

DOSAGE

Adult and Child

• TOP apply to affected area bid for 14-21 days, intertriginous lesions may require up to 28 days of therapy

$ **AVAILABLE FORMS/COST OF THERAPY**

• Cre, Sol—Top: 1%, 15, 30 g: **$12.24-$22.98**

CONTRAINDICATIONS: Hypersensitivity

PREGNANCY AND LACTATION: Pregnancy category B; excretion into breast milk unknown, problems have not been documented

SIDE EFFECTS/ADVERSE REACTIONS

SKIN: Local irritation, burning sensation, vesicle formation, erythema, scaling, itching, folliculitis, pruritus

SPECIAL CONSIDERATIONS

PATIENT/FAMILY EDUCATION

• For external use only
• Avoid contact with eyes
• Complete full course of therapy
• Notify physician if condition worsens, or if irritation, redness, swelling, stinging, or burning persists

heparin

(hep′a-rin)

Liquaemin

Chemical Class: Sulfated glycosaminoglycan

Therapeutic Class: Anticoagulant

CLINICAL PHARMACOLOGY

Mechanism of Action: Potentiates inhibitory action of antithrombin III (heparin cofactor) on several activated coagulation factors, including thrombin (factor IIa) and factors IXa, Xa, XIa, and XIIa, by forming a

H

complex with and inducing a conformational change in the antithrombin III molecule

Pharmacokinetics

IV: Onset immediate (if no loading dose is given, onset may depend on rate of inf)

SC: Onset 20-60 min

Highly bound to plasma proteins, primary route of removal from circulation via uptake by the reticuloendothelial system, also metabolized by liver, eliminated in urine usually as metabolites (50% of IV dose may be excreted unchanged), $t_{1/2}$ 90 min

INDICATIONS AND USES: Venous thrombosis, pulmonary embolism, peripheral arterial embolism; coagulopathies (e.g. disseminated intravascular coagulation); DVT/PE prophylaxis; clotting prevention in arterial and heart surgery, blood transfusions, extracorporeal circulation, dialysis and blood samples; prophylaxis of LV thrombi and CVA post MI;* evolving stroke;* adjunctive therapy of coronary occlusion with acute MI*

DOSAGE

Adult

• *DVT/PE:* IV INF 50-100 U/kg initially, then 15-25 U/kg/hr, adjusted based on aPTT results; intermittent IV 10,000 U initially, then 75-125 U/kg q4-6h; SC 10,000-20,000 units initially, then 8000-10,000 U q8h, or 15,000-20,000 U q12h

• *Prevention of DVT/PE:* SC 5000 U q8-12h until patient is ambulatory

Child

• IV INF 50 U/kg initially, then 15-25 U/kg/hr; increase dose by 2-4 U/kg/hr q6-8h based on aPTT results; intermittent IV 50-100 U/kg initially, then 50-100 U/kg q4h

$ AVAILABLE FORMS/COST OF THERAPY

• Inj, Sol—IV; SC: 40,000 U/ml: **$15.60-$22.75**

• Inj, Sol—IV: 40 U/ml, 500 ml: **$11.57-$21.30;** 50 U/ml, 500 ml: **$2.05;** 100 U/ml, 250 ml: **$10.53-$22.15;** 1000 U/ml, 10 ml: **$3.03-$64.06;** 2500 U/ml, 5 ml: **$3.41;** 5000 U/ml, 1 ml: **$1.03-$1.61;** 10,000 U/ml, 10 ml: **$7.75-$17.25;** 20,000 U/ml, 5 ml: **$7.44-$15.90**

CONTRAINDICATIONS: Hypersensitivity, severe thrombocytopenia, uncontrolled bleeding (except when due to DIC), suspected intracranial hemorrhage, shock, severe hypotension

PRECAUTIONS: IM inj (avoid due to risk for hematoma), elderly, children, diabetes, renal insufficiency, severe hypertension, subacute bacterial endocarditis, acute nephritis, peptic ulcer disease, severe renal disease

PREGNANCY AND LACTATION: Pregnancy category C; does not cross the placenta, has major advantages over oral anticoagulants as the treatment of choice during pregnancy; is not excreted into breast milk due to its high molecular weight

SIDE EFFECTS/ADVERSE REACTIONS

CNS: Headache, fever

CV: Shock, ***allergic vasospastic reactions***

EENT: Rhinitis, lacrimation

GI: Nausea, vomiting

GU: Priapism, ***hematuria***

HEME: ***Hemorrhage, thrombocytopenia, white clot syndrome (new thrombus formation associated with heparin administration)***

METAB: Suppressed aldosterone synthesis, rebound hyperlipidemia

MS: Osteoporosis (after long-term, high doses)

RESP: Asthma, ***anaphylactoid reactions***
SKIN: ***Cutaneous necrosis,*** delayed transient alopecia, local irritation, erythema, hematoma/ulceration, histamine-like reactions, chills, urticaria

▼ **DRUG INTERACTIONS**

Drugs

• *Oral anticoagulants:* Warfarin may prolong the aPTT in patients receiving heparin; heparin may prolong the PT in patients receiving warfarin
• *Salicylates:* Increased risk of bleeding

Labs

• *Increase:* T_3 uptake
• *Decrease:* Uric acid

SPECIAL CONSIDERATIONS

PATIENT/FAMILY EDUCATION

• Use soft-bristle toothbrush to avoid bleeding gums, avoid contact sports, use electric razor, avoid IM inj
• Report any signs of bleeding: gums, under skin, urine, stools

MONITORING PARAMETERS

• aPTT (usual goal is to prolong aPTT to 1.5-2.5 times normal), usually measure 6-8 hr after initiation of IV and 6-8 hr after inf rate changes; increase or decrease inf by 2-4 U/kg/hr dependent on aPTT
• For intermittent inj measure aPTT 3.5-4 hr after IV inj
• Platelet counts, signs of bleeding, Hgb, Hct

homatropine hydrobromide (optic)

(hoe-mat′ro-peen)
AK-Homatropine, Homatrine, I-Homatrine, Isopto Homatropine
Chemical Class: Belladonna alkaloid
Therapeutic Class: Mydriatic; cytoplegic; anticholinergic

CLINICAL PHARMACOLOGY

Mechanism of Action: Blocks responses of the sphincter muscle of the iris and the accommodative muscle of the ciliary body to stimulation by acetylcholine; dilation of the pupil (mydriasis) and paralysis of accommodation (cytoplegia) result

Pharmacokinetics

OPHTH: Peak ½-1 hr, duration 1-3 days

INDICATIONS AND USES: Uveitis, iritis, mydriatic, cycloplegic for refraction

DOSAGE

Adult and Child

• INSTILL 1 gtt; repeat in 5-10 min for refraction or q3-4h for uveitis; patients with heavily pigmented irides may require larger doses; use only 2% strength in children and compress the lacrimal sac for several min following instillation

$ **AVAILABLE FORMS/COST OF THERAPY**

• Sol—Ophth: 2%, 5, 15 ml: **$10.94-$15.12;** 5%, 5, 15 ml: **$10.02-$16.37**
• Sol—Ophth; Top: 5%, 1 ml units, 1 ml × 12: **$25.80**

CONTRAINDICATIONS: Hypersensitivity to belladonna alkaloids, adhesions between the iris and the lens, primary glaucoma, narrow anterior chamber angle

PRECAUTIONS: Elderly, small children, and infants

PREGNANCY AND LACTATION: Pregnancy category C; may be detectable in very small amounts in breast milk; compatible with breast-feeding

SIDE EFFECTS/ADVERSE REACTIONS

CNS: Confusion, somnolence, headache, visual hallucinations, fever

CV: Tachycardia, vasodilation

EENT: Blurred vision, photophobia, increased intraocular pressure, irritation, edema

GI: Dry mouth, abdominal distension in infants, decreased GI motility

GU: Urinary retention

SKIN: Rash, dry skin

SPECIAL CONSIDERATIONS

PATIENT/FAMILY EDUCATION

- Do not touch tip of dropper to any surface
- May cause blurred vision, do not drive or engage in any hazardous activities while pupils are dilated
- May cause sensitivity to light, protect eyes from bright light
- Wash hands immediately following instillation
- Discontinue immediately if eye pain occurs
- To minimize systemic effects, compress the lacrimal sac for several minutes following instillation

hyaluronidase

(hye-al-yoor-on′i-dase)

Wydase

Chemical Class: Protein enzyme

Therapeutic Class: Adjuvant for injectables

CLINICAL PHARMACOLOGY

Mechanism of Action: Modifies permeability of connective tissue through hydrolysis of hyaluronic acid; enhances diffusion of substances injected SC

INDICATIONS AND USES: Hypodermoclysis; subcutaneous urography; adjunct to dispersion of other drugs; enhances diffusion of locally irritating or toxic drugs in management of IV extravasation

DOSAGE

Adult and Child

- *Adjunct to dispersion of other drugs:* INJ 150 U with other drug; consult appropriate references regarding physical or chemical incompatibilities before adding hyaluronidase to sol containing other drug
- *Hypodermoclysis:* SC 150 U/1000 ml of clysis sol; for child <3 yr, limit volume of single clysis to 200 ml
- *SC urography:* SC 75 U over each scapula, then contrast medium injected at same sites

$ **AVAILABLE FORMS/COST OF THERAPY**

- Inj, Lyphl-Sol—SC: 150 U/ml, 10 ml: **$21.06**

CONTRAINDICATIONS: Hypersensitivity to bovine products, inj into infected, acutely inflamed, or cancerous area

PREGNANCY AND LACTATION: Pregnancy category C; excretion into breast milk unknown, use caution in nursing mothers

SIDE EFFECTS/ADVERSE REACTIONS

SKIN: Urticaria, rash, itching

SPECIAL CONSIDERATIONS

Prior to administration, conduct a preliminary test for sensitivity: 0.02 ml of 150 U/ml sol is injected, if wheal with pseudopods develops within 5 min and persists for 20-30 min, test is positive

hydralazine
(hye-dral'a-zeen)
Apresoline
Chemical Class: Phthalazine
Therapeutic Class: Antihypertensive; direct-acting peripheral vasodilator

CLINICAL PHARMACOLOGY
Mechanism of Action: Preferentially dilates arterioles with little effect on veins; interferes with calcium movement within vascular smooth muscle responsible for initiating or maintaining the contractile state; increases cardiac output, decreases systemic resistance, reduces afterload
Pharmacokinetics
PO: Well absorbed, undergoes first-pass metabolism, bioavailability 50% (slow acetylators) or 30% (fast acetylators), peak 60 min, onset 45 min, duration 3-8 hr
IM: Onset 5-10 min, peak 1 hr, duration 2-4 hr
IV: Onset 10-20 min, duration 3-8 hr
Metabolized by liver (genetic variation among individuals in rate of acetylation), excreted in urine, $t_{1/2}$ 0.44-0.47 hr (metabolite 2-4 hr)
INDICATIONS AND USES: Hypertension, CHF,* afterload reduction in severe aortic insufficiency and after valve replacement*
DOSAGE
Adult
- PO 10 mg qid, increase by 10-25 mg/dose q2-5d as needed to max of 300 mg/d; IM/IV 10-20 mg q4-6h, may increase to 40 mg/dose

Child
- PO 0.75-1 mg/kg/d divided bid-qid, increase over 3-4 wk to 7.5 mg/kg/d divided bid-qid if necessary; do not exceed 200 mg/d; IM/IV 0.1-0.2 mg/kg/dose q4-6h; do not exceed 20 mg/dose

$ AVAILABLE FORMS/COST OF THERAPY
- Inj, Sol—IM; IV: 20 mg/ml, 1 ml: **$28.39-$140.63**
- Tab, Uncoated—Oral: 10, 25, 50, 100 mg, 100's: **$1.65-$61.76**

CONTRAINDICATIONS: Hypersensitivity, CAD, mitral valvular rheumatic heart disease
PRECAUTIONS: Advanced renal disease, children, pulmonary hypertension
PREGNANCY AND LACTATION: Pregnancy category C; in England, hydralazine is the most commonly used antihypertensive in pregnant women; excreted into breast milk, compatible with breast feeding
SIDE EFFECTS/ADVERSE REACTIONS
CNS: Peripheral neuritis, *dizziness, tremors,* psychotic reactions, *headache, anxiety*
CV: Angina, palpitations, reflex tachycardia, flushing, edema, hypotension
EENT: Nasal congestion
GI: Anorexia, nausea, vomiting, diarrhea, constipation, paralytic ileus, hepatitis
GU: Urination difficulty
HEME: ***Anemia, leukopenia, agranulocytosis, eosinophilia***
MS: Muscle cramps, arthralgia
RESP: Dyspnea
SKIN: Rash, urticaria, pruritus
MISC: Lupus-like syndrome (arthralgia, dermatoses, fever, splenomegaly, glomerulonephritis)
▼ DRUG INTERACTIONS
Drugs
- *Diazoxide:* Severe hypotension
- *NSAIDs:* Inhibited antihypertensive response to hydralazine

SPECIAL CONSIDERATIONS
Lupus-like syndrome more common in "slow acetylators" and fol-

lowing higher doses for prolonged periods

PATIENT/FAMILY EDUCATION

• Take with meals

• Notify physician of any unexplained prolonged general tiredness or fever, muscle or joint aching, or chest pain

MONITORING PARAMETERS

• CBC and ANA titer before and during prolonged therapy

---

hydrochlorothiazide

(hye-droe-klor-oh-thye'a-zide)

Diaqua, Esidrix, Hydro-Chlor, HydroDiuril, Hydromal, Hydro-T, Oretic, Thiuretic

Chemical Class: Sulfonamide derivative

Therapeutic Class: Antihypertensive; thiazide diuretic

CLINICAL PHARMACOLOGY

Mechanism of Action: Increases urinary excretion of sodium and water by inhibiting sodium reabsorption in the early distal tubules; increases urinary excretion of potassium by increasing potassium secretion in the distal convoluted tubule and collecting ducts; decreases urinary calcium excretion

Pharmacokinetics

PO: Peak 4 hr, onset 2 hr, duration 6-12 hr, excreted unchanged in urine, $t_{1/2}$ 5.6-14.8 hr

INDICATIONS AND USES: Edema associated with CHF, hepatic cirrhosis, corticosteroid and estrogen therapy; hypertension; calcium nephrolithiasis;* osteoporosis;* diabetes insipidus*

DOSAGE

Adult

• PO 12.5-50 mg qd; max 200 mg/d; doses >50 mg/d generally not recommended due to increased incidence of hypokalemia and other metabolic disturbances

Child

• PO (<6 mo) 2-3.3 mg/kg/d divided bid; (>6 mo) 2 mg/kg/d divided bid

$ **AVAILABLE FORMS/COST OF THERAPY**

• Sol—Oral: 50 mg/5ml, 120 ml: **$4.95**

• Tab, Uncoated—Oral: 25 mg, 100's: **$1.50-$13.48;** 50 mg, 100's: **$1.88-$21.35;** 100 mg, 100's: **$4.43-$38.34**

CONTRAINDICATIONS: Anuria, renal decompensation, hypersensitivity to thiazides or related sulfonamide-derived drugs

PRECAUTIONS: Hypokalemia, renal disease, hepatic disease, gout, COPD, lupus erythematosus, diabetes mellitus, children, vomiting, diarrhea, hyperlipidemia

PREGNANCY AND LACTATION: Pregnancy category D; 1st trimester use may increase risk of congenital defects, use in later trimesters does not seem to carry this risk; other risks to the fetus or newborn include hypoglycemia, thrombocytopenia, hyponatremia, hypokalemia, and death from maternal complications; excreted into breast milk in small amounts, considered compatible with breast feeding

SIDE EFFECTS/ADVERSE REACTIONS

CNS: Drowsiness, paresthesia, depression, headache, *dizziness, fatigue, weakness*

CV: Irregular pulse, orthostatic hypotension, palpitations, volume depletion

EENT: Blurred vision

GI: Nausea, vomiting, anorexia, constipation, diarrhea, cramps, pancreatitis, GI irritation, ***hepatitis***

GU: Frequency, polyuria, ***uremia, glucosuria***

HEME: ***Aplastic anemia, hemolytic anemia, leukopenia, agranulocytosis, thrombocytopenia, neutropenia***
METAB: Hyperglycemia, hyperuricemia, increased creatinine, BUN, *hypokalemia,* hypercalcemia, hyponatremia, hypochloremia, hypomagnesemia
SKIN: Rash, urticaria, purpura, photosensitivity, fever

▼ **DRUG INTERACTIONS**

Drugs

- *Antidiabetics:* Thiazide diuretics tend to increase blood glucose, may increase dosage requirements of antidiabetic drugs
- *Cholestyramine:* Reduced serum concentrations of thiazide diuretics
- *Colestipol:* Reduced serum concentrations of thiazide diuretics
- *Diazoxide:* Hyperglycemia
- *Digitalis glycosides:* Diuretic-induced hypokalemia may increase the risk of digitalis toxicity
- *Lithium+:* Increased serum lithium concentrations, toxicity may occur

Labs

- *Increase:* BSP retention, amylase, parathyroid test
- *Decrease:* PBI, PSP

SPECIAL CONSIDERATIONS

PATIENT/FAMILY EDUCATION

- Take with food or milk
- Will increase urination, take early in the day
- Notify physician if muscle pain, weakness, cramps, nausea, vomiting, restlessness, excessive thirst, tiredness, drowsiness, increased heart rate, diarrhea, or dizziness occurs
- May cause sensitivity to sunlight, avoid prolonged exposure to the sun and other ultraviolet light
- May cause gout attacks, notify physician if sudden joint pain occurs

MONITORING PARAMETERS

- Serum electrolytes, BUN, creatinine, CBC, uric acid, glucose

hydrocodone

(hye-droe-koe'done)
Anexsia 5/500, Anexsia 7.5/650, Bancap HC, Co-Gesic, Dolacet, DuoCet, Duradyne DHC, Hydrocet, Hy-Phen, Lorcet 10/650, Lorcet-HD, Lorcet Plus, Lortab 2.5/500, Lortab 5/500, Lortab 7.5/500, Lortab Liquid, Norcet 5mg, Vicodin, Vicodin ES, Zydone
Chemical Class: Opiate, phenanthrene derivative
Therapeutic Class: Narcotic analgesic; antitussive
DEA Class: Schedule III

CLINICAL PHARMACOLOGY

Mechanism of Action: Binds to opiate receptors in CNS causing inhibition of ascending pain pathways, altering perception of and response to pain; suppresses cough by direct central action in the medulla

Pharmacokinetics

Peak 1.3 hr, duration 4.6 hr, $t_{1/2}$ 3.8 hr, metabolized in liver, excreted mainly in urine

INDICATIONS AND USES: Moderate to moderately severe pain, nonproductive cough

DOSAGE

Commercially available only in combination products

Adult

- PO 5-10 mg q4-6h prn

Child

- PO 0.6 mg/kg/d or 20 mg/m^2 d in 3-4 divided doses; do not exceed 1.25 mg/dose (<2 yr), 5 mg/dose (2-12 yr), 10 mg/dose (>12 yr)

$ **AVAILABLE FORMS/COST OF THERAPY**

- Cap, Gel—Oral: 500 mg (acetaminophen)/5 mg, 100's: **$17.99-$94.25**

• Elixir—Oral: 120 mg (acetaminophen)/2.5 mg/5 ml, 480 ml: **$45.77**

• Tab, Uncoated—Oral: 500 mg (acetaminophen)/2.5, 5, 7.5 mg, 100's: **$6.53-$46.90;** 550 mg (acetaminophen)/5 mg, 100's: **$23.88;** 650 mg (acetaminophen)/7.5, 10 mg, 100's: **$34.25-$56.89;** 750 mg (acetaminophen)/7.5 mg, 100's: **$30.83-$33.75**

CONTRAINDICATIONS: Hypersensitivity

PRECAUTIONS: Head injury, increased intracranial pressure, acute abdominal conditions, elderly, severe impairment of hepatic or renal function, hypothyroidism, Addison's disease, prostatic hypertrophy, urethral stricture, history of drug abuse

PREGNANCY AND LACTATION: Pregnancy category B (category D if used for prolonged periods or in high doses at term); withdrawal could theoretically occur in infants exposed *in utero* to prolonged maternal ingestion; excretion into breast milk unknown, use caution in nursing mothers

SIDE EFFECTS/ADVERSE REACTIONS

CNS: Drowsiness, sedation, dizziness, agitation, dependency, lethargy, restlessness

GI: Nausea, vomiting, anorexia, constipation

RESP: ***Respiratory depression, respiratory paralysis***

CV: Bradycardia, palpitations, orthostatic hypotension, tachycardia

GU: Urinary retention

SKIN: Flushing, rash, urticaria

▼ DRUG INTERACTIONS

Drugs

• *Barbiturates:* Additive CNS depression

• *Cimetidine:* Increased effect of narcotic analgesics

• *Ethanol:* Additive CNS effects

• *Neuroleptics:* Hypotension and excessive CNS depression

SPECIAL CONSIDERATIONS

PATIENT/FAMILY EDUCATION

• Report any symptoms of CNS changes, allergic reactions

• Physical dependency may result when used for extended periods

• Change position slowly, orthostatic hypotension may occur

• Avoid hazardous activities if drowsiness or dizziness occurs

• Avoid alcohol, other CNS depressants unless directed by physician

• Minimize nausea by administering with food and remain lying down following dose

hydrocortisone

(hye-dro-kor'ti-sone)

Systemic: A-Hydrocort, Anucort-HC, Cort-Dome, Cortef, Cortenema, Cortifoam, Hemorrhoidal HC, Hydrocortone, Hydrocortone Phosphate, Hydrocortone Acetate, Solu-Cortef

Topical: Acticort 100, Aeroseb-HC, Ala-Cort, Ala-Scalp, Alphaderm, Bactine Hydrocortisone, Caldecort Anti-Itch, Cetacort, Cortaid, Cortaid Maximum Strength, Cort-Dome, Cortef Feminine Itch, Cortizone-5, Cortizone-10, Cortril, Delacort, Delcort, Dermacort, Dermicort, Dermolate Anti-Itch, Dermtex HC, Hi-Cor 1.0, Hi-Cor 2.5, Hycort, HydroTex, Hytone, Lacticare-HC, Locoid, Nutracort, Penecort, 1% HC, S-T Cort, Synacort, Tega-Cort, Tega-Cort Forte, Texacort, U-Cort, Westcort

Chemical Class: Glucocorticoid, short-acting

Therapeutic Class: Corticosteroid; nonfluorinated group IV (low) potency: acetate, plain; group III (medium) potency: valerate, butyrate

CLINICAL PHARMACOLOGY

Mechanism of Action: Controls the rate of protein synthesis, depresses migrations of polymorphonuclear leukocytes and fibroblasts, reverses capillary permeability, and causes lysosomal stabilization at the cellular level to prevent or control inflammation; depresses formation, release, and activity of endogenous mediators of inflammation such as prostaglandins, kinins, histamine, liposomal enzymes, and the complement system resulting in decreased edema, erythema, and pruritus

Pharmacokinetics

PO: Onset 1-2 hr, peak 1 hr, duration 1-1½ days

IM/IV: Onset 20 min, peak 4-8 hr, duration 1-1½ days

PR: Onset 3-5 days

TOP: Absorbed through the skin (increased by inflammation and occlusive dressings), metabolized by liver, excreted in urine (17-OHCS, 17-KS)

INDICATIONS AND USES: Anti-inflammatory or immunosuppressant agent in the treatment of a variety of diseases including those of hematologic, allergic, inflammatory, neoplastic, and autoimmune origin

DOSAGE

Adult

- *Acute adrenal insufficiency:* PO 5-30 mg bid-qid; IM/IV/SC 15-240 mg q12h
- *Anti-inflammatory:* PO 5-30 mg bid-qid; IM/IV/SC 15-240 mg q12h
- *Shock:* IM/IV 500-2000 mg q2-6h
- *Rectal:* Enema 100 mg nightly for 21 days; suppository 25 mg bid-qid prn
- *Intra-articular and soft tissue (acetate):* Large joints 25 mg; small joints 10-25 mg; bursae 25-37.5 mg; tendon sheaths 5-12.5 mg; soft tissue infiltration 25-50 mg; ganglia 12.5-25 mg

Child

- *Acute adrenal insufficiency:* IM/IV/SC 1-2 mg/kg bolus, then 25-150 mg/d in divided doses (infants and younger children); 1-2 mg/kg bolus, then 150-250 mg/d in divided doses (older children)
- *Physiologic replacement:* PO 0.5-0.75 mg/kg/d or 20-25 mg/m^2/d divided q8h; IM 0.25-0.35 mg/kg/d or 12-15 mg/m^2/d qd
- *Shock:* IM/IV 50 mg/kg initially,

H

then repeated in 4 hr and/or q24h prn

Adult and Child

• TOP: Apply to affected area bid-qid; rub completely into skin

$ **AVAILABLE FORMS/COSTS OF THERAPY**

• Supp (acetate)—Rect: 25 mg, 12's: **$1.55-$35.90**

• Aerosol, Foam (acetate)—Rect: 10%, 20 g: **$45.93**

• Enema—Rect: 100 mg/60 ml: **$7.68**

• Tab, Uncoated—Oral: 5 mg, 50's: **$5.57;** 10 mg, 100's: **$19.69-$20.09;** 20 mg, 100's: **$6.50-$38.35**

• Susp (cypionate)—Oral: 10 mg/5 ml, 120 ml: **$16.40**

• Inj, Sol (sodium phosphate)—IM; IV; SC: 50 mg/ml, 10 ml: **$50.53**

• Inj, Lyph-Sol (sodium succinate)—IM; IV: 100 mg/vial, 1's: **$1.90-$3.34;** 250 mg/2 ml, 1's: **$5.00-$7.57;** 500 mg/4 ml, 1's: **$8.88-$14.72;** 1000 mg/8 ml, 1's: **$16.90-$29.31**

• Inj, Susp (acetate)—Intra-Articular; IM: 25 mg/ml, 10 ml: **$1.48-$24.70;** 50 mg/ml, 10 ml: **$2.48-$53.92**

• Cre, Oint (butyrate)—Top: 0.1%, 15, 45 g: **$12.95-$26.95**

• Sol (butyrate)—Top: 0.1%, 20, 60 ml: **$18.40-$36.80**

• Cre, Oint (valerate)—TOP: 0.2%, 15, 45, 60 g: **$12.49-$31.16**

• Cre—Top: 0.5%, 1%, 2.5%, 15, 20, 30, 45, 60, 90, 120, 454 g: **$1.50-$93.66**

• Lotion—Top: 0.25%, 0.5%, 1%, 2%, 2.5%, 30, 60, 120 ml: **$1.13-$31.06**

• Oint—Top: 1%, 2.5%, 15, 20, 30, 60, 120, 454 g: **$2.37-$124.31**

• Sol—Top: 1%, 2.5%, 30, 60 ml: **$8.00-$15.41**

• Aer—Top: 0.5%, 58 g: **$17.57**

CONTRAINDICATIONS: Systemic fungal infections, hypersensitivity, idiopathic thrombocytopenic purpura (IM)

PRECAUTIONS: Psychosis, acute glomerulonephritis, amebiasis, cerebral malaria, child <2 yr, elderly, AIDS, tuberculosis, diabetes mellitus, glaucoma, osteoporosis, ulcerative colitis, CHF, myasthenia gravis, renal disease, esophagitis, peptic ulcer, ocular herpes simplex, live virus vaccines, hypertension, use on face, groin, or axilla

PREGNANCY AND LACTATION: Pregnancy category C; chronic maternal ingestion during the 1st trimester has shown a 1% incidence of cleft palate in humans; may appear in breast milk and could suppress growth, interfere with endogenous corticosteroid production or cause unwanted effects in the nursing infant, unknown whether topical application could result in sufficient systemic absorption to produce detectable amounts in breast milk

SIDE EFFECTS/ADVERSE REACTIONS

CNS: Depression, vertigo, ***convulsions,*** headache, *mood changes*

CV: Hypertension, thrombophlebitis, ***thromboembolism,*** tachycardia, CHF

EENT: Increased intraocular pressure, blurred vision, cataract

GI: Diarrhea, nausea, abdominal distension, ***GI hemorrhage,*** increased appetite, ***pancreatitis***

METAB: Cushingoid state, growth suppression in children, HPA suppression, decreased glucose tolerance

MS: Fractures, osteoporosis, aseptic necrosis of femoral and humeral heads, weakness, muscle mass loss

SKIN: Acne, poor wound healing, ecchymosis, bruising, petechiae, striae, thin fragile skin, suppression of skin test reactions, burning, dryness, itching, irritation, acne, folliculitis, hypertrichosis, perioral dermatitis, hypopigmentation, atrophy, striae, miliaria, allergic contact dermatitis, secondary infection

▼ **DRUG INTERACTIONS**

Drugs

- *Aminoglutethamide:* Enhanced elimination of hydrocortisone; reduction in corticosteroid response
- *Amphotericin B:* Hypokalemia
- *Antidiabetics:* Increased blood glucose in patients with diabetes
- *Barbiturates:* Reduced serum concentrations of corticosteroids
- *Carbamazepine:* Reduced serum concentrations of corticosteroids
- *Cholestyramine:* Possible reduced absorption of corticosteroids
- *Estrogens:* Enhanced effects of corticosteroids
- *Isoniazid:* Reduced plasma concentrations of isoniazid
- *Phenytoin:* Reduced therapeutic effect of corticosteroids
- *Rifampin:* Reduced therapeutic effect of corticosteroids
- *Salicylates:* Enhanced elimination of salicylates; subtherapeutic salicylate concentrations possible

Labs

- *Increase:* Cholesterol, blood glucose, urine glucose
- *Decrease:* Calcium, potassium, T_4, T_3, thyroid ^{131}I uptake test
- *False negative:* Skin allergy tests

SPECIAL CONSIDERATIONS

PATIENT/FAMILY EDUCATION

- May cause GI upset, take with meals or snacks
- Take single daily doses in AM
- Notify physician if unusual weight gain, swelling of lower extremities, muscle weakness, black tarry stools, vomiting of blood, puffing of the face, menstrual irregularities, prolonged sore throat, fever, cold, or infection occurs
- Signs of adrenal insufficiency include fatigue, anorexia, nausea, vomiting, diarrhea, weight loss, weakness, dizziness, and low blood sugar; notify physician if these signs and symptoms appear following dose reduction or withdrawal of therapy
- Avoid abrupt withdrawal of therapy following high dose or long-term therapy

MONITORING PARAMETERS

- Potassium and blood sugar during long-term therapy
- Edema, blood pressure, cardiac symptoms, mental status, weight
- Observe growth and development of infants and children on prolonged therapy

H

hydroflumethiazide

(hye-droe-flu-me-thye'a-zide)

Diucardin, Saluron

Chemical Class: Sulfonamide derivative

Therapeutic Class: Antihypertensive; thiazide diuretic

CLINICAL PHARMACOLOGY

Mechanism of Action: Increases urinary excretion of sodium and water by inhibiting sodium reabsorption in the early distal tubules; increases urinary excretion of potassium by increasing potassium secretion in the distal convoluted tubule and collecting ducts; decreases urinary calcium excretion

Pharmacokinetics

PO: Onset 2 hr, peak 4 hr, duration 6-12 hr, metabolized and excreted in the urine, t½ approximately 17 hr

INDICATIONS AND USES: Edema associated with CHF, hepatic cirrhosis, corticosteroid and estrogen therapy; hypertension; calcium nephrolithiasis;* osteoporosis;* diabetes insipidus*

DOSAGE

Adult

- *Edema:* PO 50 mg qd-bid initially; maintenance 25-200 mg/d, administer in divided doses when dosage >100 mg/d

• *Hypertension:* PO 50 mg bid initially; maintenance 50-100 mg/d, do not exceed 200 mg/d

$ AVAILABLE FORMS/COST OF THERAPY

• Tab, Uncoated—Oral: 50 mg, 100's: **$45.63-$56.17**

CONTRAINDICATIONS: Anuria, renal decompensation, hypersensitivity to thiazides or related sulfonamide-derived drugs

PRECAUTIONS: Hypokalemia, renal disease, hepatic disease, gout, COPD, lupus erythematosus, diabetes mellitus, children, vomiting, diarrhea, hyperlipidemia

PREGNANCY AND LACTATION: Pregnancy category D; 1st trimester use may increase risk of congenital defects, use in later trimesters does not seem to carry this risk; other risks to the fetus or newborn include hypoglycemia, thrombocytopenia, hyponatremia, hypokalemia, and death from maternal complications; excreted into breast milk in small amounts, considered compatible with breast feeding

SIDE EFFECTS/ADVERSE REACTIONS

CNS: Drowsiness, paresthesia, depression, headache, *dizziness, fatigue, weakness*

CV: Irregular pulse, orthostatic hypotension, palpitations, volume depletion

EENT: Blurred vision

GI: Nausea, vomiting, anorexia, constipation, diarrhea, cramps, pancreatitis, GI irritation, ***hepatitis***

GU: Frequency, polyuria, ***uremia, glucosuria***

HEME: ***Aplastic anemia, hemolytic anemia, leukopenia, agranulocytosis, thrombocytopenia, neutropenia***

METAB: Hyperglycemia, hyperuricemia, increased creatinine, BUN, *hypokalemia,* hypercalcemia, hyponatremia, hypochloremia, hypomagnesemia

SKIN: Rash, urticaria, purpura, photosensitivity, fever

▼ DRUG INTERACTIONS

Drugs

• *Antidiabetics:* Thiazide diuretics tend to increase blood glucose, may increase dosage requirements of antidiabetic drugs

• *Cholestyramine:* Reduced serum concentrations of thiazide diuretics

• *Colestipol:* Reduced serum concentrations of thiazide diuretics

• *Diazoxide:* Hyperglycemia

• *Digitalis glycosides:* Diuretic-induced hypokalemia may increase the risk of digitalis toxicity

• *Lithium+:* Increased serum lithium concentrations, toxicity may occur

Labs

• *Increase:* BSP retention, amylase, parathyroid test

• *Decrease:* PBI, PSP

SPECIAL CONSIDERATIONS

PATIENT/FAMILY EDUCATION

• Take with food or milk

• Will increase urination, take early in the day

• Notify physician if muscle pain, weakness, cramps, nausea, vomiting, restlessness, excessive thirst, tiredness, drowsiness, increased heart rate, diarrhea, or dizziness occurs

• May cause sensitivity to sunlight, avoid prolonged exposure to the sun and other ultraviolet light

• May cause gout attacks, notify physician if sudden joint pain occurs

MONITORING PARAMETERS

• Serum electrolytes, BUN, creatinine, CBC, uric acid, glucose

hydromorphone

(hye-droe-mor′fone)

Dilaudid, Dilaudid HP

Chemical Class: Opiate, semisynthetic phenathrene derivative

Therapeutic Class: Narcotic analgesic; antitussive

DEA Class: Schedule II

CLINICAL PHARMACOLOGY

Mechanism of Action: Binds to opiate receptors in CNS causing inhibition of ascending pain pathways, altering perception of and response to pain; suppresses cough by direct central action in the medulla

Pharmacokinetics

PO: Peak 45 min

IM: Onset 15-30 min, peak 0.5-1½ hr, duration 4-5 hr

Metabolized by liver, excreted by kidneys

INDICATIONS AND USES: Moderate to severe pain, nonproductive cough

DOSAGE

Adult

- *Pain:* PO/IM/IV/SC 1-4 mg q4-6h prn; PR 3 mg q6-8h
- *Antitussive:* PO 1 mg q3-4h prn

Child

- *Pain:* PO 0.03-0.08 mg/kg/dose q4-6h prn, max 5mg/dose; IV 0.015 mg/kg/dose q4-6h prn
- *Antitussive:* (6-12 yr) 0.5 mg q3-4h prn

$ AVAILABLE FORMS/COST OF THERAPY

- Inj, Sol—IM; IV; SC: 1, 2, 3, 4, 10 mg/ml, 1 ml: **$0.91-$3.19**
- Sol—Oral: 1 mg/ml, 480 ml: **$84.76**
- Supp—Rect: 3 mg, 6's: **$18.78**
- Tab, Uncoated—Oral: 2 mg, 100's: **$27.98-$38.54;** 4 mg, 100's: **$39.00-$63.11;** 8 mg, 100's: **$114.85**

CONTRAINDICATIONS: Hypersensitivity, acute bronchial asthma, upper airway obstruction, obstetrical anesthesia (parenteral)

PRECAUTIONS: Head injury, increased intracranial pressure, acute abdominal conditions, elderly, severe impairment of hepatic or renal function, hypothyroidism, Addison's disease, prostatic hypertrophy, urethral stricture, history of drug abuse

PREGNANCY AND LACTATION: Pregnancy category B (category D if used for prolonged periods or in high doses at term); use during labor produces neonatal respiratory depression; excretion into breast milk unknown, use caution in nursing mothers

SIDE EFFECTS/ADVERSE REACTIONS

CNS: Drowsiness, sedation, dizziness, agitation, dependency, lethargy, restlessness

GI: Nausea, vomiting, anorexia, constipation

RESP: ***Respiratory depression, respiratory paralysis***

CV: Bradycardia, palpitations, orthostatic hypotension, tachycardia

GU: Urinary retention

SKIN: Flushing, rash, urticaria

▼ DRUG INTERACTIONS

Drugs

- *Barbiturates:* Additive CNS depression
- *Cimetidine:* Increased effect of narcotic analgesics
- *Ethanol:* Additive CNS effects
- *Neuroleptics:* Hypotension and excessive CNS depression

Labs

- *Increase:* Amylase

SPECIAL CONSIDERATIONS

PATIENT/FAMILY EDUCATION

- Report any symptoms of CNS changes, allergic reactions
- Physical dependency may result when used for extended periods

H

• Change position slowly, orthostatic hypotension may occur
• Avoid hazardous activities if drowsiness or dizziness occurs
• Avoid alcohol, other CNS depressants unless directed by physician
• Minimize nausea by administering with food and remain lying down following dose

hydroquinone

(hye-droe-kwin'own)

Esoterica, Eldopaque, Eldopaque-Forte, Eldoquin, Eldoquin-Forte, Melanex, Porcelana, Solaquin, Solaquin Forte

Chemical Class: Monobenzone derivative

Therapeutic Class: Depigmenting agent

CLINICAL PHARMACOLOGY

Mechanism of Action: Depigments hyperpigmented skin by inhibiting the enzymatic oxidation of tyrosine and suppressing other melanocyte metabolic processes, thereby inhibiting melanin formation

INDICATIONS AND USES: Temporary bleaching of hyperpigmented skin conditions (e.g., freckles, senile lentigines, chloasma and melasma, other forms of melanin hyperpigmentation)

DOSAGE

Adult and Child ≥12 yr

TOP: apply to affected skin bid

$ AVAILABLE FORMS/COST OF THERAPY

• Cre—Top: 1.5%, 90 g: **$6.09;** 2%, 30, 60, 90, 120 g: **$6.09-$20.16;** 4%, 15, 30, 60 g: **$11.25-$30.30**
• Lotion—Top: 2%, 15 ml: **$6.10**
• Gel—Top: 4%, 15, 30, 60 g: **$11.25-$30.30**
• Sol—Top: 30 mg/ml, 30 ml: **$8.70-$11.94**

CONTRAINDICATIONS: Hypersensitivity

PRECAUTIONS: Sulfite sensitivity

PREGNANCY AND LACTATION: Pregnancy category C; degree of systemic absorption unknown; excretion into breast milk unknown

SIDE EFFECTS/ADVERSE REACTIONS

SKIN: Dryness and fissuring of paranasal and infraorbital areas, erythema, stinging, irritation, sensitization, and contact dermatitis

SPECIAL CONSIDERATIONS

PATIENT/FAMILY EDUCATION

• Positive response may require 3 wk to 6 mo
• Protect the treated area from UV light by using a sunscreen, sun block, or protective clothing
• Avoid application to lips or near eyes

MONITORING PARAMETERS

• Apply small amount to an unbroken patch of skin and check in 24 hr, if vesicle formation, itching, or excessive inflammation occurs, further treatment not advised

hydroxocobalamin (vitamin B_{12})

(hye-drox'oh-co-bal'a-min)

alphaRedisol, Codroxomin, Hydrobexan, Hydro-Cobex, Hydro-Crysti-12, LA-12

Chemical Class: Cobalamin

Therapeutic Class: B complex vitamin

CLINICAL PHARMACOLOGY

Mechanism of Action: Physiologic role is associated with methylation, participating in nucleic acid and protein synthesis; participates in red blood cell formation through activation of folic acid coenzymes

Pharmacokinetics

IM: Slowly absorbed from inj site; distributed into liver, bone marrow, and other tissue; available for urinary excretion when administered parenterally in doses that exceed binding capacity of plasma, liver, and other tissues

INDICATIONS AND USES: Vitamin B_{12} deficiency (pernicious anemia, GI pathology, fish tapeworm infestation, malignancy of pancreas or bowel, gluten enteropathy, sprue, gastrectomy); increased Vitamin B_{12} requirement (pregnancy, thyrotoxicosis, hemolytic anemia, hemorrhage, malignancy, hepatic or renal disease); Schilling test for Vitamin B_{12} absorption; cyanide toxicity associated with sodium nitroprusside*

DOSAGE

Adult

- IM 30 µg/d for 5-10 days, followed by 100-200 µg qmo

Child

- IM 1-5 mg over 2 or more wk in doses of 100 µg, then 30-50 µg q4wk for maintenance

$ AVAILABLE FORMS/COST OF THERAPY

- Inj, Sol—IM: 250 mg/ml, 5 ml: **$10.90;** 1000 µg/ml, 30 ml: **$3.49-$11.85**

CONTRAINDICATIONS: Hypersensitivity to cobalt, vitamin B_{12} or any component

PRECAUTIONS: IV route, infection, uremia, bone marrow suppressant drugs, concurrent iron or folic acid deficiency, severe megaloblastic anemia, polycythemia vera, stomach carcinoma, immunodeficient patients

PREGNANCY AND LACTATION: Pregnancy category C; vitamin B_{12} is an essential vitamin and needs are increased during pregnancy; excreted into breast milk; 2.6 µg/day should be consumed during pregnancy and lactation

SIDE EFFECTS/ADVERSE REACTIONS

CV: ***Pulmonary edema, CHF,*** peripheral vascular thrombosis

GI: Mild diarrhea

HEME: Polycythemia vera

RESP: ***Anaphylactic shock***

SKIN: Pain at inj site

MISC: Feeling of swelling of the entire body

▼ DRUG INTERACTIONS

Labs

- *False positive:* Intrinsic factor

SPECIAL CONSIDERATIONS

PATIENT/FAMILY EDUCATION

- Therapy may require life-long monthly injections

MONITORING PARAMETERS

- Serum potassium for 1st 48 hr during treatment of severe megaloblastic anemia
- Reticulocyte counts, Hct, vitamin B_{12}, iron, and folic acid plasma levels prior to treatment, between days 5 and 7 of treatment, then frequently until Hct is normal
- Periodic hematologic evaluations throughout patient's lifetime

hydroxychloroquine

(hye-drox-ee-klor'oh-kwin)

Plaquenil

Chemical Class: 4-aminoquinoline derivative

Therapeutic Class: Antimalarial; disease modifying antirheumatic agent

CLINICAL PHARMACOLOGY

Mechanism of Action: Interferes with digestive vacuole function within sensitive malarial parasites by increasing pH and interfering with lysosomal degradation of Hgb; inhibits locomotion of neutrophils and chemotaxis of eosinophils; impairs complement-dependent antigen–antibody reactions

Pharmacokinetics

PO: Rapidly and completely absorbed, peak 1-6 hr, partially metabolized, slowly excreted by kidneys (parent drug and metabolites)

INDICATIONS AND USES: Prophylaxis and treatment of acute attacks of malaria due to *Plasmodium vivax, P. malariae, P. ovale,* and susceptible strains of *P. falciparum;* discoid and systemic lupus erythematosus; rheumatoid arthritis; porphyria cutanea tarda,* polymorphous light eruptions*

DOSAGE

Hydroxychloroquine sulfate 200 mg = 155 mg hydroxychloroquine base

Adult

- *Prophylaxis of malaria:* PO 400 mg qwk on same day each wk; begin 1-2 wk before exposure, continue 6-8 wk after leaving endemic area
- *Acute malaria attack:* PO 800 mg initial dose, followed by 400 mg in 6 hr on day 1, then 400 mg as single dose on days 2 and 3
- *Rheumatoid arthritis:* PO 400-600 mg qd initially, increase dose until optimal response achieved (usually 4-12 wk); maintenance dose 200-400 mg qd
- *Lupus erythematosus:* PO 400 mg qd-bid for several wk depending on response; maintenance 200-400 mg/d

Child

- *Prophylaxis of malaria:* PO 5 mg/kg (base) qwk on same day each wk; begin 1-2 wk before exposure, continue 6-8 wk after leaving endemic area; do not exceed recommended adult dose
- *Acute malaria attack:* PO 10 mg/kg (base) initial dose, followed by 5 mg/kg (base) in 6 hr on day 1, then 5 mg/kg (base) as a single dose on days 2 and 3
- *Juvenile rheumatoid arthritis/lupus erythematosus:* PO 3-5 mg/kg/d divided 1-2 times/d, max 400 mg/d

$ **AVAILABLE FORMS/COST OF THERAPY**

- Tab, Uncoated—Oral: 200 mg, 100's: **$115.94**

CONTRAINDICATIONS: Hypersensitivity, retinal or visual field changes, children (long-term therapy)

PRECAUTIONS: Psoriasis, porphyria, children, hepatic function impairment, G-6-PD deficiency

PREGNANCY AND LACTATION: Pregnancy category C; should be avoided except in suppression or treatment of malaria when in the judgment of the physician the benefit outweighs the possible hazard; excreted in breast milk, safe use during nursing has not been established

SIDE EFFECTS/ADVERSE REACTIONS

CNS: Headache, psychic stimulation, psychotic episodes, ***convulsions,*** neuropathy, decreased reflexes

CV: Hypotension, ECG changes (inversion or depression of T-wave, widening of QRS complex)

EENT: ***Nerve-type deafness*** (prolonged high doses), tinnitus, reduced hearing, ***irreversible retinal damage*** (prolonged high doses), visual disturbances, nyctalopia, scotomatous vision, misty vision, fog before eyes

GI: Anorexia, nausea, vomiting, diarrhea, abdominal cramps

HEME: Agranulocytosis, blood dyscrasias, hemolytic anemia

MS: Muscular weakness

SKIN: Pruritus, lichen planus-like eruptions, skin and mucosal pigmentary changes, pleomorphic skin eruptions (prolonged therapy)

▼ **DRUG INTERACTIONS**

Drugs

• *Digitalis glycosides:* Increased serum digoxin concentrations

SPECIAL CONSIDERATIONS

PATIENT/FAMILY EDUCATION

• Take with food to decrease GI upset

• Report any muscle weakness, visual disturbances, difficulty hearing, or ringing in ears to physician

• Use sunglasses in bright sunlight to decrease photophobia

MONITORING PARAMETERS

• Baseline and periodic ophthalmologic examinations (visual acuity, expert slit-lamp, funduscopic, and visual field tests); periodic tests of knee and ankle reflexes to detect muscular weakness

• Periodic CBCs during prolonged therapy

---

hydroxyprogesterone

(hye-drox-ee-proe-jess'te-rone)

Duralutin, Gesterol L.A. 250, Hy-Gestrone, Hylutin, Hypro-gest 250, Pro-Depo, Prodrox 250

Chemical Class: Progestin
Therapeutic Class: Long-acting progestin; antineoplastic

CLINICAL PHARMACOLOGY

Mechanism of Action. Shares the actions of the progestins; in the presence of adequate estrogen, transforms a proliferative endometrium into a secretory one; stimulates growth of mammary alveolar tissue; has some androgenic, estrogenic, and adrenocorticoid activity

Pharmacokinetics

IM: Duration 9-17 days, metabolized primarily in the liver, excreted by the kidney

INDICATIONS AND USES: Amenorrhea (primary and secondary), dysfunctional uterine bleeding, metrorrhagia, metastatic endometrial carcinoma (palliative therapy)

DOSAGE

Adult

• *Amenorrhea and uterine bleeding:* IM 375 mg, repeated q4 wk prn

• *Endometrial carcinoma:* IM 1-7 g/wk

$ **AVAILABLE FORMS/COST OF THERAPY**

• Inj, Sol—IM: 125 mg/ml, 10 ml: **$7.40;** 250 mg/ml, 5 ml: **$10.49-$15.75**

CONTRAINDICATIONS: Hypersensitivity, thrombophlebitis, thromboembolic disorders, cerebral hemorrhage, impaired liver function or disease, breast cancer, undiagnosed vaginal bleeding, missed abortion, use as a diagnostic test for pregnancy

PRECAUTIONS: Epilepsy, migraine, asthma, cardiac or renal dysfunction, depression, diabetes

PREGNANCY AND LACTATION: Pregnancy category D; ambiguous genitalia of both male and female fetuses have been reported; detectable amounts of progestins enter the breast milk, effect on the nursing infant has not been determined

SIDE EFFECTS/ADVERSE REACTIONS

CNS: Dizziness, headache, migraines, depression, fatigue

CV: Hypotension, thrombophlebitis, edema, ***thromboembolism, stroke, pulmonary embolism, MI***

EENT: Diplopia

GI: Nausea, vomiting, anorexia, cramps, increased weight, ***cholestatic jaundice***

GU: Amenorrhea, cervical erosion, breakthrough bleeding, dysmenorrhea, vaginal candidiasis, breast changes, *gynecomastia, testicular at-*

rophy, *impotence,* endometriosis, ***spontaneous abortion***

METAB: Hyperglycemia

SKIN: Rash, urticaria, acne, hirsutism, alopecia, oily skin, seborrhea, purpura, melasma, photosensitivity

▼ **DRUG INTERACTIONS**

Labs

• *Increase:* Alk phosphatase, pregnanediol, liver function tests

• *Decrease:* Glucose tolerance test, HDL

SPECIAL CONSIDERATIONS

PATIENT/FAMILY EDUCATION

• Take protective measures against exposure to UV light or sunlight

• Diabetic patients must monitor blood glucose carefully during therapy

• Notify physician of pain, swelling, warmth or redness in calves, sudden severe headache, visual disturbances, numbness in arm or leg

MONITORING PARAMETERS

Pretreatment physical exam should include breasts and pelvic organs, Pap smear

hydroxyzine

(hye-drox'i-zeen)

Anxanil, Atarax, Atarax 100, Atozine, Durel, E-Vista, Hydroxacen, Hydroxyzine HCl, Hydroxyzine Pamoate, Hyzine-50, Quiess, Vamate, Vistacon, Vistaject-25, Vistaject-50, Vistaquel 50, Vistaril, Vistazine 50

Chemical Class: Piperazine derivative

Therapeutic Class: Antianxiety, sedative hypnotic, antihistaminic, antiemetic (parenteral only)

CLINICAL PHARMACOLOGY

Mechanism of Action: Depresses subcortical levels of CNS, including limbic system, reticular formation

Pharmacokinetics

Onset 15-30 min, duration 4-6 hr, $t_{1/2}$ 3 hr

INDICATIONS AND USES: Anxiety, nausea, vomiting, to potentiate narcotic analgesics; sedation; pruritus, anxiety in alcohol withdrawal

DOSAGE

Adult

• PO 50-100 mg q4-6h; IM 25-100 mg q4-6h

Child

• PO >6 yr 50-100 mg/d in divided doses; PO <6 yr 50 mg/d in divided doses; IM 1.1 mg/kg q4-6h

$ **AVAILABLE FORMS/COST OF THERAPY**

• Tab—Oral: 10, 25, 50, 100 mg, 100's: **$2.55-$124.34**

• Inj—IM: 25 mg/ml, 10 ml: **$2.03-$11.44;** 50 mg/ml, 10 ml: **$1.66-$18.25**

• Syr—Oral: 10 mg/5ml, 120ml: **$2.06-$4.30**

CONTRAINDICATIONS: Hypersensitivity

PRECAUTIONS: Elderly, debilitated, hepatic disease, renal disease, pregnancy

PREGNANCY AND LACTATION: Pregnancy category C because of lack of clinical data but no excess in birth defects documented; safe during labor for relief of anxiety; no data on breast feeding

SIDE EFFECTS/ADVERSE REACTIONS

CNS: Dizziness, drowsiness, confusion, headache, tremors, fatigue, depression, convulsions

GI: Dry mouth

▼ **DRUG INTERACTIONS**

Drugs

• *Barbiturates, narcotics, analgesics, alcohol:* Increased CNS depressant effect

Labs
- *False increase:* 17-OHCS

hyoscyamine

(hye-oh-sye'a-meen)

Anaspaz, Cystospaz, Cystospaz-M, Gastrosed, Levsin, Levsin Drops, Levsinex Timecaps, Neoquess

Chemical Class: Belladonna alkaloid

Therapeutic Class: GI anticholinergic

CLINICAL PHARMACOLOGY

Mechanism of Action: Inhibits muscarinic actions of acetylcholine at postganglionic parasympathetic neuroeffector sites

Pharmacokinetics

PO: Duration 4-6 hr; metabolized by liver; excreted in urine; $t_{1/2}$ 3.5 hr

INDICATIONS AND USES: Irritable bowel syndrome, biliary colic, hypermotility in cystitis, adjunctive treatment of peptic ulcer disease, sinus bradycardia (parenteral)

DOSAGE

Adult
- PO/SL 0.125-0.25 mg tid-qid ac, hs; TIME REL 0.375 mg q12h; IM/SC/IV 0.25-0.5 mg q6h

Child
- 2-10 yr ½ adult dose; <2 yr ¼ adult dose

$ **AVAILABLE FORMS/COST OF THERAPY**
- Cap, Gel, Sust Action—Oral: 0.375 mg, 100's: **$44.06-$58.13**
- Tab, Uncoated—Oral; SL: 0.125 mg, 100's: **$11.25-$41.25**
- Elixir—Oral: 0.125 mg/5ml, 480 ml: **$11.45-$36.43**
- Sol—Oral: 0.125 mg/ml, 15 ml: **$8.40-$14.30**
- Inj, Sol—IM; IV; SC: 0.5 mg/ml, 1 ml: **$6.36**

CONTRAINDICATIONS: Hypersensitivity to anticholinergics, narrow angle glaucoma, GI obstruction, myasthenia gravis, paralytic ileus, GI atony, toxic megacolon, prostatic hypertrophy

PRECAUTIONS: Hyperthyroidism, CAD, dysrhythmias, CHF, ulcerative colitis, hypertension, hiatal hernia, hepatic disease, renal disease, urinary retention

PREGNANCY AND LACTATION: Pregnancy category C; excreted in breast milk, infants sensitive to anticholinergics

SIDE EFFECTS/ADVERSE REACTIONS

CNS: Confusion, stimulation in elderly, headache, insomnia, dizziness, drowsiness, anxiety, weakness, hallucination

CV: Palpitations, tachycardia

EENT: Blurred vision, photophobia, mydriasis, cycloplegia, increased ocular tension

GI: Dry mouth, constipation, paralytic ileus, heartburn, nausea, vomiting, dysphagia, absence of taste

GU: Hesitancy, retention, impotence

SKIN: Urticaria, rash, pruritus, anhidrosis, fever, allergic reactions

ibuprofen

(eye-byoo'proe-fen)

Aches-N-Pain, Advil, Children's Advil, Excedrin IS, Genpril, Haltran, Ibuprin, Ibuprohm, IBU-Tab, Medipren, Menadol, Midol-200, Motrin, Motrin IB, Nuprin, Pamprin-IB, PediaProfen, Rufen, Saleto-200, Saleto-400, Saleto-600, Saleto-800, Trendar

Chemical Class: Propionic acid derivative

Therapeutic Class: Nonsteroidal antiinflammatory drug (NSAID)

CLINICAL PHARMACOLOGY

Mechanism of Action: Inhibits prostaglandin synthesis by decreasing enzyme needed for biosynthesis; analgesic, antiinflammatory, antipyretic

Pharmacokinetics

PO: Onset ½ hour; peak 1-2 hr, $t_{1/2}$ 2-4 hr; metabolized in liver (inactive metabolites), excreted in urine (inactive metabolites) within 24 hr, does not enter breast milk, food decreases rate but not extent of absorption

INDICATIONS AND USES: Rheumatoid arthritis, osteoarthritis, primary dysmenorrhea, gout, pain, musculoskeletal disorders, fever, tocolysis in preterm labor*

DOSAGE

Adult

- PO 200-800 mg qid, not to exceed 3.2 g/d

Child

- PO 20-40 mg/kg/d divided tid or qid

$ AVAILABLE FORMS/COST OF THERAPY

- Tab—Oral: 200 mg, 100's: **$2.90-$8.95;** 300 mg, 100's: **$4.95-$15.22;** 400 mg, 100's: **$3.75-$21.57;** 600 mg, 100's: **$4.74-$28.13;** 800 mg, 100's: **$6.75-$36.93**
- Susp—Oral: 100 mg/5 ml, 120 ml: **$6.44**

CONTRAINDICATIONS: Hypersensitivity to NSAIDs (including symptoms of asthma, nasal polyps, angioedema), severe renal disease, severe hepatic disease

PRECAUTIONS: Bleeding disorders, GI disorders, cardiac disorders predisposition to fluid retention, advanced age (>65)

PREGNANCY AND LACTATION: Pregnancy category B; reduces amniotic fluid volume, constriction of the ductus arteriosus in 3rd trimester; compatible with breast feeding

SIDE EFFECTS/ADVERSE REACTIONS

CNS: Dizziness, drowsiness, fatigue, tremors, confusion, insomnia, anxiety, depression

CV: Tachycardia, peripheral edema, palpitations, dysrhythmias, hypertension

EENT: Tinnitus, hearing loss, blurred vision

GI: Nausea, anorexia, vomiting, diarrhea, jaundice, ***cholestatic hepatitis,*** constipation, flatulence, cramps, dry mouth, peptic ulcer, ***GI bleeding***

GU: ***Nephrotoxicity;*** dysuria, hematuria, oliguria, azotemia

HEME: ***Blood dyscrasias***

SKIN: Purpura, rash, pruritus, sweating

▼ DRUG INTERACTIONS

Drugs

- *Coumarin:* Increased risk of bleeding
- *Furosemide:* Reduced diuretic and antihypertensive effect
- *Lithium:* Increased lithium levels
- *Methotrexate:* Increased methotrexate toxicity

Labs

- *Increased:* Bleeding time

SPECIAL CONSIDERATIONS

- Administer with food or antacids if GI symptoms occur

---

idoxuridine

(eye-dox-your'ih-deen)

Herplex, Stoxil

Chemical Class: Pyrimidine nucleoside

Therapeutic Class: Ophthalmic antiviral

CLINICAL PHARMACOLOGY

Mechanism of Action: Inhibits viral replication by interfering with viral DNA synthesis

Pharmacokinetics

Deactivated by deaminases and nucleotidases, penetrates cornea poorly

INDICATIONS AND USES: Herpes simplex keratitis, CMV, varicella zoster alone or with corticosteroids

DOSAGE

Adult and Child

• Instill 1 gtt q1h during day and q2h during night

$ **AVAILABLE FORMS/COST OF THERAPY**

• Sol—Ophth; Top: 0.1%, 15 ml: **$13.21**

CONTRAINDICATIONS: Hypersensitivity

PRECAUTIONS: Sensitivity to iodine

PREGNANCY AND LACTATION: Pregnancy category C; crosses placenta, teratogenic in rabbits and mice; no data available for breast feeding; no problems documented in humans

SIDE EFFECTS/ADVERSE REACTIONS

EENT: Poor corneal wound healing, temporary visual haze, overgrowth of nonsusceptible organisms

▼ **DRUG INTERACTIONS**

• *Boric acid:* Precipitate formation

imipenem

(i-me-pen'em)

Primaxin

Therapeutic Class: Antibiotic

Chemical Class: Thienamycin antibiotic and renal dipeptidase inhibitor

CLINICAL PHARMACOLOGY

Mechanism of Action: Bactericidal; binds to penicillin-binding proteins which inhibits bacterial cell wall synthesis, results in cell lysis; formulated with cilastin which prevents renal metabolism of imipenem

Pharmacokinetics

IV: Onset immediate, peak ½-1 hr, $t_{1/2}$ 1 hr

IM: Peak 2 hr, $t_{1/2}$ 6-8 hr

Excreted by kidney (75%) and unknown non-renal mechanism (25%); rapidly cleared by hemodialysis; $t_{1/2}$ longer in children (2 hr in neonates, 1.2 hr in older children)

INDICATIONS AND USES: Serious infections of the lower respiratory tract, urinary tract, skin; intra-abdominal infections, gynecologic infections, septicemia, endocarditis. Antibacterial spectrum usually includes: gram-positive organisms: *Streptococcus pneumoniae,* group A beta-hemolytic streptococci, *Staphylococcus aureus,* enterococcus; gram-negative organisms: *Klebsiella, Proteus, E. coli, Acinetobacter, Serratia, Pseudomonas aeruginosa; Salmonella, Shigella*

DOSAGE

Adult

• IV 250-500 mg q6h; severe infections may require 1 g q6h; max 50 mg/kg or 4 g/d (whichever is lower)

• IM 500 or 750 mg q12h to max 1500 mg qd

• Dosage adjustment in impaired renal function: CrCl 30-70 ml/sec, 500 mg q6-8h; CrCl 20-30 ml/sec, 500 mg q8-12h; CrCl 0-20 ml/sec: 250-500 mg q12h

• Hemodialysis patients, supplemental dose after hemodialysis, unless scheduled dose within 4h

Child

• >40 kg, adult dose

• <40 kg, 60 mg/kg/d in divided doses

$ **AVAILABLE FORMS/COST OF THERAPY**

• Inj, Dry-Sol—IV: 250 mg: **$11.15;** 500 mg: **$20.60**

• Inj, Dry-Sol—IM: 500 mg: **$25.02;** 750 mg: **$37.53**

CONTRAINDICATIONS: Hypersensitivity, IM hypersensitivity to local anesthetics of the amide type

PRECAUTIONS: Elderly, hypersensitivity to penicillins, seizure disorders, renal disease, children

PREGNANCY AND LACTATION: Pregnancy category C; unknown if excreted in breast milk

SIDE EFFECTS/ADVERSE REACTIONS

CNS: Fever, somnolence, ***seizures,*** dizziness, weakness, myoclonia

CV: Hypotension, palpitations

GI: Diarrhea, nausea, vomiting, ***pseudomembranous colitis, hepatitis,*** glossitis

HEME: ***Eosinophilia, neutropenia,*** decreased Hgb, Hct

RESP: Chest discomfort, dyspnea, hyperventilation

SKIN: Rash, urticaria, pruritus, pain at inj site, phlebitis, erythema at inj site

MISC: ***Anaphylaxis***

▼ DRUG INTERACTIONS

Drugs

• *Probenecid:* Increased imipenem plasma levels

• *Ganciclovir:* Increased ganciclovir levels, increased seizure risk

Labs

• *Increase:* AST, ALT, LDH, BUN, alk phosphatase, bilirubin, creatinine

• *False positive:* Direct Coombs' test

imipramine

(im-ip'ra-meen)

Impril, ♣ Janimine, Novopramine, ♣ Tofranil, Tofranil PM

Chemical Class: Dibenzazepine—tertiary amine

Therapeutic Class: Antidepressant, tricyclic

CLINICAL PHARMACOLOGY

Mechanism of Action: Blocks reuptake of norepinephrine, serotonin into nerve endings, increasing action of norepinephrine, serotonin in nerve cells

Pharmacokinetics

PO: Steady state 2-5 days; metabolized by liver; excreted in urine, feces; crosses placenta; excreted in breast milk; $t_{1/2}$ 6-20 hr

INDICATIONS AND USES: Depression, enuresis in children

DOSAGE

Adult

• PO/IM 75-100 mg/d in divided doses, may increase by 25-50 mg to 200 mg, not to exceed 300 mg/d; may give daily dose hs

Child

• PO 25-75 mg/d

$ AVAILABLE FORMS/COST OF THERAPY

• Tab, Sugar Coated—Oral: 10, 25, 50 mg, 100's: **$2.03-$74.12**

• Cap, Gel—Oral: 75 mg, 100's: **$103.67;** 100 mg, 100's: **$136.29;** 125 mg, 100's: **$169.95;** 150 mg, 100's: **$193.73**

• Inj—IM: 25 mg/2 ml, 10's: **$22.52**

CONTRAINDICATIONS: Hypersensitivity to tricyclic antidepressants, recovery phase of MI, convulsive disorders, prostatic hypertrophy

PRECAUTIONS: Suicidal patients,

severe depression, increased intraocular pressure, narrow-angle glaucoma, urinary retention, cardiac disease, hepatic disease, hyperthyroidism, electroshock therapy, elective surgery, elderly

PREGNANCY AND LACTATION: Pregnancy category C

SIDE EFFECTS/ADVERSE REACTIONS

CNS: Dizziness, drowsiness, confusion, headache, anxiety, tremors, stimulation, weakness, insomnia, nightmares, EPS (elderly), increased psychiatric symptoms, paresthesia

CV: Orthostatic hypotension, ECG changes, tachycardia, ***hypertension,*** palpitations

EENT: Blurred vision, tinnitus, mydriasis

GI: Diarrhea, dry mouth, nausea, vomiting, ***paralytic ileus,*** increased appetite, cramps, epigastric distress, jaundice, ***hepatitis,*** stomatitis

GU: Retention, ***acute renal failure***

HEME: ***Agranulocytosis, thrombocytopenia, eosinophilia, leukopenia***

SKIN: Rash, urticaria, sweating, pruritus, photosensitivity

▼ DRUG INTERACTIONS

Drugs

- *Guanethidine, clonidine, indirect-acting sympathomimetics (ephedrine):* Decreased effects of these drugs
- *Direct-acting sympathomimetics (epinephrine), alcohol, barbiturates, benzodiazepines, CNS depressants:* Increased effects
- *MAOI:* Hyperpyretic crisis, convulsions, hypertensive episode

Labs

- *Increase:* Serum bilirubin, alk phosphatase, blood glucose
- *Decrease:* 5-HIAA, VMA, urinary catecholamines

SPECIAL CONSIDERATIONS

PATIENT/FAMILY EDUCATION

- Withdrawal symptoms (headache, nausea, vomiting, muscle pain, weakness) may occur if drug discontinued abruptly

indapamide

(in-dap'a-mide)

Lozol, Lozide ♣

Chemical Class: Indoline

Therapeutic Class: Diuretic; thiazide-like

CLINICAL PHARMACOLOGY

Mechanism of Action: Acts on proximal section of distal renal tubule by inhibiting reabsorption of sodium; may act by direct vasodilation caused by blocking of calcium channel

Pharmacokinetics

PO: Onset 1-2 hr, peak 2 hr, duration up to 36 hr; excreted in urine, feces; $t_{1/2}$ 14-18 hr

INDICATIONS AND USES: Edema, hypertension, diuresis

DOSAGE

Adult

- PO 2.5-5 mg qd in AM

Child

- Dosage not established

$ AVAILABLE FORMS/COST OF THERAPY

- Tab, Plain Coated—Oral: 1.25 mg, 100's: **$64.98;** 2.5 mg, 100's: **$65.98-$84.73**

CONTRAINDICATIONS: Hypersensitivity to indapamide or other sulfonamides, anuria

PRECAUTIONS: Hypokalemia, dehydration, ascites, hepatic disease, severe renal disease, diabetes mellitus, gout, hyperuricemia, sympathectomy

PREGNANCY AND LACTATION: Pregnancy category B; not known if excreted in breast milk

SIDE EFFECTS/ADVERSE REACTIONS

CNS: Headache, dizziness, fatigue, weakness, paresthesias, depression

CV: Orthostatic hypotension, volume depletion, palpitations, dysrhythmias

EENT: Loss of hearing, tinnitus, blurred vision, nasal congestion, increased intraocular pressure

GI: Nausea, diarrhea, dry mouth, vomiting, anorexia, cramps, constipation, pancreatitis, abdominal pain, jaundice, hepatitis

GU: Polyuria, dysuria, frequency

HEME: ***Thrombocytopenia, agranulocytosis, leukopenia, neutropenia, anemia***

METAB: Hypochloremic alkalosis, hypomagnesemia, hyperuricemia, hypercalcemia, hyponatremia, hypokalemia, hyperglycemia

MS: Cramps

SKIN: Rash, pruritus, photosensitivity, alopecia, urticaria

▼ **DRUG INTERACTIONS**

Drugs

- *Anticoagulants:* Effects of anticoagulant may either increase or decrease
- *Antihypertensives:* Antihypertensive effects increased
- *Amiodarone:* Dysrhythmias associated with hypokalemia
- *Cholestyramine and colestipol:* Decreased absorption
- *Digitalis:* Increased digitalis toxicity secondary to hypokalemia
- *Hypoglycemics:* Decreased effect
- *Lithium:* Lithium toxicity
- *NSAIDs:* Decreased hypotensive effect of indapamide
- *Steroids:* Decreased potassium
- *Sympathomimetics:* Decreased indapamide effectiveness

Labs

- *Increase:* Plasma renin activity, uric acid
- *Decrease:* Potassium, sodium

indomethacin

(in-doe-meth'a-sin)

Indocin, Indocin SR, Indocin IV

Chemical Class: Propionic acid derivative

Therapeutic Class: Nonsteroidal antiinflammatory (NSAID)

CLINICAL PHARMACOLOGY

Mechanism of Action: Inhibits prostaglandin synthesis by decreasing enzyme needed for biosynthesis; analgesic, antiinflammatory, antipyretic

Pharmacokinetics

PO: Completely absorbed, onset 1-2 hr, peak 3 hr, duration 4-6 hr; metabolized in liver, kidneys; excreted in urine, bile, feces; 99% plasma protein binding

PR: 80%-90% absorbed

IV: $t_{1/2}$ 4½ in adults; in infants inversely related to gestational age and wt (<7 days age, <1000 g $t_{1/2}$ 20-21 hr; >7 days age, >1000 g $t_{1/2}$ 12-15 hr)

INDICATIONS AND USES: Rheumatoid arthritis, ankylosing spondylitis, acute gouty arthritis, closure of patent ductus arteriosus in premature infants, psoriatic arthritis,* Reiter's disease,* rheumatic complications of Paget's disease,* non-rheumatic inflammatory conditions, fever,* dysmenorrhea,* Bartter's syndrome,* pericarditis,* vascular headache*

DOSAGE

Adult

- *Antirheumatic/Anti-inflammatory:* PO 25-50 mg bid-qid; may increase by 25 mg/d qwk, not to exceed 200 mg/d; Sus Rel 75 mg qd, may increase to 75 mg bid; PR 50 mg bid-qid
- *Gout:* PO 100 mg initially then 50 mg tid until pain relieved, then reduce dose; PR 50 mg bid-qid

Child

• *Antirheumatic/Anti-inflammatory:* PO/PR 1.5-2.5 mg/kg/d divided tid-qid to max 4 mg/kg/d or 150-200 mg qd

• *Patent ductus arteriosus:* IV (preferred)/PO/PR 200 μg/kg initial dose; may follow with 100 μg/kg (infants ≤ 48 hrs age), 200 μg/kg (infants 2-7 days age), 250 μg/kg (infants >7 days age) q12-24 hr for two doses

$ AVAILABLE FORMS/COST OF THERAPY

• Inj, Lyphl-Sol—IV: 1 mg/vial: **$25.90**

• Powder Anhydrous—IV: 1 g: **$78.30**

• Cap, Gel—Oral: 25 mg, 100's: **$2.63-$56.08;** 50 mg, 100's: **$3.75-$89.09**

• Cap, Gel, Sus Rel—Oral: 75 mg, 100's: **$73.50-$106.58**

• Supp—Rect: 50 mg, 30's: **$30.62-$46.43**

• Susp—Oral: 25 mg/5ml, 500 ml: **$61.89**

CONTRAINDICATIONS: Hypersensitivity (including nasal polyps associated with bronchospasm induced by NSAIDs, ASA), severe renal disease, severe hepatic disease, severe cardiac disease, active ulcer disease

PRECAUTIONS: Bleeding disorders, anemia, asthma, GI disorders, hypertension, CHF, edema, SLE, hypersensitivity to other NSAIDs, elderly, depression, alcoholism

PREGNANCY AND LACTATION: Pregnancy category B; crosses placenta; excreted in breast milk

SIDE EFFECTS/ADVERSE REACTIONS

CNS: Dizziness, drowsiness, fatigue, tremors, confusion, insomnia, anxiety, depression, *headache*

CV: Tachycardia, peripheral edema, palpitations, dysrhythmias, hypertension

EENT: Tinnitus, hearing loss, blurred vision

GI: Nausea, anorexia, vomiting, diarrhea, jaundice, ***cholestatic hepatitis,*** constipation, flatulence, cramps, dry mouth, peptic ulcer, ***GI bleeding***

GU: ***Nephrotoxicity: dysuria, hematuria, oliguria, azotemia***

HEME: ***Blood dyscrasias***

RESP: Asthma

SKIN: Purpura, rash, pruritus, sweating

MISC: ***Anaphylaxis,*** fever

▼ DRUG INTERACTIONS

Drugs

• *ACE inhibitors, beta blockers, hydralazine:* Inhibits antihypertensive effect

• *Aminoglycosides:* Reduced renal clearance of antibiotic

• *Lithium:* Increases lithium levels

• *Loop diuretics:* Reduced diuretic and antihypertensive effect

• *Methotrexate:* Increased toxicity of methotrexate

• *Triamterene:* Acute renal failure

• *Warfarin:* Indomethacin effects on gastric mucosa and platelet inhibition, increased risk of bleeding

SPECIAL CONSIDERATIONS

MONITORING PARAMETERS

• Liver enzymes

insulin

(in'suh-lin)

Rapid acting:

Regular Insulin: Beef Regular Iletin II, Humulin BR, Humulin R, Novolin R, Pork Regular Iletin II, Regular Purified Pork, Novolin R PenFill, Velosulin

Zinc suspension prompt: Semilente Iletin I, Semilente Insulin

Intermediate acting:

Zinc suspension: Humulin L, Lentard Monotard, ♣ Lente Iletin II, Lente Insulin, Lente Ile I, Lente Purified Pork Insulin, Novolin

Isophane Suspension (NPH): Beef NPH Iletin II, Humulin N, Iletin NPH, ♣ Insulatard NPH, NPH Iletin, Pork NPH Iletin II, Novolin N, NPH Insulin, NPH Purified Pork

Long Acting:

Zinc Suspension Extended: Ultralente, ♣ Ultralente Iletin I, Ultralente Insulin, Protamine Zinc Insulin Suspension (PZI)

Insulin Mixtures:

Isophane Insulin and Regular Insulin: Humulin 70/30, Mixtard 70/30, Mixtard Human 70/30, Novolin 70/30, Humulin 50/50

Concentrated Insulin:

Regular Concentrated Insulin: Iletin II U-500

Chemical Class: Exogenous insulin

Therapeutic Class: Antidiabetic

CLINICAL PHARMACOLOGY

Mechanism of Action: Hormone which controls storage and metabolism of carbohydrates, protein, and fats; decreases blood glucose

Pharmacokinetics

See Insulins Table, App. A, p. 890. Metabolized by liver, muscle, kidneys; excreted in urine

INDICATIONS AND USES: Type I diabetes, Type II diabetes not controlled by other means, ketoacidosis, hyperkalemia, nonketotic hyperosmolar syndrome; human insulin is insulin of choice in insulin allergy, insulin resistance, pregnancy

DOSAGE

Adult/Child

- *Ketoacidosis:* IV bolus or IM 0.1-0.25 U/kg regular insulin, then 0.1 U/kg/hr IV inf/IM q1h until blood glucose 250 mg/dl, then give SC replacement dose
- *Type I DM replacement:* SC dosage individualized by blood glucose levels; initial total daily dose based on presence of urine ketones; if ketones negative–moderate 0.5 U/kg, if ketones large 0.7 U/kg; give ⅔ total dose in AM, ⅓ in PM; use mixture regular/NPH insulin (ratio 1:2 for AM dose, 1:1 for PM dose)
- *Type II DM replacement:* SC dosage individualized by blood glucose levels; initial total daily dose 0.3 U/kg; give ⅔ total dose in AM, ⅓ in PM; use mixed insulin 70/30 or 50/50 or mixture of regular/NPH (ratio 1:2 for AM dose, 1:1 for PM dose)
- *Type II DM combination with oral agent* (unable to achieve targets on max dose oral agent, AM hyperglycemia): Decrease oral agent to ½ max dose, give as single AM dose; add insulin with evening snack SC 0.1 U/kg NPH
- *Nonketotic hyperosmolar syndrome:* IV 10-20 U regular insulin, then IV/IM 5-15 U/hr until glucose 250 mg/dl, then give SC replacement dose
- *Gestational DM:* SC dosage individualized by blood glucose levels; initial total daily dose 0.4 U/kg current wt given as mixture regular/NPH distributed as for Type I DM

• *Hyperkalemia:* Adult IV 5-10 U regular insulin with 25 g dextrose (1 ampule D_{50}); child: 0.5g/kg dextrose with 0.3 U regular insulin/g dextrose over 2 hr

$ AVAILABLE FORMS/COST OF THERAPY

Rapid-acting insulin:
• Inj, Sol—IM; IV; SC: 100 U/ml, 10 ml: **$14.34-$23.42**
• Inj, Susp—SC: 40 U/ml, 10 ml: **$5.79**

Intermediate-acting insulin:
• Inj, Susp—SC: 100 U/ml, 10 ml: **$14.34-$23.42;** 40 U/ml, 10 ml: **$5.79**

Long-acting insulin:
• Inj, Sol—SC: 100 U/ml, 10 ml: **$12.68-$13.72;** 40 U/ml, 10 ml: **$5.79**

Mixed insulin 70/30:
• Inj, Sol—SC: 100 U/ml, 10 ml: **$17.42-$21.23**

Mixed insulin 50/50:
• Inj, Susp—SC: 100 U/ml, 10 ml: **$17.42**

Concentrated insulin:
• Inj, Susp—SC: 500 U/ml, 20 ml: **$104.59**

CONTRAINDICATIONS: Hypersensitivity

PREGNANCY AND LACTATION: Pregnancy category B; insulin requirements of pregnant diabetic patients often decreased in first half and increased in the latter half of pregnancy; elevated blood glucose levels associated with congenital abnormalities; does not pass into breast milk

SIDE EFFECTS/ADVERSE REACTIONS

CNS: Headache, lethargy, tremors, weakness, fatigue, ***delirium,*** sweating
CV: Tachycardia, palpitations
EENT: Blurred vision, dry mouth
GI: Hunger, nausea
SKIN: Flushing, rash, urticaria, warmth, lipodystrophy, lipohypertrophy
META: *Hypoglycemia*
MISC: ***Anaphylaxis***

▼ DRUG INTERACTIONS

Drugs
• *MAO inhibitors, phenylbutazone, salicylates:* Hypoglycemia
• *Beta blockers:* Hypoglycemia symptoms masked, except for sweating

Labs
• *Decrease:* K, Ca, PO_4, Mg

SPECIAL CONSIDERATIONS

PATIENT/FAMILY EDUCATION
• For hypoglycemia give 1 mg glucagon or glucose 25 g IV (via dextrose 50% sol, 50 ml)
• When mixing insulins draw up regular first
• Dosage adjustment may be necessary when changing insulin products
• Use single brand/type of syringe
• Human insulin now considered insulin of choice

interferon alfa-2a/2b

(in-ter-feer′on)
Roferon-a (interferon alfa-2a), Intron-a (interferon alfa-2b)
Chemical Class: Recombinant protein product
Therapeutic Class: Miscellaneous antineoplastic

CLINICAL PHARMACOLOGY

Mechanism of Action: Altered synthesis of RNA, DNA, and cellular proteins

Pharmacokinetics

SC: Absorption >80%; $t_{1/2}$ (interferon alfa-2a) 6-8 hr, peak 7.3 hr; $t_{1/2}$ (interferon alfa-2b) 2-3 hr, peak 3-12 hr
IV: $t_{1/2}$, 4-8 hr
IM: Absorption >80%; $t_{1/2}$ (interferon alfa-2a) 6-8 hr, peak 3.8 hr;

$t_{1/2}$ (interferon alfa-2b) 2-3 hr, peak 3-12 hr

INTRALESIONAL: Minimal systemic absorption

Excreted by kidney; unknown if excreted in human breast milk

INDICATIONS AND USES: Hairy cell leukemia, condylomata acuminata, hepatitis C, chronic active hepatitis, metastatic melanoma, AIDS-associated Kaposi's sarcoma, bladder carcinoma, renal carcinoma, chronic myelocytic leukemia, laryngeal papillomatosis, non-Hodgkin's lymphoma, multiple myeloma, mycosis fungoides

DOSAGE

• A variety of dosage schedules have been used; consult medical literature prior to choosing specific dosage

Interferon alfa-2a

Adult

• *Hairy cell leukemia:* IM/SC 3 million U qd for 16-24 wk then 3 million U 3 times/wk

• *Kaposi's sarcoma:* IM/SC 36 million U qd for 10-12 wk OR 3 million U qd days 1-3 then 9 million U qd days 4-6, then 18 million U days 7-9, then 36 million U qd for remainder of 10-12 wk; maintenance with 36 million U 3 times/wk

Child

• Not established; caution in adolescent females because interferes with serum estradiol and progesterone concentration

Interferon alfa-2b

Adult

• *Hairy cell leukemia:* IM/SC 2 million U/m^2 body surface area 3 times/wk

• *Condylomata acuminata:* Intralesional, 1 million U (0.1 ml) per wart (up to five warts) 3 times/wk for 3 wk; second course may be given 12-16 wk after first course; treat more warts sequentially in groups of five

• *Kaposi's sarcoma:* IM/SC 30 million U/m^2 body surface area 3 times/wk

• *Chronic active hepatitis:* IM/SC 3 million U 3 times/wk

Child

• Not established

$ **AVAILABLE FORMS/COST OF THERAPY**

Interferon alfa-2a

• Inj, Dry-Sol—IM; SC: 9 million IU/vial: **$84.14;** IM; SC: 18 million IU/vial: **$179.20;** IM: 36 million IU/1 ml: **$358.38;** IM; SC: 3 million IU/0.5 ml: **$179.20**

Interferon alfa-2b

• Inj, Conc-Sol—IM: 5 million IU/vial: **$52.51;** IM: 25 million IU/vial: **$262.57;** IM; SC: 50 million IU/vial: **$525.12**

• Inj, Lyphl-Sol—IM: 3 million IU/vial: **$31.51**

• Inj, Lyphl-Sol—IV: 10 million IU/vial: **$105.03**

• Inj, Sol—IV: 5 million IU/ml, 2ml: **$105.02;** 6 million IU/ml, 3ml: **$189.04;** 18 million IU/vial: **$189.04**

CONTRAINDICATIONS: Hypersensitivity

PRECAUTIONS: Severe hypotension, dysrhythmia, tachycardia, severe renal or hepatic disease, seizure disorder

PREGNANCY AND LACTATION: Pregnancy category C; abortifacient in animal models; avoid breast feeding

SIDE EFFECTS/ADVERSE REACTIONS

CNS: Dizziness, confusion, numbness, paresthesias, hallucinations, ***convulsions, coma,*** amnesia, anxiety, mood changes

CV: Edema, hypotension, hypertension, chest pain, palpitations, dysrhythmias, ***CHF, MI, CVA***

EENT: Blurred vision, *dry mouth*

GI: Weight loss, taste changes, anorexia, diarrhea
GU: Impotence
HEME: ***Anemia, leukopenia, thrombocytopenia***
SKIN: Rash, dry skin, itching, alopecia, flushing
MISC: Flulike syndrome; fever, fatigue, myalgias, headache, chills

▼ **DRUG INTERACTIONS**

Drugs

• *Theophylline:* Increased theophylline levels

interferon alfa-n3

(in-ter-feer′on)

Alferon N

Chemical Class: Human leukocyte interferon

Therapeutic Class: Antineoplastic

CLINICAL PHARMACOLOGY

Mechanism of Action: Altered synthesis of RNA, DNA, and cellular proteins

Pharmacokinetics

Unable to detect by assay although some systemic effects noted

INDICATIONS AND USES: Condylomata acuminata (venereal/genital warts)

DOSAGE

Adult

• Intralesional (into base of wart): 0.05 ml (250,000 IU) per wart, given 2 times/wk for max 8 wk

Child

• Dosage not established

$ **AVAILABLE FORMS/COST OF THERAPY**

• Inj, Sol—ID; SC: 250,000 U/.05 ml, 1 ml: **$141.62**

CONTRAINDICATIONS: Hypersensitivity to interferon alfa, anaphylaxis to egg protein, neomycin, mouse IgG

PRECAUTIONS: CHF, angina (unstable), COPD, diabetes mellitus with ketoacidosis, hemophilia, pulmonary embolism, thrombophlebitis, bone marrow depression, seizure disorder

PREGNANCY AND LACTATION: Pregnancy category C; unknown if excreted in breast milk

SIDE EFFECTS/ADVERSE REACTIONS

CNS: Fever, headache, sweating, vasovagal reaction, chills, fatigue, dizziness, insomnia, sleepiness, depression
CV: ***Chest pain, hypotension***
GI: Nausea, vomiting, heartburn, diarrhea, constipation, anorexia, stomatitis, dry mouth
MS: Myalgias, arthralgia, back pain
SKIN: Pain at inj site, pruritis

▼ **DRUG INTERACTIONS**

Drugs

• *Theophylline:* Increased theophylline levels

interferon beta

(in-ter-feer′on)

Betaseron

Chemical Class: E. coli derivative

Therapeutic Class: Multiple sclerosis agent

CLINICAL PHARMACOLOGY

Mechanism of Action: Antiviral, immunoregulatory; action not clearly understood; biologic response modifying properties mediated through specific receptors on cells, inducing expression of interferon-induced gene products

Pharmacokinetics

SC: Serum levels very low or not detectable at recommended dose; at higher doses 50% bioavailable, peak 1-8 hr

INDICATIONS AND USES: Ambulatory patients with relapsing or remitting multiple sclerosis, treatment of AIDS,* AIDS-related Kaposi's sarcoma,* malignant melanoma,* metastatic renal cell carcinoma,* cutaneous T-cell lymphoma,* acute non-A, non-B hepatitis*

DOSAGE

Adult

• Relapsing/remitting multiple sclerosis: SC 0.25 mg (8 IU) qod

Child

• Not established

AVAILABLE FORMS/COST OF THERAPY

• Inj, Lyphl-Sol—SC: 0.3 mg/vial: **$72.00**

CONTRAINDICATIONS: Hypersensitivity to natural or recombinant interferon-beta or human albumin

PRECAUTIONS: Children under 18 yr, chronic progressive MS, depression, mental disorders

PREGNANCY AND LACTATION: Pregnancy category C; possible abortifacient; not known if excreted in breast milk, avoid in nursing mothers

SIDE EFFECTS/ADVERSE REACTIONS

CNS: Headache, fever, pain, chills, mental changes, hypertonia, ***suicide attempts***

CV: Migraine, palpitations, hypertension, tachycardia, peripheral vascular disorders

EENT: Conjunctivitis, blurred vision

GI: Diarrhea, constipation, vomiting, abdominal pain

GU: Dysmenorrhea, irregular menses, metrorrhagia, cystitis, breast pain

HEME: ***Decreased lymphocytes, neutrophils, lymphadenopathy***

MS: Myalgia, ***myasthenia***

RESP: Sinusitis, dyspnea

SKIN: Sweating, inj site reaction

▼ DRUG INTERACTIONS

Drugs

• *Zidovudine:* Increased levels

SPECIAL CONSIDERATIONS

MONITORING PARAMETERS

• Follow CBC, platelets, LFTs q3mo

• D/C for ANC < 750/mm^3, ALT/AST> 10 × upper limits normal, bili >5 × upper limits normal; when labs return to these levels restart at 50% reduction dose

---

interferon gamma

(in-ter-feer'on)

Actimmune

Chemical Class: Lymphokine, interleukin type

Therapeutic Class: Biologic response modifier

CLINICAL PHARMACOLOGY

Mechanism of Action: Interacts with other lymphokines (e.g., interleukin-2); activates macrophages, enhancing phagocytic function; enhances cellular cytotoxicity

Pharmacokinetics

SC: 89% dose absorbed, $t_{1/2}$ 5.9 hr, peak 7 hr

INDICATIONS AND USES: Serious infections associated with chronic granulomatous disease

DOSAGE

Adult/Child

• SC 50 μg/m^2 (1.5 million U/m^2) for patients with surface area of >0.5 m^2; 1.5 μg/kg/dose for patient with a surface area of <0.5/m^2; given 3 ×/wk

AVAILABLE FORMS/COST OF THERAPY

• Inj, Sol—SC: 100 μg (3 million U)/0.5 ml: **$140.00**

CONTRAINDICATIONS: Hypersensitivity to product or *E. coli*-derived products

PRECAUTIONS: Cardiac disease, seizure disorders, CNS disorders, myelosuppression, safety not established in children <1

PREGNANCY AND LACTATION: Pregnancy category C; possible abortifacient; not known if excreted in breast milk, not recommended in breastfeeding

SIDE EFFECTS/ADVERSE REACTIONS

CNS: Headache, fatigue, depression, fever, chills

GI: Nausea, anorexia, abdominal pain, weight loss, diarrhea, vomiting

MS: Myalgia, arthralgia

SKIN: Rash, pain at inj site

▼ **DRUG INTERACTIONS**

Drugs

- *Myelosuppressive drugs:* May potentiate myelosuppression

---

iodinated glycerol

Iophen, Organidin, Par Glycerol, R-Gen (available as other products in combination with theophylline, dextromethorphan, codeine)

Chemical Class: Iodopropylidene glycerol isomer

Therapeutic Class: Expectorant

CLINICAL PHARMACOLOGY

Mechanism of Action: Increases respiratory tract fluid by decreasing surface tension, increases removal of mucus

Pharmacokinetics

Readily absorbed, concentrated in respiratory secretions, excreted by kidneys

INDICATIONS AND USES: Mucolytic expectorant in asthma, emphysema, bronchitis, cystic fibrosis, chronic sinusitis; efficacy not proven

DOSAGE

Adult

- PO TAB 60 mg qid; ELIX 5 ml qid; SOL 20 gtt qid

Child

- PO up to half adult dose, depending on weight

$ **AVAILABLE FORMS/COST OF THERAPY**

- Elixir—Oral: 60 mg/5 ml, 120 ml: **$1.25-$6.93**
- Sol—Oral: 50 mg/ml, 30 ml: **$5.50-$27.62**
- Tab, Uncoated—Oral: 30 mg, 100's: **$10.66-$18.07**

CONTRAINDICATIONS: Hypersensitivity to iodides, pulmonary TB, hyperthyroidism, hyperkalemia, pregnancy, newborns, lactation, acute bronchitis

PRECAUTIONS: Thyroid disease, cystic fibrosis (increased goitrogenic effect in children with CF)

PREGNANCY AND LACTATION: Contraindicated in pregnancy, category X; not recommended in nursing mothers (rash and thyroid suppression in infant)

SIDE EFFECTS/ADVERSE REACTIONS

CNS: Frontal headache, *CNS depression,* fever, parkinsonism

EENT: Burning mouth, throat, eye irritation, swelling of eyelids

GI: Gastric irritation

METAB: Iodism, goiter, myxedema

RESP: Pulmonary edema

SKIN: ***Angioedema,*** rash

▼ **DRUG INTERACTIONS**

Drugs

- *Lithium, antithyroid drugs:* Increased hypothyroid effects
- *K-sparing diuretics, K-containing medication:* Dysrhythmias, hyperkalemia

iodoquinol

(eye-oh-do-kwin'ole)

Diodoquin, ♣ Yodoxin

Chemical Class: Dihalogenated derivative of 8-hydroxyquinoline

Therapeutic Class: Amebicide

CLINICAL PHARMACOLOGY

Mechanism of Action: Direct-acting amebicide; action occurs in intestinal lumen

Pharmacokinetics

Poorly absorbed, excreted in feces

INDICATIONS AND USES: Intestinal amebiasis

DOSAGE

Adult

- PO 650 mg tid after meals for 20 days, not to exceed 2 g/d

Child

- PO 30-40 mg/kg/d in 3 divided doses for 20 days, not to exceed 1.95 g/24 hr for 20 days; do not repeat treatment before 2-3 wk

$ **AVAILABLE FORMS/COST OF THERAPY**

- Powder—Oral: 25 g: **$27.98**
- Tab, Uncoated—Oral: 210 mg, 100's: **$32.80;** 650 mg, 100's: **$18.20-$40.29**

CONTRAINDICATIONS: Hypersensitivity to this drug or iodine, renal disease, hepatic disease, severe thyroid disease, preexisting optic neuropathy

PRECAUTIONS: Thyroid disease

PREGNANCY AND LACTATION: Pregnancy category C; excretion into breast milk unknown

SIDE EFFECTS/ADVERSE REACTIONS

CNS: Malaise, headache, agitation, peripheral neuropathy

EENT: Blurred vision, sore throat, retinal edema, optic neuritis, optic atrophy

GI: Anorexia, nausea, vomiting, diarrhea, epigastric distress, gastritis, constipation, abdominal cramps, rectal irritation, anal itching

HEME: ***Agranulocytosis*** (rare)

SKIN: Rash; pruritus; discolored skin, hair, nails; alopecia

MISC: Fever, chills, vertigo, thyroid enlargement

▼ **DRUG INTERACTIONS**

Labs

- *Increase:* PBI
- *Decrease:* I^{131} uptake test
- *Interfere:* Thyroid function test
- *False positive:* PKU

ipecac

(ip'e-kak)

Chemical Class: Cephaelis ipecacuanha derivative

Therapeutic Class: Emetic

CLINICAL PHARMACOLOGY

Mechanism of Action: Acts on chemoreceptor trigger zone to induce vomiting; irritates gastric mucosa

Pharmacokinetics

PO: Onset 15-30 min; minimal systemic absorption

INDICATIONS AND USES: In poisoning to induce vomiting

DOSAGE

Adult

- PO 15-30 ml, then 3-4 glasses water

Child 1-12 yr

- PO 15 ml, then 1-2 glasses water

Child <1 yr

- PO 5-10 ml, then ½-1 glass water, may repeat dose if needed

$ **AVAILABLE FORMS/COST OF THERAPY**

- Liq—Oral: 30 ml: **$1.76-$16.03**

CONTRAINDICATIONS: Hypersensitivity, unconscious/semiconscious, depressed gag reflex, poisoning with petroleum products or caustic substances, convulsions

PREGNANCY AND LACTATION: Pregnancy category C; not known if excreted in breast milk

SIDE EFFECTS/ADVERSE REACTIONS

CNS: ***Depression, convulsions, coma***

CV: ***Circulatory failure, atrial fibrillation, fatal myocarditis, dysrhythmias***

GI: Nausea, vomiting, bloody diarrhea

▼ **DRUG INTERACTIONS**

Drugs

- *Activated charcoal:* Decreased effect of ipecac; if both drugs used, give activated charcoal after emesis induced

SPECIAL CONSIDERATIONS

May not work on empty stomach. Do not confuse with ipecac fluid extract (14 times stronger)

---

ipratropium

(eye-pra-troep'ee-um)

Atrovent

Chemical Class: Synthetic quaternary ammonium compound
Therapeutic Class: Anticholinergic bronchodilator

CLINICAL PHARMACOLOGY

Mechanism of Action: Inhibits interaction of acetylcholine at receptor sites on bronchial smooth muscle, resulting in bronchodilation

Pharmacokinetics

INH: Onset 5-15 min; peak effect 1-2 hr duration of action 3-6 hr; absorption minimal; does not cross blood-brain barrier; 90% excreted in feces

INDICATIONS AND USES: Maintenance treatment of bronchospasm in COPD, bronchial asthma;* not indicated for acute bronchospasm

DOSAGE

Adult

- INH 1-2 puffs qid, not to exceed 12 puffs/24 hr
- Sol 500 μg via nebulizer q6-8 hr; can be mixed with albuterol

Child <12 yr

- Dosage not established

$ **AVAILABLE FORMS/COST OF THERAPY**

- Aer—Inh: 18 μg/inh, 14 g: **$28.14**
- Sol—Inh: 0.2 mg/ml, 2.5 ml, 500 μg/vial: **$1.87**

CONTRAINDICATIONS: Hypersensitivity to ipratropium, atropine

PRECAUTIONS: Angle closure glaucoma, prostatic hypertrophy, bladder neck obstruction, urinary retention

PREGNANCY AND LACTATION: Pregnancy category B; not known if excreted in breast milk but little systemic absorption when administered by inh

SIDE EFFECTS/ADVERSE REACTIONS

CNS: Anxiety, dizziness, headache, nervousness

CV: Palpitations

EENT: Dry mouth, blurred vision, metallic taste, stomatitis

GI: Nausea, vomiting, cramps

RESP: Cough, worsening of symptoms, ***bronchospasm***

SKIN: Rash

---

iron dextran

Hydextran, Imferon, K-Feron

Chemical Class: Ferric hydroxide complexed with dextran
Therapeutic Class: Hematinic

CLINICAL PHARMACOLOGY

Mechanism of Action: Iron is carried by transferrin to bone marrow and incorporated into hemoglobin

Pharmacokinetics

IM: Excreted in feces, urine, bile, breast milk; crosses placenta; most absorbed through lymphatics; can be gradually absorbed over weeks/ months from fixed locations

INDICATIONS AND USES: Iron deficiency anemia when oral administration not satisfactory, patients receiving epoetin therapy*

DOSAGE

- To calculate total amt of iron (in mg) required to restore hemoglobin to normal levels and replenish iron stores in iron deficient anemia: (0.3) × (weight in lb) × [100-(Hgb in g/dl × 100/14.8)]
- Divide this result by 50 to obtain dose in ml

Adult

- IM 0.5 ml as a test dose by Z-track (pull skin laterally prior to injection); wait ≥ 1 hr before giving remainder of therapeutic dose; max dose 2 ml (100 μg) qd
- IV 0.5 ml as test dose IV; give slowly, ≤ 1 ml/min; follow same protocol and dose as for IM

Child

- If <30 lb total dose is 80% of dose as calculated by above formula
- IM/IV 0.5 ml as a test dose as above then no more than the following per day: <10 lb 0.5 ml (25 mg); <20 lb 1 ml (50 mg)

$ AVAILABLE FORMS/COST OF THERAPY

- Inj, Sol—IM; IV: 50 mg/ml, 2 ml: **$36.36**

CONTRAINDICATIONS: Hypersensitivity, all anemias excluding iron deficiency anemia, hepatic disease

PRECAUTIONS: Acute renal disease, asthma, rheumatoid arthritis (IV), severe liver disease, infants <4 mo

PREGNANCY AND LACTATION: Pregnancy category C; excreted in breast milk

SIDE EFFECTS/ADVERSE REACTIONS

CNS: Headache, paresthesia, dizziness, shivering, weakness, ***seizures***

CV: Chest pain, ***shock,*** hypotension, tachycardia

GI: Nausea, vomiting, metallic taste, abdominal pain

HEME: ***Leukocytosis***

RESP: Dyspnea

SKIN: Rash, pruritus, urticaria, fever, sweating, chills, brown skin discoloration, pain at inj site, necrosis, sterile abscesses, phlebitis

MISC: ***Anaphylaxis***

▼ DRUG INTERACTIONS

Drugs

- *Oral iron:* Increased toxicity
- *Vitamin E, chloramphenicol:* Decreased reticulocyte response

SPECIAL CONSIDERATIONS

- Discontinue oral iron before giving
- Delayed reaction (fever, myalgias, arthralgias, nausea) may occur 1-2 days after administration
- When giving IM give only in gluteal muscle

isocarboxazid

(eye-soe-kar-box'a-zid)

Marplan

Chemical Class: Hydrazine

Therapeutic Class: Antidepressant, MAOI

CLINICAL PHARMACOLOGY

Mechanism of Action: Increases concentrations of endogenous epinephrine, norepinephrine, serotonin, dopamine in storage sites in CNS by inhibition of MAO; increased concentrations reduce depression

Pharmacokinetics

PO: Duration up to 2 wk; metabolized by liver; excreted by kidneys

INDICATIONS AND USES: Depression when uncontrolled by other means

DOSAGE

Adult

• PO 30 mg/d in single or divided doses; reduce dose to lowest effective dose (10-20 mg qd) when condition improves. Full effect may take 3-4 wk

$ **AVAILABLE FORMS/COST OF THERAPY**

• Tab, Uncoated—Oral: 10 mg, 100's: **$55.06**

CONTRAINDICATIONS: Hypersensitivity to MAOIs, elderly, hypertension, CHF, severe hepatic disease, pheochromocytoma, severe renal disease, severe cardiac disease

PRECAUTIONS: Suicidal patients, seizure disorders, severe depression, schizophrenia, hyperactivity, diabetes mellitus

PREGNANCY AND LACTATION: Pregnancy category C; breast feeding data not available

SIDE EFFECTS/ADVERSE REACTIONS

CNS: Dizziness, drowsiness, confusion, headache, anxiety, tremors, stimulation, weakness, hyperreflexia, mania, insomnia, fatigue

CV: ***Orthostatic hypotension, hypertension, dysrhythmias, hypertensive crisis***

EENT: Blurred vision

GI: Constipation, dry mouth, nausea, vomiting, *anorexia,* diarrhea, weight gain

GU: Change in libido, frequency

HEME: Anemia

METAB: ***SIADH-like syndrome,*** hypoglycemia

SKIN: Rash, flushing, increased perspiration, jaundice

▼ **DRUG INTERACTIONS**

Drugs

• *Antidiabetic drugs:* Hypoglycemia

• *Barbiturates:* Prolonged action of barbiturate

• *Dextromethorphan:* Agitation, seizure, increased BP, hyperpyrexia

• *Ephedrine+, amphetamines+, levodopa, phenylephrine, phenylpropanolamine, pseudoephedrine, reserpine:* Hypertension

• *Meperidine+:* Sweating, rigidity, hypertension

• *Neuromuscular blocking agents:* Prolonged effects of blocking agent

• *Selegiline:* Increased pressor response

• *Sertraline+, fluoxetine+:* CNS effects

• *Sumatriptan:* Increased sumatriptan levels

• *Tricyclic antidepressants:* Excessive sympathetic response, mania, hyperpyrexia

SPECIAL CONSIDERATIONS

PATIENT/FAMILY EDUCATION

• Phentolamine for severe hypertension

• Avoid high-tyramine foods: cheese (aged), sour cream, beer, wine, pickled products, liver, raisins, bananas, figs, avocados, meat tenderizers, chocolate, yogurt; soy sauce, caffeine

• Do not discontinue medication quickly after long-term use

isoetharine

(eye-soe-eth'a-reen)

Arm-a-Med, Beta-2, Bronkometer, Bronkosol

Chemical Class: Adrenergic beta$_2$-agonist

Therapeutic Class: Bronchodilator

CLINICAL PHARMACOLOGY

Mechanism of Action: Causes bronchodilation by beta-$_2$ stimulation, causing relaxation of bronchial smooth muscle

Pharmacokinetics

INH: Onset immediate, peak 5-15 min, duration 1-4 hr, metabolized in liver, GI tract, lungs, excreted in urine

INDICATIONS AND USES: Bronchospasm, asthma

DOSAGE

Adult

- Aerosol nebulizer 3-7 puffs undiluted q4h
- IPPB Dosage (give q4h): 1% sol 0.25-1.0 ml; 0.25% sol 2 ml; 0.2% sol 1.25-2.5 ml; 0.17% sol 3 ml; 0.167% sol 3 ml; 0.125% sol 2-4 ml; 0.1% sol 2.5-5 ml; 0.08% sol 3 ml

Child

- Dosage not established

$ AVAILABLE FORMS/COST OF THERAPY

- Sol—Inh: 0.08%, 3 ml, 25's: **$19.90;** 0.1%, 5 ml, 25's: **$19.90;** 0.125%, 4 ml, 25's: **$14.34-$24.84;** 0.17%, 3 ml, 25's: **$19.90;** 0.167%, 3 ml, 25's: **$14.34-24.84;** 0.2%, 2.5 ml, 25's: **$14.34-$24.84;** 0.25%, 2 ml, 25's: **$19.90-$24.84;** 1%, 10 ml: **$5.00-$17.49**
- Aer—Inh: 0.61%, 10 ml: **$21.75-$23.20**

CONTRAINDICATIONS: Hypersensitivity to sympathomimetics, narrow-angle glaucoma

PRECAUTIONS: Cardiac disorders, hyperthyroidism, diabetes mellitus, prostatic hypertrophy

PREGNANCY AND LACTATION: Pregnancy category C; no breast feeding data available

SIDE EFFECTS/ADVERSE REACTIONS

CNS: Tremors, anxiety, insomnia, headache, dizziness, stimulation

CV: Palpitations, tachycardia, hypertension, ***cardiac arrest, dysrhythmias***

GI: Nausea

METAB: Hyperglycemia

▼ DRUG INTERACTIONS

Drugs

- *Beta blockers:* Decreased action of isoetharine
- *MAOIs:* Hypertensive crisis
- *Other sympathomimetics:* Increased effects of both drugs

---

isoflurophate

(eye-soe-flure'oh-fate)

Floropryl

Chemical Class: Cholinesterase inhibitor, irreversible

Therapeutic Class: Miotic

CLINICAL PHARMACOLOGY

Mechanism of Action: Prevents breakdown of neurotransmitter acetylcholine, which then accumulates, causing enhancement and prolongation of its physiologic effects

Pharmacokinetics

MIOSIS: Onset 5-10 min, duration 1-4 wk

INTRAOCULAR PRESSURE: Peak 24 hr, duration 1 wk

INDICATIONS AND USES: Open-angle glaucoma, accommodative esotropia, conditions obstructing aqueous outflow

DOSAGE

Adult and Child

- *Glaucoma:* Instill ¼″ strip in conjunctival sac q8-72 hr qhs for 2 wk
- *Esotropia:* Instill ¼″ strip in conjunctival sac qhs for 2 wk

$ AVAILABLE FORMS/COST OF THERAPY

- Oint—Ophth: .025%, 3.5 g: **$8.14**

CONTRAINDICATIONS: Hypersensitivity, uveal inflammation

PRECAUTIONS: History of retinal detachment, asthma, bradycardia,

parkinsonism, peptic ulcer, recent MI, epilepsy, myasthenia gravis
PREGNANCY AND LACTATION: Pregnancy category C; no data available on breast feeding
SIDE EFFECTS/ADVERSE REACTIONS
CNS: Headache
CV: Hypotension, bradycardia, paradoxic tachycardia
EENT: Blurred vision, lacrimation, conjunctival congestion, lid muscle twitching, stinging, burning
GU: Urinary incontinence
GI: Abdominal cramps, diarrhea, increased salivation, nausea, vomiting
RESP: ***Bronchospasm,*** dyspnea, bronchoconstriction, wheezing
▼ **DRUG INTERACTIONS**
Drugs
• *Succinylcholine, systemic anticholinesterase:* Increased effects of both drugs

isometheptene
(i-so-meh-thep′tene)
Only available in combination with dichloralphenazone and acetominophen: Midrin, Midchlor, Isopap, Isocom, Migratine
Chemical Class: Sympathomimetic amine
Therapeutic Class: Analgesic, sedative, and vasoconstrictor

CLINICAL PHARMACOLOGY
Mechanism of Action: Indirect-acting sympathomimetic agent with vasoconstricting activity; vasoconstriction of cerebral blood vessels may reduce pulsation of cerebral arteries; dichloralphenazone is a mild sedative, acetominophen an analgesic
INDICATIONS AND USES: Possibly effective for relief of tension and vascular headaches
DOSAGE
• Acetominophen 325 mg/dichloralphenazone 100 mg/isometheptene mucate 65 mg
Adult
• *Tension headache:* PO 1-2 caps q4h prn to max 8 caps qd
• *Vascular headache suppressant:* PO 2 caps at start of prodrome, then 1 cap qhr prn to max 5 caps/12 hr
$ **AVAILABLE FORMS/COST OF THERAPY**
• Cap, Gel—Oral: 325 mg/100 mg/65 mg, 100's: **$14.84-$37.05**
CONTRAINDICATIONS: Glaucoma, severe renal disease, severe hepatic disease (acetominophen), organic heart disease, MAOI
PRECAUTIONS: Hypertension, peripheral vascular disease, recent CVA
PREGNANCY AND LACTATION: Data not available
SIDE EFFECTS/ADVERSE REACTIONS
CNS: Dizziness
SKIN: Rash
▼ **DRUG INTERACTIONS**
Drugs
• *MAOIs:* Hypertensive crisis

isoniazid (INH)
(eye-soe nye′a-zid)
Laniazid, Laniazid C.T., Nydrazid
Chemical Class: Synthetic isonicotinic acid derivative
Therapeutic Class: Antituberculosis agent

CLINICAL PHARMACOLOGY
Mechanism of Action: Interferes with lipid and nucleic acid biosynthesis in growing tubercle bacilli; active only against mycobacteria,

primarily those that are actively dividing

Pharmacokinetics

IM: Peak 45-60 min

PO: Peak 1-2 hr, duration 6-8 hr Widely distributed to all fluids and tissues; low protein binding; metabolized in liver, primarily by acetylation; rate of metabolism genetically determined; eliminated in urine; $t_{1/2}$ 0.5-1.6 hr (fast acetylators), 2-5 hr (slow acetylators)

INDICATIONS AND USES: Treatment and prophylaxis of tuberculosis; severe tremor in patients with multiple sclerosis*

DOSAGE

Adult

- *Treatment:* IM/PO 5 mg/kg/d (up to 300 mg total) in a single dose; use in conjunction with other effective antituberculosis agents; duration of treatment 6 mo-2 yr
- *Disseminated disease:* IM/PO 10 mg/kg/d in 1-2 divided doses
- *Prophylaxis:* IM/PO 300 mg qd

Child

- *Treatment:* IM/PO 10-20 mg/kg/d (up to 300 mg total) in 1-2 divided doses
- *Prophylaxis:* IM/PO 10 mg/kg/d qd, do not exceed 300 mg/d

$ AVAILABLE FORMS/COST OF THERAPY

- Syr—Oral: 50 mg/ml, 480 ml: **$17.50**
- Tab, Uncoated—Oral: 100 mg, 100's: **$1.18-$7.55;** 300 mg, 100's: **$2.48-$10.49**
- Inj, Sol—IM: 100 mg/ml, 10 ml: **$15.85**

CONTRAINDICATIONS: Previous isoniazid-associated hepatic injury, severe adverse reactions to isoniazid, hypersensitivity, acute liver disease of any etiology

PRECAUTIONS: Active chronic liver disease, severe renal dysfunction; malnutrition, slow acetylators, elderly, diabetes, alcoholics (increased risk of peripheral neuropathy)

PREGNANCY AND LACTATION: Pregnancy category C; the American Thoracic Society recommends use of isoniazid for tuberculosis during pregnancy; excreted in breast milk, women can safely breast feed their infants while taking isoniazid if the infant is periodically examined for signs and symptoms of peripheral neuritis or hepatitis

SIDE EFFECTS/ADVERSE REACTIONS

CNS: *Peripheral neuropathy,* ***convulsions, toxic encephalopathy,*** memory impairment, toxic psychosis, fever

EENT: Optic neuritis and atrophy

GI: Nausea, vomiting, epigastric distress, ***hepatotoxicity*** (mild and transient elevation of serum transaminases in 10%-20% does not require discontinuation; progressive liver damage rare in patients <20 yr, but is seen in as many as 2.3% of those >50 yr)

HEME: ***Agranulocytosis; hemolytic, sideroblastic or aplastic anemia; thrombocytopenia; eosinophilia***

METAB: Pyridoxine deficiency, pellagra, hyperglycemia, metabolic acidosis, gynecomastia, hypocalcemia, hypophosphatemia

SKIN: Skin eruptions, vasculitis, local irritation (IM)

MISC: Rheumatic syndrome, SLE-like syndrome

▼ DRUG INTERACTIONS

Drugs

- *Antacids:* Reduced plasma isoniazid concentrations
- *Carbamazepine+:* Increased serum carbamazepine concentrations; toxicity may occur
- *Corticosteroids:* Reduced plasma concentrations of isoniazid

• *Disulfiram:* Adverse mental changes and coordination problems
• *Phenytoin+:* Predictable increases in serum phenytoin concentrations; toxicity possible
• *Rifampin:* Increased hepatotoxicity of isoniazid in some patients; more common with slow acetylators of isoniazid, and/or pre-existing liver disease

SPECIAL CONSIDERATIONS

PATIENT/FAMILY EDUCATION

• Take on empty stomach if possible, however, may be taken with food to decrease GI upset
• Complete the full course of therapy
• Minimize daily alcohol consumption to lessen the risk of hepatitis
• Notify physician of weakness, fatigue, loss of appetite, nausea and vomiting, yellowing of skin or eyes, darkening of urine, numbness or tingling of hands and feet

MONITORING PARAMETERS

• Periodic ophthalmologic examinations even when visual symptoms do not occur
• Periodic liver function tests

isoproterenol

(eye-soe-proe-ter'e-nole)
Dispos-a-Med Isoproterenol, Isuprel Glossets, Isuprel, Isuprel Mistometer, Medihaler-Iso
Chemical Class: Catecholamine
Therapeutic Class: Bronchodilator; vasopressor

CLINICAL PHARMACOLOGY

Mechanism of Action: Stimulates β_1 and β_2-adrenergic receptors resulting in relaxation of bronchial, GI, and uterine smooth muscle, increased heart rate and contractility, vasodilation of peripheral vasculature

Pharmacokinetics

IV: Onset rapid, duration 10 min
INH: Onset immediate
SL/SC: Onset 30 min, duration up to 2 hr
Metabolized by conjugation in many tissues including the liver and lungs; $t_{1/2}$ 2½-5 min; excreted in urine (principally as sulfate conjugates)

INDICATIONS AND USES: Mild or transient episodes of heart block (not requiring electric shock or pacemaker therapy); serious episodes of heart block and Stokes-Adams attacks (except when caused by ventricular tachycardia or fibrillation); cardiac arrest (until electric shock or pacemaker is available); bronchospasm occurring during anesthesia, asthma, chronic bronchitis or emphysema; hypovolemic and septic shock, low cardiac output (hypoperfusion) states, congestive heart failure, cardiogenic shock

DOSAGE

Adult

• *Bronchospasm:* MDI 1-2 puffs 4-6 times/d; NEB 0.25-0.5 ml of a 1% sol diluted in 2-3 ml normal saline or 0.25% and 0.5% undiluted, treatment may be repeated up to 5 times/d; SL 10-20 mg q6-8h
• *Dysrhythmia/heart block:* IV 0.02-0.06 mg (1-3 ml of 1:50,000 dilution) bolus, followed by subsequent doses of 0.01-0.2 mg (0.5-10 ml of 1:50,000 dilution); IV INF 5 µg/min initially, titrate to desired response, usual range 2-20 µg/min; IM 0.2 mg (1 ml of 1:5,000 dilution) initially, subsequent doses of 0.02-1 mg (0.1-5 ml of 1:5,000 dilution); SC 0.2 mg (1 ml of 1:5,000 dilution) initially, subsequent doses of 0.15-0.2 mg (0.75-1 ml of 1:5,000 dilution); IC 0.02 mg (0.1 ml of 1:5,000 dilution); SL 10-30 mg 4-6 times/d; PR (use SL tablets) 5 mg, followed by 5-15 mg prn
• *Shock:* IV INF 0.5-5 µg/min (0.25-

2.5 ml of 1:500,000 dilution), titrate to patient response

Child

• *Bronchospasm:* MDI 1-2 puffs up to 6 times/d; NEB 0.01 ml/kg of 1% sol; min dose 0.1 ml, max dose 0.5 ml diluted in 2-3 ml normal saline; SL 5-10 mg q3-4h, max 30 mg/d

• *Shock:* IV INF 0.05-2 μg/kg/min, rate (ml/hr) = dose (μg/kg/min) × weight (kg) × 60 min/hr divided by concentration (μg/ml)

$ AVAILABLE FORMS/COST OF THERAPY

• Sol—Inh: 0.5%, 60 ml: **$93.21;** 1%, 10 ml: **$23.98**

• Aer—Inh: 0.25%, 10, 15 ml: **$15.30-$30.60**

• Aer, Spray—Inh: 0.25%, 15 ml: **$13.49-$19.85;** 2 mg/ml, 15 ml: **$20.52-$26.16**

• Inj, Sol—IV: 0.02 mg/ml, 10 ml: **$13.24;** 0.2 mg/ml, 5 ml: **$3.58-$18.45**

• Tab—SL: 10 mg, 50's: **$31.98**

CONTRAINDICATIONS: Tachydysrhythmias, tachycardia or heart block caused by digitalis intoxication, ventricular dysrhythmias requiring inotropic therapy, angina pectoris

PRECAUTIONS: Hypovolemia, CAD, coronary insufficiency, diabetes, hyperthyroidism

PREGNANCY AND LACTATION: Pregnancy category C; no reports linking isoproterenol with congenital defects have been located; excretion into breast milk unknown, use caution in nursing mothers

SIDE EFFECTS/ADVERSE REACTIONS

CNS: Mild tremors, anxiety, nervousness, headache, dizziness, weakness

CV: Tachycardia, palpitations, hypertension, hypotension, ventricular dysrhythmias, tachydysrhythmias, precordial distress, angina

GI: Nausea, vomiting

RESP: Pulmonary edema

SKIN: Flushing of skin, sweating

▼ DRUG INTERACTIONS

Drugs

• *Beta blockers:* Reduced effectiveness of isoproterenol in the treatment of asthma

SPECIAL CONSIDERATIONS

MONITORING PARAMETERS

• Heart rate, central venous pressure, systemic blood pressure, urine output, blood gases

---

isosorbide

(eye-soe-sor'bide)

Ismotic

Therapeutic Class: Osmotic diuretic; antiglaucomatous agent

CLINICAL PHARMACOLOGY

Mechanism of Action: Induces diuresis by elevating the osmolarity of glomerular filtrate, thereby hindering the tubular reabsorption of water

Pharmacokinetics

PO: Onset 10-30 min, peak 1-1½ hr, duration 5-6 hr, $t_{1/2}$ 5-9½ hr, excreted unchanged in urine

INDICATIONS AND USES: Short-term reduction of intraocular pressure prior to and after intraocular surgery; acute attack of glaucoma

DOSAGE

Adult

• PO 1.5 g/kg initially, then 1-3 g/kg bid-qid prn

$ AVAILABLE FORMS/COST OF THERAPY

• Sol—Oral: 45%, 220 ml: **$291.72**

CONTRAINDICATIONS: Well established anuria, severe dehydration, pulmonary edema, severe cardiac decompensation, hypersensitivity

PRECAUTIONS: Diseases associated with salt retention

PREGNANCY AND LACTATION: Pregnancy category B; excretion into breast milk unknown, use caution in nursing mothers

SIDE EFFECTS/ADVERSE REACTIONS

CNS: Headache, confusion, disorientation, lethargy, dizziness, lightheadedness

CV: Syncope

EENT: Vertigo

GI: Nausea, vomiting, gastric discomfort, thirst

METAB: Hypernatremia, hyperosmolarity

SKIN: Rash

MISC: Hiccoughs, irritability

SPECIAL CONSIDERATIONS

PATIENT/FAMILY EDUCATION

- Palatability may be improved if the medication is poured over cracked ice and sipped

MONITORING PARAMETERS

- Fluid and electrolyte balance; urine output

isosorbide dinitrate/mononitrate

(eye-soe-sor′bide)

Dinitrate: Dilatrate-SR, Iso-Bid, Isordil, Isordil Titradose, Isordil Tembids, Isotrate Timecelles, Sorbitrate, Sorbitrate SA; Mononitrate: Imdur, ISMO, Monoket

Chemical Class: Nitrates

Therapeutic Class: Antianginal

CLINICAL PHARMACOLOGY

Mechanism of Action: Relaxes vascular smooth muscle; the venous (capacitance) system is affected to a greater degree than arterial (resistance) system; venous pooling, decreased venous return to the heart (preload), and decreased arterial resistance (afterload) reduce intracardiac pressures and left ventricular size, thereby decreasing myocardial oxygen demand and ischemia; may also improve regional myocardial blood supply

Pharmacokinetics

Dinitrate

PO: Onset 20-40 min, duration 4-6 hr

PO SR: Onset up to 4 hr, duration 6-8 hr

SL: Onset 2-5 min, duration 1-3 hr

Metabolized by liver to 2- and 5-mononitrates (most of the clinical activity of dinitrate is attributable to mononitrate metabolites), excreted in urine as metabolites

Mononitrate

PO: Onset 30-60 min

Not subject to first-pass metabolism, <4% bound to plasma proteins, metabolized to inactive metabolites, $t_{1/2}$ 5 hr

INDICATIONS AND USES: Prevention of angina pectoris; relief of acute anginal episodes and prophylaxis prior to events likely to provoke an attack (SL dinitrate formulation only); CHF;* Hypertension (acute)*

DOSAGE

- Asymmetric dosing regimens provide a daily nitrate-free interval to minimize the development of tolerance

Adult

- *Dinitrate:* SL 2.5-5 mg initially, titrate upward until angina is relieved or side effects limit the dose; chewable 5 mg initially, titrate upward until angina is relieved or side effects limit the dose; PO 5-20 mg bid-tid initially (last dose no later than 7 PM), maintenance 10-40 mg bid-tid (last dose no later than 7 PM); PO SR 40 mg qd-bid initially (last dose no later than 2 PM), maintenance 40-80 mg qd-bid (last dose no later than 2 PM)

• *Mononitrate:* PO 5-20 mg bid (with the 2 doses 7 hr apart); PO SR 30-60 mg qd initially, increase to 120-240 mg qd prn

$ **AVAILABLE FORMS/COST OF THERAPY**

Dinitrate:

• Tab, Chewable—Oral: 5 mg, 100's: **$19.99;** 10 mg, 100's: **$22.96**

• Tab—SL: 2.5 mg, 100's: **$3.23-$22.91;** 5 mg, 100's: **$1.88-$24.49;** 10 mg, 100's: **$28.59**

• Tab, Uncoated—Oral: 5, 10, 20, 30, 40 mg, 100's: **$1.88-$54.19**

• Cap, Gel, Sust Action—Oral: 40 mg, 100's: **$5.83-$52.51**

• Tab, Coated, Sust Action—Oral: 40 mg, 100's: **$4.95-$52.51**

Mononitrate:

• Tab, Uncoated—Oral: 10 mg, 100's: **$52.50;** 20 mg, 100's: **$55.29-$65.81**

• Tab, Coated, Sust Action—Oral: 60 mg, 100's: **$90.00;** 120 mg, 100's: **$144.90**

CONTRAINDICATIONS: Hypersensitivity to nitrates, severe anemia, closed angle glaucoma, postural hypotension, head trauma or cerebral hemorrhage (may increase intracranial pressure), acute MI or CHF (mononitrate)

PRECAUTIONS: Acute MI, hypertrophic cardiomyopathy, glaucoma, volume depletion, hypotension, abrupt withdrawal, continuous delivery without nitrate-free interval (tolerance will develop)

PREGNANCY AND LACTATION: Pregnancy category C; excretion into breast milk unknown, use caution in nursing mothers

SIDE EFFECTS/ADVERSE REACTIONS

CNS: Headache, apprehension, restlessness, weakness, vertigo, *dizziness,* agitation, anxiety, confusion, insomnia, nervousness, nightmares, dyscoordination, hypoesthesia, hypokinesia

CV: Tachycardia, retrosternal discomfort, palpitations, hypotension (sometimes with paradoxical bradycardia and increased angina), syncope, ***cardiovascular collapse,*** crescendo angina, rebound hypertension, dysrhythmias, atrial fibrillation, premature ventricular contractions, *postural hypotension,* edema

EENT: Blurred vision, diplopia

GI: Nausea, vomiting, diarrhea, dyspepsia, involuntary passing of feces, abdominal pain, tenesmus

GU: Dysuria, impotence, urinary frequency, involuntary passing of urine

HEME: ***Hemolytic anemia, methemoglobinemia***

MS: Arthralgia, muscle twitching

SKIN: Rash, exfoliative dermatitis, *flushing,* crusty skin lesions, pruritis, pallor, perspiration, cold sweat

▼ **DRUG INTERACTIONS**

Labs

• *Interference:* Serum cholesterol measured by Zlatkis-Zak color reaction

SPECIAL CONSIDERATIONS

PATIENT/FAMILY EDUCATION

• Headache may be a marker for drug activity, do not try to avoid by altering treatment schedule, contact physician if severe or persistent; aspirin or acetaminophen may be used for relief

• Dissolve SL tablets under tongue, do not crush, chew, or swallow

• Do not crush chewable tablets before administering

• Avoid alcohol

• Make changes in position slowly to prevent fainting

isotretinoin

(eye-soe-tret′i-noyn)

Accutane

Chemical Class: Vitamin A derivative

Therapeutic Class: Antiacne agent; dermatological

CLINICAL PHARMACOLOGY

Mechanism of Action: Exact mechanism unknown; reduces sebaceous gland size and inhibits gland activity thereby decreasing sebum secretion; indirectly decreases the number of *Propionibacterium acnes* organisms within the follicle; exhibits anti-keratinizing and anti-inflammatory actions

Pharmacokinetics

PO: Peak 3 hr, 99.9% bound to plasma proteins (almost exclusively to albumin), metabolized in liver and possibly in gut wall to 4-oxo-isotretinoin (active), eliminated via the bile and urine, $t_{1/2}$ 10-20 hr

INDICATIONS AND USES: Severe recalcitrant cystic acne; keratinization disorders (keratosis follicularis, pityriasis rubra pilaris, lamellar ichthyosis, keratosis palmaris et plantaris, congenital ichthyosiform erythroderma, rosacea, lichen planus, psoriasis);* cutaneous T-cell lymphoma (mycosis fungoides) and leukoplakia;* prevention of skin cancer in patients with xeroderma pigmentosum;* prevention of second primary tumors in patients treated for squamous-cell carcinoma of the head and neck*

DOSAGE

Adult and Child

- PO 0.5-2 mg/kg/d divided bid for 15-20 wk or until total cyst count decreases by 70%; a second course may be initiated after ≥2 mo off therapy if warranted by persistent or recurring severe cystic acne

$ AVAILABLE FORMS/COST OF THERAPY

- Cap, Elastic—Oral: 10 mg, 100's: **$323.28;** 20 mg, 100's: **$383.38;** 40 mg, 100's: **$445.41**

CONTRAINDICATIONS: Pregnancy, hypersensitivity to parabens

PRECAUTIONS: Diabetes, obesity, family history of hypertriglyceridemia, contact lens use, inflammatory bowel disease

PREGNANCY AND LACTATION: Pregnancy category X; isotretinoin is a potent human teratogen; excretion into breast milk unknown, but based on the close relationship to vitamin A, the presence of isotretinoin in breast milk should be expected; avoid use in nursing mothers

SIDE EFFECTS/ADVERSE REACTIONS

CNS: Fatigue, headache, ***pseudotumor cerebri*** (headache, visual disturbances, papilledema), depression

CV: Palpitations, tachycardia, transient chest pain, edema, vasculitis

EENT: Epistaxis, dry nose, conjunctivitis, optic neuritis, photophobia, eyelid inflammation, corneal opacities, cataracts, visual disturbances, *dry eyes,* decreased night vision, contact lens intolerance

GI: Dry mouth, nausea, vomiting, abdominal pain, anorexia, inflammatory bowel disease, weight loss, gingival bleeding and inflammation, ***hepatotoxicity***

GU: White cells in urine, proteinuria, hematuria, abnormal menses

HEME: **Anemia, thrombocytopenia**

METAB: Hypertriglyceridemia, glucose intolerance

MS: Bone, joint and muscle pain and stiffness

SKIN: Cheilitis, dry skin, pruritis, skin fragility, facial skin desquama-

tion, drying of mucous membranes, petechiae, nail brittleness, rash, thinning of hair, peeling of palms and soles, skin infections, photosensitivity, hypo/hyperpigmentation, erythema nodosum, paronychia, urticaria, exaggerated healing response, pyogenic granuloma, bruising

▼ **DRUG INTERACTIONS**

Labs

- *Increase:* Sedimentation rate, triglycerides, liver function tests
- *Decrease:* RBC, WBC

SPECIAL CONSIDERATIONS

PATIENT/FAMILY EDUCATION

- Have patient complete consent form included with package insert prior to initiating therapy
- Administer with meals
- Avoid alcohol
- Do not take vitamin supplements containing vitamin A
- **Women of childbearing potential should practice contraception during therapy and for 1 mo before and after therapy,** a pregnancy test 2 wk prior to starting therapy is advised
- Notify physician immediately if pregnancy is suspected
- A transient exacerbation of acne may occur during the initiation of therapy
- Avoid prolonged exposure to sunlight or sunlamps
- Report visual disturbances, abdominal pain, rectal bleeding, severe diarrhea, difficulty in controlling blood sugar, decreased tolerance to contact lens wear to physician immediately
- Do not donate blood during and for 30 days after stopping therapy
- Use caution driving or operating any vehicle at night

MONITORING PARAMETERS

- CBC with differential, platelet count, baseline sed rate, serum triglycerides (baseline and biweekly for 4 wk), liver enzymes

isoxsuprine

(eye-sox'syoo-preen)

Vasodilan, Voxsuprine

Chemical Class: Nylidrin-related agent

Therapeutic Class: Peripheral vasodilator

CLINICAL PHARMACOLOGY

Mechanism of Action: Produces peripheral vasodilation by a direct effect on vascular smooth muscle, primarily within skeletal muscle with little effect on cutaneous blood flow; produces cardiac stimulation and uterine relaxation

Pharmacokinetics

PO: Onset 1 hr, partially conjugated in blood, eliminated primarily in urine, $t_{1/2}$ 1¼ hr

INDICATIONS AND USES: "Possibly effective" for cerebral vascular insufficiency, peripheral vascular disease or arteriosclerosis obliterans, thromboangiitis obliterans, and Raynaud's disease; dysmenorrhea*; threatened premature labor*

DOSAGE

Adult

- PO 10-20 mg tid-qid

$ **AVAILABLE FORMS/COST OF THERAPY**

- Tab, Uncoated—Oral: 10 mg, 100's: **$4.30-$30.10;** 20 mg, 100's: **$5.45-$48.23**

CONTRAINDICATIONS: Immediately postpartum, arterial bleeding, hypersensitivity

PREGNANCY AND LACTATION: Pregnancy category C; has been used to prevent premature labor; excretion into breast milk unknown, use caution in nursing mothers

SIDE EFFECTS/ADVERSE REACTIONS

CNS: Dizziness, weakness
CV: Hypotension, tachycardia, chest pain
GI: Nausea, vomiting, abdominal distress
SKIN: Severe rash, flushing

SPECIAL CONSIDERATIONS

PATIENT/FAMILY EDUCATION

- May cause palpitations or skin rash, notify physician if these symptoms become bothersome
- Avoid sudden changes in posture to avoid dizziness (orthostatic hypotension)

---

isradipine

(is-rad'i-peen)
DynaCirc
Chemical Class: Dihydropyridine calcium channel blocker
Therapeutic Class: Antihypertensive

CLINICAL PHARMACOLOGY
Mechanism of Action: Inhibits calcium ion influx across cell membrane in vascular smooth muscle and cardiac muscle; produces relaxation of coronary vascular smooth muscle, peripheral vascular smooth muscle; reduces total peripheral resistance (afterload); increases myocardial oxygen delivery
Pharmacokinetics
PO: Peak 1½ hr, onset 2 hr, 95% bound to plasma proteins, metabolized in liver, excreted in urine and feces (metabolites), $t_{1/2}$ 8 hr
INDICATIONS AND USES: Hypertension, chronic stable angina*
DOSAGE
Adult

- PO 2.5 mg bid initially, increase in 2-4 wk intervals prn to max of 10 mg bid

$ **AVAILABLE FORMS/COST OF THERAPY**

- Cap, Gel—Oral: 2.5 mg, 100's: **$52.14;** 5 mg, 100's: **$79.02**

CONTRAINDICATIONS: Hypersensitivity
PRECAUTIONS: CHF, hypotension, hepatic insufficiency, aortic stenosis, elderly, children
PREGNANCY AND LACTATION: Pregnancy category C; excretion into breast milk unknown, use caution in nursing mothers
SIDE EFFECTS/ADVERSE REACTIONS
CNS: Headache, fatigue, dizziness, anxiety, depression, insomnia, paresthesia, somnolence, asthenia, nervousness, malaise, tremor
*CV: **Dysrhythmia,** peripheral edema,* bradycardia, hypotension, palpitations, syncope, tachycardia
GI: Nausea, vomiting, diarrhea, gastric upset, constipation, abdominal cramps, flatulence, dry mouth
GU: Nocturia, polyuria
SKIN: Rash, pruritus, urticaria, hair loss
MISC: Flushing, nasal congestion, sweating, shortness of breath, sexual dysfunction, muscle cramps, cough, weight gain, tinnitus, epistaxis

▼ **DRUG INTERACTIONS**

Drugs

- *Barbiturates:* Reduced plasma concentrations of isradipine
- *Beta blockers:* Enhanced effects of beta blockers, hypotension
- *Calcium:* Reduced activity of isradipine
- *Cimetidine:* Increased isradipine concentrations possible
- *Neuromuscular blocking agents:* Prolongation of neuromuscular blockade

SPECIAL CONSIDERATIONS

PATIENT/FAMILY EDUCATION

- Notify physician of irregular heart beat, shortness of breath, swelling of feet and hands, pronounced dizziness, constipation, nausea, hypotension

itraconazole

(it-ra-con'a-zol)

Sporanox

Chemical Class: Triazole derivative

Therapeutic Class: Antifungal

CLINICAL PHARMACOLOGY

Mechanism of Action: Inhibits the cytochrome P-450-dependent synthesis of ergosterol, which is a vital component of fungal cell membranes

Pharmacokinetics

PO: Peak 3-5 hr, requires acid pH for absorption, distributed poorly to CSF, 98% bound to plasma proteins, metabolized in liver to hydroxyitraconazole (active) and other metabolites, excreted in urine, bile, and feces, $t_{1/2}$ 60 hr

INDICATIONS AND USES: Blastomycosis, histoplasmosis, aspergillosis, superficial mycoses (dermatophytoses, Pityriasis versicolor, sebopsoriasis, candidiasis*), onychomycosis, systemic mycoses (candidiasis,* cryptococcal infections, paracoccidioidomycosis, coccidioidomycosis),* subcutaneous mycoses (sporotrichosis, chromomycosis),* cutaneous leishmaniasis,* fungal keratitis,* alternariosis,* zygomycosis*

DOSAGE

Adult

- *Blastomycosis/histoplasmosis:* PO 200 mg qd; may increase if evidence of progressive disease to 300-400 mg/d in 2 divided doses
- *Aspergillosis:* PO 200-400 mg/d, doses >200 mg/d should be given in 2 divided doses
- *Life-threatening situations:* PO loading dose of 200 mg tid should be given for first 3 days
- *Onychomycosis:* PO 200 mg qd for at least 3 mo

$ AVAILABLE FORMS/COST OF THERAPY

- Cap, Gel—Oral: 100 mg, 30's: **$161.81**

CONTRAINDICATIONS: Hypersensitivity, coadministration of terfenadine or astemizole

PRECAUTIONS: Hypersensitivity to other azole antifungals; preexisting hepatic function abnormalities, children, hypochlorhydria (reduces drug absorption)

PREGNANCY AND LACTATION: Pregnancy category C; excreted into breast milk, do not administer to nursing mothers

SIDE EFFECTS/ADVERSE REACTIONS

CNS: Headache, dizziness, somnolence, depression, insomnia, decreased libido, fatigue, fever, malaise

CV: Hypertension, edema

GI: Nausea, vomiting, diarrhea, abdominal pain, anorexia, ***hepatitis,*** liver function test abnormality

GU: Albuminuria, impotence

METAB: Hypokalemia

SKIN: Rash (more common in patients receiving immunosupressants), pruritis

▼ DRUG INTERACTIONS

Drugs

- *Astemizole:* QT interval prolongation and dysrhythmia
- *Cisapride:* Increased cisapride concentrations; toxicity including dysrhythmias possible
- *Cyclosporine:* Increased cyclosporine serum concentrations; nephrotoxicity
- *Didanosine:* Reduced absorption of itraconazole; loss of therapeutic efficacy may result

• *Food:* Enhanced bioavailability
• *Midazolam:* Marked increase in oral midazolam plasma concentrations
• *Oral anticoagulants:* Excessive hypoprothrombinemic response to warfarin
• *Rifampin:* Reduced itraconazole plasma concentrations
• *Terfenadine:* QT interval prolongation and dysrhythmia

SPECIAL CONSIDERATIONS

PATIENT/FAMILY EDUCATION

• Take with food to ensure maximal absorption
• Report signs and symptoms of liver dysfunction: Unusual fatigue, anorexia, nausea, vomiting, jaundice, dark urine, clay-colored stool
• Avoid antacids within 2 hr of itraconazole administration

MONITORING PARAMETERS

• Liver function tests in patients with preexisting abnormalities

kanamycin

(kan-a-mye'sin)
Kantrex
Chemical Class: Aminoglycoside
Therapeutic Class: Antibiotic

CLINICAL PHARMACOLOGY

Mechanism of Action: Interferes with protein synthesis in bacterial cell by binding to 30S ribosomal subunit, which causes misreading of genetic code, inaccurate peptide sequence forms in protein chain, causing bacterial death

Pharmacokinetics

IM: Onset rapid, peak 1-2 hr
IV: Onset immediate
Plasma $t_{1/2}$ 2-3 hr, not metabolized, excreted unchanged in urine

INDICATIONS AND USES: Severe systemic infections of CNS, respiratory, GI, urinary tract, bone, skin, soft tissues caused by susceptible organisms; *Mycobacterium avium* complex infections (as part of a multiple-drug regimen),* cystic fibrosis (inhaled),* suppression of intestinal bacteria (PO), hepatic coma (PO). Antibacterial spectrum usually includes: gram-positive organisms: penicillinase and non-penicillinase-producing *Staphylococcus* sp (in general has a low order of activity against other Gram-positive organisms); gram-negative organisms: *Escherichia coli, Proteus* sp (indole-positive and indole-negative), *Providencia* sp, *Klebsiella-Enterobacter-Serratia* sp, *Acinetobacter* sp, *Citrobacter* sp, *Shigella* sp, *Yersinia pestis, Hemophilus influenzae, Neisseria* sp, *Salmonella* sp

DOSAGE

Adult

• *Severe systemic infections:* IM/IV 15 mg/kg/d divided q8-12h; do not exceed 1.5 g/d
• *Suppression of intestinal bacteria:* PO 1g q1h for 4 hr, followed by 1 g q6h for 36-72 hr
• *Hepatic coma:* PO 8-12 g/d in divided doses
• *Aerosol treatment:* 250 mg bid-qid; withdraw 250 mg (1 ml) from 500 mg vial, dilute with 3 ml normal saline and nebulize
• *Intraperitoneal:* 500 mg diluted in 20 ml sterile distilled water instilled through a polyethylene catheter into wound (absorption similar to IM use)

Child

• *Severe systemic infections:* IM/IV 15 mg/kg/d divided q8-12h; do not exceed 1.5 g/d

$ AVAILABLE FORMS/COST OF THERAPY

• Inj, Sol—IM; IV: 1 g/3 ml, 3 ml: **$9.49-$238.13;** 75 mg/2 ml, 2 ml:

$3.04-$5.06; 500 mg/2 ml, 2 ml: **$4.80-$111.25**

- Cap, Gel—Oral: 0.5 g, 100's: **$198.29**

CONTRAINDICATIONS: Hypersensitivity to aminoglycosides

PRECAUTIONS: Neonates, renal disease, myasthenia gravis, hearing deficits, Parkinson's disease, elderly, dehydration

PREGNANCY AND LACTATION: Pregnancy category D; eighth cranial nerve toxicity in the fetus has been reported; excreted into breast milk in low concentrations, poor oral availability reduces potential for ototoxicity for the infant, may modify bowel flora or interfere with interpretation of culture results if fever workup is required; compatible with breast feeding

SIDE EFFECTS/ADVERSE REACTIONS

CNS: Paresthesia, ***neuromuscular blockade,*** headache

EENT: ***Ototoxicity,*** hearing loss, deafness, loss of balance

GI: Nausea, vomiting, diarrhea

GU: ***Oliguria,*** hematuria, ***renal damage,*** azotemia, ***renal failure, nephrotoxicity***

MS: ***Acute muscular paralysis***

RESP: Apnea

SKIN: Rash

▼ **DRUG INTERACTIONS**

Drugs

- *Amphotericin B:* Synergistic nephrotoxicity
- *Cephalosporins:* Increased potential for nephrotoxicity in patients with pre-existing renal disease
- *Cyclosporine:* Additive renal damage
- *Ethacrynic acid+:* Increased risk of ototoxicity
- *Extended spectrum penicillins:* Potential for inactivation of aminoglycosides in patients with renal failure
- *Methoxyflurane:* Enhanced renal toxicity
- *Neuromuscular blocking agents+:* Potentiation of respiratory suppression produced by neuromuscular blocking agents
- *NSAIDs:* Reduced renal clearance of aminoglycosides in premature infants

SPECIAL CONSIDERATIONS

PATIENT/FAMILY EDUCATION

- Report headache, dizziness, loss of hearing, ringing, roaring in ears or feeling of fullness in head

MONITORING PARAMETERS

- Urinalysis for proteinuria, cells, casts
- Urine output
- Serum peak, drawn at 30-60 min after IV inf or 60 min after IM inj, trough level drawn just before next dose, adjust dosage per levels, especially in renal function impairment (usual therapeutic plasma levels; peak 15-30 mg/L, trough ≤ 10 mg/L)
- Serum creatinine for CrCl calculation
- Serum calcium, magnesium, sodium
- Audiometric testing, assess hearing before, during, after treatment

kaolin-pectin

(kay'o-lynn)

Kaodene, Kaopectate, K-P, Kapectolin, K-Pek, Parapectolin

Chemical Class: Kaolin: Hydrous magnesium aluminum silicate; Pectin: purified carbohydrate product

Therapeutic Class: Antidiarrheal

CLINICAL PHARMACOLOGY

Mechanism of Action: Supposedly act as adsorbents and protectants;

effects in the treatment of diarrhea remain to be clearly established

INDICATIONS AND USES: Diarrhea

DOSAGE

Adult

• PO 60-120 ml after each loose bowel movement

Child 6-12 yr

• PO 30-60 ml after each loose bowel movement

Child 3-6 yr

• PO 15-30 ml after each loose bowel movement

$ AVAILABLE FORMS/COST OF THERAPY

• Susp—Oral: 0.65 g, (kaolin)/32.4 mg (pectin)/5 ml, 120 ml: **$1.55;** 0.98 g (kaolin)/21.7 mg (pectin)/5 ml, 360 ml: **$2.85**

PRECAUTIONS: Infants, debilitated elderly patients

PREGNANCY AND LACTATION: Pregnancy category C; neither agent is systemically absorbed; should have no effect on lactation or nursing infant

SIDE EFFECTS/ADVERSE REACTIONS

GI: Constipation

▼ DRUG INTERACTIONS

Drugs

• *Lincomycin:* Reduced antibacterial efficacy of lincomycin

• *Quinidine:* Reduced plasma quinidine concentrations

SPECIAL CONSIDERATIONS

PATIENT/FAMILY EDUCATION

• Do not self-medicate diarrhea for >48 hr without consulting a physician

• Notify physician if fever develops

ketoconazole

(kee-toe-koe'na-zole)

Nizoral

Chemical Class: Imidazole

Therapeutic Class: Antifungal

CLINICAL PHARMACOLOGY

Mechanism of Action: Inhibits biosynthesis of ergosterol or other sterols, damaging the fungal cell membrane and altering its permeability with resultant loss of essential intracellular elements; inhibits several fungal enzymes resulting in build-up of toxic concentrations of hydrogen peroxide; inhibits biosynthesis of triglycerides and phospholipids by fungi

Pharmacokinetics

PO: Bioavailability decreases as gastric pH increases, peak 1-4 hr, partially metabolized by liver to inactive metabolites, excreted mainly in feces (57%) and urine (13%), $t_{1/2}$ 8 hr

INDICATIONS AND USES: Tab: candidiasis, chronic mucocutaneous candidiasis, oral thrush, candiduria, blastomycosis, coccidioidomycosis, histoplasmosis, chromomycosis, paracoccidioidomycosis; severe recalcitrant dermatophyte infections; onychomycosis;* pityriasis versicolor;* tinea corporis, pedis, capitus and cruris;* vaginal candidiasis,* advanced prostate cancer (high doses);* Cushing's syndrome (high doses);* Cream: tinea corporis, cruris and pedis; pityriasis versicolor; cutaneous candidiasis; seborrheic dermatitis; Shampoo: dandruff

DOSAGE

Adult

• PO 200 mg qd initially, increase to 400 mg qd for serious infections or if clinical response insufficient;

duration 1-2 wk (candidiasis), 6 mo (other indicated systemic mycoses)
• Cream, apply qd to affected area for 2 wk (bid for 4 wk for seborrheic dermatitis)
• Shampoo twice weekly for 4 wk with at least 3 days between each shampooing, then intermittently prn
Child >2 yr
• PO 3.3-6.6 mg/kg/d as a single dose

$ AVAILABLE FORMS/COST OF THERAPY
• Cre—Top: 20 mg/g, 15, 30, 60 g: **$13.46-$34.39**
• Shampoo—Top: 2%, 120 ml: **$16.64**
• Tab, Uncoated—Oral: 200 mg, 100's: **$270.92**

CONTRAINDICATIONS: Hypersensitivity, fungal meningitis, coadministration with terfenadine

PRECAUTIONS: Renal disease, hepatic disease, achlorhydria (drug-induced), children <2 yr, other hepatotoxic agents, sulfite sensitivity (cream)

PREGNANCY AND LACTATION: Pregnancy category C; has been used, apparently without harm, for the treatment of vaginal candidiasis during pregnancy

SIDE EFFECTS/ADVERSE REACTIONS
CNS: Headache, dizziness, somnolence
GI: Nausea, vomiting, anorexia, diarrhea, abdominal pain, ***hepatotoxicity***
GU: Gynecomastia, impotence, oligospermia (high doses)
HEME: ***Thrombocytopenia, leukopenia, hemolytic anemia***
SKIN: Pruritus, rash, dermatitis, purpura, urticaria
MISC: Anaphylaxis, fever, chills, photophobia

▼ DRUG INTERACTIONS
Drugs
• *Antacids:* Reduced ketoconazole concentrations
• *Astemizole+:* Excessive astemizole concentrations; increased risk of cardiac dysrhythmia
• *Benzodiazepines:* Increased concentrations of midazolam and triazolam
• *Cisapride:* Increased cisapride concentrations; dysrhythmias possible
• *Cyclosporine:* Increased serum cyclosporine concentrations; increased risk of renal toxicity
• *H_2-receptor antagonists:* Reduced plasma concentrations of ketoconazole
• *Methylprednisolone:* Increased methylprednisolone concentrations; enhanced suppression of cortisol secretion
• *Oral anticoagulants:* Increased hypoprothrombinemic response to warfarin
• *Rifampin:* Decreased ketoconazole concentrations; decreased rifampin concentrations
• *Terfenadine+:* Excessive terfenadine concentrations; increased risk of cardiac dysrhythmia

SPECIAL CONSIDERATIONS

PATIENT/FAMILY EDUCATION
• For shampoo, moisten hair and scalp, apply shampoo, and gently massage over entire scalp for 1 min, rinse with warm water, repeat leaving shampoo on scalp for additional 3 min
• Do not take tablets with antacids or H_2-receptor antagonists; separate doses by at least 2 hr
• Take tablets with food
• May cause dizziness, use caution driving or performing tasks requiring alertness
• Notify physician of signs and symptoms of liver toxicity: Unusual

fatigue, anorexia, nausea, vomiting, jaundice, dark urine, pale stools

MONITORING PARAMETERS

- Liver function tests at baseline and frequently during treatment

ketoprofen

(kee-toe-proe'fen)

Orudis, Oruvail

Chemical Class: Propionic acid derivative

Therapeutic Class: Nonsteroidal antiinflammatory drug (NSAID)

CLINICAL PHARMACOLOGY

Mechanism of Action: Inhibits cyclooxygenase activity and prostaglandin synthesis; other mechanisms such as inhibition of lipoxygenase, leukotriene synthesis, lysosomal enzyme release, neutrophil aggregation, and various cell-membrane functions may exist as well

Pharmacokinetics

PO: Peak 0.5-2 hr, highly bound to plasma proteins, metabolized primarily in liver, excreted in urine (60%-75%) and feces, $t_{1/2}$ 1-4 hr

INDICATIONS AND USES: Rheumatoid arthritis, osteoarthritis, mild to moderate pain, primary dysmenorrhea, juvenile rheumatoid arthritis,* sunburn,* migraine*

DOSAGE

Adult

- PO 150-300 mg in divided doses tid-qid, not to exceed 300 mg/d; PO SR 100-200 mg qd (not recommended for acute pain)

$ **AVAILABLE FORMS/COST OF THERAPY**

- Cap, Gel—Oral: 25 mg, 100's: **$65.68-$80.66;** 50 mg, 100's: **$80.62-$99.01;** 75 mg, 100's: **$89.67-$110.13**
- Cap, Gel, Sust Action—Oral: 100 mg, 100's: **$162.50;** 150 mg, 100's: **$197.50;** 200 mg, 100's:**$220.13**

CONTRAINDICATIONS: Hypersensitivity to NSAIDs or ASA

PRECAUTIONS: Bleeding tendencies, peptic ulcer, renal/hepatic function impairment, elderly, CHF, hypertension

PREGNANCY AND LACTATION: Pregnancy category B (category D if used in 3rd trimester); could cause constriction of the ductus arteriosus *in utero,* persistent pulmonary hypertension of the newborn or prolonged labor; unknown if excreted into human breast milk

SIDE EFFECTS/ADVERSE REACTIONS

CNS: Dizziness, headache, lightheadedness

CV: ***CHF, hypotension,*** hypertension, palpitation, ***arrhythmias,*** tachycardia, edema, chest pain

EENT: Visual disturbances, photophobia, dry eyes, hearing disturbances, tinnitus

GI: Nausea, vomiting, diarrhea, constipation, abdominal cramps, *dyspepsia,* flatulence, ***gastric or duodenal ulcer with bleeding or perforation,*** occult blood in stool, ***hepatitis, pancreatitis***

HEME: ***Neutropenia, eosinophilia, leukopenia, pancytopenia, thrombocytopenia, agranulocytosis***

GU: ***Acute renal failure***

METAB: Hyperglycemia, ***hypoglycemia,*** hyperkalemia, hyponatremia

RESP: Dyspnea, bronchospasm

SKIN: Rash, urticaria, photosensitivity

▼ **DRUG INTERACTIONS**

Drugs

- *ACE inhibitors:* Inhibition of antihypertensive response
- *Aminoglycosides:* Reduction of aminoglycoside clearance in premature infants

- *Beta blockers:* Reduced hypotensive effects of beta-blockers
- *Furosemide:* Reduced diuretic and antihypertensive response to furosemide
- *Hydralazine:* Reduced antihypertensive response to hydralazine
- *Lithium:* Increased plasma lithium concentrations, toxicity
- *Methotrexate:* Reduced renal clearance of methotrexate, increased toxicity
- *Oral anticoagulants:* Increased risk of bleeding due to adverse effects on GI mucosa and platelet function
- *Potassium sparing diuretics:* Acute renal failure

Labs

- *Increase:* Bleeding time

SPECIAL CONSIDERATIONS

PATIENT/FAMILY EDUCATION

- Avoid aspirin and alcoholic beverages
- Take with food, milk, or antacids to decrease GI upset
- Notify physician if edema, black stools, or persistant headache occurs

MONITORING PARAMETERS

- CBC, BUN, serum creatinine, LFTs, occult blood loss

---

ketorolac

(kee-toe'role-ak)

Acular (ophthalmic), Toradol

Chemical Class: Acetic acid

Therapeutic Class: Nonsteroidal antiinflammatory drug (NSAID)

CLINICAL PHARMACOLOGY

Mechanism of Action: Inhibits cyclooxygenase activity and prostaglandin synthesis; other mechanisms such as inhibition of lipoxygenase, leukotriene synthesis, lysosomal enzyme release, neutrophil aggregation, and various cell-membrane functions may exist as well

Pharmacokinetics

PO: Peak 0.5-1 hr

IM: Onset 10 min, duration up to 6 hr

99% bound to plasma proteins, metabolized in liver, excreted in urine (metabolites), $t_{1/2}$ 2.4-8.6 hr (increased in elderly, renal impairment)

INDICATIONS AND USES: Moderately severe acute pain; ocular itching due to seasonal allergic conjunctivitis (ophth); migraine*

DOSAGE

Adult

- IM 60 mg loading dose, may be followed by 30 mg q6h for no more than 5 days, max 120 mg/d; IV one 30 mg dose; PO (indicated only as continuation therapy for parenteral ketorolac) 20 mg as a first dose then 10 mg q4-6h for no longer than 5 days (including parenteral therapy), max 40 mg/d
- Elderly (>65 yr), renal impairment, weight <50 kg: IM 30 mg loading dose, may be followed by 15 mg q6h for no more than 5 days, max 60 mg/d; IV one 15 mg dose; PO 10 mg q4-6h for no more than 5 days (including parenteral therapy), max 40 mg/d
- Ophth: 1 gtt qid

$ AVAILABLE FORMS/COST OF THERAPY

- Inj, Sol—IM: 15 mg/ml, 1 ml: **$7.05;** 30 mg/ml, 1 ml: **$7.24;** 60 mg/ml, 1 ml: **$7.43**
- Sol—Ophth: 0.5%, 5 ml: **$27.78**
- Tab, Uncoated—Oral: 10 mg, 100's: **$118.87**

CONTRAINDICATIONS: Active peptic ulcer disease, recent GI bleeding or perforation, history of peptic ulcer disease or GI bleeding; advanced renal impairment, volume depletion; hypersensitivity; before any major surgery; suspected or confirmed cerebrovascular bleeding, hemorrhagic diathesis, incomplete hemostasis and those at high risk of bleeding; concurrent ASA or NSAIDs; neuraxial (epidural or intrathecal) administration due to its alcohol content; concomitant use of probenecid; while wearing soft contact lenses (ophth)

PRECAUTIONS: Children, bleeding disorders, GI disorders, cardiac disorders, hypersensitivity to other antiinflammatory agents

PREGNANCY AND LACTATION: Pregnancy category C; excreted into breast milk; not recommended in lactation

SIDE EFFECTS/ADVERSE REACTIONS

CNS: Dizziness, headache, lightheadedness

CV: ***CHF, hypotension,*** hypertension, palpitation, ***dysrhythmias,*** tachycardia, edema, chest pain

EENT: Visual disturbances, photophobia, dry eyes, hearing disturbances, tinnitus, *burning/stinging upon instillation*

GI: Nausea, vomiting, diarrhea, constipation, abdominal cramps, *dyspepsia,* flatulence, ***gastric or duodenal ulcer with bleeding or perforation,*** occult blood in stool, ***hepatitis, pancreatitis***

HEME: ***Neutropenia, eosinophilia, leukopenia, pancytopenia, thrombocytopenia, agranulocytosis***

GU: ***Acute renal failure***

METAB: Hyperglycemia, ***hypoglycemia,*** hyperkalemia, hyponatremia

RESP: Dyspnea, ***bronchospasm***

SKIN: Rash, urticaria, photosensitivity

▼ DRUG INTERACTIONS

Drugs

• *ACE inhibitors:* Inhibition of antihypertensive response
• *Aminoglycosides:* Reduction of aminoglycoside clearance in premature infants
• *Beta blockers:* Reduced hypotensive effects of beta blockers
• *Furosemide:* Reduced diuretic and antihypertensive response to furosemide
• *Hydralazine:* Reduced antihypertensive response to hydralazine
• *Lithium:* Increased plasma lithium concentrations, toxicity
• *Methotrexate:* Reduced renal clearance of methotrexate, increased toxicity
• *Oral anticoagulants:* Increased risk of bleeding due to adverse effects on GI mucosa and platelet function
• *Potassium sparing diuretics:* Acute renal failure

Labs

• *Increase:* Bleeding time

SPECIAL CONSIDERATIONS

PATIENT/FAMILY EDUCATION

• Not for chronic use
• Avoid aspirin and alcoholic beverages
• Take with food, milk, or antacids to decrease GI upset
• Notify physician if edema, black stools, or persistant headache occurs

MONITORING PARAMETERS

• CBC, BUN, serum creatinine, LFTs, occult blood loss

labetalol

(la-bet'a-lole)

Normodyne, Trandate

Chemical Class: Benzamide derivative

Therapeutic Class: Antihypertensive

CLINICAL PHARMACOLOGY

Mechanism of Action: Combines both selective, competitive postsynaptic α_1-adrenergic blocking and nonselective, competitive β-adrenergic blocking activity

Pharmacokinetics

PO: Onset 20 min-2 hr, peak 1-4 hr, duration 8-24 hr

IV: Onset 5 min, peak 5-15 min, duration 2-4 hr

50% bound to plasma proteins, metabolized in liver, excreted in urine and feces (metabolites), $t_{1/2}$ 5.5-8 hr

INDICATIONS AND USES: Hypertension, hypertensive emergencies (parenteral), pheochromocytoma,* clonidine withdrawal hypertension*

DOSAGE

Adult

• PO 100 mg bid initially, may increase prn q2-3d by 100 mg until desired response obtained, max 2.4 g/d; IV 20 mg initially, repeated doses of 40-80 mg may be given at 10 min intervals up to 300 mg total dose; IV INF 2 mg/min initially, titrate to response

$ AVAILABLE FORMS/COST OF THERAPY

• Inj, Sol—IV: 5 mg/ml, 20 ml: **$30.88**

• Tab, Coated—Oral: 100 mg, 100's: **$42.53;** 200 mg, 100's: **$60.32;** 300 mg, 100's: **$80.23**

CONTRAINDICATIONS: Bronchial asthma, overt cardiac failure, greater than 1st degree heart block, cardiogenic shock, severe bradycardia, hypersensitivity

PRECAUTIONS: Major surgery, diabetes mellitus, renal disease, hepatic disease, thyroid disease, well-compensated heart failure, nonallergic bronchospasm, abrupt discontinuation, children

PREGNANCY AND LACTATION: Pregnancy category C; does not seem to pose a risk to the fetus, except possibly in the 1st trimester; excreted in breast milk, compatible with breast feeding

SIDE EFFECTS/ADVERSE REACTIONS

CNS: Dizziness, mental changes, drowsiness, fatigue, headache, catatonia, depression, anxiety, nightmares, paresthesias, lethargy

CV: Orthostatic hypotension, bradycardia, ***CHF,*** chest pain, ***ventricular dysrhythmias,*** AV block

EENT: Tinnitus, visual changes, sore throat, double vision, dry burning eyes

GI: Nausea, vomiting, diarrhea

GU: Impotence, dysuria, ejaculatory failure, Peyronie's disease

HEME: ***Agranulocytosis, thrombocytopenia, purpura*** (rare)

MS: Asthenia, muscle cramps, toxic myopathy

RESP: ***Bronchospasm,*** dyspnea, wheezing

SKIN: Rash, alopecia, urticaria, pruritus, fever

▼ DRUG INTERACTIONS

Drugs

• *Antidiabetics:* Altered response to hypoglycemia, prolonged recovery of normoglycemia, hypertension, blockade of tachycardia; may increase blood glucose and impair peripheral circulation

• *Cimetidine:* Increased plasma labetolol concentrations

• *Dihydropyridines:* Additive hemodynamic effects

• *Diltiazem:* Enhanced effects of both drugs, particularly antrioventricular conduction slowing

• *Dipyridamole:* Bradycardia

• *Disopyramide:* Additive negative inotropic effects

• *Isoproterenol:* Potential reduction in effectiveness of isoproterenol in the treatment of asthma

• *Lidocaine:* Increased lidocaine concentrations possible

• *NSAIDs:* Reduced hypotensive effects of beta-blockers

• *Prazosin:* First-dose response to prazosin may be enhanced by beta-blockade
• *Tacrine:* Additive bradycardia
• *Theophylline:* Antagonistic pharmacodynamic effects
• *Verapamil:* Enhanced effects of both drugs, particularly atrioventricular conduction slowing

Labs

• *Increase:* Serum transaminases (reversible)
• *False increase:* Urinary catecholamines

SPECIAL CONSIDERATIONS

PATIENT/FAMILY EDUCATION

• Do not discontinue abruptly
• Transient scalp tingling may occur, especially when treatment is initiated
• Notify physician of shortness of breath, edema, excessive fatigue, increase in weight, pulse <50 beats/min
• Avoid hazardous activities if dizziness, drowsiness, lightheadedness are present
• May mask the symptoms of hypoglycemia, except for sweating, in diabetic patients

lactulose

(lak'tyoo-lose)

Cephulac, Cholac, Chronulac, Constilac, Constulose, Duphalac, Enulose

Chemical Class: Synthetic disaccharide analog of lactose
Therapeutic Class: Ammonia detoxicants; laxative

CLINICAL PHARMACOLOGY

Mechanism of Action: Hydrolyzed by colonic bacteria to low molecular weight acids which convert ammonia (NH_3) to ammonium ion (NH_4+), trapping it and preventing its absorption; laxative action due to increased osmotic pressure of colonic contents and increased stool water content

Pharmacokinetics

PO: Poorly absorbed, does not produce effect until reaching colon, 24-48 hr may be required to produce normal bowel movement

INDICATIONS AND USES: Constipation, portal-systemic encephalopathy

DOSAGE

Adult

• *Constipation:* PO 15-30 ml qd, increase to 60 ml qd if necessary
• *Portal-systemic encephalopathy:* PO 30-45 ml tid-qid, adjust dose to produce 2-3 soft stools/d; PR mix 300 ml lactulose with 700 ml water, instill 180 ml via rectal balloon catheter and retain for 30-60 min, repeat q4-6h

Child

• *Constipation:* PO 7.5 ml qd after breakfast
• *Portal-systemic encephalopathy:* PO 40-90 ml/d divided tid-qid, adjust dose to produce 2-3 soft stools/d

Infant

• *Portal-systemic encephalopathy:* PO 2.5-10 ml/d divided tid-qid, adjust dose to produce 2-3 soft stools/d

$ AVAILABLE FORMS/COST OF THERAPY

• Syr—Oral: 10 g/15 ml, 480 ml: **$16.03-$36.42**

CONTRAINDICATIONS: Patients requiring a low galactose diet

PRECAUTIONS: Electrocautery procedures (may spark explosion), diabetes

PREGNANCY AND LACTATION: Pregnancy category B; breast feeding risk to fetus and the newborn appears to be negligible

SIDE EFFECTS/ADVERSE REACTIONS

GI: Gaseous distension, flatulence,

belching, abdominal discomfort, diarrhea, *nausea,* vomiting

SPECIAL CONSIDERATIONS

PATIENT/FAMILY EDUCATION

• May be mixed with fruit juice, water, or milk to increase palatability

• Do not take other laxatives while on lactulose therapy

MONITORING PARAMETERS

• Serum electrolytes, carbon dioxide periodically during chronic treatment

---

lamotrigine

(la-moe-trih'jeen)

Lamictal

Chemical Class: Phenyltriazine

Therapeutic Class: Anticonvulsant

CLINICAL PHARMACOLOGY

Mechanism of Action: Precise mechanism of anticonvulsive action unknown; may inhibit voltage-sensitive sodium channels thereby stabilizing neuronal membranes and consequently modulating presynaptic transmitter release of excitatory amino acids, (e.g., glutamate and aspartate)

Pharmacokinetics

PO: Peak 1.4-4.8 hr, metabolized by glucuronic acid conjugation, eliminated in urine as unchanged drug (10%) and inactive glucuronides (86%), induces its own metabolism, $t_{1/2}$ 25.4-32.8 hr

INDICATIONS AND USES: Adjunctive therapy of partial seizures; generalized tonic-clonic, absence, atypical absence, myoclonic seizures;* Lennox-Gastaut syndrome*

DOSAGE

Adult

• Patients receiving enzyme-inducing antiepileptic drugs (AEDs) and *no* valproic acid: PO 50 mg qd for 2 wk, followed by 50 mg bid for 2 wk, then 300-500 mg/d divided bid (escalate dose by 100 mg/day qwk)

• Patients receiving enzyme-inducing AEDs *plus* valproic acid: PO 25 mg qod for 2 wk, followed by 25 mg qd for 2 wk, then 100-150 mg/d divided bid (escalate dose by 25-50 mg/d q1-2wk)

$ AVAILABLE FORMS/COST OF THERAPY

• Tab, Uncoated—Oral: 25 mg, 25's: **$39.00;** 100 mg, 100's: **$165.60;** 150 mg, 60's: **$104.40;** 200 mg, 60's: **$109.44**

CONTRAINDICATIONS: Hypersensitivity

PRECAUTIONS: Abrupt discontinuation (reduce by 50% qwk over at least 2 wk), renal/hepatic function impairment, children, cardiac function impairment

PREGNANCY AND LACTATION: Pregnancy category C; passes into breast milk, effects on infants exposed by this route are unknown

SIDE EFFECTS/ADVERSE REACTIONS

CNS: Dizziness, ataxia, somnolence, headache, fever, ***seizure exacerbation,*** chills, insomnia, tremor, depression, anxiety, irritability, speech disorder, decreased memory, confusion, sleep disorder, emotional liability, vertigo

CV: Hot flushes, palpitations

EENT: Diplopia, blurred vision, ear pain, tinnitus

GI: Nausea, vomiting, abdominal pain

GU: Dysmenorrhea, vaginitis, amenorrhea

MS: Neck pain, arthralgia, joint disorder, myasthenia

RESP: Rhinitis, pharyngitis, increased cough, dyspnea

SKIN: Rash, **Stevens-Johnson syndrome, toxic epidermal necroly-**

sis, angioedema, photosensitivity, pruritus, alopecia, acne

▼ **DRUG INTERACTIONS**

Drugs

- *Carbamazepine:* Increased carbamezepine epoxide levels
- *Carbamazepine, phenobarbital, primidone, phenytoin:* Decreased lamotrigine concentrations
- *Valproic acid:* Increased lamotrigine concentration; decreased valproic acid concentration

SPECIAL CONSIDERATIONS

PATIENT/FAMILY EDUCATION

- Notify physician if a skin rash develops
- Avoid prolonged exposure to direct sunlight

lansoprazole

(lan-soe'pray-zole)

Prevacid

Chemical Class: Substituted benzimidazole

Therapeutic Class: Proton pump inhibitor; gastrointestinal antisecretory compound

CLINICAL PHARMACOLOGY

Mechanism of Action: Suppresses gastric acid secretion by specific inhibition of the (H^+, K^+)-ATPase enzyme system at the secretory surface of the gastric parietal cell; blocks the final step of acid production

Pharmacokinetics

PO: Peak 1.7 hr, duration >24 hr, 97% bound to plasma proteins, extensively metabolized in the liver, eliminated as metabolites in urine (33%) and feces (66%), $t_{1/2}$ ½ hr (does not reflect duration of acid suppression)

INDICATIONS AND USES: Duodenal ulcer, erosive esophagitis, pathologic hypersecretory conditions (Zollinger-Ellison syndrome)

DOSAGE

Adult

- *Duodenal ulcer:* PO 15 mg qd before eating for 4 wk
- *Erosive esopohagitis:* PO 30 mg qd before eating for 8 wk
- *Zollinger-Ellison syndrome:* PO 60 mg qd initially, increase as needed up to 180 mg/day, doses >120 mg/d should be divided bid

$ **AVAILABLE FORMS/COST OF THERAPY**

- Cap, Gel, Sust Action—Oral:15 mg, 30's: **$97.51;** 30 mg, 100's: **$325.00**

CONTRAINDICATIONS: Hypersensitivity

PRECAUTIONS: Children, maintenance therapy in duodenal ulcer or erosive esophagitis

PREGNANCY AND LACTATION: Pregnancy category B; excretion into breast milk unknown

SIDE EFFECTS/ADVERSE REACTIONS

CNS: Headache

GI: Diarrhea, abdominal pain, nausea

▼ **DRUG INTERACTIONS**

Drugs

- *Food:* 50% decrease in absorption if given 30 min after food compared to the fasting condition

Labs

- *Increase:* ALT, AST

SPECIAL CONSIDERATIONS

PATIENT/FAMILY EDUCATION

- Take before eating
- Do not open, chew, or crush capsules; swallow whole

L

leucovorin

(loo-koe-vor'in)
Wellcovorin
Chemical Class: Folic acid derivative
Therapeutic Class: Antidote; blood modifier

CLINICAL PHARMACOLOGY
Mechanism of Action: Reduced form of folic acid which does not require reduction by dihydrofolate reductase and is therefore not affected by blockage of this enzyme by dihydrofolate reductase inhibitors (e.g., methotrexate)
Pharmacokinetics
PO: Peak 1.72 hr, onset 20-30 min, duration 3-6 hr
IM: Peak 0.71 hr, onset 10-20 min, duration 3-6 hr
IV: Onset <5 min, duration 3-6 hr
Metabolized by liver and intestinal mucosa to active metabolite, eliminated in the urine (80%-90%) and feces (5%-8%), $t_{1/2}$ 6.2 hr
INDICATIONS AND USES: Rescue therapy following high-dose methotrexate therapy in osteosarcoma and inadvertant overdoses of dihydrofolate reductase inhibitors (methotrexate, pyrimethamine, trimetrexate, trimethoprim); megaloblastic anemias due to folic acid deficiency; palliative therapy of advanced colorectal cancer (in combination with 5-fluorouracil)
DOSAGE
Adult and Child
- Give parenterally when individual doses are >25 mg
- *Folate deficient megaloblastic anemia:* IM 1 mg/d
- *Megaloblastic anemia secondary to congenital deficiency of dihydrofolate reductase:* IM 3-6 mg/d
- *Rescue dose:* PO/IV/IM 15 mg (approximately 10 mg/m^2) every 6 hr for 10 doses starting 24 h after the beginning of the methotrexate inf (administer parenterally in the presence of GI toxicity, nausea, or vomiting); if serum creatinine is elevated >50% 24 hr after methotrexate **or** the serum methotrexate concentration is $>5 \times 10^{-6}$M, increase dose to 100 mg/m^2/dose q3h until serum methotrexate concentration is $<1 \times 10^{-8}$M
- *Advanced colorectal cancer:* Consult current protocols

$ **AVAILABLE FORMS/COST OF THERAPY**
- Inj, Sol—IM: 3 mg/ml, 1 ml × 6: **$22.44**
- Inj, Sol—IV: 350 mg, 10's: **$1379.38**
- Inj, Lyphl-Sol—IM; IV: 50 mg/vial, 1's: **$9.74-$119.00;** 100 mg/vial, 1's: **$37.99-$56.25**
- Tab, Uncoated—Oral: 5 mg, 100's: **$275.93-$566.30;** 10 mg, 24's: **$138.33-$168.11;** 15 mg, 24's: **$195.62-$200.96;** 25 mg, 25's: **$475.07-$680.34**

CONTRAINDICATIONS: Pernicious anemia and other megaloblastic anemias secondary to the lack of vitamin B_{12}
PRECAUTIONS: Third space fluid accumulation (i.e., ascites, pleural effusion), renal insufficiency, or inadequate hydration (may increase leucovorin requirement to prevent methotrexate toxicity); administer as soon as possible following overdoses of dihydrofolate reductase inhibitors
PREGNANCY AND LACTATION: Pregnancy category C; has been used in the treatment of megaloblastic anemia during pregnancy; compatible with breast feeding

SIDE EFFECTS/ADVERSE REACTIONS

RESP: Wheezing, ***anaphylactoid reactions***

SKIN: Rash, pruritus, erythema, thrombocytosis, urticaria

▼ **DRUG INTERACTIONS**

• *5-Flurouracil:* enhanced 5-FU toxicity

SPECIAL CONSIDERATIONS

MONITORING PARAMETERS

• CBC with differential and platelets, electrolytes, and liver function tests prior to each treatment with leucovorin/5-FU combination

• Plasma methotrexate concentrations as a therapeutic guide to high-dose methotrexate therapy with leucovorin rescue; continue leucovorin until plasma methotrexate concentrations are $<1 \times 10^{-7}$M (see Dosage)

• Serum creatinine

---

leuprolide

(loo'proe-lide)

Lupron

Chemical Class: Synthetic nonapeptide analog of gonadotropin releasing hormone (GnRH)

Therapeutic Class: Androgen inhibitor; antineoplastic

CLINICAL PHARMACOLOGY

Mechanism of Action: Occupies pituitary GnRH receptors and desensitizes them; inhibits gonadotropin secretion when given continuously in therapeutic doses; after initial stimulation, chronic leuprolide results in suppression of ovarian and testicular steroidogenesis, which is reversible upon discontinuation

Pharmacokinetics

SC: Peak 3 hr

IM (depot): Peak 4 hr, duration >4 wk

7%-15% bound to plasma proteins, $t_{1/2}$ 3 hr

INDICATIONS AND USES: Advanced prostate cancer, endometriosis, central precocious puberty; breast, ovarian, and endometrial cancer,* leiomyoma uteri;* infertility;* prostatic hypertrophy*

DOSAGE

Adult

• *Advanced prostate cancer:* SC 1 mg qd; IM (depot) 7.5 mg/dose given qmo

• *Endometriosis:* IM (depot) 3.75 mg/dose given once qmo for 6 consecutive mo; repeated courses not recommended

Child

• *Precocious puberty:* SC 50 μg/kg/d, titrate upward by 10 μg/kg qd if total suppression of ovarian or testicular steroidogenesis is not achieved; IM/SC (depot) 7.5 mg q4wk (children <25 kg), 11.25 mg q4wk (children 25-37.5 kg), 15 mg q4wk (children >37.5 kg); titrate upward in 3.75 mg/dose increments q4wk until clinical or laboratory tests indicate no progression of disease

$ **AVAILABLE FORMS/COST OF THERAPY**

• Inj, Sol—SC: 1 mg/0.2 ml, 2.8 ml: **$267.50**

• Inj, Susp (Depot)—IM: 7.5 mg/vial, 1's: **$477.50**

• Kit (Depot)—IM: 3.75 mg/vial, 1's: **$381.88**

• Kit (Depot-Ped)—IM: 7.5 mg/vial, 1's: **$477.50;** 11.25 mg/vial, 1's: **$859.38;** 15 mg/vial, 1's: **$955.00**

CONTRAINDICATIONS: Pregnancy, lactation, hypersensitivity, undiagnosed vaginal bleeding

PRECAUTIONS: Edema, hepatic disease, CVA, MI, seizures, hypertension, diabetes mellitus, thromboembolic disease

PREGNANCY AND LACTATION: Pregnancy category X; spontaneous abortions or intrauterine growth retardation are theoretically possible

SIDE EFFECTS/ADVERSE REACTIONS

CNS: Insomnia, pain, headache, dizziness

CV: ***ECG changes/ischemia,*** hypertension, cardiac murmers, ***CHF,*** thrombosis, *edema*

GI: Anorexia, constipation, nausea, vomiting

GU: Vaginitis, vaginal bleeding, vaginal discharge, urinary frequency

METAB: Androgen-like effects, decreased testicular size, impotence, decreased libido

MS: Myalgia, *bone pain* (with initiation)

RESP: Dyspnea, sinus congestion

SPECIAL CONSIDERATIONS

PATIENT/FAMILY EDUCATION

- May cause increase in bone pain and difficulty urinating during first few wk of treatment for prostate cancer, may also cause hot flushes
- Continuous therapy vital for treatment of central precocious puberty
- Females may experience some menses or spotting during first 2 mo of therapy for central precocious puberty, notify physician if continues into 2nd treatment mo

MONITORING PARAMETERS

- Monitor response to therapy for prostate cancer by measuring prostate specific antigen (PSA) levels
- GnRH stimulation test and sex steroid levels 1-2 mo after starting therapy for central precocious puberty, measurement of bone age for advancement q6-12mo

levamisole

(lee-vam'i-sole)

Ergamisol

Therapeutic Class: Immunomodulator

CLINICAL PHARMACOLOGY

Mechanism of Action: Exact mechanism unknown; appears to restore depressed immune function rather than to stimulate response to above normal levels; stimulates formation of antibodies to various antigens, enhances T-cell responses by stimulating T-cell activation and proliferation, potentiates monocyte and macrophage functions including phagocytosis and chemotaxis, increases neutrophil mobility, adherence, and chemotaxis

Pharmacokinetics

PO: Peak 1½-2 hr, metabolized by the liver, metabolites excreted by the kidneys, elimination $t_{1/2}$ 3-4 hr

INDICATIONS AND USES: Duke's stage C colon cancer (adjuvant treatment in combination with fluorouracil after surgical resection)

DOSAGE

Adult

- Initial PO 50 mg q8h for 3 days (starting 7-30 days after resection); given with fluorouracil 450 mg/m^2/d IV given daily for 5 days concomitant with a 3 day course of levamisole (beginning 21-34 days after resection)
- Maintenance 50 mg q8h for 3 days q2wk for 1 yr; given with fluorouracil 450 mg/m^2/d IV push qwk starting 28 days after the initial 5 day course for 1 yr

$ **AVAILABLE FORMS/COST OF THERAPY**

- Tab, Coated—Oral: 50 mg, 36's: **$194.40**

CONTRAINDICATIONS: Hypersensitivity

PRECAUTIONS: Children

PREGNANCY AND LACTATION: Pregnancy category C

SIDE EFFECTS/ADVERSE REACTIONS

CNS: Dizziness, headache, paresthesia, somnolence, depression, anxiety, fatigue, fever, mental changes, ataxia, insomnia

CV: Chest pain, edema

EENT: Altered sense of smell

GI: Nausea, vomiting, anorexia, diarrhea, stomatitis, constipation, flatulence, dyspepsia, abdominal pain

HEME: ***Agranulocytosis***

METAB: Hyperbilirubinemia

MS: Arthralgia, myalgia

SKIN: Rash, pruritus, alopecia, dermatitis, urticaria

▼ **DRUG INTERACTIONS**

Drugs

- *Alcohol:* May produce disulfiram-like effects

SPECIAL CONSIDERATIONS

MONITORING PARAMETERS

- Baseline CBC with differential and platelets, electrolytes, liver function tests
- Repeat CBC qwk
- Repeat electrolytes and liver function tests q3mo

---

levodopa

(lee-voe-doe'pa)

Dopar, Larodopa

Chemical Class: Catecholamine

Therapeutic Class: Antiparkinson agent

CLINICAL PHARMACOLOGY

Mechanism of Action: Decarboxylated to dopamine which stimulates dopaminergic receptors in the basal ganglia, improving the balance between cholinergic and dopaminergic activity; improves modulation of voluntary nerve impulses transmitted to the motor cortex

Pharmacokinetics

PO: Peak 1-3 hr, onset 2-3 wk, duration up to 5 hr/dose, 95% converted to dopamine by L-aromatic amino acid decarboxylase enzyme in the lumen to the stomach and intestines and on first pass through the liver, <1% reaches CNS due to extensive metabolism in the periphery and liver, excreted by the kidneys as metabolites, $t_{1/2}$ 1-3 hr

INDICATIONS AND USES: Idiopathic Parkinson's disease, postencephalitic parkinsonism, symptomatic parkinsonism following injury to the nervous system by carbon monoxide or manganese intoxication, parkinsonism associated with cerebral arteriosclerosis; herpes zoster,* restless legs syndrome*

DOSAGE

Adult

- PO 0.5-1 g qd divided bid-qid with meals; may increase gradually by up to 0.75 g/d q3-7d as tolerated, do not exceed 8 g/d unless closely supervised

$ **AVAILABLE FORMS/COST OF THERAPY**

- Cap, Gel—Oral: 100 mg, 100's: **$25.80;** 250 mg, 100's: **$45.60;** 500 mg, 100's: **$68.84**
- Tab, Uncoated—Oral: 100 mg, 100's: **$22.60;** 250 mg, 100's: **$36.08;** 500 mg, 100's: **$61.98**

CONTRAINDICATIONS: Hypersensitivity, narrow-angle glaucoma, concurrent MAOI therapy, history of melanoma or suspicious undiagnosed skin lesions (can activate malignant melanoma)

PRECAUTIONS: Severe cardiovascular or pulmonary disease, bronchial asthma, occlusive cerebrovascular disease, renal/hepatic/endocrine disease, affective disorders, major psychoses, cardiac dysrhyth-

L

mias, history of peptic ulcer, wide-angle glaucoma

PREGNANCY AND LACTATION: Safety for use in pregnancy has not been established; do not use in nursing mothers

SIDE EFFECTS/ADVERSE REACTIONS

CNS: Choreiform or dystonic movements, ataxia, increase hand tremor, headache, dizziness, confusion, insomnia, nightmares, hallucinations, delusions, anxiety, euphoria, depression, mental changes, "on-off" phenomenon

CV: Palpitations, orthostatic hypotension, hypertension, phlebitis, edema

EENT: Blepharospasm, diplopia, blurred vision, dilated pupils, hoarseness, oculogyric crisis

GI: Nausea, vomiting, anorexia, abdominal pain, dry mouth, dysphagia, dysgeusia, sialorrhea, burning sensation of tongue, diarrhea, constipation, flatulence, GI bleeding

GU: Urinary incontinence, urinary retention, priapism, dark urine

HEME: ***Hemolytic anemia, leukopenia, agranulocytosis***

RESP: Bizarre breathing patterns, hiccoughs

SKIN: Flushing, rash, increased sweating, hot flushes, dark sweat, loss of hair

MISC: Weight gain

▼ DRUG INTERACTIONS

Drugs

- *Food:* High-protein diets may inhibit the efficacy of levodopa
- *Methionine, neuroleptics, papaverine, phenytoin, pyridoxine, spiramycin, tacrine:* Inhibited clinical response to levodopa
- *Moclobemide:* Increased risk of adverse effects from levodopa
- *MAOIs:* Hypertensive response

Labs

- *False positive:* Urine ketones, urine glucose, Coombs' test
- *False negative:* Urine glucose (glucose oxidase)
- *False increase:* Uric acid, urine protein
- *Decrease:* VMA

SPECIAL CONSIDERATIONS

PATIENT/FAMILY EDUCATION

- Full benefit may require up to 6 mo
- Take with food to minimize GI upset
- Use caution while driving or performing other tasks requiring alertness
- Avoid sudden changes in posture
- May cause darkening of the urine or sweat
- May interfere with urine tests for sugar or ketones
- Notify physician of uncontrollable movements of the face, eyelids, mouth, tongue, neck, arms, hands or legs; mood or mental changes; irregular heartbeats; difficult urination; severe nausea or vomiting

MONITORING PARAMETERS

- CBC, renal function, liver function, ECG, intraocular pressure

levonorgestrel

(lee-voe-nor-jess'trel)

Norplant System

Chemical Class: 19-nortestosterone derivative

Therapeutic Class: Contraceptive

CLINICAL PHARMACOLOGY

Mechanism of Action: Alters cervical mucus; exerts a progestational effect on the endometrium, apparently producing cellular changes that render the endometrium hostile to implantation by a fertilized egg; suppresses ovulation in some patients

Pharmacokinetics

IMPLANT: Max concentrations within

24 hr; duration 5 yr; concentrations show considerable interindividual variation depending on individual clearance rates, body weight, and possibly other factors; metabolized by reduction followed by conjugation

INDICATIONS AND USES: Prevention of pregnancy

DOSAGE

Adult

• IMPLANT 216 mg (6 × 36 mg caps) subdermally in the upper arm during 1st 7 days after onset of menses; implantation should be fan-like, 15 degrees apart, 8 cm (3 in) above the crease of the elbow

$ AVAILABLE FORMS/COST OF THERAPY

• Kit: 216 mg, 1 kit: **$456.25**

CONTRAINDICATIONS: Active thrombophlebitis or thromboembolic disorders, undiagnosed abnormal genital bleeding, pregnancy, acute liver disease, liver tumors, breast cancer, hypersensitivity

PRECAUTIONS: Diabetes mellitus, impaired liver function, conditions aggravated by fluid retention, history of depression, contact lens wearers

PREGNANCY AND LACTATION: Pregnancy category X; has been identified in breast milk, no significant effects on the growth or health of infants has been identified in mothers who used implants beginning 6 wk postpartum

SIDE EFFECTS/ADVERSE REACTIONS

CNS: Headache, nervousness, dizziness

CV: Edema

EENT: Contact lens intolerance

GI: Nausea, change of appetite, abdominal discomfort

GU: Many bleeding days, prolonged bleeding, spotting, amenorrhea, irregular bleeding, scanty bleeding, cervicitis, vaginitis, adnexal enlargement

METAB: Altered glucose tolerance

MS: Musculoskeletal pain

SKIN: Dermatitis, acne, hirsutism, hypertrichosis, scalp hair loss, infection at inj site, pain/itching at inj site

MISC: Breast discharge, mastalgia, weight gain

▼ DRUG INTERACTIONS

Drugs

• *Carbamazepine, phenytoin:* Decreased efficacy of levonorgestrel; pregnancy has occurred

Labs

• *Increase:* Triiodothyronine uptake

• *Decrease:* Sex hormone binding globulin, thyroxine

SPECIAL CONSIDERATIONS

PATIENT/FAMILY EDUCATION

• If vision problems occur, an ophthalmologist should be seen

• Most women can expect some variation in menstrual bleeding, these irregularities should diminish with continued use

• Capsules will be removed at any time for any reason or at the end of 5 yr

MONITORING PARAMETERS

• Annual physical exam, Pap smear

---

levorphanol

(lee-vor'fa-nole)

Levo-Dromoran

Chemical Class: Synthetic morphinan derivative

Therapeutic Class: Narcotic analgesic

DEA Class: Schedule II

CLINICAL PHARMACOLOGY

Mechanism of Action: Binds to opiate receptors in the CNS causing inhibition of ascending pain pathways, altering the perception of and response to pain; produces less nausea, vomiting, and constipation, but more sedation and smooth muscle stimulation than equianalgesic doses of morphine

Pharmacokinetics

PO/SC: Peak analgesia 1-1½ hr, duration 6-8 hr

IV: Peak analgesia 20 min, duration 6-8 hr

Metabolized by liver, excreted in urine as glucuronide conjugate, $t_{1/2}$ 11 hr

INDICATIONS AND USES: Moderate to severe pain, preoperative sedation (parenteral)

DOSAGE

Adult

• PO/SC/IV 2-3 mg q6-8h prn

$ AVAILABLE FORMS/COST OF THERAPY

• Inj, Sol—SC: 2 mg/ml, 10 ml: **$21.92**

• Tab, Uncoated—Oral: 2 mg, 100's: **$54.68-$59.84**

CONTRAINDICATIONS: Hypersensitivity, acute bronchial asthma, upper airway obstruction

PRECAUTIONS: Head injury, increased intracranial pressure, acute abdominal conditions, elderly, severe impairment of hepatic or renal function, hypothyroidism, Addison's disease, prostatic hypertrophy, urethral stricture, history of drug abuse

PREGNANCY AND LACTATION: Pregnancy category B (category D if used for prolonged periods or in high doses at term); use during labor produces neonatal depression

SIDE EFFECTS/ADVERSE REACTIONS

CNS: Drowsiness, sedation, dizziness, agitation, dependency, lethargy, restlessness

GI: Nausea, vomiting, anorexia, constipation

RESP: ***Respiratory depression, respiratory paralysis***

CV: Bradycardia, palpitations, orthostatic hypotension, tachycardia

GU: Urinary retention

SKIN: Flushing, rash, urticaria

▼ DRUG INTERACTIONS

Drugs

• *Barbiturates, ethanol:* Additive CNS depression

• *Cimetidine:* Increased effect of narcotic analgesics

• *Neuroleptics:* Hypotension and excessive CNS depression

Labs

• *Increase:* Amylase

SPECIAL CONSIDERATIONS

PATIENT/FAMILY EDUCATION

• Report any symptoms of CNS changes, allergic reactions

• Physical dependency may result when used for extended periods

• Change position slowly, orthostatic hypotension may occur

• Avoid hazardous activities if drowsiness or dizziness occurs

• Avoid alcohol, other CNS depressants unless directed by physician

• Minimize nausea by administering with food and remain lying down following dose

---

levothyroxine

(lee-voe-thye-rox′een)

Levo-T, Levothroid, Levoxine, Synthroid, Synthrox

Chemical Class: Synthetic *levo* isomer of thyroxine

Therapeutic Class: Thyroid hormone

CLINICAL PHARMACOLOGY

Mechanism of Action: Involved in normal metabolism, growth, and development, especially the development of the CNS of infants; increases the metabolic rate of body tissues

Pharmacokinetics
IV: Onset 6-8 hr
PO: Extent of absorption increased by the fasting state, peak 12-48 hr >99% bound to plasma proteins, 35% of T_4 is converted in the periphery to T_3, $t_{1/2}$ 6-7 days (3-4 days in hyperthyroidism, 9-10 days in myxedema)

INDICATIONS AND USES: Hypothyroidism (including cretinism, myxedema, non-toxic goiter), pituitary TSH suppression (thyroid nodules, Hashimoto's disease, multinodular goiter, thyroid cancer), thyrotoxicosis (with antithyroid drugs)

DOSAGE
Adult
- *Hypothyroidism:* PO 50 μg qd to start, increase by 25-50 μg/d at intervals of 2-4 wk, usual dose 100-200 μg/day; use ≤25 μg/d in patients with long-standing hypothyroidism if cardiovascular impairment present; IM/IV 50% of oral dose
- *Myxedema:* IV 200-500 μg one time, then 100-300 μg the next day prn; resume oral therapy as soon as clinical situation stabilized
- *TSH suppression:* PO larger amounts than needed for replacement are required, optimal dose determined by laboratory findings and clinical response

Child
- PO 8-10 μg/kg or 25-50 μg qd (0-6 mo); 6-8 μg/kg or 50-75 μg qd (6-12 mo); 5-6 μg/kg or 75-100 μg qd (1-5 yr); 4-5 μg/kg or 100-150 μg qd (6-12 yr); 2-3 μg/kg or ≥ 150 μg qd (>12 yr); IM/IV 50%-75% of oral dose

$ AVAILABLE FORMS/COST OF THERAPY
- Inj, Lyphl-Sol—IM; IV: 0.2, 0.5 mg/vial, 10 ml: **$9.75-$103.76**
- Tab, Uncoated—Oral: 0.025, 0.05, 0.075, 0.088, 0.1, 0.112, 0.125, 0.137, 0.15, 0.175, 0.2, 0.3 mg, 100's: **$3.89-$43.50**

CONTRAINDICATIONS: Adrenal insufficiency, MI, thyrotoxicosis, hypersensitivity

PRECAUTIONS: Cardiovascular disease, diabetes mellitus or insipidus

PREGNANCY AND LACTATION: Pregnancy category A; little or no transplacental passage at physiologic serum concentrations; excreted into breast milk in low concentrations, the effect on the nursing infant is not thought to be physiologically significant

SIDE EFFECTS/ADVERSE REACTIONS
CNS: *Tremors,* headache, nervousness, *insomnia*
CV: *Palpitations, tachycardia, cardiac dysrhythmias, angina pectoris,* ***cardiac arrest***
GI: Diarrhea, vomiting, gastric intolerance
GU: Menstrual irregularities
SKIN: Allergic skin reactions (rare)
MISC: Weight loss, sweating, heat intolerance, fever

▼ DRUG INTERACTIONS
Drugs
- *Bile acid sequestrants:* Reduced serum thyroid hormone concentrations
- *Carbamazepine, phenytoin:* Increased elimination of thyroid hormones; possible increased requirement for thyroid hormones in hypothyroid patients
- *Oral anticoagulants+:* Thyroid hormones increase catabolism of vitamin K-dependent clotting factors; an increase or decrease in clinical thyroid status will increase or decrease the hypoprothrombinemic response to oral anticoagulants

Labs
- *Increase:* CPK, LDH, AST, PBI, blood glucose

• *Decrease:* TSH, ^{131}I uptake test, uric acid, triglycerides

SPECIAL CONSIDERATIONS

PATIENT/FAMILY EDUCATION

• Notify physician of headache, nervousness, diarrhea, excessive sweating, heat intolerance, chest pain, increased pulse rate, palpitations
• Transient, partial hair loss may be experienced by children in the first few months of therapy
• Take as a single daily dose, preferably before breakfast
• Do not change from one brand of this drug to another without consulting your pharmacist or physician

MONITORING PARAMETERS

• TSH, serum T_4, resin triiodothyronine uptake (RT_3U), free thyroxine index (FTI), heart rate, blood pressure
• Clinical signs of hypo- and hyperthyroidism

---

lidocaine (local, topical)

(lye'doe-kane)

Local: Dalcaine, Dilocaine, Duo-Trach Kit, L-Caine, Lidocaine HCl, Lidoject-1, Lidoject-2, Nervocaine 1%, Nervocaine 2%, Octocaine HCl, Xylocaine HCl; Topical: Anestacon, Xylocaine, Xylocaine Viscous

Chemical Class: Aminoacyl amide

Therapeutic Class: Local/topical anesthetic

CLINICAL PHARMACOLOGY

Mechanism of Action: Prevents the generation and conduction of nerve impulses by reducing sodium permeability, increasing electrical excitation threshold, slowing nerve impulse propagation, and reducing rate of rise of the action potential

Pharmacokinetics

TOP: Peak 2-5 min, duration 30-60 min

LOCAL: Onset 0.5-1 min (5-15 min for epidural), duration 0.5-1 hr (1-3 hr for epidural)

55%-65% bound to plasma proteins, metabolized primarily in the liver, excreted in urine and bile as metabolites

INDICATIONS AND USES: Local: Infiltration anesthesia, nerve block techniques (peripheral, sympathetic, epidural [including caudal], spinal), intraperitoneal anesthesia*; Topical: Anesthesia of skin and accessible mucous membranes

DOSAGE

Adult and Child

• LOCAL varies with procedure, degree of anesthesia desired, vascularity of tissue, duration of anesthesia required, and physical condition of patient; max 4.5 mg/kg/dose, do not repeat within 2 hr
• TOP apply to affected area prn; max 3 mg/kg/dose, do not repeat within 2 hr

$ AVAILABLE FORMS/COST OF THERAPY

Top

• Jel—Top; Oral: 2%, 30 g: **$12.85**
• Jelly—Top: 2%, 5, 10, 20, 30 ml: **$7.19-$14.24**
• Oint—Top: 5%, 35 g: **$4.95-$13.13**
• Sol—Top: 4%, 50 ml: **$7.04-$15.04**
• Sol, Viscous—Top; Oral: 2%, 100 ml: **$2.44-$15.74**
• Aer, Spray—Oral; Top: 10%, 30 ml: **$44.82**

Local

• Inj, Sol: 0.5%, 50 ml: **$3.22-$9.44;** 1%, 50 ml: **$1.75-$6.60;** 1.5%, 20 ml: **$5.96-$10.46;** 2%, 50 ml: **$2.00-$6.60;** 4%, 50 ml: **$2.03-$2.53;** 10%,

10 ml: **$8.65;** 20%, 10 ml: **$11.93-$18.13**

• Kit—Intracavity; Intrathecal; Misc: 4%, 5 kits: **$38.23**

CONTRAINDICATIONS: Hypersensitivity, heart block (large doses), septicemia (spinal anesthesia), ophthalmic use (topical preparations), spinal anesthesia (preparations containing preservatives)

PRECAUTIONS: Inflammation, sepsis, shock, elderly, children, severe liver disease

PREGNANCY AND LACTATION: Pregnancy category C; has been used as a local anesthetic during labor and delivery, may produce CNS depression and bradycardia in the newborn with high serum levels; compatible with breast feeding

SIDE EFFECTS/ADVERSE REACTIONS

CNS: Anxiety, restlessness, ***convulsions, loss of consciousness,*** drowsiness, disorientation, tremors, shivering

CV: ***Myocardial depression, cardiac arrest, dysrhythmias,*** bradycardia, hypotension, hypertension

EENT: Blurred vision, tinnitus, pupil constriction

GI: Nausea, vomiting

RESP: ***Status asthmaticus, respiratory arrest, anaphylaxis***

SKIN: Rash, urticaria, allergic reactions, edema, burning, skin discoloration at inj site, tissue necrosis; rash, irritation, sensitization (top)

▼ **DRUG INTERACTIONS**

Drugs

• *Beta blockers, cimetidine:* Increased serum lidocaine concentrations

• *Phenytoin:* Reduced serum lidocaine concentrations; additive depressant effects on myocardial tissue

lidocaine (systemic)

(lye'doe-kane)

Lidopen Auto-Injector, Xylocaine IM for Cardiac Arrythmias, Xylocaine IV for Cardiac Arrhythmias

Chemical Class: Aminoacyl amide

Therapeutic Class: Antidysrhythmic (Class IB)

CLINICAL PHARMACOLOGY

Mechanism of Action: Decreases depolarization, automaticity, and excitability in the ventricles during the diastolic phase by a direct action on the tissues, especially the Purkinje network, without involvement of the autonomic system; neither contractility, systolic arterial blood pressure, atrioventricular (AV) conduction velocity, nor absolute refractory period is altered by usual therapeutic doses

Pharmacokinetics

IV: Onset immediate, duration 10-20 min

IM: Onset 5-15 min, duration 60-90 min

60%-80% bound to plasma proteins, metabolized by liver to active metabolites, eliminated in urine (10% as unchanged drug), $t_{1/2}$ 1-2 hr

INDICATIONS AND USES: Acute ventricular dysrhythmias

DOSAGE

Adult

• IV BOL 50-100 mg over 2-3 min, repeat q3-5min, not to exceed 300 mg in 1 hr, begin IV INF; IV INF 20-50 μg/kg/min (1-4 mg/min); decrease the dose in patients with CHF, acute MI, shock, or hepatic disease; IM 200-300 mg in deltoid muscle, additional doses may be given after 60-90 min if necessary; ET 2-2.5 times the IV dose

L

Child

• IV/ET/IO 1 mg/kg loading dose, repeat if needed in 10-15 min × 2 doses, begin IV INF; IV INF 20-50 µg/kg/min

AVAILABLE FORMS/COST OF THERAPY

For direct IV administration:

• Inj, Sol—IV: 1%, 5 ml: **$1.51-$23.24;** 2%, 5 ml: **$4.75-$11.78**

For IV admixture:

• Inj, Sol: 4%, 25 ml: **$1.59-$2.25;** 10%, 10 ml: **$8.65;** 20%, 10 ml: **$11.93-$18.13**

CONTRAINDICATIONS: Hypersensitivity to amide local anesthetics, Stokes-Adams syndrome, Wolff-Parkinson-White syndrome, severe heart block (in absence of a pacemaker)

PRECAUTIONS: Children, renal disease, liver disease, CHF, reduced cardiac output, digitalis toxicity accompanied by AV block, respiratory depression, genetic predisposition to malignant hyperthermia, atrial fibrillation or flutter

PREGNANCY AND LACTATION: Pregnancy category C; compatible with breast feeding

SIDE EFFECTS/ADVERSE REACTIONS

CNS: Lightheadedness, nervousness, drowsiness, *dizziness,* apprehension, confusion, mood changes, hallucinations, euphoria, twitching, tremors, ***convulsions, unconsciousness***

CV: Hypotension, bradycardia, ***cardiovascular collapse, heart block,*** edema

EENT: Tinnitus, blurred or double vision

GI: Vomiting

RESP: ***Respiratory depression and arrest***

SKIN: Rash, urticaria, swelling

MISC: Febrile response, phlebitis at inj site, ***malignant hyperthermia***

▼ DRUG INTERACTIONS

Drugs

• *Beta blockers, cimetidine:* Increased serum lidocaine concentrations

• *Phenytoin:* Reduced serum lidocaine concentrations; additive depressant effects on myocardial tissue

Labs

• *Increase:* CPK (following IM inj)

SPECIAL CONSIDERATIONS

MONITORING PARAMETERS

• Constant ECG monitoring, blood pressure

• Therapeutic serum concentrations are 1.5-6 µg/ml (concentrations >6-10 µg/ml are usually associated with toxicity)

lindane (gamma benzene hexachloride)

(lin'dane)

gBh, ✤ G-Well, Kwell, Kwellada, ✤ Lindane, Scabene

Chemical Class: Cyclic chlorinated hydrocarbon

Therapeutic Class: Scabicide/Pediculicide

CLINICAL PHARMACOLOGY

Mechanism of Action: Following absorption through the chitinous exoskeleton of arthropods, stimulates the nervous system resulting in seizures and death

Pharmacokinetics

TOP: Slowly and incompletely absorbed through intact skin, stored in body fat, metabolized by the liver, excreted in urine and feces

INDICATIONS AND USES: *Pediculus capitis* (head lice), *Pediculus pubis* (crab lice) and their ova; *Sarcoptes scabiei* (scabies)

DOSAGE

Adult and Child

- *Lotion:* (Crab lice) Apply sufficient quantity only to cover the hair and skin of the pubic area and adjacent infested areas, leave in place for 12 hr then wash thoroughly, may repeat in 7 days if necessary; treat sexual contacts concurrently; (Head lice) Apply a sufficient quantity to cover only the affected area, rub into scalp, and leave in place for 12 hr then wash thoroughly, may repeat in 7 days if necessary; (Scabies) Make total body application from neck down, leave on 8-12 hr (adults), 6-8 hr (children), 6 hr (infants); remove by thorough washing
- *Shampoo:* (Head lice and crab lice) Apply a sufficient quantity to dry hair, work thoroughly into hair and allow to remain in place for 4 min, add small quantities of water until a good lather forms, rinse hair thoroughly and towel briskly; comb with a fine-toothed comb or use tweezers to remove any remaining nits or nit shells

$ AVAILABLE FORMS/COST OF THERAPY

- Lotion—Top: 1%, 60 ml: **$1.80-$5.55**
- Shampoo—Top: 1%, 60 ml: **$2.10-$5.20**

CONTRAINDICATIONS: Premature neonates, seizure disorder, hypersensitivity

PRECAUTIONS: Children; infants; avoid contact with eyes; inflammation of skin, abrasions, or breaks in skin

PREGNANCY AND LACTATION: Pregnancy category B; use no more than twice during a pregnancy; amounts excreted in breast milk probably clinically insignificant

SIDE EFFECTS/ADVERSE REACTIONS

CNS: Stimulation, dizziness, ***convulsions***

SKIN: Eczematous eruptions due to irritation

SPECIAL CONSIDERATIONS

PATIENT/FAMILY EDUCATION

- Do not exceed prescribed dosage
- Do not apply to face
- Avoid getting in eyes
- Wear rubber gloves for application
- Notify physician if condition worsens or if itching, redness, swelling, burning, or skin rash occurs
- Treat sexual contacts concurrently

liothyronine (T3)

(lye-oh-thye'roe-neen)

Cytomel, Triostat

Chemical Class: Synthetic T_3 (triiodothyronine)

Therapeutic Class: Thyroid hormone

CLINICAL PHARMACOLOGY

Mechanism of Action: Involved in normal metabolism, growth, and development, especially the development of the CNS of infants; increases the metabolic rate of body tissues

Pharmacokinetics

PO: Peak 48-72 hr, duration following withdrawal of chronic therapy up to 72 hr, >99% bound to plasma proteins, $t_{1/2}$ 0.6-1.4 hr

INDICATIONS AND USES: Hypothyroidism (including cretinism, myxedema, non-toxic goiter), pituitary TSH suppression (thyroid nodules, Hashimoto's disease, multinodular goiter, thyroid cancer), T_3 suppression test

DOSAGE

Adult

- *Hypothyroidism:* PO 25 µg/d, increase by 12.5-25 μg q1-2 wk to max of 100 μg/d

• *T_3 suppression test:* PO 75-100 μg/d for 7 days

• *Myxedema coma:* IV 25-50 μg, repeat prn at 4-12 hr intervals

Elderly

• *Hypothyroidism:* PO 5 μg/d, increase by 5 μg/d q1-2wk; usual maintenance dose 25-75 μg/d

Child

• *Congenital hypothyroidism:* PO 5 μg/d, increase by 5 μg q3d to 20 μg/d (infants), 50 μg/d (child 1-3 yr), adult dose (child >3 yr)

$ AVAILABLE FORMS/COST OF THERAPY

• Tab, Uncoated—Oral: 5 μg, 100's: **$14.50;** 25 μg, 100's: **$17.55;** 50 μg, 100's: **$26.80**

• Inj, Sol—IV: 10 μg/ml, 1 ml × 6: **$1373.00**

CONTRAINDICATIONS: Adrenal insufficiency, MI, thyrotoxicosis, hypersensitivity

PRECAUTIONS: Cardiovascular disease, diabetes mellitus or insipidus

PREGNANCY AND LACTATION: Pregnancy category A; little or no transplacental passage at physiologic serum concentrations; excreted into breast milk in low concentrations, the effect on the nursing infant is not thought to be physiologically significant

SIDE EFFECTS/ADVERSE REACTIONS

CNS: Tremors, headache, nervousness, *insomnia*

CV: Palpitations, tachycardia, cardiac arrhythmias, angina pectoris, ***cardiac arrest***

GI: Diarrhea, vomiting, gastric intolerance

GU: Menstrual irregularities

SKIN: Allergic skin reactions (rare)

MISC: Weight loss, sweating, heat intolerance, fever

▼ DRUG INTERACTIONS

Drugs

• *Bile acid sequestrants:* Reduced serum thyroid hormone concentrations

• *Carbamazepine, phenytoin:* Increased elimination of thyroid hormones; possible increased requirement for thyroid hormones in hypothyroid patients

• *Oral anticoagulants+:* Thyroid hormones increase catabolism of vitamin K-dependent clotting factors; an increase or decrease in clinical thyroid status will increase or decrease the hypoprothrombinemic response to oral anticoagulants

Labs

• *Increase:* CPK, LDH, AST, PBI, blood glucose

• *Decrease:* TSH, ^{131}I uptake test, uric acid, triglycerides

SPECIAL CONSIDERATIONS

PATIENT/FAMILY EDUCATION

• Notify physician of headache, nervousness, diarrhea, excessive sweating, heat intolerance, chest pain, increased pulse rate, palpitations

• Transient, partial hair loss may be experienced by children in the first few months of therapy

MONITORING PARAMETERS

• TSH, heart rate, blood pressure

• Clinical signs of hypo- and hyperthyroidism

lisinopril

(lyse-in'oh-pril)

Prinivil, Zestril

Chemical Class: Enalaprilat lysine analog; angiotensin-converting enzyme (ACE) inhibitor

Therapeutic Class: Antihypertensive

CLINICAL PHARMACOLOGY

Mechanism of Action: Selectively suppresses renin-angiotensin-aldosterone system; inhibits ACE preventing the conversion of angiotensin 1 to angiotensin II; results in dilation of arterial, venous vessels

Pharmacokinetics

PO: Peak 7 hr, onset 1 hr, duration 24 hr, excreted unchanged in urine, $t_{1/2}$ 12 hr (prolonged in renal dysfunction)

INDICATIONS AND USES: Hypertension, CHF, diabetic nephropathy*

DOSAGE

Adult

- *Hypertension:* PO 10 mg qd, usual dosage range 20-40 mg/d
- *CHF:* PO 5 mg qd, usual dosage range 5-20 mg/d
- *Renal impairment:* PO initial dose 5 mg qd (serum creatinine ≥3 mg/dl); initial dose 2.5 mg qd (dialysis patients)

$ **AVAILABLE FORMS/COST OF THERAPY**

- Tab, Uncoated—Oral: 2.5 mg, 100's: **$52.50;** 5 mg, 100's: **$78.62;** 10 mg, 100's: **$81.29;** 20 mg, 100's: **$87.00;** 40 mg, 100's: **$127.08**

CONTRAINDICATIONS: Hypersensitivity to ACE inhibitors

PRECAUTIONS: Impaired renal function, dialysis patients, hypovolemia, diuretic therapy, collagen-vascular diseases, CHF, elderly, bilateral renal artery stenosis

PREGNANCY AND LACTATION: Pregnancy category C (first trimester), category D (second and third trimesters); ACE inhibitors can cause fetal and neonatal morbidity and death when administered to pregnant women, when pregnancy is detected, discontinue ACE inhibitors as soon as possible; detectable in breast milk in trace amounts, a newborn would receive <0.1% of the mg/kg maternal dose; effect on nursing infant has not been determined

SIDE EFFECTS/ADVERSE REACTIONS

CNS: Anxiety, insomnia, paresthesia, *headache, dizziness, fatigue*

CV: Hypotension, postural hypotension, syncope (especially with first dose), palpitations, angina

GI: Nausea, constipation, vomiting, melena, abdominal pain

GU: Increased BUN, creatinine, decreased libido, impotence, UTI

HEME: ***Neutropenia, agranulocytosis***

METAB: Hyperkalemia, hyponatremia

MS: Arthralgia, arthritis, myalgia

RESP: *Cough,* asthma, bronchitis, dyspnea, sinusitis

SKIN: ***Angioedema,*** rash, flushing, sweating

▼ **DRUG INTERACTIONS**

Drugs

- *Lithium:* Increased risk of serious lithium toxicity
- *Loop diuretics:* Initiation of ACE inhibitor therapy in the presence of intensive diuretic therapy results in a precipitous fall in blood pressure in some patients; ACE inhibitors may induce renal insufficiency in the presence of diuretic-induced sodium depletion
- *NSAIDs:* Inhibition of the antihypertensive response to ACE inhibitors
- *Potassium sparing diuretics:* Increased risk for hyperkalemia

SPECIAL CONSIDERATIONS

PATIENT/FAMILY EDUCATION

- Do not use salt substitutes containing potassium without consulting physician
- Rise slowly to sitting or standing position to minimize orthostatic hypotension

• Notify physician of mouth sores, sore throat, fever, swelling of hands or feet, irregular heartbeat, chest pain
• Dizziness, fainting, light-headedness may occur during 1st few days of therapy
• Persistent dry cough may occur and usually does not subside unless medication is stopped, notify physician if this effect occurs

MONITORING PARAMETERS
• BUN, creatinine (watch for increased levels that may indicate acute renal failure)
• Potassium levels, although hyperkalemia rarely occurs

lithium

(li'thee-um)

Carbolith, ✦ Cibalith-S, Duralith, Eskalith, Eskalith CR, Lithane, Lithobid, Lithonate, Lithotabs

Chemical Class: Monovalent cation

Therapeutic Class: Antimanic; psychotherapeutic agent

CLINICAL PHARMACOLOGY

Mechanism of Action: Alters sodium transport in nerve and muscle cells, and effects a shift toward intraneuronal metabolism of catecholamines; specific mechanism in mania unknown but may be secondary to effects on neurotransmitters associated with affective disorders (norepinephrine and serotonin)

Pharmacokinetics

PO: Peak ½ hr (syr), 1-3 hr (cap or tabs), 3-4 hr (ext rel formulations); onset 1-3 wk; not bound to plasma proteins; excreted unchanged in urine (95%); $t_{1/2}$ 18-36 hr

INDICATIONS AND USES: Manic episodes of bipolar affective disorder; prophylaxis of cluster headache,* premenstrual tension,* bulimia,* alcoholism,* SIADH,* tardive dyskinesia,* hyperthyroidism,* postpartum affective psychosis*

DOSAGE

Adult

• *Acute mania:* PO 600 mg tid or 900 mg bid (ext rel formulations); determine serum lithium concentrations twice weekly until stabilized
• *Maintenance:* PO 300 mg tid-qid, adjust to maintain therapeutic serum lithium concentration

Child

• PO 15-60 mg/kg/d in 3-4 divided doses; adjust to maintain therapeutic serum lithium concentration; do not exceed usual adult dose

$ **AVAILABLE FORMS/COST OF THERAPY**

• Cap, Gel—Oral: 150 mg, 100's: **$7.63;** 300 mg, 100's: **$4.28-$16.90;** 600 mg, 100's: **$13.23**
• Tab, Uncoated—Oral: 300 mg, 100's: **$6.89-$7.41**
• Tab, Coated, Sust Action—Oral: 300 mg, 100's: **$15.53-$23.69;** 450 mg, 100's: **$35.80**
• Syr—Oral: 300 mg/5 ml, 480 ml: **$16.18-$19.29**

CONTRAINDICATIONS: Hypersensitivity, severe cardiovascular or renal disease

PRECAUTIONS: Dehydration, sodium depletion, elderly, children <12 yr, concomitant infection, thyroid disease, tartrazine sensitivity, diabetes mellitus

PREGNANCY AND LACTATION: Pregnancy category D; avoid use in pregnancy if possible, especially during the 1st trimester; contraindicated in nursing mothers

SIDE EFFECTS/ADVERSE REACTIONS

CNS: Headache, drowsiness, dizziness, fine hand tremor, twitching, ataxia, ***seizure,*** slurred speech, restlessness, confusion, stupor, memory

loss, clonic movements, ***pseudotumor cerebri***
CV: Hypotension, ECG changes, ***dysrhythmias, circulatory collapse,*** edema, ***bradycardia***
EENT: Tinnitus, blurred vision
GI: Dry mouth, anorexia, nausea, vomiting, diarrhea, abdominal pain, metallic taste, excessive salivation, gastritis, flatulence
GU: Polyuria, glycosuria, proteinuria, albuminuria, urinary incontinence, polydipsia, symptoms of nephrogenic diabetes, decreased creatinine clearance, sexual dysfunction
HEME: Benign leukocytosis
METAB: Euthyroid goiter, hypothyroidism, hyperthyroidism (rare), transient hyperglycemia, hyponatremia
MS: Arthralgia
SKIN: Drying and thinning of hair, anesthesia of skin, chronic folliculitis, exacerbation of psoriasis, acne, ***angioedema,*** generalized pruritis
MISC: Thirst, excessive weight gain

▼ DRUG INTERACTIONS

Drugs

- *ACE inhibitors, methyldopa:* Increased risk of lithium toxicity
- *Calcium channel blockers, carbamazepine, fluoxetine:* Neurotoxicity
- *MAOIs:* Malignant hyperpyrexia
- *Neuroleptics:* Reduced neuroleptic response; severe neurotoxicity possible in acute manic patients receiving lithium and neuroleptics
- *NSAIDs:* Increased lithium concentrations
- *Potassium iodide:* Increased risk for hypothyroidism
- *Sodium bicarbonate:* Decreased plasma lithium concentrations
- *Sodium chloride:* High sodium intake may reduce serum lithium concentrations; sodium restriction may increase serum lithium
- *Thiazide diuretics+:* Increased lithium concentrations

Labs

- *Increase:* Potassium excretion, urine glucose, blood glucose, protein, BUN
- *Decrease:* VMA, T_3, T_4, PBI, ^{131}I

SPECIAL CONSIDERATIONS

PATIENT/FAMILY EDUCATION

- Take with meals to avoid stomach upset
- Discontinue medication and contact physician for diarrhea, vomiting, unsteady walking, coarse hand tremor, severe drowsiness, muscle weakness
- May cause drowsiness, use caution while driving or performing other tasks requiring alertness
- Drink 8-12 glasses of water or other liquid every day
- Maintain a regular diet (including salt)

MONITORING PARAMETERS

- Serum lithium concentrations drawn immediately prior to next dose (8-12 hr after previous dose), monitor biweekly until stable then q2-3mo; therapeutic range 0.8-1.2 mEq/L (acute), 0.5-1.0 mEq/L (maintenance)
- Serum creatinine, CBC, urinalysis, serum electrolytes, fasting glucose, ECG, thyroid function tests

lomefloxacin

(lome-flock'sa-sin)
Maxaquin
Chemical Class: Fluoroquinolone
Therapeutic Class: Antiinfective

CLINICAL PHARMACOLOGY

Mechanism of Action: Interferes with the enzyme DNA gyrase needed for synthesis of bacterial DNA; bactericidal

Pharmacokinetics

PO: Peak 1-2 hr, absorption decreased by coadministration with food, excreted in urine as active drug, metabolites, $t_{1/2}$ 6-8 hr

INDICATIONS AND USES: Infections of the lower respiratory tract, urinary tract; prevention of UTI in patients undergoing transurethral procedures; gonorrhea*; all approved indications caused by susceptible organisms. Antibacterial spectrum usually includes: gram-positive organisms: *Staphylococcus saprophyticus;* gram-negative organisms: *Citrobacter diversus, Enterobacter cloacae, Escherichia coli, Haemophilus influenzae, Klebsiella pneumoniae, Moraxella catarrhalis, Proteus mirabilis, Pseudomonas aeruginosa* (urinary tract only)

DOSAGE

Adult

- *Lower respiratory tract:* PO 400 mg qd for 10 days
- *Urinary tract:* PO 400 mg qd for 3-14 days
- *Prophylaxis:* PO 400 mg as a single dose 2-6 hr prior to surgery
- *Gonorrhea:* PO 400 mg as a single dose
- *Renal function impairment:* PO 400 mg loading dose, then 200 mg qd for duration of treatment (CrCl <40 ml/min/1.73 m^2)

$ AVAILABLE FORMS/COST OF THERAPY

- Tab, Uncoated—Oral: 400 mg, 20's: **$122.13**

CONTRAINDICATIONS: Hypersensitivity to quinolones, empiric treatment of acute bacterial exacerbation of chronic bronchitis likely due to *S. pneumoniae*

PRECAUTIONS: Children (potential for arthropathy and osteochondrosis), elderly, renal disease, seizure disorders

PREGNANCY AND LACTATION: Pregnancy category C; excretion into breast milk unknown, due to the potential for arthropathy and osteochondrosis use extreme caution in nursing mothers

SIDE EFFECTS/ADVERSE REACTIONS

CNS: Dizziness, headache, fatigue, somnolence, depression, insomnia, anxiety, seizures

EENT: Visual disturbances, dizziness

GI: Diarrhea, *nausea,* vomiting, anorexia, flatulence, heartburn, abdominal pain, dry mouth, increased AST, ALT, ***pseudomembranous colitis***

SKIN: Rash, pruritus, photosensitivity

▼ DRUG INTERACTIONS

Drugs

- *Antacids, iron, zinc:* Reduced serum lomefloxacin concentrations

SPECIAL CONSIDERATIONS

PATIENT/FAMILY EDUCATION

- Avoid direct exposure to sunlight (even when using sunscreen)
- Drink fluids liberally
- Do not take antacids containing magnesium or aluminum or products containing iron or zinc within 4 hr before or 2 hr after dosing
- Observe caution while driving or performing other tasks requiring alertness

loperamide

(loe-per'a-mide)

Loperamide solution, Imodium, Imodium A-D, Imodium A-D Caplet, Loperamide

Chemical Class: Piperidine derivative

Therapeutic Class: Antidiarrheal

CLINICAL PHARMACOLOGY

Mechanism of Action: Direct action on intestinal muscles to decrease GI peristalsis

Pharmacokinetics

PO: 40% absorbed, onset 30-60 min, peak 5 hr (capsule) and 2½ hr (liquid), $t_{1/2}$ 7-14 hr; metabolized in liver; excreted in feces as unchanged drug; small amount in urine

INDICATIONS AND USES: Diarrhea (acute nonspecific), chronic diarrhea (inflammatory bowel disease), reduce volume from ileostomy, traveler's diarrhea*

DOSAGE

Adult

- PO 4 mg, then 2 mg after each loose stool, max 16 mg/d

Child

- PO 80-240 μg/kg/d divided into 2 or 3 doses; or by age and weight
- <2 yr, use not recommended
- 13-20 kg PO 1 mg tid on day 1, then 0.1 mg/kg after each loose stool
- 20-30 kg PO 2 mg bid on day 1, then 0.1 mg/kg after each loose stool
- >30 kg PO 2 mg tid on day 1, then 0.1 mg/kg after each loose stool

$ AVAILABLE FORMS/COST OF THERAPY

- Cap, Gel—Oral: 2 mg, 100's: **$29.25-$79.70**
- Tab (OTC)—Oral: 2 mg, 12's: **$2.57-$5.30**
- Liq (OTC)—Oral: 1 mg/5 ml, 120 ml: **$4.71-$5.65**

CONTRAINDICATIONS: Hypersensitivity, acute diarrhea due to invasive organisms (enteroinvasive *E.coli, Salmonella, Shigella*) or pseudomembranous colitis

PRECAUTIONS: Liver disease, dehydration, severe ulcerative colitis (toxic megacolon), children (greater variability in response)

PREGNANCY AND LACTATION: Pregnancy category B; unknown if excreted in breast milk but considered compatible with breast feeding

SIDE EFFECTS/ADVERSE REACTIONS

CNS: Dizziness, drowsiness, fatigue, fever

GI: Nausea, dry mouth, vomiting, constipation, abdominal pain, anorexia, ***toxic megacolon***

RESP: ***Respiratory depression***

SKIN: Rash

L

loracarbef

(lor-a-kar'bef)

Lorabid

Chemical Class: Carbacephem (beta-lactam structurally related to cephalosporins)

Therapeutic Class: Antibiotic

CLINICAL PHARMACOLOGY

Mechanism of Action: Inhibits bacterial cell wall synthesis, which renders cell wall osmotically unstable

Pharmacokinetics

PO: Well absorbed from GI tract, slower with food; peak 1 hr (cap), ½ hr (susp), $t_{1/2}$ 1 hr; excreted in urine as unchanged drug

INDICATIONS AND USES: Infections of the upper and lower respiratory tract, urinary tract, skin infections, otitis media.

Antibacterial spectrum usually includes:

- Gram-positive organisms: *Streptococcus pneumoniae, Str. pyogenes, Staphylococcus aureus*

• Gram-negative organisms: *Haemophilus influenzae, E. coli, Proteus mirabilis, Klebsiella*

DOSAGE

Adult

• *Cystitis:* PO 200 mg q24h for 7 days

• *Pyelonephritis:* PO 400 mg q12h for 14 days

• *Upper and lower respiratory tract:* PO 200-400 mg q12h

• *Skin:* PO 200 mg q12h

Child 6 mo-12 yr

• *Acute otitis media:* PO 15 mg/kg q12h for 10 days

• *Pharyngitis, skin infections:* PO 7.5 mg/kg q12h

• *Renal function impairment:* CrCl ≥50 ml/min, use regular dose; CrCl 10-49 ml/min, use half regular dose at regular interval; CrCl <10 ml/min, use regular dose q3-5d; repeat after hemodialysis

$ AVAILABLE FORMS/COST OF THERAPY

• Cap, Gel—Oral: 200 mg, 30's: **$94.35;** 400 mg, 30's: **$118.50**

• Susp—Oral: 100 mg/5 ml, 100 ml: **$24.34;** 200 mg/5 ml, 100 ml: **$36.51**

CONTRAINDICATIONS: Hypersensitivity to cephalosporins or related antibiotics, seizures

PRECAUTIONS: Children <6 mo, renal disease

PREGNANCY AND LACTATION: Pregnancy category B; unknown if excreted in breast milk

SIDE EFFECTS/ADVERSE REACTIONS

CNS: Dizziness, headache, fatigue, paresthesia, fever, chills, confusion

GI: Diarrhea, nausea, vomiting, anorexia, dysgeusia, glossitis, bleeding, increased liver function tests, abdominal pain, loose stools, flatulence, heartburn, stomach cramps, colitis, jaundice

GU: Vaginitis, pruritus, candidiasis, increased BUN, ***nephrotoxicity, renal failure,*** pyuria, dysuria, reversible interstitial nephritis

HEME: ***Leukopenia, thrombocytopenia, agranulocytosis,*** *anemia,* ***neutropenia, lymphocytosis, eosinophilia, pancytopenia, hemolytic anemia, leukocytosis, granulocytopenia***

RESP: Dyspnea

SKIN: Rash, urticaria, dermatitis, ***anaphylaxis***

▼ DRUG INTERACTIONS

Drugs

• *Aminoglycosides, furosemide, probenecid, ethacrynic acid, vancomycin:* Increased effect/toxicity

• *Tetracyclines, erythromycins:* Decreased effects

Labs

• *False positive:* Urinary protein, direct Coombs' test, urine glucose

• *Interference:* Cross-matching

loratadine

(loer-at'i-deen)

Claritin

Chemical Class: Selective histamine (H_1) receptor antagonist

Therapeutic Class: Antihistamine

CLINICAL PHARMACOLOGY

Mechanism of Action: Binds to peripheral histamine receptors, provides antihistamine action without sedation

Pharmacokinetics

PO: Absorption limited by food; peak 1-2 hr, elimination $t_{1/2}$ 14½ hr; metabolized in liver to active metabolites, excreted in urine, $t_{1/2}$ 3-20 hr

INDICATIONS AND USES: Seasonal rhinitis

DOSAGE

Adult

• PO 10 mg qd; give qod in hepatic impairment

Child <12 yrs age
- Not established

AVAILABLE FORMS/COST OF THERAPY
- Tab, Uncoated—Oral: 10 mg, 30's: **$55.30**

CONTRAINDICATIONS: Hypersensitivity

PRECAUTIONS: Increased intraocular pressure, asthma, hepatic disease

PREGNANCY AND LACTATION: Pregnancy category B; excreted into breast milk at levels equivalent to serum levels; not recommended in nursing mothers

SIDE EFFECTS/ADVERSE REACTIONS

CNS: Sedation (more common with increased doses), insomnia

EENT: Dry mouth

▼ DRUG INTERACTIONS

Drugs
- *Erythromycin, ketoconazole:* Increased loratadine levels but no increase in toxicity reported

lorazepam

(lor-a'ze-pam)

Ativan, Alzapam, Loraz, Lorazepam, Lorazepam Intensol, Novolorazem ♣

Chemical Class: Benzodiazepine
Functional Class: Antianxiety
DEA Class: Schedule IV

CLINICAL PHARMACOLOGY

Mechanism of Action: Binds to benzodiazepine receptor sites, potentiates action of GABA

Pharmacokinetics

PO: Peak 1-3 hr, duration 3-6 hr; metabolized by liver; excreted by kidneys; crosses placenta, breast milk; $t_{1/2}$ 10-20 hr

INDICATIONS AND USES: Anxiety, irritability in psychiatric or organic disorders, preoperatively, insomnia,* acute alcohol withdrawal symptoms,* anticonvulsant,* adjunct in endoscopic procedures, chemotherapy induced nausea and vomiting*

DOSAGE

Adult
- *Anxiety:* PO 2-6 mg/d in divided doses bid-tid, largest dose at hs, not to exceed 10 mg/d
- *Insomnia:* PO 2-4 mg hs; only minimally effective after 2 wk continuous therapy
- *Elderly:* 1-2 mg/d in divided doses
- *Preoperatively:* IM 0.05 mg/kg to max 4 mg given ≥2 hr before procedure; IV 0.044-0.05 mg/kg, max 4 mg, 15-20 min before procedure

Child
- Not recommended IM/IV <18 yr, PO <12 yr

AVAILABLE FORMS/COST OF THERAPY
- Inj, Sol—IM; IV: 2 mg/ml, 1 ml: **$9.27-$277.88;** 4 mg/ml, 1 ml: **$11.49-$339.63**
- Tab, Uncoated—Oral: 0.5 mg, 100's: **$1.73-$70.64;** 1 mg, 100's: **$2.07-$85.99;** 2 mg, 100's: **$85.99-$125.20**

CONTRAINDICATIONS: Hypersensitivity to benzodiazepines, acute narrow angle glaucoma, psychosis

PRECAUTIONS: Elderly, debilitated, hepatic disease, renal disease, suicidal patients, COPD, history of drug abuse

PREGNANCY AND LACTATION: Pregnancy category D (other benzodiazepines associated with cleft lip/palate, microcephaly, pyloric stenosis); neonatal withdrawal, hypotonia; excreted into breast milk in low quantities; effect on infant unknown

SIDE EFFECTS/ADVERSE REACTIONS

CNS: Dizziness, drowsiness, confusion, headache, anxiety, tremors, stimulation, fatigue, depression, insomnia, hallucinations, weakness, unsteadiness

CV: Orthostatic hypotension, ***ECG changes, tachycardia***

EENT: Blurred vision, tinnitus, mydriasis

GI: Constipation, dry mouth, nausea, vomiting, anorexia, diarrhea

SKIN: Rash, dermatitis, itching

▼ **DRUG INTERACTIONS**

Drugs

• *Clozapine:* Cardiovascular or respiratory collapse

• *Ethanol:* Increased adverse psychomotor effects of lorazepam

• *Rifampin:* May reduce serum benzodiazepine levels

Labs

• *Increase:* LFTs

SPECIAL CONSIDERATIONS

PATIENT/FAMILY EDUCATION

• Do not discontinue abruptly after long term use as withdrawal syndrome (seizures, anxiety, insomnia, nausea/vomiting, flu-like illness, confusion, hallucinations, memory impairment) can occur

losartan

(lo-sar′tan)

Cozaar

Chemical Class: Angiotension II receptor antagonist

Therapeutic Class: Antihypertensive

CLINICAL PHARMACOLOGY

Mechanism of Action: Blocks vasoconstrictor and aldosterone-secreting effects of angiotensin II by blocking binding angiotensin II receptors

Pharmacokinetics

Converted in liver to active metabolite; peak 1 hr, 3-4 hr for metabolite; excreted in urine, bile, feces; max antihypertensive effect occurs in 3-6 wk

INDICATIONS AND USES: Hypertension

DOSAGE

Adult >18 yr

• PO 25-50 mg qd; use lower dosage in volume depleted patients, hepatic disease; range 25-100 mg qd; divide bid if effect at trough inadequate

$ **AVAILABLE FORMS/COST OF THERAPY**

• Tab, Uncoated—Oral: 25, 50 mg, 100's: **$110.00**

CONTRAINDICATIONS: Hypersensitivity

PRECAUTIONS: Hypotension, volume depleted patients, less effective in African-Americans, renal artery stenosis, CHF, liver disease

PREGNANCY AND LACTATION: Pregnancy category C (first trimester), category D (second and third trimesters); may cause fetal death; not known if excreted in breast milk

SIDE EFFECTS/ADVERSE REACTIONS

CNS: Dizziness, insomnia

GI: Diarrhea, dyspepsia, elevated liver enzymes

GU: Increased BUN, creatinine

HEME: Decreased Hct

MS: Muscle cramps, myalgia, back pain, leg pain

RESP: Nasal congestion, cough, sinus disorder

▼ **DRUG INTERACTIONS**

Drugs

• *Cimetidine:* Increased levels of losartan

• *Phenobarbital:* Decreased levels of losartan

lovastatin

(lo'va-sta-tin)
Mevacor

Chemical Class: Aspergillus terreus strain derivative
Therapeutic Class: Cholesterol-lowering agent

CLINICAL PHARMACOLOGY

Mechanism of Action: Inhibits HMG-COA reductase, necessary enzyme for cholesterol synthesis; results in lowered total cholesterol levels, decreased LDL levels, modest decrease in triglycerides and variable increase in HDL levels

Pharmacokinetics

PO: Peak 2-4 hr, metabolized in liver (metabolites), highly protein bound, excreted in urine, feces, crosses placenta, excreted in breast milk; max effect on lipid levels in 4-6 wk

INDICATIONS AND USES: As an adjunct to diet in primary hypercholesterolemia (types IIa, IIb), mixed hyperlipidemia

DOSAGE

Adult

• PO 20 mg qd with evening meal; may increase to 20-80 mg/d in single or divided doses, not to exceed 80 mg/d; dosage adjustments should be made qmo; for cholesterol levels >300 mg/dl initiate at 40 mg/d

Child

• Not recommended

$ AVAILABLE FORMS/COST OF THERAPY

• Tab, Uncoated—Oral: 10 mg, 60's: **$73.69;** 20 mg, 60's: **$125.05;** 40 mg, 60's: **$225.09**

CONTRAINDICATIONS: Active liver disease, hypersensitivity

PRECAUTIONS: Past liver disease, alcoholics, severe acute infections, trauma, hypotension, uncontrolled seizure disorders, severe metabolic disorders, electrolyte imbalances

PREGNANCY AND LACTATION: Pregnancy category X (may produce skeletal malformations); not recommended in nursing mothers

SIDE EFFECTS/ADVERSE REACTIONS

CNS: Dizziness, headache, insomnia

EENT: Blurred vision, dysgeusia, lens opacities

GI: Nausea, constipation, diarrhea, dyspepsia, flatus, abdominal pain, heartburn, ***liver dysfunction***

MS: Muscle cramps, myalgia, ***myositis, rhabdomyolysis***

SKIN: Rash, pruritus

▼ DRUG INTERACTIONS

Drugs

• *Cyclosporine, erythromycin, gemfibrozil, niacin:* Severe myopathy or rhabdomyolysis

• *Warfarin:* Increased prothrombin time

Labs

• *Increase:* CPK, liver function tests

SPECIAL CONSIDERATIONS

MONITORING PARAMETERS

• Perform liver function tests before initiating therapy and q4-6wk during first 3 mo of therapy, q6-12wk during the next year; discontinue drug if rise to >3 times normal

• Less effective in homozygous familial hypercholesterolemia (lack of functional LDL receptors); these patients also more likely to have adverse reaction of elevated transaminases

loxapine

(lox'a-peen)

Loxapax, ♣ Loxapine Succinate, Loxitane IM, Loxitane/Loxitane-C

Chemical Class: Dibenzoxazepine

Therapeutic Class: Antipsychotic/neuroleptic

CLINICAL PHARMACOLOGY

Mechanism of Action: Depresses cerebral cortex, hypothalamus, limbic system which control activity and aggression; blocks neurotransmission produced by dopamine at synapse; strong α-adrenergic, anticholinergic blocking action; mechanism for antipsychotic effects is unclear

Pharmacokinetics

PO: Onset 20-30 min, peak 2-4 hr, duration 12 hr

IM: Onset 15-30 min, peak 15-20 min, duration 12 hr

Metabolized by liver; excreted in urine; crosses placenta; enters breast milk; initial $t_{1/2}$ 5 hr; terminal $t_{1/2}$ 19 hr

INDICATIONS AND USES: Psychotic disorders

DOSAGE

Adult

• PO 10 mg bid-qid initially, may be rapidly increased depending on severity of condition, range 60-100 mg/d, reduce to maintenance 20-60 mg qd; IM 12.5-50 mg q4-6hr or more until desired response, then start PO form

$ AVAILABLE FORMS/COST OF THERAPY

• Cap, Gel—Oral: 5 mg, 100's: **$36.24-$79.07;** 10 mg, 100's: **$46.83-$88.54;** 25 mg, 100's: **$70.74-$154.39;** 50 mg, 100's: **$94.38-$213.98**

• Liq—Oral: 25 mg/ml, 120 ml: **$234.51**

• Inj, Sol—IM: 50 mg/ml, 10 ml: **$96.34**

CONTRAINDICATIONS: Hypersensitivity, blood dyscrasias, coma, child, brain damage, bone marrow depression, alcohol and barbiturate withdrawal

PRECAUTIONS: Seizure disorders, hepatic disease, cardiac disease, prostatic hypertrophy, cardiac conditions, child <16 yr

PREGNANCY AND LACTATION: Pregnancy category C; no data in lactating women

SIDE EFFECTS/ADVERSE REACTIONS

CNS: Pseudoparkinsonism, akathisia, dystonia, tardive dyskinesia, drowsiness, headache, ***seizures,*** *confusion*

CV: Orthostatic hypotension, ***cardiac arrest,*** ECG changes, tachycardia

EENT: Blurred vision, glaucoma

GI: Dry mouth, nausea, vomiting, anorexia, constipation, diarrhea, jaundice, weight gain

GU: Urinary retention, urinary frequency, enuresis, impotence, amenorrhea, gynecomastia

HEME: ***Anemia, leukopenia, leukocytosis, agranulocytosis***

RESP: ***Laryngospasm,*** dyspnea, ***respiratory depression***

SKIN: Rash, photosensitivity, dermatitis

▼ DRUG INTERACTIONS

Drugs

• *Anticholinergics:* Decreased neuroleptic effect

• *Antidepressants:* Increased toxic effects of both drugs

• *Barbiturates:* Reduced effect of both drugs

• *Bromocriptine:* Decreased lowering of protactin

• *Epinephrine:* Paradoxical decrease in blood pressure
• *Lithium:* Increased neurotoxicity
• *Narcotics:* Hypotension, CNS depression

lypressin

(lye-press'in)
Diapid
Chemical Class: Lysine vasopressin
Therapeutic Class: Pituitary hormone

CLINICAL PHARMACOLOGY
Mechanism of Action: Promotes reabsorption of water by action on renal tubular epithelium, acts as ADH
Pharmacokinetics
NASAL: Prompt onset, peak 30-120 min, duration 3-8 hr, $t_{1/2}$ 15 min; metabolized in liver, kidneys, excreted in urine
INDICATION AND USES: Neurogenic diabetes insipidus
DOSAGE
Adult
• INTRANASAL 1-2 sprays in one or both nostrils qid prn excessive urination or thirst, extra dose hs if needed; reduce time between doses if >2 sprays q4-6h needed
$ **AVAILABLE FORMS/COST OF THERAPY**
• Spray—Intranasal: 0.185 mg/ml, 8 ml: **$41.76**
PRECAUTIONS: CAD, URI symptoms (decreased effectiveness)
PREGNANCY AND LACTATION: Pregnancy category B; compatible with breast feeding
SIDE EFFECTS/ADVERSE REACTIONS
CNS: Headache
CV: ***MI***
EENT: Nasal irritation, congestion, rhinitis, conjunctivitis, rhinorrhea
GI: Nausea, heartburn, cramps
RESP: Chest tightness, cough, dyspnea (when inhaled)
▼ **DRUG INTERACTIONS**
Drugs
• *Carbamazepine, chlorpropamide:* Increased effects of lypressin

mafenide

(ma'fe-nide)
Sulfamylon
Chemical Class: Sulfonamide
Therapeutic Class: Local anti-infective

CLINICAL PHARMACOLOGY
Mechanism of Action: Inhibits cell wall synthesis; inhibits carbonic anhydrase
Pharmacokinetics
TOP: Absorbed through devascularized areas, peak concentration 24 hr after initial dose; rapidly metabolized to inactive metabolite, excreted in urine
INDICATIONS AND USES: Adjunctive treatment in burns (2nd, 3rd degree); bacteriostatic against many gram positive and gram negative organisms, including *Pseudomonas* and some anaerobes
DOSAGE
Adult and Child (>2 months)
• TOP apply thin layer (1/16") to clean and debrided affected area qd-bid, reapply if washed off
$ **AVAILABLE FORMS/COST OF THERAPY**
• Cre—Top: 60 g: **$17.50;** 120 g: **$32.50;** 435 g: **$108.50**
CONTRAINDICATIONS: Hypersensitivity, inhalation injury
PRECAUTIONS: Impaired pulmonary function, impaired renal function, G6PD deficiency, blood dyscrasias
PREGNANCY AND LACTATION: Pregnancy category C; compatible

M

with breast feeding except in G6PD deficiency and ill, jaundiced, or premature infants

SIDE EFFECTS/ADVERSE REACTIONS

HEME: ***Bone marrow suppression, fatal hemolytic anemia, eosinophilia***

METAB: Metabolic acidosis

RESP: Tachypnea

SKIN: Rash, urticaria, stinging, burning, bleeding, excoriation of new skin, superinfections, pruritus, blisters, facial edema, hives, erythema

---

magaldrate

(mag'al-drate)

Lowsium, Lowsium Plus, Riopan, Riopan Plus, Riopan Plus 2, (Plus products containing simethicone)

Chemical Class: Mixture of aluminum and magnesium hydroxide and sulfate

Therapeutic Class: Antacid

CLINICAL PHARMACOLOGY

Mechanism of Action: Neutralizes gastric acidity

Pharmacokinetics

PO: Duration 20-60 min (fasting), 1-3 hr (if given 1 hr after meals)

INDICATIONS AND USES: Antacid

DOSAGE

Adult/Child

Suspension preferred, 1-2 tabs may be substituted for susp

• *Peptic ulcer disease:* 5-10 ml 1 and 3 hr after meals and at hs for 4-6 wk

• *GE reflux:* 5-10 ml q 30-60 min for severe symptoms, or as for PUD

• *GI bleeding:* Administer q hr to keep nasogastric aspirate pH >3.5

• *Before anesthesia:* 5-10 ml 30 min before anesthesia

$ **AVAILABLE FORMS/COST OF THERAPY**

• Susp/Liq—Oral: 540 mg/5ml, 12 oz: **$2.69-$47.95**

Formulations with simethicone

• Susp/Liq—Oral: 540 magaldrate/20 mg simethicone/5 ml, 12 oz: **$2.82-$3.99**

• Susp—Oral: 1080 mg magaldrate/30 mg simethicone/5 ml, 12 oz: **$5.53**

• Tab/Chewable Tab: 480 mg/20 mg, 60's: **$3.15**

• Tab: 1080 mg/30 mg, 60's: **$4.58**

CONTRAINDICATIONS: Hypersensitivity to this drug or aluminum products

PRECAUTIONS: Elderly, fluid restriction, decreased GI motility, GI obstruction, dehydration, renal disease, Na-restricted diets, CHF, edema, cirrhosis

PREGNANCY AND LACTATION: Pregnancy category C

SIDE EFFECTS/ADVERSE REACTIONS

GI: Constipation, diarrhea

METAB: Hypermagnesemia

▼ **DRUG INTERACTIONS**

• *Allopurinol, cefpodoxime, ciprofloxacin, isoniazid, ketoconazole, quinolones, tetracyclines, digoxin, iron salts, indomethacin:* Decreased GI absorption of these drugs

• *Pseudoephedrine, enteric coated aspirin, diazepam:* Increased GI absorption of these drugs

• *Salicylates:* Increased urinary excretion of salicylates

• *Quinidine:* Increased quinidine levels

---

magnesium

Magnesium oxide: Mag-Ox 400, Maox, Uro-Mag; Magnesium hydroxide: Milk of Magnesia; Magnesium citrate: Evac-Q-Mag, Citro-Nesia, Citroma; Magnesium sulfate: Epsom Salts, Magnesium Sulfate Injection; Magnesium gluconate: Magonate

Chemical Class: Magnesium products

Therapeutic Class: Antacid; laxative; antiarrhythmic, uterine relaxant, CNS depressant, electrolyte supplement (parenteral magnesium sulfate)

CLINICAL PHARMACOLOGY

Mechanism of Action: Antacid products: Neutralize gastric acidity

Magnesium citrate: Causes osmotic retention of fluid, increases peristalsis

Magnesium sulfate: Decreases acetylcholine release at neuromuscular junction; slows rate of SA node impulse formation, prolongs conduction time

Pharmacokinetics

Magnesium citrate: Renal excretion

Magnesium hydroxide/oxide: Onset of laxative action 4-8 hr; renal excretion (30%), unabsorbed drug excreted in feces

Magnesium sulfate: PO onset of laxative action 1-2 hr; IM onset 1 hr, duration 3-4 hr; IV onset immediate, duration 30 min; excreted by kidneys and in stool

Magnesium gluconate: PO 15%-30% absorbed; renal excretion

INDICATIONS AND USES: Magnesium citrate: Bowel evacuation prior to procedures

Magnesium oxide/hydroxide/sulfate (PO): Laxative

Magnesium hydroxide/oxide: Antacid, hypomagnesemia (oxide)

Magnesium gluconate: Hypomagnesemia

Magnesium sulfate (parenteral): Hypomagnesemia, eclampsia prophylaxis, preterm labor,* cardiac dysrhythmias,* acute MI,* acute exacerbations of asthma*

DOSAGE

Adult

- Magnesium citrate: PO ½-1 full bottle
- Magnesium hydroxide: PO 30-60 ml qd (laxative); 5-15 ml or 650 mg-1.3 g tabs up to qid (antacid)
- Magnesium oxide: PO 2-4 g hs with water (laxative); 140 mg tid-qid or 400-840 mg/d (antacid)
- Magnesium gluconate: PO 1-2 tabs bid-tid
- Magnesium sulfate: IM 1-4 g q4h; IV 4 g initially then 1-4 g/hr by infusion (pre-eclampsia); PO 3 g q6h for 4 doses; IM/IV 1 g q6h for 4 doses; for severe deficiency 8-12 g/d in divided doses (hypomagnesemia); PO 10-15 g with water (laxative)

Child

- Magnesium citrate: PO (<6 yr) 0.5 ml/kg to max 200 ml repeated q 4-6 hr until clear; (6-12 yr) ⅓-½ bottle
- Magnesium hydroxide: Laxative PO (<2 yr) 0.5 ml/kg/dose, (2-5 yr) 5-15 ml/d or divided, (6-12 yr) 15-30 ml/d or divided; Antacid PO 2.5-5 ml qd-qid as needed
- Magnesium gluconate: PO 3-6 mg/kg/d divided tid-qid, max 400 mg/d
- Magnesium sulfate: Neonate IV 25-50 mg/kg/dose q 8-12 hr for 2-3 doses; child IM/IV 25-50 mg/kg/dose q 4-6 hr for 3-4 doses, max single dose 2000 mg (hypomagnesemia); PO 0.25 g/kg q 4-6 hr (laxative)

M

$ AVAILABLE FORMS/COST OF THERAPY

- Liq (citrate)—Oral: 10 oz: **$.80**
- Liq (hydroxide)—Oral: 16 oz: **$1.44-$3.60**
- Powder (hydroxide)—Oral: 500 g: **$9.75**
- Powder (oxide)—Oral: 500 g: **$14.50**
- Powder (sulfate)—Oral: 500 g: **$9.45-$21.00**
- Cap, Gel (hydroxide)—Oral: 30's: **$3.54**
- Tab (hydroxide)—Oral: 100's: **$4.09**
- Tab (gluconate)—Oral: 30 mg, 100's: **$3.56;** 500 mg, 100's: **$1.85-$2.39**
- Inj, Conc-Sol (sulfate)—IV; IM: 500 mg/ml, 10 ml: **$1.91-$18.44**
- Inj, Sol (sulfate)—IV; IM: 100 mg/ml, 20 ml: **$1.20-$5.75**
- Inj, Sol (sulfate)—IV: 2 meq/ml, 150 ml: **$1.15**
- Sol (sulfate)—IV: 1%, 100 ml: **$7.15;** 2%, 500 ml: **$7.51;** 4%, 100 ml: **$7.08;** 8%, 50 ml: **$7.08**

CONTRAINDICATIONS: Hypersensitivity, renal failure (Mg toxicity), hypermagnesemia; do not use cathartics in patients with appendicitis, impaction, intestinal obstruction, or perforation; do not use parenterally in patients with heart block, myocardial damage

PRECAUTIONS: Diarrhea, digitalized patients, impaired renal function (monitor Mg levels)

PREGNANCY AND LACTATION: Pregnancy category B; compatible with breast feeding

SIDE EFFECTS/ADVERSE REACTIONS

CNS: Weakness, lethargy, depression, ***coma,*** *depressed deep tendon reflexes*

CV: Decreased BP, increased pulse, ***heart block***

GI: (PO) Diarrhea, flatulence, cramps, belching, nausea, vomiting, impaction, ***obstruction,*** pain

METAB: Hypermagnesemia

RESP: ***Respiratory depression***

▼ DRUG INTERACTIONS

Drugs

- *Tetracyclines, digoxin, indomethacin, iron salts, glipizide:* Decreased effectiveness of these drugs with PO mg products
- *Parenteral magnesium sulfate:* nifedipine (decreased effect); aminoglycosides, CNS depressants, neuromuscular antagonists (increased toxicity of drugs); betamethasone (pulmonary edema); ritodrine (cardiotoxicity)

Labs

- *Increase:* Magnesium
- *Decrease:* Potassium

SPECIAL CONSIDERATIONS

MONITORING PARAMETERS: Parenteral magnesium: knee jerk reflexes prior to each dose (do not administer if absent), respiration rate (do not administer if <16/min), urine output (do not administer if <100 ml during 4 hr preceding each dose), serum magnesium concentrations (normal 1.5-3 mEq/L; therapeutic concentrations for preeclampsia/eclampsia/convulsions 4-7 mEq/L)

magnesium salicylate

Doan's pills, Magan, Mobidin

Chemical Class: Salicylic acid derivative

Therapeutic Class: Nonnarcotic analgesic; anti-inflammatory; antirheumatic; antipyretic

CLINICAL PHARMACOLOGY

Mechanism of Action: Inhibits prostaglandin synthesis and release; acts on the hypothalamus heat-regulating center to reduce fever; increases urinary excretion of urates at higher doses but may decrease excretion at lower doses

Pharmacokinetics

PO: Onset 15-30 min, peak 1-2 hr, duration 4-6 hr, 50%-90% bound to plasma proteins, metabolized in liver, eliminated in urine, $t_{1/2}$ 2 hr

INDICATIONS AND USES: Mild to moderate pain, rheumatoid arthritis, osteoarthritis, various inflammatory conditions

DOSAGE

Adult

- PO 650 mg q4h or 1090 mg tid; may increase to 3.6-4.8 g/d in 3-4 divided doses

$ AVAILABLE FORMS/COST OF THERAPY

- Tab, Uncoated—Oral: 325 mg, 24's: **$3.66;** 500 mg, 24's: **$4.39**
- Cap, Gel—Oral: 500 mg, 100's: **$58.00**
- Tab, Uncoated—Oral: 545 mg, 100's: **$50.95;** 600 mg, 100's: **$23.22**

CONTRAINDICATIONS: Hypersensitivity to NSAIDs, hemophilia, bleeding ulcers, hemorrhagic states, advanced chronic renal insufficiency

PRECAUTIONS: Children/teenagers with chickenpox or influenza (association with Reye's syndrome), impaired hepatic function, history of peptic ulcer disease, diabetes mellitus, gout

PREGNANCY AND LACTATION: Pregnancy category C; excreted into breast milk, use caution in nursing mothers due to potential adverse effects in nursing infant

SIDE EFFECTS/ADVERSE REACTIONS

CNS: Drowsiness, dizziness, confusion, headache

EENT: Tinnitus, reversible hearing loss, dimness of vision

GI: Nausea, dyspepsia, ***GI bleeding,*** diarrhea, heartburn, epigastric discomfort, anorexia, ***acute reversible hepatotoxicity***

HEME: ***Thrombocytopenia, leukopenia,*** prolonged bleeding time, decreased plasma iron concentration, shortened erythrocyte survival time

METAB: Hypoglycemia, hyponatremia, hypokalemia, hypermagnesemia

RESP: Wheezing, hyperpnea

SKIN: Rash, hives, angioedema, urticaria, bruising

MISC: Fever, thirst

▼ DRUG INTERACTIONS

Drugs

- *Acetazolamide:* Increased concentrations of acetazolamide, possibly leading to CNS toxicity
- *Antacids:* Decreased serum salicylate concentrations
- *Antidiabetics:* Enhanced hypoglycemic response to sulfonylureas, particularly chlorpropamide
- *Corticosteroids:* Increased incidence and/or severity of GI ulceration
- *Ethanol:* Enhanced salicylate-induced GI mucosal damage; increased ethanol concentrations
- *Heparin:* Increased risk of bleeding
- *Methotrexate+:* Increased serum methotrexate concentrations and enhanced methotrexate toxicity
- *Oral anticoagulants:* Increased risk of bleeding
- *Phenytoin:* Large doses of salicylates may reduce total serum phenytoin concentrations, but free serum concentrations do not appear to be affected
- *Probenecid:* Salicylates inhibit the uricosuric activity of probenecid
- *Sulfinpyrazone:* Salicylates inhibit the uricosuric activity of sulfinpyrazone
- *Valproic acid:* Salicylates may increase unbound serum valproic acid

M

concentrations sufficiently to result in toxicity

Labs

• *Increase:* Coagulation studies, liver function studies, serum uric acid, amylase, CO_2, urinary protein

• *Decrease:* Serum K, PBI, cholesterol, blood glucose

• *Interfere:* Urine catecholamines, pregnancy test

SPECIAL CONSIDERATIONS

PATIENT/FAMILY EDUCATION

• Administer with food

• Do not exceed recommended doses

• Notify physician if ringing in ears or persistent GI pain occurs

• Read label on other OTC drugs, many contain aspirin

• Therapeutic response may take 2 wk (arthritis)

• Avoid alcohol ingestion, GI bleeding may occur

• **Not to be given to children, Reye's syndrome may develop**

MONITORING PARAMETERS

• AST, ALT, bilirubin, creatinine, CBC, Hct if patient is on long-term therapy

malathion

(mal-a-thye'on)

Ovide

Chemical Class: Organophosphate

Therapeutic Class: Pediculicide

CLINICAL PHARMACOLOGY

Mechanism of Action: Inhibits cholinesterase exerting both lousicidal and ovicidal actions; activity selective to insects as the drug is rapidly hydrolyzed and detoxified in mammals

Pharmacokinetics

TOP: Up to 8% of applied dose may be absorbed through human skin

INDICATIONS AND USES: Treatment of head lice and their ova

DOSAGE

Adult and Child > 2 yr

• TOP Sprinkle lotion on *dry* hair and rub gently until scalp thoroughly moistened; allow to dry naturally; leave on for 8-12 hr then wash hair with nonmedicated shampoo and rinse; use fine-toothed comb to remove dead lice and eggs; may repeat in 7-9 days if required

$ AVAILABLE FORMS/COST OF THERAPY

• Lotion—Top: 0.5%, 60 ml: **$11.91**

CONTRAINDICATIONS: Hypersensitivity

PRECAUTIONS: Children <2 yr

PREGNANCY AND LACTATION: Pregnancy category B

SIDE EFFECTS/ADVERSE REACTIONS

CNS: Anxiety, confusion, dizziness, drowsiness, ***seizures***

CV: Bradycardia

GI: Abdominal cramps, diarrhea

SKIN: Irritation of scalp, contact dermatitis

SPECIAL CONSIDERATIONS

PATIENT/FAMILY EDUCATION

• Drug contains flammable alcohol, lotion and wet hair should not be exposed to open flame or electric heat, including hair driers, do not smoke while using this product

• Avoid exposure to pesticides and insecticides during therapy

• For external use only (serious toxicity may occur if ingested)

• Avoid contact with eyes

mannitol

(man'i-tall)

Osmitrol, Resectial

Chemical Class: Hexahydric alcohol

Therapeutic Class: Osmotic diuretic; genitourinary irrigant

CLINICAL PHARMACOLOGY

Mechanism of Action: Induces diuresis by elevating the osmolarity of the glomerular filtrate, thereby hindering the tubular reabsorption of water; excretion of sodium and chloride is increased

Pharmacokinetics

IV: Onset 30-60 min, peak 1 hr, duration 6-8 hr, mainly excreted unchanged in the urine, $t_{1/2}$ 15-100 min

INDICATIONS AND USES: Reduction of intracranial pressure associated with cerebral edema; reduction of intraocular pressure; improvment of renal function in oliguric phase of acute renal failure; irrigation in transurethral prostatic resection or other transurethral surgical procedures (2.5% only); promotion of urinary excretion of toxic substances

DOSAGE

Adult

- *Oliguria (prevention):* IV 50-100 g of 5%-25% sol
- *Oliguria (treatment):* IV 50-100 g of 15%-20% sol
- *Intraocular pressure/intracranial pressure:* IV 1.5-2 g/kg of 15%-25% sol over 30-60 min
- *Diuresis in drug intoxication:* IV 5%-10% sol continuously up to 200 g, while maintaining urine output of 100-500 ml/hr
- *Urologic irrigation:* Add contents of two 50 ml vials of 25% mannitol to 900 ml sterile water for inj and use as irrigation

Child

- IV 0.5-1 g/kg initially, then 0.25-0.5 g/kg q4-6hr for maintenance

$ **AVAILABLE FORMS/COST OF THERAPY**

- Inj, Sol—IV: 5%, 10%, 1000 ml: **$32.70-$68.91;** 15%, 500 ml: **$49.40-$68.92;** 20%, 250 ml: **$51.84-$56.33;** 25%, 50 ml: **$5.05-$8.51**

CONTRAINDICATIONS: Active intracranial bleeding, hypersensitivity, anuria, severe pulmonary congestion or edema, severe dehydration

PRECAUTIONS: Fluid and electrolyte imbalances, renal function impairment (consider use of 0.2 g/kg test dose followed by monitoring for increased urine flow), hepatic function impairment

PREGNANCY AND LACTATION: Pregnancy category C

SIDE EFFECTS/ADVERSE REACTIONS

CNS: Dizziness, headache, ***convulsions,*** rebound increased intracranial pressure, confusion

CV: Edema, thrombophlebitis, hypotension, hypertension, tachycardia, angina-like chest pains, ***CHF***

EENT: Loss of hearing, blurred vision, nasal congestion

GI: Nausea, vomiting, dry mouth, diarrhea

GU: Urinary retention, osmotic nephrosis

METAB: Fluid and electrolyte imbalances, acidosis, electrolyte loss, dehydration

RESP: Pulmonary congestion

SKIN: Skin necrosis, urticaria

MISC: Fever, chills

▼ **DRUG INTERACTIONS**

Labs

- *Interference:* Inorganic phosphorus, ethylene glycol

SPECIAL CONSIDERATIONS
MONITORING PARAMETERS
- Serum electrolytes, urine output

maprotiline

(ma-proe'ti-leen)
Ludiomil

Chemical Class: Dibenzo-bicyclo-octadiene derivative
Therapeutic Class: Antidepressant, tetracyclic

CLINICAL PHARMACOLOGY
Mechanism of Action: Blocks reuptake of norepinephrine at the neuronal membrane; possesses anticholinergic activity; does not appear to influence reuptake of serotonin
Pharmacokinetics
PO: Peak 9-16 hr, onset of therapeutic effect 2-3 wk, 88% bound to plasma proteins, metabolized in the liver, excreted in bile (30%) and urine (65%), $t_{1/2}$ 27-58 hr (active metabolite 60-90 hr)

INDICATIONS AND USES: Major depression, dysthymic disorder, anxiety associated with depression, depressive phase of bipolar disorder

DOSAGE
Adult
- PO 75 mg/d initially, increase by 25 mg q2wk up to 150-225 mg/d divided qd-tid; elderly may require smaller doses

Child 6-14 yr
- PO 10 mg/d, increase to max of 75 mg/d

$ **AVAILABLE FORMS/COST OF THERAPY**
- Tab, Coated—Oral: 25 mg, 100's: **$21.23-$44.34;** 50 mg, 100's: **$30.75-$65.61;** 75 mg, 100's: **$44.25-$90.10**

CONTRAINDICATIONS: Hypersensitivity, acute recovery phase of MI, concurrent use of MAOIs, seizure disorder

PRECAUTIONS: Suicidal patients, prostatic hypertrophy, psychiatric disease, severe depression, increased intraocular pressure, narrow-angle glaucoma, urinary retention, cardiac disease, hepatic/renal disease, hyperthyroidism, electroshock therapy, elective surgery, elderly, abrupt discontinuation

PREGNANCY AND LACTATION: Pregnancy category B; excreted into breast milk, M:P ratios of 1.5 and 1.3 have been reported, significance to the nursing infant unknown

SIDE EFFECTS/ADVERSE REACTIONS
CNS: Dizziness, drowsiness, confusion (especially in elderly), headache, anxiety, nervousness, panic, tremors, stimulation, weakness, fatigue, insomnia, nightmares, EPS (elderly), increased psychiatric symptoms, memory impairment, ***seizures*** (dose related)
CV: Orthostatic hypotension, ***ECG changes, tachycardia, dysrhythmias,*** hypertension, palpitations, syncope
EENT: Blurred vision, tinnitus, mydriasis, ophthalmoplegia, nasal congestion, increased intraocular pressure
GI: Constipation, dry mouth, nausea, vomiting, ***paralytic ileus,*** increased appetite, cramps, epigastric distress, jaundice, ***hepatitis,*** stomatitis, diarrhea
GU: Urinary retention
HEME: ***Agranulocytosis, thrombocytopenia, eosinophilia, leukopenia***
SKIN: Rash, urticaria, sweating, pruritus, photosensitivity

▼ **DRUG INTERACTIONS**
Drugs
- *Amphetamines:* Theoretical increase in effect of amphetamines, clinical evidence lacking

• *Anticholinergics:* Excessive anticholinergic effects
• *Barbiturates:* Reduced serum concentrations of cyclic antidepressants
• *Bethanidine:* Reduced antihypertensive effect of bethanidine
• *Carbamazepine:* Reduced cyclic antidepressant serum concentrations
• *Clonidine:* Reduced antihypertensive response to clonidine; enhanced hypertensive response with abrupt clonidine withdrawal
• *Debrisoquin:* Inhibited antihypertensive response of debrisoquin
• *Epinephrine+:* Markedly enhanced pressor response to IV epinephrine
• *Ethanol:* Additive impairment of motor skills; abstinent alcoholics may eliminate cyclic antidepressants more rapidly than nonalcoholics
• *Fluoxetine:* Marked increases in cyclic antidepressant plasma concentrations
• *Guanethidine:* Inhibited antihypertensive response to guanethidine
• *Moclobemide+:* Potential association with fatal or non-fatal serotonin syndrome
• *MAOIs:* Excessive sympathetic response, mania or hyperpyrexia possible
• *Neuroleptics:* Increased therapeutic and toxic effects of both drugs
• *Norepinephrine+:* Markedly enhanced pressor response to norepinephrine
• *Phenylephrine:* Enhanced pressor response to IV phenylephrine
• *Phenytoin:* Altered seizure control; decreased cyclic antidepressant serum concentrations
• *Propoxyphene:* Enhanced effect of cyclic antidepressants
• *Quinidine:* Increased cyclic antidepressant serum concentrations

Labs

• *Increase:* Serum bilirubin, blood glucose, alk phosphatase
• *Decrease:* VMA, 5-HIAA
• *False increase:* Urinary catecholamines

SPECIAL CONSIDERATIONS

PATIENT/FAMILY EDUCATION

• Therapeutic effects may take 2-3 wk
• Use caution in driving or other activities requiring alertness
• Do not discontinue abruptly after long-term use

MONITORING PARAMETERS

• CBC
• Weight
• ECG
• Mental status: mood, sensorium, affect, suicidal tendencies
• Determination of maprotiline plasma concentrations is not routinely recommended but may be useful in identifying toxicity, drug interactions, or noncompliance (adjustments in dosage should be made according to clinical response not plasma concentrations); therapeutic plasma levels 200-300 ng/ml (including active metabolite)

mazindol

(may′zin-dole)

Mazanor, Sanorex

Chemical Class: Imidazoisoindol derivative

Therapeutic Class: Anorexiant

DEA Class: Schedule IV

CLINICAL PHARMACOLOGY

Mechanism of Action: Acts on adrenergic and dopaminergic pathways, directly stimulating the satiety center in the hypothalamic and limbic regions; produces CNS stimulation and blood pressure elevation

Pharmacokinetics

PO: Onset 30-60 min, duration 8-15 hr, excreted primarily in urine as unchanged drug and conjugated metabolites

INDICATIONS AND USES: Exogenous obesity (as a short-term adjunct to caloric restriction)

DOSAGE

Adult

- PO 1 mg tid, 1 hr ac, or 2 mg qd, 1 hr before lunch

$ AVAILABLE FORMS/COST OF THERAPY

- Tab, Uncoated—Oral: 1 mg, 100's: **$120.12;** 2 mg, 100's: **$190.62**

CONTRAINDICATIONS: Hypersensitivity to sympathomimetic amines, glaucoma, history of drug abuse, cardiovascular disease, moderate to severe hypertension, advanced arteriosclerosis, agitated states, hyperthyroidism, within 14 days of MAOI administration

PRECAUTIONS: Diabetes mellitus, convulsive disorders, mild hypertension, children

PREGNANCY AND LACTATION: Pregnancy category C

SIDE EFFECTS/ADVERSE REACTIONS

CNS: Overstimulation, nervousness, restlessness, dizziness, insomnia, dysphoria, headache, mental depression, drowsiness, weakness, tremor, shivering, exacerbation of schizophrenia

CV: Palpitation, ***tachycardia,*** chest pain

GI: Dry mouth, nausea, constipation, diarrhea, unpleasant taste

GU: Urinary hesitancy, impotence, testicular pain

SKIN: Rash, excessive sweating, clamminess, pallor

▼ DRUG INTERACTIONS

Drugs

- *MAOIs:* Hypertensive crisis

SPECIAL CONSIDERATIONS

PATIENT/FAMILY EDUCATION

- May cause insomnia, avoid taking late in the day
- Weight reduction requires strict adherence to caloric restriction
- Notify physician if palpitations, nervousness, or dizziness occur
- Use caution while driving or performing other tasks requiring alertness, may cause dizziness or blurred vision
- Take with food if stomach upset occurs
- Do not discontinue abruptly

mebendazole

(me-ben'da-zole)

Vermox

Chemical Class: Benzimidazole derivative

Therapeutic Class: Anthelmintic

CLINICAL PHARMACOLOGY

Mechanism of Action: Causes degeneration of parasite's cytoplasmic microtubules and thereby selectively and irreversibly blocks glucose uptake in susceptible adult intestine-dwelling helminths and their tissue-dwelling larvae

Pharmacokinetics

PO: Poorly absorbed (5%-10%), peak 2-5 hr, 90%-95% bound to plasma proteins, metabolized by liver to inactive metabolites, eliminated primarily in feces (95%), $t_{1/2}$ 2.5-5.5 hr (35 hr in liver dysfunction)

INDICATIONS AND USES: Single or mixed infections due to *Trichuris trichiura* (whipworm), *Enterobius vermicularis* (pinworm), *Ascaris lumbricoides* (roundworm), *Ancylostoma duodenale* (common hookworm), *Necator americanus* (American hookworm)

DOSAGE

Adult and Child

- *Pinworms:* PO 100 mg as a single dose, may need to repeat after 3 wk
- *Whipworms, roundworms, hookworms:* PO 100 mg bid for 3 con-

secutive days; repeat course in 3-4 wk if necessary

$ AVAILABLE FORMS/COST OF THERAPY

• Tab, Chewable—Oral: 100 mg, 12's: **$58.00**

CONTRAINDICATIONS: Hypersensitivity

PRECAUTIONS: Child <2 yr

PREGNANCY AND LACTATION: Pregnancy category C; consider treatment if the parasite is causing clinical disease or may cause public health problems; it is doubtful that enough mebendazole is absorbed to be excreted into breast milk in significant quantities

SIDE EFFECTS/ADVERSE REACTIONS

CNS: Fever, dizziness

GI: Transient abdominal pain, diarrhea

▼ DRUG INTERACTIONS

Drugs

• *Phenytoin:* Decreased mebendazole concentrations; possible impairment of therapeutic effect

SPECIAL CONSIDERATIONS

PATIENT/FAMILY EDUCATION

• Chew or crush tablets and administer with food

• Parasite death and removal from digestive tract may take up to 3 days after treatment

• Consult physician if not cured in 3 wk

• For pinworms, all family members in close contact with patient should be treated

• Strict hygiene essential to prevent reinfection, disinfect toilet facilities, change and launder undergarments, bed linens, towels and nightclothes daily

mecamylamine

(mek-a-mill'a-meen)

Inversine

Chemical Class: Secondary amine

Therapeutic Class: Antihypertensive

CLINICAL PHARMACOLOGY

Mechanism of Action: Blocks transmission of impulses at both sympathetic and parasympathetic ganglia; hypotensive effect is due to reduction in sympathetic tone, vasodilation, and reduced cardiac output, and is primarily postural

Pharmacokinetics

PO: Onset 0.5-2 hr, duration 6-12 hr, mostly excreted unchanged in urine

INDICATIONS AND USES: Moderate to severe hypertension (not first line)

DOSAGE

Adult

• PO 2.5 mg bid initially, may increase in increments of 2.5 mg q2 days until desired response; usual maintenance dose 25 mg/d divided bid-qid

$ AVAILABLE FORMS/COST OF THERAPY

• Tab, Uncoated—Oral: 2.5 mg, 100's: **$13.03**

CONTRAINDICATIONS: Mild/labile hypertension; coronary insufficiency, recent MI; uremia; glaucoma; organic pyloric stenosis; hypersensitivity; patients receiving sulfonamides or antibiotics; uncooperative

PRECAUTIONS: Cerebral arteriosclerosis, recent CVA, renal insufficiency, abrupt discontinuation, prostatic hypertrophy, bladder neck obstruction, urethral stricture

M

PREGNANCY AND LACTATION: Pregnancy category C; not recommended in nursing mothers

SIDE EFFECTS/ADVERSE REACTIONS

CNS: Weakness, *fatigue, sedation,* paresthesia, tremor, choreiform movements, mental abberations, ***convulsions***

CV: Orthostatic dizziness, syncope

EENT: Dilated pupils, *blurred vision*

GI: Anorexia, dry mouth, glossitis, nausea, vomiting, constipation, ***paralytic ileus***

GU: Decreased libido, impotence, urinary retention

SPECIAL CONSIDERATIONS

PATIENT/FAMILY EDUCATION

- Take after meals
- Notify physician if tremor or signs of ileus (frequent loose stools, abdominal distention, decreased borborygmi)
- Arise slowly from reclining position
- Orthostatic changes are exacerbated by alcohol, exercise, hot weather

MONITORING PARAMETERS

- Maintenance doses should be limited to dose which causes slight faintness or dizziness in the standing position

meclizine

(mek'li-zeen)

Antivert, Antivert/25, Antivert/25 Chewable, Antivert-50, Antrizine, Bonamine, ♣ Bonine, Dizmiss, Meni-D, Ru-Vert-M

Chemical Class: Piperazine derivative

Therapeutic Class: Antiemetic; antihistamine; anticholinergic

CLINICAL PHARMACOLOGY

Mechanism of Action: Exact mechanism unknown but may be related to central anticholinergic actions; diminishes vestibular stimulation, depresses labyrinthine function; an action on medullary chemoreceptive trigger zone may also be involved in antiemetic effect; also has antihistaminic, anticholinergic, CNS depressant, and local anesthetic effects

Pharmacokinetics

PO: Onset 1 hr, duration 8-24 hr, $t_{1/2}$ 6 hr

INDICATIONS AND USES: Motion sickness, "possibly effective" in vertigo associated with diseases affecting vestibular system

DOSAGE

Adult and Child >12 yr

- *Motion sickeness:* PO 25-50 mg 1 hr prior to travel, may repeat qd for duration of journey
- *Vertigo:* PO 25-100 mg/d in divided doses

$ **AVAILABLE FORMS/COST OF THERAPY**

- Tab, Uncoated—Oral: 12.5 mg, 100's: **$2.40-$35.65;** 25 mg, 100's: **$2.97-$56.37;** 32 mg, 100's: **$54.00;** 50 mg, 100's: **$107.10**
- Tab, Chewable—Oral: 25 mg, 100's: **$2.53-$50.11**
- Cap—Oral: 30 mg, 100's: **$15.00**

CONTRAINDICATIONS: Hypersensitivity

PRECAUTIONS: Children <12 yr, glaucoma, obstructive GI/GU disease, prostatic hypertrophy

PREGNANCY AND LACTATION: Pregnancy category B; often used for treatment of nausea and vomiting during pregnancy

SIDE EFFECTS/ADVERSE REACTIONS

CNS: Drowsiness, restlessness, excitation, nervousness, insomnia, euphoria

CV: Hypotension, palpitations, tachycardia

EENT: Blurred vision, diplopia, ver-

tigo, tinnitus, auditory and visual hallucinations, dry nose, dry throat
GI: Dry mouth, anorexia, nausea, vomiting, diarrhea, constipation
GU: Urinary frequency, difficult urination, urinary retention
SKIN: Urticaria, rash

▼ **DRUG INTERACTIONS**

Labs

• *False negative:* Allergy skin test

SPECIAL CONSIDERATIONS

PATIENT/FAMILY EDUCATION

• Use caution driving or engaging in other activities requiring altertness
• Avoid alcohol or other CNS depressants

---

meclocycline

(me-kloe-si′kleen)
Meclan
Chemical Class: Tetracycline derivative
Therapeutic Class: Topical antibiotic

CLINICAL PHARMACOLOGY

Mechanism of Action: Exact mechanism of action leading to improvement of acne unknown; may involve inhibition of the growth of *Propionibacterium acnes* on the surface of the skin and reduction in the concentration of free fatty acids in sebum

Pharmacokinetics

TOP: Not systemically absorbed

INDICATIONS AND USES: Acne vulgaris

DOSAGE

Adult and Child ≥ 12 yr

• TOP apply to affected areas bid

$ **AVAILABLE FORMS/COST OF THERAPY**

• Cre—Top: 1%, 20, 45 g: **$20.40-$35.16**

CONTRAINDICATIONS: Hypersensitivity to tetracyclines

PRECAUTIONS: Hepatic/renal dysfunction (possibility of systemic absorption with prolonged use), sulfite sensitivity, formaldehyde sensitivity

PREGNANCY AND LACTATION: Pregnancy category B

SIDE EFFECTS/ADVERSE REACTIONS

SKIN: Irritation, contact dermatitis, temporary follicular staining with excessive application

SPECIAL CONSIDERATIONS

PATIENT/FAMILY EDUCATION

• Drug is for external use only, keep out of eyes, nose and mouth
• Stinging or burning may occur, but will subside in a few minutes
• Normal use of cosmetics is permissible

---

meclofenamate

(me′kloe-fen′a-mate)
Meclomen
Chemical Class: Anthranilic acid derivative
Therapeutic Class: Nonsteroidal antiinflammatory drug (NSAID)

CLINICAL PHARMACOLOGY

Mechanism of Action: Inhibits cyclooxygenase activity and prostaglandin synthesis; other mechanisms such as inhibition of lipoxygenase, leukotriene synthesis, lysosomal enzyme release, neutrophil aggregation, and various cell-membrane functions may exisit as well

Pharmacokinetics

PO: Peak 0.5-1 hr, >90% bound to plasma proteins, metabolized by liver, excreted in urine (metabolites), $t_{1/2}$ 2-3.3 hr

INDICATIONS AND USES: Rheumatoid arthritis, osteoarthritis, mild to moderate pain, primary dysmenorrhea, migraine headache,* menorrhagia*

DOSAGE

Adult

• *Mild to moderate pain:* PO 50 mg q4-6h, max 400 mg/d

• *Primary dysmenorrhea:* PO 100 mg tid for up to 6 days, start at onset of menstrual flow

• *Arthritis:* PO 200-400 mg/d in 3-4 divided doses

$ AVAILABLE FORMS/COST OF THERAPY

• Cap, Gel—Oral: 50 mg, 100's: **$15.83-$74.12;** 100 mg, 100's: **$23.93-$102.62**

CONTRAINDICATIONS: Hypersensitivity to NSAIDs or ASA

PRECAUTIONS: Bleeding tendencies, peptic ulcer, renal/hepatic function impairment, elderly, CHF, hypertension, child <14 yr

PREGNANCY AND LACTATION: Pregnancy category B (category D if used in 3rd trimester); may inhibit labor and prolong pregnancy, cause constriction of the ductus arteriosus *in utero,* or cause persistent pulmonary hypertension of the newborn

SIDE EFFECTS/ADVERSE REACTIONS

CNS: Dizziness, headache, lightheadedness

CV: ***CHF,*** hypotension, hypertension, palpitation, ***dysrhythmias,*** tachycardia, edema, chest pain

EENT: Visual disturbances, photophobia, dry eyes, hearing disturbances, tinnitus

GI: Nausea, vomiting, *diarrhea,* constipation, abdominal cramps, *dyspepsia,* flatulence, ***gastric or duodenal ulcer with bleeding or perforation,*** occult blood in stool, ***hepatitis, pancreatitis***

HEME: ***Neutropenia, eosinophilia, leukopenia, pancytopenia, thrombocytopenia, agranulocytosis***

GU: ***Acute renal failure***

METAB: Hyperglycemia, hypoglycemia, hyperkalemia, hyponatremia

RESP: Dyspnea, bronchospasm

SKIN: Rash, urticaria, photosensitivity

▼ DRUG INTERACTIONS

Drugs

• *Aminoglycosides:* Reduction of aminoglycoside clearance in premature infants

• *ACE inhibitors, beta blockers, hydralazine:* Inhibition of antihypertensive response

• *Furosemide:* Reduced diuretic and antihypertensive response to furosemide

• *Lithium:* Increased plasma lithium concentrations, toxicity

• *Methotrexate:* Reduced renal clearance of methotrexate, increased toxicity

• *Oral anticoagulants:* Increased risk of bleeding due to adverse effects on GI mucosa and platelet function

• *Potassium sparing diuretics:* Acute renal failure

SPECIAL CONSIDERATIONS

PATIENT/FAMILY EDUCATION

• Drug may cause diarrhea; notify physician if excessive

• Avoid aspirin and alcoholic beverages

• Take with food, milk, or antacids to decrease GI upset

• Notify physician if edema, black stools, or persistent headache occurs

MONITORING PARAMETERS

• CBC, BUN, serum creatinine, LFTs, occult blood loss

medroxyprogesterone

(me-drox'ee-proe-jess'te-rone)
Amen, Curretab, Cycrin, Depo-Provera, Provera

Chemical Class: 17 α-hydroxyprogesterone derivative
Therapeutic Class: Progestin; contraceptive; antineoplastic

CLINICAL PHARMACOLOGY

Mechanism of Action: Shares the actions of the progestins; in the presence of adequate estrogen, transforms a proliferative endometrium into a secretory one; stimulates growth of mammary alveolar tissue; has some androgenic and adrenocorticoid activity; inhibits secretion of pituitary gonadotropins following usual IM doses, thus preventing follicular maturation and ovulation

Pharmacokinetics

Metabolized in the liver, excreted mainly in feces

INDICATIONS AND USES: Dysfunctional uterine bleeding, secondary amenorrhea, endometrial cancer, renal cancer, contraceptive, menopause,* obesity-hypoventilation syndrome (Pickwickian syndrome),* obstructive sleep apnea,* hirsutism,* homozygous sickle-cell disease*

DOSAGE

Adult

- *Secondary amenorrhea:* PO 5-10 mg qd for 5-10 days, withdrawal bleeding usually occurs 3-7 days after therapy ends
- *Endometrial/renal cancer:* IM 400-1000 mg/wk, maintenance of improvement may require as little as 400 mg/mo
- *Uterine bleeding:* PO 5-10 mg qd for 5-10 days starting on 16th to 21st day of menstrual cycle, withdrawal bleeding usually occurs 3-7 days after therapy ends
- *Contraceptive:* IM 150 mg q3 mo
- *Menopause:* PO 10 mg qd days 16-25 of month, or 2.5 mg qd (in combination with estrogen)

$ **AVAILABLE FORMS/COST OF THERAPY**

- Tab, Uncoated—Oral: 2.5 mg, 100's: **$29.34-$35.45;** 5 mg, 100's: **$44.32-$53.49;** 10 mg, 100's: **$11.40-$66.28**
- Inj, Susp—IM: 150 mg/ml, 1 ml: **$36.90;** 400 mg/ml, 2.5 ml: **$89.37**

CONTRAINDICATIONS: Hypersensitivity, thrombophlebitis, thromboembolic disorders, cerebral hemorrhage, impaired liver function or disease, breast cancer, undiagnosed vaginal bleeding, missed abortion, use as a diagnostic test for pregnancy

PRECAUTIONS: Epilepsy, migraine, asthma, cardiac or renal dysfunction, depression, diabetes

PREGNANCY AND LACTATION: Pregnancy category D; ambiguous genitalia of both male and female fetuses and cardiovascular defects have been reported; compatible with breast feeding

SIDE EFFECTS/ADVERSE REACTIONS

CNS: Dizziness, headache, migraines, depression, fatigue

CV: Hypotension, thrombophlebitis, edema, ***thromboembolism, stroke, pulmonary embolism, MI***

EENT: Diplopia

GI: Nausea, vomiting, anorexia, cramps, increased weight, ***cholestatic jaundice***

GU: Amenorrhea, cervical erosion, breakthrough bleeding, dysmenorrhea, vaginal candidiasis, breast changes, *gynecomastia, testicular atrophy, impotence,* endometriosis, ***spontaneous abortion***

METAB: Hyperglycemia

SKIN: Rash, urticaria, acne, hirsutism, alopecia, oily skin, seborrhea, purpura, melasma, photosensitivity

▼ **DRUG INTERACTIONS**

Drugs

• *Aminoglutethimide:* Reduced plasma medroxyprogesterone concentrations

Labs

• *Increase:* Alk phosphatase, pregnanediol, liver function tests

• *Decrease:* Glucose tolerance test, HDL

SPECIAL CONSIDERATIONS

PATIENT/FAMILY EDUCATION

• Take protective measures against exposure to ultraviolet light or sunlight

• Diabetic patients must monitor blood glucose carefully during therapy

• Notify physician of pain, swelling, warmth or redness in calves, sudden severe headache, visual disturbances, numbness in arm or leg

• Take with food if GI upset occurs

• When used as contraceptive menstrual cycle may be disrupted and irregular and unpredictable bleeding or spotting results, usually decreases to the point of amenorrhea as treatment continues

MONITORING PARAMETERS

• Pretreatment physical exam should include breasts and pelvic organs, Pap smear

medrysone

(me′dri-sone)

HMS Liquifilm

Chemical Class: Corticosteroid

Therapeutic Class: Ophthalmic antiinflammatory

CLINICAL PHARMACOLOGY

Mechanism of Action: Suppresses aspects of the inflammatory process such as hyperemia, cellular infiltration, vascularization, and fibroblastic proliferation; antiinflammatory action is accomplished through potentiation of epinephrine vasoconstriction, stabilization of lysosomal membranes, retardation of macrophage movement, prevention of kinin release, inhibition of lymphocyte and neutrophil function, inhibition of prostaglandin synthesis, and decrease of antibody production (prolonged use)

Pharmacokinetics

OPHTH: Absorbed through aqueous humor, metabolized in liver, excreted in urine and feces

INDICATIONS AND USES: Steroid-responsive inflammatory conditions of the palpebral and bulbar conjunctiva, lid, cornea, and anterior segment of the globe (e.g., allergic conjunctivitis, nonspecific superficial keratitis, superficial punctate keratitis, herpes zoster keratitis, iritis, cyclitis, and selected infective conjunctivitis); corneal injury (chemical, radiation, or thermal burns or penetration of foreign bodies); graft rejection following keratoplasty

DOSAGE

Adult and Child

• Instill 1 gtt q1h during the day and q2h during the night; reduce dosage to 1 gtt q4h when a favorable response is obtained

$ AVAILABLE FORMS/COST OF THERAPY

• Susp, Top—Ophth: 1%, 5, 10 ml: **$13.63-$20.93**

CONTRAINDICATIONS: Hypersensitivity; acute superficial herpes simplex keratitis; fungal diseases of ocular structures; vaccinia, varicella, and most other viral diseases of the cornea and conjunctiva; ocular TB; following uncomplicated removal of a superficial corneal foreign body

PRECAUTIONS: Prolonged use, infections of the eye, glaucoma

PREGNANCY AND LACTATION: Pregnancy category C

SIDE EFFECTS/ADVERSE REACTIONS

EENT: ***Increased intraocular pressure,*** poor corneal wound healing, increased possibility of corneal infection, glaucoma exacerbation, ***optic nerve damage,*** decreased acuity, visual field, cataracts, transient burning/stinging

SPECIAL CONSIDERATIONS

PATIENT/FAMILY EDUCATION

- Keep bottle tightly closed and out of the reach of children
- Avoid touching tip of container to any surface
- Wash hands immediately prior to use
- Apply continuous gentle pressure on the lacrimal duct with the index finger for several seconds immediately following instillation of drops to minimize systemic absorption
- Do not discontinue use without consulting physician
- Drug may cause sensitivity to bright light, minimize by wearing sunglasses
- Notify physician if no improvement after 1 wk, if condition worsens, or if pain, itching, or swelling of the eye occurs

MONITORING PARAMETERS

- Check IOP and lens frequently during prolonged use

mefenamic acid

(me-fe-nam′ik)

Ponstel

Chemical Class: Anthranilic acid derivative

Therapeutic Class: Nonsteroidal antiinflammatory drug (NSAID)

CLINICAL PHARMACOLOGY

Mechanism of Action: Inhibits cyclooxygenase activity and prostaglandin synthesis; other mechanisms such as inhibition of lipoxygenase, leukotriene synthesis, lysosomal enzyme release, neutrophil aggregation and various cell-membrane functions may exist as well

Pharmacokinetics

PO: Peak 2-4 hr, >90% bound to plasma proteins, metabolized by liver, excreted in urine (metabolites), $t_{1/2}$ 2-4 hr

INDICATIONS AND USES: Mild to moderate pain, primary dysmenorrhea, migraine headache,* premenstrual syndrome*

DOSAGE

Adult and Child >14 yr

- *Acute pain:* PO 500 mg, then 250 mg q6h prn, not to exceed 1 wk of therapy
- *Primary dysmenorrhea:* PO 500 mg, then 250 mg q6h, start with onset of bleeding and associated symptoms

$ AVAILABLE FORMS/COST OF THERAPY

- Cap, Gel—Oral: 250 mg, 100's: **$91.51**

CONTRAINDICATIONS: Hypersensitivity to NSAIDs or ASA, active ulceration or chronic inflammation of either the upper or lower GI

PRECAUTIONS: Bleeding tendencies, peptic ulcer, renal/hepatic func-

M

tion impairment, elderly, CHF, hypertension, child <14 yr

PREGNANCY AND LACTATION: Pregnancy category C (category D if used in 3rd trimester)

SIDE EFFECTS/ADVERSE REACTIONS

CNS: Dizziness, headache, lightheadedness

CV: ***CHF,*** hypotension, hypertension, palpitation, ***dysrhythmias,*** tachycardia, edema, chest pain

EENT: Visual disturbances, photophobia, dry eyes, hearing disturbances, tinnitus

GI: Nausea, vomiting, *diarrhea,* constipation, abdominal cramps, *dyspepsia,* flatulence, ***gastric or duodenal ulcer with bleeding or perforation,*** occult blood in stool, ***hepatitis,*** pancreatitis

HEME: ***Neutropenia, eosinophilia, leukopenia, pancytopenia, thrombocytopenia, agranulocytosis***

GU: ***Acute renal failure***

METAB: Hyperglycemia, hypoglycemia, hyperkalemia, hyponatremia

RESP: Dyspnea, bronchospasm

SKIN: Rash, urticaria, photosensitivity

▼ **DRUG INTERACTIONS**

Drugs

- *Aminoglycosides:* Reduction of aminoglycoside clearance in premature infants
- *ACE inhibitors, beta blockers, hydralazine:* Inhibition of antihypertensive response
- *Furosemide:* Reduced diuretic and antihypertensive response to furosemide
- *Lithium:* Increased plasma lithium concentrations, toxicity
- *Methotrexate:* Reduced renal clearance of methotrexate, increased toxicity
- *Oral anticoagulants:* Increased risk of bleeding due to adverse effects on GI mucosa and platelet function
- *Potassium sparing diuretics:* Acute renal failure

SPECIAL CONSIDERATIONS

PATIENT/FAMILY EDUCATION

- Drug may cause diarrhea, notify physician if excessive
- Avoid aspirin and alcoholic beverages
- Take with food, milk, or antacids to decrease GI upset
- Notify physician if edema, black stools, or persistent headache occurs

MONITORING PARAMETERS

- CBC, BUN, serum creatinine, LFTs, occult blood loss

---

mefloquine

(me-flow′quine)

Lariam

Chemical Class: Quinine analog

Therapeutic Class: Antimalarial

CLINICAL PHARMACOLOGY

Mechanism of Action: Exact mechanism unknown, but may act by raising intravesicular pH in parasite acid vesicles

Pharmacokinetics

PO: 98% bound to plasma proteins, concentrated in blood erythrocytes, metabolized in liver, $t_{1/2}$ 15-33 days

INDICATIONS AND USES: Treatment and prevention of *Plasmodium falciparum* and *P. vivax* malaria infections

DOSAGE

Adult

- *Treatment:* PO 1250 mg (5 tabs) as a single dose
- *Prevention:* PO 250 mg qwk for 4 wk, then 250 mg q2wk; CDC recommends 250 mg qwk starting 1 wk prior to travel, continued weekly dur-

ing travel and for 4 wk after leaving endemic area

Child

• PO: CDC recommends following doses to be taken weekly starting 1 wk prior to travel, continued weekly during travel and for 4 wk after leaving endemic area: 15-19 kg, ¼ tab; 20-30 kg, ½ tab; 31-45 kg, ¾ tab; >45 kg, 1 tab

$ AVAILABLE FORMS/COST OF THERAPY

• Tab, Uncoated—Oral: 250 mg, 25's: **$167.64**

CONTRAINDICATIONS: Hypersensitivity

PRECAUTIONS: Children, cardiac dysrhythmias, neurologic disease

PREGNANCY AND LACTATION: Pregnancy category C; use caution during the first 12-14 wk of pregnancy; excreted in breast milk in amounts not thought to be harmful to the nursing infant, and insufficient to provide adequate protection against malaria

SIDE EFFECTS/ADVERSE REACTIONS

CNS: Dizziness, headache, syncope, anxiety, confusion, disorientation, hallucinations, ***coma, convulsions***

CV: Bradycardia, extrasystole

EENT: Tinnitus; retinal, lens, corneal abnormalities (rats only)

GI: Nausea, vomiting, loss of appetite, diarrhea, abdominal pain

HEME: ***Leukopenia, thrombocytopenia***

MS: Myalgia

SKIN: Itching, rash

▼ DRUG INTERACTIONS

Drugs

• *Metoclopramide:* Increased peak mefloquine plasma concentrations

Labs

• *Increase:* Transaminases (transient)

• *Decrease:* Hematocrit

SPECIAL CONSIDERATIONS

PATIENT/FAMILY EDUCATION

• Do not take on an empty stomach

• Take medication with at least 8 oz water

MONITORING PARAMETERS

• Liver function tests and ophthalmic examinations during prolonged therapy

---

megestrol

(me-jess'trole)

Megace

Chemical Class: Progesterone derivative; appetite stimulant

Therapeutic Class: Antineoplastic

CLINICAL PHARMACOLOGY

Mechanism of Action: Exact mechanisms of antineoplastic action or weight gain have not been determined; antineoplastic effect may result from suppression of luteinizing hormone by inhibition of pituitary function or a local effect on cancerous cells; effects on weight gain may be related to appetite-stimulant or metabolic effects

Pharmacokinetics

PO: Peak 1-5 hr, metabolized in liver, eliminated in urine and feces, $t_{1/2}$ 60 min

INDICATIONS AND USES: Anorexia, cachexia, or unexplained weight loss in patients with AIDS (suspension); advanced breast or endometrial cancer

DOSAGE

Adult

• *Breast cancer:* PO 40 mg qid for at least 2 mo

• *Endometrial cancer:* PO 40-320 mg/d in divided doses for at least 2 mo

• *Anorexia/cachexia:* PO 800 mg/d (20 ml susp/d) initially; daily doses of 400-800 mg have been shown to be effective

$ AVAILABLE FORMS/COST OF THERAPY

• Tab, Uncoated—Oral: 20 mg, 100's: **$43.13-$69.86;** 40 mg, 100's: **$76.35-$124.60**

• Susp—Oral: 40 mg/ml, 235.6 ml: **$103.65**

CONTRAINDICATIONS: As a diagnostic test for pregnancy, known or suspected pregnancy, prophylactic use to avoid weight loss, hypersensitivity

PRECAUTIONS: History of thromboembolic disease, children, HIV-infected women

PREGNANCY AND LACTATION: Pregnancy category X; not recommended during the first 4 months of pregnancy

SIDE EFFECTS/ADVERSE REACTIONS

CNS: Paresthesia, confusion, ***convulsions,*** depression, neuropathy, hypesthesia, abnormal thinking

CV: ***Cardiomyopathy,*** palpitation, edema

EENT: Amblyopia

GI: Constipation, dry mouth, hepatomegaly, increased salivation, oral moniliasis, abdominal pain

GU: Albuminuria, urinary incontinence, UTI, gynecomastia

HEME: ***Leukopenia***

RESP: Dyspnea, cough, pharyngitis, lung disorder

SKIN: Alopecia, herpes, pruritus, vesiculobullous rash, sweating, skin disorder

▼ **DRUG INTERACTIONS**

Labs

• *Increase:* Alk phosphatase, urinary N, urinary pregnanediol, plasma amino acids

• *Decrease:* HDL, glucose tolerance test

• *False positive:* Urine glucose

SPECIAL CONSIDERATIONS

PATIENT/FAMILY EDUCATION

• Use contraception while taking this medication

menadiol

(men-a-dye'ol)

Synkavite, ♣ Synkayvite

Chemical Class: Water-soluble derivative of menadione (vitamin K_3)

Therapeutic Class: Hemostatic; vitamin

CLINICAL PHARMACOLOGY

Mechanism of Action: Similar in activity to naturally occurring vitamin K, which is necessary for synthesis in the liver of blood coagulation factors II, VII, IX, and X

INDICATIONS AND USES: Vitamin K deficiency, hypoprothrombinemia

DOSAGE

Adult

• PO/IM/IV/SC 5-10 mg qd

$ AVAILABLE FORMS/COST OF THERAPY

• Inj, Sol—IM; IV; SC: 5 mg/ml, 1 ml: **$1.88;** 10 mg/ml, 1 ml: **$2.75;** 75 mg/2ml, 2 ml: **$3.79**

• Tab, Uncoated—Oral: 5 mg, 100's: **$10.69**

CONTRAINDICATIONS: Hypersensitivity, severe hepatic disease, last few weeks of pregnancy

PRECAUTIONS: Neonates, ineffective in the treatment of oral anticoagulant-induced hypoprothrombinemia, sulfite sensitivity, glucose 6-PD deficiency

PREGNANCY AND LACTATION: Pregnancy category C (category X if used in 3rd trimester or close to delivery); use close to delivery may cause hyperbilirubinemia and kernicterus; compatible with breast feeding

SIDE EFFECTS/ADVERSE REACTIONS

CNS: Headache, ***brain damage*** (neonates)

GI: Nausea

HEME: ***Hemolytic anemia, hemoglobinuria, hyperbilirubinemia***

SKIN: Rash, urticaria

▼ **DRUG INTERACTIONS**

Drugs

• *Oral anticoagulants:* Decreased sensitivity to oral anticoagulants

Labs

• *False increase:*Urinary 17-OHCS

SPECIAL CONSIDERATIONS

MONITORING PARAMETERS

• Prothrombin time

menotropins

(men-oh-troe'pins)

Humegon, Pergonal

Chemical Class: Purified preparation of the human pituitary gonadotropins, follicle-stimulating hormone (FSH) and luteinizing hormone (LH)

Therapeutic Class: Gonadotropin; fertility agent

CLINICAL PHARMACOLOGY

Mechanism of Action: In women, produces ovarian follicular growth in the absence of primary ovarian failure, does not induce ovulation; when administered to men with human chorionic gonadotropin (HCG), induces spermatogenesis in the presence of primary or secondary pituitary hypofunction in men who have achieved adequate masculinization with prior HCG therapy

Pharmacokinetics

IM: $t_{1/2}$ of FSH and LH 70 and 4 hr, respectively, 8% of dose excreted unchanged in urine

INDICATIONS AND USES: Stimulation of ovarian follicular growth prior to induction of ovulation by HCG; induction of multiple follicles in ovulatory patients participating in an in vitro fertilization program; stimulation of spermatogenesis in men with primary or secondary hypogonadotropic hypogonadism (in conjunction with HCG)

DOSAGE

Adult

• Women: IM 75 IU of FSH, LH qd for 7-12 days, followed by 10,000 IU HCG 1 day after last dose of menotropins; repeat for at least 2 more cycles if evidence of ovulation, but no pregnancy, then increase to 150 IU of FSH, LH qd for 7-12 days, followed by 10,000 U HCG 1 day after last dose of menotropins, repeat as above

• Men: IM 1 amp 3 times/wk with HCG 2000 IU 2 times/wk for 4 mo (following pretreatment with HCG alone 5000 IU 3 times/wk for 4-6 mo)

$ **AVAILABLE FORMS/COST OF THERAPY**

• Inj, Sol—IM: 75 U, 1's: **$56.65-$64.94;** 150 U, 1's: **$108.77-$124.67**

CONTRAINDICATIONS: Women: Primary ovarian failure, abnormal bleeding, thyroid/adrenal dysfunction, organic intracranial lesion, ovarian cysts, pregnancy

Men: Primary testicular failure, normal pituitary function, infertility disorder other than hyopgonadotropic hypogonadism

PREGNANCY AND LACTATION: Pregancy category X

SIDE EFFECTS/ADVERSE REACTIONS

CNS: Febrile reactions, chills, headache, malaise, dizziness, ***stroke***

CV: ***Venous/arterial thromboembolism,*** tachycardia

GI: Nausea, abdominal pain, vomiting, diarrhea, cramps, *bloating*

GU: Ovarian enlargement, ovarian cysts, adnexal torsion, ***hyperstimulation syndrome*** (sudden ovarian enlargement and ascites, with or without pain or pleural effusion), ***hemoperitoneum, ectopic pregnancy***
MS: Musculoskeletal aches, joint pains
RESP: Atelectasis, ***acute respiratory distress syndrome,*** dyspnea, tachypnea
SKIN: Pain, rash, irritation at inj site; body rashes
MISC: Gynecomastia (men)

SPECIAL CONSIDERATIONS

PATIENT/FAMILY EDUCATION

- Multiple births occur in approximately 20% of women treated with menotropins and HCG
- Couple should engage in intercourse daily, beginning on the day prior to HCG administration, until ovulation occurs

MONITORING PARAMETERS

- Urinary estrogen; do not administer HCG if >150 μg/24 hr (increased risk of hyperstimulation syndrome)

---

mepenzolate

(me-pen′zoe-late)
Cantil

Chemical Class: Aminoalcohol ester; quaternary ammonium compound
Therapeutic Class: Gastrointestinal antimuscarinic/antispasmodic

CLINICAL PHARMACOLOGY

Mechanism of Action: Inhibits GI motility and diminishes gastric acid secretion

Pharmacokinetics

PO: Onset 1 hr, duration 3-4 hr, poor lipid solubility, 3%-22% of dose excreted in urine, remainder excreted in feces (probably as unabsorbed drug)

INDICATIONS AND USES: Adjunctive treatment of peptic ulcer; functional GI disorders (diarrhea, pylorospasm, hypermotility, neurogenic colon);* irritable bowel syndrome (spastic colon, mucous colitis);* acute enterocolitis,* ulcerative colitis,* diverticulitis,* mild dysenteries,* pancreatitis,* splenic flexure syndrome*

DOSAGE

Adult

- PO 25-50 mg qid with meals, hs

$ AVAILABLE FORMS/COST OF THERAPY

- Tab, Uncoated—Oral: 25 mg, 100's: **$77.40**

CONTRAINDICATIONS: Hypersensitivity to anticholinergic drugs, narrow-angle glaucoma, obstructive uropathy, obstructive disease of the GI tract, paralytic ileus, intestinal atony, unstable cardiovascular status in acute hemorrhage, severe ulcerative colitis, toxic megacolon complicating ulcerative colitis, myasthenia gravis

PRECAUTIONS: Hyperthyroidism, CAD, dysrhythmias, CHF, ulcerative colitis, hypertension, hiatal hernia, hepatic disease, renal disease, urinary retention, prostatic hypertrophy, elderly, children, glaucoma

PREGNANCY AND LACTATION: Pregnancy category C; excretion into breast milk unknown, although would be expected to be minimal due to quaternary structure

SIDE EFFECTS/ADVERSE REACTIONS

CNS: Confusion, stimulation (especially in elderly), headache, insomnia, dizziness, drowsiness, anxiety, weakness, hallucination
CV: Palpitations, tachycardia
EENT: Blurred vision, photophobia,

mydriasis, cycloplegia, increased ocular tension

GI: Dry mouth, constipation, ***paralytic ileus,*** heartburn, nausea, vomiting, dysphagia, absence of taste

GU: Hesitancy, retention, impotence

SKIN: Urticaria, rash, pruritus, anhidrosis, fever, allergic reactions

▼ **DRUG INTERACTIONS**

Drugs

• *Anticholinergics:* Increased anticholinergic side effects

SPECIAL CONSIDERATIONS

PATIENT/FAMILY EDUCATION

• Take drug 30-60 min before a meal

• Drug may cause drowsiness, dizziness or blurred vision, use caution while driving or performing other tasks requiring alertness

• Notify physician if eye pain occurs

---

meperidine

(me-per′i-deen)

Demerol

Chemical Class: Opiate, phenylpiperidine derivative

Therapeutic Class: Narcotic analgesic

DEA Class: Schedule II

CLINICAL PHARMACOLOGY

Mechanism of Action: Binds to opiate receptors in the CNS causing inhibition of ascending pain pathways, altering perception of and response to pain

Pharmacokinetics

PO: Peak analgesia within 1 hr, duration 2-4 hr

IM: Peak analgesia 30-50 min, duration 2-4 hr

SC: Peak analgesia 40-60 min, duration 2-4 hr

60%-80% bound to plasma proteins, metabolized by liver (normeperidine is an active metabolite with half the analgesic potency but twice the CNS stimulant potency of the parent drug), eliminated in urine, $t_{1/2}$ 3-5 hr (normeperidine $t_{1/2}$ 8-21 hr, may be prolonged in renal impairment)

INDICATIONS AND USES: Moderate to severe pain, preoperative sedation (parenteral)

DOSAGE

Oral doses are about half as effective as parenteral doses

Adult

• *Analgesia:* PO/IM/IV/SC 50-150 mg q3-4h prn

• *Preoperative sedation:* IM/SC 50-100 mg 30-90 min before beginning anesthesia

Child

• *Analgesia:* PO/IM/IV/SC 1-1.5 mg/kg/dose q3-4h prn, max 100 mg/dose

• *Preoperative sedation:* IM/SC 1-2 mg/kg 30-90 min before beginning anesthesia

$ **AVAILABLE FORMS/COST OF THERAPY**

• Inj, Sol—IM; IV; SC: 10 mg per ml, 30 ml: **$1.64-$14.20;** 25, 50, 75, 100 mg/ml, 1 ml: **$0.54-$1.13**

• Syr—Oral: 50 mg/5ml, 480 ml: **$31.87-$80.71**

• Tab, Uncoated—Oral: 50 mg, 100's: **$20.15-$71.88;** 100 mg, 100's: **$29.19-$136.73**

CONTRAINDICATIONS: Hypersensitivity, acute bronchial asthma, upper airway obstruction, within 14 days of MAOI therapy

PRECAUTIONS: Head injury, increased intracranial pressure, acute abdominal conditions, elderly, renal function impairment (normeperidine may accumulate, resulting in increased CNS adverse reactions), hepatic impairment, hypothyroidism, Addison's disease, prostatic hy-

M

pertrophy, urethral stricture, history of drug abuse

PREGNANCY AND LACTATION: Pregnancy category B (category D if used for prolonged periods or in high doses at term); use during labor may produce neonatal respiratory depression; compatible with breast feeding

SIDE EFFECTS/ADVERSE REACTIONS

CNS: Drowsiness, sedation, dizziness, agitation, dependency, lethargy, restlessness, ***seizures,*** tremors, twitches, myoclonus

GI: Nausea, vomiting, anorexia, constipation

RESP: ***Respiratory depression, respiratory paralysis***

CV: Bradycardia, palpitations, orthostatic hypotension, tachycardia

GU: Urinary retention

SKIN: Flushing, rash, urticaria

▼ **DRUG INTERACTIONS**

Drugs

- *Barbiturates:* Enhanced metabolism to normeperidine, increased toxicity of meperidine
- *Cimetidine:* Enhanced respiratory and CNS depression
- *Ethanol:* Additive CNS depressive effects
- *MAOIs+:* Accumulation of CNS serotonin leading to agitation, blood pressure changes, hyperpyrexia, convulsions
- *Neuroleptics:* Hypotension, excessive CNS depression

Labs

- *Increase:* Amylase, lipase

SPECIAL CONSIDERATIONS

PATIENT/FAMILY EDUCATION

- Report any symptoms of CNS changes, allergic reactions
- Physical dependency may result when used for extended periods
- Change position slowly, orthostatic hypotension may occur
- Avoid hazardous activities if drowsiness or dizziness occurs
- Avoid alcohol, other CNS depressants unless directed by physician
- Minimize nausea by administering with food and remain lying down following dose

---

mephentermine

(me-fen′ter-meen)

Wyamine

Chemical Class: Methamphetamine derivative

Therapeutic Class: Sympathomimetic

CLINICAL PHARMACOLOGY

Mechanism of Action: Primarily an indirect sympathomimetic that releases norepinephrine from its storage sites; increases blood pressure by increasing cardiac output (positive inotropic effect) and, to a lesser degree, by increasing peripheral resistance due to vasoconstriction

Pharmacokinetics

IM: Onset 5-15 min, duration 1-4 hr

IV: Onset almost immediate, duration 15-30 min

Metabolized by liver, eliminated in urine

INDICATIONS AND USES: Hypotension during spinal anesthesia

DOSAGE

Adult

- *Prevention of hypotension during spinal anesthesia:* IM 30-45 mg 10-20 min prior to anesthesia
- *Hypotension following spinal anesthesia:* IV 30-45 mg, repeat doses of 30 mg prn to maintain blood pressure; IV INF use 0.1% sol in D_5W (1 mg/ml), titrate to patient response

$ **AVAILABLE FORMS/COST OF THERAPY**

- Inj, Sol—IM; IV: 15 mg/ml, 10 ml: **$10.83;** 30 mg/ml, 10 ml: **$17.18**

CONTRAINDICATIONS: Hypersensitivity, hypotension induced by chlorpromazine, concurrent use with any MAOI
PRECAUTIONS: Cardiovascular disease, chronically ill patients, hemorrhagic shock, hyperthyroidism, hypertension
PREGNANCY AND LACTATION: Pregnancy category C
SIDE EFFECTS/ADVERSE REACTIONS
CNS: Tremors, drowsiness, confusion, incoherence, anxiety
CV: Palpitations, tachycardia, hypertension

▼ **DRUG INTERACTIONS**
Drugs
• *Halogenated hydrocarbon anesthetics:* Sensitization of myocardium to effects of catecholamines, serious dysrhythmia may result
• *MAOIs:* Hypertensive crisis

mephenytoin

(me-fen′i-toyn)
Mesantoin
Chemical Class: Hydantoin derivative
Therapeutic Class: Anticonvulsive

CLINICAL PHARMACOLOGY
Mechanism of Action: Stabilizes neuronal membranes and decreases seizure activity by increasing efflux or decreasing influx of sodium ions across cell membranes in the motor cortex during generation of nerve impulses
Pharmacokinetics
PO: Onset 30 min, duration 24-48 hr, metabolized by liver to active metabolite, excreted in urine, $t_{1/2}$ 144 hr
INDICATIONS AND USES: Tonic-clonic, partial, Jacksonian, and psychomotor seizures in patients refractory to less toxic anticonvulsants
DOSAGE
Adult
• PO 50-100 mg/d initially, increase by 50-100 mg at weekly intervals; usual maintenance dose 200-600 mg/d divided tid; max 800 mg/d
Child
• PO 3-15 mg/kg/d divided tid; usual maintenance dose 100-400 mg/d divided tid

$ **AVAILABLE FORMS/COST OF THERAPY**
• Tab, Uncoated—Oral: 100 mg, 100's: **$27.00**
CONTRAINDICATIONS: Hypersensitivity to hydantoins
PRECAUTIONS: Abrupt withdrawal, elderly, impaired liver function, hyperglycemia, acute intermittent porphyria
PREGNANCY AND LACTATION: Pregnancy category C
SIDE EFFECTS/ADVERSE REACTIONS
CNS: Drowsiness, ataxia, dysarthria, fatigue, irritability, choreiform movements, depression, tremor, nervousness, insomnia, dizziness, mental confusion, psychotic disturbances
CV: Edema
EENT: Diplopia, nystagmus, photophobia
GI: Nausea, vomiting, ***hepatitis,*** jaundice
GU: Nephrosis
HEME: ***Leukopenia, neutropenia, agranulocytosis, thrombocytopenia, pancytopenia, anemia, hemolytic anemia, megaloblastic anemia, aplastic anemia,*** lymphadenopathy
METAB: Hyperglycemia
MS: Polyarthropathy, osteomalacia
RESP: ***Pulmonary fibrosis***
SKIN: Maculopapular, morbilliform, scarlantiniform, urticarial, purpuric, and nonspecific skin rashes; ***ex-***

M

foliative dermatitis, erythema multiforme, toxic epidermal necrolysis, alopecia

MISC: Weight gain, lupus erythematosus syndrome

▼ **DRUG INTERACTIONS**

Drugs

• *Acetazolamide:* Increased risk of otseomalacia
• *Amiodarone:* Increased mephenytoin concentrations, decreased amiodarone concentrations
• *Antidepressants:* Increased mephenytoin concentrations; reduced cyclic antidepressant concentrations
• *Antineoplastics, aspirin, diazoxide, folic acid, rifampin, salicylates:* Reduced plasma mephenytoin concentrations
• *Chloramphenicol+, cimetidine, disulfiram+, felbamate, fluconazole, fluoxetine, isoniazid+, omeprazole, phenyramidol, sulfonamides, sulthiame:* Increased serum mephenytoin concentrations
• *Corticosteroids:* Reduced therapeutic effect of corticosteroids
• *Cyclosporine:* Reduced cyclosporine concentrations
• *Digitalis glycosides:* Reduced concentrations of digitoxin
• *Disopyramide:* Reduced efficacy, increased toxicity of disopyramide
• *Doxycycline:* Reduced doxycycline concentrations
• *Lidocaine:* Reduced serum lidocaine concentrations; additive cardiac depression
• *Loop diuretics:* Reduced diuretic response
• *Mebendazole:* Reduced plasma mebendazole concentrations
• *Methadone:* Reduced serum methadone concentrations
• *Metyrapone:* Invalidated metyrapone test
• *Mexiletine:* Reduced mexiletine concentrations
• *Oral anticoagulants:* Transient increase followed by inhibition of hypoprothrombinemic response to oral anticoagulants
• *Oral contraceptives:* Inhibited effect of oral contraceptives
• *Primidone:* Enhanced conversion of primidone to phenobarbital
• *Quinidine:* Decreased serum quinidine concentrations
• *Theophylline:* Reduced serum theophylline concentrations
• *Thyroid hormones:* Increased thyroid replacement dose requirements
• *Valproic acid:* Increased, decreased, or unaltered plasma mephenytoin concentrations

SPECIAL CONSIDERATIONS

PATIENT/FAMILY EDUCATION

• Take with food
• Drug may cause drowsiness, dizziness, or blurred vision
• Avoid alcohol
• Notify physician of skin rash, severe nausea or vomiting, swollen glands, bleeding, swollen or tender gums, yellowish discoloration of skin or eyes, joint pain, unexplained fever, sore throat, persistent headache, pregnancy

MONITORING PARAMETERS

• CBC with differential and platelet count at baseline, 2 wk after dosage changes, q1 mo for 1 yr, then q3 mo thereafter
• Therapeutic serum concentrations 25-40 µg/ml (mephenytoin plus active metabolite)

mephobarbital

(me-foe-bar′bi-tal)

Mebaral

Chemical Class: Barbiturate (long acting)

Therapeutic Class: Anticonvulsant; sedative/hypnotic

DEA Class: Schedule IV

CLINICAL PHARMACOLOGY

Mechanism of Action: Depresses activity in brain cells primarily in reticular activating system in brain stem; also selectively depresses neurons in posterior hypothalamus, limbic structures; able to decrease seizure activity in subhypnotic doses by inhibition of impulses in CNS

Pharmacokinetics

PO: Onset 20-60 min, duration 10-16 hr, metabolized by the liver to phenobarbital, excreted in urine, $t_{1/2}$ 11-67 hr

INDICATIONS AND USES: Routine sedation, partial and generalized tonic-clonic and cortical focal seizures

DOSAGE

Adult

- *Sedative:* PO 32-100 mg tid-qid
- *Epilepsy:* PO 400-600 mg/d in 2-4 divided doses

Child

- *Sedative:* PO 16-32 mg tid-qid
- *Epilepsy:* PO 4-10 mg/kg/d in 2-4 divided doses

$ AVAILABLE FORMS/COST OF THERAPY

- Tab, Uncoated—Oral: 32 mg, 250's: **$41.58;** 50 mg, 250's: **$59.51;** 100 mg, 250's: **$79.76**

CONTRAINDICATIONS: Hypersensitivity to barbiturates, respiratory depression, addiction to barbiturates, severe liver impairment, porphyria, nephritic patients

PRECAUTIONS: Myasthenia gravis, myxedema, anemia, hepatic disease, renal disease, hypertension, elderly, acute/chronic pain, mental depression, history of drug abuse, abrupt discontinuation, children, hyperthyroidism, fever, diabetes

PREGNANCY AND LACTATION: Pregnancy category D; has caused major adverse effects in some nursing infants, should be given with caution to nursing women

SIDE EFFECTS/ADVERSE REACTIONS

CNS: Lethargy, drowsiness, hangover, dizziness, stimulation in the elderly and children, lightheadedness, physical dependence, CNS depression, mental depression, slurred speech, vertigo, headache

CV: Hypotension, bradycardia

GI: Nausea, vomiting, diarrhea, constipation

HEME: ***Agranulocytosis, thrombocytopenia, megaloblastic anemia*** (long-term treatment)

RESP: ***Depression, apnea, laryngospasm, bronchospasm***

SKIN: Rash, urticaria, erythema multiforme, pain, abscesses at injection site, ***angioedema,*** thrombophlebitis, ***Stevens-Johnson syndrome***

MISC: Rickets, osteomalacia (prolonged use)

▼ DRUG INTERACTIONS

Drugs

- *Acetaminophen:* Enhanced hepatotoxic potential of acetaminophen overdoses
- *Antidepressants, disopyramide, doxycycline, quinidine, theophylline:* Reduced serum concentrations
- *Beta blockers:* Reduced serum concentrations of beta blockers which are extensively metabolized
- *Calcium channel blockers:* Reduced concentrations of verapamil and nifedipine
- *Central nervous system depressants:* Excessive CNS depression
- *Chloramphenicol:* Increased barbiturate concentrations; reduced serum chloramphenicol concentrations
- *Corticosteroids:* Reduced serum concentrations of corticosteroids, may impair therapeutic effect
- *Ethanol:* Excessive CNS depression

• *Methoxyflurane:* Enhanced nephrotoxic effect
• *MAOIs:* Prolonged effect of some barbiturates
• *Narcotic analgesics:* Increased toxicity of meperidine; reduced effect of methadone; additive CNS depression
• *Neuroleptics:* Reduced effect of either drug
• *Oral anticoagulants+:* Inhibited hypoprothrombinemic response to oral anticoagulants
• *Oral contraceptives:* Reduced efficacy of oral contraceptives

SPECIAL CONSIDERATIONS

PATIENT/FAMILY EDUCATION

• Avoid driving or other activities requiring alertness
• Avoid alcohol ingestion or CNS depressants
• Do not discontinue medication abruptly after long-term use
• Notify physician of fever, sore throat, mouth sores, easy bruising or bleeding, tiny broken blood vessels under skin

MONITORING PARAMETERS

• Periodic CBC, liver and renal function tests, serum folate, vitamin D during prolonged therapy

mepivacaine

(me-piv'a-kane)
Carbocaine, Isocaine HCl, Polocaine

Chemical Class: Amide
Therapeutic Class: Local anesthetic

CLINICAL PHARMACOLOGY

Mechanism of Action: Blocks the generation and conduction of nerve impulses, presumably by increasing the threshold for electrical excitation in the nerve, slowing the propagation of the nerve impulse, and reducing the rate rise of the action potential

Pharmacokinetics

Infiltrative anesthesia: Onset 3-5 min, duration 0.75-1.5 hr
Epidural: Onset 5-15 min, duration 1-3 hr
Spinal: Duration 0.5-1.5 hr 60%-85% bound to plasma proteins, metabolized by liver, excreted in urine (metabolites)

INDICATIONS AND USES: Nerve block, caudal anesthesia, epidural anesthesia, pain relief, paracervical block in obstetrics, transvaginal block, soft tissue infiltration anesthesia, anesthesia for dental procedures

DOSAGE

Adult

• Dose varies with type of procedure, degree of anesthesia required, and individual response; max amount given per procedure should not exceed 400 mg, total dose/24 hr should not exceed 1 g
• *Nerve block:* 1% or 2% sol
• *Paracervical block:* 1% sol
• *Transvaginal block:* 1% sol
• *Caudal and epidural block:* 1%, 1.5%, or 2% sol
• *Infiltration:* 1% sol
• *Dental procedures:* 3% sol

$ AVAILABLE FORMS/COST OF THERAPY

• Inj, Sol—Dental: 30 mg/ml, 1.8 ml × 100: **$35.00**
• Inj, Sol: 1%, 30 ml: **$6.76-$11.44;** 1.5%, 30 ml: **$9.16-$14.00;** 2%, 20 ml: **$7.51-$11.53**

CONTRAINDICATIONS: Hypersensitivity to local anesthetics, heart block (large doses), septicemia (spinal anesthesia)

PRECAUTIONS: Hepatic disease, use in head and neck area, children, inflammation, sepsis, elderly; neurologic disease, spinal deformities, septicemia, severe hypertension (epidural and caudal anesthesia); impaired cardiovascular function, renal disease

PREGNANCY AND LACTATION: Pregnancy category C; epidural, caudal, or pudendal anesthesia during labor and delivery may alter the forces of parturition through changes in uterine contractility or maternal expulsive efforts

SIDE EFFECTS/ADVERSE REACTIONS

CNS: Anxiety, restlessness, ***convulsions, loss of consciousness,*** drowsiness, disorientation, tremors, shivering

CV: ***Myocardial depression, cardiac arrest, dysrhythmias,*** bradycardia, ***hypotension,*** hypertension, ***fetal bradycardia***

EENT: Blurred vision, tinnitus, pupil constriction

GI: Nausea, vomiting

RESP: ***Respiratory arrest, anaphylaxis***

SKIN: Rash, urticaria, allergic reactions, edema, burning, skin discoloration at inj site, tissue necrosis

▼ **DRUG INTERACTIONS**

Drugs

• *Beta blockers:* Hypertensive reactions possible; acute discontinuation of beta blockers before local anesthesia may increase the risk of side effects due to anesthetic

SPECIAL CONSIDERATIONS

MONITORING PARAMETERS

• Blood pressure, pulse, respiration during treatment, ECG

• Fetal heart tones if drug is used during labor

meprobamate

(me-proe'ba-mate)

Apo-Meprobamate, Equanil, Meditran, Meprospan, Miltown, Neuramate, Novomepro

Chemical Class: Carbamate derivative

Therapeutic Class: Anxiolytic; sedative/hypnotic

DEA Class: Schedule IV

CLINICAL PHARMACOLOGY

Mechanism of Action: Exact mechanism of action unknown; apparently acts at multiple sites in CNS including hypothalamus, thalamus, limbic system, and spinal cord

Pharmacokinetics

PO: Onset 1 hr, peak 1-3 hr, metabolized in liver, excreted in urine (metabolites), $t_{1/2}$ 10 hr

INDICATIONS AND USES: Anxiety disorders

DOSAGE

Adult

• PO 1.2-1.6 g/d divided tid-qid, do not exceed 2.4 g/d; SR 400-800 mg bid

Child (6-12 yr)

• PO 100-200 mg bid-tid; SR 200 mg bid

$ **AVAILABLE FORMS/COST OF THERAPY**

• Tab, Uncoated—Oral: 200 mg, 100's: **$3.98-$108.25;** 400 mg, 100's: **$4.65-$132.74;** 600 mg, 100's: **$206.81**

• Cap, Gel, Sust Action—Oral: 200 mg, 100's: **$187.51;** 400 mg, 100's: **$283.55**

CONTRAINDICATIONS: Acute intermittent porphyria, hypersensitivity

PRECAUTIONS: History of drug abuse, renal and hepatic function impairment, elderly, children <6 yr, epilepsy

PREGNANCY AND LACTATION: Pregnancy category D; excreted into breast milk in concentrations 2-4 times that of maternal plasma, effect on nursing infant unknown

SIDE EFFECTS/ADVERSE REACTIONS

CNS: *Drowsiness,* ataxia, *dizziness,* slurred speech, headache, vertigo, weakness, euphoria, overstimulation, paradoxical excitement, fast EEG activity, ***convulsions***

CV: Palpitations, ***tachycardia,*** various dysrhythmias, transient ECG changes, syncope, ***hypotensive crises***, peripheral edema

EENT: Impairment of visual accommodation

GI: Nausea, vomiting, diarrhea, stomatitis, proctitis

GU: ***Oliguria, anuria***

HEME: ***Leukopenia, eosinophilia, agranulocytosis, aplastic anemia,*** thrombocytopenic purpura

RESP: ***Bronchospasm***

SKIN: Rash, petechiae, ecchymoses, fixed drug eruption, ***erythema multiforme, exfoliative dermatitis, Stevens-Johnson syndrome***

MISC: ***Anaphylaxis, angioneurotic edema, exacerbation of porphyric symptoms***

▼ **DRUG INTERACTIONS**

Drugs

• *Ethanol:* Enhanced CNS depression

Labs

• *False increase:* 17-OHCS
• *False positive:* Phentolamine test

SPECIAL CONSIDERATIONS

PATIENT/FAMILY EDUCATION

• Notify physician if pregnant or become pregnant while taking this drug
• Drug may cause drowsiness, dizziness, or blurred vision, use caution driving or other activities requiring alertness
• Avoid alcohol
• Notify physician if skin rash, sore throat, or fever occurs
• Do not crush or chew sustained released capsules
• Do not discontinue abruptly following long-term use

MONITORING PARAMETERS

• Periodic CBC with differential and platelets during prolonged therapy

mesalamine

(mez-al'a-meen)

Asacol, Pentasa, Rowasa

Chemical Class: 5-amino derivative of salicylic acid
Therapeutic Class: GI antiinflammatory

CLINICAL PHARMACOLOGY

Mechanism of Action: Exact mechanism of action uncertain; may act by blocking cyclooxygenase and inhibiting prostaglandin production in the colon; appears to produce a local inhibitory effect on the mucosal production of arachidonic acid metabolites, which are increased in patients with chronic inflammatory bowel disease

Pharmacokinetics

PR: Poorly absorbed, excreted principally in feces

PO (tabs): Designed to release drug in terminal ileum and beyond, 28% absorbed, peak 4-12 hr

PO (caps): Designed to release drug throughout the GI tract, 20%-30% absorbed, peak 3 hr

Unabsorbed drug eliminated in feces, absorbed drug metabolized and eliminated in urine (metabolite), $t_{1/2}$ 42 min (following IV administration)

INDICATIONS AND USES: Ulcerative colitis (oral); distal ulcerative colitis, proctosigmoiditis or proctitis (rectal)

DOSAGE

Adult

• PO (tabs) 800 mg tid for 6 wk; PO (caps) 1 g qid for up to 8 wk; PR (supp) 1 supp (500 mg) bid for 3-6 wk, retain supp in rectum for 1-3 hr if possible; PR (enema) 60 ml (4 g) instilled qd, preferably hs, and retained for 8 hr, treat for 3-6 wk

$ AVAILABLE FORMS/COST OF THERAPY

• Tab, Enteric Coated—Oral: 400 mg, 100's: **$ 59.41**
• Cap, Gel, Sust Action—Oral: 250 mg, 240's: **$82.38**
• Enema—Rect: 4 g/60 ml, 60 ml × 7: **$63.87**
• Supp—Rect: 500 mg/supp, 12's: **$34.78**

CONTRAINDICATIONS: Hypersensitivity to salicylates

PRECAUTIONS: Hypersensitivity to sulfasalazine, renal function impairment, sulfite sensitivity, children

PREGNANCY AND LACTATION: Pregnancy category B; has produced adverse effects in a nursing infant and should be used with caution during breast feeding, observe nursing infant closely for changes in stool consistency

SIDE EFFECTS/ADVERSE REACTIONS

CNS: Headache, fatigue, asthenia, malaise, weakness, mental depression, insomnia

CV: Peripheral edema, ***pericarditis***

GI: Abdominal pain, cramps, discomfort; nausea, flatulence, worsening diarrhea, colitis, constipation, hemorrhoids, rectal pain, difficulty retaining enema, pain on enema insertion, extension of inflammation to entire colon (rectal), ***pancreatitis***

GU: Urinary burning

MS: Leg or joint pain, back pain

SKIN: Rash, pruritus, acne, alopecia, ***Stevens-Johnson syndrome***

MISC: Acute intolerance syndrome (cramping, abdominal pain, bloody diarrhea, fever, headache, rash)

SPECIAL CONSIDERATIONS

PATIENT/FAMILY EDUCATION

• Swallow tabs whole, do not break the outer coating
• Intact or partially intact tabs may be found in stool, notify physician if this occurs repeatedly
• Avoid excess handling of suppositories

---

mesna

(mess'na)

Mesnex

Chemical Class: Thiol

Therapeutic Class: Antidote

CLINICAL PHARMACOLOGY

Mechanism of Action: Binds with and detoxifies acrolein and other urotoxic metabolites of ifosfamide and cyclophosphamide

Pharmacokinetics

IV: Rapidly oxidized to mesna disulfide (dimesna), dimesna rapidly eliminated by kidneys, dimesna reduced to free thiol compound (mesna) in the kidney, $t_{1/2}$ 0.36 hr (dimesna 1.17 hr)

INDICATIONS AND USES: Prevention of ifosfamide-induced hemorrhagic cystitis, prevention of cyclophosphamide-induced hemorrhagic cystitis*

DOSAGE

Adult and Child

• IV Give 20% of ifosfamide dosage (by weight) at the time of ifosfamide administration and 4 and 8 hr after each dose of ifosfamide

$ AVAILABLE FORMS/COST OF THERAPY

• Inj, Sol—IV: 200 mg/ampul, 2 ml: **$222.24;** 400 mg/ampul,

4 ml: **$444.46;** 1 g/ampul, 10 ml: **$740.80**

CONTRAINDICATIONS: Hypersensitivity to thiol compounds

PRECAUTIONS: Children

PREGNANCY AND LACTATION: Pregnancy category B

SIDE EFFECTS/ADVERSE REACTIONS

CNS: Headache, fatigue

CV: Hypotension

GI: Bad taste in mouth, soft stools, diarrhea, nausea, vomiting

MS: Limb pain

▼ **DRUG INTERACTIONS**

Labs

• *False positive:* Urinary ketones

SPECIAL CONSIDERATIONS

MONITORING PARAMETERS

• Urinalysis each day prior to ifosfamide administration

• Reduction or discontinuation of ifosfamide may be initiated in patients developing hematuria (>50 rbc/hpf)

---

mesoridazine

(mez-oh-rid'a-zeen)

Serentil

Chemical Class: Alkylpiperidine derivative of phenothiazine

Therapeutic Class: Antipsychotic/neuroleptic

CLINICAL PHARMACOLOGY

Mechanism of Action: Blocks postsynaptic dopamine receptors in the basal ganglia, hypothalamus, limbic system, brain stem, and medulla; appears to act at both D_1 and D_2 receptors; also exerts anticholinergic and α-adrenergic blocking effects

Pharmacokinetics

PO: Peak 2-4 hr, onset 0.5-1 hr, duration 4-6 hr, 91%-99% bound to plasma proteins, metabolized in liver, eliminated mostly in urine, $t_{1/2}$ 24-48 hr

INDICATIONS AND USES: Psychotic disorders, behavioral problems associated with mental deficiency and chronic brain syndrome, adjunctive treatment of alcoholism, personality disorders, anxiety and tension associated with neuroses

DOSAGE

Adult

• *Psychosis:* PO 50 mg tid initially, usual range 100-400 mg/d

• *Mental deficiency/chronic brain syndrome:* PO 25 mg tid initially, usual range 75-300 mg/d

• *Alcoholism:* PO 25 mg bid initially, usual range 50-200 mg/d

• *Neuroses:* PO 10 mg tid initially, usual range 30-150 mg/d

• IM 25 mg as a single dose, may repeat in 30-60 min, if necessary; do not exceed 200 mg/day

$ **AVAILABLE FORMS/COST OF THERAPY**

• Inj, Sol—IM: 25 mg/ml, 1 ml × 20: **$86.46**

• Liq—Oral: 25 mg/ml, 120 ml: **$46.96**

• Tab, Plain Coated—Oral: 10 mg, 100's: **$53.50;** 25 mg, 100's: **$71.71;** 50 mg, 100's: **$80.88;** 100 mg, 100's: **$99.06**

CONTRAINDICATIONS: Hypersensitivity to phenothiazines, severe toxic CNS depression, coma, subcortical brain damage, bone marrow depression

PRECAUTIONS: Children <12 yr, elderly, prolonged use, severe cardiovascular disorders, epilepsy, hepatic or renal disease, glaucoma, prostatic hypertrophy, severe asthma, emphysema, hypocalcemia (increased susceptibility to dystonic reactions)

PREGNANCY AND LACTATION: Pregnancy category C; bulk of evidence indicates that phenothiazines are safe for mother and fetus; effect on nursing infant is unknown but may be of concern

SIDE EFFECTS/ADVERSE REACTIONS

CNS: EPS (pseudoparkinsonism, akathisia, dystonia, tardive dyskinesia), drowsiness, headache, ***seizures, neuroleptic malignant syndrome,*** confusion, insomnia, restlessness, anxiety, euphoria, agitation, depression, lethargy, vertigo, exacerbation of psychotic symptoms including hallucinations, catatonic-like behavioral states, heat or cold intolerance

CV: ***Tachycardia,*** hypotension, hypertension, ECG changes

EENT: Blurred vision, glaucoma, dry eyes, cataracts, retinopathy, pigmentation of retina or cornea

GI: Anorexia, constipation, diarrhea, hypersalivation, dyspepsia, *nausea,* vomiting, *dry mouth*

GU: Urinary retention, priapism

HEME: Transient leukopenia, leukocytosis, minimal decreases in red blood cell counts, anemia, ***agranulocytosis, aplastic anemia, hemolytic anemia***

METAB: Lactation, breast engorgement, mastalgia, menstrual irregularities, gynecomastia, impotence, increased libido, hyperglycemia, hypoglycemia, hyponatremia

RESP: ***Laryngospasm, bronchospasm,*** increased depth of respiration

SKIN: Maculopapular and acneiform skin reactions, photosensitivity, loss of hair, diaphoresis

▼ **DRUG INTERACTIONS**

Drugs

- *Anticholinergics:* Inhibited therapeutic response to antipsychotic; enhanced anticholinergic side effects
- *Antidepressants:* Increased serum concentrations of some cyclic antidepressants
- *Barbiturates:* Reduced effect of antipsychotic
- *Beta blockers:* Enhanced effects of both drugs
- *Bromocriptine, lithium:* Reduced effects of both drugs
- *Epinephrine:* Reversed pressor response to epinephrine
- *Guanethidine+:* Inhibited antihypertensive response to guanethidine
- *Levodopa:* Inhibited effect of levodopa on Parkinson's disease
- *Narcotic analgesics:* Excessive CNS depression, hypotension, respiratory depression
- *Orphenadrine:* Reduced serum neuroleptic concentrations, excessive anticholinergic effects
- *Phenylpropanoloamine:* Case report of patient death on combination of these two drugs

Labs

- *Increase:* Liver function tests, cardiac enzymes, cholesterol, blood glucose, prolactin, bilirubin, PBI, cholinesterase, ^{131}I
- *Decrease:* Hormones (blood, urine)
- *False positive:* Pregnancy tests, PKU
- *False negative:* Urinary steroids, 17-OHCS

SPECIAL CONSIDERATIONS

PATIENT/FAMILY EDUCATION

- Contact physician if sore throat or other signs of infection
- Arise slowly from reclining position
- Do not discontinue abruptly
- Use a sunscreen during sun exposure to prevent burns, take special precautions to stay cool in hot weather
- Concentrate may be diluted just prior to administration with distilled water, acidified tap water, orange, or grape juice

M

• May cause drowsiness

MONITORING PARAMETERS

• Observe closely for signs of tardive dyskinesia

• Periodic CBC with platelets during prolonged therapy

metaproterenol

(met-a-proe-ter′e-nole)

Alupent, Arm-a-Med Metaproterenol Sulfate, Dey-Lute Metaproterenol Sulfate, Metaprel

Chemical Class: Sympathomimetic amine

Therapeutic Class: Bronchodilator

CLINICAL PHARMACOLOGY

Mechanism of Action: Relaxes smooth muscle of the bronchial tree and peripheral vasculature by stimulating β-adrenergic receptors; greater effect on β_2-receptors than β_1-receptors compared to isoproterenol and less selectivity on β_2-receptors than albuterol

Pharmacokinetics

PO: Onset 15 min, peak 1 hr, duration 4 hr

INH: Onset 1 min (MDI), 5-30 min (NEB), peak 1 hr, duration 4 hr

Metabolized in the liver, eliminated in urine (40% as unchanged drug)

INDICATIONS AND USES: Bronchial asthma, reversible bronchospasm

DOSAGE

Adult

• PO 20 mg tid-qid; MDI 2-3 inhalations q3-4h prn; NEB 5-15 inhalations of undiluted 5% sol or 0.2-0.3 ml of 5% sol diluted in 2.5-3 ml normal saline q4-6h (can be given more frequently according to need)

Child

• PO (<2 yr) 0.4 mg/kg/dose tid-qid, in infants the dose can be given q8-12h; (2-6 yr) 1-2.6 mg/kg/d divided q6-8h; (6-9 yr) 10 mg tid-qid; NEB 0.01-0.12 ml/kg of 5% sol (min dose 0.1 ml, max dose 0.3 ml) diluted in 2-3 ml normal saline q4-6h (may be given more frequently according to need)

$ AVAILABLE FORMS/COST OF THERAPY

• Sol—Inh: 0.4%, 0.6%, 2.5 ml × 25: **$17.17-$41.76;** 5%, 30 ml: **$29.25-$40.15**

• Syr—Oral: 10 mg/5ml, 480 ml: **$8.64-$33.37**

• Tab, Uncoated—Oral: 10 mg, 100's: **$5.75-$34.20;** 20 mg, 100's: **$11.25-$48.59**

• MDI—Inh: 200 puffs: **$9.96**

CONTRAINDICATIONS: Hypersensitivity, preexisting cardiac dysrhythmias associated with tachycardia

PRECAUTIONS: Ischemic heart disease, cardiac dysrhythmias, hypertension, congestive heart failure, hyperthyroidism, seizure disorders, diabetes mellitus, excessive use

PREGNANCY AND LACTATION: Pregnancy category C; has been used to prevent premature labor; long-term evaluation of infants exposed *in utero* to β-agonists has been reported, but not specifically for metaproterenol, no harmful effects were observed

SIDE EFFECTS/ADVERSE REACTIONS

CNS: Tremors, anxiety, insomnia, headache, dizziness, stimulation, nervousness

CV: Palpitations, tachycardia, hypertension, ***dysrhythmias, cardiac arrest***

EENT: Throat irritation

GI: Nausea, vomiting, bad taste, GI distress

MS: Muscle cramps in extremities

RESP: Dyspnea, cough

▼ DRUG INTERACTIONS

Labs

- *Decrease:* Potassium

SPECIAL CONSIDERATIONS

PATIENT/FAMILY EDUCATION

- Proper inhalation technique is vital for MDIs
- Excessive use may lead to adverse effects
- Notify physician if no response to usual doses, or if palpitations, rapid heart beat, chest pain, muscle tremors, dizziness, headache

---

metaraminol

(met-ar-am′e-nol)

Aramine

Chemical Class: Sympathomimetic amine

Therapeutic Class: Vasopressor

CLINICAL PHARMACOLOGY

Mechanism of Action: Increases both systolic and diastolic blood pressure, primarily by vasoconstriction which is usually accompanied by marked reflex bradycardia; acts predominantly by a direct effect on α-adrenergic receptors; also has an indirect effect by releasing norepinephrine from its storage sites

Pharmacokinetics

IV: Onset 1-2 min, duration 20-90 min

IM: Onset 10 min, duration 20-90 min

SC: Onset 5-10 min, duration 20-90 min

Pharmacologic effect terminated principally by uptake into tissues and urinary excretion

INDICATIONS AND USES: Acute hypotensive states associated with spinal anesthesia, hemorrhage, reactions to medications, surgical complications; shock associated with brain damage resulting from trauma or tumor; "probably effective" in hypotension due to cardiogenic shock or septicemia

DOSAGE

Adult

- SC/IM 2-10 mg; IV INF dilute 15-500 mg in 500 ml of D_5W or normal saline, administer at a rate adjusted to maintain desired blood pressure; IV 0.5-5 mg as a single dose in severe shock

Child

- SC/IM 0.1 mg/kg or 3 mg/m^2, IV INF 0.4 mg/kg or 12 mg/m^2, diluted and administered at a rate adjusted to maintain desired blood pressure; IV 0.01 mg/kg or 0.3 mg/m^2 as a single dose in severe shock

$ AVAILABLE FORMS/COST OF THERAPY

- Inj, Sol—IM; IV; SC: 10 mg/ml, 10 ml: **$11.85-$126.38**

CONTRAINDICATIONS: Hypersensitivity, use with cyclopropane or halothane anesthesia

PRECAUTIONS: Prolonged administration, heart disease, thyroid disease, hypertension, diabetes, cirrhosis, extravasation (phentolamine is antidote), history of malaria, sulfite sensitivity

PREGNANCY AND LACTATION: Pregnancy category D; use could cause reduced uterine blood flow and fetal hypoxia

SIDE EFFECTS/ADVERSE REACTIONS

CNS: Headache, tremors, dizziness, apprehension

CV: ***Sinus tachycardia, ventricular tachycardia, other dysrhythmias,*** hypertension, hypotension (following cessation), ***cardiac arrest,*** palpitation, flushing

GI: Nausea

SKIN: Sweating, extravasation (abscess, tissue necrosis, sloughing at inj site)

▼ **DRUG INTERACTIONS**

Drugs

- *MAOIs+:* Severe hypertensive response
- *Cyclopropane or halothane anesthesia:* Increased cardiac irritability and risk of dysrhythmia

SPECIAL CONSIDERATIONS

MONITORING PARAMETERS

- Blood pressure, heart rate, central venous pressure
- Maximum effect is not immediately apparent, allow at least 10 min to elapse before increasing the dose

metaxalone

(me-tax-a'lone)

Skelaxin

Chemical Class: Oxazolidinone derivative

Therapeutic Class: Skeletal muscle relaxant

CLINICAL PHARMACOLOGY

Mechanism of Action: Mechanism of action unknown, but may be due to general CNS depression; has no direct action on contractile mechanism of striated muscle, the motor endplate, or nerve fiber

Pharmacokinetics

PO: Peak 2 hr, onset 1 hr, duration 4-6 hr, metabolites excreted in urine, $t_{1/2}$ 2-3 hr

INDICATIONS AND USES: Acute, painful musculoskeletal conditions

DOSAGE

Adult and Child >12 yr

- PO 800 mg tid-qid

$ **AVAILABLE FORMS/COST OF THERAPY**

- Tab, Uncoated—Oral: 400 mg, 100's: **$36.15**

CONTRAINDICATIONS: Hypersensitivity, tendency to drug-induced hemolytic or other anemia, significantly impaired renal or hepatic function

PRECAUTIONS: Liver function impairment, children

SIDE EFFECTS/ADVERSE REACTIONS

CNS: *Drowsiness,* dizziness, headache, nervousness, irritability

GI: Nausea, vomiting, GI upset, jaundice

HEME: ***Leukopenia, hemolytic anemia***

SKIN: Hypersensitivity reaction (light rash with or without pruritus)

▼ **DRUG INTERACTIONS**

Labs

- *False positive:* Benedict's test, a glucose-specific test will differentiate findings

SPECIAL CONSIDERATIONS

PATIENT/FAMILY EDUCATION

- May cause drowsiness or dizziness, use caution while driving or performing other tasks requiring alertness
- Avoid alcohol
- Notify physician if skin rash or yellowish discoloration of skin or eyes occurs

metformin

(met-for'min)

Glucophage

Chemical Class: Biguanide

Therapeutic Class: Antidiabetic agent

CLINICAL PHARMACOLOGY

Mechanism of Action: Potentiates the effect of insulin by mechanisms not fully understood; does not stimulate pancreatic β-cells to increase secretion of insulin; decreases hepatic glucose production and improves insulin sensitivity by increasing peripheral glucose uptake and utilization

Pharmacokinetics
PO: Extent and rate of absorption reduced by food, peak 2.25 hr, up to 90% of dose eliminated unchanged in urine, some fecal elimination, $t_{1/2}$ 6.2 hr

INDICATIONS AND USES: Non-insulin-dependent diabetes mellitus

DOSAGE

Adult

- PO 500 mg bid, with morning and evening meals, increase by 500 mg at weekly intervals as needed, **or** 850 mg qd with morning meal, increase by 850 mg at 14 day intervals; usual maintenance dose 500 or 850 mg bid-tid with meals; not to exceed 2250 mg/d

$ **AVAILABLE FORMS/COST OF THERAPY**

- Tab, Uncoated—Oral: 500 mg, 100's: **$46.27;** 850 mg, 100's: **$78.66**

CONTRAINDICATIONS: Renal disease/dysfunction, radiologic studies involving parenteral administration of iodinated contrast materials (discontinue temporarily), hypersensitivity, acute or chronic metabolic acidosis including diabetic ketoacidosis

PRECAUTIONS: Hypoxemia, dehydration, hepatic disease, fever, trauma, infection, megaloblastic anemia, thyroid disease

PREGNANCY AND LACTATION: Pregnancy category B; excreted into breast milk

SIDE EFFECTS/ADVERSE REACTIONS

CNS: Headache

GI: Diarrhea, nausea, vomiting, abdominal bloating, flatulence, anorexia, metallic taste

HEME: Megaloblastic anemia (impaired vitamin B_{12} absorption)

METAB: ***Lactic acidosis (diarrhea, severe muscle pain/cramping, shallow and fast breathing, unusual tiredness and weakness, unusual sleepiness),*** hypoglycemia (rare)

SKIN: Rash, dermatitis

▼ **DRUG INTERACTIONS**

Drugs

- *Cimetidine, furosemide, nifedipine:* Increased metformin concentrations

Labs

- *False positive:* Urine ketones

SPECIAL CONSIDERATIONS

PATIENT/FAMILY EDUCATION

- Administer with food
- Avoid alcohol
- Notify physician of diarrhea, severe muscle pain or cramping, shallow and fast breathing, unusual tiredness and weakness, unusual sleepiness (signs of lactic acidosis)

MONITORING PARAMETERS

- Serum vitamin B_{12} concentrations every 1-2 yr during chronic therapy
- Fasting blood glucose, Hgb A_{1c}
- Renal function tests at least annually

---

methacholine

(meth-a-ko'leen)
Provocholine
Chemical Class: β-methyl homolog of acetylcholine
Therapeutic Class: Diagnostic agent

CLINICAL PHARMACOLOGY

Mechanism of Action: Causes bronchoconstriction; when inhaled in a sodium chloride solution, patients with asthma are significantly more sensitive to methacholine-induced bronchoconstriction than are healthy individuals

INDICATIONS AND USES: Diagnosis of bronchial airway hyperreactivity in subjects who do not have clinically apparent asthma (methacholine challenge test)

DOSAGE

Adult and Child >5 yr

- INH 5 inhalations at each of 5 concentrations in ascending order as follows: 0.025 mg/ml, 0.25 mg/ml, 2.5 mg/ml, 10 mg/ml and 25 mg/ml (see monitoring parameters); administer via nebulizer that permits intermittent delivery time of 0.6 sec by either a Y-tube or a breath-actuated timing device; following the procedure, a β-agonist inhalation may be administered to help return FEV_1 to baseline and relieve patient discomfort

$ AVAILABLE FORMS/COST OF THERAPY

- Inh: 100 mg/5 ml, 15 ml: **$52.31**

CONTRAINDICATIONS: Hypersensitivity to parasympathomimetics, repeated challenge tests on the same day, use in patients receiving any β-adrenergic blocking agent

PRECAUTIONS: Epilepsy, cardiovascular disease accompanied by bradycardia, vagotonia, peptic ulcer disease, thyroid disease, urinary tract obstruction, child <5 yr; **for diagnostic purposes only**

PREGNANCY AND LACTATION: Pregnancy category C

SIDE EFFECTS/ADVERSE REACTIONS

CNS: Headache, lightheadedness
EENT: Throat irritation
SKIN: Itching

▼ DRUG INTERACTIONS

Drugs

- *Beta blockers:* Exaggerated response to methacholine challenge, prolonged recovery, poor response to treatment

SPECIAL CONSIDERATIONS

MONITORING PARAMETERS

- FEV_1 3-5 min after administration of each serial concentration; procedure is complete when there is a ≥20% reduction in FEV_1 compared to baseline (positive response) or when 5 inhalations have been administered at each concentration and FEV_1 has been reduced by ≤14% (negative response)

---

methadone

(meth'a-done)
Dolophine, Methadose
Chemical Class: Opiate, synthetic diphenylheptane derivative
Therapeutic Class: Narcotic analgesics
DEA Class: Schedule II

CLINICAL PHARMACOLOGY

Mechanism of Action: Binds to opiate receptors in the CNS causing inhibition of ascending pain pathways, altering the perception of and response to pain

Pharmacokinetics

PO: Onset 30-60 min, prolonged duration compared to parenteral therapy
IM: Onset 10-20 min, peak 30-60 min, duration 4-6 hr (22-48 hr after repeated administration)
SC: Onset 10-20 min, peak 50-90 min, duration 4-6 hr (22-48 hr after repeated administration)
Highly bound to tissue protein, metabolized by liver, eliminated in urine and feces, $t_{1/2}$ 13-47 hr

INDICATIONS AND USES: Severe pain, detoxification and maintenance of opiate dependence

DOSAGE

Adult

- *Pain:* SC/IM 2.5-10 mg q3-4h prn; PO 2.5-10 mg q6h prn; adjust dose according to severity of pain and response/tolerance of patient
- *Detoxification:* PO 15-40 mg/d should suppress withdrawal symptoms, daily reductions of 10-20% usually tolerated; treatment should not exceed 21 days and may not be

repeated earlier than 4 wk after completion of preceding course

• *Maintenance of opiate dependence:* PO 20-120 mg/d

Child

• *Pain:* PO/SC/IM 0.7 mg/kg/d divided q4-6h prn or 0.1-0.2 mg/kg q4-12h prn; max 10 mg/dose

$ AVAILABLE FORMS/COST OF THERAPY

• Conc—Oral: 10 mg/ml, 946 ml: **$69.99-$85.00**

• Sol—Oral: 1 mg/ml, 500 ml: **$27.93** 10 mg/5 ml, 500 ml: **$48.38**

• Tab, Uncoated—Oral: 5 mg, 100's: **$7.91-$8.68;** 10 mg, 100's: **$12.95-$14.10;** 40 mg, 100's: **$32.81-$35.69**

• Inj, Sol—IM; SC: 10 mg/ml, 1 ml: **$0.56-$1.97**

CONTRAINDICATIONS: Hypersensitivity, acute bronchial asthma, upper airway obstruction

PRECAUTIONS: Head injury, increased intracranial pressure, acute abdominal conditions, elderly, severe impairment of hepatic or renal function, hypothyroidism, Addison's disease, prostatic hypertrophy, urethral stricture, history of drug abuse

PREGNANCY AND LACTATION: Pregnancy category B (category D if used for prolonged periods or in high doses at term); compatible with breast feeding if mother consumes ≤20 mg/24 hr

SIDE EFFECTS/ADVERSE REACTIONS

CNS: Drowsiness, sedation, dizziness, agitation, dependency, lethargy, restlessness

GI: Nausea, vomiting, anorexia, constipation

RESP: ***Respiratory depression, respiratory paralysis***

CV: Bradycardia, palpitations, orthostatic hypotension, tachycardia

GU: Urinary retention

SKIN: Flushing, rash, urticaria, *excessive sweating*

▼ DRUG INTERACTIONS

Drugs

• *Barbiturates:* Additive CNS depression

• *Carbamazepine, phenytoin, rifampin:* Reduced serum methadone concentrations; increased symptoms associated with narcotic withdrawal

• *Cimetidine:* Increased effect of narcotic analgesics

• *Ethanol:* Additive CNS effects

• *Neuroleptics:* Hypotension and excessive CNS depression

Labs

• *Increase:* Amylase

SPECIAL CONSIDERATIONS

When used for the treatment of narcotic addiction in detoxification or maintenance programs, can only be dispensed by approved hospital pharmacies, approved community pharmacies, and maintenance programs approved by the Food and Drug Administration and the designated state authority

PATIENT/FAMILY EDUCATION

• Report any symptoms of CNS changes, allergic reactions

• Physical dependency may result when used for extended periods

• Change position slowly, orthostatic hypotension may occur

• Avoid hazardous activities if drowsiness or dizziness occurs

• Avoid alcohol, other CNS depressants unless directed by physician

• Minimize nausea by administering with food and remain lying down following dose

M

methamphetamine

(meth-am-fet′a-meen)
Desoxyn
Chemical Class: Amphetamine
Therapeutic Class: Cerebral stimulant
DEA Class: Schedule II

CLINICAL PHARMACOLOGY
Mechanism of Action: Increases release of norepinephrine from central noradrenergic neurons, at higher doses dopamine may be released in the mesolimbic system
Pharmacokinetics
PO: Duration 8-24 hr, metabolized in liver to amphetamine (4%-7%) and other metabolites, eliminated in urine, $t_{1/2}$ 12-34 hr
INDICATIONS AND USES: Short-term adjunct to caloric restriction in exogenous obesity **(high potential for abuse, use only when alternative therapies have failed),** attention deficit disorder with hyperactivity
DOSAGE
Adult
• *Obesity:* PO 5 mg 30 min before each meal; SR PO 10-15 mg qAM; treatment duration should not exceed a few weeks
Child
• *Attention deficit disorder with hyperactivity:* PO 5 mg qd-bid initially, increase in increments of 5 mg/d at weekly intervals until an optimum response is achieved, usual effective dose 20-25 mg/d
$ AVAILABLE FORMS/COST OF THERAPY
• Tab, Uncoated—Oral: 5 mg, 100's: **$66.70**
• Tab, Uncoated, Sust Action—Oral: 5 mg, 100's: **$179.06;** 10 mg, 100's: **$240.62;** 15 mg, 100's: **$306.96**

CONTRAINDICATIONS: Hypersensitivity to sympathomimetic amines, hyperthyroidism, moderate to severe hypertension, glaucoma, severe arteriosclerosis, history of drug abuse, cardiovascular disease, agitated states, within 14 days of MAOI administration
PRECAUTIONS: Mild hypertension, child <3 yr, Tourette's disorder, motor and phonic tics
PREGNANCY AND LACTATION: Pregnancy category C; use of amphetamine for medical indications does not pose a significant risk to the fetus for congenital anomalies, mild withdrawal symptoms may be observed in the newborn; illicit maternal use presents significant risks to the fetus and newborn including intrauterine growth retardation, premature delivery and the potential for increased maternal, fetal, and neonatal morbidity; concentrated in breast milk, contraindicated during breast feeding
SIDE EFFECTS/ADVERSE REACTIONS
CNS: Hyperactivity, insomnia, restlessness, talkativeness, dizziness, headache, chills, overstimulation, dysphoria, euphoria, irritability, aggressiveness, tremor, dependence, addiction, dyskinesia, changes in libido, psychotic episodes
CV: Palpitations, tachycardia, hypertension, dysrhythmias, reflex decrease in heart rate, arryhthmias (at larger doses)
GI: Nausea, vomiting, anorexia, dry mouth, diarrhea, constipation, weight loss, metallic taste, cramps
GU: Impotence
METAB: Reversible elevations in serum thyroxine (T_4) with heavy use
SKIN: Urticaria
▼ DRUG INTERACTIONS
Drugs
• *Acetazolamide:* Increased serum

amphetamine concentrations and prolonged amphetamine effects
• *Antidepressants:* Increased effect of amphetamines, clinical evidence lacking
• *Furazolidone+:* Hypertensive reactions
• *Guanadrel, guanethidine:* Inhibition of the antihypertensive response
• *MAOIs+:* Severe hypertensive reactions possible
• *Sodium bicarbonate:* Large doses of sodium bicarbonate inhibit the elimination and increase the effect of amphetamines

Labs

• *Increase:* Plasma corticosteroid
• *Altered:* Urinary steroid

SPECIAL CONSIDERATIONS

PATIENT/FAMILY EDUCATION

• Take early in the day
• Do not discontinue abruptly
• Avoid hazardous activities until stabilized on medication
• Avoid OTC preparations unless approved by physician
• Notify physician if pronounced nervousness, restlessness, insomnia, dizziness, anorexia, dry mouth, or GI disturbances occur

methantheline

(meth-an'tha-leen)

Banthine

Chemical Class: Aminoalcohol ester; quaternary ammonium compound

Therapeutic Class: Gastrointestinal antimuscarinic/antispasmodic

CLINICAL PHARMACOLOGY

Mechanism of Action: Inhibits GI motility and diminishes gastric acid secretion

Pharmacokinetics

PO: Incompletely absorbed from GI tract, excreted mainly in urine as unchanged drug and metabolites, remainder excreted in feces (probably as unabsorbed drug)

INDICATIONS AND USES: Adjunctive treatment of peptic ulcer, uninhibited or reflex neurogenic bladder

DOSAGE

Adult

• *Peptic ulcer:* PO 50-100 mg q6h initially, decrease dose by half for maintenance therapy
• *Neurogenic bladder:* PO 50-100 mg qid, adjust dose according to patient response and tolerance

Child

• PO (<1 mo) 12.5 mg bid, increased to tid if necessary; (1-12 mo) 12.5 mg qid increased to 25 mg qid if necessary; (>12 mo) 12.5-50 mg qid

$ **AVAILABLE FORMS/COST OF THERAPY**

• Tab, Uncoated—Oral: 50 mg, 100's: **$28.93**

M

CONTRAINDICATIONS: Hypersensitivity to anticholinergic drugs, narrow-angle glaucoma, obstructive uropathy, obstructive disease of the GI tract, paralytic ileus, intestinal atony, unstable cardiovascular status in acute hemorrhage, severe ulcerative colitis, toxic megacolon complicating ulcerative colitis, myasthenia gravis

PRECAUTIONS: Hyperthyroidism, CAD, dysrhythmias, CHF, ulcerative colitis, hypertension, hiatal hernia, hepatic disease, renal disease, urinary retention, prostatic hypertrophy, elderly, children, glaucoma

PREGNANCY AND LACTATION: Pregnancy category C; excretion into breast milk unknown, although would be expected to be minimal due to quaternary structure (see also atropine)

SIDE EFFECTS/ADVERSE REACTIONS

CNS: Confusion, stimulation (especially in elderly), headache, insomnia, dizziness, drowsiness, anxiety, weakness, hallucination
CV: Palpitations, tachycardia
EENT: Blurred vision, photophobia, mydriasis, cyclopegia, increased ocular tension
GI: Dry mouth, constipation, ***paralytic ileus,*** heartburn, nausea, vomiting, dysphagia, absence of taste
GU: Hesitancy, retention, impotence
SKIN: Urticaria, rash, pruritus, anhidrosis, fever, allergic reactions

SPECIAL CONSIDERATIONS

PATIENT/FAMILY EDUCATION

- Drug is usually taken 30-60 min before a meal
- Drug may cause drowsiness, dizziness, or blurred vision, use caution while driving or performing other tasks requiring alertness
- Notify physician if eye pain occurs

---

methazolamide

(meth-a-zoe'la-mide)
MZM, Neptazane
Chemical Class: Carbonic anhydrase inhibitor; sulfonamide derivative
Therapeutic Class: Antiglaucoma agent

CLINICAL PHARMACOLOGY

Mechanism of Action: Inhibitory action on carbonic anhydrase decreases the secretion of aqueous humor and results in decreased intraocular pressure

Pharmacokinetics

PO: Onset 2-4 hr, peak 6-8 hr, duration 10-18 hr, partially metabolized in liver, excreted in urine

INDICATIONS AND USES: Adjunctive treatment of open-angle glaucoma, preoperatively in acute angle-closure glaucoma when delay of surgery is desired to lower intraocular pressure

DOSAGE

Adult

- PO 50-100 mg bid-tid

$ AVAILABLE FORMS/COST OF THERAPY

- Tab, Uncoated—Oral: 25 mg, 100's: **$37.14-$53.13;** 50 mg, 100's: **$55.43-$79.30**

CONTRAINDICATIONS: Hypersensitivity to sulfonamides, severe renal disease, severe hepatic disease, hyponatremia, hypokalemia, hyperchloremic acidosis, adrenal-cortical insufficiency, cirrhosis

PRECAUTIONS: Children, severe loss of respiratory capacity, diabetes mellitus, hypercalciuria, gout

PREGNANCY AND LACTATION: Pregnancy category C

SIDE EFFECTS/ADVERSE REACTIONS

CNS: Drowsiness, sedation, headache, confusion, depression, fatigue, lassitude, malaise, irritability, nervousness, excitement, dizziness, vertigo, ***seizures,*** *paresthesia,* ataxia, tremor, flaccid paralysis
EENT: Altered smell, myopia, tinnitus
GI: Anorexia, nausea, vomiting, diarrhea, weight loss, altered taste, constipation, dry mouth, excessive thirst, abdominal distention
GU: Dysuria, crystalluria, renal colic, sulfonamide-like renal lesions, renal calculi, *urinary frequency,* ***hematuria,*** glycosuria, polyuria, phosphaturia
HEME: ***Aplastic anemia, thrombocytopenia, leukopenia, agranulocytosis, hemolytic anemia***
METAB: Hyperglycemia, increased serum uric acid, hypokalemia
MS: Muscular weakness

SKIN: Rash, skin eruptions, ***exfoliative dermatitis,*** urticaria, pruritus, photosensitivity

▼ **DRUG INTERACTIONS**

Drugs

- *Amphetamines:* Increased amphetamine serum concentrations and prolonged effects)
- *Ephedrine:* Increased ephedrine concentrations
- *Methenamine compounds:* Interference with antibacterial activity
- *Phenytoin:* Increased risk of osteomalacia with prolonged use of both agents
- *Quinidine:* Alkalinization of urine increases quinidine concentrations
- *Salicylates:* Increased concentrations of methazolamide leading to CNS toxicity

Labs

- *Increase:* Blood glucose levels, bilirubin, blood ammonia, calcium, chloride
- *Decrease:* Urine citrate, serum potassium
- *False positive:* Urinary protein, 17-OHCS

SPECIAL CONSIDERATIONS

PATIENT/FAMILY EDUCATION

- Take with food if GI upset occurs
- Avoid prolonged exposure to sunlight or sunlamps
- Drug may cause drowsiness, use caution driving or performing other tasks requiring alertness
- Notify physician of sore throat, fever, unusual bleeding or bruising, tingling or tremors in the hands or feet, flank or loin pain, skin rash

MONITORING PARAMETERS

- CBC and platelet counts at baseline and at regular intervals during therapy
- Serum electrolytes periodically

methenamine

(meth-en'a-meen)

Hiprex, Hip-Rex, 🍁 Urex, Mandameth, Mandelamine

Chemical Class: Formaldehyde precursor

Therapeutic Class: Urinary antiinfective

CLINICAL PHARMACOLOGY

Mechanism of Action: Hydrolyzed by acids to form formaldehyde and ammonia; formaldehyde is a nonspecific antibacterial agent which is bactericidal in action; acid portions of methenamine salts (hippuric acid, mandelic acid) have some nonspecific bacteriostatic activity and may enhance liberation of formaldehyde by maintaining urinary acidity

Pharmacokinetics

PO: Peak formaldehyde concentrations in acid urine in 2-8 hr, some hepatic metabolism (10%-25%), 70%-90% excreted unchanged in urine, $t_{1/2}$ 3-6 hr

INDICATIONS AND USES: Prophylaxis or suppression of recurrent UTI **(should not be used alone for acute infections)**

DOSAGE

Adult

- *Hippurate:* PO 1 g bid
- *Mandelate:* PO 1 g qid, ac and hs

Child 6-12 yr

- *Hippurate:* PO 25-50 mg/kg/d divided q12h
- *Mandelate:* PO 50-75 mg/kg/d divided q6h

$ **AVAILABLE FORMS/COST OF THERAPY**

- Tab, Uncoated (hipurrate)—Oral: 1 g, 100's: **$102.60-$103.62**
- Granule, Reconst (mandelate)—Oral: 1 g/pk, 56 pk: **$60.40**
- Susp (mandelate)—Oral: 250

M

mg/5 ml, 480 ml: **$53.88;** 500 mg/5 ml: **$37.50-$76.20**

• Tab, Enteric Coated (mandelate)—Oral: 500 mg, 100's: **$5.25-$31.36;** 1 g 100's: **$6.95-$50.12**

CONTRAINDICATIONS: Hypersensitivity, renal insufficiency, severe hepatic impairment (hippurate), severe dehydration (hippurate)

PRECAUTIONS: Tartrazine sensitivity (Hiprex tablets), patients susceptible to lipoid pneumonitis (mandelate susp)

PREGNANCY AND LACTATION: Pregnancy category C; excreted into breast milk, no adverse effects on nursing infants have been reported

SIDE EFFECTS/ADVERSE REACTIONS

CNS: Headache

CV: Edema

EENT: Tinnitus

GI: Nausea, vomiting, diarrhea, abdominal cramps, anorexia, stomatitis, transient elevations in serum AST and ALT (hippurate)

GU: Dysuria, hematuria

MS: Muscle cramps

RESP: Dyspnea, lipoid pneumonitis (mandelate suspension)

SKIN: Rash, pruritus, urticaria

▼ **DRUG INTERACTIONS**

Labs

• *Interfere:* VMA, urinary catecholamines

• *False decrease:* Urine estriol, 5HIAA

• *False increase:* 17-OHCS

SPECIAL CONSIDERATIONS

PATIENT/FAMILY EDUCATION

• Keep urine acidic (pH <5.5) by eating food that acidifies urine (meats, eggs, fish, gelatin products, prunes, plums, cranberries); may need to add ascorbic acid

• Fluids must be increased to 3 L/d to avoid crystallization in kidneys

• Take at evenly spaced intervals around clock for best results

MONITORING PARAMETERS:

• Periodic liver function tests (hippurate); urine pH

methicillin

(meth-i-sill'in)

Staphcillin

Chemical Class: Semisynthetic penicillinase-resistant penicillin

Therapeutic Class: Antibiotic

CLINICAL PHARMACOLOGY

Mechanism of Action: Inhibits biosynthesis of cell wall mucopeptide in susceptible organisms; the cell wall, rendered osmotically unstable, swells and bursts from osmotic pressure; bacteriocidal when adequate concentrations are reached; resistant to inactivation by most staphylococcal penicillinases

Pharmacokinetics

IM: Peak 30-60 min, duration 4 hr

IV: Peak 15 min, duration 2 hr

30%-50% bound to plasma proteins, not metabolized to any appreciable extent, excreted in urine, $t_{1/2}$ 0.4-.5 hr (normal renal function)

INDICATIONS AND USES: Infections of the upper and lower respiratory tract, skin and skin structures, bones and joints, urinary tract, meningitis, septicemia and endocarditis caused by penicillinase-producing staphylococci; perioperative prophylaxis*

Antibacterial spectrum usually includes: gram positive organisms: Penicillinase-producing and non-penicillinase-producing strains of *Staphylococus aureus, S. epidermis, S. saprophyticus;* groups A, B, C, and G streptococci, *Streptococcus pneumoniae,* some viridans streptococci, *Bacillus anthracis*

DOSAGE

Adult

• IM 1 g q4-6h; IV 1 g q6h

• *Endocarditis/acute or chronic osteomyelitis:* IV 1.5-2 g q4h

• Dose adjustment in renal impairment: Administer q8-12h for CrCl <10 ml/min

Child

• IM/IV 150-200 mg/kg/d divided q6h; 200-400 mg/kg/d divided q4-6h has been used for severe infections; max 12 g/d

$ **AVAILABLE FORMS/COST OF THERAPY**

• Inj, Dry-Sol—IM; IV: 4 g/vial, 1's: **$20.15;** 1 g/vial, 1's: **$5.53**

CONTRAINDICATIONS: Hypersensitivity to penicillins

PRECAUTIONS: Hypersensitivity to cephalosporins, renal insufficiency, prolonged or repeated therapy, neonates

PREGNANCY AND LACTATION: Pregnancy category B; potential exists for modification of bowel flora in nursing infant, allergy/sensitization and interference with interpretation of culture results if fever workup required

SIDE EFFECTS/ADVERSE REACTIONS

CNS: Headache, fever, chills

CV: Phlebitis, thrombophlebitis

GI: Increased AST, ALT

GU: ***Interstitial nephritis, nephropathy, hemorrhagic cystitis***

HEME: ***Eosinophilia, hemolytic anemia, neutropenia, leukopenia, granulocytopenia thrombocytopenia,*** positive Coombs' test

MS: Myalgia

RESP: ***Anaphylaxis***

SKIN: Pain at inj site, sterile abscess at inj site, rash, pruritus

MISC: Serum sickness-like reactions

▼ **DRUG INTERACTIONS**

Drugs

• *Chloramphenicol:* Inhibited antibacterial activity of methicillin, ensure adequate amounts of both agents are given and administer methicillin a few hours before chloramphenicol

• *Methotrexate:* Increased serum methotrexate concentrations

• *Oral contraceptives:* Occasional impairment of oral contraceptive efficacy, consider use of supplementary contraception during cycles in which methicillin is used

• *Tetracyclines:* Inhibited antibacterial activity of methicillin, ensure adequate amounts of both agents are given and administer methicillin a few hours before tetracycline

Labs

• *False positive:* Urine glucose, urine protein

SPECIAL CONSIDERATIONS

MONITORING PARAMETERS

• Urinalysis, BUN, serum creatinine, CBC with differential, periodic liver function tests

M

methimazole

(meth-im'a-zole)

Tapazole

Chemical Class: Thioimidazole derivative

Therapeutic Class: Antithyroid agent

CLINICAL PHARMACOLOGY

Mechanism of Action: Inhibits the synthesis of thyroid hormones by interfering with the incorporation of iodine into tyrosyl residues of thyroglobulin; inhibits the coupling of these iodotyrosyl residues to form iodothyronine; does not inhibit the action of thyroid hormones already formed and present in the thyroid gland and circulation of exogenously administered thyroid hormones

Pharmacokinetics

PO: Peak 1 hr, onset 30-40 min, excreted in urine, $t_{1/2}$ 5-13 hr

INDICATIONS AND USES: Hyperthyroidism, preparation for thyroidectomy or radioactive iodine therapy, thyrotoxic crisis

DOSAGE

Adult

• PO 15-60 mg/d divided q8h initially; 5-30 mg/d maintenance

Child

• PO 0.4 mg/kg/d in 3 divided doses initially; 0.2 mg/kg/d in 3 divided doses maintenance

• Dose adjustment in renal impairment: CrCl 10-50 ml/min, administer 75% of recommended dose; CrCl <10 ml/min, administer 50% of recommended dose

$ AVAILABLE FORMS/COST OF THERAPY

• Tab, Uncoated—Oral: 5 mg, 100's: **$13.35;** 10 mg, 100's: **$21.30**

CONTRAINDICATIONS: Hypersensitivity

PRECAUTIONS: Infection, bone marrow depression, hepatic disease

PREGNANCY AND LACTATION: Pregnancy category D; use smallest possible dose to control maternal disease; excreted into breast milk, compatible with breast feeding

SIDE EFFECTS/ADVERSE REACTIONS

CNS: Paresthesias, neuritis, *headache, vertigo, drowsiness,* neuropathies, CNS stimulation, depression

CV: Edema

GI: Nausea, vomiting, epigastric distress, loss of taste, sialadenopathy, ***hepatitis,*** jaundice

GU: ***Nephritis***

HEME: ***Agranulocytosis, granulocytopenia, thrombocytopenia, aplastic anemia, hypoprothrombinemia, leukopenia***

METAB: Insulin autoimmune syndrome (may result in hypoglycemia coma)

MS: Arthralgia, myalgia

RESP: Interstitial pneumonitis

SKIN: Skin rash, urticaria, pruritis, erythema nodosum, skin pigmentation, ***exfoliative dermatitis,*** lupus-like syndrome

MISC: Splenomegaly, *abnormal hair loss,* lymphadenopathy

▼ DRUG INTERACTIONS

Drugs

Oral anticoagulants+: Reduced hypoprothrombinemic response to oral anticoagulants

SPECIAL CONSIDERATIONS

PATIENT/FAMILY EDUCATION

• Notify physician of fever, sore throat, unusual bleeding or bruising, headache, rash, yellowing of skin, vomiting

MONITORING PARAMETERS

• Thyroid function tests periodically during therapy

---

methocarbamol

(meth-oh-kar'ba-mole)

Marbaxin, Robaxin, Robomol

Chemical Class: Carbamate derivative of guaifenesin

Therapeutic Class: Skeletal muscle relaxant

CLINICAL PHARMACOLOGY

Mechanism of Action: Mechanism of action unknown but may be due to general CNS depression; no direct action on contractile mechanism of striated muscle, motor endplate, or nerve fiber

Pharmacokinetics

PO: Peak 2 hr, onset 30 min, extensively metabolized by liver, excreted in urine and small amounts in feces, $t_{1/2}$ 1-2 hr

INDICATIONS AND USES: Painful musculoskeletal conditions, tetanus

DOSAGE

Adult

• *Musculoskeletal conditions:* PO 1.5 g qid for 2-3 days, then decrease to 4-4.5 g/d in 3-6 divided doses;

IM/IV 1 g q8h, max 3 g/d for 3 consecutive days (unless treating tetanus), may be reinstituted after 2 drug-free days

- *Tetanus:* IV 1-2 g, followed by additional 1-2 g (max 3 g total), repeat with 1-2 g q6h until NG tube or PO therapy possible; total daily dose of up to 24 g may be needed

Child

- *Tetanus:* IV 15 mg/kg/dose or 500 mg/m^2/dose, may repeat q6h prn; max 1.8 g/m^2/d for 3 days only

$ AVAILABLE FORMS/COST OF THERAPY

- Inj, Sol—IM; IV: 100 mg/ml, 10 ml: **$3.52-$7.80**
- Tab, Plain Coated—Oral: 500 mg, 100's: **$6.75-$46.29;** 750 mg, 100's: **$8.93-$66.16**

CONTRAINDICATIONS: Hypersensitivity, known or suspected renal pathology (parenteral)

PRECAUTIONS: Child <12 yr, extravasation, seizure disorder

PREGNANCY AND LACTATION: Pregnancy category C; compatible with breast feeding

SIDE EFFECTS/ADVERSE REACTIONS

CNS: Drowsiness, dizziness, lightheadedness, headache, fever, vertigo, ***seizures*** (IV administration)

CV: Flushing, syncope, hypotension, bradycardia

EENT: Blurred vision, nystagmus, diplopia, conjunctivitis, nasal congestion

GI: Nausea, anorexia, metallic taste, GI upset

HEME: ***Leukopenia*** (rare), small amount of hemolysis (IV administration)

SKIN: Rash, urticaria, pruritus, skin eruptions, extravasation (thrombophlebitis, sloughing, pain at injection site)

MISC: Muscular incoordination

▼ DRUG INTERACTIONS

Labs

- *False increase:* VMA, urinary 5-HIAA

SPECIAL CONSIDERATIONS

PATIENT/FAMILY EDUCATION

- May cause drowsiness, dizziness, or lightheadedness, use caution driving or performing other tasks requiring alertness
- Avoid alcohol
- Urine may darken to brown, black, or green

---

methotrexate

(meth-oh-trex'ate)

Folex PFS, Methotrexate LPF, Rheumatrex Dose Pack

Chemical Class: Folic acid antagonist

Therapeutic Class: Antineoplastic; antiinflammatory; antipsoriatic

CLINICAL PHARMACOLOGY

Mechanism of Action: Reversibly inhibits dihydrofolate reductase, the enzyme that reduces folic acid to tetrahydrofolic acid; limits the availability of one-carbon fragments necessary for synthesis of purines and the conversion of deoxyuridylate to thymidylate in the synthesis of DNA and cell reproduction; also has immunosuppressive activity

Pharmacokinetics

IM/IV: Peak 0.5-2 hr

PO: Peak 1-4 hr

Widely distributed into body tissues, 50% bound to plasma proteins, does not appear to be appreciably metabolized, excreted primarily by kidneys and small amounts in feces, $t_{1/2}$ 2-4 hr

INDICATIONS AND USES: Trophoblastic neoplasms, testicular choriocarcinomas (combination therapy),

M

palliation of acute leukemias, leukemic infiltration into meninges and CSF (intrathecal), severe psoriasis, rheumatoid arthritis, adjunctive therapy of nonmetastatic osteosarcoma, breast cancer, epidermoid cancers of head and neck, lung cancer (especially squamous cell and small cell types), Burkitt's lymphoma, advanced lymphosarcoma, advanced mycosis fungoides, solid tumors,* psoriatic arthritis,* systemic lupus erythematosus,* vasculitis,* dermatomyositis,* polymyositis,* Wegener's granulomatosis,* therapeutic abortion in ectopic pregnancy*

DOSAGE

Adult

- *Trophoblastic neoplasms:* PO/IM 15-30 mg qd for 5 days; repeat 3-5 times as required, with rest periods of one or more weeks interposed between courses
- *Acute lymphoblastic leukemias:* PO 3.3 mg/m^2 in combination with 60 mg/m^2 of prednisone qd for 4-6 wk to induce remission (not drug of choice for induction); IM/PO 20-30 mg/m^2 twice weekly or IV 2.5 mg/kg q14d for maintenance therapy
- *Meningeal leukemia:* IT 12 mg/m^2, max 15 mg at 2-5 day intervals until the cell count of the CSF returns to normal, then 1 additional dose (use preservative-free preparation only)
- *Burkitt's lymphoma:* PO 10-25 mg/d for 4-8 days; usually given as several courses interposed with 7-10 day rest periods
- *Mycosis fungoides:* PO 2.5-10 mg/d for weeks to months; IM 50 mg qwk or 25 mg twice weekly
- *Psoriasis:* PO/IM/IV 10-25 mg qwk or PO 2.5 mg q12h for 3 doses each wk; adjust gradually to achieve optimal clinical response; max 30 mg/wk; once response achieved reduce to lowest possible effective dose
- *Rheumatoid arthritis:* PO 7.5 mg qwk or 2.5 mg q12h for 3 doses each wk; adjust gradually to achieve an optimal response; max 20 mg/wk; once response achieved reduce to lowest possible effective dose

Child

- *Antineoplastic:* IV 10-33,000 mg/m^2 bolus dosing or continuous inf over 6-42 hr
- *Acute lymphoblastic leukemias:* Same as adult
- *Meningeal leukemia:* IT (≤3 months) 3 mg, (4-11 months) 6 mg, (1 yr) 8 mg, (2 yr) 10 mg at 2-5 day intervals until the cell count of the CSF returns to normal, then 1 additional dose (use preservative-free preparation only)
- *Rheumatoid arthritis:* PO/IM 5-15 mg/m^2/wk as a single dose or in 3 divided doses given 12 h apart

$ AVAILABLE FORMS/COST OF THERAPY

- Inj, Sol—Intra-Articular; IM; IV: 2.5 mg/ml, 2 ml: **$78.75**
- Inj, Sol—IM; IV: 25 mg/ml, 25, 50 mg: **$4.75-$13.94;** 100 mg/vial, 100 mg: **$3.02-$25.64;** 200 mg/vial, 200 mg: **$5.91;** 250 mg/vial, 10 ml: **$20.48-$673.13;** 1 g/vial, 1 g: **$61.44**
- Inj, Lyphl-Sol—Intrathecal: 20 mg/vial, 20 mg: **$2.78**
- Tab, Uncoated—Oral: 2.5 mg, 100's: **$299.39-$404.09**

CONTRAINDICATIONS: Hypersensitivity, severe renal or hepatic impairment, pre-existing profound bone marrow depression

PRECAUTIONS: Infection, peptic ulcer, ulcerative colitis, elderly, preexisting bone marrow suppression, renal or hepatic impairment, ascites, pleural effusion, dehydration

PREGNANCY AND LACTATION: Pregnancy category D; contraindicated in breast feeding

SIDE EFFECTS/ADVERSE REACTIONS

CNS: Heachache, drowsiness, dizziness, malaise, ***seizures***

EENT: Blurred vision, eye discomfort, tinnitus

GI: Gingivitis, glossitis, pharyngitis, *stomatitis,* enteritis, ulcerations and ***bleeding of the mucous membranes of the mouth or other portion of the GI tract,*** abdominal distress, *anorexia, nausea, vomiting,* hematemesis, diarrhea, melena, ***hepatotoxicity***

GU: Urinary retention, ***renal failure,*** menstrual irregularities, defective spermatogenesis, ***hematuria, azotemia, uric acid nephropathy***

HEME: ***Leukopenia, thrombocytopenia, anemia, hemorrhage, pancytopenia***

METAB: Increased serum uric acid

MS: Arthralgia, myalgia, osteoporosis

RESP: ***Pneumonitis, pulmonary fibrosis***

SKIN: Erythematous rashes, alopecia, pruritus, dermatitis, urticaria, folliculitis, vasculitis, photosensitivity, depigmentation, hyperpigmentation, petechiae, ecchymoses, telangiectasia, acne, furunculosis

MISC: Effects following IT (headache, back pain, nuchal rigidity, fever, paresis, leukoencephalopathy)

▼ **DRUG INTERACTIONS**

Drugs

- *Binding resins:* Reduced methotrexate concentrations
- *Co-trimoxazole, NSAIDs, omeprazole, penicillins, probenecid+, salicylates+:* Increased methotrexate concentrations; possible toxicity
- *Cyclosporine:* Increased toxicity of both agents
- *Phenytoin:* Reduced plasma phenytoin concentrations
- *Vaccines+:* Increased risk of infection following use of live vaccines; reduced seroconversion rate to vaccine

SPECIAL CONSIDERATIONS

PATIENT/FAMILY EDUCATION

- Notify physician of black, tarry stools, chills, fever, sore throat, bleeding, bruising, cough, shortness of breath, dark or bloody urine
- Hair may be lost during treatment
- Drink 10-12 glasses of fluid/day
- Avoid alcohol, salicylates

MONITORING PARAMETERS

- CBC with differential, platelet count, withhold drug if WBC is $<3500/mm^3$ or platelet count is $<100{,}000/mm^3$
- BUN, serum uric acid, urine ClCr, electrolytes before, during therapy
- Liver function tests before and during therapy

M

methotrimeprazine

(meth-oh-trye-mep′ra-zeen)

Levoprome, Nozinan ✤

Chemical Class: Propylamino derivative of phenothiazine

Therapeutic Class: Analgesic; anxiolytic, sedative

CLINICAL PHARMACOLOGY

Mechanism of Action: Depresses subcortical area of the brain at the levels of the thalamus, hypothalamus, and reticular and limbic systems; suppresses sensory impulses, reduces motor activity, alters temperature regulation, causes sedation and tranquilization; appears to have some analgesic effects possibly by raising pain threshold

Pharmacokinetics

IM: Onset of analgesia 20-40 min, duration 4 hr, metabolized in liver, excreted primarily in urine and feces (metabolites)

INDICATIONS AND USES: Sedative, moderate to severe pain in nonambulatory patients, preoperative sedation, analgesia and sedation during labor

DOSAGE

Adult

• *Analgesia:* IM 10-20 mg q4-6h; max 40 mg/dose

• *Preoperative sedation:* IM 2-20 mg 0.75-3 hr prior to surgery

• *Labor:* IM 15-20 mg

$ AVAILABLE FORMS/COST OF THERAPY

• Inj, Sol—IM: 20 mg/ml, 10 ml: **$226.89**

CONTRAINDICATIONS: Hypersensitivity to phenothiazines; severe renal, cardiac, or hepatic disease; seizure disorders; coma; during overdoses of CNS depressants, child <12 yr

PRECAUTIONS: Ambulatory patients (can cause substantial orthostatic hypotension), elderly, hypotension, use for >30 days, sulfite sensitivity

PREGNANCY AND LACTATION: Pregnancy category C; does not affect force, duration, and frequency of uterine contractions during labor

SIDE EFFECTS/ADVERSE REACTIONS

CNS: Drowsiness, excessive sedation, amnesia, disorientation, euphoria, headache, weakness, slurred speech, extrapyramidal reactions, ***seizures***

CV: Orthostatic hypotension (fainting, weakness, dizziness), palpitation, tachycardia, bradycardia

EENT: Nasal congestion, blurred vision

GI: Abdominal discomfort, dry mouth, nausea, vomiting, anorexia, ***hepatotoxicity,*** jaundice

GU: ***Hematuria,*** dysuria, hesitancy, retention, uterine inertia (rare)

HEME: ***Thrombocytopenia, agranulocytosis, leukopenia, neutropenia, hemolytic anemia*** (long-term, high dose)

RESP: Respiratory depression

SKIN: Pain at inj site

▼ DRUG INTERACTIONS

Drugs

• MAOIs: Coadministration with pargyline associated with fatality in 1 reported case

SPECIAL CONSIDERATIONS

MONITORING PARAMETERS

• CBC with differential and platelets, liver function tests during prolonged therapy

---

methoxamine

(meth-ox'a-meen)

Vasoxyl

Chemical Class: Synthetic sympathomimetic

Therapeutic Class: Vasopressor

CLINICAL PHARMACOLOGY

Mechanism of Action: Constricts resistance and, to a lesser degree, capacitance blood vessels by effects on α-adrenergic receptors; has virtually no stimulant effect on β-adrenergic receptors

Pharmacokinetics

IV: Onset immediate, peak 0.5-2 min, duration 5-15 min

IM: Peak 15-20 min, duration 60-90 min

Metabolic fate and route of excretion unknown

INDICATIONS AND USES: Hypotension during anesthesia, supraventricular paroxysmal tachycardia, hypotension and shock,* diagnosis of heart murmurs*

DOSAGE

Adult

• *During spinal anesthesia:* IM

10-20 mg shortly before or with spinal anesthesia, repeat prn
• *Emergencies:* IV 3-5 mg injected slowly
• *Supraventricular tachycardia:* IV 10 mg injected slowly

$ AVAILABLE FORMS/COST OF THERAPY

• Inj, Sol—IM; IV: 20 mg/ml, 1 ml ampul: **$22.19**

CONTRAINDICATIONS: Severe hypertension, hypersensitivity

PRECAUTIONS: Children, hypovolemia, extravasation (phentolamine can be used as antidote), hyperthyroidism, bradycardia, partial heart block, myocardial disease, severe arteriosclerosis, sulfite sensitivity

PREGNANCY AND LACTATION: Pregnancy category C; could reduce uterine blood flow, thereby producing fetal hypoxia and bradycardia; may also interact with oxytocics or ergot derivatives to produce severe persistent maternal hypertension; ephedrine may be a more suitable pressor agent

SIDE EFFECTS/ADVERSE REACTIONS

CNS: Headache (often severe), anxiety
CV: Excessive blood pressure elevation, ventricular ectopic beats
GI: Nausea, vomiting (often projectile)
GU: Uterine hypertonus, fetal bradycardia, urinary urgency
SKIN: Sweating, pilomotor response

▼ DRUG INTERACTIONS

Drugs

• *Halogenated hydrocarbon anesthetics:* Sensitization of myocardium to effects of catecholamines; serious dysrhythmia possible
• *Oxytocic drugs:* Severe persistent hypertension

Labs

• *Increase:* Plasma cortisol, ACTH

SPECIAL CONSIDERATIONS

MONITORING PARAMETERS

• Blood pressure, ECG

methoxsalen

(meth-ox'a-len)
8-Mop, Oxsoralen, Oxsoralen Ultra
Chemical Class: Psoralen derivative
Therapeutic Class: Pigmenting agent; antipsoriatic

CLINICAL PHARMACOLOGY

Mechanism of action: Exact mechanism unknown; may involve increased tyrosinase activity in melanin-producing cells, as well as inhibition of DNA synthesis, cell division, and epidermal turnover; successful pigmentation requires the presence of functioning melanocytes

Pharmacokinetics

PO: Peak serum concentration 1.5-6 hr (hard gelatin capsule), 0.5-4 hr (soft gelatin capsule); peak photosensitivity 3.9-4.25 hr (hard capsule), 1.5-2.1 hr (soft capsule); duration approximately 8 hr; highly protein bound; activated by long-wavelength ultraviolet light (UVA), further metabolized by liver; eliminated mainly in urine as metabolites; $t_{1/2}$ 1.1 hr (hard capsule), 2 hr (soft capsule)

INDICATIONS AND USES: Severe, refractory, disabling psoriasis, in conjunction with UVA—treatment known as PUVA (psoralen plus ultraviolet light A); repigmentation in the treatment of vitiligo (PUVA); cutaneous T-cell lymphoma (in conjunction with photopheresis with the UVAR instrument)

DOSAGE

Adult

• *Psoriasis:* PO (hard caps) admin-

M

ister 2 hr before UVA exposure, separate doses by at least 48 hr, (<30 kg) 10 mg, (30-50 kg) 20 mg, (51-65 kg) 30 mg, (66-80 kg) 40 mg, (81-90 kg) 50 mg, (91-115 kg) 60 mg, (>115 kg) 70 mg; (soft caps) administer 2 hr before UVA exposure, separate doses by at least 48 hr, (<30 kg) 10 mg, (30-50) kg) 10-20 mg, (51-65 kg) 20-30 mg, (66-80 kg) 20-40 mg, (81-90 kg) 30-50 mg, (91-115 kg) 30-60 mg, (>115 kg) 40-70 mg

• *Vitilgo:* PO 20 mg 2-4 hr before measured periods of UVA exposure, 2-3 times/wk (at least 48 hr apart); TOP apply to small, well defined lesion, then expose to UVA light once/wk or less depending on results

• *Cutaneous T-cell lymphoma:* PO (hard capsules) 0.6 mg/kg administered 2 hr before obtaining blood for extracorporeal exposure of extracted leukocytes to high-intensity UVA light

$ AVAILABLE FORMS/COST OF THERAPY

• Cap, Gel—Oral: 10 mg, 50's: **$219.69** (soft caps); **$219.69** (hard caps)

• Lotion—Top: 1%, 30 ml: **$88.75 (do not dispense to patient)**

CONTRAINDICATIONS: Hypersensitivity to psoralens, diseases associated with photosensitivity, melanoma, invasive squamous cell carcinoma, aphakia (oral)

PRECAUTIONS: Hard and soft caps not equivalent, cardiac disease, hepatic disease, children <12 yr, contains tartrazine (FD&C #5), photosensitizing agents

PREGNANCY AND LACTATION: Pregnancy category C

SIDE EFFECTS/ADVERSE REACTIONS

CNS: Nervousness, insomnia, psychological depression, dizziness, headache, malaise

CV: Edema, hypotension

EENT: Cataract formation

GI: Nausea

MS: Leg cramps

SKIN: ***Severe burns,*** basal cell epitheliomas, hypopigmentation, vesiculation and bullae formation, nonspecific rash, herpes simplex, urticaria, folliculitis, cutaneous tenderness, extension of psoriasis, *pruritus, erythema*

▼ DRUG INTERACTIONS

Drugs

• *Anthralin, coal tar, griseofulvin, phenothiazines, nalidixic acid, halogenated salicylanilides, sulfonamides, tetracyclines, thiazides:* Increased photosensitivity

SPECIAL CONSIDERATIONS

PATIENT/FAMILY EDUCATION

• Do not sunbathe during 24 hr prior to methoxsalen ingestion and UVA exposure

• Wear UVA-absorbing sunglasses for 24 hr following treatment to prevent cataract

• Avoid sun exposure for at least 8 hr after methoxsalen ingestion

• Take with food or milk

• Avoid furocoumarin-containing foods (e.g. limes, figs, parsley, parsnips, mustard, carrots, celery)

• Repigmentation may require 6-9 mo

methscopolamine

(meth-skoe-pol'a-meen)

Pamine

Chemical Class: Synthetic quaternary ammonium antimuscarinic

Therapeutic Class: Gastrointestinal antimuscarinic/antispasmodic

CLINICAL PHARMACOLOGY

Mechanism of Action: Inhibits GI

motility and diminishes gastric acid secretion

Pharmacokinetics

PO: Incompletely absorbed from GI tract, excreted mainly in urine as unchanged drug and metabolites, remainder excreted in feces (probably as unabsorbed drug)

INDICATIONS AND USES: Adjunctive treatment of peptic ulcer

DOSAGE

Adult

• PO 2.5-5 mg ½ hr ac, hs

Child

• PO 0.2 mg/kg or 6 mg/m^2 daily, given in 4 equally divided doses

$ **AVAILABLE FORMS/COST OF THERAPY**

• Tab, Uncoated—Oral: 2.5 mg, 100's: **$30.80**

CONTRAINDICATIONS: Hypersensitivity to anticholingeric drugs, narrow-angle glaucoma, obstructive uropathy, obstructive disease of the GI tract, paralytic ileus, intestinal atony, unstable cardiovascular status in acute hemorrhage, severe ulcerative colitis, toxic megacolon complicating ulcerative colitis, myasthenia gravis

PRECAUTIONS: Hyperthyroidism, CAD, dysrhythmias, CHF, ulcerative colitis, hypertension, hiatal hernia, hepatic disease, renal disease, urinary retention, prostatic hypertrophy, elderly, children, glaucoma

PREGNANCY AND LACTATION: Pregnancy category C; excretion into breast milk unknown, although would be expected to be minimal due to quaternary structure (see also atropine)

SIDE EFFECTS/ADVERSE REACTIONS

CNS: Confusion, stimulation (especially in elderly), headache, insomnia, dizziness, drowsiness, anxiety, weakness, hallucination

CV: Palpitations, tachycardia

EENT: Blurred vision, photophobia, mydriasis, cycloplegia, increased ocular tension

GI: Dry mouth, constipation, ***paralytic ileus,*** heartburn, nausea, vomiting, dysphagia, absence of taste

GU: Hesitancy, retention, impotence

SKIN: Urticaria, rash, pruritus, anhidrosis, fever, allergic reactions

SPECIAL CONSIDERATIONS

PATIENT/FAMILY EDUCATION

• Drug is usually taken 30-60 min before a meal

• Drug may cause drowsiness, dizziness, or blurred vision, use caution while driving or performing other tasks requiring alertness

• Notify physician if eye pain occurs

M

---

methsuximide

(meth-sux'i-mide)

Celontin

Chemical Class: Succinimide derivative

Therapeutic Class: Anticonvulsant

CLINICAL PHARMACOLOGY

Mechanism of Action: Increases the seizure threshold and suppresses paroxysmal spike-and-wave pattern in absence seizures; depresses nerve transmission in the motor cortex

Pharmacokinetics

PO: Peak 1-3 hr, rapidly demethylated in liver to N-desmethylmethsuximide (active), excreted in urine (metabolites), $t_{1/2}$ 2-4 hr (N-desmethylmethsuximide 26-80 hr)

INDICATIONS AND USES: Refractory absence (petit mal) seizures

DOSAGE

Adult

• PO 300 mg/d for first wk; may increase by 300 mg/d at weekly intervals up to 1.2 g/d divided bid-qid

Child

• PO 10-15 mg/kg/d divided tid-qid initially; increase weekly up to max of 30 mg/kg/d

$ AVAILABLE FORMS/COST OF THERAPY

• Cap, Gel—Oral: 150 mg, 100's: **$39.71;** 300 mg, 100's: **$70.40**

CONTRAINDICATIONS: Hypersensitivity to succinimides

PRECAUTIONS: Hepatic/renal function impairment, abrupt withdrawal

PREGNANCY AND LACTATION: Pregnancy category C

SIDE EFFECTS/ADVERSE REACTIONS

CNS: Drowsiness, ataxia, dizziness, irritability, nervousness, headache, euphoria, dream-like state, lethargy, hyperactivity, fatigue, insomnia, confusion, instability, mental slowness, depression, hypochondriacal behavior, night terrors, aggressiveness, inability to concentrate

EENT: Blurred vision, myopia, photophobia, periorbital edema

GI: Nausea, vomiting, vague gastric upset, cramps, *anorexia,* diarrhea, weight loss, epigastric and abdominal pain, constipation, swelling of tongue

GU: Urinary frequency, ***renal damage,*** vaginal bleeding, microscopic hematuria

HEME: ***Eosinophilia, granulocytopenia, leukopenia, agranulocytosis, monocytosis, pancytopenia***

MS: Muscle weakness

SKIN: Pruritus, urticaria, ***Stevens-Johnson syndrome,*** pruritic erythematous rashes, skin eruptions, erythema multiforme, systemic lupus erythematosus, alopecia, hirsutism

▼ DRUG INTERACTIONS

Drugs

• *Hydantoins:* Increased serum hydantoin concentrations

• *Primidone:* Reduced primidone and phenobarbital concentrations

Labs

• *Increase:* Coombs' test

SPECIAL CONSIDERATIONS

PATIENT/FAMILY EDUCATION

• Take with food or milk

• Do not discontinue abruptly

• Drug may cause drowsiness, use caution driving or performing other tasks requiring alertness

• Notify physician of skin rash, joint pain, unexplained fever, sore throat, unusual bleeding or bruising, drowsiness, dizziness, blurred vision

MONITORING PARAMETERS

• CBC with differential liver enzymes

• Serum N-desmethylmethsuximide concentrations at trough for efficacy (range 10-40 μg/ml) and 3 hr postdose for toxicity (range >40 μg/ml)

---

methyclothiazide

(meth-ee-cloh-thye'a-zide)

Enduron, Aquatensen

Chemical Class: Sulfonamide derivative

Therapeutic Class: Antihypertensive; thiazide diuretic

CLINICAL PHARMACOLOGY

Mechanism of Action: Increases urinary excretion of sodium and water by inhibiting sodium reabsorption in the early distal tubules; increases urinary excretion of potassium by increasing potassium secretion in the distal convoluted tubule and collecting ducts; decreases urinary calcium excretion

Pharmacokinetics

PO: Onset 2 hr, peak 6 hr, duration 24 hr, excreted unchanged in urine

INDICATIONS AND USES: Edema associated with CHF, hepatic cirrhosis, corticosteroid and estrogen therapy; hypertension; calcium nephrolithiasis,*osteoporosis*; diabetes insipidus*

DOSAGE

Adult

- *Edema:* PO 2.5-10 mg qd
- *Hypertension:* PO 2.5-5 mg qd

$ AVAILABLE FORMS/COST OF THERAPY

- Tab, Uncoated—Oral: 2.5 mg, 100's: **$7.95-$41.44;** 5 mg, 100's: **$6.21-$109.99**

CONTRAINDICATIONS: Anuria, renal decompensation, hypersensitivity to thiazides or related sulfonamide-derived drugs

PRECAUTIONS: Hypokalemia, renal disease, hepatic disease, gout, COPD, lupus erythematosus, diabetes mellitus, children, vomiting, diarrhea, hyperlipidemia

PREGNANCY AND LACTATION: Pregnancy category D; 1st trimester use may cause an increased risk of congenital defects, use in later trimesters does not seem to carry this risk; other risks to the fetus or newborn include hypoglycemia, thrombocytopenia, hyponatremia, hypokalemia, and death from maternal complications; excreted into breast milk in small amounts, considered compatiblc with breast feeding

SIDE EFFECTS/ADVERSE REACTIONS

CNS: Drowsiness, paresthesia, depression, headache, *dizziness, fatigue, weakness*

CV: Irregular pulse, orthostatic hypotension, palpitations, volume depletion

EENT: Blurred vision

GI: Nausea, vomiting, anorexia, constipation, diarrhea, cramps, pancreatitis, GI irritation, ***hepatitis***

GU: Frequency, polyuria, ***uremia, glucosuria***

HEME: ***Aplastic anemia, hemolytic anemia, leukopenia, agranulocytosis, thrombocytopenia, neutropenia***

METAB: Hyperglycemia, hyperuricemia, increased creatinine, BUN, *hypokalemia,* hypercalcemia, hyponatremia, hypochloremia, hypomagnesemia

SKIN: Rash, urticaria, purpura, photosensitivity, fever

▼ DRUG INTERACTIONS

Drugs

- *Antidiabetics:* Thiazide diuretics tend to increase blood glucose, may increase dosage requirements of antidiabetic drugs
- *Cholestyramine:* Reduced serum concentrations of thiazide diuretics
- *Colestipol:* Reduced serum concentrations of thiazide diuretics
- *Diazoxide:* Hyperglycemia
- *Digitalis glycosides:* Diuretic-induced hypokalemia may increase the risk of digitalis toxicity
- *Lithium+:* Increased serum lithium concentrations, toxicity may occur

Labs

- *Increase:* BSP retention, amylase, parathyroid test
- *Decrease:* PBI, PSP

SPECIAL CONSIDERATIONS

PATIENT/FAMILY EDUCATION

- Take with food or milk
- Drug will increase urination, take early in the day
- Notify physician if muscle pain, weakness, cramps, nausea, vomiting, restlessness, excessive thirst, tiredness, drowsiness, increased heart rate, diarrhea, or dizziness occurs
- Drug may cause sensitivity to sun-

M

light, avoid prolonged exposure to the sun and other UV light

• Drug may cause gout attacks, notify physician if sudden joint pain occurs

MONITORING PARAMETERS

• Serum electrolytes, BUN, creatinine, CBC, uric acid, glucose

methylcellulose

(meth-ill-sell'yoo-lose)

Citrucel

Chemical Class: Hydrophilic semisynthetic cellulose derivative

Therapeutic Class: Bulk laxative

CLINICAL PHARMACOLOGY

Mechanism of Action: Attracts water, expands in intestine to increase peristalsis; also absorbs excess water in stool; decreases diarrhea

Pharmacokinetics

PO: Not absorbed, onset 12-24 hr, full effect may not be apparent for 2-3 days

INDICATIONS AND USES: Constipation

DOSAGE

Adult and Child >12 yr

• PO 1 heaping tbsp in 8 oz cold water, 1-3 times daily

Child

• PO 1 level tbsp in 4 oz cold water, 1-3 times daily

$ AVAILABLE FORMS/COST OF THERAPY

• Powder—Oral: 2 g/heaping tbsp, 480 g: **$7.37**

CONTRAINDICATIONS: Nausea, vomiting or other symptom of appendicitis; acute surgical abdomen; fecal impaction; intestinal obstruction; undiagnosed abdominal pain

PRECAUTIONS: Rectal bleeding; esophageal stricture; intestinal ulcerations, stenosis, or disabling adhesions

PREGNANCY AND LACTATION: Bulk forming laxatives are the laxative of choice during pregnancy; compatible with breast feeding

SIDE EFFECTS/ADVERSE REACTIONS

GI: ***Obstruction,*** abdominal distension

SPECIAL CONSIDERATIONS

PATIENT/FAMILY EDUCATION

• Do not use in presence of abdominal pain, nausea or vomiting

• Notify physician of unrelieved constipation, rectal bleeding

• Assure adequate fluids, proper dietary fiber intake and regular exercise

methyldopa

(meth-ill-doe'pa)

Aldomet, Amodopa, Apo-Methyldopa, ♣ Dopamet, ♣ Novomedopa ♣

Chemical Class: Structurally related to the catecholamines

Therapeutic Class: Antihypertensive

CLINICAL PHARMACOLOGY

Mechanism of Action: Exact mechanism unknown; thought to involve stimulation of central α_2-adrenergic receptors by a metabolite, α-methylnorepinephrine, thus inhibiting sympathetic outflow to the heart, kidneys, and peripheral vasculature; reduced peripheral resistance and plasma renin activity levels may also contribute to its effect

Pharmacokinetics

PO: Peak 3-6 hr

IV (methyldopate): Onset 4-6 hr, duration 10-16 hr

Weakly bound to plasma proteins, extensively metabolized in GI tract and liver, eliminated in urine, $t_{1/2}$ 1-3 hr

INDICATIONS AND USES: Moderate to severe hypertension

DOSAGE

Adult

• PO 250 mg bid-tid, increase q2d prn; usual dose 1-1.5 g/d in 2-4 divided doses, max 3 g/d; IV (methyldopate) 250-1000 mg q6-8h; max 4 g/d

Child

• PO 10 mg/kg/d in 2-4 divided doses; increase q2d prn to max dose of 65 mg/kg/d; do not exceed 3 g/d; IV 2-4 mg/kg/dose; if response not seen within 4-6 hr, may increase to 5-10 mg/kg/dose; administer doses q6-8h; max daily dose 65 mg/kg or 3 g, whichever is less

• Dosing interval in renal impairment: CrCl >50 ml/min q8h; CrCl 10-50 ml/min q8-12h; CrCl <10 ml/min q12-24h

$ **AVAILABLE FORMS/COST OF THERAPY**

• Inj, Sol—IV: 50 mg/ml, 5 ml: **$1.98-$12.53** (methyldopate)

• Tab, Plain Coated—Oral: 125 mg, 100's: **$4.50-$26.89;** 250 mg, 100's: **$6.00-$34.23;** 500 mg, 100's: **$9.38-$62.53**

CONTRAINDICATIONS: Active hepatic disease, hypersensitivity, previous methyldopa-associated liver abnormalities or direct Coombs' positive hemolytic anemia

PRECAUTIONS: History of liver disease, pheochromocytoma, sulfite sensitivity, renal failure

PREGNANCY AND LACTATION: Pregnancy category C; no unusual adverse reactions or obvious teratogenic effects have been reported despite rather wide use during pregnancy; compatible with breast feeding

SIDE EFFECTS/ADVERSE REACTIONS

CNS: Sedation, headache, asthenia or weakness, *dizziness,* lightheadedness, symptoms of cerebrovascular insufficiency, paresthesias, parkinsonism, Bell's palsy, decreased mental acuity, involuntary choreoathetotic movements, psychic disturbances, verbal memory impairment

CV: Bradycardia, prolonged carotid sinus hypersensitivity, aggravation of angina pectoris, paradoxical pressor response, pericarditis, ***myocarditis,*** orthostatic hypotension, edema

EENT: Nasal stuffiness

GI: Nausea, vomiting, distension, constipation, flatus, diarrhea, colitis, mild dry mouth, sore or "black" tongue, pancreatitis, sialadenitis, abnormal liver function tests, jaundice, hepatitis, liver disorders

GU: Impotence, failure to ejaculate, decreased libido

HEME: Positive Coombs' test, ***hemolytic anemia, bone marrow depression, leukopenia, granulocytopenia, thrombocytopenia;*** positive tests for antinuclear antibody, LE cells and rheumatoid factor

METAB: Breast enlargement, gynecomastia, lactation, hyperprolactinemia, amenorrhea, galactorrhea

MS: Arthralgia, myalgia

SKIN: Rash, ***toxic epidermal necrolysis***

MISC: Lupus-like syndrome

▼ **DRUG INTERACTIONS**

Drugs

• *Beta blockers:* Hypertension during periods of catecholamine release

• *Iron:* Inhibited antihypertensive response to methyldopa

• *Lithium:* Lithium toxicity not necessarily associated with excessive lithium concentrations

Labs

• *Interfere:* Urinary uric acid, serum creatinine, AST

M

• *False increase:* Urinary catecholamines

SPECIAL CONSIDERATIONS

PATIENT/FAMILY EDUCATION

• Notify physician of unexplained prolonged general tiredness, fever, or jaundice
• Urine exposed to air after voiding may darken
• Drug may cause drowsiness, use caution driving or performing other activities requiring alertness
• Do not discontinue abruptly

MONITORING PARAMETERS

• CBC, liver function tests periodically during therapy
• Direct Coombs' test before therapy and after 6-12 mo

methylene blue

(meth'i-leen)

Urolene Blue

Chemical Class: Thiazine dye
Therapeutic Class: Antidote, cyanide; antidote, drug induced methemoglobinemia; diagnostic agent

CLINICAL PHARMACOLOGY

Mechanism of Action: In low concentrations, hastens conversion of methemoglobin to hemoglobin; has the opposite effect at high concentrations; in cyanide toxicity, combines with cyanide to form cyanmethemoglobin preventing interference of cyanide with the cytochrome system; directly inhibits calcium binding by oxalate and by organic stone matrix; also acts as a crystal poison at the interface, reducing tendency of calcium oxalate particles to aggregate; possesses weak antiseptic and tissue-staining properties

Pharmacokinetics

PO/IV: Rapidly reduced in tissues to leukomethylene blue, excreted in urine and bile

INDICATIONS AND USES: Methemoglobinemia, cyanide poisoning, urolithiasis (ineffective in dissolving previously formed stones), genitourinary antiseptic, cutaneous viral infections (in conjunction with polychromatic light),* diagnosis of gastroesophageal reflux in infants and children,* delineation of body structures and fistulas through dye effect;* diagnosis of premature rupture of membrane*

DOSAGE

Adult

• IV 1-2 mg/kg or 25-50 mg/m^2 over several min, may be repeated after 1 hr if necessary; PO 65-130 mg tid with a full glass of water

Child

• IV 1-2 mg/kg or 25-50 mg/m^2 over several min, may be repeated after 1 hr if necessary

$ AVAILABLE FORMS/COST OF THERAPY

• Inj, Sol—IV 1%, 1 ml: **$4.50-$8.06**
• Tab, Uncoated—Oral: 65 mg, 100's: **$24.12**

CONTRAINDICATIONS: Hypersensitivity, renal insufficiency, instraspinal inj

PRECAUTIONS: G-6-PD deficiency, prolonged administration

PREGNANCY AND LACTATION: Pregnancy category C (category D if inj intra-amniotically); deep blue staining of the newborn, hemolytic anemia, hyperbilirubinemia, and methemoglobinemia in the newborn may occur after inj into the amniotic fluid

SIDE EFFECTS/ADVERSE REACTIONS

CNS: Dizziness, headache, fever, mental confusion
CV: Precordial pain
GI: Blue-green stool, *nausea, vomiting,* diarrhea, *abdominal pain*

GU: Blue-green urine, bladder irritation
HEME: Methemoglobinemia (large doses)
SKIN: Profuse sweating, stains skin blue (may be removed by hypochlorite solution)

SPECIAL CONSIDERATIONS

PATIENT/FAMILY EDUCATION

- Take oral form after meals with a glass of water
- Drug may discolor urine, and sometimes the stool, blue-green

MONITORING PARAMETERS

- CBC

---

methylergonovine

(meth-ill-er-goe-noe'veen)
Methergine
Chemical Class: Ergot alkaloid
Therapeutic Class: Oxytocic

CLINICAL PHARMACOLOGY

Mechanism of Action: Partial agonist or antagonist at α-adrenergic, dopaminergic, and tryptaminergic receptors; increases the strength, duration, and frequency of uterine contractions and decreases uterine bleeding when used after placental delivery

Pharmacokinetics

IV: Onset immediate, duration 3 hr
IM: Onset 2-5 min, duration 3 hr
PO: Onset 5-10 min, duration 3 hr
Excretion partially renal and partially hepatic, $t_{1/2}$ 20-30 min

INDICATIONS AND USES: Postpartum/postabortal hemorrhage due to uterine atony

DOSAGE

Adult

- IM/IV 0.2 mg after delivery of the placenta, after delivery of the anterior shoulder, or during the puerperium; repeat q2-4h prn; PO 0.2 mg tid-qid in the puerperium for a max of 1 wk

$ AVAILABLE FORMS/COST OF THERAPY

- Inj, Sol—IM;IV: 0.2 mg/ml, 20's: **$55.02**
- Tab, Coated—Oral: 0.2 mg, 100's: **$49.86**

CONTRAINDICATIONS: Hypertension, toxemia, hypersensitivity to ergots

PRECAUTIONS: Rapid IV inf (may induce sudden hypertension and CVAs), sepsis, obliterative vascular disease, hepatic/renal involvement

PREGNANCY AND LACTATION: Pregnancy category C; small quantity appears in breast milk, adverse effects have not been described

SIDE EFFECTS/ADVERSE REACTIONS

CNS: Dizziness, headache
CV: Hypertension, palpitations, temporary chest pain
EENT: Tinnitus
GI: Nausea, vomiting
RESP: Dyspnea
SKIN: Diaphoresis

SPECIAL CONSIDERATIONS

PATIENT/FAMILY EDUCATION

- Report increased blood loss, severe abdominal cramps, increased temperature, or foul-smelling lochia

MONITORING PARAMETERS

- Blood pressure, pulse, and uterine response

---

methylphenidate

(meth-ill-fen'i-date)
Ritalin, Ritalin SR
Chemical Class: Piperidine derivative stimulant
Therapeutic Class: Cerebral stimulant
DEA Class: Schedule II

M

CLINICAL PHARMACOLOGY

Mechanism of Action: Similar to amphetamines; CNS and respiratory stimulation, weak sympathomimetic activity; main sites of CNS activity appear to be the cerebral cortex and subcortical structures including the thalamus; produces an anorexigenic effect, increases motor activity and mental alertness, diminishes sense of fatigue, brightens spirits, and causes mild euphoria

Pharmacokinetics

PO: Peak 1-3 hr (SR 4-7 hr), duration 3-6 hr (SR 8 hr), 80% metabolized to ritalinic acid, excreted in urine

INDICATIONS AND USES: Attention deficit disorders, narcolepsy, depression in elderly, cancer and post-stroke patients*

DOSAGE

Adult

• *Narcolepsy:* PO 10 mg bid-tid, 30-45 min ac, may increase up to 40-60 mg/d

Child ≥6 yr

• *Attention deficit disorder:* PO 0.3 mg/kg/dose or 2.5-5 mg/dose given before breakfast and lunch; increase by 0.1 mg/kg/dose or 5-10 mg/d at weekly intervals; usual dose 0.5-1 mg/kg/d; max 2 mg/kg/d or 60 mg/d

$ AVAILABLE FORMS/COST OF THERAPY

• Tab, Plain Coated, Sust Action—Oral: 20 mg, 100's: **$74.95-$98.41**

• Tab, Uncoated—Oral: 5 mg, 100's: **$23.95-$31.32**; 10 mg, 100's: **$34.95-$44.70;** 20 mg, 100's: **$48.95-$64.30**

CONTRAINDICATIONS: Marked anxiety, tension, and agitation; hypersensitivity; glaucoma, history of Gilles de la Tourette's syndrome

PRECAUTIONS: Severe depression, seizure disorders, hypertension, history of drug abuse, visual disturbances, children <6 yr, symptoms associated with acute stress reactions

PREGNANCY AND LACTATION: Pregnancy category C

SIDE EFFECTS/ADVERSE REACTIONS

CNS: Hyperactivity, insomnia, restlessness, talkativeness, dizziness, headache, akathisia, dyskinesia, Gilles de la Tourette's syndrome, fever

CV: Palpitations, tachycardia, B/P changes, angina, dysrhythmias, ***thrombocytopenic purpura***

GI: Nausea, anorexia, dry mouth, weight loss, abdominal pain

GU: ***Uremia***

HEME: ***Leukopenia, anemia***

METAB: Growth retardation

MS: Arthralgia

SKIN: ***Exfoliative dermatitis,*** urticaria, rash, erythema-multiforme, scalp hair loss

▼ DRUG INTERACTIONS

Drugs

• *Guanethidine:* Inhibition of guanethidine antihypertensive effect

SPECIAL CONSIDERATIONS

PATIENT/FAMILY EDUCATION

• Take early in the day
• Do not discontinue abruptly
• Avoid hazardous activities until stabilized on medication
• Avoid OTC preparations unless approved by physician
• Notify physician if pronounced nervousness, restlessness, insomnia, dizziness, anorexia, dry mouth, or GI disturbances occur
• Do not crush or chew SR formulation

MONITORING PARAMETERS

• Periodic CBC with differential and platelet count

methylprednisolone

(meth-il-pred-niss'oh-lone)

Medrol, depMedalone, Depoject, Depo-Medrol, Depopred, Depo-Predate, Duralone, Medralone, Methylone, Rep-Pred, A-methaPred, Solu-Medrol

Chemical Class: Glucocorticoid
Therapeutic Class: Corticosteroid

CLINICAL PHARMACOLOGY
Mechanism of Action: Controls rate of protein synthesis, depresses migrations of polymorphonuclear leukocytes and fibroblasts, reverses capillary permeability, and causes lysosomal stabilization at the cellular level to prevent or control inflammation

Pharmacokinetics
PO: Peak effect 1-2 hr, duration 30-36 hr
IM (acetate): Peak effect 4-8 days, duration 1-4 wk
Intra-articular: Peak effect 1 wk, duration 1-5 wk
Metabolized in liver, excreted in urine and bile, biologic $t_{1/2}$ 18-36 hr

INDICATIONS AND USES: Anti-inflammatory or immunosuppressant agent in the treatment of a variety of diseases including those of hematologic, allergic, inflammatory, neoplastic, and autoimmune origin

DOSAGE
Adult
• PO 4-48 mg/d initially, adjust until satisfactory response is noted, taper gradually if used continuously for >10 days
• *Sodium succinate:* IM/IV 10-40 mg initially, may repeat q6h prn; for acute spinal cord injury give 30 mg/kg IV over 15 min followed in 45 min by a continuous inf of 5.4 mg/kg/hr for 23 hr
• *Acetate:* IM 40-120 mg q1-2wk; intra-articular/intralesional 4-40 mg, up to 80 mg for large joints, q1-5wk

Child
• PO/IM/IV 0.12-1.7 mg/kg/d or 5-25 mg/m²/d in divided doses q6-12h
• *Status asthmaticus:* IV 2 mg/kg loading dose, then 0.5-1 mg/kg/dose q6h

$ AVAILABLE FORMS/COST OF THERAPY
• Tab, Uncoated—Oral: 4 mg, 21's: **$9.20-$15.87** (dose-pack)
• Tab, Uncoated—Oral: 4 mg, 100's: **$43.82-$97.51;** 16 mg, 50's: **$45.90-$64.14;** 24 mg, 25's: **$37.81;** 32 mg, 25's: **$46.02**
• Inj, Sol (acetate)—IM; intra-articular; intra-lesional: 20 mg/ml, 10 ml: **$6.30-$20.62;** 40 mg/ml, 10 ml: **$6.05-$34.24;** 80 mg/ml, 5 ml: **$6.05-$34.24**
• Inj, Lyphl Sol (sodium succinate)—IM;IV: 40 mg/vial, 1's: **$2.00-$4.00;** 125 mg/vial, 1's: **$7.00-$12.50;** 500 mg/vial, 1's: **$17.03-$30.40;** 1 g/vial, 1's: **$28.89-$51.67**
• Inj, Sol (sodium succinate)—IM; IV: 2 g/vial, 1's: **$54.73**

CONTRAINDICATIONS: Systemic fungal infections, hypersensitivity, idiopathic thrombocytopenic purpura (IM)

PRECAUTIONS: Psychosis, acute glomerulonephritis, amebiasis, cerebral malaria, child <2 yr, elderly, AIDS, tuberculosis, diabetes mellitus, glaucoma, osteoporosis, ulcerative colitis, CHF, myasthenia gravis, renal disease, esophagitis, peptic ulcer, ocular herpes simplex, live virus vaccines, hypertension

PREGNANCY AND LACTATION: Pregnancy category C; may appear in breast milk and could suppress

M

growth, interfere with endogenous corticosteroid production, or cause unwanted effects in the nursing infant

SIDE EFFECTS/ADVERSE REACTIONS

CNS: Depression, vertigo, ***convulsions,*** headache, *mood changes*

CV: Hypertension, thrombophlebitis, ***thromboembolism,*** tachycardia, CHF

EENT: Increased intraocular pressure, blurred vision, cataract

GI: Diarrhea, nausea, abdominal distension, ***GI hemorrhage,*** increased appetite, ***pancreatitis***

METAB: Cushingoid state, growth suppression in children, HPA suppression, decreased glucose tolerance

MS: Fractures, osteoporosis, aseptic necrosis of femoral and humeral heads, weakness, muscle mass loss

SKIN: Acne, poor wound healing, ecchymosis, bruising, petechiae, striae, thin fragile skin, suppression of skin test reactions

▼ DRUG INTERACTIONS

Drugs

- *Aminoglutethamide:* Enhanced elimination of corticosteroids; marked reduction in corticosteroid response
- *Antidiabetics:* Increased blood glucose in patients with diabetes
- *Barbiturates, carbamazepine:* Reduced serum concentrations of corticosteroids
- *Cholestyramine:* Possible reduced absorption of corticosteroids
- *Estrogens:* Enhanced effects of corticosteroids
- *Isoniazid:* Reduced plasma concentrations of isoniazid
- *Ketoconazole:* Increased methylprednisolone concentrations
- *Phenytoin, rifampin:* Reduced therapeutic effect of corticosteroids
- *Salicylates:* Enhanced elimination of salicylates; subtherapeutic salicylate concentrations possible

Labs

- *Increase:* Cholesterol, blood glucose, urine glucose
- *Decrease:* Calcium, potassium, T_4, T_3, thyroid ^{131}I uptake test
- *Fale negative:* Skin allergy tests

SPECIAL CONSIDERATIONS

PATIENT/FAMILY EDUCATION

- Drug may cause GI upset, take with meals or snacks
- Take single daily doses in A.M.
- Notify physician if unusual weight gain, swelling of lower extremities, muscle weakness, black tarry stools, vomiting of blood, puffing of the face, menstrual irregularities, prolonged sore throat, fever, cold, or infection occurs
- Signs of adrenal insufficiency include fatigue, anorexia, nausea, vomiting, diarrhea, weight loss, weakness, dizziness, and low blood sugar; notify physician if these signs and symptoms appear following dose reduction or withdrawal of therapy
- Avoid abrupt withdrawal of therapy following high dose or long-term therapy

MONITORING PARAMETERS

- Potassium and blood sugar during long-term therapy
- Edema, blood pressure, cardiac symptoms, mental status, weight
- Observe growth and development of infants and children on prolonged therapy

methyltestosterone

(meth-ill-tess-toss'teh-rone)

Android, Oreton, Testred, Virilon

Chemical Class: Synthetic androgenic anabolic steroid hormone

Therapeutic Class: Anabolic steroid; androgen

DEA Class: Schedule III

CLINICAL PHARMACOLOGY

Mechanism of Action: Promotes weight gain via retention of nitrogen, potassium, and phosphorus, increased protein anabolism and decreased amino acid catabolism; endogenous androgens are essential for normal growth and development of male sex organs and maintenance of secondary sex characteristics

Pharmacokinetics

PO: Half as potent as buccally administered tablets, metabolized in liver, excreted in urine

INDICATIONS AND USES: Males: primary hypogonadism (congenital or acquired), hypogonadotropic hypogonadism (congenital or acquired), delayed puberty; Females: palliative therapy of metastatic breast cancer, postpartum breast pain/engorgement, moderate to severe vasomotor symptoms of menopause (in conjunction with estrogens)

DOSAGE

Adult

- *Male hypogonadism:* PO 10-50 mg qd; buccal 5-25 mg qd
- *Delayed puberty:* PO 10 mg qd for 4-6 wk; buccal 5 mg qd for 4-6 wk
- *Breast cancer:* PO 50-200 mg qd; buccal 25-100 mg qd
- *Postpartum breast pain and engorgement:* PO 80 mg qd for 3-5 days after parturition; buccal 40 mg qd for 3-5 days after parturition
- *Menopause:* PO 1.25-10 mg qd (with estrogen)

$ **AVAILABLE FORMS/COST OF THERAPY**

- Cap, Gel—Oral: 10 mg, 100's: **$43.20-$130.06**
- Tab—Oral, SL: 10 mg, 100's: **$4.95**
- Tab—SL: 10 mg, 100's: **$5.00**
- Tab—Uncoated—Oral: 10 mg, 100's: **$2.80-$130.06;** 25 mg, 100's: **$6.72-$325.13**

CONTRAINDICATIONS: Hypersensitivity; serious cardiac, hepatic, or renal disease; carcinoma of breast or prostate (males); pregnancy; enhancement of athletic performance

PRECAUTIONS: Epilepsy, migraine headaches, children, BPH, acute intermittent porphyria, hypercholesterolemia

PREGNANCY AND LACTATION: Pregnancy category X; causes virilization of the external genitalia of female fetuses; excretion into breast milk unknown, use extreme caution in nursing mothers

SIDE EFFECTS/ADVERSE REACTIONS

CNS: Dizziness, headache, fatigue, tremors, paresthesias, flushing, sweating, anxiety, lability, insomnia, decreased or increased libido

CV: Increased blood pressure

EENT: Conjunctional edema, nasal congestion

GI: Nausea, vomiting, constipation, weight gain, ***cholestatic jaundice,*** stomatitis (buccal)

GU: ***Hematuria,*** *amenorrhea,* vaginitis, *clitoral hypertrophy,* testicular atrophy, excessive frequency and duration of erection, oligospermia

HEME: Suppression of clotting factors II, V, VII, and X; polycythemia

METAB: Abnormal GTT; hypercalcemia; sodium, chloride, water, po-

M

tassium, calcium and inorganic phosphate retention; increased serum cholesterol

MS: Cramps, spasms

SKIN: Rash, acneiform lesions, oily hair, skin, flushing, sweating, acne vulgaris, alopecia, hirsutism

MISC: Virilization (females), decreased breast size, gynecomastia

▼ **DRUG INTERACTIONS**

Drugs

- *Antidiabetic agents:* Enhanced hypoglycemic effects
- *Cyclosporine:* Increased cyclosporine concentrations
- *Warfarin+:* Enhanced hypoprothrombinemic response to oral anticoagulants

Labs

- *Increase:* Serum cholesterol, blood glucose, urine glucose
- *Decrease:* Serum Ca, serum K, T_4, T_3, thyroid ^{131}I uptake test, urine 17-OHCS, 17-KS, PBI, BSP

SPECIAL CONSIDERATIONS

PATIENT/FAMILY EDUCATION

- Drug may cause GI upset
- Notify physician if swelling of extremities, priapism, or jaundice occurs (males)
- Notify physician if hoarseness, deepening of voice, male-pattern baldness, hirsutism, acne, or menstrual irregularities occur (females)
- Do not swallow buccal tablets, allow to dissolve between cheek and gum
- Avoid eating, drinking, or smoking while buccal tablet in place

MONITORING PARAMETERS

- Frequent urine and serum calcium determinations (females)
- Periodic LFTs
- X-ray examinations of bone age q6 mo during treatment of prepubertal males
- Hgb and Hct periodically to check for polycythemia

methysergide

(meth-i-ser′jide)

Sansert

Chemical Class: Semisynthetic ergot alkaloid

Therapeutic Class: Antimigraine agent

CLINICAL PHARMACOLOGY

Mechanism of Action: Exact mechanism of action in preventing migraine is unknown, may be related to antiserotonin effect

Pharmacokinetics

PO: Onset of action 1-2 days, duration 1-2 days, metabolized in liver, excreted in urine (unchanged drug and metabolites), $t_{1/2}$ 10 hr

INDICATIONS AND USES: Prevention of vascular headache; diarrhea in patients with carcinoid disease*

DOSAGE

Adult

- PO 4-8 mg/d in divided doses with meals; **a drug-free interval of 3-4 wk must follow each 6 mo course**

$ **AVAILABLE FORMS/COST OF THERAPY**

- Tab, Coated—Oral: 2 mg, 100's: **$164.22**

CONTRAINDICATIONS: Peripheral vascular disease, severe arteriosclerosis, severe hypertension, CAD, phlebitis or cellulitis of lower limbs, pulmonary disease, collagen diseases or fibrotic processes, impaired liver or renal function, valvular heart disease, peptic ulcer, debilitated states, serious infections, hypersensitivity to ergot alkaloids

PRECAUTIONS: Tartrazine sensitivity, uninterrupted administration (increases risk of fibrotic complications)

PREGNANCY AND LACTATION: Contraindicated in pregnancy due to oxytocic properties; ergot derivatives in the milk of nursing mothers have caused symptoms of ergotism (e.g., vomiting, diarrhea) in the infant

SIDE EFFECTS/ADVERSE REACTIONS

CNS: Insomnia, drowsiness, mild euphoria, dizziness, ataxia, weakness, lightheadedness, hyperesthesia, unworldly feelings

CV: Vasoconstriction of small and large arteries (chest pain, abdominal pain, cold, numb, painful extremities, diminished or absent pulses), ***cardiac fibrosis,*** edema

GI: Nausea, vomiting, diarrhea, heartburn, abdominal pain, constipation, increased gastric acid

GU: ***Retroperitoneal fibrosis***

HEME: ***Neutropenia, eosinophilia***

MS: Arthralgia, myalgia

RESP: ***Pleuropulmonary fibrosis***

SKIN: Facial flush, telangiectasia, nonspecific rashes, increased hair loss

MISC: Weight gain

SPECIAL CONSIDERATIONS

PATIENT/FAMILY EDUCATION

- Drug may cause GI upset, take with food or milk
- Drug may cause drowsiness
- Continuous administration should not exceed 6 mo
- Notify physician of cold, numb, or painful extremities, leg cramps when walking, girdle, flank, or chest pain, painful urination, or shortness of breath

MONITORING PARAMETERS

- Consider baseline urography, repeated q6-12 mo during therapy

metipranolol

(met-ee-pran'oh-lol)

Optipranolol

Chemical Class: Nonselective β-adrenergic blocker

Therapeutic Class: Antiglaucoma agent

CLINICAL PHARMACOLOGY

Mechanism of Action: Reduces aqueous humor production; slight increase in outflow may be an additional mechanism; little or no effect on pupil size or accommodation

Pharmacokinetics

OPHTH: Onset ≤30 min, max effect by 2 hr, duration 12-24 hr, may be absorbed systemically

INDICATIONS AND USES: Chronic open-angle glaucoma, ocular hypertension, ocular conditions where lowering intraocular pressure would be of benefit

DOSAGE

Adult

- Instill 1 gtt in affected eye(s) bid

$ AVAILABLE FORMS/COST OF THERAPY

- Sol—Ophth: 0.3%, 10 ml: **$19.18**

CONTRAINDICATIONS: Hypersensitivity, asthma, severe COPD, sinus bradycardia, 2nd or 3rd degree AV block, cardiac failure, cardiogenic shock

PRECAUTIONS: Systemic absorption, major surgery, diabetes mellitus, hyperthyroidism, cerebrovascular insufficiency, children, angle-closure glaucoma

PREGNANCY AND LACTATION: Pregnancy category C

SIDE EFFECTS/ADVERSE REACTIONS

CNS: Headache, depression, asthenia, dizziness, anxiety

CV: ***Arrhythmia,*** syncope, heart block, ***cerebral vascular accident, cerebral ischemia, congestive heart failure,*** palpitation, hypertension, ***MI,*** angina, bradycardia
EENT: Keratitis, blepharoptosis, visual disturbances, diplopia, ptosis, transient local discomfort, conjunctivitis, eyelid dermatitis, blepharitis, tearing, browache, photophobia, rhinitis, epistaxis
GI: Nausea
METAB: Masked symptoms of hypoglycemia in diabetics
MS: Arthritis, myalgia
RESP: ***Bronchospasm, respiratory failure,*** dyspnea
SKIN: Hypersensitivity, localized and generalized rash

SPECIAL CONSIDERATIONS

PATIENT/FAMILY EDUCATION

- Transient stinging/discomfort is common, notify physician if severe
- Apply pressure to lacrimal sac for 1 min following instillation
- Do not touch dropper to eye

MONITORING PARAMETERS

- Intraocular pressure

metoclopramide

(met′oh-kloe-pra′mide)
Clopra, Emex, ♣ Maxeran, ♣ Maxolon, Octamide PFS, Reclomide, Reglan
Chemical Class: Paraminobenzoic acid derivative
Therapeutic Class: Gastrointestinal motility agent; antiemetic

CLINICAL PHARMACOLOGY

Mechanism of Action: Inhibits gastric smooth muscle relaxation produced by dopamine thus enhancing cholinergic responses of GI smooth muscle; increases resting pressure of the lower esophageal sphincter, increases amplitude of esophageal peristaltic contractions; dopamine antagonist action raises the threshold of activity in the chemoreceptor trigger zone and decreases input from afferent visceral nerves; stimulates prolactin secretion

Pharmacokinetics

PO: Onset 30-60 min, duration 1-2 hr
IM: Onset 10-15 min, duration 1-2 hr
IV: Onset 1-3 min, duration 1-2 hr
13%-22% bound to plasma proteins, partially metabolized in liver, eliminated in urine, $t_{1/2}$ 4-6 hr

INDICATIONS AND USES: Gastroesophageal reflux disease (GERD), diabetic gastroparesis, chemotherapy-induced nausea and vomiting (parenteral), facilitation of small bowel intubation, drug-related postoperative nausea and vomiting,* prevention of aspiration pneumonitis presurgery,* slow gastric emptying,* gastic stasis in preterm infants,* vascular headache,* lactation deficiency,* diabetic cystoparesis,* esophageal variceal bleeding*

DOSAGE

Adult

- *GERD/gastroparesis:* PO/IM/IV 10-15 mg 30 min ac and hs
- *Intubation of small bowel:* IV 10 mg
- *Chemotherapy-induced nausea and vomiting:* IV 1-2 mg/kg/dose q2-4 hr

Child

- *GERD:* PO/IM/IV 0.4-0.8 mg/kg/d divided qid
- *Intubation of small bowel:* IV (<6 yr) 0.1 mg/kg; (6-14 yr) 2.5-5 mg/kg
- *Chemotherapy-induced nausea and vomiting:* IV 1-2 mg/kg/dose q2-4 hr
- Dosing adjustment in renal failure: CrCl 10-50 ml/min administer 75% of recommended dose; CrCl

<10 ml/min, administer 25%-50% of recommended dose

$ AVAILABLE FORMS/COST OF THERAPY

- Inj, Sol—IM; IV: 5 mg/ml, 2 ml: **$2.93-$58.75**
- Syr—Oral: 5 mg/5ml, 480 ml: **$11.97-$46.13**
- Conc—Oral: 10 mg/ml, 30 ml: **$19.49**
- Tab, Uncoated—Oral: 5 mg, 100's: **$16.88-$39.53;** 10 mg, 100's: **$2.25-$61.76**

CONTRAINDICATIONS: GI hemorrhage, mechanical obstruction or perforation, pheochromocytoma, hypersensitivity, seizure disorder

PRECAUTIONS: History of depression, Parkinson's disease, hypertension, anastomosis or closure of the gut

PREGNANCY AND LACTATION: Pregnancy category B; has been used during pregnancy as an antiemetic and to decrease gastric emptying time; excreted into milk, use during lactation a concern because of the potent CNS effects the drug is capable of producing

SIDE EFFECTS/ADVERSE REACTIONS

CNS: Sedation, fatigue, restlessness, headache, sleeplessness, EPS (dystonia, parkinson-like symptoms, akathisia, ***tardive dyskinesia),*** dizziness, *drowsiness,* ***seizures,*** hallucinations

CV: Hypotension, hypertension, supraventricular tachycardia, bradycardia

EENT: Visual disturbances

GI: Nausea, bowel disturbances, *diarrhea*

GU: Urinary frequency, incontinence

HEME: Neutropenia, leukopenia, agranulocytosis, methemoglobinemia (especially overdoses in neonates), porphyria

METAB: Galactorrhea, amenorrhea, gynecomastia, impotence (hyperprolactinemia), elevated aldosterone

SKIN: Urticaria, rash

MISC: ***Neuroleptic malignant syndrome***

▼ DRUG INTERACTIONS

Drugs

- *Cyclosporine:* Increased bioavailability and serum concentrations of cyclosporine
- *Digitalis glycosides:* Reduced serum digoxin concentration when coadministered with generic formulations

Labs

- *Increase:* Prolactin, aldosterone, thyrotropin

SPECIAL CONSIDERATIONS

PATIENT/FAMILY EDUCATION

- Drug may cause drowsiness and dizziness, use caution driving or performing other tasks requiring alertness
- Notify physician if involuntary movements of eyes, face, or limbs occur

M

metolazone

(me-tole'a-zone)

Diulo, Mykrox, Zaroxolyn

Chemical Class: Quinazoline derivative

Therapeutic Class: Antihypertensive; thiazide diuretic

CLINICAL PHARMACOLOGY

Mechanism of Action: Increases urinary excretion of sodium and water by inhibiting sodium reabsorption in the early distal tubules and increases urinary excretion of potassium by increasing potassium secretion in the distal convoluted tubule and collecting ducts; decreases urinary calcium excretion; does not substantially decrease the glomerular filtration rate (GFR) or renal plasma flow; may produce diuresis in patients with GFR <20 ml/min

Pharmacokinetics

PO: (Mycrox) peak 2-4 hr, steady-state within 4-5 days; (Zaroxolyn) peak 8 hr; 50%-70% bound to erythrocytes, up to 33% bound to plasma proteins, 70%-95% excreted unchanged in urine by glomerular filtration and active tubular secretion, $t_{1/2}$ 8 hr

INDICATIONS AND USES: Edema associated with CHF, hepatic cirrhosis, corticosteroid and estrogen therapy (may be more effective than other thiazide-like diuretics in patients with impaired renal function); has been used concomitantly with furosemide to induce diuresis in patients who did not respond to either diuretic alone; hypertension

DOSAGE

Adult

- *Edema:* PO (Zaroxolyn) 5-10 mg qAM, up to 20 mg qd may be required for edema associated with renal disease
- *Hypertension:* PO (Zaroxolyn) 1.25-5 mg qAM; (Mykrox) 0.5-1 mg qAM

Child

- PO (Zaroxolyn) 0.2-0.4 mg/kg/d divided q12-24h

$ AVAILABLE FORMS/COST OF THERAPY

- Tab, Uncoated—Oral: 0.5 mg, 100's: **$70.80** (Mykrox)
- Tab, Uncoated—Oral: 2.5 mg, 100's: **$42.86;** 5 mg, 100's: **48.73;** 10 mg, 100's: **$58.32** (Zaroxolyn)

CONTRAINDICATIONS: Anuria, renal decompensation, hepatic coma or pre-coma, hypersensitivity to thiazides or related sulfonamide-derived drugs

PRECAUTIONS: Hypokalemia, renal disease, hepatic disease, gout, COPD, lupus erythematosus, diabetes mellitus, children, vomiting, diarrhea, hyperlipidemia

PREGNANCY AND LACTATION: Pregnancy category D; 1st trimester use may increase risk of congenital defects, use in later trimesters does not seem to carry this risk; other risks to the fetus or newborn include hypoglycemia, thrombocytopenia, hyponatremia, hypokalemia, and death from maternal complications; excreted into breast milk in small amounts, considered compatible with breast feeding

SIDE EFFECTS/ADVERSE REACTIONS

CNS: Drowsiness, paresthesia, depression, headache, *dizziness, fatigue, weakness,* chills

CV: Irregular pulse, orthostatic hypotension, palpitations, volume depletion, chest pain

EENT Blurred vision

GI: Nausea, vomiting, anorexia, constipation, diarrhea, cramps, pancreatitis, GI irritation, ***hepatitis,*** abdominal bloating

GU: Frequency, polyuria, ***uremia, glucosuria***

HEME: ***Aplastic anemia, hemolytic, anemia, leukopenia, agranulocytosis, thrombocytopenia, neutropenia***

METAB: Hyperglycemia, hyperuricemia, increased creatinine, BUN, *hypokalemia,* hypercalcemia, hyponatremia, hypochloremia, hypomagnesemia

SKIN: Rash, urticaria, purpura, photosensitivity, fever

▼ DRUG INTERACTIONS

Drugs

- *Antidiabetics:* Thiazide diuretics tend to increase blood glucose, may increase dosage requirements of antidiabetic drugs
- *Cholestyramine, colestipol:* Reduced serum concentrations of thiazide diuretics

• *Diazoxide:* Hyperglycemia
• *Digitalis glycosides:* Diuretic-induced hypokalemia may increase the risk of digitalis toxicity
• *Lithium+:* Increased serum lithium concentrations, toxicity may occur

Labs

• *Increase:* BSP retention, amylase, parathyroid test
• *Decrease:* PBI, PSP

SPECIAL CONSIDERATIONS

PATIENT/FAMILY EDUCATION

• Take with food or milk
• Drug will increase urination, take early in the day
• Notify physician if muscle pain, weakness, cramps, nausea, vomiting, restlessness, excessive thirst, tiredness, drowsiness, increased heart rate, diarrhea, or dizziness occurs
• Drug may cause sensitivity to sunlight, avoid prolonged exposure to the sun and other ultraviolet light
• Drug may cause gout attacks, notify physician if sudden joint pain occurs

MONITORING PARAMETERS

• Serum electrolytes, BUN, creatinine, CBC, uric acid, glucose

---

metoprolol

(met-oh'proe-lol)

Apo-metoprolol, ♣ Betaloc, ♣ Lopresor, ♣ Lopressor, Novometoprol, ♣ Toprol XL

Chemical Class: β_1-selective adrenergic blocking agent

Therapeutic Class: Antihypertensive; antianginal

CLINICAL PHARMACOLOGY

Mechanism of Action: Preferentially competes with β-adrenergic agonists for available β_1-receptor sites inhibiting the chronotropic and inotropic responses to β_1-adrenergic stimulation (cardioselective); slows conduction of AV node, decreases heart rate, decreases O_2 consumption in myocardium, also decreases renin-aldosterone-angiotensin system at higher doses; blocks β_2-receptors in bronchial system at higher doses; lacks intrinsic sympathomimetic (partial agonist) activity

Pharmacokinetics

PO: Peak effect 1.5-4 hr, duration 10-20 hr

IV: Peak effect 20 min, duration 5-8 hr

8%-12% bound to plasma proteins, extensively metabolized in liver, excreted in urine (3%-10% unchanged), $t_{1/2}$ 3-4 hr

INDICATIONS AND USES: Chronic stable angina pectoris, hypertension, acute MI, multifocal atrial tachycardia,* rate control in atrial fibrillation,* ventricular dysrhythmias/tachycardias,* migraine prophylaxis,* essential tremor,* aggressive behavior,* congestive heart failure*

DOSAGE

Adult

• *Hypertension:* PO 100 mg/d in single or divided doses, max 450 mg/d; SUS REL 50-100 mg qd, max 400 mg/d
• *Angina pectoris:* PO 50 mg bid, max 400 mg/d; SUS REL 100 mg qd, max 400 mg/d
• *MI:* (early treatment) IV 5 mg q2 min times 3 doses, then PO 25-50 mg q6h 15 min after last IV dose, continue for 48 hr; maintenance 100 mg bid; (late treatment) 100 mg bid as soon as clinical condition allows

$ AVAILABLE FORMS/COST OF THERAPY

• Inj, Sol—IV: 5mg/5ml, 3's: **$66.53**
• Tab, Coated—Oral: 50 mg, 100's: **$20.49-$52.05;** 100 mg, 100's: **$31.43-$78.21**

M

• Tab, Coated, Sust Action—Oral: 50 mg, 100's: **$44.63;** 100 mg, 100's: **$67.07;** 200 mg, 100's: **$134.14**

CONTRAINDICATIONS: Hypersensitivity to beta blockers, cardiogenic shock, 2nd or 3rd degree heart block, sinus bradycardia, CHF unless secondary to a tachydysrhythmia treatable with beta blockers, moderate to severe cardiac failure, treatment of MI when heart rate <45 bpm, systolic blood pressure <100 mm Hg

PRECAUTIONS: Major surgery, diabetes mellitus, renal disease, hepatic disease, thyroid disease, COPD, asthma, well-compensated heart failure, abrupt withdrawal, peripheral vascular disease, bradycardia

PREGNANCY AND LACTATION: Pregnancy category B; has been used during pregnancy for treatment of maternal hypertension and tachycardia; newborn should be closely observed during the first 24-48 hr after birth for bradycardia and other symptoms; compatible with breast feeding

SIDE EFFECTS/ADVERSE REACTIONS

CNS: Insomnia, *fatigue, dizziness,* mental changes, memory loss, hallucinations, depression, *lethargy,* drowsiness, strange dreams

CV: Profound hypotension, ***bradycardia,*** CHF, cold extremities, postural hypotension, ***2nd or 3rd degree heart block***

EENT: Sore throat, dry burning eyes, visual disturbances

GI: Nausea, diarrhea, vomiting, dry mouth, ***mesenteric arterial thrombosis, ischemic colitis***

GU: Impotence, sexual dysfunction

HEME: ***Agranulocytosis, thrombocytopenia***

METAB: Masked hypoglycemic response to insulin (sweating excepted), hyperlipidemia (increase TG, total cholesterol, LDL; decrease HDL)

RESP: ***Bronchospasm,*** dyspnea, wheezing

SKIN: Rash, pruritis, alopecia

▼ DRUG INTERACTIONS

Drugs

• *Amiodarone:* Bradycardia, cardiac arrest, or ventricular dysrhythmia
• *Antidiabetics:* Altered response to hypoglycemia, prolonged recovery of normoglycemia, hypertension, blockade of tachycardia; may increase blood glucose and impair peripheral circulation
• *Cimetidine, propafenone, propoxyphene, quinidine:* Increased plasma metoprolol concentration
• *Clonidine:* Exacerbation of rebound hypertension upon discontinuation of clonidine
• *Dihydropyridines:* Additive hemodynamic effects
• *Diltiazem, verapamil:* Enhanced effects of both drugs, particularly antrioventricular conduction slowing
• *Dipyridamole, tacrine:* Bradycardia
• *Disopyramide:* Additive negative inotropic effects
• *Epinephrine+:* Enhanced pressor response to epinephrine; less likely with cardioselective agents like metoprolol
• *Fluoxetine:* Enhanced effect of β-blocker
• *Isoproterenol:* Potential reduction in effectiveness of isoproterenol in the treatment of asthma; less likely with cardioselective agents like metoprolol
• *Lidocaine:* Increased lidocaine concentrations possible
• *Local anesthetics:* Use of local anesthetics containing epinephrine

may result in hypertensive reactions in patients taking β-blockers
• *Methyldopa:* Development of hypertension during situations resulting in release of catecholamines
• *NSAIDs:* Reduced hypotensive effects of β-blockers
• *Phenylephrine:* Enhanced pressor response to phenylephrine, particularly when it is administered IV
• *Prazosin:* First-dose response to prazosin may be enhanced by β-blockade
• *Rifampin:* Reduced plasma metoprolol concentration
• *Theophylline:* Antagonistic pharmacodynamic effects

Labs

• *Interference:* Glucose/insulin tolerance tests
• *Increase:* Serum transaminase, alkaline phosphatase and LDH

SPECIAL CONSIDERATIONS

PATIENT/FAMILY EDUCATION

• Do not discontinue drug abruptly, may precipitate angina
• Report bradycardia, dizziness, confusion, depression, fever, shortness of breath, swelling of the extremities
• Take pulse at home, notify physician if <50 beats/min
• Avoid hazardous activities if dizziness, drowsiness, lightheadedness are present
• Drug may mask symptoms of hypoglycemia, except for sweating, in diabetic patients

MONITORING PARAMETERS

• Blood pressure, pulse

metronidazole

(me-troe-ni'da-zole)

Apo-Metronidazole, ♣ Femazole, Flagyl, Metizol, Metric 21, Metro IV, Metryl, Neo-Metric, ♣ Novonidazole, ♣ PMS-Metronidazole, ♣ Protostat, Satric

Chemical Class: Nitroimidazole derivative

Therapeutic Class: Antibacterial; antiprotozoal; anthelmintic

CLINICAL PHARMACOLOGY

Mechanism of Action: Reduced metronidazole, which is cytotoxic but short-lived, interacts with DNA to cause a loss of helical structure, strand breakage, and resultant inhibition of nucleic acid synthesis and cell death

Pharmacokinetics

PO: Peak 1-3 hr

IV: Onset immediate

VAG: 20%-25% systemic bioavailability

<20% bound to plasma proteins, metabolized in liver, eliminated via urine (60%-80%) and feces (6%-15%), $t_{1/2}$ 6-8 hr

INDICATIONS AND USES: Trichomoniasis, amebiasis, giardiasis, anaerobic bacterial infections, perioperative prophylaxis during colorectal surgery, bacterial vaginosis, acne rosacea, *Helicobacter pylori* infection associated with peptic ulcer disease (as part of a multi-drug regimen),* pseudomembranous colitis,* dracunculiasis (guinea worm disease),* Crohn's disease*

Antibacterial spectrum usually includes:

• Anaerobic gram-negative bacilli: *Bacteroides* sp including the *B. fragilis* group (*B. fragilis, B. distasonis, B. ovatus, B. thetaiotaomicron, B. vulgatus*), *Fusobacterium* sp

• Anaerobic gram-positive bacilli: *Clostridium* sp, susceptible strains of *Eubacterium*

• Anaerobic gram-positive cocci: *Peptococcus* sp, *Peptostreptococcus* sp; protozoa: *Entamoeba histolytica, Trichmonas vaginalis, Giardia lamblia, Balantidium coli*

DOSAGE

Adult

• *Amebiasis:* PO 500-750 mg q8h

• *Other parasitic infections:* PO 250 mg q8h, or 2 g as a single dose

• *Anaerobic infections:* PO/IV 500 mg q8h, do not exceed 4 g/d

• *Pseudomembranous colitis:* PO 250-500 mg tid-qid for 10-14 days; IV 500 mg q8h for 10-14 days

• *Rosacea:* TOP apply to affected areas bid

• *Bacterial vaginosis:* VAG 5 g (1 applicatorful) bid for 5 days; PO 500 mg bid for 7-10 days

Child

• *Amebiasis:* PO 35-50 mg/kg/d divided q8h, do not exceed 4 g/d

• *Other parasitic infections:* PO 15-30 mg/kg/d divided q8h

• *Anaerobic infections:* PO/IV 30 mg/kg/d divided q6h, do not exceed 4 g/d

• *Pseudomembranous colitis:* PO 20 mg/kg/d divided q6h

$ **AVAILABLE FORMS/COST OF THERAPY**

• Inj, Sol—IV: 500 mg/100 ml, 100 ml: **$8.85-$28.93**

• Tab, Plain Coated—Oral: 250 mg, 100's: **$4.04-$130.58;** 500 mg, 100's: **$7.88-$237.86**

• Gel—Top: 0.75%, 28.4, 45 g: **$23.75-$31.06**

• Gel—Vag: 0.75%, 70 g: **$25.20**

CONTRAINDICATIONS: Hypersensitivity to nitroimidazole derivatives

PRECAUTIONS: History of blood dyscrasias, severe hepatic impairment, CNS disease, severe renal failure

PREGNANCY AND LACTATION: Pregnancy category B; available reports have arrived at conflicting conclusions regarding safety during pregnancy, use during the first trimester and single dose therapy should be avoided; use with caution during breast feeding, if single dose therapy is used, discontinue breast feeding for 12-24 hr to allow excretion of the drug

SIDE EFFECTS/ADVERSE REACTIONS

CNS: Peripheral neuropathy, ***seizures,*** dizziness, vertigo, headache, incoordination, ataxia, confusion, irritability, depression, weakness, insomnia, fever

CV: ECG changes

EENT: Nasal congestion

GI: Nausea, anorexia, dry mouth, metallic taste, vomiting, diarrhea, epigastric distress, abdominal discomfort, constipation, ***pancreatitis*** (rare), furry tongue, glossitis, stomatitis, pseudomembranous colitis

GU: Urethral burning, dysuria, cystitis, polyuria, incontinence, vaginal dryness, dyspareunia, decreased libido, sense of pelvic pressure, discoloration of urine (IV)

HEME: ***Transient leukopenia, thrombocytopenia***

MS: Fleeting joint pains

SKIN: Urticaria, pruritus, erythematous rash, flushing

▼ **DRUG INTERACTIONS**

Drugs

• *Disulfiram:* CNS toxicity

• *Fluorouracil:* Enhanced toxicity of fluorouracil

• *Oral anticoagulants+:* Increased hypoprothrombinemic response to warfarin

Labs

• *Decrease:* AST, ALT

SPECIAL CONSIDERATIONS
PATIENT/FAMILY EDUCATION
- Drug may cause GI upset, take with food
- Avoid alcoholic beverages during therapy and for at least 24 hr following last dose (disulfiram-like reaction possible)
- Complete full course of therapy
- Drug may cause darkening of urine
- An unpleasant metallic taste may be noticeable

MONITORING PARAMETERS
- CBC

---

metyrosine
(me-tye'roe-seen)
Demser
Chemical Class: Catecholamine synthesis inhibitor
Therapeutic Class: Antipheochromocytoma agent

CLINICAL PHARMACOLOGY
Mechanism of Action: Competitively inhibits tyrosine hydroxylase, the rate-limiting step in catecholamine synthesis; decreases endogenous catecholamine concentrations in patients with normal or increased catecholamine production
Pharmacokinetics
PO: Peak 1-3 hr, onset within first 2 days of therapy, excreted unchanged in urine, $t_{1/2}$ 3.4-7.2 hr
INDICATIONS AND USES: Pheochromocytoma (short-term and long-term management), adjunct to neuroleptics in chronic schizophrenia*
DOSAGE
Adult and Child >12 yr
- PO 250 mg qid, may increase by 250-500 mg qd up to max of 4 g/d in divided doses

$ **AVAILABLE FORMS/COST OF THERAPY**
- Cap, Gel—Oral: 250 mg, 100's: **$142.49**

CONTRAINDICATIONS: Hypersensitivity, hypertension of unknown etiology
PRECAUTIONS: Impaired hepatic or renal function, children <12 yr
PREGNANCY AND LACTATION: Pregnancy category C
SIDE EFFECTS/ADVERSE REACTIONS
CNS: Sedation, psychic stimulation upon drug withdrawal, headache, drooling, speech difficulty, tremor, trismus, parkinsonism, anxiety, depression, hallucinations, disorientation, confusion
CV: Peripheral edema
EENT: Nasal stuffiness
GI: Diarrhea, dry mouth, nausea, vomiting, abdominal pain, increased AST
GU: Crystalluria, impotence, failure to ejaculate, transient dysuria, ***hematuria***
HEME: ***Eosinophilia, anemia, thrombocytopenia, thrombocytosis***
METAB: Breast swelling, galactorrhea
MISC: Hypersensitivity reactions (urticaria, pharyngeal edema)
▼ **DRUG INTERACTIONS**
Drugs
- *Phenothiazines, haloperidol:* Potentiation of EPS

Labs
- *False increase:* Urinary catecholamines (due to presence of metyrosine metabolites)

SPECIAL CONSIDERATIONS
PATIENT/FAMILY EDUCATION
- Maintain a daily liberal fluid intake
- Avoid alcohol or CNS depressants
- Drug may cause drowsiness, use caution driving or performing tasks requiring alertness
- Notify physician of drooling,

speech difficulty, tremors, disorientation, diarrhea, painful urination

MONITORING PARAMETERS

• Blood pressure, ECG

mexiletine

(mex-il'e-teen)

Mexitil

Chemical Class: Lidocaine analog

Therapeutic Class: Antidysrhythmic (Class IB)

CLINICAL PHARMACOLOGY

Mechanism of Action: Blocks the fast sodium channel in cardiac tissues, especially the Purkinje network; reduces rate of rise and amplitude of the action potential, decreases automaticity, shortens the action potential duration and decreases the effective refractory period in Purkinje fibers; does not significantly alter conduction velocity, membrane potential, sinus node automaticity, left ventricular function, systolic arterial blood pressure, AV conduction velocity, QRS or QT intervals

Pharmacokinetics

PO: Onset 0.5-2 hr, peak 2-3 hr, 60%-75% bound to plasma proteins, metabolized in liver, eliminated via bile and urine, $t_{1/2}$ 10-12 hr (prolonged in hepatic/renal failure, reduced cardiac output, acute MI)

INDICATIONS AND USES: Documented, life-threatening ventricular dysrhythmia, diabetic neuropathy*

DOSAGE

Adult

• PO 200 mg q8h initially, adjust in 50-100 mg increments q2-3d, do not exceed 1200 mg/d

Child

• PO 1.4-5 mg/kg/dose q8h

• Dosing adjustment in renal impairment: Administer 50%-75% of normal dose if CrCl<10 ml/min

• Dosing adjustment in hepatic disease: Administer 25%-30% of normal dose

$ **AVAILABLE FORMS/COST OF THERAPY**

• Cap, Gel—Oral: 150 mg, 100's: **$69.06-$76.73;** 200 mg, 100's: **$82.22-$91.38;** 250 mg, 100's: **$95.66-$106.29**

CONTRAINDICATIONS: Cardiogenic shock, preexisting 2nd or 3rd degree AV block (if pacemaker not present), hypersensitivity

PRECAUTIONS: Structural heart disease, hepatic disease, renal function impairment, children, 1st degree AV block, preexisting sinus node dysfunction, intraventricular conduction abnormalities, hypotension, severe CHF, seizure disorder

PREGNANCY AND LACTATION: Pregnancy category C; limited data do not suggest significant risk to the fetus; compatible with breast feeding

SIDE EFFECTS/ADVERSE REACTIONS

CNS: Tremor, lightheadedness, coordination difficulties, dizziness, nervousness, changes in sleep habits, headache, paresthesias, weakness, fatigue, speech difficulties, confusion, depression, short-term memory loss, hallucinations, psychosis, ***seizures,*** fever

CV: Palpitations, chest pain, ***increased ventricular dysrhythmias/PVCs,*** angina, ***CHF,*** syncope, hypotension, bradycardia, edema, AV block, conduction disturbances, hot flashes, atrial dysrhythmias, hypertension, cardiogenic shock

EENT: Blurred vision, tinnitus

GI: Upper GI distress, nausea, heartburn, vomiting, constipation, diar-

rhea, dry mouth, changes in appetite, abdominal pain, pharyngitis, altered taste, salivary changes, dysphagia, oral mucous membrane changes, ***peptic ulcer, upper GI bleeding,*** esophageal ulceration
GU: Impotence, decreased libido, urinary hesitancy
HEME: ***Leukopenia, agranulocytosis, thrombocytopenia*** (rare)
MS: Arthralgia
RESP: Dyspnea, hiccoughs
SKIN: Rash, diaphoresis, hair loss, dry skin, ***exfoliative dermatitis***

▼ **DRUG INTERACTIONS**

Drugs

• *Phenytoin, rifampin:* Reduced mexiletine concentrations
• *Quinidine:* Elevated mexiletine concentrations
• *Theophylline:* Elevated theophylline serum concentrations and toxicity

Labs

• *Increase:* CPK

SPECIAL CONSIDERATIONS

PATIENT/FAMILY EDUCATION

• Take with food or antacid
• Notify physician if signs of liver injury or blood cell damage occur, such as unexplained general tiredness, jaundice, fever, sore throat

MONITORING PARAMETERS

• Therapeutic mexiletine concentrations 0.5-2 μg/ml
• ECG

mezlocillin

(mez-loe-sill'in)
Mezlin
Chemical Class: Semisynthetic acylaminopenicillin
Therapeutic Class: Antibiotic

CLINICAL PHARMACOLOGY

Mechanism of Action: Inhibits the biosynthesis of cell wall mucopeptide in susceptible organisms; the cell wall, rendered osmotically unstable, swells and bursts from osmotic pressure; bacterocidal when adequate concentrations are reached

Pharmacokinetics

IM: Peak 45-90 min, 16%-42% bound to plasma proteins, 15% metabolized to inactive metabolites, excreted principally in urine by tubular secretion and glomerular filtration, partly excreted via bile, $t_{1/2}$ 0.7-1.3 hr (prolonged in severe renal impairment)

INDICATIONS AND USES: Treatment of infections caused by susceptible gram-negative aerobic bacilli and mixed aerobic-anaerobic bacterial infections including serious intra-abdominal infections, UTIs, gynecologic infections, respiratory tract infections, skin and skin stucture infections, bone and joint infections and septicemia

Antibacterial spectrum usually includes:

• Gram-positive organisms: *Staphylococcus aureus* (non-penicillinase producing strains), β- hemolytic streptococci (Groups A and B), *Streptococcus pneumoniae, Str. faecalis* (enterococcus)
• Gram-negative organisms: *Escherichia coli, Klebsiella* sp (including *K. pneumoniae), Proteus mirabilis, P. vulgaris, Enterobacter* sp, *Shigella* sp, *Morganella morganii, Pseudomonas aeruginosa, Providencia rettgeri, Haemophilus influenzae, H. parainfluenzae, Providencia stuartii, Citrobacter* sp, *Neisseria* sp, many strains of *Serratia, Salmonella,* and *Acinetobacter* are also susceptible
• Anaerobes: *Peptococcus* sp, *Peptostreptococcus* sp, *Clostridium* sp, *Bacteroides* sp (including *B. fragilis* group), *Fusobacterium* sp, *Veillonella* sp, *Eubacterium* sp

M

DOSAGE

Adult

- IM/IV 3 g q4h or 4 g q6h, do not exceed 24 g/d
- *Uncomplicated UTI:* IM/IV 1.5-2 g q6h
- *Complicated UTI:* IM/IV 3 g q6h
- *Uncomplicated gonococcal urethritis:* IM/IV 1-2 g in conjunction with 1 g of probenecid
- *Perioperative prophylaxis:* IV 4 g 0.5-1.5 hr prior to surgery

Child 1 month-12 yr

- IM/IV 50 mg/kg q4h

$ **AVAILABLE FORMS/COST OF THERAPY**

- Inj, Dry-Sol—IM;IV: 1 g/vial, 25 ml: **$42.77;** 2 g/vial, 30 ml: **$82.93;** 3 g/vial, 20 ml: **$125.06**
- Inj, Dry-Sol—IV: 4 g/vial, 20 ml: **$158.11**

CONTRAINDICATIONS: Hypersensitivity to penicillins

PRECAUTIONS: Hypersensitivity to cephalosporins, renal insufficiency, prolonged or repeated therapy, sodium restricted patients

PREGNANCY AND LACTATION: Pregnancy category B; excreted into breast milk in low concentrations, no adverse effects have been observed but potential exists for modification of bowel flora in nursing infant, allergy/sensitization, and interference with interpretation of culture results if fever workup required

SIDE EFFECTS/ADVERSE REACTIONS

CNS: Headache, fever, ***seizures,*** dizziness, giddiness, fatigue, neuromuscular hyperirritability

GI: Nausea, vomiting, diarrhea, increased AST, ALT, abdominal pain, glossitis, colitis, ***pseudomembranous colitis***

GU: ***Acute interstitial nephritis,*** transient increases in serum creatinine and BUN

HEME: Anemia, ***bleeding abnormalities, bone marrow depression, granulocytopenia, leukopenia, eosinophilia***

METAB: Hypokalemia, hypernatremia

RESP: ***Anaphylaxis, respiratory distress***

SKIN: Urticaria, rash, erythema multiforme, pain at inj site

▼ **DRUG INTERACTIONS**

Drugs

- *Aminoglycosides:* Potential for inactivation of aminoglycosides in patients with severe renal impairment
- *Methotrexate:* Increased methotrexate concentrations, possible toxicity

Labs

- *False positive:* Urine glucose, urine protein

SPECIAL CONSIDERATIONS

MONITORING PARAMETERS

- Renal, hepatic, and hematological systems during prolonged therapy
- Serum electrolytes

---

miconazole

(mi-kon′a-zole)

IV: Monistat, Monistat IV

Top: Micatin, Monistat-Derm, Monistat 3, Monistat 7, Monistat Dual-Pak

Chemical Class: Imidazole

Therapeutic Class: Antifungal

CLINICAL PHARMACOLOGY

Mechanism of Action: Alters permaeability of fungal cell membrane

Pharmacokinetics

TOP: Small amounts absorbed systemically

IV: Onset immediate; distributed into inflamed joints, vitreous humor, peritoneal cavity; limited crossing of blood brain barrier terminal $t_{1/2}$ 24 h; metabolized in liver; excreted in feces, urine (inactive metabolites); >90% protein binding

INDICATIONS AND USES: *IV:* Second line drug in treatment of severe systemic fungal infections such as coccidioidomycosis, candidiasis, cryptococcoses, paracoccidioidomycosis, fungal meningitis, fungal UTI; *TOP:* Tinea pedis, tinea cruris, tinea corporis, tinea versicolor, vulvovaginal candidiasis

DOSAGE

Adult

- IV INF initial test dose of 200 mg, then 200-3600 mg/d; may be divided in 3 inf 200-1200 mg/inf for 1-20 wk
- *Fungal meningitis:* Supplement IV inf with intrathecal miconazole 20 mg q3-7d
- *Bladder mycoses:* Supplement IV inf with bladder irrigation of miconazole 200 mg bid-qid or as continuous inf
- *Vulvovaginal candidiasis:* INTRA VAG (cream) 1 applicatorful qhs for 7 days; (supp) 200 mg (1 supp) qhs for 3 days
- *Tinea, candida:* TOP apply to affected area bid for 2-4 wk

Child > 1 yr

- IV 20-40 mg/kg/d, not to exceed 15 mg/kg/dose
- *Tinea, candida:* TOP same as adult

$ AVAILABLE FORMS/COST OF THERAPY

- Inj, Sol—Intrathecal; IV: 10 mg/ml, 20 ml: **$38.50**
- Cre—Top: 2%, 45 g: **$8.00-$14.04**
- Vag Supp—Top: 200 mg, 3's: **$20.89-$24.36**
- Kit—Top Cre; Vag Supp: 200 mg: **$26.52**
- Kit—Top for nails: 2%: **$13.50-$20.25**
- Powder/Spray—Top: 3 oz: **$3.70-$5.21**
- Aer, Spray—Top: 2%, 42.5 ml: **$16.25**
- Tincture—Top: 2%, 29.57 ml: **$9.25**

CONTRAINDICATIONS: Hypersensitivity

PRECAUTIONS: Renal disease, hepatic disease

PREGNANCY AND LACTATION: Pregnancy category C (TOP category B); unknown if excreted in breast milk

SIDE EFFECTS/ADVERSE REACTIONS

CNS: Drowsiness, headache

CV: Tachycardia, dysrhythmias (rapid IV), ***hyponatremia***

GI: Nausea, vomiting, anorexia, diarrhea, cramps

GU: Vulvovaginal burning, itching, hyponatremia, pelvic cramps (topical forms)

HEME: ***Anemia, thrombocytopenia, hyperlipidemia***

METAB: Hyperlipidemia

SKIN: Pruritus, rash, fever, flushing, ***anaphylaxis,*** hives, *phlebitis*

▼ DRUG INTERACTIONS

- The base in suppository products may interfere with latex; do not use these with contraceptive diaphragms, condoms

Drugs

- *Amphotericin B:* Antagonism
- *Coumarin drugs:* Enhanced anticoagulant effect
- *Cyclosporine:* Possible increased cyclosporine levels
- *Phenytoin:* Possible alterations in levels of both drugs
- *Rifampin:* Possible decreased miconazole efficacy
- *Terfenadine, astemizole:* Adverse cardiovascular effects

Labs

- *False positive:* Urine glucose, urine protein

M

midazolam

(mid-az′zoe-lam)

Versed

Chemical Class: Benzodiazepine, short-acting

Therapeutic Class: Sedative hypnotic

DEA Class: Schedule IV

CLINICAL PHARMACOLOGY

Mechanism of Action: Benzodiazepine receptor agonist; increases activity of the inhibitory neurotransmitter gamma aminobutyric acid (GABA)

Pharmacokinetics

IM: Onset: 15 min, peak ½-1 hr

IV: Onset: 3-5 min, onset of anesthesia 1½-5 min; protein binding 97%; $t_{1/2}$ 1.2-12.3 hr; metabolized in liver; metabolites excreted in urine; crosses placenta, blood-brain barrier

INDICATIONS AND USES: Preoperative sedation, general anesthesia induction, sedation for diagnostic endoscopic procedures, intubation

DOSAGE

Adult

- *Preoperative sedation:* IM 70-80 μg/kg 30-60 min before general anesthesia
- *Induction of general anesthesia:* IV 150-350 μg/kg over 30 sec, wait 2 min, follow with 25% of initial dose if needed; use lower doses for patients who are >55 yrs age, premedicated, ASA III-IV

Child

- *Preoperative sedation:* IM 80-200 μg/kg
- *General anesthesia:* IV 50-200 μg/kg

$ AVAILABLE FORMS/COST OF THERAPY

- Inj, Sol—IM;IV: 1 mg/ml, 2 ml: **$4.34;** 5 mg/ml, 2 ml: **$17.05**

CONTRAINDICATIONS: Hypersensitivity to benzodiazepines, shock, coma, alcohol intoxication, acute narrow-angle glaucoma

PRECAUTIONS: COPD, CHF, chronic renal failure, hepatic disease, elderly, debilitated, myasthenia gravis, other muscular dystrophies and myotonias

PREGNANCY AND LACTATION: Pregnancy category D; no data on breast feeding

SIDE EFFECTS/ADVERSE REACTIONS

CNS: Retrograde amnesia, euphoria, confusion, headache, anxiety, insomnia, slurred speech, paresthesia, tremors, weakness, chills

CV: ***Hypotension, PVCs, tachycardia, bigeminy, nodal rhythm***

EENT: Blurred vision, nystagmus, diplopia, blocked ears, loss of balance

GI: Nausea, vomiting, increased salivation, hiccups

RESP: Coughing, ***apnea, bronchospasm, laryngospasm,*** dyspnea

SKIN: Urticaria, pain, swelling at inj site, rash, pruritus

▼ DRUG INTERACTIONS

Drugs

- *Calcium channel blockers, erythromycin, ketoconazole, itraconazole:* Increased midazolam levels, increased sedation, respiratory depression
- Additive effects with other CNS depressants

milrinone

(mill're-none)

Primacor

Chemical Class: Bipyridine derivative

Therapeutic Class: Inotropic/vasodilator agent with phosphodiesterase activity

CLINICAL PHARMACOLOGY

Mechanism of Action: Positive inotropic agent with vasodilator properties; reduces preload and afterload by direct relaxation of vascular smooth muscle

Pharmocokinetics

IV: Onset 2-5 min, peak 10 min, duration variable; $t_{1/2}$ 4-6 hr; metabolized in liver; excreted in urine as drug and metabolites 60%-90%

INDICATIONS AND USES: Short-term management of CHF that has not responded to other medication; can be used with digitalis

DOSAGE

Adult

• IV BOL 50 µg/kg given over 10 min; start inf of 0.375-0.75 µg/kg/min

• Reduced dose in renal impairment:

CREATININE CLEARANCE (ml/min/1.73 m 2)	INFUSION RATE (mcg/kg/min)
5	0.20
10	0.23
20	0.28
30	0.33
40	0.38
50	0.43

$ AVAILABLE FORMS/COST OF THERAPY

• Inj, Sol—IV: 1 mg/ml, 5ml: **$31.26**

CONTRAINDICATIONS: Hypersensitivity to this drug, severe aortic stenosis, severe pulmonic stenosis, acute MI

PRECAUTIONS: Children, renal disease, hepatic disease, atrial flutter/fibrillation, outflow tract obstruction in hypertrophic subaortic stenosis, elderly

PREGNANCY AND LACTATION: Pregnancy category C; unknown if excreted in breast milk

SIDE EFFECTS/ADVERSE REACTIONS

CNS: Headache, tremor

CV: ***Dysrhythmias, hypotension, chest pain,*** *hypokalemia*

GI: Nausea, vomiting, anorexia, abdominal pain, ***hepatotoxicity,*** jaundice

HEME: ***Thrombocytopenia***

minocycline

(mi-noe-sye'kleen)

Dynacin, Minocin, Minocin IV

Chemical Class: Semisynthetic tetracycline

Therapeutic Class: Antibiotic

CLINICAL PHARMACOLOGY

Mechanism of Action: Inhibits protein synthesis, phosphorylation in microorganisms by binding to 30S ribosomal subunits, reversibly binding to 50S ribosomal subunits; bacteriostatic

Pharmacokinetics

PO: Peak 2-3 hr, $t_{1/2}$ 11-17 hr; biliary and urinary excretion, crosses placenta; excreted in breast milk, 76% protein bound

INDICATIONS AND USES: Syphilis, non-gonococcal urethritis, endocervical and rectal infections caused by *C. trachomatis/U. urealyticum,* gonorrhea, lymphogranuloma venereum, rickettsial infections, inflammatory acne, skin granulomas caused by *Mycobacterium marinum,* respiratory tract infections caused by susceptible organisms, UTI, treatment of asymptomatic meningococcal carriers when rifampin contraindicated, tularemia, cholera, plague, chancroid, psittacosis, brucellosis (with streptomycin), yaws, anthrax, actinomycosis, sclerosing agent in malignant pleural effusions

Antibacterial specturm usually includes:

- Gram-positive organisms: *Streptococcus pneumoniae, Str. pyogenes,* alpha hemolytic streptococci; many strains strep resistant, demonstrate susceptibility
- Gram-negative organisms: *Bartonella bacilliformis, Brucella, Campylobacter fetus, Francisella tularensis, Haemophilus influenzae, H. ducreyi, Listeria monocytogenes, Neisseria gonorrhea, Vibrio cholera, Yersinia pestis;* some strains of *E. coli, Klebsiella, Shigella, Bacteroides, Enterobacter aerogenes, Acinetobacter;* other: *Bacillus anthracis, Balantidium coli, Borrelia recurrentis, Chlamydia psittoci, C. trachomatis, Clostridium, Fusobacterium fusiforme, Mycoplasma pneumoniae, Propionibacterium acnes, Rickeltsiae, Treponema pallidum, Ureaplasma urealyticum*

DOSAGE

Adult

- PO/IV 200 mg, then 100 mg q12h or 50 mg q6h, not to exceed 400 mg/24h IV
- *Gonorrhea* (not drug of choice): PO 200 mg, then 100 mg q12h for 4 days
- *Chlamydia trachomatis/Ureaplasma urealyticum:* PO 100 mg bid for 7 days
- *Syphilis* (PCN allergic pts): PO 200 mg, then 100 mg q12h for 10-15 days
- *Acne:* 50 mg 1-3 times/d
- *Skin granulomas from M. marinum:* 100 mg bid for 6-8 wk
- *Sclerosing agent:* 300 mg diluted with 50 ml 0.9% NaCl inj instilled via thoracostomy tube

Child >8 yrs

- PO/IV 4 mg/kg then 4 mg/kg/d PO in divided doses q12h

$ AVAILABLE FORMS/COST OF THERAPY

- Inj, Lyphl-Sol—IV: 100 mg/vial: **$32.79**
- Susp—Oral: 50 mg/5 ml, 60 ml: **$30.49**
- Cap, Gel—Oral: 50 mg, 100's: **$67.43-$163.35;** 100 mg, 50's: **$90.44-$136.06**

CONTRAINDICATIONS: Hypersensitivity to tetracyclines, children < 8 yr

PRECAUTIONS: Hepatic disease

PREGNANCY AND LACTATION: Pregnancy category D; not recommended in last half of pregnancy secondary to adverse effects on fetal teeth; not recommended in breast feeding

SIDE EFFECTS/ADVERSE REACTIONS

CNS: Dizziness, fever, light-headedness, vertigo, ***pseudotumor cerebri***

CV: Pericarditis

EENT: Dysphagia, glossitis, decreased calcification of deciduous teeth, oral candidiasis

GI: Nausea, abdominal pain, *vomiting, diarrhea,* anorexia, enterocolitis, ***hepatotoxicity,*** flatulence, abdominal cramps, epigastric burning, stomatitis

GU: Increased BUN, polyuria, polydipsia, ***renal failure, nephrotoxicity***

HEME: ***Eosinophilia, neutropenia, thrombocytopenia, hemolytic anemia***

SKIN: Rash, urticaria, photosensitivity, increased pigmentation, ***exfoliative dermatitis,*** pruritus, angioedema, blue-gray color of skin, mucous membranes

▼ **DRUG INTERACTIONS**

Drugs

• *Antacids, $NaHCO_3$, bismuth subsalicylate, iron, sodium bicarbonate, carbamazepine, phenobarbital:* Decreased effect of minocycline
• *Methoxyflurane:* Renal toxicity
• *Oral contraceptives:* Decreased contraceptive efficacy
• *Penicillins:* Antagonizes antibacterial effect of PCN

Labs

• *False negative:* Urine glucose with Clinistix or Tes-Tape

SPECIAL CONSIDERATIONS

• May take with food
• Avoid sun exposure

minoxidil

(min-nox'i-dill)
Oral: Loniten, Minodyl
Topical: Rogaine
Chemical Class: Peripheral vasodilator
Therapeutic Class: Antihypertensive (oral use), hair growth stimulant (topical use)

CLINICAL PHARMACOLOGY

Mechanism of Action: Relaxes arteriolar smooth muscle, causes vasodilation with reflex increase in heart rate, cardiac output; may increase cutaneous blood flow, stimulate hair follicles

Pharmocokinetics

PO: Onset 30 min, peak 2-3 hr, duration 24-48 hr; $t_{1/2}$ 4.2 hr; metabolized in liver; 97% renal excretion; excreted in breast milk

TOP: Small amounts absorbed (0.3%-4.5%), absorption increased through inflamed skin; onset of action min 4 mo; growth peaks at 1 yr

INDICATIONS AND USES: Severe hypertension not responsive to other therapy, in conjunction with diuretic; topically to treat alopecia androgenetica; less effective in frontal hair loss

DOSAGE

Adult/Adolescent

• PO 2.5-5 mg/d as single dose or divided bid not to exceed 100 mg/d, usual range 10-40 mg/d; double dose q3d to appropriate response; for rapid control adjust q6h, monitor closely
• TOP 1 ml (2% sol) bid regardless of size of area; max 2 ml qd

Child <12 yr

• Initial dose PO 0.2 mg/kg/d (max 5 mg); effective range 0.25-1 mg/kg/d in one or two doses; max 50 mg/d

$ **AVAILABLE FORMS/COST OF THERAPY**

• Tab, Uncoated—Oral: 2.5 mg, 100's: **$13.88-$47.25;** 10 mg, 100's: **$15.75-$56.70**
• Sol—Top: 2%, 60 ml: **$57.78**

CONTRAINDICATIONS: Acute MI, dissecting aortic aneurysm, hypersensitivity, pheochromocytoma

PRECAUTIONS: Children, renal disease, CAD, CHF

PREGNANCY AND LACTATION: Pregnancy category C; compatible with breast feeding per Am Acad Pediatrics, manufacturer does not recommend

SIDE EFFECTS/ADVERSE REACTIONS

ORAL:

CNS: Drowsiness, dizziness, sedation, headache, depression, fatigue

CV: ***Severe rebound hypertension,*** tachycardia, angina, ***CHF, pulmonary edema, pericardial effusion, pericarditis,*** edema, sodium and water retention, T wave changes (direction and magnitude)

GI: Nausea, vomiting

GU: Gynecomastia, breast tenderness
HEME: ***Thrombocytopenia, leukopenia,*** decreased Hct (hemodilution)
SKIN: Pruritus, ***Stevens-Johnson syndrome,*** rash, hypertrichosis (80% of patients, resolves 1-6 mo after discontinuation of drug)
TOPICAL:
SKIN: Hypertrichosis, irritant/contact dermatitis

▼ DRUG INTERACTIONS

Drugs

• *Guanethidine:* Orthostatic hypotension
• No known interactions with top sol

SPECIAL CONSIDERATIONS

• Must be used in conjunction with diuretic (except dialysis patients) and beta blocker (reflex tachycardia)
• Methyldopa may be used if beta blocker contraindicated

---

misoprostol

(me-soe-prost'ole)
Cytotec
Chemical Class: Prostaglandin E_1 analog
Therapeutic Class: Gastric mucosa protectant, abortifacient

CLINICAL PHARMACOLOGY

Mechanism of Action: Inhibits gastric acid secretion; may protect gastric mucosa; can increase bicarbonate, mucus production; stimulates uterine contractions

Pharmacokinetics

PO: Rapidly metabolized to active metabolite, peak 12 min, plasma steady state achieved within 2 days, excreted in urine, unknown if metabolite excreted in breast milk

INDICATIONS AND USES: Prevention of nonsteroidal antiinflammatory drug (NSAID)-induced gastric ulcers, treatment of duodenal ulcer,* abortifacient in early pregnancies (with methotrexate or RU486),* morning after treatment*

DOSAGE

Adult

• *Gastric ulcer prophylaxis:* PO 200 μg qid with food for duration of NSAID therapy; if not tolerated, decrease to 100 μg qid or 200 μg bid
• *Morning after treatment/abortifacient:* Different protocols used; consult literature

$ AVAILABLE FORMS/COST OF THERAPY

• Tab, Uncoated—Oral: 100 μg, 100's: **$50.91;** 200 μg, 100's: **$70.63**

CONTRAINDICATIONS: Allergy to prostaglandins, pregnancy (unless used as abortifacient)

PRECAUTIONS: Women of childbearing age

PREGNANCY AND LACTATION: Pregnancy category X; do not use in breast feeding (possible diarrhea in infant)

SIDE EFFECTS/ADVERSE REACTIONS

GI: *Diarrhea,* nausea, vomiting, flatulence, constipation, dyspepsia, abdominal pain
GU: Spotting, cramps, vaginal bleeding

---

moexipril

(moe-ex'a-prile)
Univasc
Chemical Class: Non sulfhydryl angiotensin-converting enzyme inhibitor
Therapeutic Class: Angiotensin converting enzyme inhibitor

CLINICAL PHARMACOLOGY

Mechanism of Action: Angiotensin converting enzyme inhibition suppresses the renin-angiotensin-aldosterone system, resulting in reduced peripheral arterial resistance; no change or an increase in cardiac output; increased renal blood flow, but no change in glomerular filtration rate; blood pressure reduction (standing and supine equally)

Pharmacokinetics

PO: Prodrug, requiring hepatic conversion to active metabolite (moexiprilat); bioavailability, 13%; fecal excretion, 50% (minimal renal excretion); $t_{1/2}$ 2-10 hr; Cp (moexiprilat), 1½ hr

INDICATIONS AND USES: Hypertension, heart failure,* left ventricular dysfunction,* diabetic nephropathy*

DOSAGE

Adult

- *Hypertension:* Initial 7.5 mg PO ½ hr ac qd; maintenance 7.5-30 mg PO qd-bid
- Renal function impairment, CrCl < 40 ml/min, 3.75-15 mg PO qd

$ AVAILABLE FORMS/COST OF THERAPY

- Tab, Uncoated—Oral: 7.5, 15 mg, 100's: **$49.69**

CONTRAINDICATIONS: Pregnancy, hypersensitivity

PRECAUTIONS: Hyperkalemia, valvular stenosis, surgery/anesthesia (hypotension), cough

PREGNANCY AND LACTATION: Pregnancy category C (first trimester); Category D (second and third trimesters)

SIDE EFFECTS/ADVERSE REACTIONS

CNS: Peripheral neuropathy, insomnia, *headache, dizziness, fatigue*

CV: Hypotension, Raynaud's syndrome, CHF, dysrhythmia

GI: Gastric irritation, apthous ulcers, *dysgeusia, weight loss, abdominal pain, vomiting, nausea,* diarrhea

GU: Proteinuria, renal insufficiency, nephrotic syndrome, polyuria

HEME: ***Neutropenia/agranulocytosis, thrombocytopenia, pancytopenia,*** *decreased hemoglobin*

METAB: Electrolyte disturbance (hyperkalemia, hyponatremia)

RESP: Cough

SKIN: Rash, pruritus, pemphigus, scalded mouth sensation, alopecia

MISC: ***Anaphylactoid reactions***

▼ DRUG INTERACTIONS

Drugs

- *Allopurinol:* Increased risk of hypersensitivity reactions including Stevens-Johnson syndrome, skin eruptions, fever, and arthralgias
- *Indomethacin:* Inhibits the antihypertensive response to ACE inhibition; other NSAIDs probably have similar effect
- *Lithium:* increased risk of lithium toxicity
- *Loop diuretics:* Initiation of ACE inhibition therapy with concurrent intensive diuretic therapy may cause significant hypotension, renal insufficiency
- *Potassium:* ACE inhibition tends to increase potassium, increased risk of hyperkalemia in predisposed patients
- *Potassium-sparing diuretics:* ACE inhibition tends to increase potassium, increased risk of hyperkalemia in predisposed patients

SPECIAL CONSIDERATIONS

- Besides the once-daily dosing advantage of other long-acting ACE inhibitors, does not possess any particular characteristic which would suggest its preference over any other ACE inhibitor; controlled comparisons are not available; low price may be major selling edge

molindone

(moe-lin'done)
Moban
Chemical Class: Oxygenated indole compound (dihydroindolone)
Therapeutic Class: Antipsychotic/neuroleptic

CLINICAL PHARMACOLOGY
Mechanism of Action: Competes for dopamine (D_2) receptor sites in the reticular activating and limbic systems in the brain, thus decreasing dopamine activity; depresses cerebral cortex, hypothalamus, limbic system, which control activity, aggression; exhibits α-adrenergic and anticholinergic actions
Pharmacokinetics
PO: Onset erratic; peak 1½ hr; duration 24-36 hr
Metabolized by liver (36 recognized metabolites), excreted in urine and feces; $t_{1/2}$, 1½ hr
INDICATIONS AND USES: Psychotic disorders
DOSAGE
Adult
• PO initial dose 50-75 mg/d increasing to 225 mg/d if needed; maintenance dose, mild, 5-15 mg tid-qid; moderate, 10-25 mg tid-qid; severe 225 mg/d may be required
$ **AVAILABLE FORMS/COST OF THERAPY**
• Conc—Oral: 20 mg/ml, 120 ml: **$118.79**
• Tab, Uncoated—Oral: 5 mg, 100's: **$55.98;** 10 mg, 100's: **$80.42;** 25 mg, 100's: **$119.95;** 50 mg, 100's: **$160.19;** 100 mg, 100's: **$214.00**
CONTRAINDICATIONS: Hypersensitivity, coma, children
PRECAUTIONS: Hypertension, hepatic disease, cardiac disease, Parkinson's disease, brain tumor, glaucoma, urinary retention, diabetes mellitus, respiratory disease, prostatic hypertrophy, geriatric patients
PREGNANCY AND LACTATION: Pregnancy category C
SIDE EFFECTS/ADVERSE REACTIONS
CNS: EPS: Pseudoparkinsonism, akathisia, dystonia, tardive dyskinesia; drowsiness, headache, seizures
CV: Orthostatic hypotension, hypertension, ***cardiac arrest,*** ECG changes, ***tachycardia***
EENT: Blurred vision, glaucoma
GI: Dry mouth, nausea, vomiting, anorexia, constipation, diarrhea, jaundice, weight gain
GU: Urinary retention, urinary frequency, enuresis, impotence, amenorrhea, gynecomastia
HEME: ***Anemia, leukopenia, leukocytosis, agranulocytosis***
RESP: ***Laryngospasm,*** dyspnea, ***respiratory depression***
SKIN: ***Rash,*** photosensitivity, dermatitis
MISC: Decreased sweating
▼ **DRUG INTERACTIONS**
Drugs
• *Anticholinergics:* May inhibit neuroleptic response; excess anticholinergic effects
• *Antidepressants:* Neuroleptics may increase serum concentrations of some antidepressants, with potential to increase both therapeutic and toxic effects
• *Beta blockers:* Increase plasma concentrations of both drugs, with accentuated pharmacologic responses of both
• *Bromocriptine:* Inhibits ability of bromocriptine to lower serum prolactin
• *Epinephrine:* Neuroleptics may inhibit the pressor response
• *Guanethidine+:* Neuroleptics may

inhibit the antihypertensive response to guanethidine

• *Levodopa:* Neuroleptics may inhibit the antiparkinsonian effects of levodopa

• *Orphenadrine:* Combinations may result in lower serum neuroleptic concentrations

SPECIAL CONSIDERATIONS

• Neuroleptic structurally different from the phenothiazines, thioxanthenes, and butyrophenones

• High potency with high incidence of EPS, but a low incidence of sedation, anticholinergic effects, and cardiovascular effects

mometasone

(mo-met′a-sone)

Elocon

Chemical Class: Substituted 17-hydroxyl group, non-fluorinated glucocorticoid

Therapeutic Class: Medium potency topical corticosteroid

CLINICAL PHARMACOLOGY

Mechanism of Action: Nonspecific antiinflammatory activity; interact with cytoplasmic receptors (dermal and intradermal), inducing phospholipase A2 inhibitory proteins; depress formation, release, and activity of endogenous mediators of inflammation (i.e., prostaglandins, kinins, histamine, complement system)

Pharmacokinetics

Absorbed systemically across stratum corneum, extent dependent on dosage form and condition of the skin; hepatic metabolism (resistant to skin metabolism)

INDICATIONS AND USES: Symptomatic relief of inflammation and/or pruritus associated with acute and chronic corticosteroid-responsive disorders

DOSAGE

Adult

• Apply qd-bid

$ AVAILABLE FORMS/COST OF THERAPY

• Cre—Top: 0.1%, 15 g: **$14.82;** 45 g: **$27.16**

• Lotion—Top: 0.1%, 30 ml: **$16.07;** 60 ml: **$30.66**

• Oint—Top: 0.1%, 15 g: **$14.82;** 45 g: **$27.16**

CONTRAINDICATIONS: Hypersensitivity

PRECAUTIONS: Skin lesions covering large surface areas or involving thin skinned areas; children, adolescents, geriatrics

PREGNANCY AND LACTATION: Pregnancy category C; systemic corticosteroids are excreted into breast milk in quantities not likely to have deleterious effects in breastfeeding infants; no information on topical steroids

SIDE EFFECTS/ADVERSE REACTIONS

CV: Hypertension

EENT: Subcapsular cataracts, glaucoma

METAB: Cushing's syndrome, hypokalemic syndrome

SKIN: Allergic contact dermatitis; folliculitis, furunculosis, pustules, pyoderma, vesiculation, hyperesthesia, skin atrophy, secondary skin infection, *acneiform eruptions, hypopigmentation, striae, hair loss*

▼ DRUG INTERACTIONS

Labs

• *Interference:* With adrenal function as assessed by corticotropin stimulation, 24-hour urine free cortisol, or 17-OHCS measurements; plasma cortisol

• *Decrease:* HPA axis function; eosinophil count

• *Increase:* Glucose

SPECIAL CONSIDERATIONS

• May represent mid-range efficacy with mild-range adverse effects liability

monobenzone

(mono-ben'zone)

Benoquin

Chemical Class: Monobenzyl ether of hydroquinone

Therapeutic Class: Depigmenting (demelanizing) agent

CLINICAL PHARMACOLOGY

Mechanism of Action: Decrease in the number of functional melanocytes and inhibition of the process of pigmentation (inhibition of tyrosinase, which catalyzes the oxidation of tyrosine to dihydroxyphenyalanine, a precursor of melanin)

Pharmacokinetics

Depigmentation is usually observed after 1-4 mo of therapy (discontinue if satisfactory results are not observed in 4 mo); complete depigmentation may require 9-12 mo

INDICATIONS AND USES: Final depigmantation in extensive vitiligo

DOSAGE

Adult

• Apply and rub into pigmented areas 2-3 times daily

Child

• Safety in children <12 not established

$ AVAILABLE FORMS/COST OF THERAPY

• Cre—Top: 20%, 37.5 g: **$43.06**

CONTRAINDICATIONS: Freckling; hyperpigmentation due to photosensitization; melasma (cholasma of pregnancy), cafe-au-lait spots; pigmented nevi, malignant melanoma; pigment resulting from pigments other than melanin (i.e., bile, silver); hypersensitivity

PREGNANCY AND LACTATION: Pregnancy category C

SIDE EFFECTS/ADVERSE REACTIONS

SKIN: Irritation, burning, *dermatitis*

SPECIAL CONSIDERATIONS

PATIENT/FAMILY EDUCATION

• Drug is not a mild cosmetic bleach; treated areas should not be exposed to sunlight (protect with a topical sunscreen)

moricizine

(mor-iss'i-zeen)

Ethmozine

Chemical Class: Phenothiazine derivative

Therapeutic Class: Antidysrhythmic, type I

CLINICAL PHARMACOLOGY

Mechanism of Action: Decreases rate of rise of action potential, prolongs refractory period, and shortens the action potential duration; depression of inward influx of sodium mediates these effects; slows atrial and AV nodal conduction; increase in resting blood pressure and heart rate; inhibits platelet aggregation; anticholinergic effects

Pharmacokinetics

PO: Peak plasma concentration, 0.5-2.2 hr; peak effect, shortening of JT interval, 6 hr; effect on VPD rates, 10-14 hr

Well absorbed; metabolized by the liver; metabolites are excreted in feces and urine, protein binding, >90%; $t_{1/2}$, 1.5-3.5 hr

INDICATIONS AND USES: Symptomatic, life-threatening ventricular dysrhythmias

DOSAGE

Adult

• PO 600-900 mg/d in 2-3 divided

doses; increase dosage in 150 mg increments at 3-day intervals up to 900 mg/d; decrease dose in patients with significant liver and renal dysfunction

$ AVAILABLE FORMS/COST OF THERAPY

• Tab, Coated—Oral: 200 mg, 100's: **$89.32;** 250 mg, 100's: **$106.63;** 300 mg, 100's: **$121.41**

CONTRAINDICATIONS: 2nd-3rd degree AV block, right bundle branch block when associated with left hemiblock (bifascicular block) unless a pacemaker is present, cardiogenic shock, hypersensitivity

PRECAUTIONS: CHF, hypokalemia, hyperkalemia, sick sinus syndrome, children, impaired hepatic and renal function, cardiac dysfunction

PREGNANCY AND LACTATION: Pregnancy category B; secreted into breast milk (one patient); potential for serious adverse effects exists

SIDE EFFECTS/ADVERSE REACTIONS

CNS: Dizziness, headache, fatigue, perioral numbness, euphoria, nervousness, sleep disorders, depression, tinnitus, fatigue

*CV: Palpitations, chest pain, **CHF,*** hypertension, syncope, disrhythmias, bradycardia, ***MI,*** thrombophlebitis

GI: Nausea, abdominal pain, vomiting, diarrhea

GU: Sexual dysfunction, difficult urination, dysuria, incontinence

RESP: Dyspnea, hyperventilation, ***apnea,*** asthma, pharyngitis, cough

MISC: Sweating, musculoskeletal pain

▼ DRUG INTERACTIONS

Labs

• *ECG changes:* Shortening of JT interval, widened QRS, PR prolongation, QT prolongation

SPECIAL CONSIDERATIONS

• Antidysrhythmic therapy has not been proven to be beneficial in terms of improving survival among patients with asymptomatic or mildly symptomatic ventricular dysrhythmias. Studied in the NHLBI's CAST (Cardiac Arrhythmia Suppression Trial, I and II) with findings of excessive cardiac mortality and no effect on long-term survival compared to placebo

morphine

(mor'feen)

Astramorph PF, Duramorph, Infumorph 200, Infumorph 500, MS Contin, MSIR, OMS Concentrate, Oramorph SR, RMS, Roxanol, Roxanol 100, Roxanol Rescudose, Roxanol SR

Chemical Class: Opiate

Therapeutic Class: Narcotic analgesic

DEA Class: Schedule II

CLINICAL PHARMACOLOGY

Mechanism of Action: Altered processes affecting both the perception of pain and the emotional response to pain, at the spinal cord level, by interacting with opioid receptors (primarily μ receptors)

Pharmacokinetics

PO: 60 mg = 10 IM morphine; duration of action: 8-12 hr (ext rel preps); 4-5 hr (other oral dosage forms)

SC: Onset, 10-30 min; peak analgesia, 50-90 min; duration, 4-5 hr

IM: Onset, 10-30 min; peak analgesia, 30-60; duration, 4.5 hr

IV: Peak analgesia, 20 min

Metabolized by liver; 85% excreted by kidneys, 7%-10% biliary; $t_{1/2}$ 2½-3 hr

INDICATIONS AND USES: Severe pain, anesthesia (adjunct), diarrhea, cough,* acute pulmonary edema

DOSAGE

Adult

• *Chronic pain:* SC/IM 4-15 mg q4h prn; PO 10-30 mg q4h prn; EXT REL 30-60 mg q8-12h; REC 10-20 mg q4h prn

• IV 4-10 mg diluted in 4-5 ml H_2O for inj, over 5 min

Child

• *Analgesia:* SC 0.1-0.2 mg/kg, not to exceed 15 mg

$ AVAILABLE FORMS/COST OF THERAPY

• Inj, Sol—Epidural; Intrathecal; IV: 0.5 mg/ml, 2 ml: **$7.68;** 10 ml (preservative free): **$9.29-$68.28;** 1 mg/ml, 2 ml (preservative free: **$8.30;** 10 ml: **$9.80-$72.79**

• Inj, Sol—IM; IV; SC: 4 mg/ml, 1 ml × 10: **$7.10-$11.30;** 5 mg/ml, 30 ml: **$17.50-$19.97;** 8 mg/ml, 1 ml×10: **$7.30-$11.64;** 10 mg/ml, 1 ml×10: **$7.81-$12.03;** 15 mg/ml, 1 ml×10: **$8.28-$12.50**

• Inj, Sol—IV: 25 mg/ml, 4 ml: **$9.44-$31.25;** 50 mg/ml, 10 ml: **$34.14-$238.85**

• Cap, Gel—Oral: 15 mg, 50's: **$14.45;** 30 mg, 50's: **$26.97**

• Conc—Oral: 100 mg/5ml, 120 ml: **$70.64**

• Powder: 5 g: **$50.06;** 25 g: **$233.78**

• Sol—Oral: 10 mg/5ml, 100 ml: **$8.78;** 20 mg/5 ml, 100 ml: **$12.50;** 20 mg/ml, 120 ml: **$40.00-$75.69**

• Supp—Rect: 5 mg, 12's:**$9.60-$14.35;** 20 mg, 12's: **$13.50-$20.56;** 30 mg, 12's: **$17.00-$28.71**

• Tab, Coated, Sust Action—Oral: 15 mg, 100's: **$64.71-$77.61;** 30 mg, 100's: **$122.98-$147.49;** 60 mg, 100's: **$239.97-$287.79;** 100 mg, 100's: **$367.51-$436.33;** 200 mg, 100's: **$799.00**

• Tab, Hypodermic—IM; IV: 30 mg, 100's: **$46.90**

• Tab, Hypodermic—IV; SC: 15 mg, 100's: **$27.95;** 10 mg, 100's: **$22.03**

• Tab, Uncoated—Oral: 15 mg, 100's: **$16.88-$25.36;** 30 mg, 100's: **$28.52-$43.05**

CONTRAINDICATIONS: Hypersensitivity, respiratory depression, hemorrhage, acute asthma attack, inflammatory bowel disease

PRECAUTIONS: Addictive personality, elderly, hepatic disease, renal disease, child <18 yr

PREGNANCY AND LACTATION: Pregnancy category B; trace amounts enter breast milk; compatible with breast feeding

SIDE EFFECTS/ADVERSE REACTIONS

CNS: Drowsiness, dizziness, confusion, headache, *sedation,* euphoria

CV: Palpitations, bradycardia, *hypotension*

EENT: Tinnitus, blurred vision, *miosis,* diplopia

GI: Nausea, vomiting, anorexia, *constipation,* cramps, biliary tract pressure

GU: Urinary retention

RESP: ***Respiratory depression***

SKIN: Rash, urticaria, bruising, flushing, diaphoresis, pruritus

MISC: Histamine release (decreased blood pressure, fast heartbeat, increased sweating, redness or flushing of face, wheezing or troubled breathing)

▼ DRUG INTERACTIONS

Drugs

• *Barbiturates:* Additive CNS depression

• *Neuroleptics:* Enhanced CNS depression and hypotension

• *Ethanol:* Additive CNS depression

• *H_2 receptor antagonists:* Inhibition of narcotic hepatic metabolism, additive CNS effect

• *Rifampin:* May reduce narcotic concentrations and precipitate withdrawal

Labs

• *Increase:* Amylase

SPECIAL CONSIDERATIONS

• Treatment of overdose: Naloxone (Narcan) 0.2-0.8 mg IV

• Remains the strong analgesic of choice for acute, severe pain, acute MI pain and the agent of choice for chronic cancer pain

PATIENT/FAMILY EDUCATION

• Change position slowly to avoid orthostasis

• Avoid alcohol and other CNS depressants

• Physical dependency may result

---

mupirocin

(mew-per'o-sen)

Bactroban

Chemical Class: Pseudomonic acid A

Therapeutic Class: Topical antiinfective

CLINICAL PHARMACOLOGY

Mechanism of Action: Inhibits bacterial protein synthesis; shows no cross-resistance with chloramphenicol, erythromycin, fusidic acid, gentamicin, lincomycin, methicillin, neomycin, novobiocin, penicillin, streptomycin, and tetracycline

Pharmacokinetics

No measurable systemic absorption

INDICATIONS AND USES: Impetigo caused by *Staphylococcus aureus* (including methicillin-resistant and β-lactamase producing strains), *S. epidermidis, S. saprophyticus,* β-hemolytic *Streptococcus, Strep. pyogenes*

DOSAGE

Apply small amount to affected area tid

$ AVAILABLE FORMS/COST OF THERAPY

• Oint—Top: 2%, 15 g: **$15.20**

CONTRAINDICATIONS: Hypersensitivity

PREGNANCY AND LACTATION: Prenancy category B

SIDE EFFECTS/ADVERSE REACTIONS

*SKIN: Burning, stinging, itching,*rash, dry skin, swelling, contact dermatitis, erythema, tenderness, increased exudate

SPECIAL CONSIDERATIONS

• Comparable efficacy to systemic semisynthetic penicillins and erythromycin in impetigo and infected wounds

---

muromonab-CD3

(mur-oo-mon'ab)

Orthoclone OKT3

Chemical Class: Murine monoclonal antibody

Therapeutic Class: Immunosuppressive

CLINICAL PHARMACOLOGY

Mechanism of Action: Blocks graft rejection by blocking T-cell function

Pharmacokinetics

IV: Trough levels after 5 mg/d rose over the first three days and then averaged 900 ng/ml on days 3 to 14; therapeutic levels >800 ng/ml block the function of cytotoxic T cells *in vitro* and *in vivo*

INDICATIONS AND USES: Acute allograft rejection in renal, cardiac/hepatic transplant patients

DOSAGE

Adult

• IV BOL 5 mg/d × 10-14 days

$ AVAILABLE FORMS/COST OF THERAPY

• Inj, Sol—IV: 5 mg/ 5ml ampule: **$535.00**

CONTRAINDICATIONS: Hypersensitivity to murine origin, fluid overload

PRECAUTIONS: Child <2 yr, fever, unstable angina, recent MI, heart failure, COPD, intravascular volume overload

PREGNANCY AND LACTATION: Pregnancy category C

SIDE EFFECTS/ADVERSE REACTIONS

CNS: Pyrexia, chills, tremor, headache

CV: Chest pain (angina/MI)

GI: Vomiting, nausea, diarrhea, abdominal pain

GU: Increased creatinine

MS: Muscle/joint aches and pains; generalized weakness

RESP: Dyspnea, wheezing, ***pulmonary edema***

MISC: Infection; cytokine release syndrome (CRS): ranges from "flu-like" illness to life-threatening shock-like syndrome

▼ **DRUG INTERACTIONS**

Drugs

- *Immunosuppressant agents:* Increased risk of infection, lymphoproliferative disorders
- *Vaccines, live virus:* Increased side effects, decreased antibody response

SPECIAL CONSIDERATIONS

- Effective for reversal of resistant renal, hepatic, cardiac, and kidney/pancreas transplant rejection and is an important alternative to retransplantation
- No advantage over other immunosuppressive agents for prevention of rejection
- Manifestations of CRS may be prevented or minimized by pretreatment with methylprednisolone (8mg/kg) 1-4 h prior to administration of the first dose

MONITORING PARAMETERS

- RFTs, transaminases, WBCs and differential with platelet counts
- Chest X-ray within 24 hr

mycophenolate

(my-co-fen′o-late)

CellCept

Chemical Class: 2-morpholinoethyl ester of mycophenolic acid

Therapeutic Class: Immunosuppressive agent

CLINICAL PHARMACOLOGY

Mechanism of Action: Mycophenolic acid (MPA), the active metabolite is a potent, selective, uncompetitive, and reversible inhibitor of inosine monophosphate dehydrogenase, which inhibits the de novo pathway of guanosine nucleotide synthesis; T- and B-lymphocytes are critically dependent on this process, thus, MPA has potent cytostatic effects on lymphocytes; has been shown to prolong the survival of allogeneic transplants (kidney, heart, liver, intestine, limb, small bowel, pancreatic islets, and bone marrow) and reverse ongoing acute rejection in renal and cardiac allograft models

Pharmacokinetics

PO: T_{max}, 6 hr; C_{max}, 2.6 μg/ml after 1.0 g bid dose

Rapid absorption (94% bioavailable); presystemic metabolism to MPA (active metabolite); immediately post-transplant (<40 days), mean AUC, C_{max} approximately 50% lower than healthy volunteers or stable renal transplant patients; food has no effect on absorption; MPA C_{max} decreased by 40%; V_d, MPA, 3.6 and 4.0 l/kg following IV and oral administration, respectively; MPA 97% bound to plasma albumin; negligible amount excreted as MPA (<1% of dose) in the urine; $t_{1/2}$, 17 hr

INDICATIONS AND USES: Primary maintenance immunosuppression and/or rescue/rejection therapy following renal, heart, and liver transplantation, rheumatoid arthritis,* psoriasis*

DOSAGE

Adult

- 1.0 g PO bid (on empty stomach) starting 72 hr after renal transplant; usually given with corticosteroids and cyclosporine; range 0.5 g-4 g/day
- With severe chronic renal impairment (GFR <25 ml/min/1.73m^2) outside of the immediate post-transplant period, doses > 1 g should be avoided

Child

- 15 mg/kg PO bid (on empty stomach)

$ **AVAILABLE FORMS/COST OF THERAPY**

- Cap, Gel—Oral: 250 mg, 100's: **$156.25**

CONTRAINDICATIONS: Hypersensitivity

PRECAUTIONS: Peptic ulcer disease, history of GI bleed, decreased renal function

PREGNANCY AND LACTATION: Pregnancy category C; mycophenolic acid excreted in milk; not recommended during breast feeding

SIDE EFFECTS/ADVERSE REACTIONS

CNS: Pain, headache,
CV: Hypertension
GI: Diarrhea, vomiting, constipation, nausea, dyspepsia, oral moniliasis
GU: UTI, hematuria
HEME: Leukopenia, anemia, thrombocytopenia, leukocytosis
METAB: Fever, peripheral edema, hypercholesteremia, hypophosphatemia, hypokalemia, hyperkalemia
MS: Back pain
RESP: Infection (opportunistic)
MISC: Sepsis, malignancy

▼ **DRUG INTERACTIONS**

Drugs

- *Acyclovir, ganciclovir:* Increased mycophenolate, increased antivirals
- *Antacids:* Decreased mycophenolate availability
- *Cholestyramine:* Decreased mycophenolate availability
- *Probenecid:* Increased mycophenolate

SPECIAL CONSIDERATIONS

- Drug can be given concurrently with cyclosporine, which may enable reduced cyclosporine doses and lower toxicity or potential cyclosporine substitute in patients develping cyclosporine toxicity
- Drug is less likely than azathioprine to induce severe bone marrow depression, and may replace azathioprine in conventional maintenance immunosuppression regimens

---

nabumetone

(nah-bume'tone)
Relafen
Chemical Class: Acetic acid derivative
Therapeutic Class: Nonsteroidal antiinflammatory agent

CLINICAL PHARMACOLOGY

Mechanism of Action: Inhibits prostaglandin synthesis by decreasing cyclooxygenase, the enzyme needed for biosynthesis; analgesic, antiinflammatory, and antipyretic activity

Pharmacokinetics

PO: Peak 2½-4 hr, plasma protein binding >90%, $t_{½}$ 22-30 hr; metabolized in liver to active metabolite; excreted in urine (metabolites)

INDICATIONS AND USES: Osteoarthritis, rheumatoid arthritis

N

DOSAGE

Adult

• PO 1 g as a single dose; may increase to 1.5-2 g/d if needed; may give qd or bid

$ AVAILABLE FORMS/COST OF THERAPY

• Tab, Uncoated—Oral: 500 mg, 100's: **$102.20;** 750 mg, 100's: **$123.15**

CONTRAINDICATIONS: Hypersensitivity to aspirin, iodides, NSAIDs; severe asthma, severe renal disease

PRECAUTIONS: Children, bleeding disorders, GI disorders, cardiac disorders, renal disorders, hepatic dysfunction, elderly

PREGNANCY AND LACTATION: Pregnancy category B (1st and 2nd trimester)

SIDE EFFECTS/ADVERSE REACTIONS

CNS: Dizziness, headache, drowsiness, fatigue, tremors, confusion, insomnia, anxiety, depression, nervousness

CV: CHF, tachycardia, peripheral edema, palpitations, dysrhythmias

EENT: Tinnitus, hearing loss, blurred vision

GI: Nausea, anorexia, vomiting, diarrhea, jaundice, ***cholestatic hepatitis,*** constipation, flatulence, cramps, dry mouth, peptic ulcer, gastritis, ***ulceration, perforation***

GU: ***Nephrotoxicity, dysuria, hematuria, oliguria, azotemia,*** cystitis

HEME: ***Blood dyscrasias***

RESP: Dyspnea, pharyngitis, ***bronchospasm***

SKIN: Purpura, rash, pruritus, sweating, photosensitivity

▼ DRUG INTERACTIONS

Drugs

• *Antidiabetics+:* Protein binding displacement potential, increased concentration of oral hypoglycemics

• *Aminoglycosides:* Reduced clearance of aminoglycosides with increased antibiotic concentrations

• *Angiotensin-converting inhibitors:* Inhibit the antihypertensive effects of ACE inhibitors

• *Beta blockers:* Reduced hypotensive effects of beta blockers

• *Binding resins:* Potential to delay absorption of NSAID

• *Cyclosporine:* Increase cyclosporine concentrations

• *Furosemide:* Reduces the diuretic and hypotensive effects of furosemide

• *Hydralazine:* Reduced hypotensive effects of hydralazine

• *Lithium:* Increased lithium concentrations

• *Methotrexate:* Potentially increase methotrexate concentrations and toxicity

• *Potassium-sparing diuretics:* Potential for acute renal failure i.e., indomethacin and triamterene

Labs

• *False positive:* Occult blood in stool (guaiac test)

• *Increase:* Liver function tests (especially transaminase activity)

SPECIAL CONSIDERATIONS

• Drug is similarly effective to other NSAIDs

• Drug may cause less gastric irritation

nadolol

(nay-doe'loll)

Corgard

Chemical Class: β-Adrenergic receptor blocker, non-selective

Therapeutic Class: Antihypertensive, antianginal

CLINICAL PHARMACOLOGY

Mechanism of Action: Long-acting, nonselective β-adrenergic receptor blocking agent

Pharmacokinetics

PO: Onset variable, peak 3-4 hr, duration 17-24 hr; $t_{1/2}$, 16-20 hr; not metabolized; excreted in urine (unchanged), bile

INDICATIONS AND USES: Chronic stable angina pectoris, mild to moderate hypertension, prophylaxis of migraine headaches

DOSAGE

Adult

• PO 40 mg qd, increase by 40-80 mg q3-7d; maintenance 40-240 mg/d for angina, 40-320 mg/d for hypertension

$ **AVAILABLE FORMS/COST OF THERAPY**

• Tab, Uncoated—Oral: 20 mg, 100's: **$72.40-$89.74;** 40 mg, 100's: **$84.67-$105.20;** 80 mg, 100's: **$116.09-$144.24;** 120 mg, 100's: **$151.68;** 160 mg, 100's: **$168.70-$209.09**

CONTRAINDICATIONS: Hypersensitivity, cardiogenic shock, 2nd or 3rd degree heart block, bronchospastic disease, sinus bradycardia, CHF, COPD

PRECAUTIONS: Diabetes mellitus, renal disease, hyperthyroidism, peripheral vascular disease, myasthenia gravis

PREGNANCY AND LACTATION: Pregnancy category C; excreted into breast milk, milk concentrations 4-5 times higher than maternal serum but infant would receive <10% of therapeutic adult dose; compatible with breast feeding

SIDE EFFECTS/ADVERSE REACTIONS

CNS: Depression, hallucinations, dizziness, fatigue, lethargy, paresthesias, headache

CV: Bradycardia, hypotension, ***CHF,*** palpitations, AV block, chest pain, peripheral ischemia, flushing, edema, vasodilation, conduction disturbances

EENT: Sore throat

GI: Nausea, vomiting, diarrhea, colitis, constipation, cramps, dry mouth, flatulence, hepatomegaly, pancreatitis, taste distortion

HEME: ***Agranulocytosis, thrombocytopenia***

RESP: Dyspnea, respiratory dysfunction, ***bronchospasm,*** cough, wheezing, nasal stuffiness, pharyngitis, ***laryngospasm***

SKIN: Rash, pruritus, fever

▼ **DRUG INTERACTIONS**

Drugs

• *Aminodarone:* Combined therapy may lead to bradycardia, cardiac arrest, or ventricular dysrhythmia

• *Anesthetics, local:* Enhanced sympathomimetic side effects, especially if anesthetic combined with epinephrine; acute discontinuation of nadolol before local anesthesia increases risk of anesthetic side effects

• *Antidiabetics:* β-blockers increase blood glucose and impair peripheral circulation; altered response to hypoglycemia by prolonging the recovery to normoglycemia, blocking tachycardia and other signs and symptoms of hypoglycemia

• *Barbiturates:* Reduced concentrations of nadolol

• *Calcium channel blockers:* Additive hypotension (kinetic and dynamic)

• *Clonidine:* Hypertension occurring upon withdrawal of clonidine may be exacerbated by nadolol

• *Disopyramide:* Additive negative inotropic cardiac effects

• *Epinephrine+:* Enhanced pressor response, hypertension and bradycardia

• *Fluoxetine:* Increased beta-

N

blocking effects with potential for cardiac toxicity

- *Isoproterenol:* Reduced isoproterenol efficacy in asthma
- *Methyldopa:* Potential for development of hypertension in the presence of increased catecholamines
- *Neuroleptics:* Increased plasma concentrations of each other, with potential for accentuated responses of both drugs
- *NSAIDs:* Reduced antihypertensive effects of nadolol
- *Phenylephrine:* Potential for hypertensive episodes when administered together
- *Prazosin:* First dose response to prazosin may be enhanced by beta-blockade
- *Rifampin:* Reduced nadolol concentrations
- *Tacrine:* Additive bradycardia
- *Theophylline:* Antagonistic pharmacodynamic effects

Labs

- *Increase:* Serum K, serum uric acid, ALT/AST, alk phosphatase, LDH blood glucose, cholesterol

SPECIAL CONSIDERATIONS

PATIENT/FAMILY EDUCATION

- Do **not** discontinue abruptly

---

nafarelin

(na-far′eh-lin)

Synarel

Chemical Class: Synthetic analog of gonadotropin-releasing hormone

Therapeutic Class: Gonadotropin

CLINICAL PHARMACOLOGY

Mechanism of Action: Stimulates release of LH and FSH resulting in a temporary increase of ovarian steroidogenesis; repeated dosing abolishes stimulatory effects on the pituitary gland with decreased secretion of gonadal steroids and consequent pseudomenopause

Pharmacokinetics

Peak, 0.6 ng/ml after 200 µg dose at 10-40 min; $t_{1/2}$, 3 hr; rapidly absorbed intranasally, 2.8% bioavailability; 80% bound to plasma proteins; 3% unchanged in urine

INDICATIONS AND USES: Endometriosis, gonadotropin-dependent precocious puberty

DOSAGE

Adult

- *Endometriosis:* 400 µg/d; 200 µg (1 spray) in 1 nostril AM, 200 µg in other nostril PM; start treatment between days 2 and 4 of menstrual cycle; may increase to 800 µg/d; recommended duration of treatment is 6 mo

Child

- *Central precocious puberty:* 1600 µg/d (2 sprays in each nostril bid)

$ **AVAILABLE FORMS/COST OF THERAPY**

- Sol—Nasal: 2 mg/ml, 10 ml: **$336.25** (30 day supply for endometriosis)

CONTRAINDICATIONS: Hypersensitivity, undiagnosed abnormal vaginal bleeding

PRECAUTIONS: Ovarian cysts, persistent menstruation, osteoporosis risk factors (chronic alcohol and/or tobacco use, strong family history of osteoporosis, or chronic use of drugs that can reduce bone mass such as anticonvulsants or corticosteroids)

PREGNANCY AND LACTATION: Pregnancy category X

SIDE EFFECTS/ADVERSE REACTIONS

CNS: Headache, flushing, depression, insomnia, emotional lability, hot flashes

EENT: Rhinitis

GU: Decreased libido, vaginal

dryness-bleeding, breast tenderness, transient breast enlargement, increased pubic hair
METAB: *Hot flashes,* bone density changes (8.7% decreased in trabecular bone density after 6 mo)
SKIN: *Acne, increased body hair*
MISC: ***Hypersensitivity*** *(shortness of breath, chest pain, urticaria pruritus), body odor, seborrhea, rhinitis*

▼ **DRUG INTERACTIONS**

Drugs

• *Decongestants, nasal/topical:* Potential interference with absorption; allow 30 min after use of nafarelin before applying a topical decongestant

Labs

• *Interference:* Gonadal and gonadotropic function tests conducted during treatment and for 4-8 wk after treatment may be misleading
• *Decrease:* Bone mineral content

SPECIAL CONSIDERATIONS

• Alternative to danazol and oophorectomy in the treatment of endometriosis; more tolerable adverse effect profile compared to danazol
• Agent of choice in patients concerned about future fertility
• Benefits temporary

nafcillin

(naf'sill'in)
Nafcil, Nallpen, Unipen, Vigopen ♣
Chemical Class: 6-β-aminopenicillanic acid derivative
Therapeutic Class: Penicillinase-resistant penicillin; bactericidal

CLINICAL PHARMACOLOGY

Mechanism of Action: Bactericidal via cell wall synthesis inhibition

Pharmacokinetics

IV: Cp (after single 500 mg dose), 30 μg/ml at 5 min
IM/PO: Peak, 30-60 min; duration, 4-6 hr; $t_{1/2}$ 1 hr
Poor/erratic oral absorption; metabolized by the liver, elimination, 30% as unchanged drug in urine, primarily eliminated by nonrenal routes (namely hepatic inactivation and excretion in bile)

INDICATIONS AND USES: Infections of the upper respiratory tract, bone, and localized skin and skin structure caused by susceptible organisms.
Antibacterial spectrum usually includes:
• Gram-positive organisms: *Staphylococcus aureus, Streptococcus pyogenes, Str. viridans, Str. faecalis, Str. bovis, Str. pneumoniae,* including those producing penicillinase

DOSAGE

Adult

• IM/IV 2-6 g/d in divided doses q4-6h; PO 2-6 g/d in divided doses q4-6h

Child

• IM 25 mg/kg q12h; PO 25-50 mg/kg/d in divided doses q6h

Neonates

• IM 10 mg/kg bid

$ **AVAILABLE FORMS/COST OF THERAPY**

• Inj, Dry-Sol—IM; IV: 1 g: **$3.62-$6.01;** 2 g: **$6.29-$11.82;** 500 mg: **$2.40-$3.26**
• Cap, Gel—Oral: 250 mg, 100's: **$104.96**

CONTRAINDICATIONS: Hypersensitivity to penicillins

PRECAUTIONS: Hypersensitivity to cephalosporins (5%-16% cross-allergenicity), neonates, liver and renal insufficiency

PREGNANCY AND LACTATION: Pregnancy category B; excreted into breast milk

SIDE EFFECTS/ADVERSE REACTIONS

CNS: Lethargy, hallucinations, anxiety, depression, twitching, ***coma, convulsions***

CV: Phlebitis or thrombophlebitis

GI: Nausea, vomiting, diarrhea, increased AST, ALT, abdominal pain, glossitis (black or hairy tongue), colitis

GU: Oliguria, ***proteinuria, hematuria,*** *vaginitis, moniliasis,* ***glomerulonephritis, interstitial nephritis***

HEME: Anemia, increased bleeding time, ***bone marrow depression, granulocytopenia***

MISC: Hypersensitivity, immediate (range from urticaria and pruritus to angioneurotic edema, laryngospasm, bronchospasm, hypotension, vascular collapse, and death) or delayed (serum-sickness-like symptoms, i.e., fever, malaise, urticaria, myalgia, arthralgia, abdominal pain; and various skin rashes)

▼ **DRUG INTERACTIONS**

Drugs

- *Aspirin, probenecid:* Increased nafcillin concentrations
- *Methotrexate:* Increased methotrexate concentrations, increased potential for toxicity
- *Oral anticoagulants:* Reduced hypoprothrombinemic effects
- *Oral contraceptives:* Impaired contraceptive efficacy
- *Tetracyclines, chloramphenicol:* Decreased antimicrobial effectiveness

Labs

- *False positive:* Urine glucose, urine protein, Coombs test

SPECIAL CONSIDERATIONS

MONITORING PARAMETERS

- Oral nafcillin absorption is erratic (consider alternate oral penicillinase-resistant penicillins)
- CBC and stain UA for eosinophils during therapy to prevent serious adverse effects

---

naftifine

(naf'te-feen)

Naftin

Chemical Class: Synthetic allylamine derivative

Therapeutic Class: Broad spectrum, topical antifungal

CLINICAL PHARMACOLOGY

Mechanism of Action: Fungicidal/fungistatic; interferes with sterol biosynthesis by inhibiting the enzyme squalene 2,3-epoxidase

Pharmacokinetics

TOP: Cream (6%), gel (4.2%) systemic absorption; excreted via urine and feces; $t_{1/2}$, 2-3 days

INDICATIONS AND USES: Topical fungal infections (i.e., tinea cruris, tinea corporis) caused by the following susceptible organisms: *Trichophyton rubrum, T. mentagrophytes, T. tonsurans, Epidermophyton floccosum, Microsporum canis, M. audouinii, M. gypseum;* fungistatic against *Candida* sp.

DOSAGE

- *TOP:* bid to affected and surrounding area × 7-14 days

$ **AVAILABLE FORMS/COST OF THERAPY**

- Cre—Top: 1%, 30 g: **$22.47**
- Gel—Top: 1%, 20 g: **$19.05**

CONTRAINDICATIONS: Hypersensitivity

PREGNANCY AND LACTATION: Pregnancy category B

SIDE EFFECTS/ADVERSE REACTIONS

SKIN: Burning, stinging, dryness, *itching,* redness, local irritation

SPECIAL CONSIDERATIONS

• First of a new class of antifungals (allylamine derivatives) unrelated to imidazoles

• Because of fungicidal activity at low concentrations may provide quicker onset of healing, enhance patient compliance with qd therapy

nalbuphine

(nal'byoo-feen)

Nubain

Chemical Class: Phenanthrene narcotic agonist-antagonist related to both naloxone and oxymorphone

Therapeutic Class: Synthetic narcotic agonist-antagonist analgesic

DEA Class: Schedule II

CLINICAL PHARMACOLOGY

Mechanism of Action: Potent analgesic at the spinal cord level; interacts with opioid receptors; agonist activity equivalent in potency to morphine on a mg basis; narcotic antagonist activity ¼ as potent as nalorphine, 10 times that of pentazocine

Pharmacokinetics

IV: Onset, 2-3 min; duration, 3-6 hr

SC/IM: Onset, <15 min; duration, 3-6 hr

Metabolized by liver, excreted by kidncys, $t_{1/2}$, 5 hr

INDICATIONS AND USES: Moderate to severe pain; supplement to balanced anesthesia, for preoperative and postoperative analgesia; obstetrical analgesia during labor and delivery

DOSAGE

Adult

• *Pain:*SC/IM/IV 10-20 mg q3-6h prn, not to exceed 160 mg/d

• *Supplement to balanced anesthesia:* Induction 0.3 mg/kg to 3.0 mg/kg IV; maintenance 0.25 mg to 0.50 mg/kg as required

$ AVAILABLE FORMS/COST OF THERAPY

• Inj, Sol—IM; IV; SC:10 mg/ml, 1 ml: **$4.10-$17.13;** 20 mg/ml, 1 ml: **$5.04-$25.38**

CONTRAINDICATIONS: Hypersensitivity, narcotic addiction

PRECAUTIONS: Addictive personality, increased intracranial pressure, MI (acute), severe heart disease, respiratory depression, hepatic disease, renal disease, sulfites sensitivity

PREGNANCY AND LACTATION: Pregnancy category B

SIDE EFFECTS/ADVERSE REACTIONS

CNS: Sedation, dizziness/vertigo, confusion, headache, euphoria, dysphoria (high doses), crying, dreams

CV: Palpitations, bradycardia, change in B/P

EENT: Tinnitus, blurred vision, miosis, diplopia

GI: Nausea, vomiting, anorexia, constipation, cramps, dry mouth

GU: Increased urinary output, dysuria, urinary retention

SKIN: Rash, urticaria, bruising, flushing, diaphoresis, pruritus

RESP: ***Respiratory depression***

MISC: Speech difficulty, urinary urgency, blurred vision, flushing/warmth

▼ DRUG INTERACTIONS

Drugs

• *Barbiturates:* Additive CNS depression

• *Neuroleptics:* Enhanced CNS depression and hypotension

• *Ethanol:* Additive CNS depression

• *H-2 receptor antagonists:* Inhibition of narcotic hepatic metabolism, additive CNS effects

• *Rifampin:* May reduce narcotic

N

concentrations and precipitate withdrawal

Labs

• *Increase:* Amylase

SPECIAL CONSIDERATIONS

• Proposed, but not significant, advantages include low abuse potential, low respiratory depressant effects, low incidence of psychomimetic toxicity, and a lower incidence of hemodynamic toxicity

nalidixic acid

(nal-i-dix'ik)

NegGram

Chemical Class: Synthetic naphthyridine derivative

Therapeutic Class: Urinary tract antiinfective

CLINICAL PHARMACOLOGY

Mechanism of Action: Inhibits DNA polymerization, primarily single-stranded DNA precursors in late stages of chromosomal replication; bactericidal

Pharmacokinetics

PO: Peak (serum), 20-40 μg/ml at 1-2 hr, peak (urine) 150-200 μg/ml at 3-4 hrs after 1 g dose; rapid absorption; 90% protein bound; metabolized in liver; excreted in urine (unchanged, hydroxynalidixic acid, similar antibacterial activity, and conjugates); serum $t_{1/2}$, 90 min; urine $t_{1/2}$, 6 hr; crosses placenta, enters breast milk

INDICATIONS AND USES: UTIs (acute/chronic) caused by *E. coli, Klebsiella, Enterobacter, Proteus mirabilis, P. vulgaris, P. morganii*

DOSAGE

Adult

• PO 1 g qid × 1-2 wk, 2 g/d for long-term treatment

Child >3 mo

• PO 55 mg/kg/d in 4 divided doses for 1-2 wk; 33 mg/kg/d in 4 divided doses for long-term treatment

$ AVAILABLE FORMS/COST OF THERAPY

• Tab, Uncoated—Oral: 250 mg, 56's: **$42.78;** 500 mg, 100's: **$43.45-$81.68;** 1 g, 100's: **$65.45-$190.39**

CONTRAINDICATIONS: Hypersensitivity, CNS damage, liver failure, infants <3 mo

PRECAUTIONS: Elderly, renal disease, hepatic disease

PREGNANCY AND LACTATION: Pregnancy category B (safe last 2 trimesters); excreted into breast milk in low concentrations; M:P ratio, 0.08-0.13; insignificant

SIDE EFFECTS/ADVERSE REACTIONS

CNS: Dizziness, headache, drowsiness, insomnia, ***convulsions; increased intracranial pressure,*** and toxic psychosis

EENT: Sensitivity to light, blurred vision, change in color perception

GI: Nausea, vomiting, abdominal pain, diarrhea

SKIN: Pruritus, rash, urticaria, photosensitivity

▼ DRUG INTERACTIONS

Drugs

• *Oral anticoagulants:* Enhanced hypoprothrombinemia effects

Labs

• *False positive:* Urinary glucose

• *False increase:* 17-OHCS, VMA

SPECIAL CONSIDERATIONS

• Resistance occurs in 2%-14% of patients during treatment

nalmefene

(nal'me-feen)

Revex

Chemical Class: 6-methylene analogue of naltrexone

Therapeutic Class: Opioid antagonist

CLINICAL PHARMACOLOGY

Mechanism of Action: Prevents or reverses the effects of opioids, including respiratory depression, sedation, and hypotension; no opioid agonist activity

Pharmacokinetics

IV: Cp at 5 min, 3.7-5.8 ng/ml; duration is as long as most opioids Completely bioavailable IM (Cp, 2.3 hr), SC (Cp, 1.5 hr) vs. IV; distribution to CNS rapidly (V_{dss} 8.6 L/kg); 45% bound to plasma proteins; metabolized by the liver; excreted in urine; $t_{1/2}$ 10.8 - 9.4 hr

INDICATIONS AND USES: Known or suspected opioid overdose (natural or synthetic) for complete or partial reversal of opioid drug effects, including respiratory depression

DOSAGE

Adult

- *Postoperative opioid depression:* 100 μg/ml dosage strength (blue label): initial dose, 0.25 μg/kg, then 0.25 μg/kg incremental doses at 2-5 min intervals, stopping as soon as the desired degree of opioid reversal is obtained; cumulative total doses above 1.0 μg/kg does not provide additional therapeutic effects
- *Management of known or suspected opioid overdose:* 1.0 mg/ml dosage strength (green label): initial 0.5 mg/70 kg, then, if needed, a second dose of 1.0 mg/70 kg, 2-5 min later; (if a total dose of 1.5 mg/70 kg has been administered without clinical response, additional drug is unlikely to have an effect)
- *Reasonable suspicion of opioid dependency:* Challenge dose of 0.1 mg/70 kg initially; if no evidence of withdrawal in 2 min, follow recommended dosing

$ AVAILABLE FORMS/COST OF THERAPY

- Inj—Sol: 100 μg/ml, 1 ml (Blue Label): **$2.50;** 1 mg/ml, 2 ml (Green Label): **$35.00**

CONTRAINDICATIONS: Hypersensitivity

PRECAUTIONS: Pre-existing cardiac disease, known risk of precipitated withdrawal; like other opioid antagonists, is known to produce acute withdrawal symptoms and, therefore, should be used with extreme caution in patients with known physical dependence on opioids or following surgery involving high doses of opioids

PREGNANCY AND LACTATION: Pregnancy category B

SIDE EFFECTS/ADVERSE REACTIONS

CNS: Postoperative pain, dizziness, headache, withdrawal syndrome

CV: Tachycardia, hypertension

GI: Nausea, vomiting

METAB: Fever, chills

SPECIAL CONSIDERATIONS:

- Longer duration of action than naloxone at fully reversing doses; agent of choice in instances where prolonged opioid effects are predicted, including overdose with longer-acting opioids (e.g., methadone, propoxyphene), patients given large doses of opioids, and those with liver disease or renal failure (eliminating the need for continuous infusions of naloxone and prolonged observation periods after outpatient procedures

N

naloxone

(nal-oks'one)

Narcan

Chemical Class: Thebaine derivative

Therapeutic Class: Opiate antagonist; antidote

CLINICAL PHARMACOLOGY

Mechanism of Action: Exact

mechanism of action not fully understood; evidence suggests that it antagonizes the opioid effects by competing for the same receptor sites; does not possess "agonistic" or morphine-like properties

Pharmacokinetics

IV: Onset 2 min

SC/IM: Onset slightly less rapid than IV

Metabolized in liver, excreted in urine, $t_{1/2}$ 64 min

INDICATIONS AND USES: Complete or partial reversal of narcotic depression, including respiratory depression; diagnosis of suspected acute opioid overdosage; reversal of alcoholic coma,* refractory shock,* Alzheimer's type dementia,* schizophrenia*

DOSAGE

Adult

• *Narcotic overdose (known or suspected):* SC/IM/IV 0.4-2 mg initially, repeat at 2-3 min intervals up to 10 mg, if no response after 10 mg reevaluate diagnosis

• *Postoperative narcotic depression (partial reversal):* IV 0.1-0.2 mg at 2-3 min intervals to desired level of reversal (adequate ventilation and alertness without significant pain or discomfort); repeat doses may be required within 1-2 hr intervals

Child

• *Narcotic overdose (known or suspected):* SC/IM/IV 0.01 mg/kg initially, give subsequent doses of 0.01 mg/kg prn at 2-3 min intervals

• *Postoperative narcotic depression (partial reversal):* IV 0.005-0.01 mg q2-3 min to desired degree of reversal

$ AVAILABLE FORMS/COST OF THERAPY

• Inj, Sol—IM; IV; SC: 0.02 mg/ml, 2 ml: **$1.23-$5.39;** 0.4 mg/ml, 1 ml: **$0.99-$5.98**

CONTRAINDICATIONS: Hypersensitivity

PRECAUTIONS: Physical narcotic dependency, preexisting cardiovascular disorders

PREGNANCY AND LACTATION: Pregnancy category B

SIDE EFFECTS/ADVERSE REACTIONS

CNS: Tremulousness, ***seizures***

CV: Tachycardia, hypotension, hypertension, ***ventricular arrhythmia***

GI: Nausea, vomiting

RESP: Pulmonary edema

SKIN: Sweating

MISC: Reversal of analgesia

SPECIAL CONSIDERATIONS

MONITORING PARAMETERS

• ECG, blood pressure, respiratory rate, mental status

• Duration of action of some narcotics may exceed that of naloxone

---

naltrexone

(nal-trex'one)

ReVia

Chemical Class: Thebaine derivative

Therapeutic Class: Opiate antagonist

CLINICAL PHARMACOLOGY

Mechanism of Action: Blocks the effects of opioids by competitive binding at opioid receptors; mechanism of action in alcoholism not understood, may block the effects of endogenous opioids; does not cause disulfiram-like reactions

Pharmacokinetics

PO: Peak 1 hr, significant first-pass metabolism, 21% bound to plasma proteins, metabolized to active metabolite (6-β-naltrexol), excreted primarily by kidney, $t_{1/2}$ 4 hr (13 hr for 6-β-naltrexol)

INDICATIONS AND USES: Alcohol dependence, narcotic addiction, eating disorders,* postconcussional syndrome*

DOSAGE

Adult

• *Alcoholism:* PO 50 mg qd

• *Narcotic dependence:* PO 25 mg initially, observe for 1 hr, administer remaining 25 mg if no withdrawal signs occur (**do not attempt treatment until patient has remained opioid-free for 7-10 days, verify by analyzing urine for opioids and performing naloxone challenge test**); maintenance 50 mg qd or 100-150 mg q2-3d

$ AVAILABLE FORMS/COST OF THERAPY

• Tab, Uncoated—Oral: 50 mg, 50's: **$227.58**

CONTRAINDICATIONS: Hypersensitivity, current use of opioid analgesics, opioid dependency, acute opioid withdrawal, positive urine screen for opioids, failed naloxone test, acute hepatitis, liver failure

PRECAUTIONS: Active liver disease, children

PREGNANCY AND LACTATION: Pregnancy category C

SIDE EFFECTS/ADVERSE REACTIONS

CNS: Difficulty sleeping, anxiety, nervousness, headache, feeling down, irritability, dizziness, chills, depression, paranoia, fatigue, restlessness, confusion, disorientation, hallucinations, nightmares

CV: Phlebitis, edema, increased blood pressure, non-specific ECG changes, palpitations, tachycardia

EENT: Nasal congestion, itching, rhinorrhea, sneezing, sore throat, excess mucus or phlegm, sinus trouble, nose bleeds, blurred vision, photophobia, clogged ears, tinnitus

GI: Abdominal pain/cramps, nausea, vomiting, loss of appetite, diarrhea, constipation, increased thirst, excessive gas, hemorrhoids, diarrhea, ***ulcer, hepatotoxicity***

GU: Delayed ejaculation, decreased potency, increased frequency, discomfort during urination, increased/decreased sexual interest

MS: Joint/muscle pain; painful shoulders, legs or knees

RESP: Heavy breathing, hoarseness, cough, shortness of breath

SKIN: Skin rash, oily skin, pruritus, acne, athlete's foot, cold sores, alopecia

MISC: Low energy, increased energy, ***suicide, attempted suicide***

▼ DRUG INTERACTIONS

Drugs

• *Opioid-containing products:* Decreased or no benefit from cough suppressants, antidiarrheals, analgesics

SPECIAL CONSIDERATIONS

PATIENT/FAMILY EDUCATION

• Wear ID tag indicating naltrexone use

• Do not try to overcome reversal of opiate effects by self-administration of large doses of narcotic

• Do not exceed recommended dose

• Notify physician if signs of liver injury appear

MONITORING PARAMETERS

• Liver function tests

nandrolone

(nan'droe-lone)

Decanoate: Androlone-D 200, Deca-Durabolin, Hybolin Decanoate, Neo-Durabolic; Phenpropionate: Durabolin, Hybolin Improved, Nandrobolic

Chemical Class: Halogenated testosterone derivative

Therapeutic Class: Anabolic steroid

DEA Class: Schedule III

CLINICAL PHARMACOLOGY

Mechanism of Action: Promotes body tissue-building processes and reverses catabolic or tissue depleting processes when administered with adequate calories and protein to achieve positive nitrogen balance; inhibits endogenous testosterone release

Pharmacokinetics

IM: Metabolized in liver, excreted in urine

INDICATIONS AND USES: Metastatic breast cancer in women (phenpropionate), anemia of renal insufficiency (decanoate)

DOSAGE

Adult

- *Breast cancer:* IM 50-100 mg qwk, based on therapeutic response (gluteal muscle preferred)
- *Anemia of renal disease:* IM 50-100 mg qwk (women); 100-200 mg qwk (men)

Child (2-13 yr)

- *Anemia of renal disease:* IM 25-50 mg q3-4 wk

$ **AVAILABLE FORMS/COST OF THERAPY**

- Inj, Sol (decanoate)—IM: 50 mg/ml, 2 ml: **$5.50-$14.05;** 100 mg/ml, 2 ml: **$6.50-$208.44;** 200 mg/ml, 1 ml: **$6.29-$208.44**
- Inj, Sol—IM: 25 mg/ml, 5 ml: **$5.00-$16.26;** 50 mg/ml, 2 ml: **$4.75-$14.15**

CONTRAINDICATIONS: Hypersensitivity, male patients with prostate or breast cancer, hypercalcemia in females with breast cancer, nephrosis, nephrotic phase of nephritis, enhancement of physical appearance or athletic performance

PRECAUTIONS: Elderly, children, cardiac disease, renal disease, hepatic disease, seizure disorder, migraine headache, diabetes

PREGNANCY AND LACTATION: Pregnancy category X

SIDE EFFECTS/ADVERSE REACTIONS

CNS: Excitation, insomnia, habituation, depression, choreiform movement

CV: Edema

EENT: Deepening of voice, hoarseness

GI: Nausea, vomiting, diarrhea, ***cholestatic jaundice, hepatic necrosis, hepatocellular neoplasms, peliosis hepatis***

GU: Amenorrhea, vaginitis, decreased breast size, clitoral hypertrophy, testicular atrophy, decreased libido

METAB: Virilization; retention of sodium, chloride, water, potassium, phosphates, calcium; decreased glucose tolerance, increased serum cholesterol, increased LDL cholesterol, decreased HDL cholesterol

MS: Premature closure of epiphyses in children

SKIN: Rash, acne, flushing, sweating, alopecia, hirsutism

▼ **DRUG INTERACTIONS**

Drugs

- *Antidiabetic agents:* Enhanced hypoglycemic effects
- *Cyclosporine:* Increased cyclosporine concentrations
- *Warfarin+:* Enhanced hypoprothrombinemic response to oral anticoagulants

Labs

- *Increase:* Serum cholesterol, blood glucose, urine glucose
- *Decrease:* Serum Ca, serum K, T_4, T_3, thyroid[131] I uptake test, urine 17-OHCS, 17-KS, PBI, BSP

SPECIAL CONSIDERATIONS

PATIENT/FAMILY EDUCATION

- Drug may cause GI upset or nausea
- Notify physician of hoarseness, deepening of voice, male-pattern baldness, hirsutism, menstrual irregularities, acne (women)

• Notify physician of nausea, vomiting, changes in skin color, ankle swelling

MONITORING PARAMETERS

• Frequent serum and urine calcium (discontinue if hypercalcemia develops)
• Liver function tests
• Growth rate in children

---

naphazoline

(naf-az'oh-leen)

AK-Con, Albalon, Allerest Eye Drops, Clear Eyes, Comfor Eye Drops, Degest 2, Nafazair, Naphcon, Naphcon Forte, Privine, VasoClear, Vasocon Regular

Chemical Class: Imidazoline derivative

Therapeutic Class: Decongestant

CLINICAL PHARMACOLOGY

Mechanism of Action: Vasoconstriction through a local adrenergic mechanism on dilated conjunctival and nasal mucosal blood vessels

Pharmacokinetics

TOP: Onset 10 min, duration 2-6 hr, some systemic absorption

INDICATIONS AND USES: Nasal congestion, superficial corneal vascularity (congestion, itching, minor irritation, hyperemia)

DOSAGE

Adult

• Nasal 2 gtt or sprays of 0.05% sol instilled into each nostril q3-6h; do not exceed 3-5 days duration
• Conjunctival 1 gtt q3-4h; do not exceed 3-4 days duration

Child 6-12 yr

• Nasal 1-2 gtt or sprays of 0.025% sol instilled into each nostril q3-6h; do not exceed 3-5 days duration

$ **AVAILABLE FORMS/COST OF THERAPY**

• Sol—Ophth: 0.012%, 15 ml: **$2.94-$10.50;** 0.02%, 15 ml: **$7.20;** 0.03%, 15 ml: **$5.63;** 0.1%, 15 ml: **$3.38-$14.00**
• Sol—Nasal: 0.05%, 20 ml: **$3.78**
• Spray—Nasal: 0.05%, 15 ml: **$3.64**

CONTRAINDICATIONS: Hypersensitivity, angle-closure glaucoma

PRECAUTIONS: Children <6 yr, hyperthyroidism, heart disease, hypertension, diabetes mellitus

PREGNANCY AND LACTATION: Pregnancy category C

SIDE EFFECTS/ADVERSE REACTIONS

CNS: Headache, nervousness, dizziness, weakness

CV: Hypertension, cardiac irregularities

EENT: Transient burning, stinging, dryness, ulceration of nasal mucosa, sneezing, anosmia; blurred vision, mild transient stinging, irritation, mydriasis, increased/decreased intraocular pressure; rebound congestion/hyperemia

GI: Nausea

SKIN: Sweating

SPECIAL CONSIDERATIONS

PATIENT/FAMILY EDUCATION

• Discontinue ophthalmic preparations if ocular pain or visual changes occur
• Drug may produce increased nasal congestion/redness of the eye if overused
• Do not use longer than 3-5 days unless under the direction of a physician

N

naproxen

(na-prox'en)

Aleve, Anaprox, Anaprox DS, EC-Naprosyn, Naprosyn

Chemical Class: Propionic acid derivative

Therapeutic Class: Nonsteroidal antiinflammatory drug (NSAID)

CLINICAL PHARMACOLOGY

Mechanism of Action: Inhibits cyclooxygenase activity and prostaglandin synthesis; other mechanisms such as inhibition of lipoxygenase, leukotriene synthesis, lysosomal enzyme release, neutrophil aggregation and various cell-membrane functions may exist as well

Pharmacokinetics

PO: Onset 1 hr, peak 1-4 hr, duration up to 7 hr, >90% bound to plasma proteins, metabolized in liver, excreted by kidney, $t_{1/2}$ 12-15 hr

INDICATIONS AND USES: Mild to moderate pain; primary dysmenorrhea; rheumatoid arthritis, osteoarthritis, ankylosing spondylitis, tendinitis, bursitis, acute gout, reduction of fever, migraine, minor aches and pains (OTC), headache,* premenstrual syndrome,* sunburn*

DOSAGE

Adult

• *Arthritis:* PO 250-500 mg (275-550 mg naproxen sodium) bid, may increase to 1.5 g/d (1.65 g/d naproxen sodium) for limited periods

• *Acute gout:* PO 750 mg (825 mg naproxen sodium), followed by 250 mg (275 mg naproxen sodium) q8h until attack subsides

• *Mild to moderate pain/primary dysmenorrhea:* PO 500 mg (550 mg naproxen sodium) at earliest symptoms of menses, followed by 250 mg (275 mg naproxen sodium) q6-8h; do not exceed 1.25 g/d (1.375 g/d naproxen sodium)

Child

• *Juvenile arthritis:* PO 10 mg/kg divided bid

$ **AVAILABLE FORMS/COST OF THERAPY**

• Tab, Uncoated—Oral: 220 mg, 100's: **$7.13;** 250 mg, 100's: **$13.47-$80.54;** 275 mg, 100's: **$18.38-$79.50;** 375 mg, 100's: **$17.37-$103.52**

• Tab, Enteric Coated—Oral: 375 mg, 100's: **$99.54;** 500 mg, 100's: **$21.20-$126.44;** 500 mg, 100's: **$121.57** 550 mg, 100's: **$28.88-$123.78**

• Susp—Oral: 125 mg/5 ml, 500 ml: **$34.75-$39.30**

CONTRAINDICATIONS: Hypersensitivity to NSAIDs or ASA

PRECAUTIONS: Bleeding tendencies, peptic ulcer, renal/hepatic function impairment, elderly, CHF, hypertension

PREGNANCY AND LACTATION: Pregnancy category B (category D if used in 3rd trimester); could cause constriction of the ductus arteriosus *in utero,* persistent pulmonary hypertension of the newborn, or prolonged labor; passes into breast milk in small quantities, compatible with breast feeding

SIDE EFFECTS/ADVERSE REACTIONS

CNS: Dizziness, headache, lightheadedness

CV: ***CHF,*** hypotension, hypertension, palpitation, dysrhythmias, tachycardia, edema, chest pain

EENT: Visual disturbances, photophobia, dry eyes, hearing disturbances, tinnitus, *burning/stinging upon instillation*

GI: Nausea, vomiting, diarrhea, constipation, abdominal cramps, *dyspepsia,* flatulence, ***gastric or duodenal ulcer with bleeding or perforation,*** occult blood in stool, ***hepatitis,*** pancreatitis

HEME: ***Neutropenia, eosinophilia, leukopenia, pancytopenia, thrombocytopenia, agranulocytosis***

GU: ***Acute renal failure***

METAB: Hyperglycemia, hypoglycemia, hyperkalemia, hyponatremia

RESP: Dyspnea, bronchospasm, pulmonary infiltrates

SKIN: Rash, urticaria, photosensitivity

▼ **DRUG INTERACTIONS**

Drugs

- *Aminoglycosides:* Reduction of aminoglycoside clearance in premature infants
- *ACE inhibitors:* Inhibition of antihypertensive response
- *Beta blockers:* Reduced hypotensive effects of beta blockers
- *Furosemide:* Reduced diuretic and antihypertensive response to furosemide
- *Hydralazine:* Reduced antihypertensive response to hydralazine
- *Lithium:* Increased plasma lithium concentrations, toxicity
- *Methotrexate:* Reduced renal clearance of methotrexate, increased toxicity
- *Oral anticoagulants:* Increased risk of bleeding due to adverse effects on GI mucosa and platelet function
- *Potassium sparing* diuretics (acute renal failure)

Labs

- *Increase:* Bleeding time

SPECIAL CONSIDERATIONS

PATIENT/FAMILY EDUCATION

- Avoid aspirin and alcoholic beverages
- Take with food, milk, or antacids to decrease GI upset
- Notify physician if edema, black stools, or persistent headache occurs

MONITORING PARAMETERS

- CBC, BUN, serum creatinine, LFTs, occult blood loss

---

natamycin

(na-ta-mye'sin)

Natacyn

Chemical Class: Tetraene polyene antibiotic

Therapeutic Class: Ophthalmic antifungal

CLINICAL PHARMACOLOGY

Mechanism of Action: Binds to fungal cell membrane altering membrane permeability; depletes essential cellular constituents

Pharmacokinetics

Systemic absorption should not occur after topical administration

INDICATIONS AND USES: Fungal blepharitis, conjunctivitis, keratitis; initial drug of choice in *Fusarium solani* keratitis

DOSAGE

Adult and Child

- *Fungal keratitis:* 1 gtt into conjunctival sac q1-2h, decrease to 1 gtt 6-8 times/d after 3-4 days; continue therapy for 14-21 days
- *Fungal blepharitis/conjunctivitis:* 1 gtt 4-6 times/d

$ **AVAILABLE FORMS/COST OF THERAPY**

- Susp—Ophth: 5%, 15 ml:**$93.75**

CONTRAINDICATIONS: Hypersensitivity

PRECAUTIONS: Fungal endophthalmitis (effectiveness as single agent not established)

PREGNANCY AND LACTATION: Pregnancy category C

N

SIDE EFFECTS/ADVERSE REACTIONS

EENT: Temporary visual haze, conjunctival chemosis, conjunctival hyperemia

SPECIAL CONSIDERATIONS

PATIENT/FAMILY EDUCATION

- Caution patient to notify physician of itching, increased redness, burning, stinging, swelling

MONITORING PARAMETERS

- Failure of keratitis to improve following 7-10 days of administration suggests infection not susceptible to natamycin

---

nedocromil

(ned-aw-kroe′mill)

Tilade

Chemical Class: Pyranoquinoline dicarboxylic acid derivative

Therapeutic Class: Inhaled antiinflammatory agent

CLINICAL PHARMACOLOGY

Mechanism of Action: Inhibits activation and release of inflammatory mediators from cells involved in asthmatic inflammation, including eosinophils, neutrophils, macrophages, mast cells, monocytes, and platelets; inhibits both early and late asthmatic responses to inhaled antigen and irritants

Pharmacokinetics

INH: Low systemic bioavailability, duration 4-6 hr, 89% bound to plasma proteins, excreted unchanged in urine, $t_{1/2}$ 80 min

INDICATIONS AND USES: Maintenance therapy in mild to moderate bronchial asthma, prevention of exercise-induced asthma,* prevention of acute bronchospasm induced by environmental pollutants*

DOSAGE

Adult and child ≥12 yr

- INH 2 inhalations qid at regular intervals; may reduce to bid-tid in patients under good control

$ **AVAILABLE FORMS/COST OF THERAPY**

- Aer—Inh: 1.75 mg/actuation, 16.2 g: **$25.28**

CONTRAINDICATIONS: Hypersensitivity

PRECAUTIONS: Acute bronchospasm (**not a bronchodilator**), children <12 yr

PREGNANCY AND LACTATION: Pregnancy category B

SIDE EFFECTS/ADVERSE REACTIONS

CNS: Dizziness, headache

CV: Chest pain

EENT: Throat irritation, rhinitis, burning eyes, nasal congestion, pharyngitis

GI: Nausea, vomiting, dyspepsia, dry mouth, abdominal pain, *unpleasant taste*

RESP: Coughing

SPECIAL CONSIDERATIONS

PATIENT/FAMILY EDUCATION

- Drug must be used regularly to achieve benefit, even during symptom-free periods
- Therapeutic effect may take up to 4 wk
- Drug is not to be used to treat acute asthmatic symptoms

---

nefazodone

(neh-faz′oh-doan)

Serzone

Chemical Class: Phenylpiperazine

Therapeutic Class: Antidepressant

CLINICAL PHARMACOLOGY

Mechanism of Action: Exact mechanism of action unknown; inhibits neuronal uptake of serotonin and norepinephrine; antagonizes α_1-adrenergic receptors which may be associated with postural hypotension

Pharmacokinetics

PO: Absolute bioavailability low (about 20%), peak 1 hr, >99% bound to plasma proteins, extensively metabolized (active metabolite hydroxynefazodone), $t_{1/2}$ 11-24 hr

INDICATIONS AND USES: Depression

DOSAGE

Adult

• PO 200 mg/d in 2 divided doses, increase in increments of 100-200 mg/d in intervals of no less than 1 wk; max dose, 600 mg/d

$ AVAILABLE FORMS/COST OF THERAPY

• Tab, Uncoated—Oral: 100, 150, 200, 250 mg, 60's: **$49.88**

CONTRAINDICATIONS: Hypersensitivity, coadministration with terfenadine or astemizole

PRECAUTIONS: Elderly, children, cardiovascular disease, cerebrovascular disease, dehydration, hypovolemia, history of mania, suicidal ideation, seizure disorder, cirrhosis

PREGNANCY AND LACTATION: Pregnancy category C

SIDE EFFECTS/ADVERSE REACTIONS

CNS: Headache, asthenia, *somnolence, dizziness,* insomnia, *lightheadedness,* confusion, memory impairment, paresthesia, abnormal dreams, ataxia, tremor

CV: Postural hypotension, peripheral edema, sinus bradycardia

EENT; Blurred vision, abnormal vision, tinnitus, taste perversion, visual field defect, pharyngitis

GI: Dry mouth, nausea, constipation, dyspepsia, diarrhea, increased appetite

GU: Urinary frequency, urinary retention, vaginitis, impotence

RESP: Cough

SKIN: Pruritus, rash

▼ DRUG INTERACTIONS

Drugs

• *Alprazolam, triazolam:* Increased benzodiazepine concentrations

• *Astemizole+, terfenadine+:* QT prolongation, arrhythmia

• *Digoxin:* Increased digoxin concentrations

• *MAOI:* Serious adverse reactions possible including hyperthermia, rigidity, myoclonus, autonomic instability, mental status changes, seizures; observe a 14 day washout period between discontinuing one drug and starting the other

SPECIAL CONSIDERATIONS

PATIENT/FAMILY EDUCATION

• Therapeutic effect may not be apparent for several weeks

• Drug may cause drowsiness, use caution driving or performing other tasks where alertness is required

---

neomycin

(nee-oh-mye'sin)

Mycifradin, Myciguent, Neo-Fradin, Neo-Tabs

Chemical Class: Aminoglycoside

Therapeutic Class: Antibiotic

CLINICAL PHARMACOLOGY

Mechanism of Action: Interferes with protein synthesis in bacterial cell by binding to 30S ribosomal subunit, which causes misreading of genetic code, inaccurate peptide sequence forms in protein chain, causing bacterial death

Pharmacokinetics

PO: Poorly absorbed, small absorbed fraction rapidly excreted via kidney, unabsorbed fraction eliminated unchanged in feces

INDICATIONS AND USES: (Oral) preoperative bowel preparation, adjunctive therapy of hepatic coma, hypercholesterolemia;* (topical) minor skin infections

DOSAGE

Adult

• *Preoperative bowel preparation:* PO 1 g q1h for 4 doses then 1 g q4h for 5 doses; or 1 g at 1,2, and 11 PM on day preceding surgery as an adjunct to cathartics, enema, and oral erythromycin; or 6 g/d divided q4h for 2-3 days

• *Hepatic coma:* PO 4-12 g/d divided q4-6h

• TOP apply to affected area qd-tid

Child

• *Preoperative bowel preparation:* PO 90 mg/kg/d divided q4h for 2 days; or 25 mg/kg at 1, 2, and 11 PM on the day preceding surgery as an adjunct to cathartics, enema, and oral erythromycin

• *Hepatic coma:* 2.5-7 g/m^2/d divided q4-6h for 5-6 days, not to exceed 12 g/d

• TOP apply to affected area qd-tid

$ AVAILABLE FORMS/COST OF THERAPY

• Tab, Uncoated—Oral: 500 mg, 100's: **$18.16-36.63**

• Sol—Oral: 87.5 mg/5ml, 480 ml: **$30.12**

• Oint—Top: 0.5%, 30 g: **$2.17-$3.35**

CONTRAINDICATIONS: Intestinal obstruction, hypersensitivity to aminoglycosides

PRECAUTIONS: Hepatic disease, renal disease, prolonged treatment, application to extensive burns or large surface area, children <18 yr, myasthenia gravis, parkinsonism

PREGNANCY AND LACTATION: Pregnancy category C; ototoxicity has not been reported as an effect of *in utero* exposure; eighth cranial nerve toxicity in the fetus is well known following exposure to other aminoglycosides and could potentially occur with neomycin

SIDE EFFECTS/ADVERSE REACTIONS

EENT: Ototoxicity (prolonged and high dose therapy)

GI: Nausea, vomiting, diarrhea, malabsorption syndrome has occurred during prolonged therapy, ***pseudomembranous colitis***

GU: ***Nephrotoxicity*** (prolonged and high dose therapy)

SKIN: Sensitization (low grade reddening with swelling, dry scaling, and itching or a failure to heal)

▼ DRUG INTERACTIONS

Drugs

• *Digitalis glycosides:* Reduced serum digoxin concentration

• *Ethacrynic acid+:* Increased risk of ototoxicity, especially in patients with renal impairment

• *Oral anticoagulants:* Enhanced hypoprothrombinemic response; more common with large doses of neomycin, dietary vitamin K deficiency, impaired hepatic function

• *Penicillin V:* Reduced concentrations of penicillin V, possible reduced efficacy

SPECIAL CONSIDERATIONS

PATIENT/FAMILY EDUCATION

• Drug may cause nausea, vomiting, or diarrhea

• Inform physician of loss of hearing, ringing or roaring in ears, or a feeling of fullness in head

• Drink plenty of fluids

• Notify physician if rash develops following use of topical preparation

MONITORING PARAMETERS

• Renal function, audiometric testing during extended therapy or with application to extensive burns or large surface area

netilmicin

(ne-til-mye'sin)

Netromycin

Chemical Class: Aminoglycoside

Therapeutic Class: Antibiotic

CLINICAL PHARMACOLOGY

Mechanism of Action: Interferes with protein synthesis in bacterial cell by binding to 30S ribosomal subunit, which causes misreading of genetic code, inaccurate peptide sequence forms in protein chain, causing bacterial death

Pharmacokinetics

IM: Onset rapid, peak 30-90 min

IV: Onset immediate, peak 30 min after a 30 min inf

<30% bound to plasma proteins, duration 6-8 hr, not metabolized, eliminated unchanged in urine via glomerular filtration, plasma $t_{1/2}$ 2-3 hr

INDICATIONS AND USES: Serious or life-threatening bacterial infections of the urinary tract, skin and skin structures, lower respiratory tract, septicemia, intraabdominal infections

Antibacterial spectrum usually includes:

- Gram-positive organisms: *Staphylococcus* sp. (including penicillinase and nonpenicillinase producing strains), *Streptococcus faecalis* (in combination with cell wall synthesis inhibitor)
- Gram-negative organisms: *Acinetobacter* sp., *Escherichia coli, Proteus* sp. (indole-positive and indole-negative), *Pseudomonas aeruginosa, Klebsiella* sp., *Enterobacter* sp., *Serratia* sp., *Citrobacter* sp., *Providencia* sp., *Salmonella* sp., *Shigella* sp., *Yersinia pestis*

DOSAGE

Use ideal body weight for dosage calculations

Adult

- *Serious systemic infections:* IM/IV 1.3-2.2 mg/kg diluted in 50-100 ml NS or D_5W and infused over 30-60 min q8h or 2-3.25 mg/kg q12h; adjust dosage based on results of netilmicin peak and trough levels
- *Complicated UTI:* IM/IV 1.5-2 mg/kg q12h

Child (6 wk-12 yr)

- IM/IV 1.8-2.7 mg/kg q8h or 2.7-4 mg/kg q12h

$ AVAILABLE FORMS/COST OF THERAPY

- Inj, Sol—IM; IV: 100 mg/ml, 1.5 ml: **$12.08**

CONTRAINDICATIONS: Hypersensitivity to aminoglycosides

PRECAUTIONS: Neonates, renal disease, myasthenia gravis, hearing deficits, Parkinson's disease, elderly, dehydration, hypokalemia

PREGNANCY AND LACTATION: Pregnancy category C; ototoxicity has not been reported as an effect of *in utero* exposure; eighth cranial nerve toxicity in the fetus is well known following exposure to other aminoglycosides and could potentially occur with netilmicin; potentiation of magnesium sulfate-induced neuromuscular weakness in neonates has been reported, use caution during the last 32 hr of pregnancy; excreted in breast milk in small amounts

SIDE EFFECTS/ADVERSE REACTIONS

CNS: Confusion, depression, numbness, tremors, ***convulsions,*** muscle twitching, ***neurotoxicity,*** dizziness, vertigo, myasthenia gravis-like syndrome

CV: Hypotension, hypertension, palpitations

EENT: Ototoxicity, deafness, visual disturbances, tinnitus

GI: Nausea, vomiting, anorexia, in-

creased ALT, AST, bilirubin, hepatomegaly, splenomegaly
GU: ***Oliguria,*** hematuria, ***renal damage, azotemia, renal failure, nephrotoxicity***
HEME: ***Agranulocytosis, thrombocytopenia, leukopenia, eosinophilia,*** anemia
METAB: Decreased serum calcium, sodium, potassium, magnesium
RESP: ***Respiratory depression***
SKIN: *Rash,* burning, urticaria, dermatitis, alopecia

▼ **DRUG INTERACTIONS**

Drugs

- *Amphotericin B:* Synergistic nephrotoxicity
- *Cephalosporins:* Increased potential for nephrotoxicity in patients with pre-existing renal disease
- *Cyclosporine:* Additive renal damage
- *Ethacrynic acid +:* Increased risk of ototoxicity
- *Extended spectrum penicillins:* Potential for inactivation of netilmicin in patients with renal failure
- *Methoxyflurane:* Enhanced renal toxicity
- *Neuromuscular blocking agents+:* Potentiation of respiratory suppression produced by neuromuscular blocking agents
- *NSAIDs:* Reduced renal clearance of aminoglycosides in premature infants

SPECIAL CONSIDERATIONS

PATIENT/FAMILY EDUCATION

- Report headache, dizziness, loss of hearing, ringing, roaring in ears, or feeling of fullness in head

MONITORING PARAMETERS:

- Urinalysis for proteinuria, cells, casts; urine output
- Serum peak, drawn at 30-60 min after IV inf or 60 min after IM inj, trough level drawn just before next dose, adjust dosage per levels (usual therapeutic plasma levels; peak 6-10 μg/ml, trough ≤2 μg/ml)
- Serum creatinine for CrCl calculation
- Serum calcium, magnesium, sodium
- Audiometric testing, assess hearing before, during, after treatment

---

niacin (vitamin B_3; nicotinic acid)

(nye'a-sin)

Nia-Bid, Niac, Niacels, Niacor, Nico-400, Nicobid, Nicolar, Nicotinex, Slo-Niacin, Tri-B3 ✤

Chemical Class: Water soluble B complex vitamin
Therapeutic Class: Nutritional supplement (vitamin); antihyperlipidemic

CLINICAL PHARMACOLOGY

Mechanism of Action: Necessary for lipid metabolism, tissue respiration, and glycogenolysis; lowers total serum cholesterol, low density lipoprotein (LDL) cholesterol and triglyceride concentrations by inhibiting the synthesis of very low density lipoproteins (VLDL), which are precursors to the formation of cholesterol; raises high density lipoprotein (HDL) cholesterol

Pharmacokinetics

PO: Readily absorbed from GI tract, peak 45 min, metabolized in liver, eliminated in urine (almost entirely as metabolites), $t_{1/2}$ 45 min

INDICATIONS AND USES: Vitamin deficiency (pellagra), hyperlipidemia

DOSAGE

Adult

- *Recommended daily allowance, PO:* Males 19-50 yr 19 mg/d; males >51 yr 15 mg/d; females 11-50 yr 15 mg/d; females >51 yr 13 mg/d;

SC/IM/IV when PO therapy not possible, administer by slow IV inj
• *Pellagra:* PO 50-100 mg tid-qid; max 500 mg/d
• *Niacin deficiency:* PO 10-20 mg/d, max 100 mg/d
• *Hyperlipidemia:* PO 1.5-6 g/d divided bid-tid with or after meals (start at 100-250 mg/d and titrate gradually)

Child
• *Recommended daily allowance PO:* 0-0.5 yr 5 mg/d; 0.5-1 yr 6 mg/d; 1-3 yr 9 mg/d; 4-6 yr 12 mg/d; 7-10 yr 13 mg/d; males 11-14 yr 17 mg/d; males 15-18 yr 20 mg/d
• *Pellagra:* PO 50-100 mg tid

$ AVAILABLE FORMS/COST OF THERAPY
• Tab, Uncoated—Oral: 50 mg, 100's: **$1.15-$2.20;** 100 mg, 100's: **$1.20-$2.55**; 500 mg, 100's: **$2.99-$64.40**
• Cap, Gel, Sust Action—Oral: 125 mg, 100's: **$3.75-$5.70;** 250 mg, 100's: **$4.43-$5.75;** 400 mg, 100's: **$3.63-$6.98;** 500 mg, 100's: **$7.80;** 750 mg, 100's: **$7.05**
• Elixir—Oral: 50 mg/5 ml, 480 ml: **$8.25**
• Inj, Sol—IM; IV; SC: 100 mg/ml, 30 ml: **$2.18**

CONTRAINDICATIONS: Hepatic dysfunction, active peptic ulcer, severe hypotension, hemorrhage, hypersensitivity

PRECAUTIONS: CAD, gallbladder disease, history of jaundice or liver disease, history of peptic ulcer, history of arterial bleeding, gout, diabetes mellitus, tartrazine sensitivity

PREGNANCY AND LACTATION: Pregnancy category A (category C if used in doses greater than RDA); actively excreted in human breast milk; RDA during lactation is 18-20 mg

SIDE EFFECTS/ADVERSE REACTIONS
CNS: Transient headache
CV: Hypotension, atrial fibrillation
EENT: Toxic amblyopia
GI: *GI distress,* activation of peptic ulcer, *nausea,* vomiting, abdominal pain, diarrhea, ***hepatotoxicity*** (more common with sustained release formulations)
METAB: Decreased glucose tolerance
SKIN: *Pruritus, severe generalized flushing, sensation of warmth,* keratosis nigricans, skin rash, dry skin, tingling

▼ DRUG INTERACTIONS
Labs
• *Increase:* Blood glucose, uric acid
• *Abnormality:* Liver function tests

SPECIAL CONSIDERATIONS

PATIENT/FAMILY EDUCATION
• Do not increase dose faster than recommended by physician
• Avoid alcohol and hot beverages (increases flushing)
• Administer with meals and 2 glasses of water
• 125-350 mg of aspirin 20-30 min prior to dose may lessen flushing
• Do not miss any doses (flushing may return)

MONITORING PARAMETERS
• Liver function tests, blood glucose frequently
• Fasting lipid profile q3-6 mo

nicardipine
(nye-card'i-peen)
Cardene, Cardene SR
Chemical Class: Dihydropyridine calcium channel blocker
Therapeutic Class: Antihypertensive; antianginal

CLINICAL PHARMACOLOGY
Mechanism of Action: Inhibits calcium ion influx across cell mem-

brane in vascular smooth muscle and cardiac muscle; produces relaxation of coronary and peripheral vascular smooth muscle; reduces total peripheral resistance (afterload); increases myocardial oxygen delivery

Pharmacokinetics

PO: Onset 20 min, peak 0.5-2 hr, >95% bound to plasma proteins, metabolized in liver, excreted in urine (60%) and feces (35%), $t_{1/2}$ 2-4 hr

INDICATIONS AND USES: Chronic stable angina (immediate release only), hypertension

DOSAGE

Adult

- *Angina:* PO 20 mg tid, may increase after 3 days to 40 mg tid
- *Hypertension:* PO 20 mg tid, may increase to 40 mg tid; SR 30 mg bid, may increase to 60 mg bid; IV INF 5 mg/hr initially, may be increased by 2.5 mg/hr q5-15 min up to maximum of 15 mg/hr; following achievement of goal blood pressure, decrease inf rate to 3 mg/hr then adjust rate as needed to maintain desired response

$ AVAILABLE FORMS/COST OF THERAPY

- Cap—Oral: 20 mg, 100's:**$42.34;** 30 mg, 100's: **$67.32**
- Cap, Gel, Sust Action —Oral: 30 mg, 100's: **$66.13;** 45 mg, 100's: **$105.04;** 60 mg, 60's: **$75.47**
- Inj, Sol—IV: 25 mg/ampul, 10's: **$206.25**

CONTRAINDICATIONS: Hypersensitivity, advanced aortic stenosis

PRECAUTIONS: CHF, hypotension, hepatic insufficiency, renal function impairment, aortic stenosis, elderly, children

PREGNANCY AND LACTATION: Pregnancy category C

SIDE EFFECTS/ADVERSE REACTIONS

CNS: Headache, fatigue, dizziness, anxiety, depression, insomnia, paresthesia, somnolence, asthenia, nervousness, malaise, tremor

CV: Dysrhythmia, *peripheral edema,* bradycardia, hypotension, palpitations, syncope, tachycardia

GI: Nausea, vomiting, diarrhea, gastric upset, constipation, abdominal cramps, flatulence, dry mouth

GU: Nocturia, polyuria

SKIN: Rash, pruritus, urticaria, hair loss

MISC: Flushing, nasal congestion, sweating, shortness of breath, sexual dysfunction, muscle cramps, cough, weight gain, tinnitus, epistaxis

▼ DRUG INTERACTIONS

Drugs

- *Barbiturates:* Reduced plasma concentrations of nicardipine
- *Beta blockers:* Enhanced effects of beta blockers, hypotension
- *Calcium:* Reduced activity of nicardipine
- *Cimetidine:* Increased nicardipine concentrations possible
- *Cyclosporine:* Increased blood cyclosporine concentrations
- *Neuromuscular blocking agents:* Prolongation of neuromuscular blockade

SPECIAL CONSIDERATIONS

PATIENT/FAMILY EDUCATION:

- Notify physician of irregular heart beat, shortness of breath, swelling of feet and hands, pronounced dizziness, constipation, nausea, hypotension

nicotine

(nik′o-teen)

Habitrol, Nicoderm, Nicotrol, ProStep (Transdermal); Nicorette, Nicorette DS (Chewing gum)

Chemical Class: Pyridine alkaloid

Therapeutic Class: Smoking deterrent

CLINICAL PHARMACOLOGY

Mechanism of Action: Acts as an agonist at the nicotinic receptors in the peripheral and central nervous systems; produces stimulant and depressant phases of action on all autonomic ganglia

Pharmocokinetics

BUCCAL: Peak 15-30 min, $t_{1/2}$ 30-60 min

TOP: Peak 4-9 hr, $t_{1/2}$ 3-4 hr

<5% bound to plasma proteins, metabolized by liver to cotinine and nicotine-N-oxide, eliminated in urine (10%-30% as unchanged drug)

INDICATIONS AND USES: Smoking cessation (temporary adjunct in conjunction with behavior modification), hemidystonia,* ulcerative colitis*

DOSAGE

Adult

• *Gum:* Chew 9-12 pieces of gum (2 mg for regular smokers, 4 mg for heavy smokers) at 1-2 hr intervals daily; do not exceed 80 mg/d; gradually reduce number of pieces/d; use longer than 3 mo is discouraged

• *Transdermal systems:* Apply qd, discard system in use and apply new system at different site; wear for 16 hr (Nicotrol) or 24 hr (Habitrol, Nicoderm, ProStep); initiate therapy at highest available dosage of nicotine for all patients except those weighing <45 kg, those who smoke <10 cigarettes/d, and/or those who have cardiovascular disease (should receive lower initial doses); maintain initial dose for 4-12 wk; reduce doses for one or more periods of therapy in patients who have abstained from smoking over next 2-8 wk

$ AVAILABLE FORMS/COST OF THERAPY

• Film, Cont Rel—Percutaneous: 5, 10, 15 mg/16 hr, 14's: **$48.05-$52.08** (Nicotrol); 7, 14,21 mg/24 hr, 14's: **$48.60-$57.18** (Nicoderm); 7,14,21 mg/24 hr, 30's: **$104.37-$115.96** (Habitrol); 11, 22 mg/24 hr, 7's: **$28.35-$30.76** (ProStep)

• Tab, Chewing Gum—Buccal: 2, 4 mg, 96's: **$38.85-$63.29**

CONTRAINDICATIONS: Initial recovery phase of MI, severe or worsening angina pectoris, life-threatening dysrhythmias, temporomandibular joint disease (chewing gum), nonsmokers, hypersensitivity to nicotine or any component of systems

PRECAUTIONS: Cardiovascular disease (history of MI, angina pectoris), serious cardiac dysrhythmias or vasospastic diseases, hypertension, hyperthyroidism, pheochromocytoma, insulin-dependent diabetes, hepatic/renal function impairment, elderly, children, oral or pharyngeal elimination (chewing gum), esophagitis, peptic ulcer disease, skin disease (transdermal), dental problems (chewing gum)

PREGNANCY AND LACTATION: Pregnancy category X (chewing gum), category D (transdermal systems); use of nicotine gum during last trimester has been associated with decreased fetal breathing movements; passes freely into breast milk, lower concentrations in milk can be expected with transdermal systems

N

than cigarette smoking, when used as directed

SIDE EFFECTS/ADVERSE REACTIONS

CNS: (Chewing gum) insomnia, dizziness, lightheadedness, headache, confusion, seizures, depression, euphoria, numbness, paresthesia, syncope, weakness; (Transdermal) *headache, insomnia, abnormal dreams, nervousness, dizziness,* somnolence, impaired concentration

CV: (Chewing gum) edema, flushing, hypertension, palpitations, tachydysrhythmias, tachycardia, ***MI, cardiac arrest, CVA;*** (Transdermal) chest pain, hypertension, ***MI***

EENT: (Chewing gum) tinnitus, pharyngitis; (Transdermal) pharyngitis, sinusitis

GI: (Chewing gum) traumatic injury to oral mucosa or teeth, jaw ache, eructation secondary to air swallowing, stomatitis, glossitis, gingivitis, aphthous ulcers, *nausea,* altered liver function tests, constipation, diarrhea, dry mouth, anorexia; (Transdermal) diarrhea, dyspepsia, constipation, nausea, abdominal pain, vomiting, dry mouth, taste perversion

GU: (Transdermal) dysmenorrhea

MS: (Transdermal) asthenia, back pain, arthralgia, myalgia

RESP: (Chewing gum) *hiccoughs,* breathing difficulty, cough, hoarseness, sneezing, wheezing; (Transdermal) increased cough

SKIN: (Chewing gum) rash, itching, erythema, urticaria; (Transdermal) *short lived erythema, pruritus, burning at application site,* sweating

▼ DRUG INTERACTIONS

Drugs

- *Coffee, cola:* Reduced absorption of nicotine from chewing gum

SPECIAL CONSIDERATIONS

PATIENT/FAMILY EDUCATION

- Chew gum slowly until burning or tingling sensation is felt, then park gum between cheek and gum until tingling sensation goes away
- Chew <30 min/piece
- Avoid coffee and cola drinks while chewing gum
- **Do not smoke while chewing gum or while wearing transdermal system**
- Apply new transdermal system daily
- Rotate sites; apply to non-hairy area on upper torso

---

nifedipine

(nye-fed'i-peen)

Adalat, Adalat CC, Procardia, Procardia XL

Chemical Class: Dihydropyridine calcium channel blocker

Therapeutic Class: Antihypertensive; antianginal

CLINICAL PHARMACOLOGY

Mechanism of Action: Inhibits calcium ion influx across cell membrane in vascular smooth muscle and cardiac muscle; produces relaxation of coronary and peripheral vascular smooth muscle, reduces total peripheral resistance (afterload); increases myocardial oxygen delivery

Pharmacokinetics

PO: Peak 30 min, onset within 20 min (1-5 min if capsule bitten and swallowed); SUST REL, peak 4-5 hr

92%-98% bound to plasma proteins, metabolized by liver to inactive metabolites, excreted by kidneys, $t_{1/2}$ 2-5 hr

INDICATIONS AND USES: Vasospastic (Prinzmetal's or variant) angina, chronic stable angina, hypertension, prevention of migraine headache,* preterm labor,* hypertensive emergencies,* primary pulmonary hypertension,* esophageal disorders*

DOSAGE

Adult

• PO 10 mg tid initially, usual range 10-20 mg tid; doses >120 mg/d are rarely necessary; PO XL 30-60 mg qd, titration to doses >120 mg/d is not recommended; PO CC 30 mg qd, titration to doses >90 mg/d not recommended

Child

• *Hypertensive emergencies:* PO 0.25-0.5 mg/kg/dose

$ AVAILABLE FORMS/COST OF THERAPY

• Cap, Gel—Oral: 10 mg, 100's: **$11.63-$60.57;** 20 mg, 100's: **$20.93-$109.02**

• Tab, Coated, Sust Action —Oral: 30 mg, 100's: **$87.04-$123.18;** 60 mg, 100's: **$150.59-$213.14;** 90 mg, 100's: **$184.47-$245.93**

CONTRAINDICATIONS: Hypersensitivity

PRECAUTIONS: CHF, hypotension, hepatic insufficiency, renal function impairment, aortic stenosis, elderly, children, high doses (>60 mg/d) of immediate release formulations following MI

PREGNANCY AND LACTATION: Pregnancy category C; has been used for tocolysis and as an antihypertensive agent in pregnant women; compatible with breast feeding

SIDE EFFECTS/ADVERSE REACTIONS

CNS: Headache, fatigue, dizziness, anxiety, depression, insomnia, paresthesia, somnolence, asthenia, nervousness, malaise, tremor

CV: Dysrhythmia, *peripheral edema,* bradycardia, hypotension, palpitations, syncope, tachycardia

GI: Nausea, vomiting, diarrhea, gastric upset, constipation, abdominal cramps, flatulence, dry mouth

GU: Nocturia, polyuria

SKIN: Rash, pruritus, urticaria, hair loss

MISC: Flushing, nasal congestion, sweating, shortness of breath, sexual dysfunction, muscle cramps, cough, weight gain, tinnitus, epistaxis

▼ DRUG INTERACTIONS

Drugs

• *Barbiturates, rifampin:* Reduced plasma concentrations of nifedipine

• *Beta blockers:* Enhanced effects of beta blockers, hypotension

• *Calcium:* Reduced activity of nifedipine

• *Cimetidine, ranitidine:* Increased nifedipine concentrations possible

• *Diltiazem:* Increased serum concentrations of nifedipine

• *Food:* Increased absorption of Adalat CC

• *Neuromuscular blocking agents:* Prolongation of neuromuscular blockade

• *Quinidine:* Reduced blood concentrations of quinidine

SPECIAL CONSIDERATIONS

PATIENT/FAMILY EDUCATION

• Notify physician of irregular heart beat, shortness of breath, swelling of feet and hands, pronounced dizziness, constipation, nausea, hypotension

• Administer Adalat CC on an empty stomach

• Do not crush or chew sustained release dosage forms

• Empty Procardia XL tablets may appear in stool, this is no cause for concern

N

nimodipine

(nye-mode'i-peen)

Nimotop

Chemical Class: Dihydropyridine calcium channel blocker

Therapeutic Class: Vasodilating agent

CLINICAL PHARMACOLOGY

Mechanism of Action: Inhibits influx of extracellular calcium ions through voltage-dependent and receptor-operated slow calcium channels in the membranes of myocardial, vascular smooth muscle, and neuronal cells; exact mechanism in patients with subarachnoid hemorrhage unknown; may be due to dilation of small cerebral resistance vessels, with resultant increase in collateral circulation, and/or direct effect involving prevention of calcium overload in neurons

Pharmacokinetics

PO: Peak 1 hr, >95% bound to plasma proteins, extensively metabolized in liver to inactive metabolites, excreted in urine (50%) and feces (32%), $t_{1/2}$ 1.7-9 hr

INDICATIONS AND USES: Recent subarachnoid hemorrhage, acute ischemic stroke,* prevention of migraine headache*

DOSAGE

Adult

• *Subarachnoid hemorrhage:* PO 60 mg q4h for 21 consecutive days beginning within 96 hr of occurrence of hemorrhage; reduce to 30 mg q4h in patients with hepatic failure; for patients unable to swallow oral capsules, the capsule may be punctured at both ends with an 18-gauge needle and the contents emptied directly into nasogastric tube which is then flushed with 30 ml of normal saline

• *Prevention of migraine headache:* PO 120 mg/d in divided doses; response may not be apparent for 1-2 mo

$ **AVAILABLE FORMS/COST OF THERAPY**

• Cap, Elastic—Oral: 30 mg, 100's: **$500.85**

CONTRAINDICATIONS: Hypersensitivity

PRECAUTIONS: Impaired hepatic/renal function, children <18 yr

PREGNANCY AND LACTATION: Pregnancy category C

SIDE EFFECTS/ADVERSE REACTIONS

CNS: Mental depression, headache, lightheadedness, dizziness

CV: Hypotension, edema, ECG abnormalities, palpitations, flushing

GI: Lower abdominal discomfort, constipation, ***hepatitis, jaundice***

HEME: ***Thrombocytopenia, anemia***

MS: Muscle pain

RESP: Dyspnea

SKIN: Rash

▼ **DRUG INTERACTIONS**

Labs

• *Increase:* Liver function tests

SPECIAL CONSIDERATIONS

MONITORING PARAMETERS

• Blood pressure

nitrofurantoin

(nye-troe-fyoor'an-toyn)

Furadantin, Macrobid, Macrodantin, Novofuran ♣

Chemical Class: Synthetic nitrofuran

Therapeutic Class: Urinary tract anti-infective

CLINICAL PHARMACOLOGY

Mechanism of Action: May inhibit acetylcoenzyme A, interfering with bacterial carbohydrate metabolism; may also disrupt bacterial cell wall formation

Pharmacokinetics

PO: Therapeutic concentrations achieved only in urine, macrocrystalline formulation slows absorption causing less GI irritation, food increases absorption, 60% bound to plasma proteins, partially inactivated in most body tissues, eliminated in urine (30%-50% unchanged), $t_{1/2}$ 20-60 min

INDICATIONS AND USES: UTIs

Antibacterial spectrum usually includes:

- Gram-positive organisms: *Staphylococcus aureus, S. saprophyticus, Enterococcus faecalis, Streptococcus agalactiae,* group D streptococci, viridans streptococci, *Corynebacterium*
- Gram-negative organisms: *Citrobacter amalonaticus, C. diversus, C. freundii, Klebsiella oxytoca, K. ozaenae, Enterobacter, Escherichia coli, Neisseria, Salmonella, Shigella*

DOSAGE

Adult

- PO 50-100 mg qid ac and hs; (Macrobid) 100 mg bid with food; for long-term suppressive therapy 50-100 mg qhs

Child >1 month

- PO 5-7 mg/kg/d divided qid; for long-term suppressive therapy 1 mg/kg/d divided qd-bid

$ AVAILABLE FORMS/COST OF THERAPY

Macrocrystals caps only

- Cap, Gel—Oral: 25 mg, 100's: **\$41.70-\$56.46;** 50 mg, 100's: **\$58.00-\$74.39;** 100 mg, 100's: **\$98.50-\$126.28**
- Tab—Oral: 50 mg, 100's: **\$2.25-\$58.19;** 100 mg, 100's: **\$6.00-\$98.79**
- Susp—Oral: 25 mg/5ml, 60 ml: **\$20.15**

CONTRAINDICATIONS: CrCl <60 ml/min (inadequate antibacterial concentrations achieved in urine), hypersensitivity, children <1 mo, during labor and delivery

PRECAUTIONS: G-6-PD deficiency, renal impairment, anemia, diabetes, electrolyte imbalance, vitamin B deficiency, debilitating disease

PREGNANCY AND LACTATION: Pregnancy category B; compatible with breast feeding

SIDE EFFECTS/ADVERSE REACTIONS

CNS: Peripheral neuropathy, headache, dizziness, nystagmus, drowsiness, asthenia, vertigo, confusion, depression euphoria, psychotic reactions (rare), chills

CV: ECG changes

GI: Anorexia, nausea, vomiting, abdominal pain, diarrhea, parotitis, ***pancreatitis, hepatitis, cholestatic jaundice, chronic active hepatitis, hepatic necrosis***

GU: Superinfection of GU tract

HEME: ***Hemolytic anemia, granulocytopenia, angranulocytosis, leukopenia, thrombocytopenia, eosinophilia, megaloblastic anemia, aplastic anemia***

MS: Arthralgia, myalgia

RESP: ***Acute and chronic pulmonary reactions*** (dyspnea, chest pain, cough, pulmonary infiltration), ***anaphylaxis***

SKIN: ***Exfoliative dermatitis, erythema multiforme,*** rash, pruritus, urticaria, angioedema, transient alopecia

▼ DRUG INTERACTIONS

Labs

- *False positive:* Urine glucose
- *Increase:* AST, ALT

SPECIAL CONSIDERATIONS

PATIENT/FAMILY EDUCATION

- Complete full course of therapy
- May cause GI upset, take with food or milk
- May cause brown discoloration of urine
- Notify physician of chills, cough,

N

chest pain, difficult breathing, skin rash, numbness or tingling of fingers or toes, intolerable GI upset

MONITORING PARAMETERS

- Periodic liver function tests during prolonged therapy
- CBC with differential and platelets

nitrofurazone

(nye-troe-fyoor'a-zone)

Furacin

Chemical Class: Synthetic nitrofuran derivative

Therapeutic Class: Local antibacterial

CLINICAL PHARMACOLOGY

Mechanism of Action: Exact mechanism of action unknown; appears to inhibit bacterial enzymes involved in carbohydrate metabolism; antibacterial action inhibited by organic matter (e.g., blood, pus, serum) and *p*-aminobenzoic acid

INDICATIONS AND USES: Topical adjunct in 2nd and 3rd degree burns when bacterial resistance is a real or potential problem; prevention of infection of skin grafts and/or donor sites prior to or following surgery

DOSAGE

Adult and child

- TOP Apply to affected area qd or every few days, depending on dressing technique; apply directly or place on gauze; flushing with sterile saline facilitates removal

$ **AVAILABLE FORMS/COST OF THERAPY**

- Oint—Top: 0.2%, 30, 454 g: **$1.51-$71.97**
- Cre—Top: 0.2%, 28 g: **$15.05**
- Sol—Top: 0.2%, 480 ml: **$6.48-$57.51**

CONTRAINDICATIONS: Hypersensitivity

PRECAUTIONS: Renal function impairment (ointment contains polyethylene glycol); children; superinfection with nonsusceptible organisms possible; no evidence of efficacy in minor burns, surface bacterial infection involving wounds, cutaneous ulcers, or the various pyodermas

PREGNANCY AND LACTATION: Pregnancy category C

SIDE EFFECTS/ADVERSE REACTIONS

SKIN: Contact dermatitis (rash, pruritus, local edema)

SPECIAL CONSIDERATIONS

PATIENT/FAMILY EDUCATION

- Notify physician if condition worsens or if rash or irritation occurs

nitroglycerin

(nye-troe-gli'ser-in)

Deponit, Minitran, Nitro-Bid Ointment, Nitro-Bid IV, Nitro-Bid Plateau Caps, Nitrocine Timecaps, Nitrodisc, Nitro-Dur, Nitrogard, Nitroglyn, Nitrol, Nitrolingual, Nitrong, Nitrostat, Transderm-Nitro, Tridil

Chemical Class: Organic nitrate

Therapeutic Class: Antianginal

CLINICAL PHARMACOLOGY

Mechanism of Action: Reduces myocardial oxygen demand by reducing left ventricular preload (predominantly) and afterload because of venous (predominantly) and arterial dilation with more efficient redistribution of blood flow within the myocardium; dilates coronary arteries and improves collateral flow to ischemic regions

Pharmacokinetics

SL: Onset 1-3 min, peak 4-8 min, duration 30-60 min

LINGUAL SPRAY: Onset 2 min, peak 4-10 min, duration 30-60 min

BUCCAL: Onset 2-5 min, peak 4-10 min, duration 2 hr

PO: Onset 20-45 min, peak 45-120 min, duration 4-8 hr
TOP: Onset 15-60 min, peak 30-120 min, duration 2-12 hr
TRANSDERMAL: Onset 40-60 min, peak 60-180 min, duration 8-24 hr
IV: Onset immediate, peak immediate, duration 3-5 min
60% bound to plasma proteins, metabolized by liver to inorganic nitrate (extensive 1st pass effect), eliminated in urine, $t_{1/2}$ 1-4 min
INDICATIONS AND USES: Acute angina (SL, translingual spray, buccal), angina prophylaxis (TOP, transdermal, translingual spray, buccal, oral), perioperative hypertension (IV), congestive heart failure associated with MI (IV), unresponsive angina pectoris (IV), acute MI (SL, TOP),* Raynaud's disease (TOP),* hypertensive crisis (IV)*
DOSAGE
Adult
- Buccal 1 mg q3-5h while awake (3 tid) initially, titrate dosage upward if angina occurs with tab in place
- PO 2.5-9 mg bid-qid, up to 26 mg qid
- IV 5 µg/min, increase by 5 µg/min q3-5 min to 20 µg/min; if no response increase by 10 µg/min q3-5 min up to 200 µg/min
- TOP 1-2″ q8h, up to 4-5″ q4h
- Transdermal 0.2-0.4 mg/hr initially, titrate to 0.4-0.8 mg/hr; tolerance is minimized by removing patch for 10-12 hr/d
- SL 0.2-0.6 mg q5min for max of 3 doses in 15 min; may also use prophylactically 5-10 min prior to activities which provoke angina attack
- Translingual 1-2 sprays under tongue q3-5 min for max of 3 doses in 15 min, may also use prophylactically 5-10 min prior to activities which provoke angina attack

Child
- IV 0.25-0.5 µg/kg/min, titrate by 0.5-1 µg/kg/min q3-5 min prn; usual dose 1-3 µg/kg/min; max 20 µg/kg/min

$ AVAILABLE FORMS/COST OF THERAPY
- Aer Spray—Oral: 0.4 mg/spr, 14.49 g: **$24.82**
- Tab—SL: 0.15 mg, 100's: **$5.46;** 0.3 mg, 100's: **$6.18;** 0.4 mg, 100's: **$6.18;** 0.6 mg, 100's: **$6.18;**
- Tab, Uncoated, Sust Action—Buccal: 1 mg, 100's: **$37.87;** 2 mg, 100's: **$40.09;** 3 mg, 100's: **$43.33;**
- Tab, Coated, Sust Action—Oral: 2.6 mg, 100's: **$29.61-$60.35;** 6.5 mg, 100's: **$37.06-$43.49;**
- Cap, Gel, Sust Action—Oral: 2.5 mg, 100's: **$5.49-$9.15;** 6.5 mg, 100's: **$6.61-$13.99;** 9 mg, 100's: **$8.25-$16.63**
- Oint—Percutaneous: 2%; 20, 30, 60 g: **$3.38-$16.33**
- Disk—Percutaneous: 16 mg/pad, 100's: **$144.94;** 32 mg/pad, 100's: **$160.52**
- Film, Continuous Release—Percutaneous: 0.1, 0.2, 0.3, 0.4, 0.5, 0.6, 0.8, 1.0 mg/hr 30's: **$32.84-$63.13**
- Inj, Sol—IV: 5 mg/ml, 10 ml: **$39.19-$375.00;** 0.1, 0.2, 0.4 mg/ml, 250 ml: **$16.01-$19.57**

CONTRAINDICATIONS: Hypersensitivity to nitrates or adhesives (transdermal systems), severe anemia, closed angle glaucoma, postural hypotension, early MI (SL), head trauma, cerebral hemorrhage, hypotension or uncorrected hypovolemia, inadequate cerebral circulation, increased intracranial pressure, constrictive pericarditis, pericardial tamponade (IV)
PRECAUTIONS: Early days of MI, hypertrophic cardiomyopathy, se-

vere hepatic/renal disease, children, glaucoma, abrupt withdrawal, continuous delivery (tolerance develops rapidly, IV excepted)

PREGNANCY AND LACTATION: Pregnancy category C; use of SL for angina during pregnancy without fetal harm has been reported

SIDE EFFECTS/ADVERSE REACTIONS

CNS: Headache, apprehension, restlessness, weakness, vertigo, *dizziness,* agitation, anxiety, confusion, insomnia, nervousness, nightmares, dyscoordination, hypoesthesia, hypokinesia

CV: Tachycardia, retrosternal discomfort, palpitations, hypotension, syncope, ***collapse,*** crescendo angina, rebound hypertension, dysrhythmias, atrial fibrillation, premature ventricular contractions, *postural hypotension*

EENT: Blurred vision

GI: Nausea, vomiting, diarrhea, dyspepsia, abdominal pain, tenesmus, tooth disorder, fecal incontinence

GU: Dysuria, impotence, urinary frequency

HEME: Hemolytic anemia, methemoglobinemia

MS: Arthralgia

SKIN: Rash, exfoliative dermatitis, *cutaneous vasodilation with flushing,* crusty skin lesions, pruritus, sweating, pallor, contact dermatitis (transdermal), allergic reactions (ointment)

▼ **DRUG INTERACTIONS**

Drugs

• *Ergot alkaloids:* Opposition to vasodilatory effects of nitrates

Labs

• *False decrease:* Cholesterol by the Zlatkis-Zak color reaction

SPECIAL CONSIDERATIONS

PATIENT/FAMILY EDUCATION

• Avoid alcohol

• Notify physician if persistent headache

• Take oral nitrates on empty stomach with full glass of water

• Keep tablets and capsules in original container, keep container closed tightly

• Dissolve SL tablets under tongue, lack of burning does not indicate loss of potency, use when seated, take at 1st sign of anginal attack, activate emergency response system if no relief after 3 tablets spaced 5 min apart

• Spray translingual spray onto or under tongue, do not inhale spray

• Place buccal tablets under upper lip or between cheek and gum, permit to dissolve slowly over 3-5 min, do not chew or swallow

• Spread thin layer of ointment on skin using applicator or dose-measuring papers, do not use fingers, do not rub or massage

• Apply transdermal systems to nonhairy area on upper torso, remove for 10-12 hr/d (usually hs)

MONITORING PARAMETERS

• Blood pressure, heart rate

---

nitroprusside

(nye-troe-pruss'ide)

Nitropress, Nipride

Chemical Class: Cyanonitrosylferrate

Therapeutic Class: Antihypertensive

CLINICAL PHARMACOLOGY

Mechanism of Action: Relaxes vascular smooth muscle and dilates peripheral arteries and veins; more active on veins than arteries; reduces left ventricular end-diastolic pressure and pulmonary capillary wedge pressure (preload); reduces systemic vascular resistance, systolic arterial pressure, and mean arterial pressure (afterload); dilates coronary arteries

Pharmacokinetics

IV: Onset immediate, rapidly metabolized by interaction with sulfhydryl groups in erythrocytes and tissues (cyanogen is produced and converted to thiocyanate in liver), eliminated via urine (metabolites)

INDICATIONS AND USES: Hypertensive crisis, controlled hypotension during surgery, severe refractory congestive heart failure (in combination with dopamine),* acute MI*

DOSAGE

Adult

- IV INF 2 μg/kg/min initially, increase in increments of 2-4 μg/kg/min (up to 20 μg/kg/min), then in increments of 10-20 μg/kg/min; cyanide toxicity more likely when >500 μg/kg is administered by prolonged infusion (>8 hr) of greater than 20 μg/kg/min

Child

- IV INF 1 μg/kg/min initially, increase in increments of 1 μg/kg/min at intervals of 20-60 min; do not exceed 10 μg/kg/min

$ AVAILABLE FORMS/COST OF THERAPY

- Inj, Lyphl-Sol—IV: 50 mg/vial, 1's: **$4.24-$8.53;**
- Inj, Sol—IV: 25 mg/ml, 2 ml: **$5.04**
- Kit—IV: 50 mg, 1's: **$11.76**

CONTRAINDICATIONS: Hypersensitivity, decreased cerebral perfusion, arteriovenous shunt or coarctation of the aorta (i.e. compensatory hypertension)

PRECAUTIONS: Hepatic disease, decreased renal function, prolonged infusion, elevated intracranial pressure, anemia, hypovolemia, poor surgical risks, hypothyroidism, hyponatremia

PREGNANCY AND LACTATION: Pregnancy category C

SIDE EFFECTS/ADVERSE REACTIONS

CNS: Dizziness, headache, apprehension, increased intracranial pressure

CV: Bradycardia, ECG changes, tachycardia, palpitations, retrosternal discomfort

GI: Ileus, abdominal pain, nausea, retching

HEME: Decreased platelet aggregation, methemoglobinemia

METAB: Hypothyroidism

MS: Muscle twitching

SKIN: Flushing, irritation at inf site, rash, diaphoresis

MISC: Thiocyanate/cyanide toxicity

▼ DRUG INTERACTIONS

Labs

- *Interfere:* Iodine uptake

SPECIAL CONSIDERATIONS

MONITORING PARAMETERS

- Blood pressure, arterial blood gases, oxygen saturation, cyanide and thiocyanate concentrations

N

---

nizatidine

(ni-za'ti-deen)

Axid

Chemical Class: Substituted ethenediamine

Therapeutic Class: Histamine-2 (H2) receptor blocker

CLINICAL PHARMACOLOGY

Mechanism of Action: Competitive, reversible inhibitor of histamine at H2 receptors

Pharmacokinetics

PO: Onset 30-60 min, peak 0.5 to 3 hr, duration 4-8 hr

Oral bioavailability 70%, protein binding 35%; metabolized in liver, 60% of drug excreted unchanged in urine, 6% eliminated in feces

INDICATIONS AND USES: Gastroesophageal reflux disease, gastric ulcer, duodenal ulcer (active and for maintenance suppression), gastritis*

DOSAGE

Adult

- *Active duodenal or benign gastric ulcer:* PO 300 mg hs or 150 mg bid
- *Maintenance of healed duodenal ulcer:* PO 150 mg hs
- *Gastroesophageal reflux disease:* PO 150 mg bid
- Dosage adjustment for renal insufficiency (active ulcer disease), CrCl 20-50 ml/min, 150 mg qd; CrCl <20 ml/min, 150 mg qod

$ AVAILABLE FORMS/COST OF THERAPY

- Cap, Gel—Oral: 150 mg, 100's: **$158.22;**
- 300 mg, 30's: **$62.12**

CONTRAINDICATIONS: Hypersensitivity to H2-receptor antagonists

PRECAUTIONS: Renal insufficiency

PREGNANCY AND LACTATION: Pregnancy category C; excreted in breast milk

SIDE EFFECTS/ADVERSE REACTIONS

CNS: Dizziness, drowsiness, headache

CV: Bradycardia, palpitation, tachycardia

EENT: Rhinitis

GI: Constipation, diarrhea, flatulence, hepatitis, nausea

HEME: Anemia, thrombocytopenia

METAB: Gynecomastia, hyperuricemia

MS: Myalgia

SKIN: Acne, pruritus, sweating, urticaria

▼ DRUG INTERACTIONS

Drugs

- *Antacids containing aluminum and magnesium hydroxide with simethicone:* Decrease absorption of nizatidine by 10%

Labs

- *False positive:* Urobilinogen by Multistix, urine protein

SPECIAL CONSIDERATIONS

- Separate antacid and nizatidine doses by 60 min

---

norepinephrine

(nor-ep-i-nef'rin)

Levophed

Chemical Class: Sympathomimetic amine

Therapeutic Class: Vasopressor

CLINICAL PHARMACOLOGY

Mechanism of Action: Stimulates β_1-adrenergic receptors and α-adrenergic receptors causing increased myocardial contractility and heart rate as well as vasoconstriction; increases blood pressure and coronary artery blood flow; marked pressor effect primarily due to increased peripheral resistance

Pharmacokinetics

IV: Onset rapid, duration 1-2 min after inf discontinued, metabolized in liver and other tissues by monoamine oxidase (MAO) and catechol-O-methyltransferase (COMT) to inactive metabolites, pharmacologic action terminated mainly by uptake and metabolism in sympathetic nerve endings, excreted in urine (metabolites)

INDICATIONS AND USES: Acute hypotensive states, adjunct in treatment of cardiac arrest and profound hypotension

DOSAGE

Adult

- IV INF 8-12 μg/min; initiate at 4 μg/min and titrate to desired response

Child

- IV INF 0.05-0.1 μg/kg/min initally, titrate to desired effect

$ AVAILABLE FORMS/COST OF THERAPY

• Inj, Sol—IV: 0.1%, 4 ml: **$11.28-$15.12**

CONTRAINDICATIONS: Hypotension from blood volume deficits (except as an emergency measure until volume replacement can be completed), mesenteric or peripheral vascular thrombosis, cyclopropane and halothane anesthesia

PRECAUTIONS: Atherosclerosis, arteriosclerosis, diabetic endarteritis, Buerger's disease, elderly, extravasation (may cause necrosis and sloughing of surrounding tissue), sulfite sensitivity

PREGNANCY AND LACTATION: Pregnancy category D

SIDE EFFECTS/ADVERSE REACTIONS

CNS: Anxiety, *headache*

CV: ***Cardiac dysrhythmias,*** palpitations, bradycardia, ***tachycardia, hypertension,*** *chest pain*

EENT: Photophobia

GI: Nausea, vomiting

RESP: Respiratory distress

SKIN: Diaphoresis, pallor, necrosis and sloughing following extravasation, ***gangrene***

MISC: Organ ischemia (due to vasocontriction of renal and mesenteric arteries)

▼ **DRUG INTERACTIONS**

Drugs

• *Cyclic antidepressants+:* Marked enhancement of pressor response to norepinephrine

SPECIAL CONSIDERATIONS

MONITORING PARAMETERS

• Blood pressure, heart rate, ECG, urine output, peripheral perfusion

norethindrone

(nor-eth'in-drone)

Micronor, Norlutin, Nor-Q.D.; Aygestin, Norlutate (acetate)

Chemical Class: 19-nortestosterone derivative

Therapeutic Class: Progestin; contraceptive

CLINICAL PHARMACOLOGY

Mechanism of Action: Shares the actions of the progestins; in the presence of adequate estrogen, transforms a proliferative endometrium into a secretory one; stimulates growth of mammary alveolar tissue; has some androgenic and adrenocorticoid activity; inhibits secretion of pituitary gonadotropins thus preventing follicular maturation and ovulation (inconsistent in continuous low-dose regimen); alters cervical mucus inhibiting sperm migration into the uterus; inhibits implantation of fertilized ovum in the uterus

Pharmacokinetics

PO: 80% bound to plasma proteins, metabolized in liver, $t_{1/2}$ 10 hr

INDICATIONS AND USES: Prevention of conception, secondary amenorrhea, abnormal uterine bleeding, endometriosis

DOSAGE

Adult and adolescents

• *Amenorrhea and abnormal uterine bleeding:* PO 5-20 mg (2.5-10 mg acetate) on days 5-25 of menstrual cycle **or** to induce optimum secretory transformation of estrogen-primed endometrium 2.5-10 mg of acetate for 5-10 days during the latter half of menstrual cycle

• *Endometriosis:* PO 10 mg (5 mg acetate) qd for 14 consecutive days; increase by 5 mg/d (2.5 mg/d acetate) at 14 day intervals until max of 30 mg/d (15 mg/d acetate) is reached; daily therapy may then be continued consecutively (no drug-free intervals) for 6-9 mo

• *Contraception:* PO 0.35 mg qd

$ **AVAILABLE FORMS/COST OF THERAPY**

• Tab, Uncoated—Oral: 0.35 mg, 28's: **$29.22;** 5 mg, 50's: **$42.88;**

• Tab, Uncoated (acetate)—Oral: 5 mg, 50's: **$51.43**

CONTRAINDICATIONS: Hypersensitivity, thrombophlebitis, thromboembolic disorders, cerebral hemorrhage, impaired liver function or disease, breast cancer, undiagnosed vaginal bleeding, missed abortion, use as a diagnostic test for pregnancy

PRECAUTIONS: Epilepsy, migraine, asthma, cardiac or renal dysfunction, depression, diabetes

PREGNANCY AND LACTATION: Pregnancy category X; compatible with breast feeding

SIDE EFFECTS/ADVERSE REACTIONS

CNS: Dizziness, headache, migraines, depression, fatigue

CV: Hypotension, thrombophlebitis, edema, ***thromboembolism, stroke, pulmonary embolism, MI***

EENT: Diplopia

GI: Nausea, vomiting, anorexia, cramps, increased weight, ***cholestatic jaundice***

GU: Amenorrhea, cervical erosion, breakthrough bleeding, dysmenorrhea, vaginal candidiasis, breast changes, endometriosis, ***spontaneous abortion***

METAB: Hyperglycemia

SKIN: Rash, urticaria, acne, hirsutism, alopecia, oily skin, seborrhea, purpura, melasma, photosensitivity

▼ **DRUG INTERACTIONS**

Labs

• *Increase:* Alkaline phosphatase, pregnanediol, liver function tests

• *Decrease:* Glucose tolerance, HDL

SPECIAL CONSIDERATIONS

PATIENT/FAMILY EDUCATION

• Take protective measures against exposure to UV light or sunlight

• Diabetics monitor blood glucose carefully during therapy

• Notify physician of pain, swelling, warmth or redness in calves, sudden severe headache, visual disturbances, numbness in arm or leg

• Take with food if GI upset occurs

• When used as contraceptive menstrual cycle may be disrupted and irregular and unpredictable bleeding or spotting results, usually decreases to the point of amenorrhea as treatment continues

MONITORING PARAMETERS

• Pretreatment physical exam should include breasts and pelvic organs, Pap smear

---

norfloxacin

(nor-flox'a-sin)

Noroxin, Chibroxin Ophthalmic

Chemical Class: Fluoroquinolone

Therapeutic Class: Urinary antiinfective

CLINICAL PHARMACOLOGY

Mechanism of Action: Interferes with the enzyme DNA gyrase needed for the synthesis of bacterial DNA; bacericidal

Pharmacokinetics

PO: Peak 1-2 hr, 10%-15% bound to plasma proteins, partially metabolized, excreted in urine (60%) and feces (30%), $t_{1/2}$ 2.3-4 hr

INDICATIONS AND USES: Complicated and uncomplicated UTIs, uncomplicated gonorrhea, gastroenteritis,* travelers' diarrhea,* conjunctivitis (ophthal sol)

Antibacterial spectrum usually in-

* = non-FDA-approved use

+ = major clinical significance

cludes: gram-positive organisms: *Enterococcus faecalis, Staphylococcus aureus, S. epidermidis, S. saprophyticus, Streptococcus agalactiae;* gram-negative organisms: *Citrobacter freundii, Enterobacter aerogenes, E. cloacae, Escherichia coli, Klebsiella pneumoniae, Neisseria gonorrhoeae, Proteus mirabilis, P. vulgaris, Pseudomonas aeruginosa, Serratia marcescens*

DOSAGE

Adult

- *Urinary tract infection:* PO 400 mg bid on an empty stomach for 3-10 days (uncomplicated) or 10-21 days (complicated)
- *Gonorrhea:* PO 800 mg as a single dose followed by doxycycline 100 mg bid for 7 days
- *Gastroenteritis:* PO 400 mg bid for 5 days
- *Travelers' diarrhea:* PO 400 mg bid for up to 3 days until symptoms resolve
- Dosage in renal impairment, administer 400 mg qd in patients with CrCl <30 ml/min/1.73 m^2
- *Conjunctivitis:* OPHTH 1 drop qid

$ **AVAILABLE FORMS/COST OF THERAPY**

- Sol—Ophth: 3 mg/ml, 5 ml: **$18.04**
- Tab, Plain Coated—Oral: 400 mg, 100's: **$254.29**

CONTRAINDICATIONS: Hypersensitivity to quinolones

PRECAUTIONS: Children (potential for arthropathy and osteochondrosis), elderly, renal disease, seizure disorders, dehydration (potential for crystalluria)

PREGNANCY AND LACTATION: Pregnancy category C; excretion into breast milk unknown, due to the potential for arthropathy and osteochondrosis use extreme caution in nursing mothers

SIDE EFFECTS/ADVERSE REACTIONS

CNS: Dizziness, headache, fatigue, somnolence, depression, insomnia, anxiety, ***seizures***

EENT: Visual disturbances

GI: Diarrhea, *nausea,* vomiting, anorexia, flatulence, heartburn, abdominal pain, dry mouth, increased AST, ALT, pseudomembranous colitis

GU: Crystalluria

HEME: ***Eosinophilia, leukopenia***

SKIN: Rash, pruritus, photosensitivity

▼ **DRUG INTERACTIONS**

Drugs

- *Antacids, didanosine, iron, sucralfate:* Reduced serum norfloxacin concentrations
- *Oral anticoagulants:* Potential excessive hypoprothrombinemic response to warfarin

SPECIAL CONSIDERATIONS

PATIENT/FAMILY EDUCATION

- Administer on an empty stomach (1 hr before or 2 hr after meals)
- Drink fluids liberally
- Do not take antacids containing magnesium or aluminum or products containing iron or zinc within 4 hr before or 2 hr after dosing
- Observe caution while driving or performing other tasks requiring alertness
- Avoid excessive exposure to sunlight

norgestrel

(nor-jess'trel)

Ovrette

Chemical Class: 19-nortestosterone derivative

Therapeutic Class: Contraceptive

CLINICAL PHARMACOLOGY

Mechanism of Action: Shares the

actions of the progestins; inhibits secretion of pituitary gonadotropins thus preventing follicular maturation and ovulation (inconsistent in continuous low-dose regimen); alters cervical mucus inhibiting sperm migration into the uterus; inhibits implantation of fertilized ovum in the uterus

Pharmacokinetics

PO: 93%-95% bound to plasma proteins, metabolized in liver, excreted in urine and feces, $t_{1/2}$ 11-45 hr

INDICATIONS AND USES: Prevention of conception

DOSAGE

Adult

• PO 0.075 mg qd

$ AVAILABLE FORMS/COST OF THERAPY

• Tab, Uncoated—Oral: 0.075 mg, 28's: **$26.27**

CONTRAINDICATIONS: Hypersensitivity, thrombophlebitis, thromboembolic disorders, cerebral hemorrhage, impaired liver function or disease, breast cancer, undiagnosed vaginal bleeding, missed abortion, use as a diagnostic test for pregnancy

PRECAUTIONS: Epilepsy, migraine, asthma, cardiac or renal dysfunction, depression, diabetes

PREGNANCY AND LACTATION: Pregnancy category X; compatible with breast feeding

SIDE EFFECTS/ADVERSE REACTIONS

CNS: Dizziness, headache, migraines, depression, fatigue

CV: Hypotension, thrombophlebitis, edema, ***thromboembolism, stroke, pulmonary embolism, MI***

EENT: Diplopia

GI: Nausea, vomiting, anorexia, cramps, increased weight, ***cholestatic jaundice***

GU: Amenorrhea, cervical erosion, breakthrough bleeding, dysmenorrhea, vaginal candidiasis, breast changes, endometriosis, ***spontaneous abortion***

METAB: Hyperglycemia

SKIN: Rash, urticaria, acne, hirsutism, alopecia, oily skin, seborrhea, purpura, melasma, photosensitivity

▼ DRUG INTERACTIONS

Labs

• *Increase:* Alk phosphatase, pregnanediol, liver function tests

• *Decrease:* Glucose tolerance, HDL

SPECIAL CONSIDERATIONS

PATIENT/FAMILY EDUCATION

• Take protective measures against exposure to UV light or sunlight

• Diabetic patients should monitor blood glucose carefully during therapy

• Notify physician of pain, swelling, warmth or redness in calves, sudden severe headache, visual disturbances, numbness in arm or leg

• Take with food if GI upset occurs

• Menstrual cycle may be disrupted and irregular and unpredictable bleeding or spotting results, usually decreases to the point of amenorrhea as treatment continues

MONITORING PARAMETERS

• Pretreatment physical exam should include breasts and pelvic organs, Pap smear

nortriptyline

(nor-trip'ti-leen)

Aventyl, Pamelor

Chemical Class: Dibenzocycloheptene derivative, secondary amine

Therapeutic Class Antidepressant, tricyclic

CLINICAL PHARMACOLOGY

Mechanism of Action: Inhibits reuptake of norepinephrine and serotonin at the presynaptic neuron prolonging neuronal activity; inhibition of histamine and acetylcholine activity; mild peripheral vasodilator effects and possible "quinidine-like" actions

Pharmacokinetics

PO: Peak 7-8.5 hr, 93%-95% bound to plasma proteins, metabolized in liver, excreted in urine, small amounts excreted in bile, $t_{1/2}$ 28-31 hr

INDICATIONS AND USES: Depression, panic disorder,* premenstrual depression,* dermatologic disorders (chronic urticaria and angioedema, nocturnal pruritis in atopic eczema),* nocturnal enuresis*

DOSAGE

Adult

• PO 25 mg qhs initially, increase at 3-5 day increments to 75-150 mg/d divided qd-qid

Elderly and adolescents

• PO 30-50 mg/d in divided doses

Child

• *Nocturnal enuresis:* PO, 6-7 yr 10 mg/d; 8-11 yr 10-20 mg/d; >11 yr 25-35 mg/d

$ **AVAILABLE FORMS/COST OF THERAPY**

• Cap, Gel—Oral: 10 mg, 100's: **$19.34-$45.54;** 25 mg, 100's: **$38.67-$90.96;** 50 mg, 100's: **$72.90-$171.48;** 75 mg, 100's: **$111.15-$261.42**

• Sol—Oral: 10 mg/5ml, 480 ml: **$44.00-$52.26**

CONTRAINDICATIONS: Hypersensitivity to tricyclic antidepressants, acute recovery phase of MI/ concurrent use of MAOIs

PRECAUTIONS: Suicidal patients, convulsive disorders, prostatic hypertrophy, psychiatric disease, severe depression, increased intraocular pressure, narrow-angle glaucoma, urinary retention, cardiac disease, hepatic disease/renal disease, hyperthyroidism, electroshock therapy, elective surgery, elderly, abrupt discontinuation

PREGNANCY AND LACTATION: Pregnancy category D; effect on nursing infant unknown but may be of concern, especially after prolonged exposure

SIDE EFFECTS/ADVERSE REACTIONS

CNS: Dizziness, confusion (especially in elderly), headache, anxiety, nervousness, panic, tremors, stimulation, weakness, fatigue, insomnia, nightmares, EPS (elderly), increased psychiatric symptoms, memory impairment

CV: Orthostatic hypotension, ***ECG changes, tachycardia, dysrhythmias,*** hypertension, palpitations, syncope, hypertensive episodes during surgery

EENT: Blurred vision, tinnitus, mydriasis, ophthalmoplegia, nasal congestion

GI: Constipation, dry mouth, nausea, vomiting, ***paralytic ileus,*** increased appetite, cramps, epigastric distress, jaundice, ***hepatitis,*** stomatitis, diarrhea

GU: Urinary retention

HEME: ***Agranulocytosis, thrombocytopenia, eosinophilia, leukopenia***

SKIN: Rash, urticaria, sweating, pruritus, photosensitivity

▼ **DRUG INTERACTIONS**

Drugs

• *Amphetamines:* Theoretical increase in effect of amphetamines, clinical evidence lacking

• *Anticholinergics:* Excessive anticholinergic effects

• *Barbiturates:* Reduced serum concentrations of cyclic antidepressants

• *Bethanidine:* Reduced antihypertensive effect of bethanidine

N

• *Carbamazepine:* Reduced cyclic antidepressant serum concentrations
• *Cimetidine:* Increased serum nortriptyline concentrations
• *Clonidine:* Reduced antihypertensive response to clonidine; enhanced hypertensive response with abrupt clonidine withdrawal
• *Debrisoquin:* Inhibited antihypertensive response to debrisoquin
• *Epinephrine+:* Markedly enhanced pressor response to IV epinephrine
• *Ethanol:* Additive impairment of motor skills; abstinent alcoholics may eliminate cyclic antidepressants more rapidly than nonalcoholics
• *Fluoxetine:* Marked increases in cyclic antidepressant plasma concentrations
• *Guanethidine:* Inhibited antihypertensive response to guanethidine
• *Moclobemide+:* Potential association with fatal or non-fatal serotonin syndrome
• *MAOI:* Excessive sympathetic response, mania or hyperpyrexia possible
• *Neuroleptics:* Increased therapeutic and toxic effects of both drugs
• *Norepinephrine+:* Markedly enhanced pressor response to norepinephrine
• *Phenylephrine:* Enhanced pressor response to IV phenylephrine
• *Phenytoin:* Altered seizure control; decreased cyclic antidepressant serum concentrations
• *Propoxyphene:* Enhanced effect of cyclic antidepressants
• *Quinidine:* Increased cyclic antidepressant serum concentrations

Labs

• *Increase:* Serum bilirubin, blood glucose, alk phosphatase
• *Decrease:* VMA, 5-HIAA
• *False increase:* Urinary catecholamines

SPECIAL CONSIDERATIONS

PATIENT/FAMILY EDUCATION

• Therapeutic effects may take 2-3 wk
• Use caution in driving or other activities requiring alertness
• Avoid rising quickly from sitting to standing, especially elderly
• Avoid alcohol and other CNS depressants
• Do not discontinue abruptly after long-term use
• Wear sunscreen or large hat to prevent photosensitivity
• Increase fluids, bulk in diet if constipation occurs
• Use gum, hard sugarless candy, or frequent sips of water for dry mouth

MONITORING PARAMETERS

• CBC, weight, ECG, mental status (mood, sensorium, affect, suicidal tendencies)
• Determination of nortriptyline plasma concentrations is not routinely recommended but may be useful in identifying toxicity, drug interactions, or noncompliance (adjustments in dosage should be made according to clinical response not plasma concentrations), therapeutic range 50-150 ng/ml

---

nystatin

(nye-stat'in)

Bio-Statin, Mycostatin, Nadostine, ✦ Nilstat, Nystat-Rx, Nystex

Chemical Class: Amphoteric polyene macrolide
Therapeutic Class: Antifungal

CLINICAL PHARMACOLOGY

Mechanism of Action: Binds to sterols in the fungal cell membrane which results in loss of potassium and other cellular constituents

Pharmacokinetics

PO: Poorly absorbed, excreted almost entirely in feces as unchanged drug

TOP: Not absorbed from intact skin or mucous membranes

INDICATIONS AND USES: Cutaneous, mucocutaneous, and oral cavity candidal infections; candidal vulvovaginitis; intestinal candidiasis

DOSAGE

Adult

- *Oral candidiasis:* PO 400,000-600,000 U susp, swish and swallow qid; Troche 200,000-400,000 U 4-5 times/d
- *Cutaneous candidal infections:* TOP apply tid-qid
- *Intestinal candidal infections:* PO 500,000-1,000,000 U q8h
- *Vaginal candidal infections:* Insert 1-2 vaginal tablets qhs for 2 wk

Child

- *Oral candidiasis:* PO 200,000 U qid or 100,000 U to each side of mouth qid
- *Cutaneous candidal infections:* TOP apply tid-qid
- *Vaginal candidal infections:* Insert 1-2 vaginal tablets qhs for 2 wk

Neonate

- *Oral candidiasis:* PO 100,000 U qid or 50,000 U to each side of mouth qid

$ AVAILABLE FORMS/COST OF THERAPY

- Cre—Top: 100,000 U/g 15, 30 g: **$1.46-$21.80**
- Oint—Top: 100,000 U/g, 15, 30 g: **$1.46-$20.86**
- Susp—Oral: 100,000 U/ml, 60 ml: **$3.29-$21.84**
- Tab, Plain Coated—Oral: 500,000 U 100's: **$11.93-$55.31;**
- Cap, Gel—Oral: 1,000,000 U 100's: **$42.00;** 300,000 U 100's: **$12.95;** 500,000 U 100's: **$28.80**
- Lozenge—Oral: 200,000 U 30's: **$30.19**
- Tab, Uncoated—Vag: 100,000 U 30's: **$14.85-$21.56**
- Powder—Top: 100,000 U/g; 15, 60 g: **$12.00-$22.30**

CONTRAINDICATIONS: Hypersensitivity

PREGNANCY AND LACTATION: Pregnancy category B; due to poor bioavailability serum and breast milk levels do not occur

SIDE EFFECTS/ADVERSE REACTIONS

GI: Nausea, vomiting, GI distress, diarrhea

SKIN: Rash, urticaria, stinging, burning

SPECIAL CONSIDERATIONS

PATIENT/FAMILY EDUCATION

- Complete full course of therapy; do not use troches in child <5 yr

---

octreotide

(ok-tree'oh-tide)

Sandostatin

Chemical Class: Octapeptide

Therapeutic Class: Long-acting somatostatin analog

CLINICAL PHARMACOLOGY

Mechanism of Action: Actions similar to somatostatin; inhibits growth hormone, glucagon, and insulin more than somatostatin; suppresses LH response to GnRH; decreases splanchnic blood flow; inhibits release of serotonin, gastrin, vasoactive intestinal peptide (VIP), insulin, glucagon, secretin, motilin, and pancreatic polypeptide

Pharmacokinetics

SC: Onset 0.4 hr, duration 12 hr; IV and SC doses bioequivalent; 65% protein bound; elimination t½ 1.7 hr; metabolized by liver, 32% of dose excreted unchanged in urine; in dialysis patients, clearance is half of normals

INDICATIONS AND USES: Acromegaly, carcinoid syndrome (associated with metastatic carcinoid tumors), vasoactive intestinal peptide tumors (VIPomas), insulinoma,* HIV-associated secretory diarrhea,* cryptosporidiosis in HIV-infected persons,* control of bleeding esophageal varices*

DOSAGE

Adult

- *Acromegaly:* SC or IV 0.05-0.1 mg tid
- *Carcinoid syndrome:* SC or IV 0.1-0.6 mg qd in 2-4 divided doses (mean daily dosage is 0.3 mg; max daily dose 1.5 mg)
- *VIPomas:* SC or IV 0.2-0.3 mg qd in 2-4 divided doses (range 0.15-0.75 mg)
- *HIV-associated diarrhea:* SC or IV 0.15-1.8 mg qd in 2-4 divided doses
- *Bleeding esophageal varices:* IV 0.05-0.1 mg bolus then 0.025-0.05 mg/hr continuous inf; 0.1 mg q8h as adjunct to sclerotherapy

Child

- SC 0.001-0.01 mg/kg qd in 2-4 divided doses
- For IV use, may be diluted in 50-200 ml of D_5NS and given IV over 15-30 min or given by IV push over 3 min

$ **AVAILABLE FORMS/COST OF THERAPY**

- Inj, Sol—IV: 0.2 mg/ml, 5 ml: **$90.54;** 1 mg/ml, 5 ml: **$445.86**
- Inj, Sol—SC: 0.05 mg/ml, 1 ml × 50: **$227.40;** 0.1 mg/ml, 1 ml × 50: **$416.58;** 0.5 mg/ml, 1 ml × 50: **$1906.26**

CONTRAINDICATIONS: Hypersensitivity

PRECAUTIONS: Gall bladder disease (stones or sludge in 48% of patients treated for 12 mo; in 2% of patients treated for 1 mo), may affect glycemic control in diabetics

PREGNANCY AND LACTATION: Pregnancy category B; breast milk excretion unknown

SIDE EFFECTS/ADVERSE REACTIONS

CNS: Dizziness, fatigue, headache, weakness

CV: ***Bradycardia*****,** ***conduction abnormalities***

GI: Abdominal discomfort, *constipation,* diarrhea, distension, flatulence, nausea, pancreatitis, vomiting

HEME: Vitamin B_{12} deficiency

METAB: Goiter, ***hyperglycemia, hypoglycemia,*** *hypothyroidism*

MS: Bell's palsy, leg cramps

SKIN: Alopecia

MISC: Local pain on inj

▼ **DRUG INTERACTIONS**

Drugs

- *Cyclosporine:* Octreotide reduces absorption

SPECIAL CONSIDERATIONS:

MONITORING PARAMETERS

- Thyroid function, serum glucose (especially in drug treated diabetics)
- Heart rate (especially in persons taking beta blockers and calcium channel blockers)

ofloxacin

(o-flox'a-sin)

Floxin, Ocuflox

Chemical Class: Fluoroquinolone

Therapeutic Class: Antibiotic

CLINICAL PHARMACOLOGY

Mechanism of Action: Interferes with the enzyme DNA gyrase needed for the synthesis of bacterial DNA; bactericidal

Pharmacokinetics

PO: Peak 1-2 hr, 32% bound to plasma proteins, excreted primarily unchanged in urine $t_{1/2}$ 5-10 hr

INDICATIONS AND USES: Lower respiratory tract infections, uncomplicated urethral and cervical gonorrhea, nongonococcal urethritis/cervicitis, skin and skin structure infections, UTIs, prostatitis; superficial ocular infections involving the conjunctiva or cornea (ophthalmic preparation)

Antibacterial spectrum usually includes:

• Gram-positive organisms: *Staphylococcus aureus, S. epidermidis, S. saprophyticus, Enterococcus faecalis*

• Gram-negative organisms: *Acinetobacter* sp, *Aeromonas* sp, *Campylobacter* sp, *Citrobacter* sp, *Enterobacter* sp, *Escherichia coli, Haemophilus influenzae, H. parainfluenzae, Klebsiella pneumoniae, Klebsiella* sp, *Legionella* sp, *Listeria monocytogenes, Moraxella catarrhalis, Morganella morganii, Neisseria gonorrhoeae, N. meningitidis, Plesiomonas shigelloides, Proteus mirabilis, P. vulgaris, Providencia rettgeri, P. stuartii, Pseudomonas aeruginosa, P. fluorescens, Salmonella* sp, *Serratia* sp, *Shigella* sp, *Vibro* sp, *Xanthomonas maltophilia, Yersinia enterocolitica*

DOSAGE

Adult

• *Lower respiratory tract infection:* PO/IV 400 mg q12h for 10 days

• *Uncomplicated gonorrhea:* PO 400 mg as a single dose plus doxycycline 100 mg bid for 7 days

• *Nongonococcal urethritis/cervicitis:* PO/IV 300 mg q12h for 7 days

• *Skin and skin structure infections:* PO/IV 400 mg q12h for 10 days

• *UTI:* PO/IV 200 mg q12h for 3-10 days

• *Prostatitis:* PO/IV 300 mg q12h for 6 wk (do not continue IV therapy for >10 days, switch to PO)

• *Renal function impairment:* CrCl 10-50 ml/min use 24 hr dosage interval; CrCl <10 ml/min, 50% of recommended dose given q24h

• *Superficial ocular infections:* OPHTH 1 gtt q2-4h for first 2 days, then qid for additional 5 days

Child >1 yr

• *Superficial ocular infections:* OPHTH 1 gtt q2-4h for first 2 days, then qid for additional 5 days

$ AVAILABLE FORMS/COST OF THERAPY

• Inj, Sol—IV: 4 mg/ml, 50 ml: **$13.80;** 20 mg/ml, 20 ml: **$26.40;** 40 mg/ml, 10 ml: **$26.40**

• Sol—Ophth: 0.3%, 5 ml: **$18.28**

• Tab, Plain Coated—Oral: 200, 300, 400 mg, 100's: **$307.81-$383.71**

CONTRAINDICATIONS: Hypersensitivity to quinolones

PRECAUTIONS: Children (potential for arthropathy and osteochondrosis), elderly, renal disease, seizure disorders

PREGNANCY AND LACTATION: Pregnancy category C; excreted into breast milk in quantities approximating maternal plasma concentrations, due to the potential for arthropathy and osteochondrosis, use extreme caution in nursing mothers

SIDE EFFECTS/ADVERSE REACTIONS

CNS: Dizziness, headache, fatigue, somnolence, depression, insomnia, anxiety, seizures

EENT: Visual disturbances, dizziness

GI: Diarrhea, *nausea,* vomiting, anorexia, flatulence, heartburn, abdominal pain, dry mouth, increased AST, ALT, pseudomembranous colitis

SKIN: Rash, pruritus, photosensitivity

▼ DRUG INTERACTIONS

Drugs

• *Antacids, didanosine, sucralfate food:* Reduced serum ofloxacin concentrations

O

SPECIAL CONSIDERATIONS

PATIENT/FAMILY EDUCATION

- Administer on an empty stomach (1 hr before or 2 hr after meals)
- Drink fluids liberally
- Do not take antacids containing magnesium or aluminum or products containing iron or zinc within 4 hr before or 2 hr after dosing
- Observe caution while driving or performing other tasks requiring alertness
- Avoid excessive exposure to sunlight

---

olsalazine

(ohl-sal'ah-zeen)

Dipentum

Chemical Class: Salicylate derivative

Therapeutic Class: GI antiinflammatory

CLINICAL PHARMACOLOGY

Mechanism of Action: Bioconverted by colonic bacteria to 5-aminosalicylic acid (mesalamine) which may act by blocking cyclooxygenase and inhibiting prostaglandin production in the colon; appears to produce a local inhibitory effect on the mucousal production of arachidonic acid metabolites, which are increased in patients with chronic inflammatory bowel disease

Pharmacokinetics

PO: Limited systemic bioavailability (2.4% of 1 g dose absorbed), peak 1 hr, >99% bound to plasma proteins, <1% recovered in urine, serum $t_{1/2}$ 0.9 hr

INDICATIONS AND USES: Maintenance of remission of ulcerative colitis in patients intolerant of sulfasalazine

DOSAGE

Adult

- PO 1 g/d in 2 evenly divided doses

$ AVAILABLE FORMS/COST OF THERAPY

- Cap, Gel—Oral: 250 mg, 100's: **$61.88**

CONTRAINDICATIONS: Hypersensitivity to salicylates

PRECAUTIONS: Children, pre-existing renal disease

PREGNANCY AND LACTATION: Pregnancy category C; mesalamine has produced adverse effects in a nursing infant and should be used with caution during breast feeding, observe nursing infant closely for changes in stool consistency

SIDE EFFECTS/ADVERSE REACTIONS

CNS: Headache, drowsiness, depression

GI: Diarrhea, cramping, nausea, dyspepsia, bloating, anorexia, vomiting, stomatitis

MS: Arthralgia

SKIN: Rash, itching

SPECIAL CONSIDERATIONS

PATIENT/FAMILY EDUCATION

- Take with food. Notify physician if diarrhea occurs

MONITORING PARAMETERS

- BUN, urinalysis, serum creatinine in patients with pre-existing renal disease

---

omeprazole

(om-eh-pray'zole)

Prilosec

Chemical Class: Substituted benzimidazole

Therapeutic Class: Gastric acid secretion inhibitor

CLINICAL PHARMACOLOGY

Mechanism of Action: Irreversibly inactivates proton pump in gastric parietal cells which blocks the final step in secretion of hydrochloric acid; acid secretion is inhibited until additional enzyme is synthesized; inhibits basal and stimulated gastric acid secretion

Pharmacokinetics

PO: Peak 0.5-3½ hr, 95% bound to plasma proteins, metabolized in liver to inactivate metabolites, excreted in urine (77%) and feces (23%), $t_{1/2}$ ½-1 hr

INDICATIONS AND USES: Active duodenal ulcer, gastroesophageal reflux disease (GERD), pathological hypersecretory conditions (e.g. Zollinger-Ellison syndrome, multiple endocrine adenomas, systemic mastocytosis), gastric ulcer,* NSAID induced gastric ulcer*

DOSAGE

Adult

- *Active duodenal ulcer:* PO 20 mg qd for 4-8 wk
- *GERD:* PO 20 mg qd for 4-8 wk
- *Pathological hypersecretory conditions:* PO 60 mg qd initially, doses up to 120 mg tid have been administered (administer doses >80 mg/d in divided doses)

$ AVAILABLE FORMS/COST OF THERAPY

- Cap, Gel, Sust Action—Oral: 20 mg, 30's: **$108.90**

CONTRAINDICATIONS: Hypersensitivity

PRECAUTIONS: Not for maintenance therapy of duodenal ulcer or GERD; elderly; children; symptomatic response does not preclude gastric malignancy

PREGNANCY AND LACTATION: Pregnancy category C; suppression of gastric acid secretion is potential effect in nursing infant, clinical significance unnown

SIDE EFFECTS/ADVERSE REACTIONS

CNS: Headache, dizziness, asthenia

GI: Diarrhea, abdominal pain, nausea, constipation, flatulence

MS: Back pain

RESP: Cough

SKIN: Rash

▼ DRUG INTERACTIONS

Drugs

- *Methotrexate:* Case report of elevated methotrexate concentration
- *Phenytoin:* Increased phenytoin concentration

SPECIAL CONSIDERATIONS

PATIENT/FAMILY EDUCATION

- Take before eating
- Swallow capsule whole, do not open, chew, or crush

---

ondansetron

(on-dan-seh'tron)

Zofran

Chemical Class: Carbazole derivative

Therapeutic Class: Antiemetic

CLINICAL PHARMACOLOGY

Mechanism of Action: Selectively blocks the action of serotonin at $5\text{-}HT_3$ receptors; cytotoxic chemotherapy appears to be associated with release of serotonin from enterochromaffin cells of the small intestine which may stimulate vagal afferents through $5\text{-}HT_3$ receptors initiating the vomiting reflex

Pharmacokinetics

IV: Peak immediate

PO: Peak 1.7-2 hr, bioavailability 56%

70%-76% bound to plasma proteins, extensively metabolized, excreted in urine and feces (metabolites), $t_{1/2}$ 4 hr (2-3 hr in children <15 yr)

INDICATIONS AND USES: Prevention of nausea and vomiting associated with emetogenic cancer chemotherapy, total body irradiation,

O

and postoperative nausea and vomiting

DOSAGE

Adult

- PO 8 mg 30 min before chemotherapy; repeat 4 and 8 hr after initial dose; IV 0.15 mg/kg/dose infused 30 min before start of chemotherapy; repeat 4 and 8 hr after initial dose; or single 32 mg dose beginning 30 min before chemotherapy

Child

- PO 4 mg 30 min before chemotherapy; repeat 4 and 8 hr after initial dose; IV 0.15 mg/kg/dose infused 30 min before start of chemotherapy; repeat 4 and 8 hr after initial dose

$ AVAILABLE FORMS/COST OF THERAPY

- Inj, Sol—IV: 2 mg/ml, 20 ml: **$233.02;** 32 mg/50 ml, 50 ml: **$196.76**
- Tab Coated—Oral: 4 mg, 3's: **$33.67;** 8 mg, 3's: **$56.11**

CONTRAINDICATIONS: Hypersensitivity

PRECAUTIONS: Abdominal surgery (may mask ileus or gastric distension), children ≤3 yr

PREGNANCY AND LACTATION: Pregnancy category B; has been used in the treatment of hyperemesis gravidarum

SIDE EFFECTS/ADVERSE REACTIONS

CNS: Lightheadedness, ***seizures,*** headache

CV: Tachycardia, bradycardia, angina, syncope

EENT: Blurred vision

GI: Diarrhea, constipation, transient elevation in liver enzymes

METAB: Hypokalemia

RESP: ***Bronchospasm***

SKIN: Rash

opium

(oh'pee-um)

Opium Tincture Deodorized, Pantopon

Chemical Class: Mixture of several alkaloids including morphine, codeine, and papaverine

Therapeutic Class: Narcotic analgesic; antidiarrheal

DEA Class: Schedule II (tincture, inj)

CLINICAL PHARMACOLOGY

Mechanism of Action: Increases smooth muscle tone of GI tract, inhibits GI motility and propulsion, diminishes digestive secretions; binds to opiate receptors in the CNS causing inhibition of ascending pain pathways, altering the perception of and response to pain

Pharmacokinetics

Variably absorbed from GI tract, metabolized in liver, excreted in urine

INDICATIONS AND USES: Symptomatic treatment of diarrhea; relief of severe pain in place of morphine

DOSAGE

Adult

- IM/SC 5-20 mg q4-5h; PO (tincture) 0.6 ml qid

Child

- PO (tincture) for diarrhea 0.005-0.01 ml/kg/dose q3-4h; for analgesia 0.01-0.02 ml/kg/dose q3-4h

$ AVAILABLE FORMS/COST OF THERAPY

- Inj, Sol—IM; SC: 20 mg/ml, 1 ml: **$3.41**
- Tincture—Oral: 10%, 120 ml: **$42.10**

CONTRAINDICATIONS: Hypersensitivity, acute bronchial asthma, upper airway obstruction

PRECAUTIONS: Head injury, increased intracranial pressure, acute abdominal conditions, elderly, severe impairment of hepatic or renal function, hypothyroidism, Addison's disease, prostatic hypertrophy, urethral stricture, history of drug abuse

PREGNANCY AND LACTATION: Pregnancy category B (category D if used for prolonged periods or in high doses at term); compatible with breast feeding

SIDE EFFECTS/ADVERSE REACTIONS

CNS: Drowsiness, sedation, dizziness, agitation, dependency, lethargy, restlessness

CV: Bradycardia, palpitations, orthostatic hypotension, tachycardia

GI: Nausea, vomiting, anorexia, constipation

GU: Urinary retention

RESP: ***Respiratory depression, respiratory paralysis***

SKIN: Flushing, rash, urticaria

▼ **DRUG INTERACTIONS**

Drugs

- *Barbiturates:* Additive CNS depression
- *Cimetidine:* Increased effect of narcotic analgesics
- *Ethanol:* Additive CNS effects
- *Neuroleptics:* Hypotension and excessive CNS depression

SPECIAL CONSIDERATIONS

PATIENT/FAMILY EDUCATION

- Avoid alcohol
- May cause drowsiness, impair judgment or coordination
- Drug may be addicting if used for prolonged periods

oral contraceptives

Monophasic: Genora 1/50, Nelova 1/50M, Norethin 1/50M, Norinyl 1+50, Ortho-Novum 1/50, Ovcon-50, Demulen 1/50, Ovral, Genora 1/35, N.E.E. 1/35, Nelova 1/35E, Norethin 1/35E, Norinyl 1+35, Ortho-Novum 1/35, Brevicon, Genora 0.5/35, Modicon, Nelova 0.5/35E, Ovcon-35, Ortho-Cyclen, Demulen 1/35, Loestrin Fe 1.5/30, Lo/Ovral, Desogen, Ortho-Cept, Levlen, Levora, Nordette, Loestrin Fe 1/20; Biphasic: Jenest-28, Nelova 10/11, Ortho-Novum 10/11; Triphasic: Tri-Norinyl, Ortho-Novum 7/7/7, Tri-Levlen, Triphasil, Ortho Tri-Cyclen

Chemical Class: Synthetic estrogen/progestin combinations

Therapeutic Class: Contraceptives

CLINICAL PHARMACOLOGY

Mechanism of Action: Inhibit ovulation by suppressing the gonadotropins, FSH and LH; alter cervical mucus (inhibiting sperm penetration) and endometrium (reducing likelihood of implantation)

Pharmacokinetics

- *Estrogens*

PO: Ethinyl estradiol (EE) peak 1-2 hr; mestranol demethylated to ethinyl estradiol; 98% bound to plasma proteins; metabolized in liver; excreted in urine and bile; undergoes some enterohepatic recirculation; $t_{1/2}$ 6-20 hr

- *Progestins*

PO: Bound both to albumin (79%-95%) and sex hormone binding globulin; metabolized in liver, excreted in urine and bile, $t_{1/2}$ norethindrone 5-14 hr, levonorgestrel 11-45 hr, desogestrel metabolite 38±20 hr, norgestimate metabolite 12-30 hr

INDICATIONS AND USES: Prevention of pregnancy; postcoital contraception or "morning after" pill (Ovral);* dysmenorrhea;* dysfunctional uterine bleeding,* endometriosis*

DOSAGE

Adult and Adolescent

• *21-day regimen:* PO 1 tab qd for 21 days beginning (a) first Sunday after menstruation begins or (b) day 5 of cycle, or (c) day 1 of cycle (consult instructions on dispensers or packs); no tabs are taken for next 7 days (withdrawal flow will normally occur about 3 days following last tab)

• *28-day regimen:* PO 1 tab qd for 28 days continuously beginning (a) first Sunday after menstruation begins, or (b) day 5 of cycle, or (c) day 1 of cycle (consult instructions on dispensers or packs); start new pack of tabs after completing 28-day course

$ **AVAILABLE FORMS/COST OF THERAPY**

• Tab, Uncoated—Oral: 35μg EE/1 mg ethynodiol diacetate, 28's: **$24.46** (Demulen 1/35); 50 μg/1 mg, 28's: **$27.76** (Demulen 1/50)

• Tab, Uncoated—Oral: 0.03 mg EE/ 0.15 mg levonorestrel, 28's: **$20.39-$25.60** (Levora, Nordette, Levlen); 0.03 mg/0.05, 0.075, 0.125 mg, 28's: **$19.73-$25.32** (Tri-Levlen, Triphasil)

• Tab, Uncoated—Oral: 0.035 mg EE/0.5, 1 mg norethindrone, 28's: **$13.97-$25.52** (Nelova 10/11, Ortho-Novum 10/11, Jenest-28); 0.035 mg/0.5 mg, 28's: **$10.71-$25.52** (Nelova 0.5/35E, Brevicon, Modicon, Genora 0.5/35); 0.035 mg/ 1mg, 28's: **$10.72-$23.27** (Norinyl 1+35, Genora 1/35, Nelova 1/35E, Ortho-Novum 1/35, N.E.E. 1/35, Norethin 1/35E); 0.035 mg/0.4 mg, 28's: **$24.61** (Ovcon-35); 0.05 mg/1 mg, 28's: **$27.17** (Ovcon-50); 0.05 mg/2.5 mg, 21's: **$23.92** (Norlestrin 2.5/50); 0.035 mg/0.5, 1, 0.5 mg, 28's: **$21.59** (Tri-Norinyl); 0.035 mg/0.5, 0.75, 1 mg, 28's: **$23.41** (Ortho-Novum 7/7/7)

• Tab, Uncoated—Oral: 0.02 mg EE/1 mg norethindrone acetate, 28's: **$25.24** (Loestrin Fe 1/20); 0.03 mg/ 1.5 mg, 28's: **$25.24** (Loestrin Fe 1.5/30)

• Tab, Uncoated—Oral: 0.03 mg EE/ 0.3 mg norgestrel, 28's: **$26.52** (Lo/ Ovral; 0.05 mg/0.5 mg, 28's: **$40.60** (Ovral)

• Tab, Uncoated—Oral: 0.035 mg EE/0.25 mg norgestimate, 28's: **$23.41** (Ortho-Cyclen); 0.035 mg/ 0.18, 0.215, 0.25 mg, 28's: **$23.41** (Ortho Tri-Cyclen)

• Tab, Uncoated—Oral: 0.03 mg EE/ 0.15 mg desogestrel, 28's: **$19.55-$23.41** (Desogen, Ortho-Cept)

• Tab, Uncoated—Oral: 0.05 mg mestranol/1 mg norethindrone, 28's: **$10.72-$23.27** (Genora 1/50, Nelova 1/50M, Norethin 1/50M, Ortho-Novum 1/50, Norinyl 1+50)

CONTRAINDICATIONS: Thrombophlebitis, thromboembolic disorders, history of deep-vein thrombophlebitis, cerebrovascular disease, MI, CAD, known or suspected breast carcinoma or estrogen-dependent neoplasia, carcinoma of endometrium, hepatic adenomas/carcinomas, past or present angina pectoris, undiagnosed abnormal vaginal bleeding, cholestatic jaundice

PRECAUTIONS: Depression, hypertension, renal disease, seizure disorder, lupus erythematosus, rheumatic disease, migraine headache, amenorrhea, irregular menses, fibrocystic breast disease, gallbladder disease, diabetes mellitus, cigarette smoking (especially if age >35

yr), sickle cell disease, hyperlipidemia

PREGNANCY AND LACTATION: Pregnancy category X; may shorten duration of lactation, decrease milk production, and decrease composition of nitrogen and protein content of milk; these changes may be of nutritional importance in malnourished mothers, otherwise compatible with breast feeding

SIDE EFFECTS/ADVERSE REACTIONS

CNS: Migraine headache, mental depression

CV: Edema, ***thrombophlebitis, venous thrombosis, pulmonary embolism, coronary thrombosis, MI, cerebral thrombosis, arterial thromboembolism, cerebral hemorrhage,*** hypertension

EENT: Contact lens intolerance, ***retinal thrombosis,*** optic neuritis

GI: Nausea, vomiting, abdominal cramps, bloating, ***cholestatic jaundice, gallbladder disease, hepatic adenomas or benign liver tumors, hepatocellular carcinoma, mesenteric thrombosis***

GU: Breakthrough bleeding, spotting, change in menstrual flow, amenorrhea, change in cervical secretions, cervical cancer, vaginal candidiasis

METAB: Decreased carbohydrate tolerance

SKIN: Melasma, rash

MISC: Weight change, breast tenderness, breast enlargement

▼ DRUG INTERACTIONS

Drugs

- *Barbiturates, carbamazepine, griseofulvin, phenytoin, penicillins, rifampin, tetracyclines:* Reduced efficacy of oral contraceptives
- *Chlordiazepoxide, diazepam, triazolam:* Increased benzodiazepine concentrations
- *Corticosteroids:* Enhanced effect of corticosteroids
- *Cyclosporine:* Elevated cyclosporine concentrations
- *Smoking+:* Increased risk of oral contraceptive-induced adverse cardiovascular events

Labs

- *Increase:* Sulfobromophthalein retention, prothrombin, factors VII, VIII, IX, X, thyroid binding globulin, transcorin, triglycerides, ceruloplasmin, aldosterone, amylase, γ-glutamyltranspeptidase, iron binding capacity, transferrin, prolactin, renin activity, vitamin A
- *Decrease:* Antithrombin III, free T_3 resin uptake, response to metyrapone test, folate, glucose tolerance, albumin, cholinesterase, haptoglobin, zinc, vitamin B_{12}

SPECIAL CONSIDERATIONS

PATIENT/FAMILY EDUCATION

- Take at same time each day. Take with food
- Notify physician if breakthrough bleeding/spotting lasts more than a few days or occurs in >1 cycle
- Use additional methods of birth control until after the first week of administration in the initial cycle or for entire cycle if diarrhea or vomiting occurs
- Does not protect against STDs
- Notify physician immediately of severe headache, chest pain, abdominal pain, eye pain or blurred vision, calf pain

MONITORING PARAMETERS

- Blood pressure, Pap smear, fasting lipid panel, fasting glucose

orphenadrine

(or-fen'a-dreen)

Banflex, Flexoject, Flexon, Marflex, Myolin, Myotrol, Neocyten, Norflex, O-Flex, Orphenate

Chemical Class: Tertiary amine antimuscarinic

Therapeutic Class: Skeletal muscle relaxant

CLINICAL PHARMACOLOGY

Mechanism of Action: Mechanism of action unknown but may be due to central action at brain stem; does not directly relax tense skeletal muscle; possesses anticholinergic actions

Pharmacokinetics

PO: Peak 2 hr, duration 4-6 hr, metabolized to 8 known metabolites, excreted in urine and feces, $t_{1/2}$ 14 hr

INDICATIONS AND USES: Painful acute musculoskeletal conditions, quinine-resistant leg cramps*

DOSAGE

Adult

• PO 100 mg bid; IM/IV 60 mg, may repeat q12h prn

$ AVAILABLE FORMS/COST OF THERAPY

• Inj, Sol—IM; IV: 30 mg/ml, 10 ml: **$6.25-$22.65**

• Tab, Plain Coated, Sust Action—Oral: 100 mg, 100's: **$149.94**

CONTRAINDICATIONS: Hypersensitivity, glaucoma, pyloric or duodenal obstruction, stenosing peptic ulcer, prostatic hypertrophy, obstruction of bladder neck, cardiospasm, myasthenia gravis

PRECAUTIONS: Children, cardiac decompensation, coronary insufficiency, cardiac dysrhythmia, tachycardia, sulfite sensitivity

PREGNANCY AND LACTATION: Pregnancy category C

SIDE EFFECTS/ADVERSE REACTIONS

CNS: Weakness, headache, *dizziness, lightheadedness,* confusion, hallucinations, agitation, tremor, *drowsiness*

CV: ***Tachycardia,*** palpitation, transient syncope

EENT: Blurred vision, pupil dilation, increased ocular tension

GI: Nausea, vomiting, *constipation,* gastric irritation, *dry mouth*

GU: Urinary hesitancy, urinary retention

HEME: ***Aplastic anemia*** (rare)

SKIN: Urticaria and other dermatoses

▼ DRUG INTERACTIONS

Drugs

• *Neuroleptics:* Lower serum neuroleptic concentrations, excessive anticholinergic effects

SPECIAL CONSIDERATIONS

PATIENT/FAMILY EDUCATION

• May cause drowsiness

• Use caution driving or performing other tasks requiring alertness

• Avoid alcohol

• Notify physician of difficult urination, fainting, rapid heart rate, palpitation, mental confusion

oxacillin

(ox-a-sill'in)

Bactrocill, Prostaphlin

Chemical Class: Semisynthetic penicillinase-resistant penicillin

Therapeutic Class: Antibiotic

CLINICAL PHARMACOLOGY

Mechanism of Action: Inhibits the biosynthesis of cell wall mucopeptide in susceptible organisms; the cell wall, rendered osmotically unstable, swells and bursts from osmotic pressure; bacterocidal when adequate concentrations are reached;

resistant to inactivation by most staphylococcal penicillinases

Pharmacokinetics

PO: Peak 0.5-2 hr, duration 4-6 hr

IM: Peak 30 min, duration 4-6 hr

89%-94% bound to plasma proteins, partially metabolized to active and inactive metabolites, rapidly excreted in urine, $t_{1/2}$ 0.3-0.8 hr

INDICATIONS AND USES: Infections of the upper and lower respiratory tract, skin and skin structures, bones and joints, urinary tract, meningitis, septicemia, and endocarditis caused by penicillinase-producing staphylococci; perioperative prophylaxis*

Antibacterial spectrum usually includes:

- Gram positive organisms: penicillinase-producing and nonpenicillinase-producing strains of *Staphylococus aureus, S. epidermidis, S. saprophyticus,* groups A, B, C, and G streptococci, *Streptococcus pneumoniae,* some viridans streptococci, *Bacillus anthracis*

DOSAGE

Adult

- PO 500-1000 mg q4-6h; IM/IV 250-1000 mg q4-6h; max 12 g/d

Child

- PO/IM/IV 50-100 mg/kg/d divided q4-6h; max 300 mg/kg/d

$ AVAILABLE FORMS/COST OF THERAPY

- Powder, Reconst—Oral: 250 mg/5 ml, 100 ml: **$5.25-$14.58**
- Cap, Gel—Oral: 250 mg, 100's: **$21.75-$30.50;** 500 mg, 100's: **$41.93-$57.05**
- Inj, Dry-Sol—IM; IV: 1 g/vial, 1 g: **$3.82-$11.50;** 2 g/vial, 2 g: **$6.29-$8.67;** 4 g, 1's: **$41.13**

CONTRAINDICATIONS: Hypersensitivity to penicillins

PRECAUTIONS: Hypersensitivity to cephalosporins, renal insufficiency, prolonged or repeated therapy, neonates

PREGNANCY AND LACTATION: Pregnancy category B; potential exists for modification of bowel flora in nursing infant, allergy/sensitization, and interference with interpretation of culture results if fever workup required

SIDE EFFECTS/ADVERSE REACTIONS

CNS: Headache, fever, chills

CV: Phlebitis, thrombophlebitis

GI: Increased AST, ALT

GU: ***Intersitial nephritis, nephropathy, hemorrhagic cystitis***

HEME: ***Eosinophilia, hemolytic anemia, neutropenia, leukopenia, granulocytopenia thrombocytopenia,*** positive Coombs' test

MS: Myalgia

RESP: ***Anaphylaxis***

SKIN: Pain at inj site, sterile abscess at inj site, rash, pruritus

MISC: Serum sickness-like reactions

▼ DRUG INTERACTIONS

Drugs

- *Chloramphenicol:* Inhibited antibacterial activity of oxacillin, ensure adequate amounts of both agents are given and administer oxacillin a few hours before chloramphenicol
- *Methotrexate:* Increased serum methotrexate concentrations
- *Oral contraceptives:* Occasional impairment of oral contraceptive efficacy, consider use of supplementary contraception during cycles in which oxacillin is used
- *Tetracyclines:* Inhibited antibacterial activity of oxacillin, ensure adequate amounts of both agents are given and administer oxacillin a few hours before tetracycline

Labs

- *False positive:* Urine glucose, urine protein

O

SPECIAL CONSIDERATIONS

• Sodium content of 1 g = 2.8-3.1 mEq

PATIENT/FAMILY EDUCATION

• Complete entire course of medication
• Administer on an empty stomach (1 hr before or 2 hr after meals)
• Administer at even intervals
• Report sore throat, fever, fatigue, excessive diarrhea, skin rash, itching, hives, shortness of breath, wheezing
• Shake oral suspensions well before administering, discard after 14 days

MONITORING PARAMETERS

• Urinalysis, BUN, serum creatinine, CBC with differential, periodic liver function tests

---

oxamniquine

(ox-am′ni-kwin)

Vansil

Chemical Class: Tetrahydroquinoline derivative
Therapeutic Class: Anthelmintic

CLINICAL PHARMACOLOGY

Mechanism of Action: Dislodges schistosomes from usual site of residence in mesenteric veins to liver where they are retained and subsequently killed by host tissue reactions; causes contraction and paralysis of musculature and subsequent immobilization of the worm's suckers; laying of eggs by females ceases within 24-48 hr substantially reducing egg load and eliminating principal cause of pathology associated with schistosomal infection

Pharmacokinetics

PO: Peak 1-1½ hr, extensively metabolized to inactive metabolites, excreted in urine, $t_{1/2}$ 1-2½ hr

INDICATIONS AND USES: All stages of *Schistosoma mansoni* infection, single dose treatment of neurocysticercosis (in combination with praziquantel)*

DOSAGE

Adult

• PO 12-15 mg/kg as a single dose (Western Hemisphere strains of *Schistosoma mansoni*); 30-60 mg/kg given in 2-4 equally divided doses of 15 mg/kg bid for 1-2 days (African and Middle Eastern strains of *Schistosoma mansoni*)

Child (<30 kg)

• PO 20 mg/kg given in 2 divided doses of 10 mg/kg with 2-8 hr between doses

$ AVAILABLE FORMS/COST OF THERAPY

• Cap, Gel—Oral: 250 mg, 24's: **$122.53**

CONTRAINDICATIONS: Hypersensitivity

PRECAUTIONS: Seizure disorder

PREGNANCY AND LACTATION: Pregnancy category C

SIDE EFFECTS/ADVERSE REACTIONS

CNS: Dizziness, drowsiness, headache, ***convulsions*** (rare)
GI: Nausea, vomiting, abdominal pain, anorexia, mild to moderate liver enzyme elevations
GU: Orange-red discoloration of urine
SKIN: Urticaria

▼ DRUG INTERACTIONS

Labs

• *Interference:* Urinalysis based on spectrometry or color reactions

SPECIAL CONSIDERATIONS

PATIENT/FAMILY EDUCATION

• Take with food
• May cause orange-red discoloration of urine

oxandrolone

(ox-an′droe-lone)

Oxandrin

Chemical Class: Halogenated testosterone derivative

Therapeutic Class: Anabolic steroid

DEA Class: Schedule III

CLINICAL PHARMACOLOGY

Mechanism of Action: Promotes body tissue-building processes and reverses catabolic or tissue-depleting processes when administered with adequate calories and protein to achieve positive nitrogen balance; inhibits endogenous testosterone release

Pharmacokinetics

PO: Metabolized in liver, excreted in urine

INDICATIONS AND USES: Promotion of weight gain following extensive surgery, chronic infection, or severe trauma; protein catabolism associated with prolonged administration of corticosteroids; bone pain associated with osteoporosis; alcololic hepatitis;* short stature associated with Turner syndrome;* HIV wasting syndrome and HIV-associated muscle weakness;* constitutional delay of growth and puberty*

DOSAGE

Adult

• PO 2.5 mg bid-qid for 2-4 wk; repeat intermittently prn; range of effective doses 2.5-20 mg/d

Child

• PO total daily dose is ≤0.1 mg/kg or ≤0.045 mg/lb; repeat intermittently prn

$ AVAILABLE FORMS/COST OF THERAPY

• Tab, Uncoated—Oral: 2.5 mg, 100's: **$375.00**

CONTRAINDICATIONS: Hypersensitivity, male patients with prostate or breast cancer, hypercalcemia in females with breast cancer, nephrosis, nephrotic phase of nephritis, enhancement of physical appearance or athletic performance

PRECAUTIONS: Elderly, children, cardiac disease, renal disease, hepatic disease, seizure disorder, migraine headache, diabetes

PREGNANCY AND LACTATION: Pregnancy category X

SIDE EFFECTS/ADVERSE REACTIONS

CNS: Excitation, insomnia, habituation, depression, choreiform movement

CV: Edema

EENT: Deepening of voice, hoarseness

GI: Nausea, vomiting, diarrhea, ***cholestatic jaundice, hepatic necrosis, hepatocellular neoplasms, peliosis hepatis***

GU: Amenorrhea, vaginitis, decreased breast size, clitoral hypertrophy, testicular atrophy, decreased libido

METAB: Virilization; retention of sodium, chloride, water, potassium, phosphates, calcium; decreased glucose tolerance, increased serum cholesterol, increased LDL cholesterol, decreased HDL cholesterol

MS: Premature closure of epiphyses in children

SKIN: Rash, acne, flushing, sweating, alopecia, hirsutism

▼ DRUG INTERACTIONS

Drugs

• *Antidiabetic agents:* Enhanced hypoglycemic effects

• *Cyclosporine:* Increased cyclosporine concentrations

• *Warfarin+:* Enhanced hypoprothrombinemic response to oral anticoagulants

Labs

• *Increase:* Serum cholesterol, blood glucose, urine glucose

• *Decrease:* Serum Ca, serum K, T_4 T_3, thyroid ^{131}I uptake test, urine 17-OHCS, 17-KS, PBI, BSP

SPECIAL CONSIDERATIONS

PATIENT/FAMILY EDUCATION

• May cause GI upset or nausea

• Notify physician of hoarseness, deepening of voice, male-pattern baldness, hirsutism, menstrual irregularities, acne (women)

• Notify physician of nausea, vomiting, changes in skin color, ankle swelling

• Adequate dietary intake of calories and protein essential for successful treatment

MONITORING PARAMETERS

• Frequent serum and urine calcium (discontinue if hypercalcemia develops)

• Liver function tests

• Growth rate in children

---

oxaprozin

(ox-a-pr'ozin)

Daypro

Chemical Class: Propionic acid derivative

Therapeutic Class: Nonsteroidal antiinflammatory drug (NSAID)

CLINICAL PHARMACOLOGY

Mechanism of Action: Inhibits cyclooxygenase activity and prostaglandin synthesis; other mechanisms such as inhibition of lipoxygenase, leukotriene synthesis, lysosomal enzyme release, neutrophil aggregation and various cell-membrane functions may exist as well

Pharmacokinetics

PO: Peak 3-5 hr, 99.9% bound to plasma proteins, metabolized in liver to inactive metabolites, excreted in urine (65%) and feces (35%), $t_{1/2}$ 42-50 hr

INDICATIONS AND USES: Rheumatoid and osteoarthritis

DOSAGE

Adult

• PO 600-1200 mg qd, individualize dosage to lowest effective dose; max 1800 mg/d or 26 mg/kg/d, whichever is lower

$ **AVAILABLE FORMS/COST OF THERAPY**

• Tab, Uncoated—Oral: 600 mg, 100's: **$121.17**

CONTRAINDICATIONS: Hypersensitivity to NSAIDs or ASA

PRECAUTIONS: Bleeding tendencies, peptic ulcer, renal/hepatic function impairment, elderly, CHF, hypertension, children

PREGNANCY AND LACTATION: Pregnancy category C (category D if used in 3rd trimester); could cause constriction of the ductus arteriosus *in utero,* persistent pulmonary hypertension of the newborn, or prolonged labor

SIDE EFFECTS/ADVERSE REACTIONS

CNS: Dizziness, headache, lightheadedness

CV: ***CHF,*** hypotension, hypertension, palpitation, dysrhythmias, tachycardia, edema, chest pain

EENT: Visual disturbances, photophobia, dry eyes, hearing disturbances, tinnitus

GI: Nausea, vomiting, diarrhea, constipation, abdominal cramps, *dyspepsia,* flatulence, ***gastric or duodenal ulcer with bleeding or perforation,*** occult blood in stool, ***hepatitis,*** pancreatitis

HEME: ***Neutropenia, eosinophilia, leukopenia, pancytopenia, thrombocytopenia, agranulocytosis***

GU: ***Acute renal failure***

METAB: Hyperglycemia, hypoglycemia, hyperkalemia, hyponatremia

RESP: Dyspnea, bronchospasm, pulmonary infiltrates

SKIN: Rash, urticaria, photosensitivity

▼ **DRUG INTERACTIONS**

Drugs

- *ACE inhibitors:* Inhibition of antihypertensive response
- *Beta blockers:* Reduced hypotensive effects of beta blockers
- *Furosemide:* Reduced diuretic and antihypertensive response to furosemide
- *Hydralazine:* Reduced antihypertensive response to hydralazine
- *Lithium:* Increased plasma lithium concentrations, toxicity
- *Methotrexate:* Reduced renal clearance of methotrexate, increased toxicity
- *Oral anticoagulants:* Increased risk of bleeding due to adverse effects on GI mucosa and platelet function
- *Potassium sparing diuretics:* Acute renal failure

Labs

- *Increase:* Bleeding time

SPECIAL CONSIDERATIONS

PATIENT/FAMILY EDUCATION

- Avoid aspirin and alcoholic beverages
- Take with food, milk, or antacids to decrease GI upset
- Notify physician if edema, black stools, or persistent headache occurs

MONITORING PARAMETERS

CBC, BUN, serum creatinine, LFTs, occult blood loss

oxazepam

(ox-a'ze-pam)

Apo-Oxazepam, ✤ Novoxapam, ✤ Ox-Pam, ✤ Serax, Zapex ✤

Chemical Class: Benzodiazepine

Therapeutic Class: Anxiolytic

DEA Class: Schedule IV

CLINICAL PHARMACOLOGY

Mechanism of Action: Facilitates the inhibitory effect of γ-aminobutyric acid (GABA) on neuronal excitability by increasing membrane permeability to chloride ions

Pharmacokinetics

PO: Peak 2-4 hr, onset of action intermediate compared to other benzodiazepines, 86%-96% bound to plasma proteins, metabolized via conjugation to inactive metabolites, excreted in urine as unchanged drug (50%) and metabolites, $t_{1/2}$ 5-15 hr

INDICATIONS AND USES: Anxiety disorders; management of anxiety, tension, agitation, irritability in older patients; alcohol withdrawal; irritable bowel*

DOSAGE

Adult

- PO 10-30 mg tid-qid

$ **AVAILABLE FORMS/COST OF THERAPY**

- Cap, Gel—Oral: 10 mg, 100's: **$6.03-$67.19;** 15 mg, 100's: **$7.50-$84.45;** 30 mg, 100's: **$9.75-$122.15**
- Tab, Uncoated—Oral: 15 mg, 100's: **$27.98-$84.45**

CONTRAINDICATIONS: Hypersensitivity to benzodiazepines, narrow angle glaucoma, psychosis

PRECAUTIONS: Elderly, debilitated, hepatic disease, renal disease, history of drug abuse, abrupt withdrawal, respiratory depression

PREGNANCY AND LACTATION: Pregnancy category D; may cause fetal damage when administered during pregnancy; excreted into breast milk, may accumulate in breast-fed infants and is therefore not recommended

SIDE EFFECTS/ADVERSE REACTIONS

CNS: Somnolence, asthenia, hypokinesia, hangover, abnormal thinking, anxiety, agitation, amnesia, apathy, emotional lability, hostility, seizure, sleep disorder, stupor, twitch, ataxia, decreased libido, decreased reflexes, neuritis

CV: Dysrhythmia, syncope

EENT: Ear pain, eye irritation/pain/swelling, photophobia, pharyngitis, rhinitis, sinusitis, epistaxis

GI: Dyspepsia, decreased/increased appetite, flatulence, gastritis, enterocolitis, melena, mouth ulceration, abdominal pain, increased AST

GU: Frequent urination, menstrual cramps, urinary hesitancy/urgency, vaginal discharge/itching, hematuria, nocturia, oliguria, penile discharge, urinary incontinence

HEME: ***Agranulocytosis***

MS: Lower extremity pain, back pain,

RESP: Cold symptoms, asthma, cough, dyspnea, hyperventilation

SKIN: Urticaria, acne, dry skin, photosensitivity

▼ **DRUG INTERACTIONS**

Drugs

- *Clozapine:* Cardiorespiratory collapse
- *Ethanol:* Enhanced adverse psychomotor effects of benzodiazepines

Labs

- *Increase:* AST/ALT, serum bilirubin
- *False increase:* 17-OHCS
- *Decrease:* RAIU

SPECIAL CONSIDERATIONS

PATIENT/FAMILY EDUCATION

- Avoid alcohol and other CNS depressants
- Do not discontinue abruptly after prolonged therapy
- May cause drowsiness or dizziness
- Use caution while driving or performing other tasks requiring alertness
- Inform physician if planning to become pregnant, pregnant, or becomes pregnant while taking this medicine
- May be habit forming

MONITORING PARAMETERS

- Periodic CBC, U/A, blood chemistry analyses during prolonged therapy

---

oxiconazole

(ox-i-con'a-zole)

Oxistat

Chemical Class: Synthetic imidazole derivative

Therapeutic Class: Antifungal

CLINICAL PHARMACOLOGY

Mechanism of Action: Inhibits fungal ergosterol synthesis, which is needed for cytoplasmic membrane integrity

Pharmacokinetics

TOP: Low systemic absorption

INDICATIONS AND USES: Tinea pedis (athlete's foot), tinea cruris (jock itch), and tinea corporis (ringworm) due to *Trichophyton rubrum, T. mentagrophytes,* and *Epidermophyton floccosum*

DOSAGE

Adult and Child

- TOP apply to affected area(s) qd-bid for 2 wk (jock itch, ringworm) or 4 wk (athlete's foot)

$ **AVAILABLE FORMS/COST OF THERAPY**

- Cre—Top: 1%, 15, 30, 60 g: **$13.03-$32.11**
- Lotion—Top: 1% 30 ml: **$21.76**

CONTRAINDICATIONS: Hypersensitivity

PREGNANCY AND LACTATION: Pregnancy category B; excreted in breast milk

SIDE EFFECTS/ADVERSE REACTIONS

SKIN: Pruritus, burning, stinging, irritation, contact dermatitis, scaling, tingling, pain, dyshidrotic eczema, folliculitis, erythema, papules, rash, nodules, maceration, fissuring

SPECIAL CONSIDERATIONS

PATIENT/FAMILY EDUCATION

- For external use only, avoid contact with eyes or vagina

---

oxtriphylline

(ox-trye'fi-lin)

Choledyl, Choledyl SA, Novotriphyl ♣

Chemical Class: Xanthine derivative (64% theophylline)

Therapeutic Class: Bronchodilator

CLINICAL PHARMACOLOGY

Mechanism of Action: Directly relaxes the smooth muscle of bronchi and pulmonary blood vessels, stimulates respiration, and increases diaphragmatic contractility; the exact mode of action remains unsettled but may involve inhibition of extracellular adenosine (which causes bronchoconstriction), stimulation of endogenous catecholamines, antagonism of prostaglandins, direct effect on mobilization of intracellular calcium, and inhibition of cGMP metabolism (inhibition of phosphodiesterase with resultant increases in cAMP does not occur to an appreciable extent at therapeutic concentrations)

Pharmacokinetics

PO: Peak 1-2 hr (SA 4 hr), metabolized by liver; excreted in urine, $t_{1/2}$ 3-12 hr, $t_{1/2}$ increased in geriatric patients, hepatic disease, cor pulmonale, and CHF, decreased in children and smokers

INDICATIONS AND USES: Asthma, reversible bronchospasm associated with COPD

DOSAGE

Adult

- PO 4.7 mg/kg q8h; for total daily doses approximating 800 or 1200 mg, 400 or 600 mg SA q12h may be substituted; smokers may require 4.7 mg/kg q6h

Child

- PO 9-16 yr 4.7 mg/kg q6h; 1-9 yr 6.2 mg/kg q6h

$ **AVAILABLE FORMS/COST OF THERAPY**

- Tab, Coated, Sust Action—Oral: 400 mg, 100's: **$34.18;** 600 mg, 100's: **$41.00**
- Tab, Enteric Coated—Oral: 100 mg, 100's: **$22.67;** 200 mg, 100's: **$28.87**
- Elixir—Oral: 100 mg/5ml, 480 ml: **$7.50**

CONTRAINDICATIONS: Hypersensitivity to xanthines, active peptic ulcer, underlying seizure disorder (not on anticonvulsant therapy)

PRECAUTIONS: Elderly, CHF, cor pulmonale, hepatic disease, preexisting dysrhythmias, hypertension, infants <1 yr, hypoxemia, sustained high fever, history of peptic ulcer, alcoholism

PREGNANCY AND LACTATION: Pregnancy category C; pharmacokinetics of theophylline may be altered during pregnancy, monitor serum concentrations carefully; excreted into breast milk, may cause irritability in the nursing infant, otherwise compatible with breast feeding

SIDE EFFECTS/ADVERSE REACTIONS

CNS: Anxiety, restlessness, insom-

nia, *dizziness,* ***convulsions,*** headache, lightheadedness, muscle twitching, reflex hyperexcitability
CV: Palpitations, sinus tachycardia, hypotension, flushing, ventricular dysrhythmias, circulatory failure, extrasystoles
GI: Nausea, vomiting, anorexia, diarrhea, bitter taste, dyspepsia, epigastric pain, hematemesis, esophageal reflux
GU: Urinary frequency, proteinuria
METAB: Hyperglycemia
RESP: Tachypnea
SKIN: Urticaria, alopecia

▼ DRUG INTERACTIONS

Drugs

- *Allopurinol, cimetidine,+ ciprofloxacin, disulfiram, enoxacin, fluvoxamine, mexiletine, pefloxacin, pentoxifylline, propafenone, radioactive iodine, thiabendazole, ticlopidine, troleandomycin:* Increased serum theophylline concentrations
- *Barbiturates, carbamazepine, rifampin:* Reduced serum theophylline concentrations
- *Beta blockers:* Antagonistic pharmacologic effects, propranolol increases serum theophylline concentrations in a dose-dependent manner
- *Calcium channel blockers:* Increased serum theophylline concentrations with verapamil and possibly diltiazem
- *Erythromycin:* Increased serum theophylline concentrations; reduced erythromycin concentrations
- *Interferon:* Increased serum theophylline concentrations, especially in smokers and other patients with high pre-existing theophylline clearance
- *Lithium:* Reduced lithium concentrations
- *Phenytoin:* Reduced serum theophylline concentrations; decreased serum phenytoin concentrations
- *Smoking:* Increased theophylline dosing requirements

SPECIAL CONSIDERATIONS

PATIENT/FAMILY EDUCATION

- Take doses as prescribed
- Do not change doses without consulting physician
- Avoid large amounts of caffeine-containing products (tea, coffee, chocolate, colas)
- If GI upset occurs, patient may take with 8 oz water
- Notify physician if nausea, vomiting, insomnia, jitteriness, headache, rash, palpitations occur

MONITORING PARAMETERS

- Serum theophylline concentrations (therapeutic level is 8-20 μg/ml); toxicity may occur with small increase above 20 μg/ml, especially in the elderly

---

oxybutynin

(ox-i-byoo'ti-nin)
Ditropan
Chemical Class: Synthetic tertiary amine
Therapeutic Class: Genitourinary muscle relaxant

CLINICAL PHARMACOLOGY

Mechanism of Action: Exerts direct antispasmodic effect on smooth muscle and inhibits action of acetylcholine at postganglionic cholinergic sites; increases bladder capacity and delays initial desire to void by reducing number of motor impulses reaching the detrusor muscle

Pharmacokinetics

PO: Peak 3-6 hr, onset ½-1 hr, duration 6-10 hr, metabolized in liver, eliminated via kidneys

INDICATIONS AND USES: Antispasmodic in uninhibited neurogenic or reflex neurogenic bladder, primary nocturnal enuresis,* antispasmodic in various GI disorders*

DOSAGE

Adult

- PO 5 mg bid-tid; do not exceed 5 mg qid

Child

- PO 1-5 yr 0.2 mg/kg/dose divided bid-qid; >5 yr 5 mg bid, up to 5 mg tid

$ AVAILABLE FORMS/COST OF THERAPY

- Tab, Uncoated—Oral: 5 mg, 100's: **$19.73-$45.56**
- Syr—Oral: 5 mg/5 ml, 480 ml: **$49.38**

CONTRAINDICATIONS: Angle-closure glaucoma, myasthenia gravis, partial or complete obstruction of the GI tract, adynamic ileus, megacolon, severe colitis, intestinal atony, obstructive uropathy, unstable cardiovascular status

PRECAUTIONS: Elderly, autonomic neuropathy, hepatic or renal disease, hyperthyroidism, CHD, prostatic hypertrophy, reflux esophagitis, ulcerative colitis

PREGNANCY AND LACTATION: Pregnancy category B; may suppress lactation

SIDE EFFECTS/ADVERSE REACTIONS

CNS: Drowsiness, hallucinations, insomnia, restlessness, asthenia, dizziness

CV: Tachycardia, palpitations, vasodilation

EENT: Decreased lacrimation, mydriasis, amblyopia, cycloplegia, blurred vision

GI: Dry mouth, nausea, vomiting, constipation, decreased GI motility

GU: Urinary hesitancy and retention, impotence

METAB: Suppression of lactation

SKIN: Decreased sweating, rash

SPECIAL CONSIDERATIONS

PATIENT/FAMILY EDUCATION

- May cause drowsiness, dizziness, or blurred vision;
- Use caution driving or engaging in other activities requiring alertness
- May cause dry mouth
- Avoid prolonged exposure to hot environments, heat prostration may result

oxycodone

(ox-ee-koe'done)

Supeudol, ✤ Roxicodone

Chemical Class: Opiate, synthetic phenanthrene derivative

Therapeutic Class: Narcotic analgesic

DEA Class: Schedule II

CLINICAL PHARMACOLOGY

Mechanism of Action: Binds to opiate receptors in the CNS causing inhibition of ascending pain pathways, altering the perception of and response to pain

Pharmacokinetics

PO: Onset 10-15 min, peak 30-60 min, duration 3-6 hr, metabolized in liver and kidney, excreted primarily in urine

INDICATIONS AND USES: Moderate to moderately severe pain

DOSAGE

Adult

- PO 5 mg q6h prn

Child

- PO 6-12 yr 1.25 mg q6h prn; >12 yr 2.5 mg q6h prn

$ AVAILABLE FORMS/COST OF THERAPY

- Sol—Oral: 5 mg/5 ml, 500 ml: **$40.44;** 20 mg/ml, 30 ml: **$39.38**
- Tab, Uncoated—Oral: 5 mg, 100's: **$30.14**

CONTRAINDICATIONS: Hypersensitivity, acute bronchial asthma, upper airway obstruction

PRECAUTIONS: Head injury, increased intracranial pressure, acute abdominal conditions, elderly, severe impairment of hepatic or renal function, hypothyroidism, Addison's disease, prostatic hypertrophy, urethral stricture, history of drug abuse

PREGNANCY AND LACTATION: Pregnancy category B (category D if used for prolonged periods or in high doses at term); excreted into breast milk

SIDE EFFECTS/ADVERSE REACTIONS

CNS: *Drowsiness, sedation,* dizziness, agitation, dependency, lethargy, restlessness

CV: Bradycardia, palpitations, orthostatic hypotension, tachycardia

GI: *Nausea, vomiting, anorexia, constipation*

GU: Urinary retention

RESP: ***Respiratory depression, respiratory paralysis***

SKIN: Flushing, rash, urticaria

▼ **DRUG INTERACTIONS**

Drugs

- *Barbiturates:* Additive CNS depression
- *Cimetidine:* Increased effect of narcotic analgesics
- *Ethanol:* Additive CNS effects
- *Neuroleptics:* Hypotension and excessive CNS depression

Labs

- *Increase:* Amylase, lipase

SPECIAL CONSIDERATIONS

PATIENT/FAMILY EDUCATION

- Report any symptoms of CNS changes, allergic reactions
- Physical dependency may result when used for extended periods
- Change position slowly, orthostatic hypotension may occur
- Avoid hazardous activities if drowsiness or dizziness occurs
- Avoid alcohol, other CNS depressants unless directed by physician
- Minimize nausea by taking with food and lying down following dose

oxymetazoline

(ox-ee-met-az'oh-leen)

Nasal: Afrin, Afrin Children's Nose Drops, 12 Hour Nasal, Allerest 12 Hour Nasal, Chlorphed-LA, Dristan Long Lasting, Duramist Plus, Duration, 4-Way Long Lasting Nasal, Genasal, Nasal Relief, Neo-Synephrine 12 Hour, Nostrilla, NTZ Long Acting Nasal, 12 Hour Sinarest, Sinex Long-Acting, Twice-A-Day

Ophthalmic: Ocu-Clear, Visine L.R.

Chemical Class: Imidazoline derivative

Therapeutic Class: Decongestant

CLINICAL PHARMACOLOGY

Mechanism of Action: Vasoconstriction through a local adrenergic mechanism on dilated conjunctival and nasal mucosal blood vessels

Pharmacokinteics

TOP: Onset 5-10 min, duration 5-6 hr, some systemic absorption

INDICATIONS AND USES: Nasal congestion, eye redness due to minor eye irritations

DOSAGE

Adult and Child ≥6 yr

- Nasal 2-3 gtt or sprays of 0.05% sol instilled into each nostril bid; do not exceed 3-5 days duration
- Conjunctival 1 gtt q6h; do not exceed 3-4 days duration

Child 2-5 yr

- Nasal 2-3 gtt of 0.025% sol instilled into each nostril bid; do not exceed 3-5 days duration

$ AVAILABLE FORMS/COST OF THERAPY

• Sol—Ophth: 0.025%, 15, 30 ml: **$3.07-$5.33**

• Sol—Nasal: 0.025%, 20 ml: **$3.35;** 0.05%, 15, 20, 30 ml: **$1.46-$7.24**

CONTRAINDICATIONS: Hypersensitivity, angle-closure glaucoma

PRECAUTIONS: Children <2 yr, hyperthyroidism, heart disease, hypertension, diabetes mellitus

PREGNANCY AND LACTATION: Pregnancy category C

SIDE EFFECTS/ADVERSE REACTIONS

CNS: Headache, nervousness, dizziness, weakness

CV: Hypertension, cardiac irregularities

EENT: Transient burning, stinging, dryness, ulceration of nasal mucosa, sneezing, anosmia; blurred vision, mild transient stinging, irritation, mydriasis, increased/decreased intraocular pressure; rebound congestion/hyperemia

GI: Nausea

SKIN: Sweating

SPECIAL CONSIDERATIONS

PATIENT/FAMILY EDUCATION

• Discontinue ophthal preparations if ocular pain or visual changes occur

• May produce increased nasal congestion/redness of the eye if overused

• Do not use longer than 3-5 days unless under the direction of a physician

oxymetholone

(ox-ee-meth'oh-lone)

Anadrol-50, Anapolon 50 ♣

Chemical Class: Halogenated testosterone derivative

Therapeutic Class: Anabolic steroid

DEA Class: Schedule III

CLINICAL PHARMACOLOGY

Mechanism of Action: Promotes body tissue-building processes and reverses catabolic or tissue depleting processes when administered with adequate calories and protein to achieve positive nitrogen balance; inhibits endogenous testosterone release

Pharmacokinetics

PO: Metabolized in liver, excreted in urine

INDICATIONS AND USES: Anemias caused by deficient red cell production, acquired or congenital aplastic anemia, myelofibrosis and hypoplastic anemias due to administration of myelotoxic drugs

DOSAGE

Adult

• PO 1-5 mg/kg/d

$ AVAILABLE FORMS/COST OF THERAPY

• Tab, Uncoated—Oral: 50 mg, 100's: **$88.06**

CONTRAINDICATIONS: Hypersensitivity, male patients with prostate or breast cancer, hypercalcemia in females with breast cancer, nephrosis, nephrotic phase of nephritis, enhancement of physical appearance or athletic performance

PRECAUTIONS: Elderly, children, cardiac disease, renal disease, hepatic disease, seizure disorder, migraine headache, diabetes

PREGNANCY AND LACTATION: Pregnancy category X

SIDE EFFECTS/ADVERSE REACTIONS

CNS: Excitation, insomnia, habituation, depression, choreiform movement

CV: Edema

EENT: Deepening of voice, hoarseness

GI: Nausea, vomiting, diarrhea, ***cholestatic jaundice, hepatic necrosis, hepatocellular neoplasms, peliosis hepatis***

GU: Amenorrhea, vaginitis, decreased breast size, clitoral hypertrophy, testicular atrophy, decreased libido

HEME: ***Leukemia*** (observed in several patients with aplastic anemia, role of oxymetholone unclear)

METAB: Virilization; retention of sodium, chloride, water, potassium, phosphates, calcium; decreased glucose tolerance, increased serum cholesterol, increased LDL cholesterol, decreased HDL cholesterol

MS: Premature closure of epiphyses in children

SKIN: Rash, acne, flushing, sweating, alopecia, hirsutism

▼ **DRUG INTERACTIONS**

Drugs

- *Antidiabetic agents:* Enhanced hypoglycemic effects
- *Cyclosporine:* Increased cyclosporine concentrations
- *Warfarin:* Enhanced hypoprothrombinemic response to oral anticoagulants

Labs

- *Increase:* Serum cholesterol, blood glucose, urine glucose
- *Decrease:* Serum Ca, serum K, T_4, T_3, thryroid ^{131} uptake test, urine 17-OHCS, 17-KS, PBI, BSP

SPECIAL CONSIDERATIONS

PATIENT/FAMILY EDUCATION

- May cause GI upset or nausea
- Notify physician of hoarseness, deepening of voice, male-pattern baldness, hirsutism, menstrual irregularities, acne (women)
- Notify physician of nausea, vomiting, changes in skin color, ankle swelling
- Response is often not immediate, needs to be taken for a minimum trial of 3-6 mo

MONITORING PARAMETERS

- Frequent serum and urine calcium (discontinue if hypercalcemia develops)
- Liver function tests
- Growth rate in children

---

oxymorphone

(ox-ee-mor'fone)

Numorphan

Chemical Class: Opiate, semisynthetic phenanthrene derivative

Therapeutic Class: Narcotic analgesic

DEA Class: Schedule II

CLINICAL PHARMACOLOGY

Mechanism of Action: Binds to opiate receptors in the CNS causing inhibition of ascending pain pathways, altering perception of and response to pain

Pharmacokinetics

PR: Onset 15-30 min, duration 3-6 hr

IV: Onset 5-10 min, duration 3-6 hr

SC/IM: Onset 10-15 min, duration 3-6 hr

Metabolized primarily in liver, excreted mainly in urine

INDICATIONS AND USES: Moderate to severe pain, preoperative sedation, analgesia during labor, pulmonary edema (not arising from chemical respiratory irritant)

DOSAGE

Adult

- SC/IM 1-1.5 mg q4-6h prn; IV 0.5 mg; PR 5 mg q4-6h prn

• *Analgesia during labor:* IM 0.5-1 mg

$ AVAILABLE FORMS/COST OF THERAPY

• Inj, Sol—IM; IV; SC: 1 mg/ml, 1 ml: **$3.73;** 1.5 mg/ml, 1 ml: **$4.88**
• Supp—Rect: 5 mg, 6's: **$30.56**

CONTRAINDICATIONS: Hypersensitivity, acute bronchial asthma, upper airway obstruction

PRECAUTIONS: Head injury, increased intracranial pressure, acute abdominal conditions, elderly, severe impairment of hepatic or renal function, hypothyroidism, Addison's disease, prostatic hypertrophy, urethral stricture, history of drug abuse, children

PREGNANCY AND LACTATION: Pregnancy category B (category D if used for prolonged periods or in high doses at term); use during labor produces neonatal respiratory depression

SIDE EFFECTS/ADVERSE REACTIONS

CNS: Drowsiness, sedation, dizziness, agitation, dependency, lethargy, restlessness

CV: Bradycardia, palpitations, orthostatic hypotension, tachycardia

GI: Nausea, vomiting, anorexia, constipation

GU: Urinary retention

RESP: ***Respiratory depression, respiratory paralysis***

SKIN: Flushing, rash, urticaria

▼ DRUG INTERACTIONS

Drugs

• *Barbiturates:* Additive CNS depression
• *Cimetidine:* Increased effect of narcotic analgesics
• *Ethanol:* Additive CNS effects
• *Neuroleptics:* Hypotension and excessive CNS depression

Labs

• *Increase:* Amylase, lipase

SPECIAL CONSIDERATIONS

PATIENT/FAMILY EDUCATION

• Report any symptoms of CNS changes, allergic reactions
• Physical dependency may result when used for extended periods
• Change position slowly, orthostatic hypotension may occur
• Avoid hazardous activities if drowsiness or dizziness occurs
• Avoid alcohol, other CNS depressants unless directed by physician

oxytetracycline

(ox'ee-tet-tra-sye'kleen)

Terramycin, Uri-Tet

Chemical Class: Tetracycline

Therapeutic Class: Broad-spectrum antibiotic

CLINICAL PHARMACOLOGY

Mechanism of Action: Inhibits protein synthesis in microorganisms by binding at the 30S ribosomal subunit; bacteriostatic

Pharmacokinetics

PO: Peak 2-4 hr

Absorption 50%; food decreases; 20%-40% protein bound; $t_{1/2}$ 6-10 hr; excreted in urine, bile, feces in active form

INDICATIONS AND USES: Treatment of infections caused by the following susceptible organisms:

• Gram positive organisms: *Streptococcus* species (44%-74% resistant), *Diplococcus pneumoniae*
• Gram negative organisms: *E. coli, Enterobacter aerogenes, Shigella* sp, *Actinobacter calcoaceticus, Haemophilus influenzae, H. ducreyi, Klebsiella* sp, *Yersinia pestis, Francisella tularensis, Bartonella bacilliformis, Bacteroides* sp, *Campylobacter fetus, Brucella* sp (in conjunction with streptomycin)
• Miscellaneous organisms: *Treponema pallidum, T. pertenue* (syph-

O

ilis and yaws); *Chlamydia trachomatis,* agents of lymphogranuloma venereum and granuloma inguinale, rickettsial infections, agents of psittacosis and ornithosis, *Mycoplasma pneumoniae, Borrelia recurrentis, Neisseria gonorrhoeae, N. meningitidis* (IV only), *Listeria monocytogenes, Clostridium* sp, *Bacillus anthracis, Fusobacterium fusiforme, Actinomyces* sp

DOSAGE

Adult

- *Moderate to severe infections:* PO 250-500 mg q6h; IM 100 mg q8h or 150 mg q12h; IV 250-500 mg q12h, 250 mg q24h
- *Gonorrhea:* PO 1.5 g, then 500 mg qid for a total of 9 g
- *Chlamydia trachomatis:* PO 500 mg qid times 7 days
- *Syphilis:* PO 2-3 g in divided doses × 10-15 days up to 30-40 g total
- *Acne:* PO 250 mg qid × 2 weeks; then 250-500 mg qd

Child >8 yr

- *Moderate to severe infections:* PO 25-50 mg/kg/d in divided doses q6h; IM 15-25 mg/kg/d in divided doses q8-12h; IV 10-20 mg/kg/d in divided doses q12h
- Dosage adjustment necessary in renal impairment

$ AVAILABLE FORMS/COST OF THERAPY

- Inj, Sol—IM: 50 mg/ml, 5's: **$47.18**
- Inj, Powder—IV: 500 mg, 5's: **$34.08**
- Cap—Oral: 250 mg, 100's: **$12.75-$75.10**
- Oint—Ophth: 5 mg/g, 3.5 g: **$8.23**

CONTRAINDICATIONS: Hypersensitivity to tetracyclines, children <8 yr

PRECAUTIONS: Renal disease, hepatic disease, last trimester of pregnancy, neonatal period and early childhood, direct sunlight exposure, outdated products, sulfite sensitivity, hiatal hernia

PREGNANCY AND LACTATION: Pregnancy category D; excreted into breast milk; M:P ratio: 0.6-0.8; theoretically, may cause dental staining, but usually undetectable in infant serum (<0.05 μg/ml)

SIDE EFFECTS/ADVERSE REACTIONS

CNS: Fever, pseudotumor cerebri

CV: Pericarditis

EENT: Dysphagia, glossitis, decreased calcification of deciduous teeth, oral candidiasis

GI: Nausea, abdominal pain, *vomiting, diarrhea,* anorexia, enterocolitis, ***hepatotoxicity, fatty liver,*** flatulence, abdominal cramps, epigastric burning, stomatitis, sore throat, black hairy tongue, dysphagia, proctitis, pruritus ani

GU: Increased BUN

HEME: ***Eosinophilia, neutropenia, thrombocytopenia, leukocytosis, hemolytic anemia***

SKIN: Rash, urticaria, photosensitivity, increased pigmentation, ***exfoliative dermatitis,*** pruritus, angioedema, pain at inj site, onycholysis and discoloration of nails

MISC: Tooth discoloration

▼ DRUG INTERACTIONS

Drugs

- *Antacids+, bismuth salts:* Decreased effect of tetracyclines
- *Food+:* Reduced absorption, decreased effect of tetracyclines
- *Iron:* Reduced absorption, decreased effect of tetracyclines
- *Methoxyflurane+:* Increased risk of nephrotoxicity
- *Oral contraceptives:* Interruption of enterohepatic circulation of estrogens, reduced oral contraceptive effectiveness
- *Penicillin:* May impair the efficacy of penicillins

- *Sodium bicarbonate+:* Reduction of tetracycline serum concentrations
- *Zinc:* Inhibit absorption, decreased effect of tetracyclines

Labs

- *False negative:* Urine glucose with Clinistix or Tes-Tape
- *False increase:* Urinary catecholamines

SPECIAL CONSIDERATIONS:

- Offers no significant advantage over tetracycline; shares similar spectrum of activity (maybe slightly less active than tetracycline and has longer dosage interval)

PATIENT/FAMILY EDUCATION

- Avoid milk products, take with a full glass of water

---

oxytocin

(ox-ee-toe'sin)

Pitocin, Syntocinon

Chemical Class: Synthetic polypeptide posterior pituitary gland hormone

Therapeutic Class: Oxytocic, galactokinetic

CLINICAL PHARMACOLOGY

Mechanism of Action: Acts directly on myofibrils to augment the number of contracting myofibrils, producing uterine contraction; stimulates smooth muscle contraction in myoepithelial elements surrounding the alveoli of breast inducing milk ejection (not production)

Pharmacokinetics

IM: Onset, 3-5 min; duration 3-5 hr

IV: Onset, immediate; duration, 30-60 min

INTRANASAL: Onset prompt (min); duration, 20 min

Not absorbed orally; $t_{1/2}$<10 min; elimination via liver, kidneys, and oxytocinase

INDICATIONS AND USES: Induction and augmentation of labor; missed or incomplete abortion; postpartum bleeding; postpartum breast engorgement,* initial milk letdown; antepartum fetal heart rate testing (oxytocin challenge test)*

DOSAGE

Adult

- *Labor induction:* IV dilute 10 U/L of 0.9% NS or D_5NS, run at 1-2 mU/min at 15-30 min intervals to begin normal labor
- *Augmentation of labor:* IV INF in D_5W or 0.9% NaCl at 1-2 mU/min; may increase q15-30 min, not to exceed 20 mU/min
- *Incomplete abortion:* IV INF 10 U/500 ml D_5W or 0.9% NaCl given at 20-40 mU/min
- *Control of postpartum bleeding:* IV dilute 10-40 U/L, run at 10-20 mU/min; adjust rate as needed
- *Initiate milk letdown:* Nasal spray 1 spray into one or both nostrils q2-3 min before breast feeding; nasal drops 3 gtt into one or both nostrils q2-3 min before breast feeding

O

$ **AVAILABLE FORMS/COST OF THERAPY**

- Inj, Sol—IM; IV: 10 U/ml, 1 ml: **$0.97-$9.49**
- Liq, Nasal Spray—40 U/ml, 2 ml: **$31.68**

CONTRAINDICATIONS: Hypersensitivity, cephalopelvic disproportion, fetal distress, hypertonic uterus

PRECAUTIONS: Cervical/uterine surgery, uterine sepsis, primipara >35 yr, 1st, 2nd stage of labor, fetal distress, partial placenta previa, prematurity, history of uterine sepsis, traumatic delivery, cyclopropane anesthesia, water intoxication

PREGNANCY AND LACTATION: Nasal oxytocin contraindicated during pregnancy; only minimal amounts pass into breast milk

SIDE EFFECTS/ADVERSE REACTIONS

CNS: Hypertension, ***convulsions, tetanic contractions***

CV: Hypotension, dysrhythmias, increased pulse, bradycardia, tachycardia, PVC

FETUS: Dysrhythmias, jaundice, hypoxia, ***intracranial hemorrhage***

GI: Anorexia, nausea, vomiting, constipation

GU: ***Abruptio placentae, decreased uterine blood flow***

HEME: Increased hyperbilirubinemia

METAB: Water intoxication: confusion, anuria, drowsiness, headache

RESP: Asphyxia

SKIN: Rash

SPECIAL CONSIDERATIONS

- Routinely used for the induction of labor at term and post-partum for the control of uterine bleeding; not the drug of choice for induction of labor for abortion

MONITORING PARAMETERS

- Continuous monitoring necessary for IV use (length, intensity, duration of contractions; FHTs—acceleration, deceleration, fetal distress

---

pamidronate

(pam-id′drow-nate)

Aredia

Chemical Class: Bisphosphonate

Therapeutic Class: Inhibition of bone resorption

CLINICAL PHARMACOLOGY

Mechanism of Action: Blocks hydroxyapatite crystal dissolution (“crystal poison”); inhibits bone resorption

Pharmacokinetics

Taken up by bones (49% of dose); 51% excreted unchanged in urine within 72 hr; biphasic $t_{1/2}$, 1.6/27.2 hr

INDICATIONS AND USES: Paget’s disease; hypercalcemia of malignancy

DOSAGE

Adult

- *Severe hypercalcemia of malignancy:* IV INF 90 mg over 24 hr
- *Moderate hypercalcemia of malignancy:* IV INF 60-90 mg over 24 hr
- *Paget’s disease:* IV INF 30 mg over 4 hr on 3 consecutive days (total 90 mg)

$ **AVAILABLE FORMS/COST OF THERAPY**

- Inj, Sol—IV: 30 mg, 4’s: **$708.95;** 60 mg, 1’s: **$354.47;** 90 mg, 1’s: **$531.71**

CONTRAINDICATIONS: Hypersensitivity to bisphophonates

PRECAUTIONS: Renal dysfunction

PREGNANCY AND LACTATION: Pregnancy category C

SIDE EFFECTS/ADVERSE REACTIONS

CNS: Seizures, headache

CV: Hypertension

EENT: Uveitis, iritis

GI: Abdominal pain, anorexia, constipation, nausea, vomiting

GU: UTI, fluid overload

METAB: Anemia, hypokalemia, hypomagnesemia, hypophosphatemia, hyperpyrexia

MS: Bone pain

SKIN: Redness, swelling, induration, pain on palpitation at site of catheter insertion

SPECIAL CONSIDERATIONS

- “Second-generation” bisphosphonate which offers potential advantages over etidronate (like alendronate) in that it inhibits bone resorption at doses that do not impair bone mineralization, and is less likely than etidronate to produce osteomalacia

pancrelipase

(pan-kre-li'pase)

Cotazym, Cotazym-S, Creon, Ilozyme, Ku-Zyme HP, Pancrease, Pancrease MT, Protilase, Ultrase MT, Viokase, Zymase

Chemical Class: Pancreatic enzymes, bovine/porcine; mixture of lipase/protease/amylase

Therapeutic Class: Digestant

CLINICAL PHARMACOLOGY

Mechanism of Action: Pancreatic enzymes: hydrolyze fats to glycerol and fatty acids; changes protein to proteoses; converts starch into dextrins and sugars

INDICATIONS AND USES: Exocrine pancreatic secretion insufficiency, cystic fibrosis (digestive aid), chronic pancreatitis, post pancreatectomy, ductal obstructions caused by cancer

DOSAGE

Adult

- 4000-48,000 U lipase with each meal/snack; powder 0.7 g with meals/snacks

Child

- 6 mo-1 yr, 2000 U lipase per meal
- 1-6 yr, 400-8000 U lipase with each meal; 4000 U with snacks
- 7-12 yr, 4000-12,000 U lipase with each meal and snacks

$ AVAILABLE FORMS/COST OF THERAPY

- Cap, Enteric Coated—Oral: 20,000 U lipase/4000 U protease/ 25,000 U amylase, 100's: **$25.84;** 8000/30,000/30,000: **$18.58;** 12,000/24,000/24,000: **$52.30;** 16,000/48,000/48,000: **$103.70;** 20,000/65,000/65,000: **$71.82;** 24,000/78,000/78,000: **$79.38**

CONTRAINDICATIONS: Hypersensitivity to pork, acute pancreatitis and exacerbations of chronic pancreatic disease

PREGNANCY AND LACTATION: Pregnancy category C

SIDE EFFECTS/ADVERSE REACTIONS

GI: Anorexia, nausea, vomiting, diarrhea, glossitis, anal soreness

EENT: Buccal soreness

METAB: Hyperuricuria, hyperuricemia

SKIN: Rash, hypersensitivity

SPECIAL CONSIDERATIONS

- Substitution at dispensing should be avoided
- Enteric-coated pancreatic enzymes are more effective than regular formulations; individual variations may require trials with several enzymatic preparations
- For patients who do not respond appropriately, adding antacid or H_2 antagonist may provide better results
- Preparations high in lipase concentration seem to be more effective for reducing steatorrhea

PATIENT/FAMILY EDUCATION

- Advise patient to take before or with meals
- Protect enteric coating, advise patient not to crush or chew microspheres in caps or tabs

papaverine

(pa-pav'er-een)

Cerespan, Genabid, Pavabid HP, Pavabid Plateau, Pavarine Spancaps, Pavased, Pavatine, Pavatym, Paverolan Lanacaps, Pavusule

Chemical Class: Non-narcotic opium alkaloid (no narcotic activity)

Therapeutic Class: Peripheral vasodilator

CLINICAL PHARMACOLOGY

Mechanism of Action: Relaxes all smooth muscle; inhibits cyclic nucleotide phosphodiesterase, which increases intracellular cAMP, causing vasodilation; increases cerebral blood flow and decreases cerebral vascular resistance in normal subjects

Pharmacokinetics

PO: Onset 30 sec, peak 1-2 hr, duration 3-4 hr

SUS REL: Poor and erratic absorption

Oral bioavailability 54%; 90% bound to plasma proteins, metabolized in liver, excreted in urine (inactive metabolites)

INDICATIONS AND USES: Arterial spasm resulting in cerebral and peripheral ischemia;* myocardial ischemia associated with vascular spasm or dysrhythmias;* angina pectoris;* peripheral and pulmonary embolism;* visceral spasm as in ureteral, biliary, GI colic; PVD;* with phentolamine or alprostadil intracavernously for impotence*

DOSAGE

Adult

• PO 100-300 mg 3-5 times/day; sus rel 150-300 mg q8-12h;

• IM/IV 30-120 mg q3h prn (IV slowly over 1-2 min)

$ AVAILABLE FORMS/COST OF THERAPY

• Cap, Gel, Sust Action—Oral: 150 mg, 100's: **$6.65-$27.31**

• Inj, Sol—IM; IV: 30 mg/ml, 2 ml: **$4.50-$12.00**

• Tablet, Uncoated—Oral: 100 mg, 100's: **$11.76;** 300 mg, 100's: **$7.95**

CONTRAINDICATIONS: Hypersensitivity, complete AV heart block

PRECAUTIONS: Cardiac dysrhythmias, glaucoma, hepatic hypersensitivity

PREGNANCY AND LACTATION: Pregnancy category C

SIDE EFFECTS/ADVERSE REACTIONS

CNS: Headache, dizziness, drowsiness, sedation, vertigo, malaise

CV: ***Tachycardia,*** increased B/P

GI: Nausea, anorexia, abdominal pain, constipation, diarrhea, jaundice, altered liver enzymes, ***hepatotoxicity***

GU: Priapism (intracavernously)

RESP: Increased depth of respirations

SKIN: *Flushing, sweating,* rash

▼ DRUG INTERACTIONS

Drugs

• *Levodopa:* Papaverine may inhibit the clinical response to levodopa in parkinsonian

SPECIAL CONSIDERATIONS

• No objective evidence of *any* therapeutic value

paraldehyde

(par-al'de-hyde)

Paral

Chemical Class: Cyclic ether; polymer of acetaldehyde

Therapeutic Class: Anticonvulsant

DEA Class: Schedule V

CLINICAL PHARMACOLOGY

Mechanism of Action: CNS depressant

Pharmacokinetics

PO: Sleep onset 10-15 min, peak 1-2 hr, duration 8-12 hr

RECT: Onset slower, duration 4-6 hr

80% metabolized by liver; excreted by kidneys, lungs; crosses placenta; $t_{1/2}$ 7.5 hr

INDICATIONS AND USES: Refractory seizures, status epilepticus, sedation, insomnia, alcohol withdrawal, tetanus, eclampsia

DOSAGE

Adult

• *Seizures:* IM 5-10 ml; divide 10 ml into 2 inj; IV 0.2-0.4 ml/kg in NS
• *Alcohol withdrawal:* PO/REC 5-10 ml, not to exceed 60 ml; IM 5 ml q4-6h × 24 hr, then q6h on following days, not to exceed 30 ml
• *Sedation:* PO/REC 4-10 ml; IM 5 ml; IV 3-5 ml to be used in emergency only
• *Tetanus:* IV 4-5 ml or 12 ml by gastric tube q4h diluted with water; IM 5-10 ml prn

Child

• *Seizures:* IM 0.15 ml/kg; REC 0.3 ml/kg q4-6h or 1 ml/yr of age, not to exceed 5 ml; may repeat in 1 hr prn; IV 5 ml/90 ml NS inj; begin inf at 5 ml/hr; titrate to patient response
• *Sedation:* PO/RECT/IM 0.15 ml/kg

$ AVAILABLE FORMS/COST OF THERAPY

• Inj, Sol—Oral: 100%, 30 ml: **$6.00-$24.50**

CONTRAINDICATIONS: Bronchopulmonary disease, hepatic insufficiency, gastroenteritis with ulceration

PRECAUTIONS: Hepatic impairment, mucous membrane irritation

PREGNANCY AND LACTATION: Pregnancy category C

SIDE EFFECTS/ADVERSE REACTIONS

CNS: Stimulation, drowsiness, dizziness, confusion, ***convulsion,*** headache, flushing, hallucinations, coma; addiction syndrome resembling alcoholism

CV: Pulmonary edema, ***pulmonary hemorrhage, circulatory collapse***

GI: Foul breath, irritation, hepatitis

GU: Nephrosis

HEME: ***Thrombocytopenia, agranulocytosis, leukopenia, neutropenia, hemolytic anemia,*** increased prothrombin time

METAB: Metabolic acidosis

RESP: ***Respiratory depression***

SKIN: Rash, erythema, local pain, sloughing, fat necrosis

▼ DRUG INTERACTIONS

Labs

• *False positive:* Ketones (serum, urine)
• *Interference:* 17-OHCS

SPECIAL CONSIDERATIONS

• Benzodiazepines preferred for rapid sedation
• Not considered anticonvulsant therapy of choice for any seizure type
• Injectable form no longer commercially available; Oral/Rectal product may be used, however, can cause local tissue damage

---

paregoric

(par-e-gor′ik)

Paregoric, Paregique ♣

Chemical Class: Opiate (most preparations also contain camphor and ethanol)

Therapeutic Class: Antidiarrheal

DEA Class: Schedule III

P

CLINICAL PHARMACOLOGY

Mechanism of Action: Direct effect on circular smooth muscle of the bowel that prolongs GI transit time; reduces GI secretions

Pharmacokinetics

PO: Onset 20-30 min, peak 60 min, duration 4 hr; metabolized in liver by glucuronidation; metabolites excreted in urine (90% within 24 hr), 10% excreted in bile

INDICATIONS AND USES: Antidiarrheal, neonatal opioid withdrawal syndrome*

DOSAGE

Adult

• PO 5-10 ml up to qid

Child

- *Antidiarrheal:* Age >2 yr, PO 0.25-0.5 ml/kg up to qid
- *Opioid withdrawal syndrome:* Neonate, PO 0.2 ml q3h, increase dose by 0.05 ml q3h until symptoms controlled (max dose of 0.7 ml)
- Note: 4 ml of paregoric equal to 2.5 mg diphenoxylate, 1.6 mg morphine sulfate

$ AVAILABLE FORMS/COST OF THERAPY

- Liq—Oral: 0.4 mg/ml, 480 ml: **$3.25-$11.30**

CONTRAINDICATIONS: Diarrhea due to poisoning, hypersensitivity, infectious diarrhea

PRECAUTIONS: Respiratory disease, elderly patients

PREGNANCY AND LACTATION: Pregnancy category B; excreted in breast milk

SIDE EFFECTS/ADVERSE REACTIONS

CNS: Depression, *dizziness, drowsiness,* fatigue, restlessness, withdrawal syndrome (with prolonged use at high dose)

CV: ***Hypotension,*** orthostatic hypotension

EENT: Miosis

GI: Abdominal cramping, *constipation*

GU: Urinary retention

RESP: Respiratory depression

SKIN: Pruritus

▼ DRUG INTERACTIONS

Drugs

- *Barbiturates, rifampin:* Increase metabolism of paregoric
- *Cimetidine:* Decrease metabolism of paregoric

SPECIAL CONSIDERATIONS

- Contains ethanol

paromomycin

(par-oh-moe-mye'sin)

Humatin

Chemical Class: Aminoglycoside antibiotic

Therapeutic Class: Amebicide, antibacterial

CLINICAL PHARMACOLOGY

Mechanism of Action: Direct action in intestinal lumen

Pharmacokinetics

PO: Poor absorption; 100% excreted in feces

INDICATIONS AND USES: Intestinal amebiasis, adjunct in hepatic coma, other parasitic infections* *(Dientamoeba fragilis, Diphyllobothrium latum, Taenia saginata, T. solium, Dipylidium caninum, Hymenolepis nana)*

DOSAGE

Adult

- *Intestinal amebiasis:* PO 25-35 mg/kg/d in 3 divided doses × 5-10 days pc
- *Hepatic coma:* 4 g qd in divided doses × 5-6 days

Child

- *Intestinal amebiasis:* PO 25-35 mg/kg/d in 3 divided doses × 5-10 days pc

$ AVAILABLE FORMS/COST OF THERAPY

- Cap, Gel—Oral: 250 mg, 100's: **$197.88**

CONTRAINDICATIONS: Hypersensitivity, GI obstruction

PRECAUTIONS: GI ulcerations, superinfection

PREGNANCY AND LACTATION: Pregnancy category C; poor oral bioavailability and lipid solubility limit passage into breast milk

SIDE EFFECTS/ADVERSE REACTIONS

EENT: Ototoxicity

GI: Nausea, vomiting, diarrhea, epigastric distress, anorexia, steatorrhea, pruritus ani
GU: ***Nephrotoxicity, hematuria***

▼ DRUG INTERACTIONS

Drugs

• *Amphotericin B:* Synergistic nephrotoxicity
• *Cephalosporins:* Increased potential for nephrotoxicity in patients with pre-existing renal disease
• *Cyclosporine:* Additive renal damage
• *Ethacrynic acid+:* Increased risk of ototoxicity
• *Methoxyflurane:* Enhanced renal toxicity
• *Neuromuscular blocking agents+:* Potentiation of respiratory suppression produced by neuromuscular blocking agents

Labs

• *Decrease:* Serum cholesterol

paroxetine

(par-ox'e-teen)
Paxil
Chemical Class: Phenyl piperidine derivative
Therapeutic Class: Antidepressant, serotonin reuptake inhibitor (SSRI)

CLINICAL PHARMACOLOGY

Mechanism of Action: Inhibits CNS neuron uptake of serotonin (5HT)

Pharmacokinetics

PO: Peak 5.2 hr; bioavailability, 100%; protein binding, 93%-95%; metabolized in liver (CYP2D6), unchanged drugs and metabolites excreted in feces (36%) and urine (64%); $t_{1/2}$, 21 hr

INDICATIONS AND USES: Major depressive disorder

DOSAGE

Adult

• PO 20 mg qd in AM; after 4 wk if no clinical improvement is noted, dose may be increased by 10 mg/d qwk to desired response, not to exceed 50 mg/d

$ AVAILABLE FORMS/COST OF THERAPY

• Tab, Uncoated—Oral: 20 mg, 100's: **$189.90;** 30 mg, 30's: **$58.65**

CONTRAINDICATIONS: Hypersensitivity, patients taking MAOIs (or within 14 days of discontinuing an MAOI)

PRECAUTIONS: History of mania, renal and hepatic disease

PREGNANCY AND LACTATION: Pregnancy category B; limited information; milk concentrations similar to plasma following a single oral dose; thus <1% of the daily dose would be transferred to a breast-feeding infant

SIDE EFFECTS/ADVERSE REACTIONS

CNS: Headache, nervousness, insomnia, *anxiety,* tremor, dizziness, fatigue, asthenia, euphoria, hallucinations, delusions, psychosis, myoclonus, agitation
CV: Vasodilation, postural hypotension, palpitations
EENT: Visual changes, pharyngitis
GI: Nausea, diarrhea, dry mouth, *anorexia,* dyspepsia, constipation, cramps, vomiting, taste changes, flatulence, *decreased appetite*
GU: Urinary frequency, *abnormal ejaculation*
MS: Pain, arthritis, myalgia, myopathy, myasthenia
RESP: Infection, pharyngitis, nasal congestion, sinus headache, sinusitis, cough, dyspnea
SKIN: Sweating, rash
MISC: Fever

P

▼ **DRUG INTERACTIONS**

Drugs

- *Dextromethorphan:* Metabolized by CYP2D6, inhibited by paroxetine, increased risk of adverse effects
- *Oral anticoagulants:* Increased risk of bleeding

Labs

- *Increase:* Serum bilirubin, blood glucose, alk phosphatase
- *Decrease:* VMA, 5-HIAA
- *False increase:* Urinary catecholamines

SPECIAL CONSIDERATIONS

- Minimal clinical data comparing paroxetine with other serotonin uptake inhibitors

---

pemoline

(pem'oh-leen)

Cylert

Chemical Class: Oxazolidinone derivative

Therapeutic Class: Cerebral stimulant

DEA Class: Schedule IV

CLINICAL PHARMACOLOGY

Mechanism of Action: Cerebral stimulation via dopaminergic mechanisms; minimal sympathomimetic effects

Pharmacokinetics

PO: Peak 2-4 hr duration 8 hr; gradual onset of action (3-4 wk to effect) 50% protein bound; metabolized (50%) by liver, excreted (40%) by kidneys, $t_{1/2}$ 12 hr

INDICATIONS AND USES: Attention deficit disorder with hyperactivity, narcolepsy*

DOSAGE

Child >6 yr

- *Attention deficit disorder:* 37.5 mg in AM, increasing by 18.75 mg/wk, not to exceed 112.5 mg/d

$ **AVAILABLE FORMS/COST OF THERAPY**

- Tab, Chewable—Oral: 37.5 mg, 100's: **$128.97**
- Tabl, Uncoated—Oral: 18.75 mg, 100's: **$75.28;** 37.5 mg, 100's: **$118.31;** 75 mg, 100's: **$204.31**

CONTRAINDICATIONS: Hypersensitivity, hepatic insufficiency

PRECAUTIONS: Renal disease, drug abuse, child <6 yrs

PREGNANCY AND LACTATION: Pregnancy category B

SIDE EFFECTS/ADVERSE REACTIONS

CNS: Hyperactivity, insomnia, restlessness, dizziness, depression, headache, stimulation, irritability, aggressiveness, hallucinations, ***seizures, Gilles de la Tourette's disorder,*** drowsiness, dyskinetic movements

GI: Nausea, anorexia, diarrhea, abdominal pain, increased liver enzymes, hepatitis, jaundice

MISC: Rashes, growth suppression in children

▼ **DRUG INTERACTIONS**

Drugs

- *Albuterol:* Exacerbate cardiovascular adverse effects
- *Phenothiazines and related compounds:* Inhibit central effects of sympathomimetics, reversing the anorexigenic effects and other effects
- *Furazolidone:* Increase in α-adrenergic effects of sympathomimetics
- *Procarbazine:* Hypertensive reactions

SPECIAL CONSIDERATIONS

MONITORING PARAMETERS

- LFT's periodically

penbutolol

(pen-bute'o-loll)
Levatol
Chemical Class: Non-selective β-receptor antagonist
Therapeutic Class: β-receptor antagonist, antihypertensive

CLINICAL PHARMACOLOGY
Mechanism of Action: Competitive, non-selective, β-receptor antagonist; some intrinsic sympathomimetic activity; no membrane stabilizing activity; high lipid solubility
Pharmacokinetics
PO: Peak 1½-3 hr; duration, >20 hr
Absorption, 100% bioavailability; hepatic conjugation and oxidation; 80%-98% protein bound; excreted unchanged (17% as conjugate); $t_{1/2}$ 5 hrs
INDICATIONS AND USES: Hypertension, angina pectoris,* cardiac dysrhythmias,* MI,* pheochromocytoma,* migraine,* essential tremor,* alcohol withdrawal syndrome,* aggressive behavior,* antipsychotic-induced akathisia*
DOSAGE
Adult
• *Hypertension:* 20 mg qd (flat dose-response curve)
$ AVAILABLE FORMS/COST OF THERAPY
• Tab, Uncoated—Oral: 20 mg, 100's: **$97.32**
CONTRAINDICATIONS: Cardiogenic shock, sinus bradycardia, second and third degree atrioventricular conduction block, asthma, and hypersensitivity
PRECAUTIONS: Anesthesia and major surgery; diabetes mellitus; abrupt withdrawal with concurrent CAD or thyrotoxicosis
PREGNANCY AND LACTATION: Pregnancy category C
SIDE EFFECTS/ADVERSE REACTIONS
CNS: Dizziness, fatigue, headache, insomnia
CV: Bradycardia
GI: Diarrhea, nausea, dyspepsia
GU: Sexual impotence
RESP: Cough, dyspnea
SKIN: Excessive sweating
▼ **DRUG INTERACTIONS**
• *Amiodarone:* Potentially inhibits metabolism: bradycardia/ventricular dysrhythmia
• *Anesthetics, local:* Enhanced sympathomimetic effects, hypertension due to unopposed alpha-receptor stimulation
• *Antidiabetics:* Delayed recovery from hypoglycemia, hyperglycemia, attenuated tachycardia during hypoglycemia, hypertension during hypoglycemia
• *Calcium channel blockers:* Bradycardia, hypotension
• *Clonidine:* Hypertension exacerbated upon withdrawal of clonidine
• *Disopyramide:* Additive negative inotropic effects
• *Epinephrine:* Enhanced pressor response resulting in hypertension
• *Methyldopa:* Hypertension
• *Neuroleptics:* Increased serum levels of both resulting in accentuated pharmacologic response to both drugs
• *NSAIDs:* Reduced hypotensive effects
• *Phenylephrine:* Acute hypertensive episodes
• *Prazosin:* First-dose hypotensive response enhanced
• *Tacrine:* Additive bradycardia
• *Theophylline:* Antagonist pharmacodynamics
SPECIAL CONSIDERATIONS
• Exacerbation of ischemic heart disease following abrupt withdrawal

P

due to hypersensitivity to catecholamines possible

• Comparative trials indicate that penbutolol is as effective as propranolol and atenolol in the treatment of hypertension; may have fewer CNS adverse effects than propranolol

penicillamine

(pen-i-sill'a-meen)

Cuprimine, Depen, Distamine, ✤ Pendramine ✤

Chemical Class: Chelating agent (thiol compound)

Therapeutic Class: Heavy metal antagonist, disease modifying antirheumatic

CLINICAL PHARMACOLOGY

Mechanism of Action: Binds with ions of lead, mercury, copper, iron, zinc to form a water-soluble complex excreted by kidneys; improvement of lymphocyte function, markedly reduces IgM rheumatoid factor and immune complexes, depresses T-cell but not B-cell activity; combines chemically with cystine to form disulfide, which is more soluble

Pharmacokinetics

PO: Peak 1 hr, onset of action (Wilson's disease, 1-3 mo; rheumatoid arthritis, 2-3 mo) metabolized in liver; renal and fecal elimination

INDICATIONS AND USES: Wilson's disease, rheumatoid arthritis, cystinuria, lead poisoning

DOSAGE

Adult

• *Wilson's disease:* 250 mg qid ac

• *Rheumatoid arthritis:* 125-250 mg/d, increase 250 mg q2-3 mo prn, max 1 g/d

• *Cystinuria:* PO 250 mg qid ac, not to exceed 5 g/d

Child

• *Chelating agent and cystinuria:* 20-30 mg/kg/d in divided doses qid ac

$ AVAILABLE FORMS/COST OF THERAPY

• Cap, Gel—Oral: 125 mg, 100's: **$64.88;** 250 mg, 100's: **$92.63**

• Tab, Coated—Oral: 250 mg, 100's: **$141.85**

CONTRAINDICATIONS: Hypersensitivity to penicillins, anuria, agranulocytosis, severe renal disease, pregnancy (except Wilson's disease or certain cases of cystinuria)

PRECAUTIONS: Renal insufficiency

PREGNANCY AND LACTATION: Pregnancy category D (continued therapy in Wilson's Disease and cystinuria probably OK, not rheumatoid arthritis)

SIDE EFFECTS/ADVERSE REACTIONS

CV: Hypotension, tachycardia

EENT: Tinnitus, optic neuritis

GI: Diarrhea, abdominal cramping, nausea, vomiting, ***hepatotoxicity,*** anorexia, pain, peptic ulcer

GU: ***Proteinuria, nephrotic syndrome, glomerulonephritis***

HEME: ***Thrombocytopenia, granulocytopenia, leukopenia, hemolytic anemia, aplastic anemia, eosinophilia,*** lupus syndrome, increased sedimentation rate

MS: Arthralgia

RESP: Pneumonitis, ***asthma, pulmonary fibrosis***

SKIN: Urticaria, erythema, pruritus, fever, ecchymosis, alopecia

MISC: ***Anaphylaxis***

▼ DRUG INTERACTIONS

• *Iron:* Oral iron substantially reduces plasma penicillamine concentration, with reduced therapeutic response

SPECIAL CONSIDERATIONS

PATIENT/FAMILY EDUCATION

• Should be administered on empty

stomach, ½-1 hr before meals or at least 2 hr after meals
- Urine discoloration (red)
- Teach patient that therapeutic effect may take 1-3 mo

MONITORING PARAMETERS
- Hepatic, renal, studies: CBC, urinalysis, skin for rash

penicillin

(pen-i-sill'in)

Benzathine: Bicillin L-A, Megacillin, Permapen, Bicillin C-R, Bicillin C-R 900/300

Pencillin G Potassium (Aqueous Pen G): Acrocillin, Burcillin-G, Deltapen, Megacillin, Novopen G, Pentids, Pfizerpien

Penicillin V Potassium: Pen-Vee K, Deltapen-VK, V-Cillin K, Veetids, PVFK, Apo-Pen-VK, Novop VK, Ledercillin-VK, Uticillin-VK, Betapen-VK, Penapar-VK, Robicillin-V

Penicillin G Procaine: Crysticillin A.S., Duracillin A.s., Wycillin, Pfizerpen-AS

Pencillin G Sodium: Crystapen, Pfizerpen

Chemical Class: Natural penicillin

Therapeutic Class: Antibiotic

CLINICAL PHARMACOLOGY

Mechanism of Action: Interferes with cell wall replication of susceptible organisms; osmotically unstable cell wall swells, bursts from osmotic pressure

Pharmacokinetics

Excreted in urine and breast milk, crosses placenta
- *Benzathine:* IM very slow absorption, duration 21-28 days, $t_{1/2}$ 30-60 min
- *Pen G Potassium:* IV immediate peak; IM peak 15-30 min; PO duration 6 hr, peak 1 hr
- *Pen V Potassium:* PO peak 30-60 min, duration 6-8 hr, $t_{1/2}$ 30 min
- *Pen G Procaine:* IM peak 1-4 hr, duration 15 hr
- *Pen G Sodium:* IM peak 1-3 hr, duration 6 hr

INDICATIONS AND USES: Respiratory infections, scarlet fever, erysipelas, otitis media, pneumonia, skin and soft tissue infections, gonorrhea

Antibacterial spectrum includes non-penicillinase producing strains of:
- Gram-positive: *Staphylococcus aureus, Streptococcus pyogenes, Str. viridans, Str. faecalis, Str. bovis, Str. pneumoniae, Bacillus anthracis, Listeria monocytogenes, Corynebacterium diphtheriae*
- Gram-negative: *Neisseria gonorrhoeae, N. meningitidis, E. coli, Proteus mirabilis, Salmonella, Shigella, Enterobacter, S. moniliformis;* anaerobes: *Clostrid ium* sp, *Peptococcus* sp, *Peptostreptococcus* sp, *Bacteroides* sp, (except *B. fragilis*), *Fusobacterium* sp, *Eubacterium* sp, *Treponema pallidum, Actinomyces bovis*

DOSAGE

Benzathine

Adult
- *Early syphilis:* IM 2.4 million U in single dose
- *Syphilis >1 yr duration:* IM 2.4 million U in single dose
- *Neurosyphilis:* To follow up treatment with Pen G Procaine or Pen G Potassium as below
- *Group A strep URI:* IM 1.2 million U in single dose, PO 400,000-600,000 U q4-6h
- *Rheumatic fever:* IM 1.2 million U in single dose qmo or 600,000 U q2wk

Child
- *Congenital syphilis (<2 yr):* IM 50,000 U/kg in single dose

• *Rheumatic fever/glomerulonephritis prophylaxis (<60lb):* IM 600,000 U in single dose
• *Group A strep URI (>27 kg):* IM 900,000 U in single dose; (<27 kg) 50,000 U/kg in single dose

Pen G Potassium

Adult

• *Pneumococcal/streptococcal infections:* PO 400,000-500,000 U q6-8h for 10 days
• *Rheumatic fever prophylaxis:* PO 200,000-250,000 U bid continuously
• *Meningococcal meningitis:* IM 1-2 million U q2h; IV 20-30 million U/d continuous drip for 14 d or until afebrile for 7 d
• *Pneumococcal empyema:* IV 5-24 million U/d in divided doses q4-6h
• *Pneumococcal meningitis:* IV 20-24 million U/d for 14 d
• *Pasturella infections:* IV 4-6 million U/d for 2 wk
• *Listeria infections:* IV 15-20 million U/d for 2 wk (meningitis) or 4 wk (endocarditis)
• *Neurosyphilis:* IV 2-4 million U q4h for 10-14 days (many recommend following with Benzathine Pen G 2.4 million U IM qwk for 3 doses)

Child

• *Pneumococcal/streptococcal infections:* PO 25,000-90,000 U/kg/d in 3-6 divided doses
• *Rheumatic fever prophylaxis:* PO 25,000-90,000 U/kg/d in 3-6 divided doses; IV 100,000-250,000 U/kg/d in divided doses q4h

Infant (use larger doses for meningitis)

• >7 days and >2000 g, IV 100,000-200,000 U/kg/d in divided doses q6h
• >7 days and <2000 g, IV 75,000-150,000 U/kg/d in divided doses q8h
• <7 days and >2000 g, IV 50,000-150,000 U/kg/d in divided doses q8h
• <7 days and <2000 g, IV 50,000-100,000 U/kg/d in divided doses q12h

Pen V Potassium

Adult

• *Pneumococcal infections:* PO 250-500 mg q6h
• *Streptococcal infections:* 125-250 mg q6-8h for 10 days
• *Rheumatic fever prophylaxis:* PO 125-250 mg bid continuously

Child

• PO 15-50 mg/kg/d in divided doses q6h

Pen G Procaine

Adult

• *Moderate to severe infections:* IM 600,000-1.2 million U/d in divided doses
• *Gonorrhea:* IM 4.8 million U in two inj given 30 min after probenecid 1 g
• *Syphilis (primary, secondary, latent with neg CSF):* 600,000 U/d for 8 days
• *Neurosyphilis:* 2-4 million U/d with probenecid 500 mg qid for 10-14 days (many recommend following with benzathine Pen G 2.4 million U qwk for 3 doses)

Child

• *Moderate to severe infections:* Child same as adult; avoid in newborn (risk procaine toxicity, sterile abscess)
• *Congenital syphilis:* IM 50,000 U/kg qd for 10-14 days

Pen G Sodium

Adult

• *Moderate to severe infections:* IM/IV 12-30 million U/d in divided doses q4h
• *Endocarditis prophylaxis:* IM/IV 2 million U 30-60 min before dental procedure; 1 million U 6 hr after procedure

Child

• *Moderate to severe infections:* IM/IV 25,000-300,000 U/d in divided doses q4-12h

AVAILABLE FORMS/COST OF THERAPY

Benzathine/procaine combined

• Inj, Susp—IM: 150,000 unit/150,000 unit/ml, 10 ml: **$14.36;** 300,000 unit/300,000 unit/ml, 2 ml: **$9.96;** 900,000 unit/300,000 unit/2 ml, 2 ml: **$10.36**

Benzathime

• Inj, Susp—IM: 300,000 unit/ml, 10 ml: **$21.24;** 600,000 unit/ml, 1 ml: **$7.21**

Penicillin G Potassium

• Inj, Sol—IV: 1,000,000 U/vial, 10 ml: **$1.32;** 2,000,000 U/vial, 50 ml: **$13.52;** 3,000,000 U/vial, 50 ml: **$14.03;** 5,000,000 U/vial, 50 ml: **$4.00;** 10,000,000 U/vial, 50 ml: **$7.00;** 20,000,000 U/vial, 1 ml: **$7.57**

• Powder, Reconst—Oral: 200,000 U/5ml, 100 ml: **$1.90;** 400,000 U/5ml, 100 ml: **$2.46**

• Tab, Uncoated—Oral: 200,000 U, 100's: **$7.70;** 250,000 U, 100's: **$6.95-$8.78;** 400,000 U, 100's: **$7.50-$12.39;** 800,000 U, 100's: **$18.59**

Penicillin V Potassium

• Tab, Uncoated—Oral: 125 mg, 100's: **$10.86;** 250 mg, 100's: **$4.17-$41.70;** 500 mg, 100's: **$7.50-$87.95**

• Powder, Reconst—Oral: 125 mg/5 ml, 100 ml: **$1.21-$2.51;** 250 mg/5 ml, 100 ml: **$1.67-$5.07**

Penicillin G Procaine

• Inj, Sol—IM: 600,000 U/ml, 1 ml: **$2.90;** 300,000 U/ml, 10 ml: **$1.83**

Penicillin G Sodium

• Inj, Dry-Sol—IM; IV: 5,000,000 U/vial: **$6.60**

CONTRAINDICATIONS: Hypersensitivity to penicillins

PRECAUTIONS: Hypersensitivity to cephalosporins

PREGNANCY AND LACTATION: Pregnancy category B; may cause diarrhea, candidiasis, or allergic response in nursing infant

SIDE EFFECTS/ADVERSE REACTIONS

CNS: Lethargy, hallucinations, anxiety, depression, twitching, ***coma, convulsions***

GI: Nausea, vomiting, diarrhea, abdominal pain, glossitis, colitis

GU: ***Oliguria, proteinuria, hematuria,*** vaginitis, ***glomerulonephritis***

HEME: Anemia, increased bleeding time, ***bone marrow depression, granulocytopenia***

METAB: Hyperkalemia, hypokalemia, alkalosis, hypernatremia

SKIN: Rash

MISC: ***Anaphylaxis***

▼ DRUG INTERACTIONS

Drugs

• *Chloramphenicol:* May reduce bactericidal effect of penicillin

• *Methotrexate:* Increased methotrexate levels

• *Neomycin:* Oral, reduces absorption of oral penicillin

• *Tetracyclines:* Decreased penicillin efficacy

P

pentaerythritol tetranitrate

(pen-ta-er-ith'ri-tole teh-tra-nye'trate)

Duotrate, Duotrate 45, Pentylan, Peritrate, Peritrate SA, P.E.T.N

Chemical Class: Organic nitrate
Therapeutic Class: Antianginal

CLINICAL PHARMACOLOGY

Mechanism of Action: Relaxes vascular smooth muscle; the venous (capacitance) system is affected to a greater degree than arterial (resistance) system; venous pooling, decreased venous return to the heart (preload), and decreased arterial resistance (afterload) reduce intracardiac pressures and left ventricular size, thereby decreasing myocardial oxygen demand and ischemia; may also improve regional myocardial blood supply

Pharmacokinetics

PO: Onset 20-60 min, duration 4-5 hr (SR 12 hr), metabolized to active and inactive metabolites, excreted in urine and to lesser extent in feces

INDICATIONS AND USES: Long-term prophylactic management of angina pectoris

DOSAGE

Adult

• PO 10-20 mg tid-qid initially, titrate to 40 mg qid on an empty stomach; give in individualized doses up to 160 mg/d; PO SR 1 cap or tab q12h on an empty stomach

$ **AVAILABLE FORMS/COST OF THERAPY**

• Tab, Uncoated—Oral: 10 mg, 100's: **$16.02;** 20 mg, 100's: **$3.20-$21.18;** 40 mg, 100's: **$37.81**

• Tab, Uncoated, Sust Action—Oral: 80 mg, 100's: **$51.29**

• Cap, Sust Action—Oral: 45 mg, 100's: **$74.69**

CONTRAINDICATIONS: Hypersensitivity to nitrates, severe anemia, closed angle glaucoma, postural hypotension, head trauma or cerebral hemorrhage (may increase intracranial pressure)

PRECAUTIONS: Acute MI, hypertrophic cardiomyopathy, glaucoma, volume depletion, hypotension, abrupt withdrawal, continuous delivery without nitrate-free interval (tolerance will develop)

PREGNANCY AND LACTATION: Pregnancy category C

SIDE EFFECTS/ADVERSE REACTIONS

CNS: Headache, apprehension, restlessness, weakness, vertigo, *dizziness,* agitation, anxiety, confusion, insomnia, nervousness, nightmares, dyscoordination, hypoesthesia, hypokinesia

CV: Tachycardia, retrosternal discomfort, palpitations, hypotension (sometimes with paradoxical bradycardia and increased angina), syncope, ***collapse,*** crescendo angina, rebound hypertension, dysrhythmias, atrial fibrillation, premature ventricular contractions, *postural hypotension,* edema

EENT: Blurred vision, diplopia

GI: Nausea, vomiting, diarrhea, dyspepsia, involuntary passing of feces, abdominal pain, tenesmus, tooth disorder

GU: Dysuria, impotence, urinary frequency, involuntary passing of urine

HEME: ***Hemolytic anemia, methemoglobinemia***

MS: Arthralgia, muscle twitching

SKIN: Rash, exfoliative dermatitis, *flushing,* crusty skin lesions, pruritis, pallor, perspiration, cold sweat

▼ **DRUG INTERACTIONS**

Labs

• *Interference:* Serum cholesterol measured by Zlatkis-Zak color reaction

SPECIAL CONSIDERATIONS

PATIENT/FAMILY EDUCATION

• Headache may be a marker for drug activity

• Try to avoid headache by altering treatment schedule, contact physician if severe or persistent

• Aspirin or acetaminophen may be used for relief

• Do not crush or chew sustained release tablets before administering

• Avoid alcohol

• Make changes in position slowly to prevent fainting

pentamidine

(pen-tam'i-deen)

Pentam 300, Pentacarinat, ♣ NebuPent

Chemical Class: Aromatic diamidine derivative

Therapeutic Class: Antiprotozoal

CLINICAL PHARMACOLOGY

Mechanism of Action: Interferes with protozoal nuclear metabolism and inhibits RNA/DNA, phospholipid, and protein synthesis

Pharmacokinetics

INH: Systemic accumulation does not appear to occur

IM: Well absorbed

69% bound to plasma proteins, 33%-66% excreted in urine unchanged, $t_{1/2}$ 6.4-9.4 hr

INDICATIONS AND USES: Treatment of *Pneumocystis carinii* pneumonia (PCP) (inj); prevention of PCP in high-risk, HIV-infected patients with a history of ≥1 episode of PCP and/or peripheral CD4+ lymphocyte count ≤200/mm^3 (inhal); trypanosomiasis;* visceral leishmaniasis*

DOSAGE

Adult

- *Treatment:* IM/IV 4 mg/kg qd for 14 days (reduce dosage, use a longer infusion time, or extend dosing interval in renal failure)
- *Prevention:* INH 300 mg q4 wk via Respirgard II nebulizer by Marquest

Child

- *Treatment:* IM/IV 4 mg/kg qd for 10-14 days
- *Prevention:* IM/IV 4 mg/kg q2-4 wk; INH (≥5 yr) 300 mg q3 wk via Respirgard II nebulizer

$ AVAILABLE FORMS/COST OF THERAPY

- Aer—Inh: 300 mg, 1's: **$98.75**
- Inj, Sol—IV: 300 mg, 1's: **$98.75-$113.54**

CONTRAINDICATIONS: Hypersensitivity

PRECAUTIONS: Children (inh), hypertension, hypotension, hypoglycemia, hyperglycemia, hypocalcemia, leukopenia, thrombocytopenia, anemia, hepatic/renal dysfunction, ventricular tachycardia, pancreatitis, Stevens-Johnson syndrome

PREGNANCY AND LACTATION: Pregnancy category C; since aerosolized pentamidine results in very low systemic concentrations, fetal exposure to the drug is probably negligible; breast milk levels following aerosolized administration are likely nil

SIDE EFFECTS/ADVERSE REACTIONS

CNS: (Inj) Fever, confusion/hallucination, dizziness, neuralgia; (Inh) *Fatigue, dizziness, chills,* headache, tremors, confusion, anxiety, memory loss, seizure, neuropathy, paresthesia, insomnia, drowsiness, emotional lability, vertigo, paranoia, neuralgia, hallucination, depression, unsteady gait

CV: (Inj) Hypotension, ***ventricular tachycardia;*** (Inhal) *Chest pain/congestion, edema,* tachycardia, hypotension, hypertension, palpitations, syncope, ***CVA,*** vasodilation, vasculitis

EENT: (Inh) Eye discomfort, conjunctivitis, blurred vision, blepharitis, loss of taste/smell, *pharyngitis*

GI: (Inj) Nausea, anorexia, bad taste in mouth, diarrhea, elevated liver function tests; (Inh) *Nausea,* diarrhea, abdominal pain, gingivitis, dyspepsia, oral ulcer, gastritis, gastric ulcer, hypersalivation, dry mouth, splenomegaly, melena, hematochezia, esophagitis, colitis, ***pancreatitis, hepatitis, hepatomegaly, hepatic dysfunction***

P

GU: (Inj) *Increased serum creatinine;* ***renal failure,*** flank pain, nephritis
HEME: (Inj and inh) ***Leukopenia, thrombocytopenia, anemia***
METAB: (Inj) Hypoglycemia, hypocalcemia, hyperkalemia
MS: (Inh) Arthralgia, myalgia
RESP: (Inh) *Shortness of breath, cough,* ***bronchospasm,*** pneumothorax, hyperventilation, hemoptysis, pneumonitis, pleuritis, cyanosis, tachypnea, rales
SKIN: (Inj) ***Stevens-Johnson syndrome,*** rash, sterile abscess and pain at IM inj site; (Inh) Pruritis, erythema, dry skin, desquamation, urticaria, rash

SPECIAL CONSIDERATIONS

MONITORING PARAMETERS

- BUN, serum creatinine, blood glucose daily
- CBC and platelets, liver function tests, including bilirubin, alkaline phosphatase, AST and ALT, and serum calcium before, during, and after therapy
- ECG at regular intervals

---

pentazocine

(pen-taz'oh-seen)
Talwin, Talwin NX
Chemical Class: Synthetic opiate
Therapeutic Class: Narcotic analgesic
DEA Class: Schedule IV

CLINICAL PHARMACOLOGY

Mechanism of Action: Has analgesic and very weak opiate antagonistic effects; binds to opiate receptors in the CNS causing inhibition of ascending pain pathways, altering the perception of and response to pain; believed to be a competitive antagonist at μ opiate receptors and an agonist at κ and σ opiate receptors

Pharmacokinetics

PO: Onset 15-30 min, duration 4-5 hr
IM/SC: Onset 15-30 min, duration 2-3 hr
IV: Onset 2-3 min, duration 2-3 hr
61% bound to plasma proteins, large first-pass effect, metabolized in liver, eliminated mainly in urine, small amounts eliminated in feces, $t_{1/2}$ 2-3 hr (prolonged in hepatic failure)

INDICATIONS AND USES: Moderate to severe pain

DOSAGE

Adult

- PO 50 mg q3-4h prn, may increase to 100 mg/dose prn, do not exceed 600 mg/d; IM/SC 30-60 mg q3-4h prn, do not exceed 360 mg/d; IV 30 mg q3-4h prn, do not exceed 360 mg/d

Child

- PO (>12 yr) same as adult; IM/SC 5-8 yr 15 mg; 8-14 yr 30 mg

$ **AVAILABLE FORMS/COST OF THERAPY**

- Tab, Uncoated—Oral: 50 mg pentazocine/0.5 mg naloxone, 100's: **$83.08**
- Inj, Sol—IV; IM; SC: 30 mg/ml, 10 ml: **$31.49**

CONTRAINDICATIONS: Hypersensitivity

PRECAUTIONS: Head injury, increased intracranial pressure, acute abdominal conditions, elderly, severe impairment of hepatic or renal function, hypothyroidism, Addison's disease, prostatic hypertrophy, urethral stricture, history of drug abuse, impaired respiration, bronchial asthma, cyanosis, obstructive respiratory conditions, acute MI, chronic opiate use (may precipitate withdrawal symptoms), children

PREGNANCY AND LACTATION: Pregnancy category B (category D if used for prolonged periods or in high doses at term); use during labor may produce neonatal respiratory depression

SIDE EFFECTS/ADVERSE REACTIONS

CNS: Drowsiness, sedation, dizziness, euphoria, agitation, dependency, lethargy, restlessness

CV: Tachycardia, circulatory depression, ***shock,*** increased blood pressure

EENT: Blurred vision, nystagmus, diplopia, miosis

GI: Nausea, vomiting, anorexia, constipation

GU: Urinary retention

HEME: ***Leukopenia, granulocytopenia, eosinophilia***

RESP: ***Respiratory depression, respiratory paralysis***

SKIN: Flushing, rash, urticaria

▼ **DRUG INTERACTIONS**

Drugs

• *Smoking:* Increased dosage requirements for pentazocine

Labs

• *Increase:* Amylase

SPECIAL CONSIDERATIONS

• Naloxone 0.5 mg added to oral tablets to discourage misuse via parenteral inj

PATIENT/FAMILY EDUCATION

• Report any symptoms of CNS changes, allergic reactions
• Physical dependency may result when used for extended periods
• Change position slowly, orthostatic hypotension may occur
• Avoid hazardous activities if drowsiness or dizziness occurs
• Avoid alcohol, other CNS depressants unless directed by physician
• Minimize nausea by administering with food and lying down following dose

pentobarbital

(pen-toe-bar′bi-tal)

Nembutal, Nova-Rectal, ♣ Pentogen ♣

Chemical Class: Barbiturate (short-acting)

Therapeutic Class: Sedative/hypnotic; anticonvulsant

DEA Class: Schedule II (oral, parenteral), schedule III (rectal)

CLINICAL PHARMACOLOGY

Mechanism of Action: Depresses activity in brain cells primarily in reticular activating system in brain stem; also selectively depresses neurons in posterior hypothalamus, limbic structures; able to decrease seizure activity in subhypnotic doses by inhibition of impulses in CNS

Pharmacokinetics

PO: Onset 15-60 min, peak 30-60 min, duration 1-4 hr

IM: Onset 10-25 min

IV: Onset 1 min, duration 15 min

35%-45% bound to plasma proteins, metabolized in liver, excreted in urine (metabolites), $t_{1/2}$ 22-50 hr

INDICATIONS AND USES: Insomnia (short-term), status epilepticus, facilitation of intubation and anesthesia, increased intracranial pressure,* cerebral ischemia*

DOSAGE

Adult

• *Hypnotic:* PO 100-200 mg hs or 20 mg tid-qid for daytime sedation; IM 150-200 mg; IV 100 mg initially, may repeat q1-3 min up to 200-500 mg total; PR 120-200 mg hs
• *Preoperative sedation:* IM 150-200 mg
• *Pentobarbital coma for increased intracranial pressure:* IV 10-15 mg/kg over 1-2 hr loading dose,

then 1 mg/kg/hr inf, increase to 2-3 mg/kg/hr if necessary; maintain burst suppression on EEG

Child

• *Sedative:* PO 2-6 mg/kg/d divided tid; max 100 mg/d

• *Hypnotic:* IM 2-6 mg/kg; max 100 mg/dose; PR <4 yr 3-6 mg/kg/dose, >4 yr 1.5-3 mg/kg/dose

• *Preoperative sedation:* PO/IM/PR 2-6 mg/kg; max 100 mg/dose; IV 1-3 mg/kg to a max of 100 mg until asleep

• *Pentobarbital coma for increased intracranial pressure:* Same as adult

$ AVAILABLE FORMS/COST OF THERAPY

• Cap, Gel—Oral: 50 mg, 100's: **$33.31;** 100 mg, 100's: **$52.16**

• Elixir—Oral: 20 mg/5 ml, 480 ml: **$64.74**

• Supp—Rect: 30 mg, 12's: **$41.46;** 60 mg, 12's: **$48.65;** 120 mg, 12's: **$54.24;** 200 mg, 12's: **$66.69**

• Inj, Sol—IM; IV: 50 mg/ml, 2 ml: **$2.21-$25.89**

CONTRAINDICATIONS: Hypersensitivity to barbiturates, respiratory depression, addiction to barbiturates, severe liver impairment, porphyria, nephritic patients

PRECAUTIONS: Myasthenia gravis, myxedema, anemia, hepatic disease, renal disease, hypertension, elderly, acute/chronic pain, mental depression, history of drug abuse, abrupt discontinuation, children, hyperthyroidism, fever, diabetes

PREGNANCY AND LACTATION: Pregnancy category D; excreted in breast milk, effect on nursing infant unknown

SIDE EFFECTS/ADVERSE REACTIONS

CNS: Lethargy, drowsiness, hangover, dizziness, stimulation in the elderly and children, light-headedness, physical dependence, CNS depression, mental depression, slurred speech, vertigo, headache

CV: Hypotension, bradycardia

GI: Nausea, vomiting, diarrhea, constipation

HEME: ***Agranulocytosis, thrombocytopenia, megaloblastic anemia*** (long-term treatment)

RESP: ***Depression, apnea, laryngospasm, bronchospasm***

SKIN: Rash, urticaria, erythema multiforme, pain, abscesses at inj site, ***angioedema,*** thrombophlebitis, ***Stevens-Johnson syndrome***

MISC: Rickets, osteomalacia (prolonged use)

▼ DRUG INTERACTIONS

Drugs

• *Acetaminophen:* Enhanced hepatotoxic potential of acetaminophen overdoses.

• *Antidepressants, disopyramide, doxycycline, quinidine, theophylline:* Reduced serum concentrations

• *Beta blockers:* Reduced serum concentrations of beta blockers which are extensively metabolized

• *Calcium channel blockers:* Reduced concentrations of verapamil and nifedipine

• *Chloramphenicol:* Increased barbiturate concentrations; reduced serum chloramphenicol concentrations

• *CNS depressants, ethanol:* Excessive CNS depression

• *Corticosteroids:* Reduced serum concentrations of corticosteroids, may impair therapeutic effect

• *MAOIs:* Prolonged effect of some barbiturates

• *Methoxyflurane:* Enhanced nephrotoxic effect

• *Narcotic analgesics:* Increased toxicity of meperidine; reduced effect of methadone; additive CNS depression

• *Neuroleptics:* Reduced effect of either drug

• *Oral anticoagulants+:* Inhibited hypoprothrombinemic response to oral anticoagulants
• *Oral contraceptives:* Reduced efficacy of oral contraceptives

SPECIAL CONSIDERATIONS

PATIENT/FAMILY EDUCATION

• Avoid driving or other activities requiring alertness
• Avoid alcohol ingestion or CNS depressants
• Do not discontinue medication abruptly after long-term use
• Notify physician of fever, sore throat, mouth sores, easy bruising or bleeding, tiny broken blood vessels under skin

MONITORING PARAMETERS

• Periodic CBC, liver and renal function tests, serum folate, vitamin D during prolonged therapy

---

pentoxifylline

(pen-tox'i-fi-leen)

Trental

Chemical Class: Dimethylxanthine derivative

Therapeutic Class: Hemorheologic agent

CLINICAL PHARMACOLOGY

Mechanism of Action: Exact mechanism unknown; thought to improve blood flow by decreasing blood viscosity and improving erythrocyte flexibility; increases blood flow to affected microcirculation, enhancing tissue oxygenation

Pharmacokinetics

PO: Peak 1 hr, undergoes first-pass metabolism in liver to active metabolites, excreted mainly in urine (95%) and feces (5%), $t_{1/2}$ 24-48 min (metabolites 60-96 min)

INDICATIONS AND USES: Intermittant claudication, cerebrovascular insufficiency,* diabetic angiopathies and neuropathies,* transient ischemic attack,* leg ulcers,* sickle cell thalassemias,* stroke,* high-altitude sickness,* asthenozoospermia,* acute and chronic hearing disorders,* eye circulation disorders,* Raynaud's phenomenon*

DOSAGE

Adult

• PO 400 mg tid with meals, decrease to 400 mg bid if GI and CNS side effects occur

$ AVAILABLE FORMS/COST OF THERAPY

• Tab, Coated, Sust Action—Oral: 400 mg, 100's: **$56.55**

CONTRAINDICATIONS: Hypersensitivity to methylxanthines (i.e., caffeine, theophylline, theobromine)

PRECAUTIONS: Impaired renal function, children, chronic occlusive arterial disease of limbs

PREGNANCY AND LACTATION: Pregnancy category C; excreted in breast milk

SIDE EFFECTS/ADVERSE REACTIONS

CNS: Dizziness, headache, tremor, anxiety, confusion

CV: Angina/chest pain, edema, hypotension, dyspnea

EENT: Epistaxis, laryngitis, nasal congestion, blurred vision, conjunctivitis, scotomata, earache, sore throat, swollen neck glands

GI: Dyspepsia, nausea, vomiting, belching, flatus, bloating, anorexia, cholecystitis, constipation, dry mouth, thirst, bad taste, excessive salivation

HEME: ***Leukopenia***

SKIN: Brittle fingernails, pruritus, rash, urticaria

MISC: Malaise, weight change

▼ DRUG INTERACTIONS

Drugs

• *Theophylline:* Increased plasma theophylline concentrations

P

SPECIAL CONSIDERATIONS

PATIENT/FAMILY EDUCATION

- Therapeutic effect may require 2-4 wk

pergolide

(per'go-lide)

Permax

Chemical Class: Ergot derivative

Therapeutic Class: Antiparkinsonian agent

CLINICAL PHARMACOLOGY

Mechanism of Action: Potent dopamine receptor agonist at both D_1 and D_2 receptor sites; directly stimulates postsynaptic dopamine receptors in nigrostriatal system

Pharmacokinetics

PO: 90% bound to plasma proteins, metabolized to at least 10 metabolites (some with dopamine agonist activity), excreted by kidney

INDICATIONS AND USES: Parkinson's disease (adjunct to levodopa/carbidopa)

DOSAGE

Adult

- PO 0.05 mg qd for first 2 days; increase gradually by 0.1 or 0.15 mg/d every 3rd day over next 12 days; subsequent increases by 0.25 mg/d every 3rd day until optimal therapeutic response obtained; divide total daily dose tid; doses >5 mg/day have not been systematically evaluated

$ AVAILABLE FORMS/COST OF THERAPY

- Tab, Uncoated—Oral: 0.05 mg, 30's: **$12.13;** 0.25 mg, 100's: **$84.03;** 1 mg, 100's: **$278.99**

CONTRAINDICATIONS: Hypersensitivity to ergot derivatives

PRECAUTIONS: Hypotension, children, cardiac dysrhythmia, preexisting dyskinesia; coadministration with drugs affecting protein binding

PREGNANCY AND LACTATION: Pregnancy category B; may interfere with lactation

SIDE EFFECTS/ADVERSE REACTIONS

CNS: Dyskinesia, dizziness, hallucination, dystonia, confusion, somnolence, *insomnia,* anxiety, personality disorder, psychosis, akathisia, incoordination,

CV: Postural hypotension, vasodilation, palpitation, hypotension, syncope, hypertension, peripheral edema

EENT: Rhinitis, epistaxis

GI: Nausea, constipation, diarrhea, *dyspepsia,* anorexia, dry mouth

GU: Hematuria

RESP: Dyspnea, hiccoughs, abnormal vision

SKIN: Rash

MISC: Pain

SPECIAL CONSIDERATIONS

PATIENT/FAMILY EDUCATION

- Be aware of risk for hypotension

permethrin

(per-meth'ren)

Elimite, Nix

Chemical Class: Synthetic pyrethroid

Therapeutic Class: Pediculicide; scabicide

CLINICAL PHARMACOLOGY

Mechanism of Action: Acts on parasite nerve cell membranes; disrupts sodium channel current, delays repolarization and paralyzes pest

Pharmacokinetics

TOP: Less than 2% of amount applied systemically absorbed, rapidly metabolized to inactive metabolites, excreted in urine, residual detectable on hair for at least 10 days following single application

INDICATIONS AND USES: Single application treatment of infestation with *Pediculus humanus capitis* (head louse) and its nits, or *Sarcoptes scabiei* (scabies)

DOSAGE

Adult and Child

- *Head lice:* TOP after hair has been shampooed, rinsed, and towel dried, apply sufficient volume of liquid to saturate hair and scalp; leave on hair for 10 min before rinsing with water; remove remaining nits; may repeat in 1 wk if necessary (1 application generally sufficient)
- *Scabies:* TOP apply cream from head to toe; leave on for 8-14 hr before washing off with water; may repeat in 1 wk if live mites reappear

$ AVAILABLE FORMS/COST OF THERAPY

- Cre—Top: 5%, 60 g: **$17.09**
- Liq—Top: 1%, 60 ml: **$11.63**

CONTRAINDICATIONS: Hypersensitivity to chrysanthememus, or any synthetic pyrethroid or pyrethrin

PRECAUTIONS: Children <2 months

PREGNANCY AND LACTATION: Pregnancy category B

SIDE EFFECTS/ADVERSE REACTIONS

SKIN: Pruritus (difficult to distinguish from infestation itself), transient burning/stinging, tingling, numbness, transient erythema, rash, edema

SPECIAL CONSIDERATIONS

PATIENT/FAMILY EDUCATION

- For external use only
- Avoid contact with eyes, mucous membranes
- Itching, redness, or swelling of scalp may occur
- Notify physician if irritation persists
- Itching may be temporarily aggravated following application
- Do not repeat administration sooner than 1 wk
- Itching may persist for several weeks even though infestation is cured

---

perphenazine

(per-fen'a-zeen)

Apo-Perphenazine, ♣ Phenazine, ♣ Trilafon

Chemical Class: Piperazine phenothiazine derivative

Therapeutic Class: Antipsychotic/neuroleptic; antiemetic

CLINICAL PHARMACOLOGY

Mechanism of Action: Blocks postsynaptic dopamine receptors in the basal ganglia, hypothalamus, limbic system, brain stem and medulla; appears to act at both D_1 and D_2 receptors; also exerts anticholinergic and α-adrenergic blocking effects

Pharmacokinetics

PO: Onset ½-1 hr, peak 4-8 hr

IM: Onset 10 min, peak 1-2 hr, duration 6 hr

90% bound to plasma proteins, metabolized in liver, excreted in urine and bile, $t_{1/2}$ 9 hr

INDICATIONS AND USES: Psychotic disorders, severe nausea and vomiting, intractable hiccoughs, hemiballismus*

DOSAGE

Adult

- *Psychosis:* PO 4-16 mg bid-qid; do not exceed 64 mg/d; IM 5 mg q6h up to 15 mg/d in ambulatory patients, 30 mg/d in hospitalized patients
- *Nausea/vomiting:* PO 8-16 mg/d in divided doses up to 24 mg/d; IM 5-10 mg q6h up to 15 mg/d in ambulatory patients, 30 mg/d in hos-

P

pitalized patients; IV 1 mg at 1-2 min intervals up to 5 mg total

Child

• Not established <12 yrs. Use lowest adult dose >12 yrs

• *Nausea/vomiting:* IM 5 mg q6h

$ AVAILABLE FORMS/COST OF THERAPY

• Tab, Coated—Oral: 2 mg, 100's: **$30.75-$45.50;** 4 mg, 100's: **$41.93-$87.42;** 8 mg, 100's: **$50.25-$106.08;** 16 mg, 100's: **$69.00-$142.73**

• Liq—Oral: 16 mg/5 ml, 120 ml: **$36.40**

• Inj, Sol—IM; IV: 5 mg/ml, 1 ml: **$5.42**

CONTRAINDICATIONS: Hypersensitivity to phenothiazines, severe toxic CNS depression, coma, subcortical brain damage, bone marrow depression

PRECAUTIONS: Children <12 yr, elderly, prolonged use, severe cardiovascular disorders, epilepsy, hepatic or renal disease, glaucoma, prostatic hypertrophy, severe asthma, emphysema, hypocalcemia (increased susceptibility to dystonic reactions)

PREGNANCY AND LACTATION: Pregnancy category C; has been used as an antiemetic during normal labor without producing any observable effect on newborn; excreted into human breast milk, effects on nursing infant unknown, but may be of concern

SIDE EFFECTS/ADVERSE REACTIONS

CNS: EPS (pseudoparkinsonism, akathisia, dystonia, ***tardive dyskinesia****), drowsiness, headache,* ***seizures, neuroleptic malignant syndrome,*** confusion, insomnia, restlessness, anxiety, euphoria, agitation, depression, lethargy, vertigo, exacerbation of psychotic symptoms including hallucinations, catatonic-like behavioral states, heat or cold intolerance

CV: ***Tachycardia,*** hypotension, hypertension, ECG changes

EENT: Blurred vision, glaucoma, dry eyes, cataracts, retinopathy, pigmentation of retina or cornea

GI: Anorexia, constipation, diarrhea, hypersalivation, dyspepsia, *nausea,* vomiting, *dry mouth*

GU: Urinary retention, priapism

HEME: Transient leukopenia, leukocytosis, minimal decreases in red blood cell counts, anemia, ***agranulocytosis, aplastic anemia, hemolytic anemia***

METAB: Lactation, breast engorgement, mastalgia, menstrual irregularities, gynecomastia, impotence, increased libido, hyperglycemia, hypoglycemia, hyponatremia

RESP: Laryngospasm, bronchospasm, increased depth of respiration

SKIN: Maculopapular and acneiform skin reactions, photosensitivity, loss of hair, diaphoresis

▼ DRUG INTERACTIONS

Drugs

• *Anticholinergics:* Inhibited therapeutic response to antipsychotic; enhanced anticholinergic side effects

• *Antidepressants:* Increased serum concentrations of some cyclic antidepressants

• *Barbiturates:* Reduced effect of antipsychotic

• *Beta blockers:* Enhanced effects of both drugs

• *Bromocriptine, lithium:* Reduced effects of both drugs

• *Epinephrine:* Reversed pressor response to epinephrine

• *Guanethidine+:* Inhibited antihypertensive response to guanethidine

• *Levodopa:* Inhibited effect of levodopa on Parkinsons disease

• *Narcotic analgesics:* Excessive

CNS depression, hypotension, respiratory depression
• *Orphenadrine:* Reduced serum neuroleptic concentrations, excessive anticholinergic effects
Labs
• *Increase:* Liver function tests, cardiac enzymes, cholesterol, blood glucose, prolactin, bilirubin, PBI, cholinesterase, ^{131}I
• *Decrease:* Hormones (blood, urine)
• *False positive:* Pregnancy tests, PKU
• *False negative:* Urinary steroids, 17-OHCS

SPECIAL CONSIDERATIONS

PATIENT/FAMILY EDUCATION
• Contact physician if sore throat or other signs of infection
• Arise slowly from reclining position
• Do not discontinue abruptly
• Use a sunscreen during sun exposure to prevent burns, take special precautions to stay cool in hot weather
• Concentrate may be diluted just prior to administration with distilled water, acidified tap water, orange or grape juice
• May cause drowsiness

MONITORING PARAMETERS
• Observe closely for signs of tardive dyskinesia
• Periodic CBC with platelets during prolonged therapy

phenacemide

(fe-nass'e-mide)
Phenurone
Chemical Class: Substituted acetylurea derivative
Therapeutic Class: Anticonvulsant

CLINICAL PHARMACOLOGY
Mechanism of Action: Stabilizes neuronal membranes and decreases seizure activity by increasing efflux or decreasing influx of sodium ions across cell membranes in the motor cortex during generation of nerve impulses
Pharmacokinetics
PO: Duration 5 hr, metabolized in liver, excreted by kidneys

INDICATIONS AND USES: Severe epilepsy, particularly mixed forms of complex partial (psychomotor) seizures refractory to other drugs

DOSAGE
May produce serious toxic effects, keep dosage at minimum amount necessary to achieve adequate therapeutic effect
Adult
• PO 500 mg tid initially, increase by 500 mg at weekly intervals if seizures uncontrolled and drug is well tolerated; do not exceed 5 g/d
Child (5-10 yr)
• PO ½ the adult dose at the same intervals; do not exceed 1.5 g/d

$ **AVAILABLE FORMS/COST OF THERAPY**
• Tab, Uncoated—Oral: 500 mg, 100's: **$52.86**

CONTRAINDICATIONS: Hypersensitivity

PRECAUTIONS: Personality disorder, hepatic function impairment, children <5yr, history of allergies

PREGNANCY AND LACTATION: Pregnancy category D; can cause fetal harm

SIDE EFFECTS/ADVERSE REACTIONS
CNS: Drowsiness, headache, insomnia, dizziness, paresthesias, *psychic changes*
CV: Palpitations
GI: GI disturbance, anorexia, weight loss, ***hepatitis***
GU: Abnormal urinary findings, ***nephritis***

HEME: ***Leukopenia, aplastic anemia***
MS: Muscle pain
SKIN: Rash
MISC: Fatigue, fever

SPECIAL CONSIDERATIONS

PATIENT/FAMILY EDUCATION

- Notify physician of jaundice, abdominal pain, pale stools, darkened urine, fever, sore throat, mouth sores, unusual bleeding or bruising, loss of appetite, skin rash
- May produce dizziness or drowsiness
- Use caution driving or performing other tasks requiring alertness
- Report personality changes
- Do not discontinue abruptly

MONITORING PARAMETERS

- CBC at baseline and monthly thereafter
- Urinalysis at regular intervals
- Liver function tests at baseline and at regular intervals

---

phenazopyridine

(fen-az'o-peer'i-deen)

Azo-Standard, Baridium, Eridium, Geridium, Phenazo, ✤ Phenazodine, Pyridiate, Pyridium, Urodine, Urogesic

Chemical Class: Azo dye
Therapeutic Class: Urinary tract analgesic

CLINICAL PHARMACOLOGY

Mechanism of Action: Exerts topical analgesic effect on urinary tract mucosa

Pharmacokinetics

PO: Rapidly excreted by kidneys, 65% excreted unchanged in urine

INDICATIONS AND USES: Symptomatic relief of urinary burning, itching, frequency, and urgency associated with UTI, or following urologic procedures

DOSAGE

Adult

- PO 100-200 mg tid after meals; do not exceed 2 days when used concomitantly with antibacterial agents for UTI

Child

- PO 12 mg/kg/d divided tid after meals

$ AVAILABLE FORMS/COST OF THERAPY

- Tab, Coated—Oral: 95 mg, 180's: **$30.63;** 100 mg, 100's: **$5.50-$52.76;** 200 mg, 100's: **$6.55-$101.69**

CONTRAINDICATIONS: Hypersensitivity, renal insufficiency

PRECAUTIONS: Chronic use in undiagnosed urinary tract pain, children <12 yr

PREGNANCY AND LACTATION: Pregnancy category B

SIDE EFFECTS/ADVERSE REACTIONS

CNS: Headache
EENT: Yellowish tinge of sclera, staining of contact lenses
GI: GI disturbances, ***jaundice, hepatitis***
GU: Orange-red discoloration of urine, ***transient acute renal failure,*** renal stones
HEME: ***Methemoglobinemia, hemolytic anemia***
SKIN: Rash, pruritus, yellowish tinge of skin
MISC: ***Anaphylactoid-like reaction***

▼ DRUG INTERACTIONS

Labs

- *Interference:* Urinalysis based on spectrometry or color reactions

SPECIAL CONSIDERATIONS

PATIENT/FAMILY EDUCATION

- May cause GI upset
- Take after meals
- May cause reddish-orange discoloration of urine, may stain fabric, may also stain contact lenses

phendimetrazine

(fen-dye-me'tra-zeen)

Adipost, Adphen, Anorex, Bacarate, Bontril PDM, Dyrexan-OD, Melfiat, Metra, Obalan, Obeval, Phenzine, Plegine, Prelu-2, Slyn-LL, Statobex, Trimcaps, Trimstat, Trimtabs, Wehless, Weightrol,

Chemical Class: Amphetamine congener

Therapeutic Class: Anorexiant

DEA Class: Schedule III

CLINICAL PHARMACOLOGY

Mechanism of Action: Acts on adrenergic and dopaminergic pathways, directly stimulating the satiety center in the hypothalamic and limbic regions

Pharmacokinetics

PO: Onset 30 min, peak 1-3 hr, duration 4-20 hr, metabolized by liver, excreted by kidneys, $t_{1/2}$ 2-10 hr

INDICATIONS AND USES: Exogenous obesity (as a short-term adjunct to caloric restriction)

DOSAGE

Adult

• PO 35 mg bid-tid, 1 hr ac, not to exceed 70 mg tid; PO SR 105 mg QAM before breakfast

$ **AVAILABLE FORMS/COST OF THERAPY**

• Cap, Gel—Oral: 35 mg, 1000's: **$19.00-$53.00**

• Cap, Gel, Sust Rel—Oral: 105 mg, 1000's: **$75.00-$350.00**

• Tab, Uncoated—Oral: 35 mg, 1000's: **$15.75-$110.30**

CONTRAINDICATIONS: Diabetes mellitus, convulsive disorders, mild hypertension, children, hypersensitivity to sympathomimetic amines, glaucoma, history of drug abuse, cardiovascular disease, moderate to severe hypertension, advanced arteriosclerosis, agitated states, hyperthyroidism, within 14 days of MAOI administration

PRECAUTIONS: Diabetes mellitus, convulsive disorders, mild hypertension, children

PREGNANCY AND LACTATION: Pregnancy category C

SIDE EFFECTS/ADVERSE REACTIONS

CNS: Overstimulation, nervousness, restlessness, dizziness, insomnia, dysphoria, headache, mental depression, drowsiness, weakness, tremor, shivering, exacerbation of schizophrenia

CV: Palpitation, ***tachycardia,*** chest pain

GI: Dry mouth, nausea, constipation, diarrhea, unpleasant taste

GU: Urinary hesitancy, impotence, testicular pain

SKIN: Rash, excessive sweating, clamminess, pallor

▼ **DRUG INTERACTIONS**

Drugs

• *MAOIs:* Hypertensive crisis

SPECIAL CONSIDERATIONS

PATIENT/FAMILY EDUCATION

• May cause insomnia, avoid taking late in the day

• Weight reduction requires strict adherence to caloric restriction

• Notify physician if palpitations, nervousness, or dizziness occur

• Use caution while driving or performing other tasks requiring alertness, may cause dizziness or blurred vision

• Do not discontinue abruptly

P

phenelzine

(fen′el-zeen)

Nardil

Chemical Class: Hydrazine derivative

Therapeutic Class: Monoamine oxidase (MAO) inhibitor antidepressant

CLINICAL PHARMACOLOGY

Mechanism of Action: Inhibit the activity of MAO resulting in increased endogenous concentrations of serotonin, norepinephrine, epinephrine, and dopamine in the CNS; chronic administration results in down regulation (desensitization) of α_2- or β-adrenergic and serotonin receptors which may correlate with antidepressant activity

Pharmacokinetics

PO: Onset of action 4-8 wk, duration of MAO inhibition at least 10 days, peak serum concentration 2-4 hr, metabolized in liver, excreted in urine as metabolites and unchanged drug

INDICATIONS AND USES: Treatment-resistant depression, including patients characterized as atypical, nonendogenous, or neurotic

DOSAGE

Adult

- PO 15 mg tid initially, increase as tolerated to 60-90 mg/d; following achievement of maximal benefit, reduce dosage slowly over several weeks to lowest effective dose that maintains response

$ AVAILABLE FORMS/COST OF THERAPY

- Tab, Sugar Coated—Oral: 15 mg, 100's: **$40.24**

CONTRAINDICATIONS: Hypersensitivity, pheochromocytoma, congestive heart failure, liver disease, severe renal function impairment, cerebrovascular defect, cardiovascular disease, hypertension, history of headache, age >60 yr

PRECAUTIONS: Children <16 yr, hypotension, bipolar affective disorder, agitation, schizophrenia, hyperactivity, diabetes mellitus, seizure disorder, angina, hyperthyroidism, suicidal ideation

PREGNANCY AND LACTATION: Pregnancy category C

SIDE EFFECTS/ADVERSE REACTIONS

CNS: Dizziness, vertigo, headache, overactivity, hyperreflexia, tremors, muscle twitching, mania, hypomania, jitteriness, confusion, memory impairment, sleep disturbance, weakness, myoclonic movements, fatigue, *drowsiness,* restlessness, overstimulation, agitation, akathisia, ataxia, coma, euphoria, neuritis, palilalia, chills, seizures

CV: Edema, palpitations, tachycardia, *orthostatic hypotension,* ***hypertension, dysrhythmias***

EENT: Blurred vision, glaucoma, nystagmus

GI: Constipation, nausea, diarrhea, abdominal pain, dry mouth, elevated transaminases, anorexia, black tongue, hepatitis

GU: Dysuria, incontinence, urinary retention, sexual disturbance

HEME: Anemia, ***agranulocytosis, thrombocytopenia,*** spider telangiectases

METAB: ***Hypernatremia,*** hypermetabolic syndrome, ***SIADH-like syndrome***

SKIN: Hyperhydrosis, rash, photosensitivity

MISC: Weight gain

▼ DRUG INTERACTIONS

Drugs

- *Amphetamines,+ ephedrine,+ alcoholic beverages containing ty-*

ramine, levodopa, metaraminol,+ phenylephrine,+ phenylpropanolamine,+ pseudoephedrine,+ tyramine: Severe hypertensive reaction
- *Antidepressants:* Excessive sympathetic response, mania, hyperpyrexia
- *Barbiturates:* Prolonged effect of some barbiturates
- *Dextromethorphan, meperidine+:* Agitation, blood pressure changes, hyperpyrexia, convulsions)
- *Fluoxetine,+ sertraline+:* Hypomania, confusion, hypertension, tremor
- *Food+:* Foods containing large amounts of tyramine can result in hypertensive reactions
- *Insulin:* Excessive hypoglycemia
- *Lithium:* Malignant hyperpyrexia
- *Neuromuscular blocking agents:* Prolonged muscle relaxation caused by succinylcholine
- *Sumatriptan:* Increased sumatriptan plasma concentrations

SPECIAL CONSIDERATIONS

PATIENT/FAMILY EDUCATION

- Do not discontinue or alter dosage without consulting physician
- Avoid tyramine-containing foods, beverages, and certain OTC products
- May cause drowsiness, dizziness, blurred vision
- Use caution driving or performing other tasks requiring alertness
- Arise slowly from reclining position
- Therapeutic effect may require 4-8 wk
- Notify physician of severe headache, rash, darkening of urine, pale stools, jaundice

phenobarbital

(fee-noe-bar'bi-tal)

Barbita, Luminal, Solfoton

Chemical Class: Barbiturate (long-acting)

Therapeutic Class: Sedative/ hypnotic; anticonvulsant

DEA Class: Schedule IV

CLINICAL PHARMACOLOGY

Mechanism of Action: Depresses activity in brain cells primarily in reticular activating system in brain stem; also selectively depresses neurons in posterior hypothalamus, limbic structures; able to decrease seizure activity in subhypnotic doses by inhibition of impulses in CNS

Pharmacokinetics

PO: Onset 20-60 min, peak 1-6 hr, duration 6-10 hr

IV: Onset within 5 min, peak effect within 30 min, duration 4-10 hr

20%-50% bound to plasma proteins, metabolized in liver, excreted in urine (20%-50% unchanged), $t_{1/2}$ 53-140 hr (prolonged in overdose)

INDICATIONS AND USES: Routine and preoperative sedation, tonic-clonic (grand mal) seizures, partial seizures, prevention of febrile seizures (controversial), status epilepticus (not first line), neonatal hyperbilirubinemia,* congenital nonhemolytic unconjugated hyperbilirubinemia,* chronic intrahepatic cholestasis*

DOSAGE

Adult

- *Anticonvulsant:* PO/IV 1-3 mg/kg/d in divided doses or 50-100 mg bid-tid
- *Status epilepticus:* IV 300-800 mg initially followed by 120-240 mg at 20 min intervals until seizures are controlled or a total dose of 1-2 g

P

• *Sedation:* PO/IM 30-120 mg/d in 2-3 divided doses
• *Hypnotic:* PO/IM/IV/SC 100-320 mg/kg hs
• *Preoperative sedation:* IM 100-200 mg 1-1½ hr before procedure

Child

• *Anticonvulsant:* PO/IV neonates 2-4 mg/kg/d in 1-2 divided doses; infants 5-8 mg/kg/d in 1-2 divided doses; 1-5 yr 6-8 mg/kg/d in 1-2 divided doses; 5-12 yr 4-6 mg/kg/d in 1-2 divided doses
• *Status epilepticus:* IV neonates 15-20 mg/kg in a single or divided dose; infants and children 10-20 mg/kg in a single or divided dose, may give additional 5 mg/kg/dose q15-30 min until seizure is controlled or a total dose of 40 mg/kg is reached
• *Sedation:* PO 2 mg/kg tid
• *Hypnotic:* IM/IV/SC 3-5 mg/kg hs
• *Preoperative sedation:* PO/IM/IV 1-3 mg/kg 1-1½ hr before procedure

$ AVAILABLE FORMS/COST OF THERAPY

• Inj, Sol—IM; IV: 30 mg/ml, 1 ml: **$2.12-$2.50;** 60 mg/ml, 1 ml: **$0.93-$2.74;** 130 mg/ml, 1 ml: **$1.10-$3.18**
• Tab, Uncoated—Oral: 15, 30, 60, 100 mg, 100's: **$2.66-$6.25**
• Cap, Gel—Oral: 16 mg, 100's: **$10.50**
• Elixir—Oral: 20 mg/5 ml, 480 ml: **$4.00-$11.13**

CONTRAINDICATIONS: Hypersensitivity to barbiturates, respiratory depression, addiction to barbiturates, severe liver impairment, porphyria, nephritic patients

PRECAUTIONS: Myasthenia gravis, myxedema, anemia, hepatic disease, renal disease, hypertension, elderly, acute/chronic pain, mental depression, history of drug abuse, abrupt discontinuation, children, hyperthyroidism, fever, diabetes

PREGNANCY AND LACTATION: Pregnancy category D; risks to fetus include minor congenital defects, hemorrhage at birth, addiction; risk to mother may be greater if seizure control is lost due to stopping drug; use at lowest possible level to control seizures; excreted into breast milk, has caused major adverse effects in some nursing infants, use caution in nursing women

SIDE EFFECTS/ADVERSE REACTIONS

CNS: Lethargy, drowsiness, hangover, dizziness, stimulation in the elderly and children, light-headedness, physical dependence, CNS depression, mental depression, slurred speech, vertigo, headache
CV: Hypotension, bradycardia
GI: Nausea, vomiting, diarrhea, constipation
HEME: ***Agranulocytosis, thrombocytopenia, megaloblastic anemia*** (long-term treatment)
RESP: ***Depression, apnea, laryngospasm, bronchospasm***
SKIN: Rash, urticaria, erythema multiforme, pain, abscesses at injection site, ***angioedema,*** thrombophlebitis, ***Stevens-Johnson syndrome***
MISC: Rickets, osteomalacia (prolonged use)

▼ DRUG INTERACTIONS

Drugs

• *Acetaminophen:* Enhanced hepatotoxic potential of acetaminophen overdoses
• *Antidepressants, disopyramide, doxycycline, quinidine, theophylline:* Reduced serum concentrations of these drugs
• *Beta blockers:* Reduced serum concentrations of beta blockers which are extensively metabolized
• *Calcium channel blockers:* Re-

duced concentrations of verapamil and nifedipine
• *Chloramphenicol:* Increased barbiturate concentrations; reduced serum chloramphenicol concentrations
• *CNS depressants, ethanol:* Excessive CNS depression
• *Corticosteroids:* Reduced serum concentrations of corticosteroids, may impair therapeutic effect
• *MAOIs:* Prolonged effect of some barbiturates
• *Methoxyflurane:* Enhanced nephrotoxic effect
• *Narcotic analgesics:* Increased toxicity of meperidine; reduced effect of methadone; additive CNS depression
• *Neuroleptics:* Reduced effect of either drug
• *Oral anticoagulants+:* Inhibited hypoprothrombinemic response to oral anticoagulants
• *Oral contraceptives:* Reduced efficacy of oral contraceptives
• *Valproic acid:* Increased serum phenobarbital concentrations

SPECIAL CONSIDERATIONS

PATIENT/FAMILY EDUCATION
• Avoid driving or other activities requiring alertness
• Avoid alcohol ingestion or CNS depressants
• Do not discontinue medication abruptly after long-term use
• Notify physician if fever, sore throat, mouth sores, easy bruising or bleeding, tiny broken blood vessels under skin

MONITORING PARAMETERS
• Periodic CBC, liver and renal function tests, serum folate, vitamin D during prolonged therapy
• Serum phenobarbital concentration (therapeutic range for seizure disorders 20-40 μg/ml)

phenoxybenzamine

(fen-ox-ee-ben′za-meen)
Dibenzyline
Chemical Class: Haloalkylamine
Therapeutic Class: Sympatholytic

CLINICAL PHARMACOLOGY
Mechanism of Action: Irreversible pre- and postsynaptic α-adrenergic receptor blocking agent; produces and maintains "chemical sympathectomy;" increases blood flow to skin, mucosa and abdominal viscera; lowers both supine and standing blood pressure
Pharmacokinetics
PO: Onset gradual over several hours, duration 3-4 days, metabolized via dealkylation, excreted in urine and bile, $t_{1/2}$ 24 hr

INDICATIONS AND USES: Pheochromocytoma (control of episodes of hypertension and sweating), micturition disorders (neurogenic bladder, functional outlet obstruction, partial prostatic obstruction),* peripheral vasospastic disorders*

DOSAGE
Adult
• PO 10 mg bid initially, increase dosage qod until optimal response obtained as judged by blood pressure; usual dosage range 20-40 mg bid-tid
Child
• PO 1-2 mg/kg/d divided q6-8h

$ AVAILABLE FORMS/COST OF THERAPY
• Cap, Gel—Oral: 10 mg, 100's: **$62.40**

CONTRAINDICATIONS: Hypersensitivity, conditions where a fall in blood pressure may be undesirable

PRECAUTIONS: Marked cerebral or coronary arteriosclerosis, renal damage, respiratory infection

PREGNANCY AND LACTATION: Pregnancy category C; indicated in hypertension secondary to pheochromocytoma during pregnancy, especially after 24 wk gestation when surgical intervention is associated with high rates of maternal and fetal mortality; no adverse fetal effects due to this treatment have been observed

SIDE EFFECTS/ADVERSE REACTIONS

CNS: Drowsiness, sedation, *dizziness,* confusion

CV: Postural hypotension, tachycardia, palpitations

EENT: Nasal congestion, miosis

GI: GI irritation, nausea, vomiting

GU: Inhibition of ejaculation

MISC: Fatigue

▼ DRUG INTERACTIONS

Drugs

- *Epinephrine:* Exaggerated hypotensive response, tachycardia

SPECIAL CONSIDERATIONS

PATIENT/FAMILY EDUCATION

- Avoid alcohol; avoid sudden changes in posture, dizziness may result
- Avoid cough, cold, or allergy medications containing sympathomimetics

---

phensuximide

(fen-sux'i-mide)

Milontin Kapseals

Chemical Class: Succinimide derivative

Therapeutic Class: Anticonvulsant

CLINICAL PHARMACOLOGY

Mechanism of Action: Increases seizure threshold and suppresses paroxysmal spike-and-wave pattern in absence seizures; depresses nerve transmission in the motor cortex

Pharmacokinetics

PO: Peak 1-4 hr, excreted in urine (some as hydroxylated metabolite), $t_{1/2}$ 4 hr

INDICATIONS AND USES: Absence (petit mal) seizures

DOSAGE

Adult

- PO 500-1000 mg bid-tid; usual dosage range 1-3 g/d

$ AVAILABLE FORMS/COST OF THERAPY

- Cap, Gel—Oral: 0.5 g, 100's: **$72.23**

CONTRAINDICATIONS: Hypersensitivity to succinimides

PRECAUTIONS: Hepatic/renal function impairment, abrupt withdrawal, grand mal seizures (may increase frequency when used as monotherapy), acute intermittent porphyria

PREGNANCY AND LACTATION: Pregnancy category D

SIDE EFFECTS/ADVERSE REACTIONS

CNS: Drowsiness, ataxia, dizziness, irritability, nervousness, headache, euphoria, dream-like state, lethargy, hyperactivity, fatigue, insomnia, confusion, instability, mental slowness, depression, hypochondriacal behavior, night terrors, aggressiveness, inability to concentrate

EENT: Blurred vision, myopia, photophobia, periorbital edema

GI: Nausea, vomiting, vague gastric upset, cramps, *anorexia,* diarrhea, weight loss, epigastric and abdominal pain, constipation, swelling of tongue

GU: Urinary frequency, ***renal damage,*** vaginal bleeding, ***hematuria***

HEME: ***Eosinophilia, granulocytopenia, leukopenia, agranulocytosis, monocytosis, pancytopenia***

MS: Muscle weakness

SKIN: Pruritus, urticaria, ***Stevens-***

Johnson syndrome, pruritic erythematous rashes, skin eruptions, erythema multiforme, systemic lupus erythematosus, alopecia, hirsutism

▼ **DRUG INTERACTIONS**

Drugs

• *Hydantoins:* Increase serum hydantoin concentrations

• *Primidone:* Reduced primidone and phenobarbital concentrations

SPECIAL CONSIDERATIONS

PATIENT/FAMILY EDUCATION

• Take with food or milk

• Do not discontinue abruptly

• May cause drowsiness

• Use caution driving or performing other tasks requiring alertness

• Notify physician of skin rash, joint pain, unexplained fever, sore throat, unusual bleeding or bruising, drowsiness, dizziness, blurred vision

MONITORING PARAMETERS

• CBC with differential, liver enzymes

phentermine

(fen′ter-meen)

Adipex-P, Dapex 37.5, Fastin, Ionamin, Obephen, Obe-Nix, Obermine, Obestin-30, Phentride, Phentrol, T-Diet

Chemical Class: Amphetamine congener

Therapeutic Class: Anorexiant

DEA Class: Schedule IV

CLINICAL PHARMACOLOGY

Mechanism of Action: Acts on adrenergic and dopaminergic pathways, directly stimulating the satiety center in the hypothalamic and limbic regions

Pharmacokinetics

PO; SR: Duration 10-14 hr, metabolized by liver, excreted by kidney

INDICATIONS AND USES: Exogenous obesity (as a short-term adjunct to caloric restriction)

DOSAGE

Adult

• PO 8 mg tid, ½ hr ac, or 15-37.5 mg as single daily dose before breakfast or 10-14 hr before retiring

$ **AVAILABLE FORMS/COST OF THERAPY**

• Cap, Gel—Oral: 15 mg, 100's: **$3.91;** 18.75 mg, 100's: **$7.33-$35.00;** 30 mg, 100's: **$4.43-$98.90;** 37.5 mg, 100's: **$13.62-$104.26**

• Tab, Uncoated—Oral: 8 mg, 100's: **$28.42;** 37.5 mg, 100's: **$7.43-$102.43**

CONTRAINDICATIONS: Hypersensitivity to sympathomimetic amines, glaucoma, history of drug abuse, cardiovascular disease, moderate to severe hypertension, advanced arteriosclerosis, agitated states, hyperthyroidism, within 14 days of MAOI administration

PRECAUTIONS: Diabetes mellitus, convulsive disorders, mild hypertension, children

PREGNANCY AND LACTATION: Pregnancy category C

SIDE EFFECTS/ADVERSE REACTIONS

CNS: Overstimulation, nervousness, restlessness, dizziness, insomnia, dysphoria, headache, mental depression, drowsiness, weakness, tremor, shivering, exacerbation of schizophrenia

CV: Palpitation, ***tachycardia,*** chest pain

GI: Dry mouth, nausea, constipation, diarrhea, unpleasant taste

GU: Urinary hesitancy, impotence, testicular pain

SKIN: Rash, excessive sweating, clamminess, pallor

▼ **DRUG INTERACTIONS**

Drugs

• *MAOIs:* Hypertensive crisis

SPECIAL CONSIDERATIONS
PATIENT/FAMILY EDUCATION

• May cause insomnia, avoid taking late in the day
• Weight reduction requires strict adherence to caloric restriction
• Notify physician if palpitations, nervousness or dizziness occur
• Use caution while driving or performing other tasks requiring alertness, may cause dizziness or blurred vision
• Do not discontinue abruptly

phentolamine

(fen-tole'a-meen)
Regitine, Rogitine ♣
Chemical Class: Alpha-adrenergic blocker
Therapeutic Class: Antihypertensive

CLINICAL PHARMACOLOGY
Mechanism of Action: Binds to α-adrenergic receptors which causes vasodilation, decreased peripheral vascular resistance, decreased blood pressure
Pharmacokinetics
IV: Onset of action immediate, duration 10-15 min
IM: Onset 15-20 min, duration 3-4 hr
Metabolized in liver; excreted in urine (10% as unchanged drug)
INDICATIONS AND USES: Diagnosis of and treatment of hypertension associated with pheochromocytoma, treatment of dermal necrosis following extravasation of α-adrenergic drugs (norepinephrine, epinephrine, dobutamine, dopamine), hypertensive crises secondary to MAOI/sympathomimetic amine interactions and rebound hypertension on withdrawal of antihypertensives,* with papaverine as intracavernous injection for impotence*

DOSAGE
Adult
• *Diagnosis of pheochromocytoma:* IM/IV 5 mg
• *Hypertension, surgery for pheochromocytoma:* IM/IV 5 mg 1-2 hr before procedure, repeat q2-4h as needed
• *Drug extravasation:* Dilute 5-10 mg in 10 ml NS, infiltrate area with sol within 12 hr (Blanching resolves within 1 hr if successful)
Child
• *Diagnosis of pheochromocytoma:* IM/IV 0.05-0.1 mg/kg/dose, max single dose 5 mg
• *Hypertension, surgery for pheochromocytoma:* IM/IV 0.05-0.1 mg/kg/dose 1-2 hr before procedure, repeat q2-4h as needed
• *Drug extravasation:* 0.1-0.2 mg/kg diluted in 10 ml NS infiltrated into area of extravasation within 12 hr

$ AVAILABLE FORMS/COST OF THERAPY
• Inj, Conc, w/Buffer—IM; IV: 5 mg, 2 vials: **$58.53**
CONTRAINDICATIONS: Hypersensitivity, angina, MI
PRECAUTIONS: Peptic ulcer disease (may exacerbate)
PREGNANCY AND LACTATION: Pregnancy category C; unknown if excreted in breast milk
SIDE EFFECTS/ADVERSE REACTIONS
CNS: Dizziness, flushing, weakness, severe headache, ***cerebrovascular occlusion***
CV: Hypotension, reflex tachycardia, angina, ***dysrhythmias, MI***
EENT: Nasal congestion
GI: Dry mouth, nausea, vomiting, diarrhea, abdominal pain

▼ DRUG INTERACTIONS
Drugs
• *Epinephrine, ephedrine:* Antagonizes vasoconstrictive/hypertensive effects

SPECIAL CONSIDERATIONS

- Urinary catecholamines preferred over phentolamine for screening for pheochromocytomaa

phenylbutazone

(fen-ill-byoo′ta-zone)

Butazolidin, Phenylbutazone

Chemical Class: Pyrazolone derivative

Therapeutic Class: Nonsteroidal antiinflammatory

CLINICAL PHARMACOLOGY

Mechanism of Action: Inhibits prostaglandin synthesis by decreasing an enzyme needed for biosynthesis; analgesic, antiinflammatory, antipyretic

Pharmacokinetics

PO: Peak 2 hr, $t_{1/2}$ 3-3½ hr; metabolized in liver, excreted in urine (metabolites), excreted in breast milk, 98% protein binding

INDICATIONS AND USES: Mild to moderate pain, osteoarthritis, rheumatoid arthritis, acute gouty arthritis

DOSAGE

Adult

- *Pain:* PO 100-200 mg tid-qid, then after desired response 100 mg tid-qid, not to exceed 600 mg/d
- *Acute Arthritis:* PO 400 mg, then 100 mg q4h for days or until desired response

$ **AVAILABLE FORMS/COST OF THERAPY**

- Cap, Gel—Oral: 100 mg, 100's: **$15.95**
- Tab, Uncoated—Oral: 100 mg, 100's: **$19.29-$19.80**

CONTRAINDICATIONS: Hypersensitivity, asthma, severe renal disease, severe hepatic disease, ulcer disease

PRECAUTIONS: Children, bleeding disorders, GI disorders, cardiac disorders, hypersensitivity to other antiinflammatory agents

PREGNANCY AND LACTATION: Pregnancy category C (D if used in 3rd trimester); compatible with breast feeding

SIDE EFFECTS/ADVERSE REACTIONS

CNS: Dizziness, drowsiness, fatigue, tremors, confusion, insomnia, anxiety, depression

CV: Tachycardia, peripheral edema, palpitations, ***dysrhythmias, pericarditis, myocarditis, cardiac decompensation***

EENT: Tinnitus, hearing loss, blurred vision

GI: Nausea, anorexia, vomiting, diarrhea, jaundice, ***cholestatic hepatitis,*** constipation, flatulence, cramps, dry mouth, peptic ulcer

GU: ***Nephrotoxicity: dysuria, hematuria, oliguria, azotemia***

HEME: ***Bone marrow suppression***

SKIN: Purpura, rash, pruritus, sweating

▼ **DRUG INTERACTIONS**

Drugs

- *Lithium:* Increased lithium levels
- *Methotrexate:* Severe methotrexate toxicity
- *Sulfonylurea hypoglycemic drugs+:* Increased hypoglycemic action
- *Warfarin+:* Enhanced anticoagulant response, severe bleeding

phenylephrine (systemic)

(fen-ill-ef′rin)

Neo-Synephrine

Chemical Class: Substituted phenylethylamine

Therapeutic Class: Adrenergic, direct acting

CLINICAL PHARMACOLOGY

Mechanism of Action: Selective α_1 receptor agonist; causes vasoconstriction, with increase in blood pressure; reflex bradycardia occurs

Pharmacokinetics

Excreted in urine; $t_{1/2}$ 2½ hr

IV: Duration 20-30 min

IM/SC: Duration 45-60 min

INDICATIONS AND USES: Hypotension, shock, paroxysmal supraventricular tachycardia (PSVT), prolongation of spinal anesthesia, vasoconstriction in regional analgesia

DOSAGE

Adult

- *Hypotension:* SC/IM 2-5 mg, may repeat q10-15 min if needed; IV 0.1-0.5 mg, may repeat q10-15 min if needed; IV INF 10 mg/500 ml D_5W given 100-180 gtt/min (based on 20 gtt/ml), then 40-60 gtt/min titrated to B/P
- *PSVT:* IV BOL 0.5 mg given rapidly, subsequent doses should not exceed previous dose by > 0.1-0.2 mg; max single dose 1 mg
- *Prolongation of spinal anesthesia:* Add 2-5 mg to anesthetic solution; increases duration of block by 50%
- *Prevention of hypotension in spinal anesthesia:* SC/IM 2-3 mg 3-4 min before anesthetic inj
- *Vasoconstriction in regional anesthesia:* Add 1 mg to 20 ml anesthetic sol

Child

- *Hypotension:* SC/IM 0.1 mg/kg/dose q1-2h (max 5 mg); IV BOL 5-20 μg/kg/dose q 10-15 min; IV INF 0.1-0.5 μg/kg/min
- *PSVT:* IV 5-10 μg/kg/dose over 20-30 sec
- *Prevention of hypotension in spinal anesthesia:* SC/IM 0.05-0.1 mg/kg/dose

$ **AVAILABLE FORMS/COST OF THERAPY**

- Inj, Sol—IM; IV; SC: 10 mg/ml, 1 ml: **$2.27-$7.71**

CONTRAINDICATIONS: Hypersensitivity, ventricular fibrillation/tachycardia, pheochromocytoma, narrow-angle glaucoma, severe hypertension

PRECAUTIONS: Arterial embolism, peripheral vascular disease, elderly, hyperthyroidism, bradycardia, myocardial disease, severe arteriosclerosis

PREGNANCY AND LACTATION: Pregnancy category C; unknown if excreted in breast milk

SIDE EFFECTS/ADVERSE REACTIONS

CNS: Headache, anxiety, tremor, insomnia, dizziness

CV: ***Palpitations, tachycardia, hypertension, ectopic beats, angina,*** reflex bradycardia

GI: Nausea, vomiting

SKIN: Necrosis, tissue sloughing with extravasation, ***gangrene***

▼ **DRUG INTERACTIONS**

Drugs

- *Beta blockers, debrisoquin, MAOIs+:* Acute hypertensive episodes
- *Cyclic antidepressants, oxytocic drugs:* Enhanced pressor response

SPECIAL CONSIDERATIONS

- Antidote to extravasation: 5-10 ml phentolamine in 10-15 ml saline infiltrated throughout ischemic area
- Not indicated for hypotension secondary to hypovolemia

phenylephrine (topical)

(fen-ill-ef′rin)

Nasal: Alconefrin, Alconefrin-25, Alconefrin-50, Duration, Neo-Synephrine, Nostril, Rhinall-10, Sinex, St. Joseph Measured Dose

Ophthalmic: Ak-Dilate, Ak-Nefrin, Dilatair, I-Phrine, Isopto Frin, Mydfrin, Neo-Synephrine, Ocugestrin, Ocu-Phrin Sterile Eye Drops/Ophthalmic Solution, Prefrin Liquifilm, Relief Eye Drops for Red Eyes

Chemical Class: Sympathomimetic amine

Therapeutic Class: Nasal decongestant (nasal); mydriatic and decongestant (ophthalmic)

CLINICAL PHARMACOLOGY

Mechanism of Action: Produces vasoconstriction (rapid, long-acting) of arterioles, decreasing fluid exudate, mucosal engorgement; acts on α-adrenergic receptors of the dilator muscle of the pupil, producing contraction

Pharmacokinetics

NASAL: May be systemically absorbed; duration of action 30 min-4 hr

OPHTH: Peak effect of mydriasis 15-60 min (2.5% sol), 10-90 min (10% sol); duration of action 3 hr (2.5% sol), 3-7 hr (10% sol)

INDICATIONS AND USES: Nasal congestion; mydriasis, uveitis with synechiae, and ocular decongestion

DOSAGE

Adult

- *Nasal:* INSTILL 2-3 gtt or sprays to nasal mucosa bid (0.25% sol, use 0.5%-1% sol in resistant only)
- *Ophth:* Mydriasis, 1 gtt to conjunctival sac (2.5% or 10% sol) after giving top anesthetic; ocular decongestant: 1 gtt to conjunctiva q3-4 hr as needed (0.12% sol)

Child

- *Nasal:* 6-12 yr INSTILL 1-2 gtt or sprays (0.25%) q3-4h prn; <6 yr INSTILL 2-3 gtt or sprays (0.125%) q3-4h prn
- *Ophth:* 1 gtt of 2.5% sol to conjunctiva; ocular decongestant: 1 gtt to conjunctiva q3-4 hr as needed (0.08%-0.12% sol)

$ **AVAILABLE FORMS/COST OF THERAPY**

- Sol—Nasal: 1% drops, 0.5 oz: **$3.79;** 1% spray, 15 ml: **$4.13;** 0.5% spray, 15 ml: **$4.66;** 0.25% drops, 15 ml, **$3.28;** 0.25% spray, 15 ml: **$3.52;** 0.125% drops, 15 ml: **$3.28**
- Sol—Ophth: 10%, 5 ml: **$4.20-$19.13;** 2.5%, 5 ml: **$2.30-$11.25**
- Liq—Ophth: 0.12%, 0.7 oz: **$9.06**

CONTRAINDICATIONS: Hypersensitivity to sympathomimetic amines; 10% ophth sol not recommended in infants (hypertension)

PRECAUTIONS: Child <6 yr, elderly, diabetes, CVD, hypertension, hyperthyroidism, increased ICP, prostatic hypertrophy, glaucoma

PREGNANCY AND LACTATION: Pregnancy category C; no breast feeding data, use caution

SIDE EFFECTS/ADVERSE REACTIONS

CNS: Anxiety, restlessness, tremors, weakness, insomnia, dizziness, fever, headache

EENT: Irritation, burning, sneezing, stinging, dryness, rebound congestion, visual blurring (ophth)

GI: Nausea, vomiting, anorexia

SKIN: Contact dermatitis

▼ **DRUG INTERACTIONS**

Drugs

See interactions under systemic phenylephrine; interactions less

P

likely than with systemic administration if given in proper dosage

SPECIAL CONSIDERATIONS

• Do not administer for more than 3-5 days (nasal product) or 2-3 days (ocular product used as decongestant) due to rebound congestion

phenylpropanolamine

(fen-ill-pro-pa-nole'a-mine)

Acutrim, Control, Dex-A-Diet, Dexatrim, Diet-Aid-Efed II Yellow, Phenyldrine, Prolamine, Propagest, Rhindecon, Stay Trim Diet Gum, Unitrol

Chemical Class: α-Adrenergic; sympathomimetic

Therapeutic Class: Appetite suppressant, nasal decongestant

CLINICAL PHARMACOLOGY

Mechanism of Action: Suppresses appetite control center in hypothalamus, acts on α-adrenergic receptors to produce mucosal vasoconstriction of respiratory tract,* stimulates α-adrenergic receptors, causing contraction of bladder neck and urethral smooth muscle

Pharmacokinetics

PO: Onset 15-30 min, duration of action 3 hr (cap, tab), 12-16 hr (extended-release)

Readily absorbed, hepatic metabolism, renal excretion

INDICATIONS AND USES: Exogenous obesity (short-term use, 6-12 wk, with diet, exercise, behavior modification), nasal congestion, urinary incontinence*

DOSAGE

Adult

• *Appetite suppressant:* PO 25 mg tid (tab, cap, gum); 75 mg qd (extended-release)

• *Decongestant:* PO 25 mg qid (tab, cap), 75 mg q12h (extended-release)

• *Urinary incontinence:* PO 50-150 mg/d in divided doses

Child

• *Decongestant:* PO 6.25 mg q4h, max 37.5 mg/d (2-6 yr); 12.5 mg q4h, max 75 mg/d (6-12 yr)

$ **AVAILABLE FORMS/COST OF THERAPY**

• Cap, Gel, Sust Action—Oral: 75 mg, 60's: **$12.00**

• Tab—Oral: 50 mg, 100's: **$1.95;** 37.5 mg, 100's: **$3.13;** 25 mg, 100's: **$1.80**

CONTRAINDICATIONS: Hypersensitivity, severe CAD, severe hypertension, dysrhythmias, within 14 days of MAOI use, renal disease, glaucoma, depression

PRECAUTIONS: Postpartum women and children (increased psychiatric side effects), mild hypertension, hyperthyroidism, prostatic hypertrophy

PREGNANCY AND LACTATION: Pregnancy category C; possible increase in minor malformations with first trimester use; no data on breast feeding available

SIDE EFFECTS/ADVERSE REACTIONS

CNS: Headache, confusion, ***convulsions,*** hallucinations, nervousness, insomnia, dizziness

CV: ***Hypertension, chest tightness, dysrythmias***

EENT: Dryness of nose/mouth

GI: Abdominal pain, nausea, vomiting

GU: Difficulty, pain with urination, ***renal failure***

▼ **DRUG INTERACTIONS**

Drugs

• *Bromocriptine:* Hypertension and seizures

• *MAOIs:* Severe hypertension

• *Neuroleptics:* Single report of death

SPECIAL CONSIDERATIONS

Present in combination in many otc products. Some products may contain tartrazine, which may cause asthma in susceptible individuals (e.g., patients with aspirin sensitivity)

---

phenytoin

(fen'i-toy-in)

Dilantin, Dilantin Capsules, Di-Phen, Diphenylan, Phenytoin Oral Suspension

Chemical Class: Hydantoin

Therapeutic Class: Anticonvulsant

CLINICAL PHARMACOLOGY

Mechanism of Action: Inhibits spread of seizure activity in motor cortex

Pharmacokinetics

PO: Slow and variable absorption among products; peak 1½-3 hr (prompt cap), 4-12 hr (extended cap)

IV: Immediate onset

IM: Slow but complete (92%) absorption

$t_{1/2}$ changes with dose and serum concentration secondary to saturation of hepatic metabolic enzyme systems; biotransformation increased in younger children, pregnant women, trauma; metabolites excreted in urine

INDICATIONS AND USES: Generalized tonic-clonic seizures; simple or complex partial seizures (psychomotor or temporal lobe); status epilepticus; nonepileptic seizures associated with Reye's syndrome or after head trauma; migraines; trigeminal neuralgia;* Bell's palsy; ventricular dysrhythmias, especially related to digitalis toxicity;* epidermolysis bullosa*

DOSAGE

Adult

• *Seizures:* IV loading dose 15-20 mg/kg based on recent dosing history and serum levels, followed by 100 mg PO or IV q6-8h; PO loading dose 1 g divided 400 mg, 300 mg, 300 mg given q2h; if load not necessary may give 100 mg tid, follow levels; maintenance dose: 300 mg/d or 5-6 mg/kg/d in divided doses; once dosage established may use extended caps and dose qd

• *Neuritic pain:* PO 200-400 mg/d

Child

• *Seizures:* IV loading dose 15-20 mg/kg in divided doses of 5-10 mg/kg; PO 5 mg/kg/d in 2 or 3 divided doses to max 300 mg/d; daily maintenance dose 4-8 mg/kg

$ **AVAILABLE FORMS/COST OF THERAPY**

• Inj, Sol—IM; IV: 50 mg/ml, 2 ml: **$2.43-$78.13**

• Susp—Oral: 125 mg/5 ml, 240 ml: **$28.25;** 30 mg/5 ml, 240 ml: **$18.94**

• Tab, Chewable—Oral: 50 mg, 100's: **$19.48-$27.62**

• Cap, Gel—Oral: 30 mg, 100's: **$18.78;** 100 mg, 100's: **$6.80-$20.84**

CONTRAINDICATIONS: Hypersensitivity, bradycardia, second and third degree AV block, Stokes-Adams syndrome, sino-atrial block

PRECAUTIONS: Hepatic disease, renal disease, diabetes mellitus

PREGNANCY AND LACTATION: Pregnancy category D (risk of congenital defects increased 2-3 times; fetal hydantoin syndrome includes craniofacial abnormalities, hypoplasia, ossification of distal phalanges; may also be transplacental carcinogen); compatible with breast feeding

SIDE EFFECTS/ADVERSE REACTIONS

CNS: Drowsiness, *dizziness,* insomnia, paresthesias, *psychiatriac changes,* headache, confusion, *slurred speech,* nystagmus, ataxia, fatigue

CV: ***Hypotension, CV collapse*** (when drug administered too rapidly IV), ***ventricular fibrillation***

EENT: Nystagmus, diplopia, blurred vision, *gingival hyperplasia*

GI: Nausea, vomiting, constipation, anorexia, weight loss, ***hepatitis,*** jaundice

GU: ***Nephritis***

HEME: ***Agranulocytosis, leukopenia, aplastic anemia, thrombocytopenia, megaloblastic anemia,*** lymphadenopathy

METAB: Hyperglycemia

SKIN: Rash, ***lupus erythematosus, Stevens-Johnson syndrome,*** hirsutism, alopecia

▼ DRUG INTERACTIONS

Drugs

- *Acetozolamide:* Osteomalacia
- *Amiodarone:* Increased phenytoin levels, decreased amiodarone levels
- *Antineoplastics, aspirin, cimetidine, diazoxide, folate, rifampin:* Decreased phenytoin levels
- *Chloramphenicol, disulfiram, fluconazole, felbamate, fluoxetine, isoniazid, omeprazole, sulfonamides:* Increased phenytoin levels
- *Corticosteroids:* Decreased therapeutic effect of steroids
- *Cyclic antidepressants:* Increased antidepressant levels
- *Cyclosporine:* Reduced cyclosporine levels
- *Dicumarol:* Increased anticoagulant effect, increased phenytoin levels
- *Digitalis glycosides:* Lower digitalis levels
- *Disopyramide:* Reduced efficacy, increased toxicity of disopyramide
- *Doxycycline:* Reduced doxycycline concentrations
- *Furosemide:* Decreased diuretic effect
- *Levodopa:* Decreased antiparkinsonian effect
- *Lidocaine:* Reduced lidocaine levels but with increased cardiac depressant effects
- *Mebendazole in high doses:* Decreased mebendazole levels
- *Methadone:* Withdrawal
- *Metyrapone:* Invalidates test
- *Mexiletine:* Decreased mexiletine levels
- *Oral contraceptives:* Decreased contraceptive effect
- *Primidone:* Enhanced conversion to phenobarbital
- *Quinidine:* Decreased quinidine levels
- *Theophylline:* Reduced theophylline levels
- *Thyroid hormone:* Increased thyroid replacement dose requirements
- *Valproic acid:* Variable effects on phenytoin levels, decreased valproic acid levels
- *Warfarin:* Transient increased hypoprothrombinemic response followed by inhibition of hypoprothrombinemic response

Labs

- *Interference:* Metyrapone and dexamethasone tests
- *Decrease:* Serum thyroxine and free thyroxine levels

SPECIAL CONSIDERATIONS

- Therapeutic range 10-20 μg/ml; nystagmus appears at 20 μg/ml, ataxia at 30 μg/ml, dysarthria and lethargy at levels above 40 μg/ml; lethal dose 2-5 g

physostigmine

(fi-zoe-stig'meen)

Ophthalmic: Isopto Eserine Solution, Eserine Sulfate Ointment, Eserine Salicylate, Fisostin

Systemic: Antilirium

Chemical Class: Cholinesterase inhibitor

Therapeutic Class: Miotic (ophth); antidote to anticholinergics (systemic)

CLINICAL PHARMACOLOGY

Mechanism of Action: Inactivates acetylcholinesterase, potentiates acetylcholine at sites of cholinergic transmission; results in miosis, decreased intraocular pressure; antagonizes anticholinergics

Pharmacokinetics

OPHTH: Onset 20-30 min, duration 12-36 hr (miosis); peak 2-6 hr, duration 12-36 hr (intraocular pressure)

PARENTERAL: IV/IM crosses blood brain barrier; peak effect 20-30 min (IM), 5 min (IV); duration of action 30-60 min; destroyed in body by hydrolysis, very small amounts excreted in urine

INDICATIONS AND USES: Wide-angle glaucoma (ophth), treatment of anticholinergic toxicity (systemic, including tricyclic antidepressants)

DOSAGE

Adult

- *Glaucoma:* INSTILL OINT ¼ in. strip of 0.25% oint in conjunctival sac qd-tid; INSTILL SOL 1 gtt of a 0.25%-0.5% sol in conjunctival sac qd-qid
- *Anticholinergic toxicity:* IM/IV 0.5 mg-2 mg given at rate not greater than 1 mg/min; repeat q 20-30 min, max single dose 4 mg, as needed

Child

- *Glaucoma:* See adult
- *Anticholinergic toxicity:* IV .02 mg (20 μg)/kg over at least 1 min; may repeat q5-10min; max dose 2 mg

$ AVAILABLE FORMS/COST OF THERAPY

- Inj, Sol—IM; IV: 1 mg/ml, 2 ml: **$6.95-$37.58**
- Sol—Ophth: 0.25%, 15 ml: **$11.87;** 0.5%, 15 ml: **$12.50**
- Oint—Ophth: 0.25%, 3.5 g: **$2.85-$13.44**

CONTRAINDICATIONS: Hypersensitivity, inflammatory disease of iris or ciliary body, newborn (parenteral solution contains benzyl alcohol, toxic to neonate), organophosphate poisoning, intestinal or urogenital tract obstruction, asthma, diabetes mellitus, patients receiving choline esters or depolarizing neuromuscular blocking agents (decamethonium, succinylcholine)

PRECAUTIONS: Epilepsy, parkinsonism, bradycardia, bronchitis, CV disease

PREGNANCY AND LACTATION: Pregnancy category C; no data on breast feeding available

SIDE EFFECTS/ADVERSE REACTIONS

CNS: ***Convulsions,*** headache, anxiety, delirium, disorientation, hallucinations, hyperactivity

CV: ***Hypertension, hypotension, bradycardia, irregular pulse***

EENT: Blurred vision, conjunctivitis, rhinorrhea, salivation, lacrimation, twitching of eyelids, decreased secretion in salivary and sweat glands, decreased secretions in pharynx, nasal passages

GI: Nausea, vomiting, abdominal cramps, diarrhea

RESP: ***Bronchospasm,*** dyspnea,

P

pulmonary edema, decreased bronchial secretions
MISC: ***Hyperpyrexia***

▼ **DRUG INTERACTIONS**

Drugs

- *Organophosphate insecticides:* Increased toxicity of physostigmine
- *Succinylcholine:* Respiratory and CV collapse
- *Systemic anticholinesterases:* Additive effects

SPECIAL CONSIDERATIONS

- Atropine is antidote

---

phytonadione (vitamin k_1)

(fye-toe-na-dye'one)
AquaMEPHYTON, Konakion, Mephyton, Synkayvite
Chemical Class: Fat soluble vitamin
Therapeutic Class: Nutritional supplement, antihemorrhagic

CLINICAL PHARMACOLOGY

Mechanism of Action: Normally synthesized by intestinal flora; promotes hepatic formation of clotting factors II, VII, IX, and X

Pharmacokinetics

PO; INJ: Readily absorbed from normal duodenum, bile salts required; rapid hepatic metabolism; onset of action 6-12 hr oral, 1-2 hr parenteral; prothrombin time normalizes in 12-14 hr parenteral; excreted in urine, bile

INDICATIONS AND USES: Vit K malabsorption, hypoprothrombinemia, hemorrhagic disease of the newborn (prophylaxis); does not reverse hypoprothrombinemia due to hepatocellular damage

DOSAGE

Adult

- *Hypoprothrombinemia:* PO 2.5-10 mg (up to 25 mg) may repeat in 12 hr; IM/SC 2.5-10 mg (up to 25 mg), may repeat in 6-8 hr
- *Hypoprothrombinemia prevention during total parenteral nutrition:* IM 5-10 mg qwk

Child

- *Hypoprothrombinemia:* PO/IM/SC 5-10 mg
- *Hypoprothrombinemia prevention during total parenteral nutrition:* IM 2-5 mg qwk

Infants

- *Hypoprothrombinemia:* PO/IM/SC 1-2 mg
- *Prevention of hemorrhagic disease of the newborn (HDN):* IM/SC 0.5-1 mg after birth, repeat in 6-8 hr if required (e.g., mother received anticonvulsants, rifampin, isoniazid during pregnancy)

$ **AVAILABLE FORMS/COST OF THERAPY**

- Inj, Emulsion—IM; IV; SC: 1 mg/0.5 ml, 0.5 ml: **$2.36-$5.00;** 10 mg/ml, 1 ml: **$4.75-$5.76**
- Tab, Uncoated—Oral: 5 mg, 100's: **$52.20**

CONTRAINDICATIONS: Hypersensitivity, severe hepatic disease

PRECAUTIONS: G6PD deficiency; premature infants

PREGNANCY AND LACTATION: Pregnancy category C; oral supplementation of women on anticonvulsants during last 2 weeks of pregnancy has been done to prevent HDN but effectiveness unproven; compatible with breast feeding

SIDE EFFECTS/ADVERSE REACTIONS

CNS: Headache, ***kernicterus*** (premature infants, high doses)
HEME: ***Hemolytic anemia, hemoglobinuria, hyperbilirubinemia*** (newborn)
SKIN: Rash, urticaria, flushing sensation
MISC: ***Anaphylaxis***

▼ **DRUG INTERACTIONS**
Drugs
- *Mineral oil:* Decreased vitamin K absorption from GI tract
- *Oral anticoagulants:* Decreased anticoagulant effect

pilocarpine

(pye-loe-kar'peen)
Ophthalmic: Adsorbocarpine, Akarpine, Isopto Carpine, Miocarpine, Ocu-Carpine, Ocusert Pilo-20, Ocusert Piol-40, Pilagan, ♣ Pilocar, Pilocarpine HCl, Pilopine HS, Piloptic-1, Piloptic-2, Pilostat
Oral: Salagen
Chemical Class: Cholinergic parasympathomimetic agonist
Therapeutic Class: Direct-acting miotic (ophthalmic), stimulation of saliva production (oral)

CLINICAL PHARMACOLOGY
Mechanism of Action: Produces pupillary constriction by duplicating muscarinic effects of acetylcholine; increases aqueous humor outflow, intraocular pressure (IOP) decreases; orally increases exocrine gland secretion
Pharmacokinetics
OPHTH: Onset 10-30 min, duration 4-8 hr (sol, gel); Ocusert system onset 1½-2 hr, duration 7 days
ORAL: Onset 20 min, peak 1 hr, duration 3-5 hr; excreted in urine
INDICATIONS AND USES: Ophth: Open-angle glaucoma, chronic angle-closure glaucoma, acute angle-closure glaucoma (in combination with other agents to decrease IOP before surgery), reversal of mydriasis, pre- and postoperative increased IOP; Oral: Xerostomia from salivary gland hypofunction secondary to radiotherapy for head and neck cancer

DOSAGE
Adult
- *Glaucoma:* INSTILL SOL 1-2 gtt of 1% or 2% sol in eye q6-8h; INSTILL 20-40 µg/hr (Ocusert) in cul-de-sac of eye, replace q7d; INSTILL GEL 0.5″ ribbon in conjunctival sac qhs
- *Xerostomia:* PO 5-10 mg tid

$ **AVAILABLE FORMS/COST OF THERAPY**
- Tab, Coated—Oral: 5 mg, 100's: **$107.40**
- Gel—Ophth: 4%, 5 g: **$21.25**
- Sol, Ophth: 0.25%, 0.5%, 1.0%, 2.0%, 3.0%, 4.0%, 6.0%, 8.0%, 10.0%, 15 ml: **$2.34-$18.75**
- Insert—Ophth: 20 µg/hr, 8's: **$34.20;** 40 µg/hr, 8's: **$34.20**

CONTRAINDICATIONS: Hypersensitivity, acute iritis, or other condition where acute miosis undesirable
PRECAUTIONS: Bronchial asthma, hypertension, bradycardia, hyperthyroidism, CV disease, biliary disease, renal colic (nephrolithiasis), epilepsy, parkinsonism, asthma
PREGNANCY AND LACTATION: Pregnancy category C; no data available on breast feeding
SIDE EFFECTS/ADVERSE REACTIONS
CNS: Headache
CV: ***Hypotension, tachycardia, AV block, bradycardia, hypertension, shock, dysrhythmia***
EENT: Blurred vision, twitching of eyelids, eye pain with change in focus, conjunctival irritation (Ocusert), tearing, stinging, retinal detachment
GI: Nausea, vomiting, abdominal cramps, diarrhea
GU: Bladder tightness, urgency, frequency
RESP: ***Bronchospasm***

P

DRUG INTERACTIONS

Drugs (oral interactions)

- *Anticholinergics:* Antagonism of anticholinergic
- *Beta blockers:* Conduction disturbances

SPECIAL CONSIDERATIONS

- Antidote is atropine

PATIENT/FAMILY EDUCATION

- Miotics cause poor dark adaptation, use caution with night driving

pimozide

(pi′moe-zide)

Orap

Chemical Class: Derivative of meperidine-like analgesics, butyrophenone analog

Therapeutic Class: Antipsychotic, antidyskinetic

CLINICAL PHARMACOLOGY

Mechanism of Action: Blocks dopamine receptors in CNS

Pharmacokinetics

PO: $t_{1/2}$ 19-39 hr, peak 4-12 hr

50% absorbed, hepatic metabolism, excreted in urine and stool

INDICATIONS AND USES: Gilles de la Tourette's syndrome (patients non-responsive to haloperidol), chronic schizophrenia without excitement, agitation or hyperactivity*

DOSAGE

Adult

- *Tourette's:* PO 1-2 mg qd in divided doses, increase qod as needed (usual dose 200 µg/kg/d or 10 mg qd, whichever is less); max 300 µg/kg/d or 20 mg qd
- *Psychotic disorders:* PO 2-4 mg qd, increase qwk by 2-4 mg qd

$ AVAILABLE FORMS/COST OF THERAPY

- Tab, Uncoated—Oral: 2 mg, 100's: **$70.70**

CONTRAINDICATIONS: Hypersensitivity, simple tics other than Tourette's, history of cardiac dysrhythmias

PRECAUTIONS: Breast cancer (increased prolactin levels), liver disease, renal disease, hypokalemia (dysrythmias), sensitivity to other neuroleptics

PREGNANCY AND LACTATION: Pregnancy category C; unknown if excreted in breast milk

SIDE EFFECTS/ADVERSE REACTIONS

CNS: Akathisia, extra-pyramidal effects, parkinsonism, mood or behavior changes, *tardive dyskinesia,* ***neuroleptic malignant syndrome,*** *drowsiness,* dizziness, headache

CV: ***Ventricular dysrythmias, prolonged QT interval,*** *tachycardia,* ***hypotension***

EENT: Blurred vision, dryness of mouth

GI: Obstructive jaundice, *constipation,* anorexia, nausea, vomiting, diarrhea

GU: Loss of bladder control

HEME: ***Blood dyscrasias***

SKIN: Rash, itching

MISC: Mastalgia, galactorrhea

DRUG INTERACTIONS

Drugs

- *Anticonvulsants:* Lowered seizure threshold
- *CNS depressants:* Potentiation of CNS effects
- *Phenothiazines, tricyclic antidepressants, or antidysrhythmic agents:* Additive effect on QT interval

pindolol

(pin'doe-loll)

Visken

Chemical Class: Nonselective β-adrenergic blocker

Therapeutic Class: Antihypertensive

CLINICAL PHARMACOLOGY

Mechanism of Action: Competitively blocks stimulation of β-adrenergic receptors (nonselectively); inhibits chronotropic, inotropic responses to β-adrenergic tone (decreases rate of SA node discharge, increases recovery time), slows conduction of AV node, decreases heart rate, which decreases O_2 consumption in myocardium; also decreases renin-aldosterone-angiotensin system; intrinsic sympathomimetic activity (ISA) manifests with smaller reduction in resting cardiac output and in the resting heart rate than are seen with drugs without ISA

Pharmacokinetics

PO: Peak effect, 1-2 hr

90%-100% absorption; 40% protein bound; 60%- 65% metabolized by liver; $t_{1/2}$ 3-4 hr; excreted 30%-45% unchanged

INDICATIONS AND USES: Hypertension

DOSAGE

Adult

- Hypertension: PO 5 mg bid, usual dose 15 mg/d (5 mg tid), may increase by 10 mg/d q3-4 wk to a max of 60 mg/d

$ AVAILABLE FORMS/COST OF THERAPY

- Tab, Uncoated—Oral: 5 mg, 100's: **$32.93-$79.98;** 10 mg, 100's: **$45.75-$105.90**

CONTRAINDICATIONS: Hypersensitivity to β-blockers, cardiogenic shock, 2nd, 3rd degree heart block, sinus bradycardia, CHF, cardiac failure, bronchial asthma

PRECAUTIONS: Major surgery, diabetes mellitus, renal disease, thyroid disease, COPD, well-compensated heart failure, nonallergic bronchospasm; abrupt withdrawal may precipitate CAD or sudden death, peripheral vascular disease, thyrotoxicosis

PREGNANCY AND LACTATION: Pregnancy category B; no reports available; other members of this class are excreted into milk, expect pindolol to do the same

SIDE EFFECTS/ADVERSE REACTIONS

CNS: Insomnia, dizziness, hallucinations, anxiety, fatigue

CV: Hypotension, bradycardia, ***CHF,*** edema, chest pain, palpitation, claudication, tachycardia, ***AV block***

EENT: Visual changes, sore throat, *double vision,* dry burning eyes

GI: Nausea, vomiting, ***ischemic colitis,*** diarrhea, *abdominal pain,* ***mesenteric arterial thrombosis***

GU: Impotence, frequency

HEME: ***Agranulocytosis, thrombocytopenia, purpura***

RESP: ***Bronchospasm,*** *dyspnea,* cough, rales

SKIN: Rash, alopecia, pruritus

MISC: Joint pain, muscle pain, fever

▼ DRUG INTERACTIONS

Drugs

- *Amiodarone:* Potentially inhibits pindolol's metabolism: bradycardia/ventricular dysrhythmia
- *Anesthetics, local:* Enhanced sympathomimetic effects, hypertension due to unopposed α-receptor stimulation
- *Antidiabetics:* Delayed recovery from hypoglycemia, hyperglycemia, attenuated tachycardia during hypoglycemia, hypertension during hypoglycemia

• *Calcium channel blockers:* Bradycardia, hypotension
• *Clonidine:* Hypotension exacerbated upon withdrawal
• *Disopyramide:* Additive negative inotropic effects
• *Epinephrine+:* Enhanced pressor response resulting in hypertension
• *Methyldopa:* Hypertension
• *Neuroleptics:* Increased serum levels of both resulting in accentuated pharmacologic response to both drugs
• *Nonsteroidal anti-inflammatory drugs:* Reduced hypotensive effects
• *Phenylephrine:* Acute hypertensive episodes
• *Prazosin:* First-dose hypotensive response enhanced
• *Tacrine:* Additive bradycardia
• *Theophylline:* Antagonist pharmacodynamics

Labs
• *Increase:* Liver function tests, renal function tests

SPECIAL CONSIDERATIONS
• Abrupt discontinuation may precipitate angina; taper over 1-2 wk
• Effective antihypertensive and probably antianginal agent (though not approved for this indication), especially for patients who develop symptomatic bradycardia with beta-blockade

piperacillin; piperacillin/tazobactam

(pi-per'a-sill-in; taz'o-bac-tam)
Pipracil; Zosyn
Chemical Class: Extended-spectrum penicillin
Therapeutic Class: Broad-spectrum antibiotic; β-lactamase inhibitor

CLINICAL PHARMACOLOGY
Mechanism of Action: Interferes with cell wall replication of susceptible organisms; bactericidal
Pharmacokinetics
IM: Peak 30-50 min
IV: Peak 20-30 min
$t_{1/2}$, 0.7-1.33 hr; 33% protein bound; excreted in urine, bile; crosses placenta

INDICATIONS AND USES: Infections of the respiratory, skin, genitourinary tract, bone caused by susceptible organisms; combination effective against piperacillin-resistant, β-lactamase producing strains
Antibacterial spectrum usually includes:
• Gram-positive organisms: *Staphylococcus aureus, Streptococcus pyogenes, Str. viridans, Str. faecalis, Str. bovis, Str. pneumoniae, Clostridium perfringens, C. tetani*
• Gram-negative organisms: *Neisseria gonorrhoeae, N. meningitidis, Bacteroides, Fusobacterium nucleatum, E. coli, Klebsiella, P. vulgaris, Proteus mirabilis, Morganella morganii, Enterobacter, Citrobacter, Pseudomonas aeruginosa, Serratia, Acinetobacter, Peptococcus, Peptostreptococcus, Eubacterium*
• Anaerobes: *Bacteroides* sp, *Clostridium difficile*

DOSAGE
Adult
• *Systemic infections:* Piperacillin IM/IV 100-300 mg/kg/d in divided doses q4-6h; piperacillin/tazobactam IV INF 12-15 g/d given 3.375 g q6hr over 30 min × 7-10 days
• *Prophylaxis of surgical infections:* IV 2 g ½-1 hr before procedure; may be repeated during surgery or after surgery
Child (>12 yrs)
• *Systemic infections:* IM/IV 100-300 mg/kg/d in divided doses q4-6h

$ AVAILABLE FORMS/COST OF THERAPY

Piperacillin:

• Inj, Lyphl-Sol—IM;IV: 2 g/vial: **$11.15;** 3 g/vial: **$16.97;** 4 g/vial: **$22.62**

• Inj, Sol—IM;IV: 40 g/vial: **$190.51**

Piperacillin/tazobactam:

• Inj, Sol—IV: 2 g/0.25 mg: **$9.87;** 3 g/0.375 mg: **$14.81;** 4 g/0.5 mg: **$19.74**

CONTRAINDICATIONS: Hypersensitivity to penicillins; neonates

PRECAUTIONS: Hypersensitivity to cephalosporins; CHF

PREGNANCY AND LACTATION: Pregnancy category B; excreted in breast milk in small concentrations

SIDE EFFECTS/ADVERSE REACTIONS

CNS: Lethargy, hallucinations, anxiety, depression, twitching, ***coma, convulsions***

GI: Nausea, vomiting, diarrhea, increased AST, ALT, abdominal pain, glossitis, colitis

GU: ***Oliguria, proteinuria, hematuria,*** *vaginitis, moniliasis,* ***glomerulonephritis***

HEME: Anemia, increased bleeding time, ***bone marrow depression***

METAB: Hypokalemia, hypernatremia

▼ DRUG INTERACTIONS

Drugs

• *Aminoglycosides IV:* Decreased antimicrobial effect of piperacillin

• *Aspirin:* Increased piperacillin concentrations

• *Erythromycins:* Decreased antimicrobial effect of piperacillin

• *Probenecid:* Increased piperacillin concentrations

• *Tetracyclines:* Decreased antimicrobial effect of piperacillin

Labs

• *Increase:* Platelet count, eosinophils, serum creatinine, PTT, AST, ALT, alk phosphatase, bilirubin, BUN, electrolytes

• *Decrease:* Hct, Hgb, WBC, electrolytes

• *False positive:* Urine glucose, urine protein, Coombs' test

SPECIAL CONSIDERATIONS

• Preferred over mezlocillin, more effective against *Pseudomonas;* reserve for carbenicillin or ticarcillin-resistant *P. aeruginosa* infections in combination with an aminoglycoside

---

piperazine

(pi-per'a-zeen)

Vermizine

Therapeutic Class: Anthelmintic

CLINICAL PHARMACOLOGY

Mechanism of Action: Causes paralysis in worm, leading to expulsion by normal peristalsis

Pharmacokinetics

PO: Readily absorbed; partially degraded *in vivo;* excreted in urine (unchanged); wide range between effective therapeutic and clinically toxic doses

INDICATIONS AND USES: Pinworm, roundworm

DOSAGE

Adult and Child

• *Pinworm:* PO 65 mg/kg/d × 7 days, not to exceed 2.5 g/d

• *Roundworm:* PO 75 mg/kg/d in a single dose × 2 days

$ AVAILABLE FORMS/COST OF THERAPY

• Tab—Oral: 250 mg, 100's: **$2.57**

• Syr—Oral: 500 mg/5 ml, 120 ml: **$1.68**

CONTRAINDICATIONS: Hypersensitivity, renal disease, hepatic disease, seizures

PRECAUTIONS: Severe malnutrition, seizure disorders, anemia

P

PREGNANCY AND LACTATION: Pregnancy category B; reportedly excreted in breast milk, recommendations include dosing after breast feeding and discard next 8 h of milk

SIDE EFFECTS/ADVERSE REACTIONS

CNS: Dizziness, headache, paresthesias, convulsions, fever, headache, ataxia

EENT: Blurred vision, nystagmus, strabismus, cataracts, rhinorrhea

GI: Nausea, vomiting, anorexia, diarrhea, abdominal cramps

HEME: ***Hemolytic anemia***

RESP: ***Bronchospasm***

SKIN: Rash, urticaria, photosensitivity

▼ **DRUG INTERACTIONS**

Drugs

• *Pyrantel:* Antagonistic

Labs

• *Decrease:* Serum uric acid

SPECIAL CONSIDERATIONS

• Alternative to mebendazole or pyrantel pamoate for ascariasis (roundworms); particularly useful in combined ascariasis and oxyuriasis

• Alternative to pyrantel, mebendazole, or albendazole for enterobiasis (pinworms) as requires multiple day dosing

PATIENT/FAMILY EDUCATION

• Tell patient that urine may turn orange or red

pirbuterol

(purr-byoo′ter-ole)

Maxair

Chemical Class: β-adrenergic agonist

Therapeutic Class: Bronchodilator

CLINICAL PHARMACOLOGY

Mechanism of Action: Bronchodilation with little effect on heart rate acts on β-receptors, causing increased cAMP and relaxation of smooth muscle; β-2 selective

Pharmacokinetics

INH: Onset 3 min, peak ½-1 hr, duration 5 hr

INDICATIONS AND USES: Reversible airway disease; bronchospasm (prevention, treatment)

DOSAGE

Adult and child >12 yr

Aerosol 1-2 inh (0.4 mg) q4-6h; not to exceed 12 inh/d

$ **AVAILABLE FORMS/COST OF THERAPY**

• Aer—Inh: 0.2 mg, 2.8 g: **$9.60;** 14 g: **$34.14;** 25.6 g: **$24.42**

CONTRAINDICATIONS: Hypersensitivity to sympathomimetics, tachycardia

PRECAUTIONS: Cardiac disorders, hyperthyroidism, diabetes mellitus, prostatic hypertrophy

PREGNANCY AND LACTATION: Pregnancy category C

SIDE EFFECTS/ADVERSE REACTIONS

CNS: Tremors, anxiety, insomnia, headache, dizziness, stimulation, restlessness, hallucinations, drowsiness, irritability

CV: Palpitations, tachycardia, hypertension, angina, hypotension, dysrhythmias

EENT: Dry nose and mouth, irritation of nose, throat

GI: Gastritis, nausea, vomiting, anorexia

MS: Muscle cramps

RESP: ***Bronchospasm,*** dyspnea, coughing

SPECIAL CONSIDERATIONS

• Initial and periodic reviews of metered dose inhaler technique

• No significant advantage over the other selective beta-2 agonists

piroxicam
(peer-ox'i-kam)
Feldene
Chemical Class: Oxicam derivative
Therapeutic Class: Nonsteroidal antiinflammatory agent

CLINICAL PHARMACOLOGY
Mechanism of Action: Inhibits prostaglandin synthesis by decreasing the enzyme (cyclo-oxygenase) needed for biosynthesis; possesses analgesic, antiinflammatory, antipyretic properties
Pharmacokinetics
PO: Peak concentration 3-5 hr, analgesic onset 1 hr, duration 48-72 hr, antirheumatic onset 7-12 days, peak 2-3 wk
$t_{1/2}$ 30-86 hr; metabolized in liver; excreted in urine (metabolites); excreted in breast milk; 99% protein binding
INDICATIONS AND USES: Osteoarthritis, rheumatoid arthritis
DOSAGE
Adult
• 20 mg qd or 10 mg bid
$ AVAILABLE FORMS/COST OF THERAPY
• Cap, Gel—Oral: 10 mg, 100's: **$12.53-$150.33;** 20 mg, 100's: **$19.40-$257.24**
CONTRAINDICATIONS: Hypersensitivity, asthma, severe renal disease, severe hepatic disease, ulcer disease, cardiac disease
PRECAUTIONS: Children, bleeding disorders, GI disorders, cardiac disorders, hypersensitivity to other antiinflammatory agents
PREGNANCY AND LACTATION: Pregnancy category B; excreted into breast milk, approximately 1% of mothers serum levels, should not present a risk to nursing infant
SIDE EFFECTS/ADVERSE REACTIONS
CNS: Dizziness, *drowsiness,* fatigue, tremors, confusion, insomnia, anxiety, depression, *headache*
CV: Tachycardia, peripheral edema, palpitations, dysrhythmias
EENT: Tinnitus, hearing loss, blurred vision
GI: Nausea, anorexia, vomiting, diarrhea, jaundice, ***cholestatic hepatitis,*** constipation, flatulence, cramps, dry mouth, ***bleeding, ulceration, perforation***
GU: ***Nephrotoxicity: dysuria, hematuria, oliguria, azotemia***
HEME: ***Blood dyscrasias***
SKIN: Purpura, rash, pruritus, sweating, photosensitivity
▼ DRUG INTERACTIONS
Drugs
• *ACE inhibitors:* Inhibit antihypertensive effect
• *Antidiabetics+:* Displacement, increased hypoglycemic effects
• *Beta blockers:* Reduced antihypertensive effect
• *Binding resins:* Reduced efficacy of NSAID
• *Coumarin, phenytoin, sulfonamides:* Increased action of these drugs
• *Cyclosporine:* Many NSAIDs increase nephrotoxicity
• *Furosemide:* Reduced/inhibited diuretic effect
• *Hydralazine:* Reduced antihypertensive effect
• *Lithium:* Increased risk of lithium toxicity
• *Methotrexate:* Many NSAIDs increase methotrexate toxicity
• *Oral anticoagulants:* Increased hypoprothrombinemic effects
• *Potassium sparing diuretics:* Hyperkalemia
• *Salicylates:* Reduced piroxicam concentrations

P

SPECIAL CONSIDERATIONS

- Similar in efficacy to the other NSAIDs but has the advantage of an extended $t_{1/2}$; no significant advantage over other agents

plicamycin (mithramycin)

(plik-a-mi'sin)

Mithracin

Chemical Class: Crystalline aglycone

Therapeutic Class: Antineoplastic antibiotic

CLINICAL PHARMACOLOGY

Mechanism of Action: Inhibits DNA, RNA, protein synthesis; derived from *Streptomyces plicatus;* replication is decreased by binding to DNA; demonstrates Ca-lowering effect not related to its tumoricidal activity; also acts on osteoclasts and blocks action of parathyroid hormone; visicant properties

Pharmacokinetics

Rapidly cleared from blood in 2 hr; 90% excretion in 24 hr; crosses blood-brain barrier

INDICATIONS AND USES: Testicular cancer, hypercalcemia, hypercalciuria

DOSAGE

Adult

- *Testicular tumors:* IV 25-30 μg/kg/d × 8-10 days, not to exceed 30 μg/kg/d
- *Hypercalcemia/hypercalciuria:* IV 25 μg/kg/d × 3-4 days, repeat at intervals of 1 wk

$ **AVAILABLE FORMS/COST OF THERAPY**

- Inj, Lyphl-Sol—IV: 500 μg/ml, 5 ml: **$822.71**

CONTRAINDICATIONS: Hypersensitivity, thrombocytopenia, bone marrow depression, bleeding disorders

PRECAUTIONS: Renal disease, hepatic disease, electrolyte imbalances

PREGNANCY AND LACTATION: Pregnancy category X

SIDE EFFECTS/ADVERSE REACTIONS

CNS: Drowsiness, weakness, lethargy, headache, flushing, fever, depression

GI: Nausea, vomiting, anorexia, diarrhea, stomatitis, increased liver enzymes

GU: Increased BUN, creatinine, proteinuria

HEME: ***Hemorrhage, thrombocytopenia, neutropenia***

METAB: Decreased serum Ca, P, K

SKIN: Rash, cellulitis, ***extravasation,*** facial flushing

▼ **DRUG INTERACTIONS**

Drugs

- *Bisphosphonates:* Additive hypocalcemic effect
- *Calcitonin:* Additive hypocalcemic effects
- *Foscarnet:* Additive effect on decreased ionized calcium
- *Glucagon:* Additive hypocalcemic effect

Labs

- *Increase:* Prothrombin time, clot retraction test, alanine aminotransferase, LDH, alk phosphatase, bilirubin, ornithine carbamyl transferase, isocitric dehydrogenase, BUN, serum creatinine
- *Decrease:* Calcium, hemoglobin, phosphate, potassium

SPECIAL CONSIDERATIONS

- Effective but toxic, hence use limited; additive with other calcium lowering therapies

MONITORING PARAMETERS

- CBC, differential, platelet count qwk; withhold drug if WBC is <4000/mm^3 or platelet count is <50,000/mm^3

• Renal function studies: BUN, serum uric acid, urine CrCl, electrolytes, I&O ratio
• Liver function tests: bilirubin, AST, ALT, alk phosphatase before and during therapy

podofilox

(po-doe-fil′ox)
Condylox
Chemical Class: Synthesized from *Coniferae* and *Berberidaceae* (e.g., species of Juniperus and Podophyllum)
Therapeutic Class: Topical antimitotic

CLINICAL PHARMACOLOGY
Mechanism of Action: Exact mechanism unknown; results in necrosis of visible wart tissue
Pharmacokinetics
TOP: Application of 0.1-1.5 ml yields peak serum levels of 1-17 ng/ml in 1-2 hr; $t_{1/2}$ 1-4½ hr; no accumulation with multiple applications
INDICATIONS AND USES: Condyloma acuminatum
DOSAGE
Adult
• TOP Apply (cotton-tipped applicator) q12h for 3 consecutive days, then hold for 4 days; repeat 1 week cycle until wart gone; if incomplete response after 4 cycles, consider alternate treatment; limit treatment to <10 cm^2 of wart tissue
$ AVAILABLE FORMS/COST OF THERAPY
• Sol—Top: 5 mg/ml, 3.5 ml: **$52.44**
CONTRAINDICATIONS: Hypersensitivity, perianal or mucous membrane warts
PRECAUTIONS: External use only
PREGNANCY AND LACTATION: Pregnancy category C
SIDE EFFECTS/ADVERSE REACTIONS
CNS: Insomnia, tingling, dizziness
GI: Vomiting
GU: Hematuria
HEME: Bleeding
SKIN: Burning, pain, inflammation, erosion, itching, tenderness, chafing, scarring, vesicle formation, crusting, edema, ulceration
MISC: Pain with intercourse, malodor
SPECIAL CONSIDERATIONS
• Safety preferred over podophyllum resin

podophyllum

(poe-dah′fil-um)
Podoben, Podocon, Podofilm, ♣ Pododerm
Chemical Class: Podophyllum derivative
Therapeutic Class: Keratolytic

CLINICAL PHARMACOLOGY
Mechanism of Action: Arrests mitosis in metaphase by binding to tubulin, protein subunit of spindle microtubules
INDICATIONS AND USES: Venereal warts, keratoses, multiple superficual epitheliomatoses
DOSAGE
Adults
• *Warts:* TOP cover wart, cover with wax paper, bandage for 1-4 hr, wash, may repeat qwk if needed
• *Keratosis/epitheliomatoses:* TOP apply qd with applicator, let dry, remove tissue, may reapply if needed
$ AVAILABLE FORMS/COST OF THERAPY
• Liq—Top: 25%, 15 ml: **$26.00-$33.65**
• Powder: 25 g: **$94.39**
CONTRAINDICATIONS: Hypersensitivity, bleeding warts or moles, birthmarks, moles with hair grow-

P

ing from them, poor blood circulation, diabetes

PRECAUTIONS: Avoid application on inflamed or irritated tissue

PREGNANCY AND LACTATION: Pregnancy category X

SIDE EFFECTS/ADVERSE REACTIONS

CNS: Peripheral neuropathy, paresthesia, confusion, dizziness, ***stupor, convulsions, coma, death***

HEME: ***Thrombocytopenia, leukopenia***

SKIN: Irritation of unaffected areas

MISC: Nausea, vomiting, diarrhea, abdominal pain

SPECIAL CONSIDERATIONS

- Not to be dispensed to the patient, professional application only
- Because of the potential for toxicity, cryotherapy should be attempted first or podofilox substituted

---

polymyxin B

(pol-ee-mix'in)

Aerosporin, Poly-Rx

Chemical Class: Polymyxin

Therapeutic Class: Antibacterial

CLINICAL PHARMACOLOGY

Mechanism of Action: Interferes with membrane phospholipids and increases membrane permeability; bactericidal

Pharmacokinetics

PO: Not absorbed from the GI tract

IM/IV/IT: Repeated injections accumulate; tissue diffusion poor; does not cross blood-brain barrier; $t_{1/2}$ 4½-6 hr, excreted slowly in urine unchanged (60%)

INDICATIONS AND USES: Serious infections (bacteremia) caused by susceptible strains of *Pseudomonas aeruginosa, E. aerogenes, Klebsiella pneumoniae, E. coli, Haemophilus influenzae* when other antibiotics cannot be used; in meningeal infections, polymyxin B must be given intrathecally; TOP OPHTH: superficial external ocular infections

DOSAGE

Adult

- IV INF 15,000-25,000 U/kg/d in divided doses q12h, or 25,000 U/kg/d in divided doses q4-8h
- IM pain at inj site; reconst with procaine 1%; 25,000-30,000 U/kg/d q4-6h; reduce dosage with renal dysfunction
- IT 50,000 U qd for 3-4 days, then 50,000 qod for 2 wk after cultures negative and CSF glucose normalized
- TOP OPHTH: Instill 1-2 gtt bid-qid × 7-10 days
- TOP: Apply bid-qid

Child

- IV INF 15,000-25,000 U/kg/d in divided doses q12h, or 25,000 U/kg/d in divided doses q4-8h; infants <2 yr, up to 40,000 U/d
- IM not recommended; severe pain at inj site; reconstitute with procaine 1%; 25,000-30,000 U/kg/d q4-6h; reduce dosage with renal dysfunction; infants <2 yr up to 40,000 U/d
- IT 50,000 U qd for 3-4 days, then 50,000 qod for 2 wk after cultures negative and CSF glucose normalized; infants <2 yr up to 20,000 U/d
- TOP OPHTH: Instill 1-2 gtt bid-qid × 7-10 days

$ **AVAILABLE FORMS/COST OF THERAPY**

- Inj, Dry-Sol—IM;IT;IV: 500,000 U/vial: **$5.32-$25.16**
- Sol, Dry-Powder—Ophth: 500,000 U/7.5 ml: **$7.60**

Many combination products available containing polymyxin B (both ophthalmic and topical applications) including neomycin and bacitracin (Neosporin); neomycin, bacitracin,

and hydrocortisone (Cortisporin); oxytetracycline (Terramycin w/ polymyxin B); trimethoprim (Polytrim); neomycin and dexamethasone (Maxitrol); chloramphenicol and hydrocortisone (Ophthocort)
CONTRAINDICATIONS: Hypersensitivity, severe renal disease
PRECAUTIONS: Renal dysfunction, neurologic or neuromuscular deficits
PREGNANCY AND LACTATION: Pregnancy category B
SIDE EFFECTS/ADVERSE REACTIONS
SKIN: Urticaria
CNS: Dizziness, confusion, weakness, drowsiness, paresthesia, slurred speech, ***coma, seizures,*** headache, stiff neck
EENT: Poor corneal wound healing, temporary visual haze, overgrowth of non-susceptible organisms
RESP: ***Apnea*** (concurrent use of other neurotoxic drugs or inadvertant overdosage)
GU: Proteinuria, hematuria, azotemia, leukocyturia

▼ DRUG INTERACTIONS
Drugs
- *Aminoglycosides:* Increased nephrotoxicity, neurotoxicity
- *Anesthetics:* Increased skeletal muscle relaxation
- *Neuromuscular blockers (tubocurarine, succinylcholine, gallamine, etc.):* Increased skeletal muscle relaxation

SPECIAL CONSIDERATIONS
- Generally replaced by the aminoglycosides or extended-spectrum penicillins for serious infections; still used for bladder irrigation and gut decontamination; used in combination with other antibiotics and/or corticosteroids topically to treat infections of the eye and skin

MONITORING PARAMETERS
- I&O, BUN, creatinine, urinalysis

polythiazide
(poly-thi'a-zide)
Renese
Chemical Class: Benzothiazide (thiazide) family
Therapeutic Class: Diuretic/antihypertensive agent

CLINICAL PHARMACOLOGY
Mechanism of Action: Increase renal excretion of sodium and chloride via tubular reabsorption inhibition in distal segment of nephron; some carbonic anhydrase activity due to sulfonamide moiety; increase potassium excretion; decrease calcium and uric acid excretion; decrease peripheral vascular resistance
Pharmacokinetics
PO: Onset 2 hr; peak 6 hr; duration 24-48 hr, $t_{1/2}$ 25.7 hr
INDICATIONS AND USES: Edema (CHF, hepatic cirrhosis, corticosteroid and estrogen therapy, renal dysfunction, i.e., nephrotic syndrome, acute glomerulonephritis), hypertension, calcium nephrolithiasis,* osteoporosis,* diabetes insipidus*
DOSAGE
Adult
- 1-4 mg qd; equivalent hydrochlorothiazide dose 2 mg = 50 mg

$ AVAILABLE FORMS/COST OF THERAPY
- Tab, Uncoated—Oral: 1 mg, 100's: **$41.24;** 2 mg, 100's: **$53.97;** 4 mg, 100's: **$90.21**

CONTRAINDICATIONS: Anuria, hypersensitivity
PRECAUTIONS: Imbalance of fluid and electrolytes, including calcium, potassium; gout, diabetes, tartrazine sensitivity
PREGNANCY AND LACTATION: Pregnancy category D; excreted in breast milk in low concentrations; compatible with breast feeding

SIDE EFFECTS/ADVERSE REACTIONS

CNS: Dizziness, vertigo, paresthesias, headache, xanthopsia

CV: Orthostatic hypotension

GI: Anorexia, gastric irritation, nausea, vomiting, cramping, diarrhea, constipation, jaundice (intrahepatic cholestatic jaundice), pancreatitis

HEME: ***Leukopenia, agranulocytosis, thrombocytopenia, aplastic anemia***

METAB: Hyperglycemia, glycosuria, hyperuricemia

MS: Muscle spasm, weakness

SKIN: Purpura, photosensitivity, rash, urticaria, necrotizing angitis, vasculitis, cutaneous vasculitis

▼ **DRUG INTERACTIONS**

Drugs

• *Antidiabetics:* Increased dosage requirements due to increased glucose levels

• *Carbenoxolone:* Additive potassium wasting, severe hypokalemia

• *Cholistyramine/colestipol:* Reduced absorption

• *Diazoxide:* Hyperglycemia

• *Digitalis glycosides:* Diuretic-induced hypokalemia increases risk of digitalis toxicity

• *Lithium+:* Increased lithium levels, potential toxicity

Labs

• *Increase:* BSP retention, Ca, cholesterol, triglycerides, amylase

• *Decrease:* PBI, PSP, parathyroid test

potassium iodide

Pima, SSKI, Iosat, Strong Iodine Solution (Lugol's Solution), Thyro-Block

Chemical Class: Iodine product

Therapeutic Class: Expectorant; antithyroid agent

CLINICAL PHARMACOLOGY

Mechanism of Action: Reduces viscosity of mucus by increasing respiratory tract secretions; inhibits the release and synthesis of thyroid hormone

Pharmacokinetics

PO: Accumulates in thyroid gland, onset (antithyroid effects) 24-48 hr, peak effect (antithyroid effects) 10-15 days after continuous therapy, excreted mainly by the kidney

INDICATIONS AND USES: Expectorant, preoperative reduction of thyroid gland vascularity prior to thyroidectomy, thyrotoxic crisis (in conjunction with other antithyroid agents), persistent or recurrent hyperthyroidism, radiation emergencies (to prevent uptake of radioactive isotopes of iodine), cutaneous sporotrichosis*

DOSAGE

Adult

• *Expectorant:* PO 300-650 mg tid-qid

• *Preoperative thyroidectomy:* PO 50-250 mg (1-5 gtt SSKI; 3-5 gtt Lugol's solution) tid for 10-14 days prior to surgery

• *Thyrotoxic crisis:* PO 300-500 mg (6-10 gtt SSKI; 1 ml Lugol's solution) tid

• *Cutaneous sporotrichosis:* PO 65-325 mg tid

• *Radiation emergency:* PO mg qd for 10 days

Child

• *Expectorant:* PO 60-250 mg qid; max 500 mg/dose

• *Preoperative thyroidectomy:* PO 50-250 mg (1-5 gtt SSKI; 3-5 gtt Lugol's solution) tid for 10-14 days prior to surgery

• *Thyrotoxic crisis:* PO <1 yr 65 mg qd for 10 days; older children 130 mg qd for 10 days

• *Radiation emergency:* PO <1 yr, 65 mg qd for 10 days; older children, 130 mg qd for 10 days

$ AVAILABLE FORMS/COST OF THERAPY

• Sol—Oral: 15 g/15 ml, 30 ml: **$2.25-$12.10**

• Sol—Oral: 5% iodine/10% potassium iodide, 120 ml: **$1.80-$3.83**

• Syr—Oral: 325 mg/5 ml, 480 ml: **$15.00**

CONTRAINDICATIONS: Hypersensitivity, tuberculosis, acute bronchitis, hyperkalemia

PRECAUTIONS: Hypocomplementemic vasculitis, goiter, autoimmune thyroid disease, sulfite sensitivity (increased risk for iodine-induced adverse effects)

PREGNANCY AND LACTATION: Pregnancy category D; use of iodides as expectorants during pregnancy is contraindicated; concentrated in breast milk, may affect infant's thyroid activity but considered compatible with breast feeding

SIDE EFFECTS/ADVERSE REACTIONS

CNS: Fever, headache

CV: ***Angioedema***

EENT: Rhinitis

GI: Metallic taste, *GI upset,* soreness of teeth and gums

HEME: Cutaneous and mucosal hemorrhage, eosinophilia

METAB: Goiter, hypothyroidism

MS: Arthralgia

SKIN: Urticaria, acne

MISC: Lymph node enlargement

▼ DRUG INTERACTIONS

Drugs

• *Lithium:* Increased likelihood of hypothyroidism

SPECIAL CONSIDERATIONS

PATIENT/FAMILY EDUCATION

• Dilute sol with water or fruit juice to improve taste, drink sol through straw

• Notify physician of fever, rash, metallic taste, swelling of throat, burning of mouth and throat, sore gums and teeth, head cold symptoms, severe GI distress, enlargement of thyroid gland

• Administer with food or milk

MONITORING PARAMETERS

• Thyroid function tests if used for thyroid-related conditions

potassium salts

(po-taah'see-um)

Potassium chloride:
Cena-K, Kaochlor, Kay Ciel, Klorvess, Potasalan, Rum-K, Kaon-Cl, K+ Care, K-lor, gen K, Kato, Klor-Con, Micro-K LS, Slow-K, K+10, Klotrix, K-tab, K-Dur, Ten-K, Micro-K, K-Lease, K-Norm

Potassium gluconate:
Kaon, Kaylizer, K-G Elixer

Combinations of potassium salts:
Effer-K, K-Lyte, K-Lyte DS, Klor-Con EF (as bicarbonate, citrate), Tri-K, (as acetate, bicarbonate, citrate), Twin-K (as gluconate, citrate), Kolyum (as chloride, gluconate), Klorvess Effervescent Granules (as bicarbonate, chloride, citrate), K-Lyte/Cl (as bicarbonate, chloride)

Chemical Class: Potassium salt
Therapeutic Class: Electrolyte

CLINICAL PHARMACOLOGY

Mechanism of Action: Principal intracellular cation of most body tissues; necessary for maintenance of intracellular tonicity and proper relationships with sodium across cell membranes; needed for adequate nerve transmission, cardiac, skeletal, and smooth muscle contration, renal function, and acid-base balance; normal serum potassium level 3.5-5.0 mEq/L (higher, to 7.7 mEq/L in neonates)

Pharmacokinetics

PO/IV: Primarily renal excretion (90%); fecal (10%)

INDICATIONS AND USES: Prevention and treatment of hypokalemia; with alkalosis (i.e., due to diuretics), use potassium chloride salt; when acidosis present, use potassium acetate, bicarbonate, citrate, or gluconate salts; hypertension*

DOSAGE

• Individualize dosage up to 400 mEq/d (usually not more than 3 mEq/kg/d): 16-30 mEq/d for prevention; 40-100 mEq/d for treatment

mEq/g of potassium salts

K+ Salt	mEq/g
gluconate	4.3
citrate	9.8
bicarbonate	10
acetate	10.2
chloride	13.4

Adult

• *Potassium acetate:* Serum potassium >2.5 mEq/L: IV INF, up to 200 mEq/d in concentration <30 mEq/L at rate of 10 mEq/hr; serum potassium <2.0 mEq/L: IV INF, up to 400 mEq/day in concentration and rate up to 20 mEq/hr

• *Potassium bicarbonate:* PO dissolve 25-50 mEq in water qd-bid up to 100 mEq/d

• *Potassium chloride:* PO 40-100 mEq in divided doses bid-tid; IV serum potassium>2.5 mEq/l, IV up to 200 mEq/d in <30 mEq/L conc at a rate not exceeding 10 mEq/hr; serum potassium <2.0 mEq/L; IV up to 400 mEq/d at conc and rate of 20 mEq/hr

• *Potassium gluconate:* PO 20 mEq in divided doses bid-qid

• *Potassium phosphate:* IV 1 mEq/hr in sol of 60 mEq/L, not to exceed 150 mEq/d

Child

• *Potassium acetate:* IV up to 3 mEq/kg or 40 mEq/m^2 per day

• *Potassium chloride:* PO sol 15-40 mEq/m2 or 1-3 mEq/kg/d in divided doses diluted in water or juice; IV up to 3 mEq/kg or 40 mEq/m^2 per day

• *Potassium gluconate:* PO 20-40 mEq/m^2 or 2-3 mEq/kg per day in divided doses

$ AVAILABLE FORMS/COST OF THERAPY

Potassium acetate

• Granules—Oral: 500 g: **$18.20**

• Inj, Sol—IV: 2 mEq/ml, 20 ml: **$4.75;** 4mEq/ml, 50 ml: **$5.56**

Potassium bicarbonate

• Liq—Oral: 45 mEq/15 ml, 480 ml: **$8.85-$11.74**

• Tab, Effervescent—Oral: 25 mEq, 30's: **$5.31-$45.94**

Potassium chloride

• Cap, Gel, Sust Action—Oral: 8 mEq, 100's: **$9.23-$19.21;** 10 mEq, 100's: **$14.20-$20.21**

• Tab, Coated, Sust Action—Oral: 8 mEq, 100's: **$7.28-$16.96;** 10 mEq, 100's: **$7.80-$33.75;** 6.7 mEq, 100's: **$28.00;** 20 mEq, 100's: **$39.21**

• Tab, Effervescent—Oral: 20 mEq, 30's: **$5.13-$28.00;** 50 mEq, 30's **$50.41**

• Liq—Oral: 10%, 480 ml: **$2.20-$46.61;** 20%, 480 ml: **$2.52-$26.94**

• Powder, Reconst—Oral: 15 mEq, 30's: **$6.06-$23.31;** 20 mEq/pkg, 30's: **$3.95-$50.71;** 25 mEq/pkg, 30's: **$7.41**

• Inj, Conc—Sol: 1.5 mEq/ml, 10 ml: **$4.36-$5.19;** 2 mEq/ml, 10 ml: **$2.74-$7.59;** 3 mEq/ml, 30 ml: **$1.50**
Potassium gluconate
• Elixir—Oral: 20 mEq/15 ml, 480 ml: **$5.00-$27.34**
• Inj, Susp—IM; Oral: 4.68 g/15 ml, 473 ml: **$6.00**
Potassium phosphate
• Inj, Conc-Sol—IV: 236 mg/224 mg, 5 ml: **$3.27**

CONTRAINDICATIONS: Renal disease (severe), severe hemolytic disease, Addison's disease, hyperkalemia, acute dehydration, extensive tissue breakdown

PRECAUTIONS: Cardiac disease, K-sparing diuretic therapy, systemic acidosis

SIDE EFFECTS/ADVERSE REACTIONS

CNS: Confusion
CV: Bradycardia, ***cardiac depression, dysrhythmias, arrest, peaking T waves, lowered R and depressed RST, prolonged P-R interval, widened QRS complex***
GI: Nausea, vomiting, cramps, pain, *diarrhea,* ulceration of small bowel
GU: Oliguria
SKIN: Cold extremities, rash

▼ DRUG INTERACTIONS

• *Potassium sparing diuretics:* Hyperkalemia
• *ACE inhibitors:* Hyperkalemia

SPECIAL CONSIDERATIONS

• Avoid use of compressed tablets or enteric-coated tablets (i.e., nonsustained release or effervescent tablets for sol) due to significant ulcerogenic tendency and propensity to cause significant local tissue destruction
• Sol, powder, and oral susp: dilute or dissove in 120 ml cold water or juice
• Ext-rel cap and tab: do not crush; take with food; swallow with full glass of liquid
• Injectable potassium products must be diluted prior to administration; direct inj of potassium concentrate may be fatal

pralidoxime

(pra-li-dox'eem)
Protopam Chloride
Chemical Class: Quaternary ammonium oxime
Therapeutic Class: Antidote

CLINICAL PHARMACOLOGY

Mechanism of Action: Reactivates cholinesterase inactivated by exposure to organophosphate pesticides or related compounds by displacing the enzyme from its receptor sites; most effective if administered within 24 hr of exposure

Pharmacokinetics

IM/IV: Peak 5-15 min, not bound to plasma proteins, metabolized in liver, excreted rapidly in urine (metabolite and unchanged drug), $t_{1/2}$ 1.7 hr (repeated doses may be needed)

INDICATIONS AND USES: Antidote in poisonings due to organophosphate pesticides and related compounds, control of overdosage by anticholinesterase drugs used to treat myasthenia gravis

DOSAGE

Use in conjunction with atropine

Adult

• *Organophosphate poisoning:* IM/IV 1-2 g, repeat in 1-2 hr if muscle weakness has not resolved, then at 10-12 hr intervals of cholinergic signs reappear
• *Anticholinesterase overdosage:* IV 1-2 g, followed by 250 mg q5min until desired response

Child

• *Organophosphate poisoning:* IM/IV 20-50 mg/kg/dose, repeat in 1-2

P

hr if muscle weakness has not resolved, then at 10-12 hr intervals if cholinergic signs reappear

$ **AVAILABLE FORMS/COST OF THERAPY**

• Inj, Lyphl-Sol—IM; IV; SC: 50 mg/ml, 20 ml: **$28.86**

CONTRAINDICATIONS: Hypersensitivity

PRECAUTIONS: Rapid IV inj, impaired renal function, myasthenia gravis, carbamate poisoning (less effective than with organophosphate poisoning)

PREGNANCY AND LACTATION: Pregnancy category C

SIDE EFFECTS/ADVERSE REACTIONS

CNS: Dizziness, headache, drowsiness

CV: Tachycardia

EENT: Blurred vision, diplopia, impaired accommodation

GI: Transaminase elevations (return to normal within 2 wk), nausea

MS: Muscular weakness

RESP: Hyperventilation

SKIN: Pain at inj site (IM)

SPECIAL CONSIDERATIONS

MONITORING PARAMETERS

• RBCs, plasma cholinesterase activity may help confirm diagnosis and follow course of illness

pramoxine

(pra-mox'een)

Fleet Relief, Itch-X, PrameGel, Prax, ProctoFoam, Tronolane, Tronothane

Chemical Class: Structurally similar to dyclonine

Therapeutic Class: Topical anesthetic

CLINICAL PHARMACOLOGY

Mechanism of Action: Decreases the neuronal membrane's permeability to sodium ions thus inhibiting depolarization; blocks initiation and conduction of nerve impulses

Pharmacokinetics

TOP: Onset 2-5 min, duration may be several days

INDICATIONS AND USES: Temporary relief of pain and itching associated with dermatoses, minor burns, anogenital pruritus or irritation, anal fissures, hermorrhoids

DOSAGE

Adult

• TOP apply tid-qid; PR apply up to 5 times daily; apply 1 applicatorful of aerosol foam bid-tid after bowel movements

$ **AVAILABLE FORMS/COST OF THERAPY**

• Supp—Rect: 1%, 10's: **$3.41**

• Oint—Rect: 1%, 30 g: **$2.63**

• Aer Foam Susp—Rect; Top: 1%, 15 g: **$13.92**

• Cre—Rect; Top: 1%, 30, 60 g: **$3.05-$5.21**

• Cre—Top: 1%, 30 g: **$8.46**

• Gel—Top: 1%, 35.4, 120 g: **$2.94-$6.15**

• Lotion—Top: 1%, 15, 120, 240 ml: **$3.25-$13.40**

CONTRAINDICATIONS: Hypersensitivity

PRECAUTIONS: Prolonged use, rectal bleeding, children, denuded skin

PREGNANCY AND LACTATION: Pregnancy category C

SIDE EFFECTS/ADVERSE REACTIONS

SKIN: Burning, stinging, rash, irritation

SPECIAL CONSIDERATIONS

• Cross-sensitization with other local anesthetics unlikely

PATIENT/FAMILY EDUCATION

• Do not use near eyes or nose

• Contact physician if condition fails to improve after 3-4 days or worsens

- Do not apply to large areas
- Do not apply to unaffected areas

pravastatin

(prav-i-sta'tin)

Pravachol

Chemical Class: Mevinic acid derivative

Therapeutic Class: Antilipemic

CLINICAL PHARMACOLOGY

Mechanism of Action: Competitively inhibits 3-hydroxy-3-methylglutaryl-coenzyme A (HMG-CoA) reductase which catalyzes the early rate-limiting step in cholesterol biosynthesis; increases HDL cholesterol, decreases LDL cholesterol; modestly decreases triglycerides

Pharmacokinetics

PO: Peak 1-1½ hr, absolute bioavailability 17%, 50% bound to plasma proteins, metabolized in liver, excreted in urine (20%) and feces (70%), $t_{1/2}$ 77 hr

INDICATIONS AND USES: Hypercholesterolemia (Types IIa and IIb)

DOSAGE

Adult

- PO 10-20 mg qhs, may increase to 40 mg qhs if needed

$ AVAILABLE FORMS/COST OF THERAPY

- Tab, Uncoated—Oral: 10 mg, 90's: **$157.99;** 20 mg, 90's: **$170.11;** 40 mg, 90's: **$287.57**

CONTRAINDICATIONS: Hypersensitivity, active liver disease, unexplained persistent elevated liver function tests

PRECAUTIONS: History of liver disease, renal function impairment, elderly, children <18 yr, alcoholism; risk factors predisposing to the development of renal failure secondary to rhabdomyolysis (severe acute infection, trauma, hypotension, uncontrolled seizure disorder, severe metabolic disorders, electrolyte imbalance)

PREGNANCY AND LACTATION: Pregnancy category X; small amounts excreted in breast milk, should probably not be used by women who are nursing

SIDE EFFECTS/ADVERSE REACTIONS:

CNS: Headache, dizziness

CV: Chest pain

GI: Nausea, vomiting, abdominal pain, constipation, flatulence, heartburn, ***pancreatitis, hepatitis, cholestatic jaundice, fatty change in liver, cirrhosis,*** anorexia, increased liver function tests

GU: Loss of libido, erectile dysfunction

MS: Localized pain, myalgia, myopathy, ***rhabdomyolysis,*** arthralgia

SKIN: Rash, pruritus, alopecia, photosensitivity

MISC: Fatigue, gynecomastia

▼ DRUG INTERACTIONS

Labs

- *Increase:* CPK, liver function tests

SPECIAL CONSIDERATIONS

PATIENT/FAMILY EDUCATION

- Avoid prolonged exposure to sunlight and other UV light
- Promptly report any unexplained muscle pain, tenderness, or weakness, especially if accompanied by fever or malaise
- Strictly adhere to low cholesterol diet

MONITORING PARAMETERS

- Liver function tests at baseline, q4-6 wk during first 3 mo, q6-12 wk during next 12 mo, then periodically thereafter (discontinue if elevations persist at >3 times upper limit of normal)
- CPK in any patient complaining of diffuse myalgia, muscle tenderness, or weakness
- Fasting lipid profile

prazepam

(pra'ze-pam)

Centrax

Chemical Class: Benzodiazepine
Therapeutic Class: Anxiolytic
DEA Class: Schedule IV

CLINICAL PHARMACOLOGY

Mechanism of Action: Facilitates the inhibitory effect of γ-aminobutyric acid (GABA) on neuronal excitability by increasing membrane permeability to chloride ions

Pharmacokinetics

PO: Peak 6 hr, slow onset, metabolized in liver to active metabolite, eliminated in urine, $t_{1/2}$ 30-100 hr (active metabolite)

INDICATIONS AND USES: Anxiety

DOSAGE

Adult

- PO 30 mg/d in divided doses (range 20-60 mg/d); may also be administered as single hs dose starting at 20 mg/night (range 20-40 mg/night)

Elderly

- PO 10-15 mg/d in divided doses

$ **AVAILABLE FORMS/COST OF THERAPY**

- Cap, Gel—Oral: 5 mg, 100's: **$28.05-$65.68;** 10 mg, 100's: **$32.65-$76.33;** 20 mg, 100's: **$124.82**
- Tab, Uncoated—Oral: 10 mg, 100's: **$53.78**

CONTRAINDICATIONS: Hypersensitivity to benzodiazepines, narrow angle glaucoma, psychosis

PRECAUTIONS: Elderly, debilitated, hepatic disease, renal disease, history of drug abuse, abrupt withdrawal, respiratory depression, children <18 yr

PREGNANCY AND LACTATION: Pregnancy category D; may cause fetal damage when administered during pregnancy; excreted into breast milk, may accumulate in breast-fed infants and is therefore not recommended

SIDE EFFECTS/ADVERSE REACTIONS

CNS: Somnolence, asthenia, hypokinesia, hangover, abnormal thinking, anxiety, agitation, amnesia, apathy emotional lability, hostility, seizure, sleep disorder, stupor, twitch, ataxia, decreased reflexes, neuritis

CV: Dysrhythmia, syncope

EENT: Ear pain, eye irritation/pain/swelling, photophobia, pharyngitis, rhinitis, sinusitis, epistaxis

GI: Dyspepsia, decreased/increased appetite, flatulence, gastritis, enterocolitis, melena, mouth ulceration, abdominal pain, increased AST

GU: Frequent urination, menstrual cramps, urinary hesitancy/urgency, vaginal discharge/itching, hematuria, nocturia, oliguria, penile discharge, urinary incontinence, decreased libido

HEME: ***Agranulocytosis***

MS: Lower extremity pain, back pain

RESP: Cold symptoms, asthma, cough, dyspnea, hyperventilation

SKIN: Urticaria, acne, dry skin, photosensitivity

▼ **DRUG INTERACTIONS**

Drugs

- *Cimetidine:* Increased plasma concentrations of prazepam

Labs

- *Increase:* AST/ALT, serum bilirubin
- *Decrease:* RAIU
- *False increase:* 17-OHCS

SPECIAL CONSIDERATIONS

PATIENT/FAMILY EDUCATION

- Avoid alcohol and other CNS depressants
- Do not discontinue abruptly after prolonged therapy

• May cause drowsiness or dizziness
• Use caution while driving or performing other tasks requiring alertness
• Inform your physician if you are planning to become pregnant, you are pregnant, or if you become pregnant while taking this medicine
• May be habit forming

MONITORING PARAMETERS
• Periodic CBC, urinalysis, blood chemistry analyses during prolonged therapy

praziquantel

(pray-zi-kwon'tel)
Biltricide
Chemical Class: Pyrazinoisoquinoline derivative
Therapeutic Class: Anthelmintic

CLINICAL PHARMACOLOGY
Mechanism of Action: Increases cell membrane permeability in susceptible worms causing a loss of intracellular calcium, massive contractions and paralysis of worm musculature leading to detachment of suckers from blood vessel walls and dislodgment; also results in vacuolization and disintegration of the schistosome in tegument, followed by attachment of phagocytes and death
Pharmacokinetics
PO: Rapidly absorbed, peak 1-3 hr, significant first-pass biotransformation, metabolites excreted primarily in urine, $t_{1/2}$ 0.8-1½ hr

INDICATIONS AND USES: Schistosomiasis caused by *Schistosoma* sp pathogenic to humans, clonorchiasis and opisthorchiasis (liver flukes), cysticercosis,* tissue fluke infections,* intestinal fluke infections,* intestinal cestode (tapeworm) infections*

DOSAGE
Adult and Child
• *Schistosomiasis:* PO 20 mg/kg/dose 2-3 times/d for 1 day at 4-6 hr intervals
• *Clonorchiasis and opisthorchiasis:* PO 75 mg/kg/d divided q8h for 1-2 days
• *Cysticercosis:* PO 50 mg/kg/d divided q8h for 14 days (administer steroids prior to starting praziquantel for neurocysticercosis)
• *Cestodes:* PO 10-20 mg/kg as a single dose (25 mg/kg for *Hymenolepsis nana*)

$ AVAILABLE FORMS/COST OF THERAPY
• Tab, Plain Coated—Oral: 600 mg, 6's: **$61.88**

CONTRAINDICATIONS: Hypersensitivity, ocular cysticercosis

PRECAUTIONS: Children <4 yr, cerebral cysticercosis (hospitalize patient for duration of therapy)

PREGNANCY AND LACTATION: Pregnancy category B; do not nurse on day of treatment and during the subsequent 72 hr

SIDE EFFECTS/ADVERSE REACTIONS
CNS: Headache, dizziness, fever, drowsiness
GI: Abdominal discomfort, minimal increases in liver enzymes
SKIN: Urticaria
MISC: Malaise

SPECIAL CONSIDERATIONS

PATIENT/FAMILY EDUCATION
• Swallow tablets unchewed with some liquid during meals
• May cause drowsiness
• Use caution driving or performing other tasks requiring alertness

P

prazosin

(pra'zoe-sin)
Minipress
Chemical Class: Quinazoline derivative
Therapeutic Class: Antihypertensive

CLINICAL PHARMACOLOGY

Mechanism of Action: Competitively inhibits postsynaptic α_1-adrenergic receptors; produces both arterial and venous dilation; reduces peripheral vascular resistance and blood pressure; blockade of α_1-adrenoceptors in bladder neck and prostate relaxes smooth muscle improving urine flow rates in benign prostatic hypertrophy

Pharmacokinetics

PO: Oral bioavailability 48%-68%, peak 1-3 hr, duration of antihypertensive effect 10 hr, 92%-97% bound to plasma proteins, extensively metabolized to active metabolites, excreted in bile (90%) and urine (10%), $t_{1/2}$ 2-3 hr

INDICATIONS AND USES: Hypertension, benign prostatic hypertrophy,* Raynaud's vasospasm,* refractory congestive heart failure*

DOSAGE

Adult

• PO 1 mg bid-tid, give first dose at bedtime; increase as needed to 6-15 mg/d in divided doses; doses >20 mg/d usually do not increase efficacy

Child

• PO 0.5-7 mg tid

$ **AVAILABLE FORMS/COST OF THERAPY**

• Cap, Gel—Oral: 1 mg, 100's: **$6.38-$48.28;** 2 mg, 100's: **$7.43-$66.52;** 5 mg, 100's: **$11.93-$112.47**

CONTRAINDICATIONS: Hypersensitivity to quinazolines

PRECAUTIONS: Children, hepatic disease

PREGNANCY AND LACTATION: Pregnancy category C

SIDE EFFECTS/ADVERSE REACTIONS

CNS: Depression, *dizziness,* nervousness, paresthesia, somnolence, anxiety, insomnia, asthenia, ataxia, hypertonia, *headache,* fever

CV: Palpitations, postural hypotension, tachycardia, dysrhythmia, chest pain, edema, flushing, ***"first-dose" syncope***

EENT: Abnormal vision, tinnitus, vertigo

GI: Nausea, vomiting, dry mouth, diarrhea, constipation, abdominal discomfort, flatulence

GU: Incontinence, polyuria

MS: Arthralgia, myalgia

RESP: Dyspnea

SKIN: Rash, pruritus

▼ **DRUG INTERACTIONS**

Drugs

• *Beta blockers:* Enhanced first-dose response to prazosin

Labs

• *Increase:* VMA

• *False positive:* Screening tests for pheochromocytoma

SPECIAL CONSIDERATIONS

PATIENT/FAMILY EDUCATION

• Alert patients to the possibility of syncopal and orthostatic symptoms, especially with the first dose ("first-dose syncope")

• Take initial dose at bedtime, arise slowly from reclining position

• Report dizziness or palpitations to physician

• Use caution when driving or operating heavy machinery

prednisolone

(pred-niss'oh-lone)

Delta-Cortef, Prelone; (acetate) Articulose, Key-Pred, Predaject, Predalone, Predcor, Predicort; (sodium phosphate) Hydeltrasol, Key-Pred-SP, Pediapred; (tebutate) Hydeltra-T.B.A., Predalone T.B.A., Prednisol TBA; Ophthalmic: (acetate) Econopred, Econopred Plus, Pred Mild, Pred Forte; (sodium phosphate) AK-Pred, Inflamase Mild, Inflamase Forte

Chemical Class: Glucocorticoid
Therapeutic Class: Corticosteroid

CLINICAL PHARMACOLOGY

Mechanism of Action: Controls the rate of protein synthesis, depresses the migrations of polymorphonuclear leukocytes and fibroblasts, reverses capillary permeability, and causes lysosomal stabilization at the cellular level to prevent or control inflammation

Pharmacokinetics

PO: Peak 1-2 hr, duration 2 days
IM: Peak 3-45 hr

Metabolized in most tissues but primarily in liver, excreted in urine, $t_{1/2}$ 115-212 min (biologic 18-36 hr)

INDICATIONS AND USES: Antiinflammatory or immunosuppressant agent in the treatment of a variety of diseases including those of hematologic, allergic, inflammatory, neoplastic, and autoimmune origin; (ophth) steroid-responsive inflammatory conditions of the palpebral and bulbar conjunctiva, lid, cornea, and anterior segment of the globe, corneal injury (chemical, radiation, or thermal burns or penetration of foreign bodies)

DOSAGE

Adult

- PO 5-60 mg/d; IM (acetate) 4-60 mg/d; IM/IV (sodium phosphate) 4-60 mg/d; Intra-articular/intralesional/soft tissue (acetate) 4 mg, up to 100 mg; (tebutate) large joints 20-30 mg, small joints 8-10 mg, bursae 20-30 mg, tendon sheaths 4-10 mg, ganglia 10-20 mg; (sodium phosphate) large joint 10-20 mg, small joints 4-5 mg, bursae 10-15 mg, tendon sheaths 2-5 mg, soft tissue infiltration 10-30 mg, ganglia 5-10 mg
- *Multiple sclerosis (acute exacerbations):* PO 200 mg qd for 1 wk, followed by 80 mg qod for 1 mo
- *Ophth:* 1gtt q1h during day, q2h during night until favorable response, then 1 gtt q4h

Child

- *Acute asthma:* PO 1-2 mg/kg/d divided 1-2 times/d for 3-5 days; IV 2-4 mg/kg/d divided tid-qid
- *Antiinflammatory/immunosuppressive:* PO/IV 0.1-2 mg/kg/d divided qd-qid
- *Ophth:* 1 gtt q1h during day, q2h during night until favorable response, then 1 gtt q4h

$ AVAILABLE FORMS/COST OF THERAPY

- Syr—Oral: 15 mg/5 ml, 240 ml: **$49.06**
- Liq—Oral (sodium phosphate): 5 mg/5 ml, 120 ml: **$14.89**
- Tab, Uncoated—Oral: 5 mg, 100's: **$2.04-$19.18**
- Susp, Top—Ophth (acetate): 0.12%, 5, 10 ml: **$13.84-$19.70**
- Susp—Ophth (acetate): 0.125%, 5, 10 ml: **$14.06-$21.25,** 1%, 1, 5, 10, 15 ml: **$4.69-$34.04**
- Sol—Ophth (sodium phosphate): 0.125%, 5, 10 ml: **$2.70-$18.30;** 1%, 5, 10, 15 ml: **$5.48-$25.56**
- Inj, Susp—Intra-Articular; Intra-

P

synovial (tebutate): 20 mg/ml, 5 ml: **$4.00-$20.49**

• Inj, Sol—IV (sodium phosphate): 20 mg/ml, 5 ml: **$3.50-$35.64**

• Inj, Susp—IM (acetate): 25 mg/ml, 30 ml: **$6.50-$12.98;** 50 mg/ml, 30 ml: **$7.49-$18.55**

CONTRAINDICATIONS: Systemic fungal infections, hypersensitivity, idiopathic thrombocytopenic purpura (IM); (ophth) hypersensitivity; acute superficial herpes simplex keratitis; fungal diseases of ocular structures; vaccinia, varicella and most other viral diseases of the cornea and conjunctiva; ocular TB; following uncomplicated removal of a superficial corneal foreign body

PRECAUTIONS: Psychosis, acute glomerulonephritis, amebiasis, cerebral malaria, child <2 yr, elderly, AIDS, tuberculosis, diabetes mellitus, glaucoma, osteoporosis, ulcerative colitis, CHF, myasthenia gravis, renal disease, esophagitis, peptic ulcer, ocular herpes simplex, live virus vaccines, hypertension; (ophthal) prolonged use, infections of the eye, glaucoma

PREGNANCY AND LACTATION: Pregnancy category B; compatible with breast feeding

SIDE EFFECTS/ADVERSE REACTIONS

CNS: Depression, vertigo, ***convulsions,*** headache, *mood changes*

CV: Hypertension, thrombophlebitis, ***thromboembolism,*** tachycardia, CHF

EENT: Increased intraocular pressure, blurred vision, cataract; (ophth) poor corneal wound healing, increased possibility of corneal infection, glaucoma exacerbation, ***optic nerve damage,*** decreased acuity, visual field, cataracts, transient burning/stinging

GI: Diarrhea, nausea, abdominal distension, ***GI hemorrhage,*** increased appetite, ***pancreatitis***

METAB: Cushingoid state, growth suppression in children, HPA axis suppression, decreased glucose tolerance

MS: Fractures, osteoporosis, aseptic necrosis of femoral and humeral heads, weakness, muscle mass loss

SKIN: Acne, poor wound healing, ecchymosis, bruising, petechiae, striae, thin fragile skin, suppression of skin test reactions

▼ DRUG INTERACTIONS

Drugs

• *Aminoglutethamide:* Enhanced elimination of corticosteroids; marked reduction in corticosteroid response

• *Antidiabetics:* Increased blood glucose in patients with diabetes

• *Barbiturates, carbamazepine:* Reduced serum concentrations of corticosteroids

• *Cholestyramine:* Possible reduced absorption of corticosteroids

• *Estrogens:* Enhanced effects of corticosteroids

• *Isoniazid:* Reduced plasma concentrations of isoniazid

• *Phenytoin, rifampin:* Reduced therapeutic effect of corticosteroids

• *Salicylates:* Enhanced elimination of salicylates; subtherapeutic salicylate concentrations possible

Labs

• *Increase:* Cholesterol, blood glucose, urine glucose

• *Decrease:* Calcium, potassium, T_4, T_3, thyroid ^{131}I uptake test

• *False negative:* Skin allergy tests

SPECIAL CONSIDERATIONS

PATIENT/FAMILY EDUCATION

• May cause GI upset

• Take with meals or snacks

• Take single daily doses in AM

• Notify physician if unusual weight gain, swelling of lower extremities, muscle weakness, black tarry stools, vomiting of blood, puffing of the face, menstrual irregularities, prolonged sore throat, fever, cold, or infection occurs

- Signs of adrenal insufficiency include fatigue, anorexia, nausea, vomiting, diarrhea, weight loss, weakness, dizziness, and low blood sugar
- Notify physician if these signs and symptoms appear following dose reduction or withdrawal of therapy
- Avoid abrupt withdrawal of therapy following high dose or long-term therapy; not to discontinue ophthal use without consulting physician
- May cause sensitivity to bright light; minimize by wearing sunglasses
- Notify physician if no improvement after 1 wk, if condition worsens, or if pain, itching, or swelling of the eye occurs

MONITORING PARAMETERS

- Potassium and blood sugar during long-term therapy
- Edema, blood pressure, cardiac symptoms, mental status, weight
- Observe growth and development of infants and children on prolonged therapy
- Ophth, check intraocular pressure and lens frequently during prolonged use

prednisone

(pred'ni-sone)

Deltasone, Liquid Pred, Meticorten, Orasone, Panasol-S, Prednicen-M, Prednisone Intensol Concentrate, Sterapred, Sterapred OS

Chemical Class: Glucocorticoid
Therapeutic Class: Corticosteroid

CLINICAL PHARMACOLOGY

Mechanism of Action: Controls the rate of protein synthesis, depresses the migrations of polymorphonuclear leukocytes and fibroblasts, reverses capillary permeability, and causes lysosomal stabilization at the cellular level to prevent or control inflammation

Pharmacokinetics

PO: Absorption 78%, must be metabolized to prednisolone for activity, excreted in urine, $t_{1/2}$ 60 min (biologic 18-36 hr)

INDICATIONS AND USES: Antiinflammatory or immunosuppressant agent in the treatment of a variety of diseases including those of hematologic, allergic, inflammatory, neoplastic, and autoimmune origin

DOSAGE

Adult

- PO 5-60 mg/d divided qd-qid
- *Physiologic replacement:* PO 4-5 mg/m^2/d

Child

- *Antiinflammatory/immunosuppressive:* PO 0.05-2 mg/kg/d divided qd-qid
- *Acute asthma:* PO 1-2 mg/kg/d divided qd-bid for 3-5 days
- *Asthma long-term therapy:* PO <1 yr 10 mg qod, 1-4 yr 20 mg qod, 5-13 yr 30 mg qod, >13 yr 40 mg qod
- *Physiologic replacement:* PO 4-5 mg/m^2/d

$ AVAILABLE FORMS/COST OF THERAPY

- Sol—Oral: 5 mg/5 ml, 480 ml: **$11.90-$17.22;** 30 ml **$14.02**
- Tab, Uncoated—Oral: 1, 2.5, 5, 10, 20, 25, 50 mg, 100's: **$2.51-$27.69**
- Syr—Oral: 5 mg/5 ml, 240 ml: **$25.27**

CONTRAINDICATIONS: Systemic fungal infections, hypersensitivity

PRECAUTIONS: Psychosis, acute glomerulonephritis, amebiasis, ce-

P

rebral malaria, child <2 yr, elderly, AIDS, tuberculosis, diabetes mellitus, glaucoma, osteoporosis, ulcerative colitis, CHF, myasthenia gravis, renal disease, esophagitis, peptic ulcer, ocular herpes simplex, live virus vaccines, hypertension

PREGNANCY AND LACTATION: Pregnancy category B; compatible with breast feeding

SIDE EFFECTS/ADVERSE REACTIONS

CNS: Depression, vertigo, ***convulsions,*** headache, *mood changes*

CV: Hypertension, thrombophlebitis, ***thromboembolism,*** tachycardia, CHF

EENT: Increased intraocular pressure, blurred vision, cataract

GI: Diarrhea, nausea, abdominal distension, ***GI hemorrhage,*** increased appetite, ***pancreatitis***

METAB: Cushingoid state, growth suppression in children, HPA axis suppression, decreased glucose tolerance

MS: Fractures, osteoporosis, aseptic necrosis of femoral and humeral heads, weakness, muscle mass loss

SKIN: Acne, poor wound healing, ecchymosis, bruising, petechiae, striae, thin fragile skin, suppression of skin test reactions

▼ **DRUG INTERACTIONS**

Drugs

- *Aminoglutethamide:* Enhanced elimination of corticosteroids; marked reduction in corticosteroid response
- *Antidiabetics:* Increased blood glucose in patients with diabetes
- *Barbiturates, carbamazepine:* Reduced serum concentrations of corticosteroids
- *Cholestyramine:* Possible reduced absorption of corticosteroids
- *Estrogens:* Enhanced effects of corticosteroids
- *Isoniazid:* Reduced plasma concentrations of isoniazid
- *Phenytoin, rifampin:* Reduced therapeutic effect of corticosteroids
- *Salicylates:* Enhanced elimination of salicylates; subtherapeutic salicylate concentrations possible

Labs

- *Increase:* Cholesterol, blood glucose, urine glucose
- *Decrease:* Calcium, potassium, T_4, T_3, thyroid I^{131} uptake test
- *False negative:* Skin allergy tests

SPECIAL CONSIDERATIONS

PATIENT/FAMILY EDUCATION

- May cause GI upset, teach patient to take with meals or snacks
- Take single daily doses in AM
- Notify physician if unusual weight gain, swelling of lower extremities, muscle weakness, black tarry stools, vomiting of blood, puffing of the face, menstrual irregularities, prolonged sore throat, fever, cold, or infection occurs
- Signs of adrenal insufficiency include fatigue, anorexia, nausea, vomiting, diarrhea, weight loss, weakness, dizziness, and low blood sugar
- Notify physician if these signs and symptoms appear following dose reduction or withdrawal of therapy
- Avoid abrupt withdrawal of therapy following high dose or long-term therapy

MONITORING PARAMETERS

- Potassium and blood sugar during long-term therapy
- Edema, blood pressure, cardiac symptoms, mental status, weight
- Observe growth and development of infants and children on prolonged therapy

primaquine

(prim'a-kwin)

Primaquine phosphate

Chemical Class: 8-aminoquinoline derivative

Therapeutic Class: Antimalarial

CLINICAL PHARMACOLOGY

Mechanism of Action: Exact mechanism unknown; appears to interfere with plasmodial DNA function

Pharmacokinetics

PO: Peak 1-3 hr, widely distributed in the body, rapidly metabolized in liver, excreted in urine (metabolites), $t_{1/2}$ 3.7-9.6 hr

INDICATIONS AND USES: Radical cure of vivax malaria, prevention of relapse in vivax malaria, following termination of chloroquine phosphate suppressive therapy in areas where vivax malaria is endemic, *Pneumocystis carinii* pneumonia (PCP) associated with AIDS (with clindamycin)*

DOSAGE

Adult

- *Vivax malaria:* PO 26.3 mg (15 mg base) qd for 14 days; patients suffering an attack of vivax malaria or having parasitized red blood cells should also receive a course of chloroquine phosphate; as follow-up therapy in areas where vivax malaria is endemic, begin therapy during the last 2 wk of, or following a course of, suppression with chloroquine or a comparable drug
- *PCP associated with AIDS:* PO 26.3-52.6 mg (15-30 mg base) qd (with clindamycin IV 1.8-3.6 g/d divided tid-qid or PO 1.2-3.6 g/d divided tid-qid) for 21 days

Child

- PO 0.5 mg/kg/d (0.3 mg base/kg/d; max 15 mg base/dose) for 14 days

$ AVAILABLE FORMS/COST OF THERAPY

- Tab, Uncoated—Oral: 26.3 mg, 100's: **$64.84**

CONTRAINDICATIONS: Concomitant administration with quinacrine, acutely ill patients with a tendency to granulocytopenia (rheumatoid arthritis, systemic lupus erythematosus), concurrent administration of other potentially hemolytic drugs or bone marrow suppressants, hypersensitivity

PRECAUTIONS: G-6-PD deficiency, NADH methemoglobin reductase deficiency, large doses

PREGNANCY AND LACTATION: Pregnancy category C; if possible, withhold until after delivery, however, if prophylaxis or treatment is required, primaquine should not be withheld

SIDE EFFECTS/ADVERSE REACTIONS

CNS: Headache

EENT: Interference with visual accommodation

GI: Nausea, vomiting, epigastric distress, abdominal cramps

HEME: ***Leukopenia, hemolytic anemia in G-6-PD deficient patients, methemoglobinemia in NADH methemoglobin reductase deficient patients***

SKIN: Pruritus

▼ DRUG INTERACTIONS

Drugs

- *Quinacrine:* Increased toxicity of primaquine; do not administer primaquine to patients who recently received quinacrine

SPECIAL CONSIDERATIONS

PATIENT/FAMILY EDUCATION

- Complete full course of therapy
- Take with food if GI upset occurs, notify physician if GI distress continues

P

• Notify physician if urine turns dark

MONITORING PARAMETERS

• CBC periodically during therapy, discontinue if marked darkening of urine or sudden decrease in hemoglobin concentrations or leukocyte count occurs

probenecid

(proe-ben'e-sid)

Benemid, Benuryl, ♣ Probalan

Chemical Class: Sulfonamide derivative

Therapeutic Class: Uricosuric; antigout agent

CLINICAL PHARMACOLOGY

Mechanism of Action: Inhibits the tubular reabsorption of urate; increases urinary excretion of uric acid, decreases serum uric acid concentrations; reduces miscible urate pool, retards urate deposition, promotes resorption of urate deposits; inhibits tubular secretion of most penicillins and cephalosporins, increases plasma concentrations

Pharmacokinetics

PO: Peak 2-4 hr, 85%-95% bound to plasma proteins, hydroxylated in liver to active metabolites, excreted in urine (metabolites), $t_{1/2}$ 4-17 hr

INDICATIONS AND USES: Hyperuricemia associated with gout and gouty arthritis, elevation and prolongation of plasma penicillin and cephalosporin concentrations

DOSAGE

Adult

• *Hyperuricemia:* PO 250 mg bid for 1 wk; increase to 500 mg bid; increase q4 wk prn to max of 2-3 g/d; begin therapy 2-3 wk following acute gout attack

• *Penicillin or cephalosporin therapy:* PO 500 mg qid

Child 2-14 yr

• *Penicillin or cephalosporin therapy:* PO 25 mg/kg/dose initially; 40 mg/kg/d divided qid as maintenance dose

$ **AVAILABLE FORMS/COST OF THERAPY**

• Tab, Plain Coated—Oral: 500 mg, 100's: **$11.54-$30.60**

CONTRAINDICATIONS: Hypersensitivity, children <2 yr, blood dyscrasias, uric acid kidney stones, initiation of therapy during acute gouty attack, moderate to severe renal impairment (CrCl <10 ml/min)

PRECAUTIONS: History of peptic ulcer

PREGNANCY AND LACTATION: Pregnancy category B; has been used during pregnancy without causing adverse effects in fetus or infant

SIDE EFFECTS/ADVERSE REACTIONS

CNS: Headache, dizziness

GI: Anorexia, nausea, vomiting, sore gums, ***hepatic necrosis***

GU: Urinary frequency, ***nephrotic syndrome,*** uric acid stones, renal colic, costovertebral pain, ***hematuria***

HEME: ***Anemia, hemolytic anemia (possibly related to G-6-PD deficiency), aplastic anemia***

METAB: Exacerbation of gout

SKIN: Flushing, rash

MISC: Hypersensitivity reactions

▼ **DRUG INTERACTIONS**

Drugs

• *Aminosalicylic acid:* Increased serum aminosalicylic acid concentrations

• *Dapsone:* Increased serum dapsone concentrations

• *Dyphylline:* Increased serum dyphylline concentrations

• *Ketoprofen:* Increased serum ketoprofen concentrations

• *Methotrexate+:* Marked increases

in serum methotrexate concentrations

- *Salicylates:* Inhibited uricosuric activity of probenecid
- *Sulfinpyrazone:* Increased serum sulfinpyrazone concentrations
- *Zidovudine:* Increased plasma zidovudine concentrations

Labs

- *False positive:* Glycosuria
- *False increase:* Theophylline concentrations using Schack and Waxler technique
- *Decrease:* Urinary excretion of phenolsulfonphthalein (PSP), 17 KS, sulfobromophthalein (BSP)

SPECIAL CONSIDERATIONS

PATIENT/FAMILY EDUCATION

- Avoid aspirin or other salicylates
- Take with food or antacids
- Drink plenty of water to prevent development of kidney stones

MONITORING PARAMETERS

- Serum uric acid concentrations, continue the probenecid dose that maintains normal concentrations
- Renal function tests

probucol

(proe'byoo-kole)

Lorelco

Chemical Class: Substituted bisphenol

Therapeutic Class: Antilipemic

CLINICAL PHARMACOLOGY

Mechanism of Action: Increases fractional rate of low density lipoprotein (LDL) cholesterol catabolism; inhibits early stages of cholesterol synthesis and slightly inhibits absorption of dietary cholesterol; lowers serum cholesterol with relatively little effect of serum triglycerides, decreases LDL and high density lipoprotein (HDL) cholesterol fractions

Pharmacokinetics

PO: Absorption <10% and variable (increased and less variable when administered with food), eliminated via bile and feces, $t_{1/2}$ 20 days

INDICATIONS AND USES: Primary hypercholesterolemia (elevated LDL)

DOSAGE

Adult

- PO 500 mg bid with AM and PM meals

$ AVAILABLE FORMS/COST OF THERAPY

- Tab, Film Coated—Oral: 250 mg, 120's: **$80.46;** 500 mg, 100's: **$116.04**

CONTRAINDICATIONS: Hypersensitivity, recent or progressive myocardial damage, ventricular dysrhythmias, unexplained syncope, abnormally long QT interval

PRECAUTIONS: Children, hypokalemia, hypomagnesemia, severe bradycardia due to intrinsic heart disease or drug effects

PREGNANCY AND LACTATION: Pregnancy category B; nursing not recommended

SIDE EFFECTS/ADVERSE REACTIONS

CNS: Headache, dizziness, paresthesia, *insomnia,* peripheral neuritis

CV: ***Prolongation of QT interval on ECG, syncope, ventricular dysrhythmias, sudden death,*** angioneurotic edema

EENT: Tinnitus, conjunctivitis, tearing, blurred vision

GI: Diarrhea, flatulence, abdominal pain, *nausea, vomiting,* indigestion, ***GI bleeding,*** anorexia, transient elevations of liver function tests

GU: Impotence, nocturia

HEME: ***Eosinophilia, anemia, thrombocytopenia***

METAB: Enlargement of multinodular goiter

SKIN: Rash, pruritis, ecchymosis, petechiae, hyperhidrosis, fetid sweat

▼ **DRUG INTERACTIONS**

Labs

• *Increase:* Liver function studies, CPK, blood glucose, uric acid, BUN

SPECIAL CONSIDERATIONS

PATIENT/FAMILY EDUCATION

• Take with meals

MONITORING PARAMETERS

• Fasting lipid profile

---

procainamide

(proe-kane'a-mide)

Procan SR, Promine, Pronestyl, Pronestyl-SR, Sub-Quin, Rhythmin

Chemical Class: Procaine amide analog

Therapeutic Class: Antidysrhythmic (Class IA)

CLINICAL PHARMACOLOGY

Mechanism of Action: Decreases myocardial excitability and conduction velocity; may depress myocardial contractility; increases threshold potential of ventricle, His-Purkinje system; prolongs effective refractory period and increases action potential duration in atrial and ventricular muscle; possesses anticholinergic properties which may modify direct myocardial effects

Pharmacokinetics

IM: Onset 10-30 min, peak 15-60 min

PO: Peak 0.75-2.5 hr

15%-20% bound to plasma proteins, metabolized via acetylation in liver to N-acetyl procainamide (NAPA) which is a Class III antidysrhythmic, excreted in urine (25% as NAPA), $t_{1/2}$ 2.5-4.7 hr (NAPA 6-8 hr)

INDICATIONS AND USES: Life-threatening ventricular dysrhythmias, less severe but symptomatic ventricular dysrhythmias in select patients, maintenance of sinus rhythm following cardioversion in atrial fibrillation and/or flutter,* suppression of recurrent paroxysmal atrial fibrillation*

DOSAGE

Adult

• PO 250-500 mg q3-6h; PO SR 500-1000 mg q6h; usual dose 50 mg/kg/24 hr; max 4 g/24hr; IM 0.5-1 g q4-8h until PO therapy possible; IV 1 g inf over 25-30 min or 100-200 mg/dose repeated q5 min as needed to total dose of 1 g as a loading dose; followed by continuous inf of 1-6 mg/min, titrate to patient response

Child

• PO 15-50 mg/kg/24 hr divided q3-6h; max 4 g/24 hr; IM 20-30 mg/kg/24 hr divided q4-6h; max 4 g/24 hr; IV 3-6 mg/kg inf over 5 min not to exceed 100 mg/dose as a loading dose; then 20-80 µg/kg/min as a continuous inf; max 4 g/24 hr

$ **AVAILABLE FORMS/COST OF THERAPY**

• Cap, Gel—Oral: 250 mg, 100's: **$6.53-$53.93;** 375 mg, 100's: **$7.43-$74.79;** 500 mg, 100's: **$8.48-$97.10**

• Tab, Sugar Coated—Oral: 250 mg, 100's: **$12.70-$53.93;** 375 mg, 100's: **$74.79;** 500 mg, 100's: **$97.10**

• Tab, Coated, Sust Action—Oral: 250 mg, 100's: **$11.03-$53.93;** 500 mg, 100's: **$14.73-$66.84;** 750 mg, 100's: **$23.93-$94.60;** 1000 mg, 100's: **$121.04**

• Inj, Sol—IM; IV: 100 mg/ml, 10 ml: **$4.00-$36.44;** 500 mg/ml, 2 ml: **$4.00-$36.44**

CONTRAINDICATIONS: Complete heart block, hypersensitivity, lupus erythematosus, torsade de pointes

PRECAUTIONS: Following MI,

first-degree AV block (unless ventricular rate controlled by pacemaker), asymptomatic premature ventricular contractions, digitalis intoxication, CHF, myasthenia gravis, renal insufficiency, children

PREGNANCY AND LACTATION: Pregnancy category C; compatible with breast feeding, however long-term effects in nursing infant unknown

SIDE EFFECTS/ADVERSE REACTIONS

CNS: Dizziness, giddiness, weakness, mental depression, psychosis, hallucinations, headache

CV: Hypotension, ***second-degree heart block***

GI: Anorexia, nausea, vomiting, abdominal pain, bitter taste, diarrhea, ***hepatomegaly***

HEME: ***Neutropenia, thrombocytopenia, hemolytic anemia (rare), agranulocytosis***

SKIN: ***Angioneurotic edema,*** urticaria, pruritus, flushing, rash

MISC: Lupus erythematosus-like syndrome (arthralgia, pleural or abdominal pain, arthritis, pleural effusion, pericarditis, fever, chills, rash)

▼ **DRUG INTERACTIONS**

Drugs

- *Amiodarone, cimetidine, trimethoprim:* Increased procainamide concentrations
- *Cholinergic drugs:* Antagonism of cholinergic actions on skeletal muscle

SPECIAL CONSIDERATIONS

PATIENT/FAMILY EDUCATION

- Strict compliance to dosage schedule imperative
- Report any symptoms of arthralgia, myalgia, fever, chills, skin rash, easy bruising, sore throat or sore mouth, infections, dark urine, icterus, wheezing, muscular weakness, chest or abdominal pain, palpitations, nausea, vomiting, anorexia, diarrhea, hallucinations, dizziness, depression. Empty wax core from sustained release tablets may appear in stool, this is harmless and not cause for concern

MONITORING PARAMETERS

- CBC with differential and platelets qwk for first 3 mo, periodically thereafter
- ECG
- ANA titer increases may precede clinical symptoms of lupoid syndrome
- Serum creatinine, urea nitrogen
- Plasma procainamide concentration (therapeutic range 3-10 μg/ml; 10-30 μg/ml NAPA)

procaine

(proe′kane)

Novocaine, Unicaine

Chemical Class: Ester, *p*-aminobenzoic acid derivative

Therapeutic Class: Local anesthetic

CLINICAL PHARMACOLOGY

Mechanism of Action: Blocks the generation and conduction of nerve impulses, presumably by increasing the threshold for electrical excitation in the nerve, slowing the propagation of the nerve impulse, and reducing the rate rise of the action potential; the progression of anesthesia is related to the diameter, myelination, and conduction velocity of affected nerve fibers, the order of loss of nerve function is as follows: (1) pain, (2) temperature, (3) touch, (4) proprioception, and (5) skeletal muscle tone

Pharmacokinetics

INJ: Onset 2-5 min (15-25 min epidural), duration 0.25-1 hr (0.5-1.5 epidural), rapidly hydrolyzed by plasma pseudocholinesterase to *p*-aminobenzoic acid and diethylaminoethanol, excreted in urine, $t_{1/2}$ 7.7 min

INDICATIONS AND USES: Infiltration anesthesia, peripheral or sympathetic nerve block, spinal anesthesia, intractable pain (IV),* pruritus caused by jaundice (IV)*

DOSAGE

Dose varies with procedure, depth of anesthesia, vascularity of tissues, duration of anesthesia, and condition of patient

Adult

- *Spinal anesthesia:* Inj usual rate 1 ml/5 sec; anesthesia of perineum 0.5 ml of 10% mixed with equal vol of diluent; anesthesia of perineum and lower extremities 1 ml of 10% mixed with equal vol of diluent; anesthesia extending to costal margin 2 ml of 10% mixed with 1 ml of diluent
- *Infiltration anesthesia:* Inj 350-600 mg of 0.25%-0.5%
- *Peripheral nerve block:* Inj up to 200 ml of 0.5% or 100 ml of 1% or 50 ml of 2%

$ AVAILABLE FORMS/COST OF THERAPY

- Inj, Sol—Infiltration: 1%, 2%, 30 ml: **$0.68-$14.13**
- Inj, Sol—IV: 10%, 2 ml: **$6.87**

CONTRAINDICATIONS: Hypersensitivity to ester-type local anesthetics, myasthenia gravis (IV), severe shock, impaired cardiac conduction, inj into inflamed or infected tissue

PRECAUTIONS: Cardiac disease, hyperthyroidism, endocrine disease, liver disease, elderly, low plasma pseudocholinesterase concentrations, sulfite sensitivity, use in head and neck area, retrobulbar blocks

PREGNANCY AND LACTATION: Pregnancy category C

SIDE EFFECTS/ADVERSE REACTIONS

CNS: Anxiety, restlessness, ***convulsions, loss of consciousness,*** drowsiness, disorientation, tremors, shivering

CV: ***Myocardial depression, cardiac arrest, dysrhythmias,*** bradycardia, hypotension, hypertension, fetal bradycardia

EENT: Blurred vision, tinnitus, pupil constriction

GI: Nausea, vomiting

RESP: ***Respiratory arrest, anaphylaxis***

SKIN: Rash, urticaria, allergic reactions, edema, burning, skin discoloration at inj site, tissue necrosis

▼ DRUG INTERACTIONS

Drugs

- *Echothiophate:* Increased effect of procaine
- *Succinylcholine:* IV procaine may enhance effect of succinylcholine

SPECIAL CONSIDERATIONS

MONITORING PARAMETERS

- Blood pressure, pulse, respiration during treatment, ECG
- Fetal heart tones if drug is used during labor

prochlorperazine

(proe-klor-per'a-zeen)

Compazine, Stemetil ♣

Chemical Class: Propylpiperazine derivative of phenothiazine

Therapeutic Class: Antiemetic; antipsychotic

CLINICAL PHARMACOLOGY

Mechanism of Action: Precise antiemetic action unclear; has been shown to directly affect medullary chemoreceptor trigger zone (CTZ), apparently by blocking dopamine receptors in CTZ; antipsychotic effects similar to those of chlorpromazine; weak anticholinergic effects, moderate sedative effects, strong extrapyramidal effects

Pharmacokinetics

PO: Onset 30-40 min, duration 3-4 hr (extended release 10-12 hr)
IM: Onset 10-20 min, duration 12 hr
PR: Onset 60 min, duration 3-4 hr
Metabolized in liver, excreted in urine and through enterohepatic circulation

INDICATIONS AND USES: Severe nausea and vomiting, psychotic disorders

DOSAGE

Adult

- *Antiemetic:* PO 5-10 mg tid-qid; usual max 40 mg/d; PO extended release 10 mg bid or 15 mg qd; IM 5-10 mg q3-4h; usual max 40 mg/d; IV 2.5-10 mg q3-4h; max 10 mg/dose, 40 mg/d; PR 25 mg bid
- *Psychosis:* PO 5-10 mg tid-qid; increase dose prn; max 150 mg/d; IM 10-20 mg q4h prn; convert to PO as soon as possible

Child

- *Antiemetic:* PO/PR 9-14 kg: 2.5 mg q12-24h, max 7.5 mg/d; 14-18 kg: 2.5 mg q8-12h, max 10 mg/d; 18-39 kg: 2.5 mg q8h or 5 mg q12h, max 15 mg/d; IM 0.1-0.15 mg/kg/dose; convert to PO as soon as possible; IV not recommended
- *Psychosis:* PO/PR 2-12 yr: 2.5 mg bid-tid, increase dose prn, max 20 mg/day; 2-5 yr: 25 mg/day; IM 6-12 yr: 0.13 mg/kg/dose, convert to PO as soon as possible

$ AVAILABLE FORMS/COST OF THERAPY

- Inj, Sol—IM; IV: 5 mg/ml, 2 ml: **$2.59-$5.97**
- Supp—Rect: 2.5 mg, 12's: **$24.90;** 5 mg, 12's: **$27.70;** 25 mg, 12's: **$23.12-$34.30**
- Syr—Oral: 5 mg/5 ml, 120 ml: **$18.95**
- Tab, Plain Coated—Oral: 5 mg, 100's: **$34.43-$57.90;** 10 mg, 100's: **$51.98-$86.95;** 25 mg, 100's: **$104.85**
- Cap, Gel, Sust Action—Oral: 10 mg, 50's: **$53.05;** 15 mg, 50's: **$78.85**

CONTRAINDICATIONS: Hypersensitivity to phenothiazines, severe toxic CNS depression, coma, subcortical brain damage, bone marrow depression, severe liver or cardiac disease, narrow-angle glaucoma, pediatric surgery

PRECAUTIONS: Children <5 yr, elderly, prolonged use, cardiovascular disease, epilepsy, hepatic or renal disease, glaucoma, prostatic hypertrophy, severe asthma, emphysema, hypocalcemia (increased susceptibility to dystonic reactions), thyrotoxicosis, tartrazine sensitivity

PREGNANCY AND LACTATION: Pregnancy category C; majority of evidence indicates safety for both mother and fetus if used occasionally in low doses; excretion into breast milk should be expected, sedation is a possible effect in nursing infant

SIDE EFFECTS/ADVERSE REACTIONS

CNS: EPS (pseudoparkinsonism, akathisia, dystonia, ***tardive dyskinesia),*** *drowsiness, headache,* ***seizures, neuroleptic malignant syndrome,*** confusion, insomnia, restlessness, anxiety, euphoria, agitation, depression, lethargy, vertigo, exacerbation of psychotic symptoms including hallucinations, catatonic-like behavioral states, heat or cold intolerance

CV: ***Tachycardia,*** hypotension, hypertension, ECG changes

EENT: Blurred vision, glaucoma, dry eyes, cataracts, retinopathy, pigmentation of retina or cornea

GI: Anorexia, constipation, diarrhea, hypersalivation, dyspepsia, *nausea,* vomiting, *dry mouth*

GU: Urinary retention, priapism

HEME: Transient leukopenia, leukocytosis, minimal decreases in red blood cell counts, anemia, ***agranulocytosis, aplastic anemia, hemolytic anemia***

METAB: Lactation, breast engorgement, mastalgia, menstrual irregularities, gynecomastia, impotence, increased libido, hyperglycemia, hypoglycemia, hyponatremia

RESP: Laryngospasm, bronchospasm, increased depth of respiration

SKIN: Maculopapular and acneiform skin reactions, photosensitivity, loss of hair, diaphoresis

▼ **DRUG INTERACTIONS**

Drugs

• *Anticholinergics:* Inhibited therapeutic response to antipsychotic; enhanced anticholinergic side effects
• *Antidepressants:* Increased serum concentrations of some cyclic antidepressants
• *Barbiturates:* Reduced effect of antipsychotic
• *Beta blockers:* Enhanced effects of both drugs
• *Bromocriptine, lithium:* Reduced effects of both drugs
• *Epinephrine:* Reversed pressor response to epinephrine
• *Guanethidine*+: Inhibited antihypertensive response to guanethidine
• *Levodopa:* Inhibited effect of levodopa on Parkinson's disease
• *Narcotic analgesics:* Excessive CNS depression, hypotension, respiratory depression
• *Orphenadrine:* Reduced serum neuroleptic concentrations, excessive anticholinergic effects

Labs

• *Increase:* Liver function tests, cardiac enzymes, cholesterol, blood glucose, prolactin, bilirubin, PBI, cholinesterase, ^{131}I
• *Decrease:* Hormones (blood, urine)
• *False positive:* Pregnancy tests, PKU
• *False negative:* Urinary steroids, 17-OHCS

SPECIAL CONSIDERATIONS

PATIENT/FAMILY EDUCATION

• Contact physician if sore throat or other signs of infection
• Arise slowly from reclining position
• Do not discontinue abruptly
• Use a sunscreen during sun exposure to prevent burns, take special precautions to stay cool in hot weather
• May cause drowsiness

MONITORING PARAMETERS

• Observe closely for signs of tardive dyskinesia
• Periodic CBC with platelets during prolonged therapy

---

procyclidine

(proe-sye'kli-deen)

Kemadrin, Procyclid ♣

Chemical Class: Synthetic tertiary amine antimuscarinic

Therapeutic Class: Antiparkinsonian agent

CLINICAL PHARMACOLOGY

Mechanism of Action: Blocks striatal cholinergic receptors which helps balance cholinergic and dopaminergic activity

Pharmacokinetics

PO: Peak 1.1-2 hr, $t_{1/2}$ 11.5-12.6 hr

INDICATIONS AND USES: Adjunctive treatment of all forms of Parkinson's disease; drug-induced EPS

DOSAGE

Adult

• *Parkinsonism:* PO 2.5 mg tid after meals initially, increase to 5 mg tid gradually; may occasionally administer additional dose hs if necessary
• *Drug-induced EPS:* PO 2.5 mg tid initially, increase by 2.5 mg/d in-

crements until relief of symptoms obtained; usual dose 10-20 mg/d

AVAILABLE FORMS/COST OF THERAPY

- Tab, Uncoated—Oral: 5 mg, 100's: **$41.66**

CONTRAINDICATIONS: Hypersensitivity, narrow-angle glaucoma, myasthenia gravis, GI/GU obstruction, peptic ulcer, megacolon, prostatic hypertrophy

PRECAUTIONS: Elderly, tachycardia, liver, kidney disease, drug abuse history, dysrhythmias, hypotension, hypertension, psychiatric patients, children, tardive dyskinesia

PREGNANCY AND LACTATION: Pregnancy category C

SIDE EFFECTS/ADVERSE REACTIONS

CNS: Confusion, anxiety, restlessness, irritability, delusions, hallucinations, headache, sedation, depression, incoherence, dizziness, memory loss

CV: Palpitations, tachycardia, hypotension, mild bradycardia, postural hypotension, flushing

EENT: Blurred vision, photophobia, dilated pupils, difficulty swallowing, dry eyes, mydriasis, increased intraocular tension, angle-closure glaucoma

GI: Dry mouth, constipation, nausea, vomiting, abdominal distress, ***paralytic ileus,*** epigastric distress

GU: Hesitancy, retention, dysuria, erectile dysfunction

MS: Muscular weakness, cramping

SKIN: Rash, urticaria, other dermatoses

MISC: Increased temperature, decreased sweating, hyperthermia, heat stroke, numbness of fingers

SPECIAL CONSIDERATIONS

PATIENT/FAMILY EDUCATION

- Do not discontinue this drug abruptly
- Avoid driving or other hazardous activities, drowsiness may occur
- Use hard candy, frequent drinks, sugarless gum to relieve dry mouth
- Advise patient to administer with or after meals to prevent GI upset
- Use caution in hot weather, drug may increase susceptibility to heat stroke
- May cause constipation, increase fluids, bulk, exercise if this occurs

---

progesterone

(proe-jess'ter-one)

Gesterol 50, Progestaject, Progestasert

Chemical Class: Naturally occurring progestin

Therapeutic Class: Progestin; contraceptive

CLINICAL PHARMACOLOGY

Mechanism of Action: Shares the actions of the progestins; in the presence of adequate estrogen, transforms a proliferative endometrium into a secretory one; stimulates growth of mammary alveolar tissue; has some androgenic, estrogenic, and adrenocorticoid activity

Pharmacokinetics

Hepatic metabolism

INDICATIONS AND USES: Amenorrhea, abnormal uterine bleeding; contraception in women with at least 1 child in stable, mutually monogamous relationships, without history of PID (intrauterine system)

DOSAGE

Adult

- *Amenorrhea:* IM 5-10 mg qd for 6-8 days; if ovarian activity has produced a proliferative endometrium, expect withdrawal bleeding 48-72 hr after last inj; spontaneous normal cycles may follow
- *Abnormal uterine bleeding:* IM 5-10 mg qd for 6 doses; bleeding

should cease within 6 days; when used with estrogen, begin progesterone after 2 wk of estrogen therapy; discontinue inj when menstrual flow begins

• *Contraception:* Insert 1 system into uterine cavity; replace after 1 yr

AVAILABLE FORMS/COST OF THERAPY

• Inj, Sol—IM: 50 mg/ml, 10 ml: **$8.99-$36.30**

• Insert, Sust Action—Intrauterine: 38 mg, 6's: **$450.00**

CONTRAINDICATIONS: Hypersensitivity, thrombophlebitis, thromboembolic disorders, cerebral hemorrhage, impaired liver function or disease, breast cancer, undiagnosed vaginal bleeding, missed abortion, use as a diagnostic test for pregnancy; (intrauterine system) pregnancy or suspected pregnancy, previous ectopic pregnancy, history of PID, multiple sexual partners (patient or partner), sexually transmitted disease, postpartum endometritis, infected abortion, pelvic surgery, uterine distortion, uterine or cervical malignancy, unresolved abnormal Pap smear, undiagnosed genital bleeding, vaginitis or cervicitis, incomplete involution of uterus following abortion or childbirth, previous IUD still in place, genital actinomycosis, increased susceptibility to infection (e.g., leukemia, diabetes, AIDS), IV drug use

PRECAUTIONS: Epilepsy, migraine, asthma, cardiac or renal dysfunction, depression, diabetes; (intrauterine system) history of menorrhagia or hypermenorrhea, valvular or congenital heart disease

PREGNANCY AND LACTATION: Use in pregnancy not recommended

SIDE EFFECTS/ADVERSE REACTIONS

CNS: Dizziness, headache, migraines, depression, fatigue

CV: Hypotension, thrombophlebitis, edema, ***thromboembolism, stroke, pulmonary embolism, MI***

EENT: Diplopia

GI: Nausea, vomiting, anorexia, cramps, increased weight, ***cholestatic jaundice***

GU: Amenorrhea, cervical erosion, breakthrough bleeding, dysmenorrhea, vaginal candidiasis, breast changes, *gynecomastia, testicular atrophy, impotence,* endometriosis, ***spontaneous abortion.*** Intrauterine system: endometritis, ***spontaneous abortion, septic abortion, septicemia, perforation of uterus and cervix, pelvic infection, ectopic pregnancy,*** uterine embedment, difficult removal, intermenstrual spotting, prolongation of menstrual flow, anemia, amenorrhea or delayed menses, pain, cramping, dyspareunia

METAB: Hyperglycemia

SKIN: Rash, urticaria, acne, hirsutism, alopecia, oily skin, seborrhea, purpura, melasma, photosensitivity, pain at inj site, irritation at inj site, sterile abscess formation at inj site

DRUG INTERACTIONS

Labs

• *Increase:* Alk phosphatase, pregnanediol, liver function tests

• *Decrease:* Glucose tolerance test, HDL

SPECIAL CONSIDERATIONS

PATIENT/FAMILY EDUCATION

• Take protective measures against exposure to UV light or sunlight

• Diabetic patients must monitor blood glucose carefully during therapy

• Notify physician of pain, swelling, warmth or redness in calves, sudden severe headache, visual disturbances, numbness in arm or leg

• Notify physician of abnormal or excessive bleeding, severe cramping, abnormal or odorous vaginal discharge, fever or flu-like symptoms, pain, genital lesions or sores, missed period

MONITORING PARAMETERS

- Pretreatment physical exam should include breasts and pelvic organs, Pap smear

---

promethazine

(proe-meth'a-zeen)

Anergan, Pentazine, Phenameth, Phenazine, Phenergan, Phenoject-50, Pro 50, Prometh-50, Prorex, Prothiazine, V-Gan

Chemical Class: Ethylamino derivative of phenothiazine

Therapeutic Class: Antihistamine; antiemetic; sedative; antivertigo/antimotion sickness agent; antitussive

CLINICAL PHARMACOLOGY

Mechanism of Action: Blocks the effects of histamine by competing with histamine for H_1-receptor sites of effector cells; prevents but does not reverse responses mediated by histamine alone; antiemetic effects probably mediated via inhibition of the medullary chemoreceptor trigger zone (CTZ); antivertigo/motion sickness effects through central anticholinergic effect on vestibular apparatus and the integrative vomiting center and the CTZ; sedative effects via indirect reduction of stimuli to the brain stem reticular system

Pharmacokinetics

PO/IM/PR: Onset 20 min, duration 6-12 hr (sedative effects 2-8 hr)

IV: Onset 3-5 min, duration 6-12 hr (sedative effects 2-8 hr)

Metabolized in liver, excreted in urine and feces (inactive metabolites)

INDICATIONS AND USES: Symptomatic treatment of various allergic conditions; active and prophylactic treatment of motion sickness; preoperative, postoperative, or obstetric sedation; nausea and vomiting associated with anesthesia and surgery; adjunct to analgesic for control of postoperative pain

DOSAGE

Adult

- *Antihistamine:* PO/PR 12.5 tid and 25 mg qhs; IM/IV 25 mg, repeated in 2 hr if necessary; convert to PO as soon as possible
- *Antiemetic:* PO/IM/IV/PR 12.5-25 mg q4h prn
- *Motion sickness:* PO/PR 25 mg 30-60 min prior to departure, then q12h prn
- *Sedation:* PO/IM/IV/PR 25-50 mg/dose

Child

- *Antihistamine:* PO/PR 0.1 mg/kg/dose q6h during the day and 0.5 mg/kg qhs prn
- *Antiemetic:* PO/IM/IV/PR 0.25-1 mg/kg q4-6h prn
- *Motion sickness:* PO/PR 0.5 mg/kg/dose 30-60 min prior to departure, then q12h prn
- *Sedation:* PO/IM/IV/PR 0.5-1 mg/kg/dose q6h prn

P

$ **AVAILABLE FORMS/COST OF THERAPY**

- Inj, Sol—IM; IV: 25 mg/ml, 10 ml: **$1.80-$10.60;** 50 mg/ml, 10 ml: **$4.25-$18.25**
- Supp—Rect: 12.5 mg, 12's: **$27.21;** 25 mg, 12's: **$31.22;** 50 mg, 12's: **$26.50-$45.00**
- Syr—Oral: 6.25 mg/5 ml, 120 ml: **$0.84-$5.85;** 25 mg/5 ml, 480 ml: **$11.00-$45.47**
- Tab, Uncoated—Oral: 12.5 mg, 100's: **$6.50-$18.11;** 25 mg, 100's: **$2.55-$31.99;** 50 mg, 100's: **$4.65-$49.03**

CONTRAINDICATIONS: Hypersensitivity to phenothiazines, narrow-angle glaucoma

PRECAUTIONS: Acute asthma, bladder neck obstruction, prostatic hypertrophy, predisposition to urinary retention, cardiovascular disease, glaucoma, hepatic function impairment, hypertension, history of peptic ulcer, seizure disorder, intestinal obstruction

PREGNANCY AND LACTATION: Pregnancy category C; passage of drug into breast milk should be expected

SIDE EFFECTS/ADVERSE REACTIONS

CNS: Dizziness, drowsiness, poor coordination, fatigue, anxiety, euphoria, confusion, paresthesia, neuritis

CV: Hypotension, palpitations, tachycardia

EENT: Blurred vision, dilated pupils, tinnitus, nasal stuffiness, dry nose

GI: Constipation, dry mouth, nausea, vomiting, anorexia, diarrhea

GU: Urinary retention, dysuria

HEME: ***Thrombocytopenia, agranulocytosis, hemolytic anemia***

RESP: Increased thick secretions, wheezing, chest tightness

SKIN: Photosensitivity, rash, urticaria

▼ **DRUG INTERACTIONS**

Drugs

• *CNS depressants:* Additive sedative action

Labs

• *False positive:* Immunologic urinary pregnancy tests

• *Interference:* Blood grouping in the ABO system, flare response in intradermal allergen tests

SPECIAL CONSIDERATIONS

PATIENT/FAMILY EDUCATION

• Avoid prolonged exposure to sunlight

• May cause drowsiness, use caution driving or performing other tasks requiring alertness

• Avoid alcohol

propafenone

(proe-pa-fen'one)

Rythmol

Chemical Class: 3-Phenylpropiophenone

Therapeutic Class: Antidysrhythmic (Class IC)

CLINICAL PHARMACOLOGY

Mechanism of Action: Has local anesthetic effects, and a direct stabilizing action on myocardial membranes; reduces upstroke velocity (Phase O) of the monophasic action potential; reduces fast inward current carried by sodium ions in Purkinje fibers, and to a lesser extent myocardial fibers; increases diastolic excitability threshold, prolongs effective refractory period, reduces spontaneous automaticity and depresses triggered activity; weak beta blocking activity

Pharmacokinetics

PO: Bioavailability 3.4%-10.6%, metabolized in liver to 5-hydroxypropafenone and N-depropylpropafenone (active), excreted in urine, $t_{1/2}$ 2-10 hr (10-32 hr in slow metabolizers)

INDICATIONS AND USES: Documented life-threatening ventricular dysrhythmias (e.g., sustained ventricular tachycardia), supraventricular tachycardias including atrial fibrillation and flutter,* dysrhythmias associated with Wolff-Parkinson-White syndrome*

DOSAGE

Adult

• PO 150 mg q8h initially; increase at 3-4 day intervals to 225 mg q8h and, if necessary to 300 mg q8h; do not exceed 900 mg/d

$ **AVAILABLE FORMS/COST OF THERAPY**

• Tab, Coated—Oral: 150 mg, 100's:

$83.82; 225 mg, 100's: **$119.48;** 300 mg, 100's: **$152.08**

CONTRAINDICATIONS: Uncontrolled CHF, cardiogenic shock, disorders of impulse generation or conduction in the absence of an artificial pacemaker, bradycardia, marked hypotension, bronchospastic disorders, manifest electrolyte imbalance, hypersensitivity

PRECAUTIONS: Non-life-threatening dysrhythmias, recent MI, hepatic and renal function impairment, elderly, children

PREGNANCY AND LACTATION: Pregnancy category C

SIDE EFFECTS/ADVERSE REACTIONS

CNS: Dizziness, headache, anxiety, ataxia, drowsiness, fatigue, insomnia, tremor

CV: AV block, ***congestive heart failure,*** *intraventricular conduction delay,* angina, atrial fibrillation, bradycardia, bundle branch block, chest pain, hypotension, palpitations, ***prodysrhythmia,*** premature ventricular contractions, widened QRS complex, syncope, ***ventricular tachycardia,*** edema

EENT: Blurred vision

GI: Nausea, vomiting, unusual taste, constipation, dyspepsia, anorexia, abdominal pain, diarrhea, dry mouth, flatulence, liver abnormalities

HEME: Positive ANA, ***agranulocytosis, anemia, granulocytopenia,*** increased bleeding time, ***leukopenia,*** purpura, ***thrombocytopenia***

MS: Weakness, arthralgia

RESP: Dyspnea

SKIN: Diaphoresis, rash

▼ **DRUG INTERACTIONS**

Drugs

- *Beta blockers:* Increased metoprolol or propranolol concentrations
- *Digitalis glycosides:* Increased serum digoxin concentrations
- *Food:* Increased peak serum propafenone concentrations
- *Oral anticoagulants:* Increased serum warfarin concentrations, prolonged protime
- *Rifampin:* Reduced serum propafenone concentrations
- *Theophylline:* Increased plasma theophylline concentrations

SPECIAL CONSIDERATIONS

PATIENT/FAMILY EDUCATION

- Signs of overdosage include hypotension, excessive drowsiness, decreased heart rate, or abnormal heartbeat
- Notify physician if signs of infection develop such as fever, sore throat, chills, or unusual bruising or bleeding

MONITORING PARAMETERS

- ECG, consider dose reduction in patients with significant widening of the QRS complex or 2nd- or 3rd-degree AV block
- ANA, carefully evaluate abnormal ANA test, consider discontinuation if persistent or worsening ANA titers are detected

propantheline

(proe-pan'the-leen)

Banlin, ✤ Pro-Banthine

Chemical Class: Synthetic quaternary ammonium antimuscarinic

Therapeutic Class: GI anticholinergic; antispasmodic

CLINICAL PHARMACOLOGY

Mechanism of Action: Inhibits GI motility and diminishes gastric acid secretion

Pharmacokinetics

PO: Incompletely absorbed, extensive metabolism in upper small intestine prior to absorption, peak 2-6 hr, metabolized in GI tract/liver, excreted in urine, $t_{1/2}$ 1.6-9 hr

INDICATIONS AND USES: Adjunctive treatment of peptic ulcer disease, irritable bowel syndrome,* urinary incontinence due to uninhibited hypertonic neurogenic bladder*

DOSAGE

Adult

• PO 7.5-15 mg 30 min ac and 30 min hs

Child

• *Antisecretory:* PO 1.5 mg/kg/d divided tid-qid

• *Antispasmodic:* PO 2-3 mg/kg/d divided q4-6h and hs

$ **AVAILABLE FORMS/COST OF THERAPY**

• Tab, Sugar Coated—Oral: 15 mg, 100's: **$16.92-$64.99;** 7.5 mg, 100's: **$42.66**

CONTRAINDICATIONS: Hypersensitivity to anticholinergic drugs, narrow-angle glaucoma, obstructive uropathy (e.g., bladder neck obstruction due to prostatic hypertrophy), obstructive disease of the GI tract (e.g., pyloroduodenal stenosis), paralytic ileus, intestinal atony, unstable cardiovascular status in acute hemorrhage, severe ulcerative colitis, toxic megacolon complicating ulcerative colitis, myasthenia gravis

PRECAUTIONS: Hyperthyroidism, CAD, dysrhythmias, CHF, ulcerative colitis, hypertension, hiatal hernia, hepatic disease, renal disease, urinary retention, prostatic hypertrophy, elderly

PREGNANCY AND LACTATION: Pregnancy category C; excretion into breast milk unknown, although would be expected to be minimal due to quaternary structure

SIDE EFFECTS/ADVERSE REACTIONS

CNS: Confusion, stimulation (especially in elderly), headache, insomnia, dizziness, drowsiness, anxiety, weakness, hallucination

CV: Palpitations, tachycardia

EENT: Blurred vision, photophobia, mydriasis, cycloplegia, increased ocular tension

GI: Dry mouth, constipation, ***paralytic ileus,*** heartburn, nausea, vomiting, dysphagia, absence of taste

GU: Hesitancy, retention, impotence

SKIN: Urticaria, rash, pruritus, anhidrosis, fever, allergic reactions

▼ **DRUG INTERACTIONS**

Drugs

• *Digitalis glycosides:* Increased digoxin concentrations when slowly dissolving dosage forms are used; digoxin caps do not seem to be affected

SPECIAL CONSIDERATIONS

PATIENT/FAMILY EDUCATION

• Avoid driving or other hazardous activities until stabilized on medication

• Avoid alcohol or other CNS depressants

• Avoid hot environments, heat stroke may occur

• Use sunglasses when outside to prevent photophobia, may cause blurred vision

---

proparacaine

(proe-pare'a-kane)

AK-Taine, Alcaine, Kainair, Ocu-Caine, Ophthaine, Ophthetic

Chemical Class: Ester, benzoic acid derivative

Therapeutic Class: Ophthalmic local anesthetic

CLINICAL PHARMACOLOGY

Mechanism of Action: Blocks the generation and conduction of nerve impulses, presumably by increasing the threshold for electrical excitation in the nerve, slowing the propagation of the nerve impulse, and reducing the rate rise of the action potential

Pharmacokinetics

OPHTH: Onset 20 sec, duration 15 min or longer

INDICATIONS AND USES: Corneal anesthesia of short duration for tonometry, gonioscopy, removal of foreign bodies and sutures; short corneal and conjunctival procedures; cataract surgery; conjunctival and corneal scraping for diagnostic purposes; paracentesis of anterior chamber

DOSAGE

Adult

- *Deep anesthesia (e.g., cataract extraction):* 1 gtt q5-10 min for 5-7 doses
- *Removal of sutures/foreign bodies, tonometry:* 1-2 gtt 2-3 min before procedure

$ **AVAILABLE FORMS/COST OF THERAPY**

- Sol—Ophth: 0.5%, 15 ml: **$4.29-$16.52**

CONTRAINDICATIONS: Hypersensitivity to ester-type local anesthetic, prolonged use, self-medication

PRECAUTIONS: Debilitated, elderly, acutely ill patients, reduced plasma esterase, cardiac disease, hyperthyroidism, children

PREGNANCY AND LACTATION: Pregnancy category C

SIDE EFFECTS/ADVERSE REACTIONS

EENT: Local irritation, stinging, hyperallergic corneal reaction, pupillary dilation (rare), cycloplegia (rare), conjunctival congestion and hemorrhage, softening and erosion of corneal epithelium

SPECIAL CONSIDERATIONS

- Because "blink" reflex is temporarily eliminated, covering eye with patch following instillation is recommended

PATIENT/FAMILY EDUCATION

- Avoid touching or rubbing eye until anesthesia has worn off, inadvertent damage to conjunctiva and cornea may occur

---

propoxyphene

(proe-pox'i-feen)

Darvon, Darvon-N, Dolene

Chemical Class: Synthetic opiate structurally related to methadone

Therapeutic Class: Narcotic analgesic

DEA Class: Schedule IV

CLINICAL PHARMACOLOGY

Mechanism of Action: Binds to opiate receptors in the CNS causing inhibition of ascending pain pathways; alters perception of and response to pain

Pharmacokinetics

PO: Onset 15-60 min, peak 2-2½ hr (3 hr napsylate), duration 4-6 hr, metabolized in liver (25% to norpropoxyphene), excreted in urine, $t_{1/2}$ 6-12 hr

INDICATIONS AND USES: Mild to moderate pain

DOSAGE

Adult

- PO 65 mg (100 mg napsylate) q4h prn; max 390 mg/d (600 mg/d napsylate)

$ **AVAILABLE FORMS/COST OF THERAPY**

- Cap, Gel—Oral: 65 mg, 100's: **$4.88-$34.38**
- Tab, Uncoated—Oral: 100 mg, 100's: **$50.03**

CONTRAINDICATIONS: Hypersensitivity

PRECAUTIONS: History of drug

abuse, suicidal ideation, hepatic or renal function impairment, children

PREGNANCY AND LACTATION: Pregnancy category C (category D if used for prolonged periods or in high doses at term); withdrawal could theoretically occur in infants exposed *in utero* to prolonged maternal ingestion; compatible with breast feeding

SIDE EFFECTS/ADVERSE REACTIONS

CNS: Dizziness, sedation, lightheadedness, headache, euphoria, dysphoria

EENT: Visual disturbances

GI: Nausea, vomiting, constipation, abdominal pain, abnormal liver function, reversible jaundice (rare)

RESP: Respiratory depression

SKIN: Rashes

MISC: Weakness

▼ **DRUG INTERACTIONS**

Drugs

- *Antidepressants:* Increased cyclic antidepressant serum concentrations
- *Beta blockers:* Increased concentrations of highly metabolized beta blockers
- *Carbamazepine:* Marked increases in plasma carbamazepine concentrations
- *Ethanol:* Acute alcohol intoxication increases lethality of propoxyphene
- *MAOIs:* Potentiation of propoxyphene effects in animals; little human evidence to support interaction

Labs

- *Increase:* Amylase

SPECIAL CONSIDERATIONS

PATIENT/FAMILY EDUCATION

- May cause drowsiness, dizziness or blurred vision
- Use caution driving or engaging in other activities requiring alertness
- Avoid alcohol
- May take with food to reduce GI upset
- Notify physician if shortness of breath or difficulty breathing occurs

---

propranolol

(proe-pran'oh-lole)

Inderal, Inderal LA

Chemical Class: Nonselective β-adrenergic blocking agent

Therapeutic Class: Antihypertensive; antianginal; antimigraine agent; antidysrhythmic (Class II)

CLINICAL PHARMACOLOGY

Mechanism of Action: Competes with β-adrenergic agonists for available β_1- and β_2-receptor sites inhibiting the responses to β_1- and β_2-adrenergic stimulation; slows conduction of AV node; decreases blood pressure, heart rate, and myocardial contractility; decreases myocardial O_2 consumption

Pharmacokinetics

PO: Peak 60-90 min (LA 6 hr), extensive first-pass effect

IV: Onset immediate

High lipid solubility, >90% bound to plasma proteins, metabolized in liver to active and inactive metabolites, excreted in urine, $t_{1/2}$ 4-6 hr (LA 8-11 hr)

INDICATIONS AND USES: Hypertension, cardiac dysrhythmias, MI, hypertrophic subaortic stenosis, adjunctive therapy of pheochromocytoma, migraine prophylaxis, angina pectoris, essential tremor, alcohol withdrawal syndrome,* aggressive behavior,* antipsychotic-induced akathisia,* esophageal varices,* situational anxiety,* thyrotoxicosis symptoms*

DOSAGE

Adult

- *Hypertension:* PO 40 mg bid (LA 80 mg qd) initially, usual range 120-

240 mg/d divided bid-tid (LA 120-160 mg qd); max 640 mg/d

- *Dysrhythmias:* PO 10-30 mg tid-qid; IV (reserve for life-threatening situations or dysrhythmias occurring during anesthesia) 0.5-3 mg, a 2nd dose may be administered after 2 min prn; additional doses at intervals no less than 4 hr until desired response obtained
- *Angina pectoris:* PO 10-20 mg tid-qid (LA 80 mg qd) initially, usual range 160-240 mg/d divided tid-qid; maximum 320 mg/day
- *Hypertrophic subaortic stenosis:* PO 20-40 mg tid-qid (LA 80-160 mg qd)
- *Pheochromocytoma:* PO 30 mg/d in divided doses (in conjunction with α-adrenergic blocking agent)
- *Migraine prophylaxis:* PO 80 mg/d in divided doses (LA 80 mg qd) initially, increase to optimal prophylaxis, usual range 160-240 mg/d
- *MI:* PO 180-240 mg/d divided bid-qid beginning 5-21 days after MI
- *Essential tremor:* PO 40 mg bid initially, usual range 120-320 mg/d divided tid

Child

- *Dysrhythmias:* PO 0.5-1 mg/kg/d divided q6-8h, increase dose at 3-7 day intervals, usual range 2-4 mg/kg/d; max 16 mg/kg/d or 60 mg/d; IV 0.01-0.1 mg/kg slowly over 10 min; max 1 mg
- *Hypertension:* PO 0.5-1 mg/kg/d divided q6-12h, increase dose at 3-7 day intervals, usual range 1-5 mg/kg/d
- *Migraine prophylaxis:* PO 0.6-1.5 mg/kg/d in divided doses

$ AVAILABLE FORMS/COST OF THERAPY

- Tab, Uncoated—Oral: 10, 20, 40, 60, 80, 90 mg, 100's: **$1.43-$91.79**
- Tab, Uncoated—Oral: 90 mg, 100's: **$16.25-$23.16**
- Cap, Gel, Sust Action—Oral:60 mg, 100's: **$59.93-$80.50;** 80 mg, 100's: **$72.75-$94.11;** 120 mg, 100's: **$89.93-$116.66;** 160 mg, 100's: **$118.43-$152.75**
- Sol—Oral: 20 mg/5 ml, 500 ml: **$31.50;** 40 mg/5 ml, 500 ml: **$45.01;** 80 mg/ml, 30 ml: **$30.48**
- Inj, Sol—IV: 1 mg/ml, 1 ml: **$4.31-$156.25**

CONTRAINDICATIONS: Hypersensitivity to beta blockers, cardiogenic shock, 2nd or 3rd degree heart block, sinus bradycardia, CHF unless secondary to a tachydysrhythmia treatable with beta blockers, bronchial asthma or bronchospasm, severe COPD, cardiac failure

PRECAUTIONS: Major surgery, diabetes mellitus, renal disease, hepatic disease, thyroid disease, well-compensated heart failure, abrupt withdrawal, peripheral vascular disease, bradycardia

PREGNANCY AND LACTATION: Pregnancy category C; has been used during pregnancy for maternal and fetal indications without teratogenesis, but neonatal toxicity may occur; closely observe neonate during first 24-48 hr after birth for bradycardia, hypoglycemia, and other symptoms of beta blockade; compatible with breast feeding

SIDE EFFECTS/ADVERSE REACTIONS

CNS: Insomnia, *fatigue, dizziness,* mental changes, memory loss, hallucinations, depression, *lethargy,* drowsiness, strange dreams

CV: Profound hypotension, ***bradycardia,*** CHF, cold extremities, postural hypotension, ***2nd or 3rd degree heart block***

EENT: Sore throat, dry burning eyes, visual disturbances

GI: Nausea, diarrhea, vomiting, dry mouth, ***mesenteric arterial thrombosis, ischemic colitis***

GU: Impotence, sexual dysfunction

HEME: ***Agranulocytosis, thrombocytopenia***
METAB: Masked hypoglycemic response to insulin (sweating excepted), hyperlipidemia (increase TG, total cholesterol, LDL; decrease HDL)
RESP: ***Bronchospasm,*** dyspnea, wheezing
SKIN: Rash, pruritis, alopecia

▼ **DRUG INTERACTIONS**

Drugs

- *Amiodarone:* Bradycardia, cardiac arrest, ventricular dysrhythmia shortly after initiation of beta blocker
- *Antidiabetics:* Masked symptoms of hypoglycemia, prolonged recovery of normoglycemia
- *Barbiturates, rifampin:* Reduced concentrations of propranolol
- *Calcium channel blockers:* Increased concentrations of propranolol; increase bioavailability of nifedipine
- *Cimetidine, etintidine, fluoxetine, food, propoxyphene, propafenone, quinidine:* Increased propranolol concentrations
- *Clonidine:* Exacerbation of hypertension upon withdrawal of clonidine
- *Disopyramide:* Additive negative inotropic effects
- *Epinephrine:* Enhanced pressor response to epinephrine
- *Lidocaine:* Increased lidocaine concentrations
- *Local anesthetics:* Enhanced sympathomimetic side effects of epinephrine-containing local anesthetics
- *Methyldopa:* Development of hypertension during periods of catecholamine release
- *Neuroleptics:* Increased plasma concentrations of both drugs
- *NSAIDs:* Reduced hypotensive effect of propranolol
- *Phenylephrine:* Predisposition to acute hypertensive episodes
- *Prazosin:* Enhanced first-dose response to prazosin
- *Theophylline:* Increased theophylline concentrations; antagonistic pharmacodynamic effects

Labs

- *Increase:* BUN in severe heart disease; serum transaminase, alk phosphatase, LDH

SPECIAL CONSIDERATIONS

PATIENT/FAMILY EDUCATION

- Do not discontinue drug abruptly, may precipitate angina
- Report bradycardia, dizziness, confusion, depression, fever, shortness of breath, swelling of the extremities
- Take pulse at home, notify physician if less than 50 beats/min
- Avoid hazardous activities if dizziness, drowsiness, lightheadedness are present
- May mask the symptoms of hypoglycemia, except for sweating, in diabetic patients

MONITORING PARAMETERS

- Blood pressure, pulse

propylthiouracil (PTU)

(proe-pill-thye-of-yoor′a-sill)
Propyl-Thyracil 🍁
Chemical Class: Thioamide
Therapeutic Class: Antithyroid agent

CLINICAL PHARMACOLOGY

Mechanism of Action: Inhibits synthesis of thyroid hormones by interfering with the incorporation of iodine into tyrosyl residues of thyroglobulin; inhibits the coupling of these iodotyrosyl residues to form iodothyronine; does not inhibit action of thyroid hormones already formed and present in the thyroid gland and circulation or exogenously administered thyroid hormones; partially inhibits peripheral conversion of T_4 to T_3

Pharmacokinetics

PO: Bioavailability 80%-95%, 75%-80% bound to plasma proteins, metabolized in liver, excreted in urine (35% unchanged), $t_{1/2}$ 1-2 hr

INDICATIONS AND USES: Hyperthyroidism, preparation for thyroidectomy or radioactive iodine therapy, thyrotoxic crisis, alcoholic liver disease*

DOSAGE

Adult

• PO 300-450 mg/d divided q8h initially (doses of 600-1200 mg/d may be required); maintenance dose 100-150 mg/d divided q8-12h

Child

• PO 5-7 mg/kg/d divided q8h initially; maintenance dose ⅓-⅔ of initial dose divided q8-12h

• Dose in renal impairment: PO CrCl 10-50 ml/min, decrease recommended dose by 25%; CrCl <10 ml/min, decrease recommended dose by 50%

$ AVAILABLE FORMS/COST OF THERAPY

• Tab, Uncoated—Oral: 50 mg, 100's: **$4.79-$8.75**

CONTRAINDICATIONS: Hypersensitivity

PRECAUTIONS: Infection, bone marrow depression, hepatic disease, children (hepatotoxicity has occurred)

PREGNANCY AND LACTATION: Pregnancy category D; considered drug of choice for medical treatment of hyperthyroidism during pregnancy; excreted into breast milk in low amounts, compatible with breast feeding

SIDE EFFECTS/ADVERSE REACTIONS

CNS: Paresthesias, neuritis, *headache, vertigo, drowsiness,* neuropathies, CNS stimulation, depression

CV: Edema

GI: Nausea, vomiting, epigastric distress, loss of taste, sialadenopathy, ***hepatitis,*** jaundice

GU: ***Nephritis***

HEME: ***Agranulocytosis, granulocytopenia, thrombocytopenia, aplastic anemia, hypoprothrombinemia, leukopenia***

METAB: Insulin autoimmune syndrome (may result in ***hypoglycemia, coma***)

MS: Arthralgia, myalgia

RESP: Interstitial pneumonitis

SKIN: Skin rash, urticaria, pruritis, erythema nodosum, skin pigmentation, ***exfoliative dermatitis,*** lupus-like syndrome

MISC: Splenomegaly, *abnormal hair loss,* lymphadenopathy

▼ DRUG INTERACTIONS

Drugs

• *Oral anticoagulants:* Reduced hypoprothrombinemic response to oral anticoagulants

SPECIAL CONSIDERATIONS

PATIENT/FAMILY EDUCATION

• Notify physician of fever, sore throat, unusual bleeding or bruising, headache, rash, yellowing of skin, vomiting

MONITORING PARAMETERS

• Thyroid function tests periodically during therapy

protamine

(proe'ta-meen)

Chemical Class: Strongly basic low molecular weight protein

Therapeutic Class: Heparin antagonist

CLINICAL PHARMACOLOGY

Mechanism of Action: Forms a stable salt with heparin (strongly

P

acidic) resulting in loss of anticoagulant activity of both drugs

Pharmacokinetics

IV: Rapid onset of action, heparin neutralized within 5 min, duration 2 hr, metabolic fate of heparin-protamine complex unknown

INDICATIONS AND USES: Heparin overdose

DOSAGE

Adult and Child

• IV 1 mg neutralizes 90 USP units of lung tissue-derived heparin and 115 USP units of intestinal mucosa-derived heparin; administer slowly over 10 min (for SC heparin overdose, a portion of the total protamine dose should be administered by continuous inf over 8-16 hr), do not exceed 50 mg in a 10 min period; dose requirement decreases rapidly with time elapsed since IV heparin inj; guide dosage by blood coagulation studies

$ **AVAILABLE FORMS/COST OF THERAPY**

• Inj, Sol—IV: 10 mg/ml, 5 ml: **$4.06-$104.06**

CONTRAINDICATIONS: Hypersensitivity

PRECAUTIONS: Rapid administration (hypotension, anaphylactoid reactions), previous protamine exposure, fish allergy

PREGNANCY AND LACTATION: Pregnancy category C

SIDE EFFECTS/ADVERSE REACTIONS

CNS: Lassitude

CV: Hypotension, bradycardia, flushing, ***circulatory collapse***

GI: Nausea, vomiting

RESP: ***Pulmonary edema, pulmonary hypertension,*** dyspnea

MISC: Hypersensitivity reactions

SPECIAL CONSIDERATIONS

MONITORING PARAMETERS

• Activated partial thromboplastin time (APTT) or protamine activated clotting time (ACT) 15 min after dose, then in several hr

protriptyline

(proe-trip'ti-leen)

Triptil, ♣ Vivactil

Chemical Class: Dibenzolcycloheptene derivative, secondary amine

Therapeutic Class: Antidepressant, tricyclic

CLINICAL PHARMACOLOGY

Mechanism of Action: Inhibits the reuptake of norepinephrine and serotonin at the presynaptic neuron prolonging neuronal activity; inhibition of histamine and acetylcholine activity; mild peripheral vasodilator effects and possible quinidine-like actions

Pharmacokinetics

PO: Peak 24-30 hr, therapeutic response 2-4 wk, metabolized by liver, excreted by kidneys, $t_{1/2}$ 67-89 hr

INDICATIONS AND USES: Depression, obstructive sleep apnea*

DOSAGE

Adult

• PO 15-40 mg/d divided tid-qid; may increase to 60 mg/d

Geriatric/Adolescent

• PO 5 mg tid, increase gradually if needed; use caution if dose >20 mg/d

$ **AVAILABLE FORMS/COST OF THERAPY**

• Tab, Plain Coated—Oral: 5 mg, 100's: **$46.49**; 10 mg, 100's: **$67.36**

CONTRAINDICATIONS: Hypersensitivity to tricyclic antidepressants, acute recovery phase of MI; concurrent use of MAOIs

PRECAUTIONS: Suicidal patients, convulsive disorders, prostatic hypertrophy, psychiatric disease, severe depression, increased intraocular pressure, narrow-angle glaucoma, urinary retention, cardiac disease, hepatic/renal disease, hyperthyroidism, electroshock therapy, elective surgery, elderly, abrupt discontinuation

PREGNANCY AND LACTATION: Pregnancy category C

SIDE EFFECTS/ADVERSE REACTIONS

CNS: Dizziness, confusion (especially in elderly), headache, anxiety, nervousness, panic, tremors, stimulation, weakness, fatigue, insomnia, nightmares, EPS (elderly), increased psychiatric symptoms, memory impairment, sedation

CV: Orthostatic hypotension, ***ECG changes, tachycardia, dysrhythmias,*** hypertension, palpitations, syncope, hypertensive episodes during surgery

EENT: Blurred vision, tinnitus, mydriasis, ophthalmoplegia, nasal congestion

GI: Constipation, dry mouth, nausea, vomiting, ***paralytic ileus,*** increased appetite, cramps, epigastric distress, jaundice, ***hepatitis,*** stomatitis, diarrhea

GU: Urinary retention

HEME: ***Agranulocytosis, thrombocytopenia, eosinophilia, leukopenia***

SKIN: Rash, urticaria, sweating, pruritus, photosensitivity

▼ **DRUG INTERACTIONS**

Drugs

- *Amphetamines:* Theoretical increase in effect of amphetamines, clinical evidence lacking
- *Barbiturates:* Reduced serum concentrations of cyclic antidepressants
- *Bethanidine:* Reduced antihypertensive effect of bethanidine
- *Carbamazepine:* Reduced cyclic antidepressant serum concentrations
- *Clonidine:* Reduced antihypertensive response to clonidine; enhanced hypertensive response with abrupt clonidine withdrawal
- *Debrisoquin:* Inhibited antihypertensive response of debrisoquin
- *Epinephrine+:* Markedly enhanced pressor response to IV epinephrine
- *Ethanol:* Additive impairment of motor skills; abstinent alcoholics may eliminate cyclic antidepressants more rapidly than nonalcoholics
- *Fluoxetine:* Marked increases in cyclic antidepressant plasma concentrations
- *Guanethidine:* Inhibited antihypertensive response to guanethidine
- *MAOIs:* Excessive sympathetic response, mania, or hyperpyrexia possible
- *Moclobemide+:* Potential association with fatal or non-fatal serotonin syndrome
- *Neuroleptics:* Increased therapeutic and toxic effects of both drugs
- *Norepinephrine+:* Markedly enhanced pressor response to norepinephrine
- *Phenylephrine:* Enhanced pressor response to IV phenylephrine
- *Phenytoin:* Altered seizure control; decreased cyclic antidepressant serum concentrations
- *Propoxyphene:* Enhanced effect of cyclic antidepressants
- *Quinidine:* Increased cyclic antidepressant serum concentrations

Labs

- *Increase:* Serum bilirubin, blood glucose, alk phosphatase
- *Decrease:* VMA, 5-HIAA
- *False increase:* Urinary catecholamines

SPECIAL CONSIDERATIONS

PATIENT/FAMILY EDUCATION

- Therapeutic effects may take 2-3 wk
- Use caution in driving or other activities requiring alertness
- Avoid rising quickly from sitting to standing, especially elderly

P

• Avoid alcohol and other CNS depressants
• Do not discontinue abruptly after long-term use
• Wear sunscreen or large hat to prevent photosensitivity

MONITORING PARAMETERS

• CBC, weight, ECG, mental status (mood, sensorium, affect, suicidal tendencies)

---

pseudoephedrine

(soo-doe-e-fed'rin)

Cenafed, Congestion Relief, Decofed Syrup, DeFed-60, Dorcol Children's Decongestant, Efidac 24, Genaphed, Halofed, Kidkare Decongestant Drops, PediaCare Infant's Decongestant Pseudo, Pseudo-Gest, Seudotabs, Sudafed, Uni Sed

Chemical Class: Sympathomimetic alkaloid, stereoisomer of ephedrine
Therapeutic Class: Decongestant

CLINICAL PHARMACOLOGY

Mechanism of Action: Directly stimulates α-adrenergic receptors in respiratory tract mucosa causing vasoconstriction; direct stimulation of β-adrenergic receptors causes increased heart rate and contractility

Pharmacokinetics

PO: Onset 15-30 min, duration 4-6 hr (extended release 12 hr); partially metabolized in liver to inactive metabolite, excreted in urine (55%-75% unchanged)

INDICATIONS AND USES: Nasal decongestion associated with common cold, allergies, and sinusitis; promotes nasal or sinus drainage

DOSAGE

Adult

• PO 60 mg q4-6h; PO SR 120 mg q12h or 240 mg qd (Efidac 24); max 240 mg/d

Child

• PO 6-11 yr 30 mg q4-6h, max 120 mg/d; 2-5 yr 15 mg q4-6h, max 60 mg/d; <2 yr 4 mg/kg/d divided q6h

$ **AVAILABLE FORMS/COST OF THERAPY**

• Liq—Oral: 15 mg/5 ml, 120 ml: **$3.96**
• Syr—Oral: 30 mg/5 ml, 120 ml: **$0.90-$6.40**
• Drops—Oral: 7.5 mg/0.8 ml, 15 ml: **$4.12**
• Tab, Uncoated—Oral: 30 mg, 100's: **$1.35-$10.84**; 60 mg, 100's: **$3.36-$24.95**
• Tab, Ext-Rel—Oral: 120 mg, 10's: **$3.94**; 240 mg, 12's: **$6.77**

CONTRAINDICATIONS: Hypersensitivity to sympathomimetics, severe hypertension, severe CAD

PRECAUTIONS: Heart disease, coronary insufficiency, dysrhythmias, angina, hyperthyroidism, diabetes mellitus, prostatic hypertrophy, increased intracranial pressure, hypovolemia, mild to moderate hypertension

PREGNANCY AND LACTATION: Pregnancy category C; compatible with breast feeding

SIDE EFFECTS/ADVERSE REACTIONS

CNS: Tremors, anxiety, insomnia, headache, dizziness, confusion, hallucinations, drowsiness
CV: Palpitations, tachycardia, chest pain, ***dysrhythmias***
GI: Anorexia, nausea, vomiting
GU: Dysuria, urinary retention
METAB: Hyperglycemia

▼ **DRUG INTERACTIONS**

Drugs

• *Antacids:* Sodium bicarbonate doses sufficient to alkalinize urine can inhibit elimination of pseudoephedrine

• *MAOIs+:* Severe hypertension

SPECIAL CONSIDERATIONS

PATIENT/FAMILY EDUCATION

• May cause wakefulness or nervousness
• Take last dose 4-6 hr prior to hs, notify physician of insomnia, dizziness, weakness, tremor, or irregular heart beat

psyllium

(sill'ee-yum)

Effer-Syllium, Fiberall, Hydrocil, Konsyl, Metamucil, Modane Bulk, Perdiem, Reguloid, Serutan, Siblin, Syllact, V-Lax

Chemical Class: Psyllium colloid

Therapeutic Class: Bulk forming laxative

CLINICAL PHARMACOLOGY

Mechanism of Action: Adsorbs water in the intestine; promotes peristalsis and reduces transit time through the GI tract

Pharmacokinetics

PO: Generally not absorbed, onset 12-24 hr (may be as long as 2-3 days)

INDICATIONS AND USES: Constipation, irritable bowel syndrome, diverticular disease, spastic colon, hemorrhoids, hypercholesterolemia*

DOSAGE

Adult

• PO 1-2 rounded teaspoonfuls or 1-2 packets in 8 oz glass of liquid 1-4 times/d; 1-2 wafers with 8 oz glass of liquid 1-4 times/d

Child 6-11 yr

• PO ½ to 1 rounded teaspoonful in 4 oz glass of liquid 1-3 times/d

$ **AVAILABLE FORMS/COST OF THERAPY**

• Granules—Oral: 2.5-4.03 g/rounded teaspoon; 100, 180, 250, 480, 540 g: **$5.22-$11.45**
• Powder—Oral: 50% psyllium and 50% dextrose/dose, 120, 396, 420, 630 g: **$3.50-$8.86**
• Powder, Effervescent—Oral: 3.4 g/dose, 30's (packets) and 300 g (bulk): **$5.83-$7.60**
• Powder, Hydrophilic—Oral: 3.5 g/rounded teaspoon; 210, 300, 420, 630 g: **$5.83-$9.22**
• Wafer, Chewable—Oral: 1.7-3.4 g; 14's, 24's, 48's: **$3.92-$7.63**

CONTRAINDICATIONS: Hypersensitivity, intestinal obstruction, fecal impaction

PRECAUTIONS: Phenylketonurics (sugar free preparations may contain aspartame), abdominal pain, nausea or vomiting

PREGNANCY AND LACTATION: Pregnancy category C; not systemically absorbed, exposure of fetus or nursing infant unlikely

SIDE EFFECTS/ADVERSE REACTIONS

GI: ***Esophageal or bowel obstruction,*** *nausea, vomiting, anorexia,* diarrhea, constipation, bloating, cramping

SPECIAL CONSIDERATIONS

PATIENT/FAMILY EDUCATION

• Maintain adequate fluid consumption
• Do not use in presence of abdominal pain, nausea, or vomiting
• Avoid inhaling dust from powder preparations, can cause runny nose, watery eyes, wheezing

P

pyrantel

(pye-ran'tel)

Antiminth, Combantrin, ♣ Pin-Rid, Pin-X, Reese's Pinworm

Chemical Class: Pyrimidine derivative

Therapeutic Class: Anthelmintic

CLINICAL PHARMACOLOGY
Mechanism of Action: Spasmic paralysis of worm results from depolarizing neuromuscular blockade; also inhibits cholinesterases; worms are expelled via normal peristalsis; active against *Enterobius vermicularis* (pinworm), *Ascaris lumbricoides* (roundworm), and hookworm
Pharmacokinetics
PO: Poorly absorbed, achieves low systemic levels of unchanged drug, 50% excreted unchanged in feces, ≤7% found in urine (unchanged drug and metabolites)
INDICATIONS AND USES: Ascariasis (roundworm infection), enterobiasis (pinworm infection), hookworm infection,* trichostrongyliasis*
DOSAGE
Adult and Child
• *Roundworm, pinworm, trichostrongyliasis:* PO 11 mg/kg as a single dose; max 1 g/dose; repeat in 2 wk for pinworm infection
• *Hookworm:* PO 11 mg/kg qd for 3 days
$ AVAILABLE FORMS/COST OF THERAPY
• Susp—Oral: 50 mg/ml, 30, 60 ml: **$5.62-$40.43**
CONTRAINDICATIONS: Hepatic disease, hypersensitivity
PRECAUTIONS: Child <2 yr
PREGNANCY AND LACTATION: Pregnancy category C
SIDE EFFECTS/ADVERSE REACTIONS
CNS: Headache, dizziness, drowsiness, insomnia
GI: Anorexia, nausea, vomiting, abdominal cramps, diarrhea, elevated liver enzymes
SKIN: Rash
SPECIAL CONSIDERATIONS
PATIENT/FAMILY EDUCATION
• Take with food or milk
• Using a laxative to facilitate expulsion of worms is not necessary
• All family members in close contact with patient should be treated
• Strict hygiene is essential to prevent reinfection
• Shake suspension well before pouring

pyrazinamide
(pye-ra-zin'a-mide)
Tebrazid ♣
Chemical Class: Niacinamide derivative
Therapeutic Class: Antituberculosis agent

CLINICAL PHARMACOLOGY
Mechanism of Action: Exact mechanism unknown; converted to pyrazinoic acid (POA) by susceptible strains of *Mycobacterium tuberculosis;* POA has specific antimycobacterial activity against *M. tuberculosis* and may lower environmental pH below that which is necessary for growth of the organism
Pharmacokinetics
PO: Peak 2 hr (POA 4-8 hr), 17% bound to plasma proteins, widely distributed in body tissues and fluids, metabolized in liver to POA (active), excreted in urine (4%-14% unchanged), $t_{1/2}$ 9-10 hr
INDICATIONS AND USES: Active tuberculosis (as part of a 6 mo regimen consisting of isoniazid, rifampin, and pyrazinamide given for 2 mo, followed by isoniazid and rifampin for 4 mo); after treatment failure with other primary drugs in any form of active tuberculosis
DOSAGE
Adult
• PO 15-30 mg/kg qd for first 2 mo of 6 mo regimen with isoniazid and rifampin or as part of an individu-

alized regimen for drug-resistant disease; max 2 g/d; alternatively 50-70 mg/kg can be given twice weekly to improve compliance (base dosage calculations on lean body wt)

Child

• PO 15-40 mg/kg/d divided q12-24 hr; max 2 g/d; alternatively 50-70 mg/kg twice weekly; max 2 g/dose

$ **AVAILABLE FORMS/COST OF THERAPY**

• Tab, Uncoated—Oral: 500 mg, 100's: **$87.38-$112.38**

CONTRAINDICATIONS: Hypersensitivity, severe liver disease, acute gout

PRECAUTIONS: History of gout, renal and hepatic function impairment, alcoholism, elderly, HIV infection (may require longer courses of therapy), diabetes mellitus

PREGNANCY AND LACTATION: Pregnancy category C; excreted into human milk

SIDE EFFECTS/ADVERSE REACTIONS

CNS: Fever

GI: ***Hepatotoxicity,*** nausea, vomiting, anorexia

GU: Dysuria, interstitial nephritis (rare)

HEME: Porphyria, ***thrombocytopenia, sideroblastic anemia,*** increased serum iron concentration, blood clotting abnormalities

METAB: Gout, hyperuricemia

MS: Arthralgia, myalgia

SKIN: Rash, urticaria, pruritus, acne, photosensitivity

▼ **DRUG INTERACTIONS**

Labs

• *Increase:* Liver function tests

• *Interference:* Urine ketone tests

SPECIAL CONSIDERATIONS

PATIENT/FAMILY EDUCATION

• Compliance with full course is essential

• Notify physician of fever, loss of appetite, malaise, nausea and vomiting, darkened urine, yellowish discoloration of skin and eyes, pain or swelling of joints

MONITORING PARAMETERS

• Liver function tests, serum uric acid at baseline and periodically throughout therapy

---

pyridostigmine

(peer-id-oh-stig'meen)

Mestinon, Regonol

Chemical Class: Synthetic quaternary ammonium compound

Therapeutic Class: Cholinergic, anticholinesterase

CLINICAL PHARMACOLOGY

Mechanism of Action: An acetylcholinesterase inhibitor; inhibits destruction of acetylcholine, which increases concentration at sites where acetylcholine is released, facilitating transmission of impulses across myoneural junction

Pharmacokinetics

PO: Poorly absorbed, onset 30-45 min, duration 3-6 hr

IV: Onset 2-5 min, duration 2-3 hr

IM: Onset 15 min

Hydrolyzed by cholinesterases and metabolized by microsomal enzymes in liver, excreted in urine

INDICATIONS AND USES: Myasthenia gravis, reversal of nondepolarizing neuromuscular blocking agents after surgery

DOSAGE

Adult

• *Myasthenia gravis:* PO 600 mg/d divided to provide max relief; usual range 60-1500 mg/d, individualize dosage; PO SR 180-540 mg qd-bid, individualize dosage, use dosage intervals of at least 6 hr; IM/IV 1/30th PO dose, inj IV very slowly

• *Reversal of nondepolarizing neuromuscular blockade:* IV 10-20 mg; give atropine 0.6-1.2 mg IV imme-

P

diately prior to pyridostigmine to minimize side effects

Child

- *Myasthenia gravis:* PO 7 mg/kg/d divided into 5-6 doses; IM/IV 0.05-0.15 mg/kg/dose; max 10 mg/dose, inj IV very slowly
- *Reversal of nondepolarizing neuromuscular blockade:* IV 0.1-0.25 mg/kg/dose preceded by atropine or glycopyrrolate

$ AVAILABLE FORMS/COST OF THERAPY

- Inj, Sol—IM; IV: 5 mg/ml, 2 ml: **$1.32-$5.25**
- Syr—Oral: 60 mg/5 ml, 480 ml: **$33.43**
- Tab, Uncoated—Oral: 60 mg, 100's: **$39.19**
- Tab, Coated, Sust Action—Oral: 180 mg, 100's: **$85.75**

CONTRAINDICATIONS: Mechanical obstruction of intestinal or urinary tracts, hypersensitivity to pyridostigmine or bromides (pyridostigmine bromide)

PRECAUTIONS: Seizure disorder, bronchial asthma, bradycardia, recent coronary occlusion, vagotonia, hyperthyroidism, cardiac dysrhythmias, peptic ulcer, large oral doses in megacolon and decreased GI motility (accumulation and toxicity may occur when motility is restored), anticholinesterase insensitivity (reduce or withhold dosages until patient again becomes sensitive)

PREGNANCY AND LACTATION: Pregnancy category C; would not be expected to cross the placenta because it is ionized at physiologic pH; although apparently safe for the fetus, may cause transient muscle weakness in the newborn; compatible with breast feeding

SIDE EFFECTS/ADVERSE REACTIONS

CNS: Dizziness, headache, ***convulsions,*** incoordination, ***paralysis, loss of consciousness,*** drowsiness

CV: Tachycardia, ***dysrhythmias,*** bradycardia, hypotension, AV block, nodal rhythm, nonspecific ECG changes, ***cardiac arrest,*** syncope

EENT: Miosis, blurred vision, lacrimation, visual changes, spasm of accommodation, diplopia, conjunctival hyperemia

GI: Nausea, diarrhea, vomiting, cramps, increased salivation, increased gastric secretions, dysphagia, increased peristalsis, flatulence

GU: Frequency, incontinence, urgency

MS: Weakness, fasciculation, muscle cramps and spasms, arthralgia

RESP: ***Respiratory depression, bronchospasm, laryngospasm, respiratory arrest,*** increased secretions, dyspnea

SKIN: Rash, urticaria, sweating

SPECIAL CONSIDERATIONS

PATIENT/FAMILY EDUCATION

- Take drug exactly as prescribed
- Notify physician if nausea, vomiting, diarrhea, sweating, increased salivation, irregular heartbeat, muscle weakness, severe abdominal pain, or difficulty in breathing occurs
- Do not crush or chew sustained release preparations

MONITORING PARAMETERS

- Therapeutic response: increased muscle strength, improved gait, absence of labored breathing (if severe)
- Appearance of side effects (narrow margin between first appearance of side effects and serious toxicity)

pyridoxine (vitamin B_6)

(peer-i-dox'een)

Beesix, Nestrex, Rodex TD, Hexa-Betalin

Chemical Class: Water soluble B complex vitamin

Therapeutic Class: Vitamin; antidote

CLINICAL PHARMACOLOGY

Mechanism of Action: Acts as a coenzyme in metabolism of protein, carbohydrates, and fat

Pharmacokinetics

PO: Readily absorbed, metabolized in liver to 4-pyridoxic acid, excreted in urine, biologic $t_{1/2}$ 15-20 days

INDICATIONS AND USES: Pyridoxine deficiency including inadequate diet and drug-induced (e.g., isoniazid, hydralazine, penicillamine, cycloserine, oral contraceptives); inborn errors of metabolism such as B_6-dependent seizures or B_6-responsive anemia; hydralazine or isoniazid poisoning,* premenstrual syndrome (PMS),* hyperoxaluria type I (and oxalate kidney stones); nausea and vomiting in pregnancy*

DOSAGE

Adult

- *Dietary deficiency:* PO 10-20 mg qd for 3 wk, then 2-5 mg/d
- *Drug induced deficiency:* PO 100-200 mg/d
- *Prophylaxis of drug induced deficiency:* PO 25-100 mg/d
- *Recommended daily allowance (RDA):* PO 1.6-2 mg
- *Isoniazid poisoning:* IV 4 g followed by 1 g IM q30min to equal amount of isoniazid consumed; doses of 70-357 mg/kg have been administered without incident

Child

- *Dietary deficiency:* PO 5-25 mg/d for 3 wk, then 1.5-2.5 mg/d
- *Drug induced deficiency:* PO 10-50 mg/d
- *Prophylaxis of drug induced deficiency:* PO 1-2 mg/kg/d
- *Recommended daily allowance (RDA):* PO 1-3 yr 0.9 mg; 4-6 yr 1.3 mg; 7-10 yr 1.6 mg

$ **AVAILABLE FORMS/COST OF THERAPY**

- Inj, Sol—IM; IV: 100 mg/ml, 10 ml: **$2.80-$6.74**
- Tab—Oral: 25, 50, 100 mg, 100's: **$0.94-$12.50**
- Tab, Timed Release—Oral: 200 mg, 60's: **$2.60**

CONTRAINDICATIONS: Hypersensitivity

PREGNANCY AND LACTATION: Pregnancy category A (category C if used in doses above RDA); deficiency during pregnancy is common in unsupplemented women; excreted in human breast milk, RDA for lactating women is 2.3-2.5 mg

SIDE EFFECTS/ADVERSE REACTIONS

CNS: Sensory neuropathic syndromes, unstable gait, numb feet, awkwardness of hands, perioral numbness, decreased sensation to touch/temperature/vibration, paresthesia, somnolence, ***seizures*** (following very large IV doses), headache

GI: Nausea, increased AST

HEME: Low serum folic acid levels

RESP: Respiratory distress

SKIN: Burning or stinging at inj site

MISC: Allergic reactions

▼ **DRUG INTERACTIONS**

Drugs

- *Levodopa:* Inhibited antiparkinsonian effect of levodopa; concurrent use of carbidopa negates the interaction

P

SPECIAL CONSIDERATIONS

PATIENT/FAMILY EDUCATION

- Avoid doses exceeding RDA unless directed by physician

MONITORING PARAMETERS

- Respiratory rate, heart rate, blood pressure during large IV doses

---

pyrilamine

(pye-rill'a-meen)
Nisaval
Chemical Class: Ethylenediamine derivative
Therapeutic Class: Antihistamine

CLINICAL PHARMACOLOGY

Mechanism of Action: Competes with histamine for H_1-receptor sites on effector cells in the GI tract, blood vessels, and respiratory tract; antagonizes most of pharmacological effects of histamine; also has anticholinergic, antipruritic, and sedative effects

Pharmacokinetics

PO: Well absorbed, onset 15-30 min, peak 1-2 hr, duration 4-6 hr, metabolized in liver, excreted in urine

INDICATIONS AND USES: Perennial and seasonal allergic rhinitis and other allergic symptoms

DOSAGE

Adult

- PO 25-50 mg tid-qid

$ **AVAILABLE FORMS/COST OF THERAPY**

- Tab—Oral: 25 mg, 1000's: **$17.00**

CONTRAINDICATIONS: Hypersensitivity, narrow-angle glaucoma, bladder neck obstruction

PRECAUTIONS: Liver disease, elderly, increased intraocular pressure, hyperthyroidism, cardiovascular disease, hypertension, urinary retention, renal disease, stenosed peptic ulcers

PREGNANCY AND LACTATION: Pregnancy category C

SIDE EFFECTS/ADVERSE REACTIONS

CNS: Dizziness, drowsiness, poor coordination, fatigue, anxiety, euphoria, confusion, paresthesia, neuritis

CV: Hypotension, palpitations, tachycardia

EENT: Blurred vision, dilated pupils, tinnitus, nasal stuffiness, dry nose, throat

GI: Dry mouth, nausea, vomiting, anorexia, *constipation,* diarrhea

GU: Retention, dysuria, frequency, impotence

HEME: ***Thrombocytopenia, agranulocytosis, hemolytic anemia***

RESP: Increased thick secretions, wheezing, chest tightness

SKIN: Photosensitivity

▼ **DRUG INTERACTIONS**

Labs

- *False negative:* Skin allergy tests

SPECIAL CONSIDERATIONS

PATIENT/FAMILY EDUCATION

- Notify physician if confusion, sedation, hypotension occurs
- Avoid driving or other hazardous activities if drowsiness occurs
- Avoid use of alcohol or other CNS depressants while taking drug
- Use hard candy, gum, frequent rinsing of mouth for dryness

---

pyrimethamine

(pye-ri-meth'a-meen)
Daraprim
Chemical Class: Synthetic aminopyrimidine derivative
Therapeutic Class: Antimalarial

CLINICAL PHARMACOLOGY

Mechanism of Action: Inhibits dihydrofolate reductase which catalyzes the reduction of dihydrofolate to tetrahydrofolate; highly selective against plasmodia and *Toxoplasma gondii*

Pharmacokinetics

PO: Peak 2-6 hr, 87% bound to plasma proteins, metabolized in liver, excreted in urine, $t_{1/2}$ 4 days (suppressive concentrations are maintained for approximately 2 wk)

INDICATIONS AND USES: Chemoprophylaxis of malaria due to susceptible strains of plasmodia; toxoplasmosis (in combination with sulfonamide); combination therapy with quinine and sulfadiazine for uncomplicated attack of chloroquine-resistant *P. falciparum* malaria; initiation of transmission control and suppressive cure in conjunction with fast-acting schizonticide

DOSAGE

Adult

- *Malaria prophylaxis:* PO 25 mg qwk; begin 2 wk before entering areas where chloroquine-resistant *P. falciparum* exists, continue for at least 6-10 wk after leaving endemic area
- *Chloroquine-resistant P. falciparum malaria (with quinine and sulfadiazine):* PO 25 mg bid for 3 days
- *Toxoplasmosis (with sulfadiazine):* PO 50-75 mg/d with 1-4 g of sulfonamide for 1-3 wk, reduce dose by 50% and continue for 4-5 wk; alternatively 25-50 mg/d for 3-4 wk

Child

- *Malaria prophylaxis:* PO 0.5 mg/kg qwk, do not exceed 25 mg/dose; begin 2 wk before entering areas where chloroquine-resistant *P. falciparum* exists, continue for at least 6-10 wk after leaving endemic area
- *Chloroqine-resistant P. falciparum malaria (with quinine and sulfadiazine):* PO <10 kg, 6.25 mg qd for 3 days; 10-20 kg 12.5 mg qd for 3 days; 20-40 kg 25 mg qd for 3 days
- *Toxoplasmosis (with sulfadiazine):* PO 2 mg/kg/d divided q12h for 3 days followed by 1 mg/kg/d divided qd-bid for 4 wk

$ **AVAILABLE FORMS/COST OF THERAPY**

- Tab, Uncoated—Oral: 25 mg, 100's: **$37.67**

CONTRAINDICATIONS: Hypersensitivity, documented megaloblastic anemia secondary to folate deficiency

PRECAUTIONS: Malabsorption syndrome, alcoholism, pregnancy (increased risk for folate deficiency); renal or hepatic function impairment; seizure disorder; glucose-6-PD deficiency

PREGNANCY AND LACTATION: Pregnancy category C; most studies have found pyrimethamine to be safe in pregnancy, folic acid supplementation should be given to prevent folate deficiency; compatible with breast feeding

SIDE EFFECTS/ADVERSE REACTIONS

CNS: Insomnia, headache, lightheadedness, fever, depression, ***seizures***

CV: Cardiac rhythm disturbance (large doses)

EENT: Dry throat

GI: Anorexia, nausea, vomiting, atrophic glossitis, diarrhea, dry mouth

GU: ***Hematuria***

HEME: ***Megaloblastic anemia, leukopenia, thrombocytopenia, pancytopenia, hemolytic anemia,*** decreased folic acid

RESP: Pulmonary eosinophilia

SKIN: Dermatitis, abnormal skin pigmentation

▼ **DRUG INTERACTIONS**

Drugs

- *Folic acid:* Decreased efficacy of pyrimethamine
- *Methotrexate, sulfonamides, co-*

P

trimoxazole: Increased risk of bone marrow suppression

SPECIAL CONSIDERATIONS

PATIENT/FAMILY EDUCATION

• Take with food

• Discontinue at first sign of skin rash

• Notify physician of sore throat, pallor, purpura, glossitis

MONITORING PARAMETERS

• CBC with platelets semiweekly during therapy for toxoplasmosis, less frequently for malaria-related indications

---

quazepam

(kway'ze-pam)

Doral

Chemical Class: Benzodiazepine derivative

Therapeutic Class: Hypnotic

DEA Class: Schedule IV

CLINICAL PHARMACOLOGY

Mechanism of Action: Facilitates the inhibitory effect of γ-amino butyric acid (GABA) on neuronal excitability by increasing membrane permeability to chloride ions

Pharmacokinetics

PO: Peak 2 hr, 95% bound to plasma proteins, metabolized in liver to 2-oxoquazepam and N-desalkyl-2-oxoquazepam (both active), excreted in urine (31%) and feces (23%), $t_{1/2}$ 25-41 hr (metabolites 40-114 hr)

INDICATIONS AND USES: Short-term management of insomnia

DOSAGE

Adult

• PO 7.5-15 mg hs; reduce dose after 1-2 nights if possible

$ AVAILABLE FORMS/COST OF THERAPY

• Tab, Coated—Oral: 7.5 mg, 100's: **$104.47;** 15 mg, 100's: **$114.17**

CONTRAINDICATIONS: Hypersensitivity to benzodiazepines, narrow-angle glaucoma, psychosis, pregnancy

PRECAUTIONS: Elderly, debilitated, hepatic disease, renal disease, history of drug abuse, abrupt withdrawal, respiratory depression, prolonged use

PREGNANCY AND LACTATION: Pregnancy category D; may cause fetal damage when administered during pregnancy; excreted into breast milk, may accumulate in breast-fed infants and is therefore not recommended

SIDE EFFECTS/ADVERSE REACTIONS

CNS: Somnolence, asthenia, hypokinesia, hangover, abnormal thinking, anxiety, agitation, amnesia, apathy, emotional lability, hostility, seizure, sleep disorder, stupor, twitch, ataxia, decreased libido, decreased reflexes, neuritis

CV: Dysrhythmia, syncope

EENT: Ear pain, eye irritation/pain/swelling, photophobia, pharyngitis, rhinitis, sinusitis, epistaxis,

GI: Dyspepsia, decreased/increased appetite, flatulence, gastritis, enterocolitis, melena, mouth ulceration, abdominal pain, increased AST

GU: Frequent urination, menstrual cramps, urinary hesitancy or urgency, vaginal discharge/itching, hematuria, nocturia, oliguria, penile discharge, urinary incontinence

HEME: ***Agranulocytosis***

MS: Lower extremity pain, back pain

RESP: Cold symptoms, asthma, cough, dyspnea, hyperventilation

SKIN: Urticaria, acne, dry skin, photosensitivity

▼ DRUG INTERACTIONS

Drugs

• *Cimetidine:* Increased plama levels of quazepam

• *Clozapine:* Isolated cases of cardiorespiratory collapse have been reported; causal relationship to benzodiazepines has not been established

- *Disulfiram:* Increased serum quazepam concentrations
- *Ethanol:* Enhanced adverse psychomotor side effects of benzodiazepines
- *Rifampin:* Reduced serum quazepam concentrations

Labs

- *Increase:* AST/ALT, serum bilirubin
- *Decrease:* RAIU

SPECIAL CONSIDERATIONS

PATIENT/FAMILY EDUCATION

- Avoid alcohol and other CNS depressants
- Do not discontinue abruptly after prolonged therapy
- May cause daytime sedation, use caution while driving or performing other tasks requiring alertness
- Inform physician if planning to become pregnant, or are pregnant, or if you become pregnant while taking this medicine
- May be habit forming

quinapril

(kwin′na-pril)

Accupril

Chemical Class: Angiotensin-converting enzyme (ACE) inhibitor

Therapeutic Class: Antihypertensive

CLINICAL PHARMACOLOGY

Mechanism of Action: Selectively suppresses renin-angiotensin-aldosterone system; inhibits ACE preventing conversion of angiotensin I to angiotensin II; results in dilation of arterial, venous vessels

Pharmacokinetics

PO: Onset 1 hr, duration 24 hr, has little pharmacologic activity until metabolized to active metabolite (quinaprilat), exreted in urine (60%) and feces (37%), $t_{1/2}$ (quinaprilat) 2 hr

INDICATIONS AND USES: Hypertension, CHF, diabetic nephropathy*

DOSAGE

Adult

- *Hypertension:* PO 10 mg qd initially; adjust dose at 2 wk intervals according to blood pressure response; max 80 mg/d divided qd-bid
- *CHF:* PO 5 mg bid initially; adjust dose at weekly intervals to desired effect; usual range 20-40 mg/d divided bid; in renal impairment (CrCl 10-30 ml/min) initiate at 2.5 mg bid

$ **AVAILABLE FORMS/COST OF THERAPY**

- Tab, Uncoated—Oral: 5, 10, 20, 40 mg, 90's: **$81.82**

CONTRAINDICATIONS: Hypersensitivity to ACE inhibitors

PRECAUTIONS: Impaired renal and liver function, dialysis patients, hypovolemia, diuretic therapy, collagen-vascular diseases, congestive heart failure, elderly, bilateral renal artery stenosis

PREGNANCY AND LACTATION: Pregnancy category D; ACE inhibitors can cause fetal and neonatal morbidity and death when administered to pregnant women, when pregnancy is detected, discontinue ACE inhibitors as soon as possible

SIDE EFFECTS/ADVERSE REACTIONS

CNS: Anxiety, insomnia, paresthesia, *headache, dizziness, fatigue*

CV: Hypotension, postural hypotension, syncope (especially with first dose), palpitations, angina

GI: Nausea, constipation, vomiting, melena, abdominal pain, impaired taste sensation

GU: Increased BUN, creatinine, decreased libido, impotence, UTI

HEME: ***Neutropenia, agranulocytosis, thrombocytopenia***
METAB: Hyperkalemia, hyponatremia
MS: Arthralgia, arthritis, myalgia
RESP: *Cough,* asthma, bronchitis, dyspnea, sinusitis
SKIN: ***Angioedema,*** rash, flushing, sweating

▼ DRUG INTERACTIONS

Drugs

• *Lithium:* Increased risk of serious lithium toxicity
• *Loop diuretics:* Initiation of ACE inhibitor therapy in the presence of intensive diuretic therapy results in a precipitous fall in blood pressure in some patients; ACE inhibitors may induce renal insufficiency in the presence of diuretic-induced sodium depletion
• *NSAIDs:* Inhibition of the antihypertensive response to ACE inhibitors
• *Potassium:* Increased risk for hyperkalemia
• *Potassium sparing diuretics:* Increased risk for hyperkalemia

SPECIAL CONSIDERATIONS

PATIENT/FAMILY EDUCATION

• Do not use salt substitutes containing potassium without consulting physician
• Rise slowly to sitting or standing position to minimize orthostatic hypotension
• Notify physician of mouth sores, sore throat, fever, swelling of hands or feet, irregular heartbeat, chest pain
• Dizziness, fainting, light-headedness may occur during 1st few days of therapy
• May cause altered taste perception or cough, notify physician if these persist

MONITORING PARAMETERS

• BUN, creatinine (watch for increased levels that may indicate acute renal failure)
• Potassium levels, although hyperkalemia rarely occurs

---

quinestrol

(kwin-ess'trol)
Estrovis
Chemical Class: Synthetic estrogen
Therapeutic Class: Estrogen

CLINICAL PHARMACOLOGY

Mechanism of Action: Affects release of pituitary gonadotropins, conserves calcium and phosphorous and encourages bone formation; alleviates or prevents symptoms caused by decreased estrogens produced by the ovaries after natural or surgical menopause or other estrogen-deficiency states

Pharmacokinetics

PO: Extensive distribution into and slow release from adipose tissue, metabolized in liver to ethinyl estradiol (has no estrogenic activity until dealkylated to estinyl estradiol), excreted in urine and bile, $t_{1/2}$ 120 hr

INDICATIONS AND USES Symptoms associated with menopause, female hypogonadism, female castration, primary ovarian failure

DOSAGE

Adult

• PO 100 μg qd for 7 days as a loading dose, then 100 μg qwk beginning 2 wk after initiation of therapy (i.e., day 15 of therapy); may increase to 200 μg qwk if necessary and tolerated; 7 or more days of progestin should be administered each 4 wk cycle in women with an intact uterus to prevent endometrial hyperplasia

$ AVAILABLE FORMS/COST OF THERAPY

• Tab, Uncoated—Oral: 100 μg, 100's: **$141.71**

CONTRAINDICATIONS: Breast cancer, estrogen-dependent neoplasia, pregnancy, undiagnosed abnormal genital bleeding, active thrombophlebitis or thromboembolic disorders, past history of thrombophlebitis, thrombosis, or thromboembolic disorders associated with previous estrogen use

PRECAUTIONS: Hypertension, asthma, blood dyscrasias, gallbladder disease, CHF, diabetes mellitus, bone disease, depression, migraine headache, convulsive disorders, hepatic disease, renal disease, family history of cancer of breast or reproductive tract

PREGNANCY AND LACTATION: Pregnancy category X; no reports of adverse effects from estrogens in the nursing infant have been located; potential exists for decreased milk volume and decreased nitrogen and protein content

SIDE EFFECTS/ADVERSE REACTIONS

Because quinestrol is distributed extensively into and released slowly from adipose tissue, adverse reactions may persist for variable periods following its discontinuation

CNS: Headache, migraine, dizziness, mental depression, chorea, ***convulsions***

CV: Edema, ***thromboembolism, stroke, pulmonary embolism, MI***

EENT: Steepening of corneal curvature, intolerance to contact lenses

GI: Nausea, vomiting, abdominal cramps, bloating, ***cholestatic jaundice,*** colitis, acute pancreatitis

GU: Breakthrough bleeding, spotting, change in menstrual flow, dysmenorrhea, premenstrual-like syndrome, amenorrhea, increase in size of uterine fibromyomata, vaginal candidiasis, change in cervical erosion and degree of cervical secretion, cystitis-like syndrome, hemolytic uremic syndrome, endometrial cystic hyperplasia

HEME: Aggravation of porphyria

METAB: Reduced carbohydrate tolerance, increased triglycerides

SKIN: Chloasma or melasma, erythema nodosum/multiforme, hemorrhagic eruption, scalp hair loss, hirsutism, urticaria, dermatitis

MISC: Changes in libido, *breast tenderness, breast enlargement*

▼ **DRUG INTERACTIONS**

Drugs

• *Corticosteroids:* Excessive corticosteroid effects

SPECIAL CONSIDERATIONS

PATIENT/FAMILY EDUCATION

• For missed dose, resume therapy the same day it is determined that dose was missed

• Notify physician of pain in groin or calves, sharp chest pain or sudden shortness of breath, abnormal vaginal bleeding, lumps in breast, sudden severe headache, dizziness or fainting, vision or speech disturbance, weakness or numbness in an arm or leg, severe abdominal pain, yellowing of the skin or eyes, severe depression

• Take with food to minimize GI side effects

MONITORING PARAMETERS

• Pretreatment physical exam with reference to blood pressure, breasts, pelvic, and Pap smear

• Baseline glucose, triglycerides, cholesterol, liver function tests, calcium; repeat yearly

quinidine

(kwin'i-deen)

Quinaglute Dura-Tabs, Quinalan (gluconate); Cardioquin (polygalacturonate); Quinidex Extentabs, Quinora (sulfate)

Chemical Class: Dextrorotatory isomer of quinine

Therapeutic Class: Antidysrhythmic (Class IA)

CLINICAL PHARMACOLOGY

Mechanism of Action: Decreases the rate of rise of diastolic (Phase 4) depolarization, thereby depressing automaticity, particularly in ectopic foci; slows depolarization, repolarization, and amplitude of the action potential leading to an increase in the refractoriness of atrial and ventricular tissue; exerts indirect anticholinergic effects through blockade of vagal innervation which may facilitate conduction in the atrioventricular junction

Pharmacokinetics

PO: Peak 3-4 hr (gluconate), 1-1½ hr (sulfate), 6 hr (polygalacturonate); duration 6-8 hr (ext-rel tab 12 hr)
IM: Peak ½-1½ hr
80%-90% bound to plasma proteins, metabolized in liver, excreted in urine (10%-50% unchanged), $t_{1/2}$ 6 hr

INDICATIONS AND USES: PO Premature ventricular contractions, ventricular tachycardia (when not associated with complete heart block), junctional (nodal) dysrhythmias, AV junctional premature complexes, paroxysmal junctional tachycardia, premature atrial contractions, paroxysmal atrial tachycardia, atrial flutter, atrial fibrillation (chronic and paroxysmal); IM/IV when PO therapy not feasible or when rapid therapeutic effect is required, life-threatening *Plasmodium falciparum* malaria

DOSAGE

Adult

- Give 200 mg test dose PO/IM several hr before full dosage to determine possibility of idiosyncratic reaction
- PO (sulfate) 100-600 mg q4-6h, initiate at 200 mg/dose and adjust dose to maintain desired therapeutic effect; max 3-4 g/d; SR 300-600 mg q8-12h
- PO (gluconate) 324-972 mg q8-12h
- PO (polygalacturonate) 275 mg q8-12h
- IM 400 mg q4-6h
- IV 200-400 mg diluted and infused at a rate ≤10 mg/min

Child

- Give 2 mg/kg test dose PO/IM several hr before full dosage to determine possibility of idiosyncratic reaction
- PO (sulfate) 15-60 mg/kg/d divided into 4-5 doses or 6 mg/kg q4-6h; usual 30 mg/kg/d or 900 mg/m^2/d given in 5 doses/d

$ AVAILABLE FORMS/COST OF THERAPY

- Tab, Uncoated—Oral (sulfate): 200 mg, 100's: **$8.93-$22.66:** 300 mg, 100's: **$14.93-$29.84**
- Tab, Coated, Sust Action—Oral (sulfate): 300 mg, 100's:**$64.85-$78.95**
- Tab, Uncoated, Sust Action—Oral (gluconate): 324 mg, 100's: **$17.25-$53.75**
- Tab, Uncoated—Oral (polygalacturonate): 275 mg, 100's: **$103.10**
- Inj, Sol—IM;IV (gluconate): 80 mg/ml, 10 ml: **$13.77**

CONTRAINDICATIONS: Hypersensitivity or idiosyncrasy, digitalis intoxication manifested by A-V condition disorders, complete A-V block with an A-V nodal or idioventricular pacemaker, left bundle branch block or other severe intraventricular condition defects with marked QRS widening, ectopic impulses and abnormal rhythms due to escape mechanisms, history of drug-induced torsade de pointes, history of long QT syndrome, myasthenia gravis

PRECAUTIONS: Treatment of atrial flutter without prior medication to control ventricular rate (e.g., digoxin, verapamil, diltiazem, beta blocker), marginally compensated cardiovascular disease, incomplete A-V block, digitalis intoxication, hyperkalemia, renal, or hepatic insufficiency

PREGNANCY AND LACTATION: Pregnancy category C; use during pregnancy has been classified in reviews of cardiovascular drugs as relatively safe for the fetus, high doses can produce oxytocic properties and potential for abortion; excreted in breast milk, compatible with breast feeding

SIDE EFFECTS/ADVERSE REACTIONS

CNS: Fever, *headache, dizziness,* vertigo, apprehension, excitement, confusion, delirium, dementia, ataxia, depression

CV: Ventricular extrasystoles, widening of the QRS complex, prolonged Q-T interval, ***complete A-V block, ventricular tachycardia and fibrillation,*** ventricular flutter, ***torsade de pointes,*** arterial embolism, *hypotension, bradycardia,* syncope, angioedema

EENT: Disturbed hearing (tinnitus, decreased auditory acuity), disturbed vision (mydriasis, blurred vision, disturbed color perception, photophobia, diplopia, night blindness, scotomata), optic neuritis, reduced visual field

GI: Nausea, vomiting, abdominal pain, *diarrhea,* anorexia, esophagitis, ***hepatotoxicity***

HEME: ***Thrombocytopenia,*** thrombocytopenic purpura, ***agranulocytosis, acute hemolytic anemia, neutropenia***

MS: Increase in serum skeletal muscle creatine phosphokinase, arthralgia, myalgia

RESP: ***Acute asthmatic arrest***

SKIN: Cutaneous flushing with intense pruritus, photosensitivity, urticaria, rash, eczema, exfoliative eruptions, psoriasis, abnormalities of pigmentation, purpura, vasculitis

MISC: Systemic lupus erythematosus, lupus nephritis

▼ **DRUG INTERACTIONS**

Drugs

- *Acetazolamide, antacids, sodium bicarbonate:* Alkalinization of urine increases plasma quinidine concentrations
- *Amiodarone, cimetidine, verapamil:* Increased plasma quinidine concentrations
- *Barbiturates, nifedipine, kaolin-pectin, phenytoin, rifampin:* Decreased plasma quinidine concentrations
- *Beta blockers:* Increased concentrations of metoprolol, propranolol, and timolol
- *Cholinergic agents:* Reduced therapeutic effects of cholinergic drugs
- *Cyclic antidepressants:* Increased imipramine and desipramine concentrations
- *Dextromethorphan:* Increased dextromethorphan concentrations, toxicity may result
- *Digitalis glycosides+:* Increased digoxin and digitoxin concentrations, toxicity may result
- *Encainide:* Increased encainide serum concentrations in rapid encainide metabolizers
- *Mexiletine:* Increased mexiletine concentrations

Q

• *Neuromuscular blocking agents:* Enhanced effects of neuromuscular blocking agents
• *Nifedipine:* Increased serum nifedipine concentrations

Labs

• *Increase:* CPK

SPECIAL CONSIDERATIONS

• 267 mg gluconate=275 mg polygalacturonate=200 mg sulfate

PATIENT/FAMILY EDUCATION

• Take with food to decrease GI upset
• Notify physician of ringing in ears, visual disturbances, dizziness, headache, nausea, skin rash, or breathing difficulty
• Do not crush or chew sustained release tablets

MONITORING PARAMETERS

• Plasma quinidine concentration (therapeutic range 2-6 μg/ml)
• ECG
• Liver function tests during the first 4-8 weeks
• CBC periodically during prolonged therapy

quinine

(kwye′nine)

Chemical Class: Cinchona alkaloid

Therapeutic Class: Antimalarial

CLINICAL PHARMACOLOGY

Mechanism of Action: Exact antimalarial mechanism of action unknown, appears to interfere with plasmodial DNA function; increases the refractory period of skeletal muscle by direct action on the muscle fiber, decreases the excitability of the motor end-plate, and affects the distribution of calcium within the muscle fiber

Pharmacokinetics

PO: Peak 1-3 hr, 70% bound to plasma proteins, metabolized in liver, excreted in urine, $t_{1/2}$ 4-5 hr

INDICATIONS AND USES: Chloroquine-resistant falciparum malaria (alone or in combination with pyrimethamine and a sulfonamide or with a tetracycline),* alternative for chloroquine-sensitive strains of *P. falciparum, P. malariae, P. ovale* and *P. vivax,** nocturnal leg cramps* (marketing for this indication banned by FDA in 1995)

DOSAGE

Adult

• *Chloroquine-resistant malaria:* PO 650 mg q8h for 5-7 days
• *Chloroquine-sensitive malaria:* PO 600 mg q8h for 5-7 days
• *Nocturnal leg cramps:* PO 260-300 mg hs

Child

• *Chloroquine-resistant malaria:* PO 25 mg/kg/d divided q8h for 5-7 days
• *Chloroquine-sensitive malaria:* PO 10 mg/kg q8h for 5-7 days

$ **AVAILABLE FORMS/COST OF THERAPY**

• Cap, Gel—Oral: 325 mg, 100's: **$8.20-$17.85**

CONTRAINDICATIONS: Hypersensitivity, G-6-PD deficiency, optic neuritis, tinnitus, history of blackwater fever, thrombocytopenic purpura (associated with previous quinine ingestion), pregnancy

PRECAUTIONS: Cardiac dysrhythmias, myasthenia gravis

PREGNANCY AND LACTATION: Pregnancy category X; excreted into breast milk, compatible with breast feeding; use caution in infants at risk for G-6-PD deficiency

SIDE EFFECTS/ADVERSE REACTIONS

CNS: Vertigo, headache, fever, apprehension, restlessness, confusion

CV: Syncope, anginal symptoms

EENT: Visual disturbances, *blurred vision,* photophobia, *diplopia,* di-

minished visual fields, disturbed color vision, tinnitus, deafness
GI: Nausea, vomiting, epigastric pain, ***hepatitis***
HEME: ***Acute hemolysis, disseminated intravascular coagulation, thrombocytopenic purpura, agranulocytosis, hypoprothrombinemia***
RESP: Asthmatic symptoms
SKIN: Cutaneous rashes, pruritus, flushing, sweating, edema of the face
MISC: Cinchonism (tinnitus, headache, nausea, disturbed vision)

▼ **DRUG INTERACTIONS**

Drugs

- *Barbiturates:* Increased phenobarbital concentration, toxicity possible
- *Carbamazepine:* Increased serum carbamazepine concentrations, toxicity possible
- *Smoking:* Reduced serum quinine concentrations

Labs

- *Increase:* 17-KS
- *Interference:* 17-OHCS

SPECIAL CONSIDERATIONS

PATIENT/FAMILY EDUCATION

- Take with food
- May cause blurred vision, use caution driving
- Discontinue drug if flushing, itching, rash, fever, stomach pain, difficult breathing, ringing in ears, visual disturbances

ramipril

(ra-mi′pril)
Altace
Chemical Class: Angiotensin-converting enzyme (ACE) inhibitor
Therapeutic Class: Antihypertensive

CLINICAL PHARMACOLOGY

Mechanism of Action: Selectively suppresses renin-angiotensin-aldosterone system; inhibits ACE preventing the conversion of angiotensin I to angiotensin II; results in dilation of arterial, venous vessels

Pharmacokinetics

PO: Onset 1-2 hr, duration 24 hr, 73% bound to plasma proteins, has little pharmacologic activity until metabolized to active metabolite (ramiprilat), excreted in urine (60%) and feces (40%), $t_{1/2}$ (ramiprilat) 13-17 hr

INDICATIONS AND USES: Hypertension, congestive heart failure, diabetic nephropathy*

DOSAGE

Adult

- *Hypertension:* PO 2.5 mg qd initially; adjust dose at 2 wk intervals according to blood pressure response; usual range 2.5-20 mg/d divided qd-bid; in renal impairment (CrCl <40 ml/min/1.73 m^2 initiate at 1.25 mg qd; max 5 mg/d)
- *Congestive heart failure:* PO 2.5 mg bid; titrate as tolerated to target dose of 5 mg bid; in renal impairment (CrCl <40 ml/min/1.73 m^2 initiate at 1.25 mg qd; max 2.5 mg bid)

$ **AVAILABLE FORMS/COST OF THERAPY**

- Cap, Gel—Oral: 1.25 mg, 100's: **$59.08;** 2.5 mg, 100's: **$69.31;** 5 mg, 100's: **$74.18;** 10 mg, 100's: **$86.00**

CONTRAINDICATIONS: Hypersensitivity to ACE inhibitors

PRECAUTIONS: Impaired renal and liver function, dialysis patients, hypovolemia, diuretic therapy, collagen-vascular diseases, congestive heart failure, elderly, bilateral renal artery stenosis

PREGNANCY AND LACTATION: Pregnancy category D; ACE inhibitors can cause fetal and neonatal morbidity and death when administered to pregnant women, when

R

pregnancy is detected, discontinue ACE inhibitors as soon as possible

SIDE EFFECTS/ADVERSE REACTIONS

CNS: Anxiety, insomnia, paresthesia, *headache, dizziness, fatigue*

CV: Hypotension, postural hypotension, syncope (especially with first dose), palpitations, angina

GI: Nausea, constipation, vomiting, melena, abdominal pain, impaired taste sensation

GU: Increased BUN creatinine, decreased libido, impotence, UTI

HEME: ***Neutropenia, agranulocytosis, thrombocytopenia***

METAB: Hyperkalemia, hyponatremia

MS: Arthralgia, arthritis, myalgia

RESP: *Cough,* asthma, bronchitis, dyspnea, sinusitis

SKIN: ***Angioedema,*** rash, flushing, sweating

▼ DRUG INTERACTIONS

Drugs

- *Lithium:* Increased risk of serious lithium toxicity
- *Loop diuretics:* Initiation of ACE inhibitor therapy in the presence of intensive diuretic therapy results in a precipitous fall in blood pressure in some patients; ACE inhibitors may induce renal insufficiency in the presence of diuretic-induced sodium depletion
- *NSAIDs:* Inhibition of the antihypertensive response to ACE inhibitors
- *Potassium, potassium sparing diuretics:* Increased risk for hyperkalemia

SPECIAL CONSIDERATIONS

PATIENT/FAMILY EDUCATION

- Do not use salt substitutes containing potassium without consulting physician
- Rise slowly to sitting or standing position to minimize orthostatic hypotension
- Notify physician of mouth sores, sore throat, fever, swelling of hands or feet, irregular heartbeat, chest pain
- Dizziness, fainting, light-headedness may occur during 1st few days of therapy
- May cause altered taste perception or cough, notify physician if these persist
- Capsules may be opened and contents sprinkled on small amount of applesauce or mixed in apple juice or water prior to consuming

MONITORING PARAMETERS

- BUN, creatinine (watch for increased levels that may indicate acute renal failure)
- Potassium levels, although hyperkalemia rarely occurs

---

ranitidine

(ra-ni′ti-deen)

Zantac

Chemical Class: Aminoalkyl-substituted furan derivative

Therapeutic Class: H_2-receptor antagonist

CLINICAL PHARMACOLOGY

Mechanism of Action: Competitive, reversible inhibitor of the action of histamine at the histamine H_2-receptors, including receptors on gastric parietal cells; inhibits both daytime and nocturnal basal gastric acid secretion

Pharmacokinetics

PO: Peak 1-3 hr

IM: Peak 0.25 hr

15% bound to plasma proteins, metabolized in liver, excreted in urine (30% of PO dose, 70% of IV dose unchanged), and bile, $t_{1/2}$ 2-2½ hr (prolonged in renal impairment)

INDICATIONS AND USES: Duodenal ulcer, pathological hypersecretory conditions (e.g., Zollinger-Ellison syndrome, systemic mastocytosis), benign gastric ulcer, gastroesophageal reflux disease (GERD), erosive esophagitis, stress ulcer prophylaxis,* chronic idiopathic urticaria (in combination with H_1-receptor antagonists),* acute upper GI bleeding*

DOSAGE

Adult

- *Duodenal and gastric ulcer:* PO 150 mg bid or 300 mg qhs for 4-8 wk; maintenance 150 mg qhs
- *GERD:* PO 150 mg bid
- *Erosive esophagitis:* PO 150 mg qid, maintenance 150 mg bid
- *Pathological hypersecretory conditions:* PO 150 mg bid initially, titrate to desired response up to 6 g/d; IV INF start at 1 mg/kg/hr, increase by 0.5 mg/kg/hr intervals q4h prn up to 2.5 mg/kg/hr; IM/IV 50 mg q6-8h; do not exceed 400 mg/d; IV INF 6.25 mg/hr

Child

- PO 1.25-2.5 mg/kg q12h; max 300 mg/d; IM/IV 0.75-1.5 mg/kg q6-8h; max 6 mg/kg/d or 300 mg/d; IV INF 0.1-0.25 mg/kg/hr
- Dose in renal failure (CrCl <50 ml/min): PO 150 mg q24h; IM/IV 50 mg q18-24h

$ AVAILABLE FORMS/COST OF THERAPY

- Tab, Coated—Oral: 150 mg, 60's: **$99.20;** 300 mg, 30's: **$90.06**
- Tab, Effervescent—Oral: 150 mg, 60's: **$95.66**
- Cap, Gel—Oral: 150 mg, 60's: **$95.66;** 300 mg, 30's: **$86.27**
- Granule, Effervescent—Oral: 150 mg, 60's: **$95.66**
- Syr—Oral: 15 mg/ml, 480 ml: **$186.74**
- Inj, Sol—IM; IV: 25 mg/ml, 2 ml:**$3.99**

CONTRAINDICATIONS: Hypersensitivity

PRECAUTIONS: Renal and hepatic function impairment, elderly, gastric malignancy, rapid IV administration, immunocompromised patients

PREGNANCY AND LACTATION: Pregnancy category B; compatible with breast feeding

SIDE EFFECTS/ADVERSE REACTIONS

CNS: Malaise, dizziness, somnolence, insomnia, vertigo

CV: Tachycardia, bradycardia, atrioventricular block, premature ventricular beats

GI: Constipation, diarrhea, nausea, vomiting, abdominal discomfort/pain, pancreatitis (rare), increased liver function tests, ***hepatitis***

HEME: ***Leukopenia, granulocytopenia, thrombocytopenia***

MS: Arthralgias, myalgias

SKIN: Rash, ***erythema multiforme*** (rare), alopecia

MISC: Hypersensitivity reactions

▼ DRUG INTERACTIONS

Drugs

- *Enoxacin:* Decreased plasma enoxacin concentrations
- *Ketoconazole:* Decreased plasma ketoconazole concentrations
- *Nifedipine, nitrendipine:* Increased bioavailability of nifedipine and nitrendipine

Labs

- *Increase:* AST/ALT, alk phosphatase, creatinine, LDH, bilirubin
- *False positive:* Urine protein using Multistix

SPECIAL CONSIDERATIONS

PATIENT/FAMILY EDUCATION

- Stagger doses of ranitidine and antacids
- Avoid alcohol
- Complete prescribed course of therapy

MONITORING PARAMETERS

- Intragastric pH when used for stress ulcer prophylaxis, titrate dose to maintain pH >4

R

reserpine

(re-ser'peen)

Novoreserpine ♣

Chemical Class: Rauwolfia alkaloid

Therapeutic Class: Antihypertensive

CLINICAL PHARMACOLOGY

Mechanism of Action: Depletes stores of catecholamines and 5- hydroxytryptamine in many organs; depression of sympathetic nerve function results in decreased heart rate and lowering of arterial blood pressure; sedative and tranquilizing properties are thought to be related to depletion of catecholamines and 5-hydroxytryptamine from the brain

Pharmacokinetics

PO: Peak 3.5 hr, slow onset of action, sustained duration of effect, 96% bound to plasma proteins, $t_{1/2}$ 33 hr

INDICATIONS AND USES: Hypertension, agitated psychotic states in patients unable to tolerate phenothiazines

DOSAGE

Adult

- *Hypertension:* PO 0.5 mg qd for 1-2 wk, then 0.1-0.25 mg qd; higher doses increase incidence of mental depression and serious side effects
- *Psychotic states:* PO 0.5 mg qd, range 0.1-1 mg/d

Child

- PO 20 mcg/kg/d, max 0.25 mg/d

$ **AVAILABLE FORMS/COST OF THERAPY**

- Tab, Uncoated—Oral: 0.1 mg, 100's: **$2.95-$5.50;** 0.25 mg, 100's: **$3.50-$7.65**

CONTRAINDICATIONS: Hypersensitivity, mental depression or history of mental depression, active peptic ulcer, ulcerative colitis, patients receiving electroconvulsive therapy

PRECAUTIONS: History of peptic ulcer, history of gallstones, renal function impairment, children

PREGNANCY AND LACTATION: Pregnancy category C; excreted into breast milk, no clinical reports of adverse effects in nursing infants have been located

SIDE EFFECTS/ADVERSE REACTIONS

CNS: Parkinsonian syndrome and other extrapyramidal tract symptoms (rare), *dizziness,* headache, paradoxical anxiety, depression, nervousness, nightmares, dull sensorium, *drowsiness, fatigue, lethargy*

CV: Dysrhythmias (particularly when used concurrently with digitalis or quinidine), syncope, angina-like symptoms, *bradycardia,* edema

EENT: Epistaxis, nasal congestion, deafness, optic atrophy, glaucoma, uveitis, conjunctival injection

GI: Vomiting, diarrhea, nausea, anorexia, dryness of mouth, hypersecretion

GU: Impotence, dysuria, decreased libido

METAB: Pseudolactation, gynecomastia, breast engorgement, weight gain

MS: Muscular aches

RESP: Dyspnea

SKIN: Purpura, rash, pruritus

SPECIAL CONSIDERATIONS

PATIENT/FAMILY EDUCATION

- May cause drowsiness or dizziness, use caution driving or participating in other activities requiring alertness
- Therapeutic effect may take 2-3 wk

ribavirin

rye-ba-vye'rin

Virazole

Chemical Class: Synthetic nucleoside

Therapeutic Class: Antiviral agent

CLINICAL PHARMACOLOGY

Mechanism of Action: Inhibits RNA and/or DNA synthesis by respiratory syncytial virus (RSV), influenza virus (types A and B), and many other RNA and DNA viruses

Pharmacokinetics

PO: Onset 30 min, peak 1-2 hr, well absorbed

INH: Aerosol has systemic absorption; respiratory tract secretion concentration much higher than plasma concentration; $t_{1/2}$ in respiratory tract secretion 1.4-2.5 hr

Metabolized in liver and erythrocytes; plasma $t_{1/2}$ 9.5 hr; accumulates in erythrocytes, concentration plateaus at 4 days; elimination $t_{1/2}$ from erythrocytes 40 days; excreted in urine and feces

INDICATIONS AND USES: Severe lower respiratory tract infection by RSV in children (if begun within first 3 days of infection), influenza A,* influenza B,* hepatitis C,* Lassa fever,* hantavirus-associated hemorrhagic fever*

DOSAGE

Adult

- *Influenza A or B:* INH sol of 6 g in 300 ml additive free sterile water administered by small particle aerosol generator for 18 hr then 4 hr tid per day for 3 days
- *Lassa fever:* Treatment, IV 30 mg/kg load, then in 6 hr, 16 mg/kg q6h for 4 days, then 8 mg/kg q8h for 6 days; prevention in high risk contacts, PO 500 mg q6h for 7-10 days
- *Hantavirus-associated hemorrhagic fever:* Treatment, IV 33 mg/kg (max 2000 mg) load, then in 6 hr, 16 mg/kg (max 1000 mg) q6h for 15 doses, then 8 mg/kg (max 500 mg) q8h for 9 doses

Child

- *RSV infection:* INH sol of 6 g in 300 ml additive free sterile water administered by small particle aerosol generator for 12-18 hr per day for 3-7 days
- *Lassa fever:* Prevention in high risk contacts, age >9 yr, PO 500 mg q6h for 7-10 days; age 6-9 yr, PO 400 mg q6h for 7-10 days

$ AVAILABLE FORMS/COST OF THERAPY

- Aer, Sol—Inh: 6 g, 4's: **$5499.38**

CONTRAINDICATIONS: Pregnancy and females of childbearing age

PRECAUTIONS: Patients receiving mechanical ventilation

PREGNANCY AND LACTATION: Pregnancy category X; contraindicated in lactating women

SIDE EFFECTS/ADVERSE REACTIONS

CNS: Headache, ***seizures (systemic administration only)***

CV: ***Cardiac arrest, hypotension, digitalis toxicity***

EENT: Conjunctivitis

GI: Nausea, anorexia, increased transaminases (systemic administration only)

HEME: Reticulocytosis, anemia

RESP: ***Worsening of respiratory status,*** bacterial pneumonia, pneumothorax, ***apnea***

SKIN: Rash

▼ DRUG INTERACTIONS

Drugs

- *Zalcitabine, zidovudine:* Ribavirin inhibits effect

SPECIAL CONSIDERATIONS

PATIENT/FAMILY EDUCATION

- Female health care workers who

are pregnant or may become pregnant should avoid exposure to ribavirin

MONITORING PARAMETERS

- Respiratory function
- Hematocrit

riboflavin (vitamin B_2)

(rye'bo-flay-vin)

Chemical Class: Water soluble B complex vitamin

Therapeutic Class: Vitamin

CLINICAL PHARMACOLOGY

Mechanism of Action: Functions as a coenzyme in numerous tissue respiration systems

INDICATIONS AND USES: Treatment and prevention of riboflavin deficiency

DOSAGE

Adult and Child

- PO 5-25 mg qd

$ AVAILABLE FORMS/COST OF THERAPY

- Tab—Oral: 5 mg, 100's: **$12.95;** 10, 25, 50, 100 mg, 100's: **$1.40-$4.00**

PRECAUTIONS: Riboflavin deficiency rarely occurs alone and is often associated with deficiency of other B vitamins and protein

PREGNANCY AND LACTATION: Pregnancy category A (category C if used in doses above RDA); compatible with breast feeding

SIDE EFFECTS/ADVERSE REACTIONS

GU: Yellow/orange discoloration of urine

SPECIAL CONSIDERATIONS

PATIENT/FAMILY EDUCATION

- Large doses may cause bright yellow/orange discoloration of urine

rifabutin

(rif'a-byoo-ten)

Mycobutin

Chemical Class: Semisynthetic spiropiperidyl derivative of rifamycin S

Therapeutic Class: Antimycobacterial agent

CLINICAL PHARMACOLOGY

Mechanism of Action: Inhibits DNA-dependent RNA polymerase in susceptible strains of *Escherichia coli* and *Bacillus subtilis* but not in mammalian cells; it is not known if DNA-dependent RNA polymerase is inhibited in *M. avium* complex (MAC) (*Mycobacterium avium* and *M. intracellulare*)

Pharmacokinetics

PO: Peak 2-4 hr, high lipophilicity, 85% bound to plasma proteins, metabolized to active and inactive metabolites, excreted in feces (30%) and urine (53%), $t_{1/2}$ 45 hr

INDICATIONS AND USES: Prevention of disseminated MAC disease in patients with advanced HIV infection

DOSAGE

Adult

- PO 300 mg qd; if GI upset occurs can be administered 150 mg bid with food

Child

- PO 5 mg/kg/d has been administered to small numbers of HIV positive children

$ AVAILABLE FORMS/COST OF THERAPY

- Cap, Gel—Oral: 150 mg, 100's: **$370.50**

CONTRAINDICATIONS: Hypersensitivity to rifamycins

PRECAUTIONS: Active tuberculosis (may lead to resistant strains), children

PREGNANCY AND LACTATION: Pregnancy category B

SIDE EFFECTS/ADVERSE REACTIONS

CNS: Headache, fever, asthenia, insomnia

CV: Chest pain

GI: Abdominal pain, *anorexia, nausea, vomiting,* diarrhea, dyspepsia, eructation, flatulence, taste perversion, increased liver function tests, ***hepatitis***

GU: Discolored urine

HEME: ***Anemia, eosinophilia, leukopenia, neutropenia, thrombocytopenia***

MS: Mylagia

SKIN: Rash

▼ **DRUG INTERACTIONS**

Drugs

- Has liver enzyme-inducing properties similar to rifampin although less potent
- Dosage adjustment of other drugs may be necessary, refer to rifampin monograph
- Does not appear to alter the acetylation of isoniazid

SPECIAL CONSIDERATIONS

PATIENT/FAMILY EDUCATION

- May discolor bodily secretions brown-orange, soft contact lenses may be permanently stained
- May take with food if GI upset occurs

MONITORING PARAMETERS

- Periodic CBC with differential and platelets
- Liver function tests

---

rifampin

(rye'fam-pin)

Rifadin, Rimactane, Rofact ♣

Chemical Class: Semisynthetic derivative of rifamycin B

Therapeutic Class: Antituberculosis agent

CLINICAL PHARMACOLOGY

Mechanism of Action: Suppresses initiation of chain formation for RNA synthesis in susceptible bacteria by inhibiting DNA-dependent RNA polymerase

Pharmacokinetics

PO: Peak 2-4 hr, widely distributed into most body tissues and fluids, 84%-91% bound to plasma proteins, metabolized in liver to active metabolite, excreted mainly in bile, $t_{1/2}$ 3 hr

INDICATIONS AND USES: All forms of tuberculosis (in combination with at least one other antituberculosis drug), asymptomatic *Neisseria meningitidis* carriers, prophylaxis of meningitis due to *Hemophilus influenzae,** infections caused by *Staphylococcus aureus* and *S. epidermidis,** legionella when not responsive to erythromycin,* leprosy (in combination with dapsone)*

Antibacterial spectrum usually includes: *Mycobacterium tuberculosis, M. bovis, M. marinum, M. kansasii,* some strains of *M. fortuitum, M. avium* and *M. intracellulare, Staphylococcus aureus, Haemophilus influenzae, Legionella pneumophilia*

DOSAGE

Adult

- *Tuberculosis:* PO/IV 600 mg in a single daily dose for 6-9 mo (in combination with at least one other antituberculosis agent)
- *Meningococcal carriers:* PO 600 mg bid for 2 days
- *H. influenzae prophylaxis:* PO 600 mg q24h for 4 days

Child

- *Tuberculosis:* PO/IV 10-20 mg/kg not to exceed 600 mg/d
- *Meningococcal carriers:* PO (>1 mo) 10 mg/kg q12h for 2 days; (<1 mo) 5 mg/kg q12h for 2 days

R

• *H. influenzae prophylaxis:* PO (<1 mo) 10 mg/kg q24h for 4 days; (>1 month) 20 mg/kg q24h for 4 days; do not exceed 600 mg/dose

$ **AVAILABLE FORMS/COST OF THERAPY**

• Cap, Gel—Oral: 150 mg, 30's: **$44.70;** 300 mg, 100's: **$160.83-$211.20**

• Inj, Sol—IV: 600 mg/vial, 1's: **$79.38**

CONTRAINDICATIONS: Hypersensitivity to rifamycins

PRECAUTIONS: Hepatic dysfunction, porphyria, avoid extravasation

PREGNANCY AND LACTATION: Pregnancy category C; compatible with breast feeding

SIDE EFFECTS/ADVERSE REACTIONS

CNS: Headache, fever, drowsiness, fatigue, ataxia, dizziness, inability to concentrate, mental confusion, behavioral changes, rare reports of myopathy have also been observed

EENT: Visual disturbances

GI: Heartburn, epigastric distress, anorexia, nausea, vomiting, jaundice, flatulence, cramps, diarrhea, ***pseudomembranous colitis, hepatitis,*** abnormal liver function tests

GU: Menstrual disturbances, elevations in BUN, hemolysis, hemoglobinuria, ***hematuria, interstitial nephritis, renal insufficiency, acute renal failure***

HEME: ***Thrombocytopenia, transient leukopenia, hemolytic anemia***

METAB: Elevations in serum uric acid

MS: Muscular weakness, pains in extremities, generalized numbness

SKIN: Pruritus, urticaria, rash, pemphigoid reaction

MISC: "Flu" syndrome (fever, chills, headache, dizziness, bone pain)

▼ **DRUG INTERACTIONS**

Drugs

• *Aminosalicylic acid:* Reduced serum concentrations of rifampin

• *Antidiabetics:* Diminished hypoglycemic activity of sulfonylureas

• *Benzodiazepines, beta blockers, calcium channel blockers, chloramphenicol, cyclosporine, digitalis glycosides, disopyramide, itraconazole, ketoconazole, methadone, mexiletine, phenytoin+, pirmenol, propafenone, quinidine, theophylline, zidovudine:* Reduced serum concentrations

• *Corticosteroids:* Reduced effect of corticosteroids

• *Isoniazid:* Increased hepatotoxic potential of isoniazid in slow acetylators or patients with pre-existing liver disease

• *Oral anticoagulants+:* Reduced hypoprothrombinemic effect of oral anticoagulants

• *Oral contraceptives:* Menstrual irregularities, ovulation, and occasional contraceptive failure

Labs

• *Increase*: Liver function tests

• *Interference*: Folate, vitamin B_{12}, BSP, gallbladder studies

SPECIAL CONSIDERATIONS

PATIENT/FAMILY EDUCATION

• Take on empty stomach, at least 1 hr before or 2 hr after meals

• May cause reddish-orange discoloration of bodily secretions, may permanently discolor soft contact lenses

MONITORING PARAMETERS

• Liver function tests at baseline and q2-4 wk during therapy

• CBC with differential and platelets at baseline and periodically throughout treatment

rimantadine

(ri-man'ti-deen)

Flumadine

Chemical Class: Substituted amine

Therapeutic Class: Antiviral agent

CLINICAL PHARMACOLOGY

Mechanism of Action: Inhibits growth of influenza A virus, possibly by inhibiting the uncoating of the virus

Pharmacokinetics

PO: Onset 3 hr, peak 5-7 hr, 40% protein bound; metabolized by liver ($t_{1/2}$ doubled in severe hepatic dysfunction), 25% of dose excreted in urine as unchanged drug; $t_{1/2}$ 19-31 hr (20-48 hr if age >70 yr)

INDICATIONS AND USES: Prevention and treatment (within 48 hr of onset of illness) of influenza A

DOSAGE

Adult

- *Prevention:* PO 100 mg bid; if age >65 yr or with severe hepatic or renal dysfunction (CrCl ≤ 10 ml/min), reduce dose to 100 mg qd
- *Treatment:* PO 100 mg bid; if age >65 yr or with severe hepatic or renal dysfunction (CrCl ≤ 10 ml/min), reduce dose to 100 mg qd

Child

- *Prevention:* Age >10 yr, PO 100 mg bid; age <10 yr, 5 mg/kg qd as single dose (max dose 150 mg)

$ AVAILABLE FORMS/COST OF THERAPY

- Syr—Oral: 50 mg/5 ml, 240 ml: **$25.80**
- Tab, Plain Coated—Oral: 100 mg, 100's: **$127.57**

CONTRAINDICATIONS: Hypersensitivity to rimantadine or amantadine

PRECAUTIONS: Resistant strains may develop during treatment (10%-30%), lactation

PREGNANCY AND LACTATION: Pregnancy category C; concentrated in breast milk

SIDE EFFECTS/ADVERSE REACTIONS

CNS: Asthenia, dizziness, headache, insomnia

CV: Orthostatic hypotension

EENT: Tinnitis

GI: Abdominal pain, anorexia, diarrhea, dry mouth, nausea, vomiting

GU: Urinary retention

RESP: Skin

▼ DRUG INTERACTIONS

Drugs

- *Acetaminophen:* Reduces rimantadine peak concentration by 10%
- *Aspirin:* Reduces rimantadine peak concentration by 10%

risperidone

(ris-per'i-done)

Risperdal

Chemical Class: Benzisoxazole derivative

Therapeutic Class: Antipsychotic

R

CLINICAL PHARMACOLOGY

Mechanism of Action: Antipsychotic activity mediated by dopamine type 2 and serotonin type 2 receptor antagonism

Pharmacokinetics

PO: Peak level 1 hr; metabolized by liver to active metabolite, 9-hydroxyrisperidone, (8% of Caucasians are poor metabolizers); mean elimination $t_{1/2}$ of total risperidone and 9-hydroxyrisperidone 20 hr; excreted in urine and feces; protein binding 85%

INDICATIONS AND USES: Psychotic disorders

DOSAGE

Adult

• PO: 1 mg bid, increase to 2 mg bid on second day and 3 mg bid on third day, then increase weekly as needed (usual effective dose 4-8 mg daily; max daily dose 16 mg); initial dose 0.5 mg bid increasing to 1.5 mg bid by third day in elderly or those with severe renal or hepatic impairment

$ **AVAILABLE FORMS/COST OF THERAPY**

• Tab, Coated—Oral: 1 mg, 100's: **$189.60;** 2 mg, 100's: **$315.60;** 3 mg, 100's: **$394.80;** 4 mg, 100's: **$525.60**

CONTRAINDICATIONS: Hypersensitivity

PRECAUTIONS: Neuroleptic malignant syndrome, tardive dyskinesia, prolonged QT interval, seizures

PREGNANCY AND LACTATION: Pregnancy category C; excreted in breast milk

SIDE EFFECTS/ADVERSE REACTIONS

CNS: Aggressive reaction, *anxiety, decreased libido,* dizziness, *EPS (frequency is dose related), increased dream activity,* insomnia, *somnolence*

CV: Orthostatic hypotension, tachycardia

EENT: Abnormal vision (accommodation), *dry mouth*

GI: Abdominal pain, *constipation, dyspepsia,* nausea, vomiting

GU: Menorrhagia, polyuria, sexual (erectile and orgasmic) dysfunction, urinary retention, *vaginal dryness*

HEME: Anemia

METAB: Amenorrhea, galactorrhea, gynecomastia, hyponatremia

MS: Arthralgia, back pain, chest pain

RESP: Cough, dyspnea, pharyngitis, *rhinitis,* sinusitis

SKIN: Dry skin, *increased pigmentation, photosensitivity,* rash, seborrhea

MISC: Fatigue, fever

▼ **DRUG INTERACTIONS**

Drugs

• *Carbamazepine:* Increases risperidone clearance

• *Clozapine:* Decreases risperidone clearance

• *Levodopa and dopamine agonists:* Risperidone antagonizes effect

SPECIAL CONSIDERATIONS

PATIENT/FAMILY EDUCATION

• Risk of orthostatic hypotension, especially during the period of initial dose titration

• Do not operate machinery during dose titration period

---

salicylic acid

(sal-i-sill'ik)

Compound W, Dr Scholl's Wart Remover, DuoFilm, DuoPlant, Fostex, Freezone, Gordofilm, Keralyt, Maximum Strength Wart Remover, Mediplast, Mosco, Occlusal-HP, Off-Ezy Wart Remover, P&S Shampoo, Panscol, PediaPatch, Sal-Acid, Salactic Film, Sal-Plant, Trans-Planter, Trans-Ver-Sal, Wart-Off, Wart Remover

Chemical Class: Salicylate

Therapeutic Class: Keratolytic

CLINICAL PHARMACOLOGY

Mechanism of Action: Produces desquamation of hyperkeratotic epithelium; dissolves intracellular cement substance

Pharmacokinetics

TOP: Peak 5 hr when occlusive dressing used, 50%-80% bound to plasma proteins, metabolized and excreted in urine

INDICATIONS AND USES: Removal of excessive keratin in hyperkeratotic skin disorders, common and plantar warts, psoriasis, calluses, corns, dandruff

DOSAGE

Adult and Child

- Lotion, cream, gel: TOP Apply thin layer to affected area(s) qd-bid
- Plaster: TOP Cut to size that covers corn or callus, apply and leave in place for 48 hr; do not exceed 5 applications over 2 wk period
- Shampoo: TOP Apply qd or qod; 1-2 applications/wk will usually maintain control
- Sol: TOP Apply thin layer directly to wart qd as directed for 1 wk or until wart is removed

$ AVAILABLE FORMS/COST OF THERAPY

- Gel—Top: 6%, 1 oz: **$15.56;** 27%, 15 g: **$11.19**
- Plaster, Adhesive—Top: 40%, 25's: **$24.06;** 50%, 8's: **$3.25**
- Sol—Top: 13.6%, 9.3 ml: **$3.22;** 17%, 10, 13.5 ml: **$5.00-$13.92**
- Lotion—Top: 3%, 120 ml: **$10.81**
- Oint—Top: 3%, 90 g: **$9.49**
- Cre—Top: 2%, 120 g: **$8.12**
- Shampoo—Top: 2%, 120 ml: **$6.60**

CONTRAINDICATIONS: Hypersensitivity; prolonged use; diabetes; impaired circulation; use on moles, birthmarks, or warts with hair growing from them; genital or facial warts; warts on mucous membranes; irritated skin; infected skin

PRECAUTIONS: Children

PREGNANCY AND LACTATION: Pregnancy category C

SIDE EFFECTS/ADVERSE REACTIONS

SKIN: Local irritation, burning

MISC: Salicylism (tinnitus, hearing loss, dizziness, confusion, headache, hyperventilation)

SPECIAL CONSIDERATIONS

PATIENT/FAMILY EDUCATION

- For external use only; avoid contact with face, eyes, genitals, mucous membranes, and normal skin surrounding warts
- May cause reddening or scaling of skin
- Soaking area in warm water for 5 min prior to application may enhance effect (remove any loose tissue with brush, washcloth, or emery board and dry thoroughly prior to application)

---

salmeterol

(sal-me′te-rol)

Serevent

Chemical Class: Sympathomimetic

Therapeutic Class: Bronchodilator

CLINICAL PHARMACOLOGY

Mechanism of Action: Produces long-lasting relaxation of smooth muscle in the bronchial tree by stimulating β_2-adrenergic receptors; approximately 50 times more selective for β-$_2$-adrenergic receptors than albuterol

Pharmacokinetics

INH: Onset within 20 min, peak effect 2 hr, duration 12 hr, low systemic absorption, 94%-98% bound to plasma proteins, metabolized in liver, eliminated in feces, $t_{1/2}$ 3-4 hr

INDICATIONS AND USES: Maintenance of bronchodilation and prevention of symptoms of asthma, including nocturnal asthma; prevention of exercise-induced bronchospasm

DOSAGE

Adult and Child >12 yr

- *Asthma:* INH 2 inhalations q12h
- *Exercise-induced asthma:* 2 inhalations 30-60 min before exercise; do not repeat earlier than 12 hr following initial dose

$ AVAILABLE FORMS/COST OF THERAPY

• Aer, Metered—Inh: 25 μg/inh, 13 g: **$50.30**

CONTRAINDICATIONS: Hypersensitivity, significantly worsening or acutely deteriorating asthma, acute symptoms

PRECAUTIONS: Cardiovascular disorders, coronary insufficiency, cardiac dysrhythmias, hypertension, convulsive disorders, thyrotoxicosis, children <12 yr, psychosis, diabetes, history of stroke

PREGNANCY AND LACTATION: Pregnancy category C

SIDE EFFECTS/ADVERSE REACTIONS

CNS: Tremors, anxiety, insomnia, headache, dizziness, stimulation, nervousness

CV: Palpitations, tachycardia, hypertension, dysrhythmias, ***cardiac arrest,*** lengthened Q-T segment

EENT: Throat irritation

GI: Nausea, vomiting, bad taste, GI distress

METAB: Hypokalemia, hyperglycemia

MS: Muscle cramps in extremities

RESP: Dyspnea, cough, ***paradoxical bronchospasm***

▼ DRUG INTERACTIONS

Labs

• *Decrease:* Potassium

SPECIAL CONSIDERATIONS

PATIENT/FAMILY EDUCATION

• Proper inhalation technique is vital

• Excessive use may lead to adverse effects

• Notify physician if no response to usual doses, or if palpitations, rapid heart beat, chest pain, muscle tremors, dizziness, headache

• **Do not use to treat acute symptoms or on an as needed basis**

salsalate

(sal'sa-late)

Amigesic, Argesic-SA, Artha-G, Disalcid, Mono-Gesic, Salflex, Salsitab

Chemical Class: Salicylic acid derivative

Therapeutic Class: Nonnarcotic analgesic; anti-inflammatory; antirheumatic

CLINICAL PHARMACOLOGY

Mechanism of Action: Inhibits prostaglandin synthesis and release which reduces pain and inflammation; increases urinary excretion of urates at higher doses but may decrease excretion at lower doses; does not inhibit platelet aggregation

Pharmacokinetics

PO: Onset of anti-inflammatory action 3-4 days, 75%-90% bound to plasma proteins, hydrolyzed in liver to salicylic acid (active), excreted in urine, $t_{1/2}$ 7-8 hr

INDICATIONS AND USES: Mild to moderate pain, rheumatoid arthritis, osteoarthritis, related rheumatic disorders

DOSAGE

Adult

• PO 3 g/d divided bid-tid

$ AVAILABLE FORMS/COST OF THERAPY

• Cap, Gel—Oral: 500 mg, 100's: **$12.59-$44.64;** 750 mg, 100's: **$15.10**

• Tab, Coated—Oral: 500 mg, 100's: **$7.84-$42.78;** 750 mg, 100's: **$9.38-$54.78**

• Tab, Coated, Sust Action—Oral: 500 mg, 100's: **$16.80**

CONTRAINDICATIONS: Hypersensitivity to NSAIDs, hemophilia, bleeding ulcers, hemorrhagic states

PRECAUTIONS: Children/teenagers with chickenpox or influenza (association with Reye's syndrome), impaired hepatic or renal function, history of peptic ulcer disease, diabetes mellitus, gout, anemia, diabetes

PREGNANCY AND LACTATION: Pregnancy category C; excreted into breast milk, use caution in nursing mothers due to potential adverse effects in nursing infant

SIDE EFFECTS/ADVERSE REACTIONS

CNS: Drowsiness, dizziness, confusion, headache

EENT: Tinnitus, reversible hearing loss, dimness of vision

GI: Nausea, dyspepsia, ***GI bleeding,*** diarrhea, heartburn, epigastric discomfort, anorexia, ***acute reversible hepatotoxicity***

HEME: ***Thrombocytopenia, leukopenia,*** decreased plasma iron concentration, shortened erythrocyte survival time

METAB: Hypoglycemia, hyponatremia, hypokalemia, hypermagnesemia

RESP: Wheezing, hyperpnea

SKIN: Rash, hives, angioedema, urticaria, bruising

MISC: Fever, thirst

▼ **DRUG INTERACTIONS**

Drugs

- *Acetazolamide:* Increased concentrations of acetazolamide, possibly leading to CNS toxicity
- *Antacids:* Decreased serum salicylate concentrations
- *Antidiabetics:* Enhanced hypoglycemic response to sulfonylureas, particularly chlorpropamide
- *Corticosteroids:* Increased incidence and/or severity of GI ulceration
- *Ethanol:* Enhanced salicylate-induced GI mucosal damage; increased ethanol concentrations
- *Heparin:* Increased risk of bleeding
- *Methotrexate+:* Increased serum methotrexate concentrations and enhanced methotrexate toxicity
- *Oral anticoagulants:* Increased risk of bleeding
- *Phenytoin:* Large doses of salicylates may reduce total serum phenytoin concentrations, but free serum concentrations do not appear to be affected
- *Probenecid:* Salicylates inhibit the uricosuric activity of probenecid
- *Sulfinpyrazone:* Salicylates inhibit the uricosuric activity of sulfinpyrazone
- *Valproic acid:* Salicylates may increase unbound serum valproic acid concentrations sufficiently to result in toxicity

Labs

- *Increase:* Coagulation studies, liver function studies, serum uric acid, amylase, CO_2, urinary protein
- *Decrease:* Serum K, PBI, cholesterol, blood glucose
- *Interference:* Urine catecholamines, pregnancy test

SPECIAL CONSIDERATIONS

PATIENT/FAMILY EDUCATION

- Administer with food
- Do not exceed recommended doses
- Notify physician if ringing in ears or persistent GI pain occurs
- Read label on other OTC drugs, many contain aspirin
- Therapeutic response may take 2 wk (arthritis)
- Avoid alcohol ingestion, GI bleeding may occur
- **Not to be given to children, Reye's syndrome may develop**

MONITORING PARAMETERS

- AST, ALT, bilirubin, creatinine, CBC, hematocrit if patient is on long-term therapy

scopolamine

(skoe-pol'a-meen)
Transdermal: Transderm-Scop
Ophth: Isopto Hyoscine
Chemical Class: Belladonna alkaloid
Therapeutic Class: Systemic: Anticholinergic (parasympatholytic); Ophth: Mydriatic, cycloplegic

CLINICAL PHARMACOLOGY
Mechanism of Action: Cholinergic receptor blocker decreases production of GI secretions and stomach acid; central muscarinic receptor blocker decreases involuntary movements; inhibition of vestibular input to the CNS, inhibits vomiting reflex; direct inhibitory effect on vomiting center in brain stem; ophth blocks cholinergic response of iris sphincter and accommodation of ciliary body to cholinergic stimulation resulting in dilation, paralysis of accommodation

Pharmacokinetics
PO: Onset 30-60 min, duration 4-6 hr
SC/IM: Onset 30 min, duration 4 hr
IV: Peak 10-15 min, duration 4 hr
TRANSDERMAL: Onset 3 hr, duration, up to 72 hr
OPHTH: Peak 20-30 min, duration 3-7 days
Excreted in urine, bile, feces (unchanged), $t_{1/2}$ 8 hr

INDICATIONS AND USES: Systemic: Reduction of secretions before surgery, calm delirium, motion sickness, vertigo, nausea and vomiting;* Ophth: Uveitis, iritis, cycloplegia, mydriasis

DOSAGE Note: geriatric and pediatric patients more sensitive to anticholinergic effects

Adult
- SC 0.4-0.6 mg
- Ophth INSTILL 1-2 gtt before refraction or 1-2 gtt qd-tid for iritis or uveitis
- *Parkinson symptoms:* IM/SC/IV 0.3-0.6 mg tid-qid diluted using dilution provided
- *Preoperatively:* SC 0.4-0.6 mg
- *Motion Sickness:* PATCH 1 placed behind ear 4-5 hr before travel; replace q72h prn

Child
- Ophth: INSTILL 1 gtt bid × 2 days before refraction
- *Parkinson symptoms:* SC 0.006 mg/kg tid-qid or 0.2 mg/m^2

$ AVAILABLE FORMS/COST OF THERAPY
- Inj, Sol—IM;IV;SC: 0.4 mg/ml, 1 ml, 1 mg/ml, 1 ml × 25: **$30.00-$35.00**
- Sol—Ophth: 0.25%, 5 ml: **$11.25**
- Film, Cont Rel—Percutaneous: 0.5 mg, 4 discs × 3: **$44.95**

CONTRAINDICATIONS: Hypersensitivity, narrow-angle glaucoma, increased intraocular pressure, adhesions between iris and lens, unstable cardiovascular status (tachycardia, myocardial ischemia), myasthenia gravis, GI/GU obstruction, hypersensitivity to belladonna, barbiturates

PRECAUTIONS: Children, elderly, blondes, prostatic hypertrophy, Down's syndrome, debilitated COPD, asthma, CHF, hypertension, dysrhythmia, hiatal hernia

PREGNANCY AND LACTATION: Pregnancy category C; no reports of adverse effects reported; compatible with breast feeding

SIDE EFFECTS/ADVERSE REACTIONS
CNS: Confusion, anxiety, restlessness, irritability, delusions, hallucinations, headache, sedation, depression, incoherence, dizziness, excite-

ment, delirium, flushing, weakness, drowsiness
CV: Palpitations, tachycardia, postural hypotension, paradoxical bradycardia
EENT: Blurred vision, nasal congestion, photophobia, dilated pupils, difficulty swallowing, mydriasis, cycloplegia
GI: Dryness of mouth, constipation, nausea, vomiting, abdominal distress, ***paralytic ileus***
GU: Hesitancy, retention
METAB: Fever, decreased sweating
SKIN: Urticaria
MISC: Suppression of lactation, nasal congestion

▼ **DRUG INTERACTIONS**

Drugs

• *Antihistamines, phenothiazines, tricyclics:* Increased anticholinergic effect
• *CNS depressants:* Additive CNS depression
• *Parenteral benzodiazepines:* Additive sedation, hallucinations, irrational behavior

Labs

• *Interference:* Phenolsulfonphthalein (PSP) excretion test, radionuclide gastric emptying studies (delayed gastric emptying), gastric acid secretory studies (antagonizes effects of pentagastrin and histamine), neuroradiological tests (residual cycloplegia and mydriasis interference)

SPECIAL CONSIDERATIONS

PATIENT/FAMILY EDUCATION

• Hard candy, frequent drinks, sugarless gum to relieve dry mouth
• Avoid abrupt discontinuation (taper off over 1 wk)
• Avoid driving or other hazardous activities; drowsiness may occur
• Avoid OTC medication: cough, cold preparations with alcohol, antihistamines
• Wash hands thoroughly after handling transdermal patches before contacting eyes

---

secobarbital

(see-koe-bar′bi-tal)
Secogen, ✤ Seconal, Seral, ✤ Secretin-Ferring
Chemical Class: Barbiturate
Therapeutic Class: Sedative/hypnotic (short acting)
DEA Class: Controlled Substance Schedule II

CLINICAL PHARMACOLOGY

Mechanism of Action: Nonselective CNS depressant; activity related to ability to enhance the inhibitory synaptic action of γ-aminobutyric acid (GABA); induce all levels of hypnosis: mild sedation, hypnosis, deep coma, anesthesia; decreases seizure activity by inhibition of epileptic activity in CNS

Pharmacokinetics

IM: Onset 10-15 min, duration 3-4 hr
Metabolized by liver, excreted by kidneys (metabolites); $t_{1/2}$ 15-40 hr

INDICATIONS AND USES: Sedative, hypnotic, preanesthetic medication, status epilepticus,* acute tetanus convulsions*

DOSAGE

Adult

• *Insomnia:* PO/IM 100-200 mg hs
• *Sedation/preoperatively:* PO 200-300 mg 1-2 hr preoperatively
• *Status epilepticus:* IM/IV 250-350 mg
• *Acute psychotic agitation:* IM/IV 5.5 mg/kg q3-4h

Child

• *Insomnia:* IM 3-5 mg/kg, not to exceed 100 mg
• *Sedation/preoperatively:* PO 50-100 mg 1-2 hr preoperatively
• *Status epilepticus:* IM/IV 250-350 mg

S

• *Acute psychotic agitation:* IM/IV 5.5 mg/kg q3-4h

$ **AVAILABLE FORMS/COST OF THERAPY**

• Cap, Gel—Oral: 50 mg, 100's: **$10.68;** 100 mg, 100's: **$2.00-$24.46**

• Inj, Sol—IM; IV: 50 mg/ml, 2 ml:**$2.73**

CONTRAINDICATIONS: Hypersensitivity, respiratory depression, severe liver impairment, porphyria

PRECAUTIONS: Anemia, hepatic disease, renal disease, hypertension, elderly, acute/chronic pain (paradoxical reaction to pain possible)

PREGNANCY AND LACTATION: Pregnancy category D; small amounts excreted in breast milk, drowsiness in infant reported; compatible with breast feeding

SIDE EFFECTS/ADVERSE REACTIONS

CNS: Lethargy, drowsiness, hangover, dizziness, paradoxical stimulation in the elderly and children, light-headedness, dependency, CNS depression, mental depression, slurred speech, ataxia, nightmares,

CV: Hypotension, bradycardia

GI: Nausea, vomiting, diarrhea, constipation

HEME: ***Agranulocytosis, thrombocytopenia, megaloblastic anemia*** (long-term treatment)

RESP: Hypoventilation, ***apnea, laryngospasm, bronchospasm***

SKIN: Rash, urticaria, pain, abscesses at inj site, angioedema, thrombophlebitis, ***Stevens-Johnson syndrome***

MISC: Dependence, withdrawal symptoms, minor (anxiety, muscle twitching, tremor, weakness, dizziness, distortion in visual perception, nausea, vomiting, insomnia, orthostatic hypotension), major (convulsions, delirium)

▼ **DRUG INTERACTIONS**

Drugs

• *Acetaminophen:* Barbiturates may enhance the hepatotoxic potential of overdoses and possibly large therapeutic doses of acetaminophen

• *Antidepressants:* Barbiturates reduce serum concentrations of cyclic antidepressants with reduced therapeutic response in most patients

• *Antihistamines:* Additive CNS depression

• *Beta blockers:* Barbiturates stimulate metabolism of beta blockers that are extensively metabolized i.e., propranolol, metoprolol

• *CNS depressants:* Additive CNS depression

• *Chloramphenicol:* Chloramphenicol can increase barbiturate concentrations and barbiturates can reduce serum chloramphenicol concentrations

• *Corticosterioids:* Reduced serum concentrations of steroids with impaired therapeutic effect

• *Ethanol:* Additive CNS depression

• *Haloperidol:* Hyperpyrexia of sedative-hypnotic withdrawal enhanced by haloperidol's ability to interfere with thermoregulation

• *MAOIs:* Prolonged effect of barbiturates

• *Meperidine:* Increased toxicity of meperidine

• *Methadone:* Reduced effect of methadone

• *Methoxyflurane:* Enhanced nephrotoxic potential of methoxyflurane

• *Narcotic analgesics:* Additive CNS depression

• *Neuroleptics:* Barbiturates reduce neuroleptic levels

• *Oral anticoagulants:* Inhibition of hypoprothrombinemic response to oral anticoagulants

• *Oral contraceptives:* Reduced efficacy of oral contraceptives with menstrual irregularities and unintended pregnancies possible

• *Quinidine:* Reduced quinidine concentrations
• *Theophylline:* Reduced serum concentrations of theophylline with reduced therapeutic response

Labs

• *False increase:* Sulfobromophthalein

SPECIAL CONSIDERATIONS

• Compared to the benzodiazepine sedative hypnotics, secobarbital is more lethal in overdosage, has a higher tendency for abuse and addiction, and is more likely to cause drug interactions via induction of hepatic microsomal enzymes; few advantages if any in safety or efficacy over benzodiazepines

PATIENT/FAMILY EDUCATION

• Avoid driving and other dangerous activities
• Withdrawal insomnia may occur after short-term use; do not start using drug again, insomnia will improve in 1-3 nights
• May experience increased dreaming

---

selegiline

(seh-leg′ill-ene)

Eldepryl

Chemical Class: Levorotatory acetylenic derivative of phenethylamine, i.e., L-deprenyl

Therapeutic Class: Antiparkinson agent

CLINICAL PHARMACOLOGY

Mechanism of Action: Inhibition of monoamine oxidase, type B, which blocks the catabolism of dopamine, increasing the net amount of dopamine available; other less well understood mechanisms also lead to an increase in dopaminergic activity

Pharmacokinetics: Rapidly absorbed, peak ½-2 hr; rapidly metabolized (active metabolites: N-desmethyldeprenyl $t_{1/2}$, 2 hr; amphetamine $t_{1/2}$, 17.7 hr, methamphetamine, $t_{1/2}$, 20 ½ hr), metabolites excreted in urine (45% in 48 hr)

INDICATIONS AND USES: Adjunct management of Parkinson's disease in patients being treated with levodopa/carbidopa who have had a poor response to therapy; early Parkinson's disease to delay progression;* atypical depression,* Alzheimer's disease*

DOSAGE

Adult

• *Parkinson's disease:* PO 10 mg/d in divided doses 5 mg at breakfast and lunch; after 2-3 days begin to reduce the dose of concurrent levodopa/carbidopa 10%-30%

$ AVAILABLE FORMS/COST OF THERAPY

• Tab, Uncoated—Oral: 5 mg, 60's: **$129.54**

CONTRAINDICATIONS: Hypersensitivity, concurrent use with meperidine

PRECAUTIONS: Doses above 10 mg/d (doses in the 30-40 mg/d range are associated with nonselective MAO inhibition)

PREGNANCY AND LACTATION: Pregnancy category C

SIDE EFFECTS/ADVERSE REACTIONS

CNS: Increased tremors, chorea, restlessness, blepharospasm, increased bradykinesia, grimacing, tardive dyskinesia, dystonic symptoms, involuntary movements, increased apraxia, hallucinations, dizziness, mood changes, nightmares, delusions, lethargy, apathy, overstimulation, sleep disturbances, headache, migraine, numbness, muscle cramps, confusion, anxiety, tiredness, vertigo, personality change, back/leg pain

CV: Orthostatic hypotension, hypertension, ***dysrhythmia,*** palpitations, ***angina pectoris, hypotension,*** tachycardia, edema, sinus bradycardia, syncope
EENT: Diplopia, dry mouth, blurred vision, tinnitus
GI: Nausea, vomiting, constipation, weight loss, anorexia, diarrhea, heartburn, rectal bleeding, poor appetite, dysphagia, abdominal pain
GU: Slow urination, nocturia, prostatic hypertrophy, hesitation, retention, frequency, sexual dysfunction
RESP: Asthma, shortness of breath
SKIN: Increased sweating, alopecia, hematoma, rash, photosensitivity, facial hair

▼ DRUG INTERACTIONS

Drugs

- *Fluoxetine+:* ***Death***
- *Meperidine+:* Stupor, muscular rigidity, severe agitation, elevated temperature, hallucinations, and death
- *MAOIs+:*Increased pressor effect of tyramine
- *Tyramine:* Food containing large amounts of tyramine can result in hypertensive reactions in patients taking MAOIs

Labs

- *Decrease:* VMA
- *False positive:* Urine ketones, urine glucose
- *False negative:* Urine glucose (glucose oxidase)
- *False increase:* Uric acid, urine protein

SPECIAL CONSIDERATIONS

- At low doses, irreversible type B MAOI; at higher doses is metabolized to amphetamine, inhibiting both A and B subtypes of MAO
- Several placebo-controlled studies have demonstrated a significant delay in the need to initiate levodopa therapy in patients who receive selegiline in the early phase of the disease
- May have significant benefit in slowing the onset of the debilitating consequences of Parkinson's disease

selenium sulfide

(see-leen'ee-um)
Exsel, Head and Shoulders Intensive Treatment, Selsun, Selsun Blue
Chemical Class: Trace metal
Therapeutic Class: Antiseborrheic; antifungal

CLINICAL PHARMACOLOGY

Mechanism of Action: Antimitotic action reducing turnover of epidermal cells; additional local irritant, antibacterial, and antifungal activity

Pharmacokinetics

- Absorption may be increased if applied to inflamed skin

INDICATIONS AND USES: Dandruff, seborrheic dermatitis; tinea versicolor

DOSAGE

Adult and child

- *Seborrheic dermatitis:* TOP wash hair with 1-2 tsp, leave on 2-3 min, rinse; repeat; 2 applications/wk for control or as needed for maintenance
- *Tinea versicolor:* TOP apply to affected area (perhaps with small amount of water), allow to remain on skin for 10 min, rinse thoroughly; repeat daily × 7 days; repeat as needed for maintenance

$ AVAILABLE FORMS/COST OF THERAPY

- Lotion/Shampoo—Top: 2.5%, 4 oz: **$2.81-$12.86**

CONTRAINDICATIONS: Hypersensitivity to sulfur preparations

PRECAUTIONS: Infants, inflamed skin

PREGNANCY AND LACTATION: Pregnancy category C

SIDE EFFECTS/ADVERSE REACTIONS

SKIN: Oiliness of hair/scalp, alopecia, discoloration of hair (minimized with thorough rinsing) *skin irritation*

SPECIAL CONSIDERATIONS

PATIENT/FAMILY EDUCATION

- External use only; avoid contact with eyes
- May damage jewelry (remove before using)

---

senna

(sen′na)

Black Draught, Dr. Caldwell's Senna Laxative, Fletcher's Castoria, Gentlax, Senexon, Senna-Gen, Senokot, Senokot Xtra, Senolax

Chemical Class: Anthraquinone derivatives; sennosides A and B

Therapeutic Class: Irritant or stimulant laxative

CLINICAL PHARMACOLOGY

Mechanism of Action: Stimulates peristalsis by action on intramural nerve plexi; alters water and electrolyte secretion

Pharmacokinetics

PO: Onset 6-8 hr

PR: Onset 0.5-1 hr

Minimal absorption; metabolized by liver; fecal and/or renal elimination

INDICATIONS AND USES: Constipation; bowel evacuation or preparation for surgery or examination

DOSAGE

Adult

- PO up to 1600 mg/d; tabs (187-600 mg), 1-8 tabs/d; granules (163-1600 mg/½ tsp), ¼-½ tsp/d; SYR (218 mg/5 ml), 5-20 ml/d; LIQ (33.3 mg/ml), 10-15 ml/d
- PR up to 1600 mg/d; supp (652 mg), 1-2/d

Child (>6 yr; >27 kg)

- Do not use Black Draught (granules) for children
- PO up to 800 mg/d; tabs (187-600 mg), 1-4 tabs/d; syr (218 mg/5 ml), 10-30 ml/d; liq (33.3 mg/ml), 15-30 ml/d

Child 2-5 yr

- PO up to 300-400 mg/d; liq 5-10 ml/d

Child 1 mo-1 yr

- PO up to 300-400 mg/d; syr 1.25-5 ml/d

$ **AVAILABLE FORMS/COST OF THERAPY**

- Tab—Oral: 187 mg, 100's: **$2.55-$14.35;** 217 mg, 100's: **$3.85-$4.85;** 374 mg, 12's: **$3.78**
- Granules—Oral: 326 mg/tsp, 168 g: **$13.67**
- Supp—Rect: 652 mg, 6's: **$12.06**
- Syr—Oral: 218 mg/5 ml, 240 ml: **$15.94**

CONTRAINDICATIONS: Hypersensitivity, GI bleeding, obstruction, fecal impaction, abdominal pain, nausea/vomiting, symptoms of appendicitis, acute surgical abdomen

PRECAUTIONS: Fluid and electrolyte imbalance with abuse, abuse/dependency, children

PREGNANCY AND LACTATION: Pregnancy category C; not excreted into breast milk; compatible with breast feeding

SIDE EFFECTS/ADVERSE REACTIONS

GI: Nausea, vomiting, anorexia, cramps, diarrhea

METAB: Hypocalcemia, enteropathy, alkalosis, hypokalemia, ***tetany***

▼ **DRUG INTERACTIONS**

Drugs

- *Anticoagulants:* By speeding the contents of oral anticoagulants through the GI tract, may lessen the hypoprothrombinemic response; sig-

S

nificant only with large quantities of laxatives on a frequent basis

Labs

• *Interference:* Colorimetric diagnostic urine tests may discolor urine yellowish brown, turning red with increasing pH

SPECIAL CONSIDERATIONS

• Proposed laxative of choice for narcotic-induced constipation

sertraline

(sir'trall-een)

Zoloft

Chemical Class: Unrelated to tricyclic, tetracyclic, or other heterocyclic antidepressants

Therapeutic Class: Selective serotonin reuptake antidepressant (SSRI)

CLINICAL PHARMACOLOGY

Mechanism of Action: Inhibits serotonin neuronal reuptake

Pharmacokinetics

PO: Peak 4.5-8.4 hr

Extensive first pass metabolism; plasma protein binding 99%, elimination $t_{1/2}$ 26-65 hr, metabolite excreted in urine

INDICATIONS AND USES: Major depression, obsessive-compulsive disorder*

DOSAGE

Adult

• PO 50 mg qd; may increase to a max of 200 mg/d; do not change dose at intervals of <1 wk; administer qd in AM or PM

• Reduce dose for hepatic or renal dysfunction

$ **AVAILABLE FORMS/COST OF THERAPY**

• Tab, Uncoated—Oral: 50 mg, 100's: **$202.20;** 100 mg, 100's: **$208.05**

CONTRAINDICATIONS: Hypersensitivity

PRECAUTIONS: Weight loss, hepatic or renal disease, epilepsy

PREGNANCY AND LACTATION: Pregnancy category B

SIDE EFFECTS/ADVERSE REACTIONS

CNS: Insomnia, agitation, *somnolence, dizziness, headache, tremor, fatigue,* paresthesia, twitching, confusion, ataxia

CV: Palpitations, chest pain, hypotension

EENT: Vision abnormalities

GU: Male sexual dysfunction, micturition disorder

GI: Diarrhea, nausea, constipation, anorexia, *dry mouth,* dyspepsia, vomiting, flatulence

▼ **DRUG INTERACTIONS**

Drugs

• *MAOIs+:* Mental status changes such as memory changes, confusion and irritability, chills, pyrexia, and muscle rigidity

Labs

• *Increase:* Serum bilirubin, blood glucose, alk phosphatase

• *Decrease:* VMA, 5-HIAA

• *False increase:* Urinary catecholamines

SPECIAL CONSIDERATIONS

• SSRI of choice based on intermediate length $t_{1/2}$, linear pharmacokinetics, absence of appreciable age effect on clearance, substantially less effect on P450 enzymes, reducing potential for drug interactions

• Splitting 100 mg tablets to yield 50 mg dose cuts costs

silver nitrate

Chemical Class: Heavy metal

Therapeutic Class: Antiinfective

CLINICAL PHARMACOLOGY

Mechanism of Action: Germicidal

action via liberated silver ions which precipitate bacterial proteins; also antiseptic, astringent, local epithelial stimulant, and caustic

INDICATIONS AND USES: Prevention, treatment of gonorrheal ophthalmia neonatorum; treat indolent wounds, ulcers, and fissures; cauterize vesicular, bullous, or aphthous lesions; styptic action; wet dressing in burns and acute dermatitis*

DOSAGE

Adult

• TOP (as wet dressing or irrigant) apply to affected area for approximately 5 days prn

Neonate

• *Gonorrheal ophthalmia neonatorum:* Instill 2 gtt of 1% sol into each eye; do *not* follow with irrigation

$ AVAILABLE FORMS/COST OF THERAPY

• Crystals: 25 g: **$22.28**
• Applicators—Top: 12's: **$1.20**
• Sol—Ophth: 1%, 100's: **$136.16**
• Sol—Top: 960 ml, 12's: **$5.28**

CONTRAINDICATIONS: Hypersensitivity

PRECAUTIONS: Antibiotic hypersensitivity; *not* effective for neonatal chlamydial conjunctivitis; caustic and irritating to skin

SIDE EFFECTS/ADVERSE REACTIONS

EENT: Redness, discharge, edema, swelling (chemical conjunctivitis)
METAB: Sodium and chloride depletion with chronic wet dressings
SKIN: Discoloration

SPECIAL CONSIDERATIONS

PATIENT/FAMILY EDUCATION

• Stains skin and utensils (removable with iodine tincture followed by sodium thiosulfate solution)

silver sulfadiazine

(sul-fa-dye'a-zeen)
Silvadene, SSD, SSD AF
Therapeutic Class: Local anti-infective
Chemical Class: Sulfonamide

CLINICAL PHARMACOLOGY

Mechanism of Action: Interferes with bacterial cell wall synthesis (bactericidal); broad antimicrobial activity including many gram-negative and gram-positive bacteria and yeast; *not* a carbonic anhydrase inhibitor and may be useful in situations where such agents are contraindicated

Pharmacokinetics

TOP: Absorption varies depending on surface area covered and integrity of skin; appreciable serum concentrations obtainable with extensive use (8-12 mcg/ml)

INDICATIONS AND USES: Burns (2nd, 3rd degree); prevention of wound sepsis; bacterial skin infections; dermal ulcers

DOSAGE

Adult and Child

• TOP apply to affected area qd-bid

$ AVAILABLE FORMS/COST OF THERAPY

• Cre—Top: 1%, 25 g: **$2.96-$3.31;** 50 g: **$4.20-$9.25;** 400 g: **$21.00-$47.40;** 1000 g: **$43.32-$118.50**

CONTRAINDICATIONS: Hypersensitivity, child <2 mo

PRECAUTIONS: Impaired hepatic or renal function

PREGNANCY AND LACTATION: Pregnancy category B; caution in neonates (kernicterus)

SIDE EFFECTS/ADVERSE REACTIONS

GU: Crystalluria
HEME: Reversible leukopenia

SKIN: Rash, urticaria, stinging, burning, itching, pain, skin necrosis, erythema, brownish-gray skin discoloration

▼ **DRUG INTERACTIONS**

Drugs

• *Cimetidine:* Increased risk of leukopenia

• *Proteolytic enzymes:* Silver may inactivate enzymes

SPECIAL CONSIDERATIONS

• Prior to application, burn wounds should be cleansed and debrided (following control of shock and pain)

• Use sterile glove and tongue blade to apply medication; thin layer (1.5 mm) to completely cover wound; dressing as required only

• Continue until no chance of infection

---

simethicone

(si-meth'i-kone)

Extra Strength Gas-X, Gas-X, Mylicon, Mylicon 80, Ovol, ♣ Phazyme, Phazyme 95, Phazyme 125

Therapeutic Class: Antiflatulent

CLINICAL PHARMACOLOGY

Mechanism of Action: Defoaming action, disperses and prevents formation of gas pockets in GI system

Pharmacokinetics

PO: Fecal elimination, unchanged

INDICATIONS AND USES: Flatulence, infant colic,* adjunctive for air swallowing,* dyspepsia,* peptic ulcer,* spastic or irritable colon,* diverticulitis* and for colonoscopy* and bowel radiography*

DOSAGE

Adult

• PO 40-125 mg qid pc, hs

Child 2-12 yr

• PO 40 mg qid

Child <2 yr

• PO 20 mg pc, hs (up to 240 mg/d)

$ AVAILABLE FORMS/COST OF THERAPY

• Tab, Chewable—Oral: 40 mg, 100's: **$10.06;** 80 mg, 12's: **$1.56;** 100's: **$3.80;** 125 mg, 18's: **$3.12**

• Tab—Oral: 60 mg, 100's: **$13.18**

• Cap—Oral: 125 mg, 50's: **$9.78**

• Liq—Oral: 40 mg/0.6 ml, 30 ml: **$2.77-$7.50**

CONTRAINDICATIONS: Hypersensitivity

PREGNANCY AND LACTATION: Pregnancy category C

SIDE EFFECTS/ADVERSE REACTIONS

GI: Belching, rectal flatus

SPECIAL CONSIDERATIONS

• Commonly prescribed, little evidence for any beneficial effect

---

simvastatin

(sim'va-sta-tin)

Zocor

Chemical Class: HMG-CoA reductase inhibitor

Therapeutic Class: Antihyperlipidemic

CLINICAL PHARMACOLOGY

Mechanism of Action: Inhibits HMG-CoA reductase enzyme, which catalyzes the rate-limiting step in cholesterol biosynthesis (increases HDL-cholesterol mildly, dramatically decreases total cholesterol and LDL-cholesterol)

Pharmacokinetics

PO: Peak 1-2½ hr

85% absorbed, extensive first-pass metabolism (active metabolites), highly protein bound, excreted primarily in bile, feces (60%)

INDICATIONS AND USES: Hypercholesterolemia (types IIa, IIb, i.e., elevated total and LDL-cholesterol) as an adjunct to diet; reverse the progression of coronary atherosclerosis

DOSAGE

Adult

• PO 5-10 mg qd in PM initially; usual range 5-40 mg/d qd in PM, not to exceed 40 mg/d; dosage adjustments may be made in 4-wk intervals

$ **AVAILABLE FORMS/COST OF THERAPY**

• Tab, Plain Coated—Oral: 5 mg, 60's: **$106.84;** 10 mg, 60's: **$112.77;** 20 mg, 60's: **$204.38;** 40 mg, 60's: **$206.25**

CONTRAINDICATIONS: Hypersensitivity, active liver disease

PRECAUTIONS: Past liver disease, alcoholism, severe acute infections, trauma, hypotension, uncontrolled seizure disorders, severe metabolic disorders, electrolyte imbalances

PREGNANCY AND LACTATION: Pregnancy category X; breast milk excretion unknown; other drugs in this class are excreted in small amounts; manufacturer recommends against breast feeding

SIDE EFFECTS/ADVERSE REACTIONS

CNS: Headache, tremor, vertigo, dizziness, peripheral neuropathy, memory loss, insomnia

GI: Nausea, vomiting, constipation, diarrhea, dyspepsia, flatus, abdominal pain, heartburn, ***liver dysfunction,*** cholestatic jaundice, chronic active hepatitis, hepatic necrosis, pancreatitis

GU: Gynecomastia, loss of libido, erectile dysfunction

MS: Muscle cramps, myalgia, ***myositis, rhabdomyolysis***

SKIN: Rash, pruritus, alopecia

MISC: Hypersensitivity reactions, one or more of the following features: anaphylaxis, angioedema, lupus erythematous-like syndrome, polymyalgia rheumatica, vasculitis, purpura, thrombocytopenia, leukopenia, hemolytic anemia, positive ANA, ESR increase, eosinophilia, arthritis, arthralgia, urticaria, asthenia, photosensitivity, fever, chills, flushing, malaise, dyspnea, toxic epidermal necrolysis, erythema multiforme, including Stevens-Johnson syndrome

▼ **DRUG INTERACTIONS**

Drugs

• *Cyclosporine, gemfibrozil, niacin, erythromycin:* Increased myalgia, myositis

• *Oral anticoagulants:* Slight increased effects of warfarin

Labs

• *Increase:* Transaminases, alk phosphatase, μ-glutamyl transpeptidase, bilirubin (5%)

• *Interference:* Thyroid function tests

SPECIAL CONSIDERATIONS

• Superior to fibrates, cholestyramine, and probucol in lowering total and LDL cholesterol levels

• No advantage over other lovastatin, pravastatin; base HMG-CoA selection on cost and availability

PATIENT/FAMILY EDUCATION

• Take with evening meal

sodium bicarbonate

Chemical Class: Monosodium salt of carbonic acid ($NaHO_3$)
Therapeutic Class: Alkalinizer (systemic; urinary); antacid; electrolyte

CLINICAL PHARMACOLOGY

Mechanism of Action: Orally neutralizes gastric acid, which forms water, NaC1, CO_2; increases plasma bicarbonate, buffers H^+ ion concentration, raises pH; reverses acidosis

Pharmacokinetics

Excreted in urine and by lungs (CO_2)

S

INDICATIONS AND USES: Metabolic acidosis (renal disease, cardiac arrest, circulatory insufficiency); systemic/urinary alkalinization (renal calculi, treatment of drug intoxications; antacid) electrolyte replacement (diarrhea); sickle-cell anemia treatment*

DOSAGE

Adult

- *Acidosis:* IV INF 100-350 mEq over 4-8 hr depending on CO_2 and pH
- *Cardiac arrest:* IV BOL 1 mEq/kg, then 0.5 mEq/kg q10min prn while arrest continues (based on ABGs)
- *Alkalinization:* PO 325 mg-2 g qid
- *Antacid:* PO 300 mg-2 g chewed, taken with H_2O qd-qid

Child 6-12 yr

- *Acidosis:* IV INF 2-5 mEq/kg over 4-8 hr depending on CO_2 and pH
- *Cardiac arrest:* IV BOL 1 mEq/kg, then 0.5 mEq/kg q10 min, then doses based on ABGs
- *Alkalinization:* PO 12-120 mg/kg/d
- *Antacid:* 520 mg; may repeat in 30 min

Infant

Acidosis: IV INF not to exceed 8 mEq/kg/d based on ABGs (4.2% sol)

$ **AVAILALE FORMS/COST OF THERAPY**

- Granules, Effervescent—Oral: 3 g: **$1.80**
- Inj, Sol—IV: 4.2%, 10 ml: **$7.44-$14.30;** 5%, 500 ml: **$39.23;** 7.5%, 50 ml: **$7.46-$19.72;** 8.4%, 10 ml: **$7.44-$14.13**
- Tab, Coated—Oral: 325 mg, 100's: **$1.15-$2.30;** 650 mg, 100's: **$6.23-$12.75**

CONTRAINDICATIONS: Continued losses from vomiting or GI suction; diuretic induced hypochloremic alkalosis

PRECAUTIONS: CHF, cirrhosis, hypertension, hypocalcemia, toxemia, renal disease

PREGNANCY AND LACTATION: Pregnancy category C

SIDE EFFECTS/ADVERSE REACTIONS

CNS: Irritability, headache, confusion, stimulation, tremors, *twitching, hyperreflexia,* ***tetany,*** weakness, ***convulsions*** caused by alkalosis

CV: Irregular pulse, ***cardiac arrest,*** water retention, edema, weight gain

GI: Flatulence, cramps, *belching, distension,* ***paralytic ileus,*** acid rebound, increased thirst

GU: Calculi

METAB: Alkalosis, hypercalcemia/milk-alkali syndrome, hypokalemia

RESP: Shallow, slow respirations, cyanosis, ***apnea***

▼ **DRUG INTERACTIONS**

Drugs

- *Amphetamines:* Sodium bicarbonate inhibits the elimination and increases the effects of amphetamines
- *Ephedrine:* Large doses of sodium bicarbonate increase the serum concentrations of ephedrine
- *Lithium:* Sodium bicarbonate may lower lithium plasma concentrations
- *Methenamine compound:* Sodium bicarbonate induced urinary pH changes interfere with antibacterial activity of methenamine compounds
- *Pseudoephedrine:* Sodium bicarbonate induced urinary pH changes may markedly inhibit the elimination of pseudoephedrine
- *Quinidine:* Sodium bicarbonate induced urinary pH changes may increase quinidine concentrations
- *Salicylates:* Sodium bicarbonate induced urinary pH changes can decrease serum salicylate concentrations

• *Tetracycline+:* Reduction in tetracycline serum concentrations

Labs

• *Increase:* Urinary urobilinogen
• *False positive:* Urinary protein, blood lactate

SPECIAL CONSIDERATIONS

• Milk-alkali syndrome: confusion, headache, nausea, vomiting, anorexia, urinary stones, hypercalcemia

MONITORING PARAMETERS

• Electrolytes, blood pH, PO_2, HCO_3, during treatment
• ABGs frequently during emergencies

---

sodium chloride

Nasal: SalineX, Pretz, Afrin Saline Mist, Dristan Saline, Ayr, Breathe Free, HuMist, NaSal, Ocean, SeaMist
Ophth: Adsorbonac Ophthalmic Solution, AK-NaC1, Dey-Pak Sodium Chloride 3% and 10%, Muro-128 Ophthalmic, Muroptic-S
Chemical Class: Sodium ion
Therapeutic Class: Electrolyte

CLINICAL PHARMACOLOGY

Mechanism of Action: Major electrolytes necessary for the maintenance of plasma tonicity; moisturizes dry mucous membranes; reduces corneal edema by osmosis of water through the semipermeable corneal epithelium

INDICATIONS AND USES: Electrolyte replacement, flushing IV catheters, extracellular fluid replacement, abortifacient; prevention of muscle cramps and heat prostration; GU irrigation; nasal mucous moisturization; diluent for IV, IM, or SQ injections; Ophth: corneal edema

DOSAGE

Adult

• *Electrolyte replacement:* IV Sodium deficiency (mEq/kg) = [% dehydration (L/kg)/100 × 70 (mEq/L)] + [0.6(L/kg) × (140 – serum sodium)(mEq/L)]
• *Severe hyponatremia:* mEq sodium = [desired sodium (mEq/L] – [actual sodium (mEq/L) × 0.6 × wt (kg)]; for acute correction, use 125 mEq as the desired serum sodium; acutely correct serum sodium in 5 mEq/L dose increments; more gradual correction in increments of 10 mEq/L/d is indicated in the asymptomatic patient
• *Chloride maintenance electrolyte requirement in parenteral nutrition:* 2-4 mEq/kg/24 hr or 25-40 mEq/1000 kcal/24 hr; max 100-150 mEq/24 hr
• *Sodium maintenance electrolyte requirement in parenteral nutrition:* 3-4 mEq/kg/24 hr or 25-40 mEq/1000 kcal/24 hr; max 100-150 mEq/24 hr
• *Heat cramps:* PO 0.5-1 g with full glass of water (up to 4.8 g/d)
• *GU irrigant:* 1-3 L/d
• *Nasal:* prn
• *Corneal edema:* Instill 1-2 gtt q3-4h or ointment hs
• *Abortifacient:* 20% (250 ml) transabdominal intra-amniotic instillation

Child

• *Electrolyte replacement:* IV Sodium deficiency (mEq/kg) = [% dehydration (L/kg)/100 × 70 (mEq/L)] + [0.6(L/kg) × (140 – serum sodium)(mEq/L)]
• *Nasal:* prn
• *Corneal edema:* Instill 1-2 gtt q3-4h or ointment hs

Newborn

• *Electrolyte requirement:* Premature, 2-8 mEq/kg/24 hr; Term, 0-48

S

hr 0-2 mEq/kg/24 hr; >48 hr 1-4 mEq/kg/24 hr

$ AVAILABLE FORMS/COST OF THERAPY

- Sol, bacteriostatic diluent: 0.9%, 30 ml: **$1.57**
- Sol, electrolyte—IV: 0.45%, 1000 ml: **$0.77;** 0.9%, 1000 ml: **$0.81;** 3%, 500 ml: **$0.65;** 5%, 500 ml: **$0.81;** 14.6%, 20 ml (for dilution): **$2.02;** 23.4%, 30 ml (for dilution): **1.43**
- Tab, electrolyte—Oral: 1 g, 100's: **$3.00-$7.55;** 2.25 g, 100's: **$5.37**
- Sol-Genitourinary irrigant: 0.9% (isotonic), 1000 ml: **$2.21;** 0.45%, 1000 ml (hypotonic): **$2.21**
- Sol—Nasal: 45 ml-50 ml: **$1.95-$2.34**
- Sol, isotonic—Inh: 0.9%, 3 ml × 100: **$16.40-$24.20;** 0.45%, 3 ml × 100: **$24.20**
- Sol—Ophth: 2%, 15 ml: **$9.49;** 5%, 15 ml: **$9.98**
- Oint—Ophth: 5%, 3.5 g: **$4.99**

CONTRAINDICATIONS: Hypersensitivity, hypernatremia, bacteriostatic solutions in newborns

PRECAUTIONS: Uncompensated cardiovascular, cirrhotic, or nephrotic disease, circulatory insufficiency, hypoproteinemia, hypervolemia, urinary tract obstruction, CHF, patients with concurrent edema and sodium retention, those receiving corticosteroids and those retaining salt

PREGNANCY AND LACTATION: Pregnancy category C

SIDE EFFECTS/ADVERSE REACTIONS

CNS: Irritability, restlessness, weakness, ***obtundation, convulsions, coma***

CV: Hypervolemia, ***CHF***

EENT: Stinging

GI: Nausea, vomiting, diarrhea, abdominal cramps

METAB: Sodium, chloride excess or deficit

RESP: ***Pulmonary edema***

MISC: Rapid infusion may cause local pain at inj site

▼ DRUG INTERACTIONS

Drugs

- *Lithium:* (high sodium intake may reduce serum lithium concentrations, while restriction of sodium tends to increase serum lithium

SPECIAL CONSIDERATIONS

- One g of sodium chloride provides 17.1 mEq sodium and 17.1 mEq chloride

sodium citrate and citric acid
sodium citrate and potassium citrate

Sodium citrate and citric acid: Modified Shohl's solution, Bicitra, Citra pH, Oracit

Sodium citrate and potassium citrate: Citrolith, Polycitra, Polycitra-LC, Polycitra-K

Therapeutic Class: Oral alkalizers

CLINICAL PHARMACOLOGY

Mechanism of Action: Sodium citrate is absorbed and metabolized to sodium bicarbonate, thus acting as a systemic alkalinizer; the effects of these salts are essentially those of chlorides before absorption and those of bicarbonates subsequently

Pharmacokinetics

PO: <5% of citrate is excreted unchanged

INDICATIONS AND USES: Alkalinizing agent; useful where long-term maintenance of an alkaline urine is desirable; alleviation of chronic metabolic acidosis (i.e., chronic renal insufficiency or the syndrome of renal tubular acidosis); buffers/neutralizes gastric acid

DOSAGE

Adult

- *Systemic alkalinization:* Sodium citrate and citric acid, PO 10 to 30 ml diluted pc, hs; sodium citrate and potassium citrate, PO 15-30 ml diluted pc, hs
- *Neutralizing buffer:* PO 15 ml diluted taken as a single dose

Child

- *Systemic alkalinization:* Sodium citrate and citric acid, PO 5 to 15 ml diluted pc, hs; sodium citrate and potassium citrate, PO 5-15 ml diluted pc, hs

$ **AVAILABLE FORMS/COST OF THERAPY**

Sodium Citrate/Citric acid

- Sol—Oral:15 ml × 100: **$59.00-$75.00**

Sodium Citrate/Potassium citrate

- Liq—Oral: 480 ml: **$14.50**
- Syr—Oral: 480 ml: **$14.44**

CONTRAINDICATIONS: Sodium-restricted diets or with severe renal impairment

PRECAUTIONS: Low urinary output; patients with cardiac failure, hypertension, impaired renal function, peripheral and pulmonary edema, and toxemia of pregnancy

▼ **DRUG INTERACTIONS**

Drugs

- *Amphetamines:* Sodium bicarb inhibits the elimination and increases the effects of amphetamines
- *Ephedrine:* Large doses of sodium bicarb increase serum concentrations of ephedrine
- *Lithium:* Sodium bicarb may lower lithium plasma concentrations
- *Methenamine compound:* Sodium bicarb induced urinary pH changes interfere with antibacterial activity of methenamine compounds
- *Pseudoephedrine:* Sodium bicarb induced urinary pH changes may markedly inhibit the elimination of pseudoephedrine
- *Quinidine:* Sodium bicarb-induced urinary pH changes may increase quinidine concentrations
- *Salicylates:* Sodium bicarb-induced urinary pH changes can decrease serum salicylate concentrations
- *Tetracycline+:* Reduction in tetracycline serum concentrations

SPECIAL CONSIDERATIONS

PATIENT/FAMILY EDUCATION

- Sugar free
- Dilute adequately with water and, preferably, take each dose after meals to avoid saline laxative effect

MONITORING PARAMETERS

- Serum electrolytes, particularly serum bicarb level

sodium fluoride

Acidulated Phosphate Fluoride, ACT, Altaflor; Audifluor; ✤ Checkmate, Fluor-A-Day, ✤ En-DeKay; ✤ Fluoen, ✤ Fluorabon, Fluorigard, ✤ Fluorineed, Fluorinse, Fluoritab, Fluorodex, Fluotic, ✤ Flura, Gel II, Gel-Kam, Gel-Tin, Karidium, Karigel, Karigel-N, Liqui-Flur, Listermint with Fluoride, Loz-Tabs, Luride, Minute-Gel, Nafrinse, Neutracare, Pediadent, Pediaflor, Pharmaflur, Phos-Flur, Point-Two, Prevident, Solu-Flur, Thera-Flur, Vinafluor, ✤ Zymafluor ✤

Chemical Class: Fluoride ion

Therapeutic Class: Trace element

CLINICAL PHARMACOLOGY

Mechanism of Action: Systemic action, before tooth eruption and topically post eruption; needed for hard tooth enamel and for resistance to periodontal disease; reduces acid production by dental bacteria; acidulation provides greater topical fluoride uptake by dental enamel than neutral solutions; phosphate protects enamel from demineralization by the acidulated formulation (common ion effect); potent stimulator of bone formation—increases bone mass in intermediate doses

Pharmacokinetics

PO: Absorption related to solubility; sodium fluoride almost completely absorbed; calcium or magnesium delays absorption; 50% deposited in bone and teeth; excreted in urine, feces, and breast milk; crosses placenta

INDICATIONS AND USES: Prevention of dental caries; osteoporosis*

DOSAGE

Note: 2.2 mg sodium fluoride equivalent to 1 mg of fluoride ion

Adult and child >12 yr

• *Dental rinse or gel:* TOP 10 ml 0.2% sol qd after brushing teeth, rinse mouth for >1 min with sol

• *Osteoporosis:* PO 8-80 mg/d (slow release formulation pending FDA approval)

Child

• *Systemic protection from periodontal disease:* In areas where fluoride content of drinking water <0.3 ppm, 6 mo-3 yr 0.25 mg fluoride, 3-6 yr 0.5 mg fluoride, 6-16 yr 1 mg fluoride; in areas where fluoride content of drinking water is 0.3-0.6 ppm, 3-6 yr 0.25 mg fluoride, 6-16 yr 0.25-0.75 mg fluoride

$ AVAILABLE FORMS/COST OF THERAPY

• Gel—Dental: 1.1%, 25-125 ml: **$2.20-$51.54**

• Liq—Dental: 0.275 mg/ml, 22.8 ml-50 ml: **$1.65-$12.86**

• Lozenge—Oral: 1 mg, 1000's: **$12.50**

• Mouthwash, Dental—Top: 0.2%, 500-1000 ml: **$6.00-$89.86**

• Powder: 454 g: **$23.39**

• Sol, Dental, Top—Oral: 0.2%, 30 ml: **$4.25;** 0.5%, 50 ml: **$6.00;** 1%, 30 ml: **$2.00**

• Tab, Chewable—Oral: 0.25, 0.5, 1, 2.2 mg, 100's: **$1.50**

CONTRAINDICATIONS: Hypersensitivity

PRECAUTIONS: Drinking water with >0.7 ppm fluoride

PREGNANCY AND LACTATION: Administration from 3rd-9th mo of gestation safe (no information on teratogenicity); small amounts excreted into breast milk, inadequate therapeutically due to small amount of excretion and complexation with calcium

SIDE EFFECTS/ADVERSE REACTIONS

GI: Black tarry stools, ***hematemesis,*** diarrhea, increased salivation, stomatitis, constipation, loss of appetite, nausea, weight loss, discoloration of teeth

EENT: Watery eyes

METAB: Hypocalcemia

MS: ***Tetany, osteomalacia,*** articular and juxta-articular pain, stress fractures

RESP: Decreased respiration, ***respiratory arrest***

▼ DRUG INTERACTIONS

Drug

• *Aluminum, calcium:* Decreased fluoride absorption

SPECIAL CONSIDERATIONS

• Therapy begun prenatally and continued through age 16 is effective in reducing the number of decayed, missing, or filled surfaces and teeth; especially beneficial in areas where fluoride content of drinking water is below 0.7 ppm

• Treatment of osteoporosis, combined with one or more of the following—calcium, estrogen, or vitamin D—increases bone density, reduces rate of new vertebral fractures, if correct dose and in slow release preparation; role in steroid-induced osteoporosis being investigated, reports to date indicate a poor response rate

PATIENT/FAMILY EDUCATION

• Avoid use with dairy products

sodium polystyrene sulfonate

(pol-ee-stye'reen)

Kayexalate, SPS Suspension

Chemical Class: Cation exchange resin

Therapeutic Class: Potassium-removing resin

CLINICAL PHARMACOLOGY

Mechanism of Action: Removes potassium by exchanging sodium for potassium in body; occurs primarily in large intestine

Pharmacokinetics

PO/PR: Not absorbed from the GI tract

INDICATIONS AND USES: Hyperkalemia in conjunction with other measures

DOSAGE

Administer in approx 25% sorbitol susp or concurrently treat with 70% oral sorbitol syrup 10-20 mL q2h to produce 1 or 2 watery stools/d or mild laxative

Adult

• PO 15 g qd-qid

• PR 30-50 g/100 ml of sorbitol warmed to body temp q6h

Child

• PO/PR 1g/kg q6h

$ AVAILABLE FORMS/COST OF THERAPY

• Powder—Oral: 454 g: **$164.58**

• Susp—Rect: 15 g/60 ml, 60 ml: **$5.85-$8.65**

CONTRAINDICATIONS: Hypokalemia

PRECAUTIONS: Renal failure, CHF, severe edema, severe hypertension

PREGNANCY AND LACTATION: Pregnancy category C; excretion in breast milk not expected

SIDE EFFECTS/ADVERSE REACTIONS

GI: Constipation, anorexia, nausea, vomiting, diarrhea (sorbitol), fecal impaction, gastric irritation

METAB: Hypocalcemia, hypokalemia, hypomagnesemia, Na retention

▼ DRUG INTERACTIONS

Drugs

• *Antacids:* Combined use of magnesium- or calcium-containing antacids with resin may result in systemic alkalosis

• *Sorbitol:* Necrosis of the colon has been reported following use of Kayexalate-sorbitol enemas

SPECIAL CONSIDERATIONS

• Exchange efficacy of resin is approx 33% (i.e., each gram of resin contains 4.1 mEq of sodium, 15 g of resin bind about 46.5 mEq of potassium in exchange for the release of an equal amount of sodium); 1 g of resin exchanges approximately 1 mEq of potassium

• Rectal route is less effective than oral administration

PATIENT/FAMILY EDUCATION

• Don't mix with orange juice

MONITORING PARAMETERS

• Serum K, Ca, Mg, Na, acid-base balance, bowel function, possibly ECG

somatropin somatrem

(soe-ma-troe'-pin)

Somatropin: Humatrope, Nutropin

Somatrem: Protropin

Chemical Class: Recombinant DNA product; somatropin is identical to human growth hormone, somatrem contains an additional amino acid

Therapeutic Class: Growth hormone

CLINICAL PHARMACOLOGY

Mechanism of Action: Stimulates skeletal growth in growth hormone deficiency, reduces fat stores, induces insulin resistance

Pharmacokinetics

SC: Peak 7.5 hr, localizes to highly perfused organs, metabolized by kidney, liver

INDICATIONS AND USES: Pituitary growth hormone deficiency, growth failure associated with chronic renal insufficiency (somatropin only), Turner's syndrome*

DOSAGE

Child

• *Somatropin:* SC/IM up to 0.06 (0.16 IU) mg/kg/d 3 times/wk

• *Somatrem:* SC/IM up to 0.1 (0.26 IU) mg/kg/d 3 times/wk

• May double dose for 6 mo if growth is <1 inch/6 mo

$ **AVAILABLE FORMS/COST OF THERAPY**

Somatropin:

• Inj, Dry-Sol—IM: 5 mg (13 IU)/vial: **$420.00;** 10 mg (26 IU)/vial: **$840.00**

Somatrem:

• Inj, Lyphl-Sol—IM; SC: 10 mg/vial: **$420.00**

• Kit—IM: 5 mg/vial: **$210.00**

CONTRAINDICATIONS: Hypersensitivity to benzyl alcohol, closed epiphyses, intracranial lesions

PRECAUTIONS: Diabetes mellitus, hypothyroidism

PREGNANCY AND LACTATION: Pregnancy category C; excretion into breast milk unknown

SIDE EFFECTS/ADVERSE REACTIONS

CNS: Headache, ***intracranial hypertension***

HEME: ***Leukemia*** (uncertain relationship)

METAB: Mild hyperglycemia, ***ketosis, hypothyroidism,*** hypercalciuria, glycosuria

SKIN: Rash, urticaria, pain, inflammation at inj site

MISC: Antibodies to growth hormone

▼ **DRUG INTERACTIONS**

Drugs

• *Glucocorticoids, androgens:* Inhibition of growth effect

SPECIAL CONSIDERATIONS

MONITORING PARAMETERS

• Check for hypothyroidism, malnutrition, antibodies if no response to initial dose

• TSH

• Evaluate if child limps

• Follow with fundoscopy (papilledema)

sorbitol

(sor'bi-tole)

Chemical Class: Hexitol, polyalcoholic sugar

Therapeutic Class: Non-electrolyte sol, laxative, diuretic, sweetening agent

CLINICAL PHARMACOLOGY

Mechanism of Action: Hyperosmolar; acts as diuretic, laxative

Pharmacokinetics

PO/PR: Absorption poor; onset of

action 15-60 min; when used as urologic irrigant variable systemic absorption occurs; metabolized to CO_2 and dextrose by liver or excreted by kidneys

INDICATIONS AND USES: Irrigant sol during transurethral prostatic surgery, laxative, facilitate passage of sodium polystyrene sulfonate through intestinal tract

DOSAGE

Adult

• *Laxative:* PO 30-150 ml (70% sol)
• *Rectal enema:* 120 ml (25%-30% sol)
• *Adjunt to polystyrene sulfonate:* 15 ml (70% sol) until diarrhea, or 20-100 ml as oral vehicle for the resin
• *Irrigant:* TOP 3%-3.3% sol

Child (2-11 yr)

• *Laxative:* PO 2 ml/kg (70% sol)
• *Rectal enema:* 30-60 ml (25%-30% sol)

$ AVAILABLE FORMS/COST OF THERAPY

• Sol—Irrigation: 3.3%, 4000 ml: **$6.10**; 30 mg/ml, 3000 ml: **$20.34**
• Sol: 70%, 480 ml: **$2.15**

CONTRAINDICATIONS: Anuria

PRECAUTIONS: Significant cardiopulmonary, renal dysfunction, diabetes mellitus, hyponatremia, hypovolemia

SIDE EFFECTS/ADVERSE REACTIONS

CNS: ***Seizures,*** vertigo
CV: ***CHF, hypotension, angina***
EENT: Blurred vision, rhinitis, thirst
GI: Nausea, vomiting, diarrhea
GU: Fluid retention, acidosis, diuresis, urinary retention, edema
METAB: ***Acidosis, hyponatremia, hyperglycemia, hypernatremia***
MISC: Chills, urticaria

▼ DRUG INTERACTIONS

Drugs

• *Sodium polystyrene sulfonate resin:* Colonic necrosis described in uremic patients who received Kayexalate-sorbitol enemas
• *Vitamin B_{12}:* Decreased absorption

---

sotalol

(soe'ta-lole)
Betaspace
Chemical Class: β-adrenergic blocking agent
Therapeutic Class: Antidysrhythmic

CLINICAL PHARMACOLOGY

Mechanism of Action: Non-selectively blocks β_1 (cardiac muscle) and β_2 receptors (bronchial and vascular musculature), inhibiting the chronotropic, ionotropic, and vasodilator responses to β-adrenergic stimulation

Pharmacokinetics

PO: Onset 1-2 hr, peak effect 3-4 hr, $t_{1/2}$ 12 hr, excreted unchanged by kidney; low lipid solubility, not protein bound; absorption decreased 20%-30% by meals

INDICATIONS AND USES: Treatment of life-threatening ventricular dysrhythmias (e.g., sustained ventricular tachycardia); not recommended in less severe dysrhythmias

DOSAGE

• PO initial dose 80 mg bid; may increase to 240-320 mg/d adjusting dose q2-3d; some patients require doses up to 480-640 mg qd
• Renal failure adjustment: CRCl > 60 mL/min administer q12h; CRCl 30-60 mL/min administer q24h; CRCl 10-30 mL/min administer q36-48h; individualize dose for CRCl < 10 mL/min
• Increase dose q 5-6 doses

$ AVAILABLE FORMS/COST OF THERAPY

• Tab, Coated—Oral: 80 mg, 100's: **$161.35-$164.20;** 160 mg, 100's:

$269.00-$271.80; 240 mg, 100's: **$349.70-$352.50**

CONTRAINDICATIONS: Uncompensated CHF, cardiogenic shock, bradycardia, heart block > 1°, pulmonary edema, asthma, long QT syndrome

PRECAUTIONS: CHF, peripheral vascular disease, hypokalemia, hypomagnesemia, renal dysfunction, sick-sinus syndrome

PREGNANCY AND LACTATION: Pregnancy category B; concentrated in breast milk (levels 3-5 times those of plasma); symptoms of beta blockade possible in infant but considered compatible with breast feeding

SIDE EFFECTS/ADVERSE REACTIONS

CNS: Depression, confusion, anxiety, hallucinations, dizziness, drowsiness, nightmares, insomnia, weakness, fatigue

CV: ***Bradycardia, CHF, chest pain, hypotension, ventricular dysrhythmias including torsade de points,*** Raynaud's phenomena

GI: Constipation, diarrhea, nausea, vomiting, stomach discomfort

GU: Sexual dysfunction

HEME: ***Agranulocytosis***

RESP: ***Bronchospasm,*** *dyspnea, cough*

▼ **DRUG INTERACTIONS**

Drugs

- *Amiodarone:* Bradycardia, cardiac arrest, ventricular dysrhythmia shortly after initiation of beta blocker
- *Antidiabetics:* Masked symptoms of hypoglycemia, prolonged recovery of normoglycemia
- *Calcium channel blockers:* Hypotension
- *Clonidine:* Exacerbation of hypertension upon withdrawal of clonidine
- *Disopyramide:* Additive negative inotropic effects
- *Epinephrine:* Enhanced pressor response to epinephrine
- *Lidocaine:* Increased lidocaine concentrations
- *Local anesthetics:* Enhanced sympathomimetic side effects of epinephrine-containing local anesthetics
- *Methyldopa:* Development of hypertension during periods of catecholamine release
- *Neuroleptics:* Increased plasma concentrations of both drugs
- *NSAIDs:* Reduced hypotensive effect of beta blocker
- *Phenylephrine:* Predisposition to acute hypertensive episodes
- *Prazosin:* Enhanced first-dose response to prazosin
- *Theophylline:* Increased theophylline concentrations; antagonistic pharmacodynamic effects

SPECIAL CONSIDERATIONS

PATIENT/FAMILY EDUCATION

- Do not discontinue abruptly

MONITORING PARAMETERS

- Because of prodysrythmic risk, begin and increase drug in setting with cardiac rhythm monitoring
- QT intervals; discontinue or reduce dose if QT > 550 msec
- Withdraw any previous antidysrhythmic therapy, allowing for at least 2-3 half lives
- After discontinuation of amiodarone, do not initiate sotalol until QT normalized

---

spectinomycin

(spek-ti-noe-mye'sin)

Trobicin

Chemical Class: Aminocyclitol, related to aminoglycosides

Therapeutic Class: Antibiotic

CLINICAL PHARMACOLOGY

Mechanism of Action: Inhibits bacterial synthesis by binding to 30S

subunit on ribosomes, bacteriostatic
Pharmacokinetics
IM: Peak 1-2 hr, duration 8 hr, $t_{1/2}$ 1-3 hr (10-30 hr if CrCl < 20 ml/min), excreted in urine (unchanged); poor distribution into saliva
INDICATIONS AND USES: Gonorrhea, except pharyngeal infection, in patients who cannot take ceftriaxone
DOSAGE
Adult
• IM 2-4 g as single dose, 2 g q12h for days of disseminated infection
Child <45 kg
• IM 30-40 mg/kg as single dose
$ AVAILABLE FORMS/COST OF THERAPY
• Inj, Dry-Susp—IM: 400 mg/ml, 2 g: **$16.86**
CONTRAINDICATIONS: Hypersensitivity, infants (diluent contains benzyl alcohol)
PRECAUTIONS: Children
PREGNANCY AND LACTATION: Pregnancy category B; excretion into breast milk unknown
SIDE EFFECTS/ADVERSE REACTIONS
CNS: Dizziness, chills, fever, insomnia, headache, anxiety
GI: Nausea, vomiting
GU: Decreased urine output
HEME: Anemia
SKIN: Pain at inj site, urticaria, rash, pruritus, fever
SPECIAL CONSIDERATIONS
• Follow with doxycycline 100 mg bid for 7 days (erythromycin if pregnant or allergic)
• Ineffective against syphilis and may mask symptoms
• Give in gluteal muscle, dose not > 2 g at one site

spironolactone
(speer-on-oh-lak'tone)
Aldactone, Novospiroton ♣
Chemical Class: Aldosterone antagonist
Therapeutic Class: Potassium-sparing diuretic

CLINICAL PHARMACOLOGY
Mechanism of Action: Competes with aldosterone at receptor sites in distal tubule, resulting in excretion of sodium chloride, water, retention of potassium, phosphate; has antiandrogenic effect
Pharmacokinetics
PO: Onset 24-48 hr, peak 48-72 hr; metabolized in liver, excreted in urine, crosses placenta
INDICATIONS AND USES: Edema, hypertension, diuretic-induced hypokalemia, primary hyperaldosteronism, nephrotic syndrome, cirrhosis of the liver with ascites, polycystic ovary disease,* female hirsutism*
DOSAGE
Adult
• *Edema/hypertension:* PO 25-200 mg/d in single or divided doses
• *Hypokalemia:* PO 25-100 mg/d in single or divided doses
• *Primary hyperaldosteronism diagnosis:* PO 400 mg/d for 4 days (short test) or 4 wk (long test), then 100-400 mg/d maintenance
• *Polycystic ovary disease/hirsutism:* PO 100-200 mg/d
Child
• *Diuretic/antihypertensive/ascites:* PO 1-3 mg/kg/d in single or divided doses
$ AVAILABLE FORMS/COST OF THERAPY
• Tab, Plain Coated—Oral: 25 mg, 100's: **$4.53-$38.64;** 50 mg, 100's:

$67.86-$71.08; 100 mg, 100's: **$113.78-$119.29**

CONTRAINDICATIONS: Hypersensitivity, anuria, severe renal disease, hyperkalemia

PRECAUTIONS: Dehydration, hepatic disease, hyponatremia, renal insufficiency, patients receiving other potassium-sparing diuretics or potassium supplements, diabetic nephropathy, menstrual abnormalities, gynecomastia, acidosis, elderly

PREGNANCY AND LACTATION: Pregnancy category D; active metabolite excreted in breast milk, compatible with breast feeding

SIDE EFFECTS/ADVERSE REACTIONS

CNS: Headache, confusion, drowsiness, lethargy, ataxia

CV: ***Bradycardia, hypotension, CHF***

GI: Diarrhea, cramps, ***bleeding,*** gastritis, *vomiting,* anorexia, nausea, constipation

GU: Impotence, gynecomastia, irregular menses, amenorrhea, postmenopausal bleeding, hirsutism, deepening voice

METAB: Hyperchloremic metabolic acidosis, ***hyperkalemia, hyponatremia***

SKIN: Rash, pruritus, urticaria

▼ **DRUG INTERACTIONS**

Drugs

- *ACE inhibitors, potassium sparing diuretics, potassium supplements and salt substitutes:* Increased serum K
- *Digoxin:* Possible true increased serum level of digoxin, see lab below

Labs

- *False increase:* Digoxin, cortisol

stanozolol

(stan-oh'zoe-lole)

Winstrol

Chemical Class: Halogenated testosterone derivative

Therapeutic Class: Androgenic anabolic steroid

DEA Class: Schedule III

CLINICAL PHARMACOLOGY

Mechanism of Action: Promotes protein anabolism, stimulates appetite; increases erythropoetin; increases C1 esterase inhibitor and resulting C2 and C4 concentrations; androgenic

INDICATIONS AND USES: Prevention of hereditary angioedema (adult) and during an attack (child), possibly effective for aplastic anemia

DOSAGE

Adult

- *Aplastic anemia:* PO 2 mg tid
- *Angioedema:* PO 2 mg tid, then decrease q1-3mo to 2 mg qd or qod

Child

- *Aplastic anemia:* PO up to 2 mg tid (6-12 yr); PO 1 mg bid (< 6 yr)
- *Angioedema:* PO up to 2 mg qd (6-12 yr); PO 1 mg qd (< 6 yr)

$ **AVAILABLE FORMS/COST OF THERAPY**

- Tab, Uncoated—Oral: 2 mg, 100's: **$65.87**

CONTRAINDICATIONS: Severe renal disease, severe cardiac disease, severe hepatic disease, hypersensitivity, genital bleeding (abnormal), prostate cancer, male breast cancer, female breast cancer with hypercalcemia, nephrosis

PRECAUTIONS: Diabetes mellitus, CV disease, MI

PREGNANCY AND LACTATION: Pregnancy category X (masculinization); excretion into breast milk unknown

SIDE EFFECTS/ADVERSE REACTIONS

CNS: Dizziness, headache, fatigue, tremors, paresthesias, flushing, sweating, anxiety, lability, insomnia, carpal tunnel syndrome

CV: Increased B/P

EENT: Conjunctival edema, nasal congestion, deepening of voice in women

GI: Nausea, vomiting, diarrhea, weight gain, ***cholestatic jaundice, hepatocellular necrosis***

GU: ***Hematuria,*** menstrual irregularities, vaginitis, decreased libido, decreased breast size, gynecomastia, clitoral hypertrophy, testicular atrophy, phallic enlargement in prepubertal males, impotence, priapism, epididymitis, oligospermia

METAB: Abnormal glucose tolerance

MS: Cramps, spasms

SKIN: Rash, acneiform lesions, oily hair, skin, flushing, sweating, acne vulgaris, alopecia, hirsutism and male pattern baldness in women

▼ **DRUG INTERACTIONS**

Drugs

- *Anticoagulants:* Enhanced hypoprothrombinemic response
- *Cyclosporine:* Increased cyclosporine concentrations
- *HMB-CoA reductase inhibitors:* Myositis
- *Oral hypoglycemics:* Enhanced hypoglycemic response

Labs

- *Increase:* Serum cholesterol and LDLs, blood glucose, urine glucose, T_4
- *Decrease:* Serum Ca, serum K, serum HDL cholesterol, T_3 uptake, thyroid ^{131}I uptake test, urine 17-OHCS

stavudine

stav'yoo-deen

Zerit (d4T)

Chemical Class: Nucleoside (thymidine) analog

Therapeutic Class: Antiretroviral agent

CLINICAL PHARMACOLOGY

Mechanism of Action: Phosphorylated intracellularly to stavudine triphosphate which inhibits HIV reverse transcriptase by competing with deoxythymidine triphosphate and inhibits viral DNA synthesis by causing DNA chain termination

Pharmacokinetics

PO: Peak level 1 hr, bioavailability 85% (not affected by food); plasma $t_{1/2}$ 1½ hr, intracellular $t_{1/2}$ 3½ hr; not protein bound; only slightly metabolized; renal clearance by filtration and tubular secretion; urinary excretion of unchanged drug over 24 hr after oral dose 40%

INDICATIONS AND USES: Adults with advanced HIV infection who are intolerant of approved therapies or who deteriorate during these therapies; indication is based on evaluation of surrogate end point responses (CD_4 lymphocyte counts)

DOSAGE

Adult

- *PO:* 40 mg q12h if weight ≥60 kg, 30 mg q12h if weight <60 kg; reduce dose by half if resuming therapy after resolution of side effect (neuropathy, transaminitis); adjust dose for renal insufficiency: CrCl 26-50 ml/min, 20 mg q12h if weight ≥60 kg, 15 mg q12h if weight < 60 kg, CrCl 10-25 ml/min, 20 mg q24h if weight ≥60 kg, 15 mg q24h if weight <60 kg

$ AVAILABLE FORMS/COST OF THERAPY

- Cap, Gel—Oral: 15 mg, 60's:

$207.47; 20 mg, 60's: **$215.76;** 30 mg, 60's: **$225.10;** 40 mg, 60's: **$233.40**

CONTRAINDICATIONS: Hypersensitivity to nucleoside analogs

PRECAUTIONS: Peripheral neuropathy, pancreatitis, renal insufficiency, folate or vitamin B_{12} deficiency

PREGNANCY AND LACTATION: Pregnancy category C; excreted in breast milk

SIDE EFFECTS/ADVERSE REACTIONS

CNS: Dementia, headache, insomnia, *neuropathy*

GI: Abdominal pain, diarrhea, *increased transaminases,* nausea, ***pancreatitis***

HEME: ***Neutropenia***

MS: Myalgia

SKIN: Rash

MISC: Asthenia, fever

SPECIAL CONSIDERATIONS

PATIENT/FAMILY EDUCATION

- Report neuropathic symptoms (numbness, tingling, or pain in the feet or hands)

MONITORING PARAMETERS

- CBC, SGOT, SGPT

---

streptokinase

(strep-toe-kye'nase)

Kabikinase, Streptase

Chemical Class: Beta-hemolytic streptococcus filtrate (purified)

Therapeutic Class: Thrombolytic enzyme

CLINICAL PHARMACOLOGY

Mechanism of Action: Activates conversion of plasminogen to plasmin; plasmin degrades fibrin clots, fibrinogen, other plasma proteins

Pharmacokinetics

IV/IC: Onset immediate, $t_{1/2}$ of streptokinase activator complex 23 min, mechanism of elimination unknown; no metabolites identified

INDICATIONS AND USES: Acute evolving transmural MI, pulmonary embolism, deep venous thrombosis, arterial thrombosis, or embolism, arteriovenous cannulae occlusion not responsive to heparin flush

DOSAGE

Adult

- *Acute evolving transmural MI:* IV INF 1,500,000 IU diluted to a volume of 45 ml; give within 1 hr; IC (intracardiac infusion) dilute 250,000 IU vial to total volume of 125 ml, give 20,000 IU (10 ml) by bolus followed by 2000 IU/min for 60 min for total dose 140,000 IU
- *Thrombosis/embolism:* IV INF 250,000 IU over ½ hr, then 100,000 IU/hr for 72 hr for deep thrombosis; 100,000 IU/hr over 24 hr for pulmonary embolism
- *Arteriovenous cannula occlusion:* IV INF 250,000 IU/2 ml sol into occluded limb of cannula run over 30 min; clamp for 2 hr; aspirate contents; flush with saline sol and reconnect

$ AVAILABLE FORMS/COST OF THERAPY

- Inj, Lyphl-Sol—IC; IV: 1,500,000 U/vial: **$511.75;** 750,000 U/vial: **$255.86;** 600,000 U/vial: **$160.00;** 250,000 U/vial: **$115.93**

CONTRAINDICATIONS: Hypersensitivity, active internal bleeding; recent (within 2 mo) CVA, intracranial or intraspinal surgery, intracranial neoplasm, severe uncontrolled hypertension

PRECAUTIONS: Recent (within 10 days) surgery, obstetrical delivery, organ biopsy, recent trauma including CPR, likelihood of left heart thrombus (e.g., mitral stenosis with atrial fibrillation), subacute bacterial endocarditis, hemostatic defects, age ≥ 75 yrs, diabetic hemorrhagic retinopathy, septic thrombophlebitis or infected occluded AV cannula

PREGNANCY AND LACTATION: Pregnancy category C; no data available for breast feeding

SIDE EFFECTS/ADVERSE REACTIONS

CNS: Headache, fever

CV: ***Hypotension, reperfusion, dysrhythmias***

EENT: Periorbital edema

GI: Nausea, vomiting

HEME: Anemia, ***bleeding (GI, GU, intracranial, retroperitoneal,*** *surface*)

RESP: Altered respirations, SOB, ***bronchospasm, noncardiogenic pulmonary edema***

SKIN: Rash, urticaria, phlebitis at IV inf site, itching, flushing

MISC: ***Anaphylaxis,*** chills, sweating

▼ **DRUG INTERACTIONS**

Labs

Increase: PT, APTT, TT

---

streptomycin

(strep-toe-mye'sin)

Chemical Class: Aminoglycoside

Therapeutic Class: Antibiotic

CLINICAL PHARMACOLOGY

Mechanism of Action: Interferes with protein synthesis in bacterial cell by binding to ribosomal sub unit, causing inaccurate peptide sequence to form in protein chain, causing bacterial death

Pharmacokinetics

IM: Onset rapid, peak 1-2 hr; plasma $t_{1/2}$ 2-2½ hr; not metabolized, excreted unchanged in urine, crosses placenta

INDICATIONS AND USES: In combination with other drugs (INH, rifampin, pyrazinamide) in the treatment of TB unless likelihood of INH or rifampin resistance very low; also indicated when one or more of the above drugs contraindicated; reassess need when susceptibility testing results known; part of multidrug treatment for *Mycobacterium avium* complex;* not usually used for long term therapy secondary to nephrotoxicity and ototoxicity; secondary choice for nontubercular infections caused by sensitive strains of gram-negative organisms: *Hemophilus influenzae* (with another agent); *H. ducreyi* (chancroid); *Klebsiella pneumoniae* pneumonia (with another agent); *Yersinia pestis* (plague); *Brucella* sp; *Francisella tularensis* (tularemia); UTIs caused by *E. coli, Proteus* sp, *Klebsiella pneumonia;* gram-positive organisms: *Streptococcus viridans* endocarditis; *Enterococcus faecalis* (UTI and endocarditis)

DOSAGE

Adult

- *Tuberculosis:* IM 15 mg/kg/d (max 1 g qd), should ultimately be discontinued or reduced to 1 g 2-3 ×/wk; given in combination with other antitubercular drugs
- *Streptococcal endocarditis:* IM 1 g q12h for 1 wk with penicillin, then 500 mg bid for 1 wk; if > 60 years give 500 mg bid for entire 2 wk
- *Enterococcal endocarditis:* IM 1 g q12h for 2 wk, then 500 mg q12h for 4 wk with penicillin
- *Tularemia:* IM 1-2 g qd in divided doses for 7-14 days or until afebrile for 5-7 days
- *Plague:* IM 2-4 g qd in divided doses until afebrile for 3 days
- *Moderate to severe infections:* 1-2 g qd in divided doses q6-12h, max 2 g qd

Child

- *Tuberculosis:* IM 20-40 mg/kg/d in divided doses q6-12h given with

S

other antitubercular drugs, max 1 g/d

$ AVAILABLE FORMS/COST OF THERAPY

- Inj, Sol—IM: 1 g: **$3.95**

CONTRAINDICATIONS: Severe renal disease, hypersensitivity

PRECAUTIONS: Neonates (renal immaturity) and especially those born to mothers on magnesium sulfate therapy (respiratory arrest), mild renal disease, hearing deficits, elderly

PREGNANCY AND LACTATION: Pregnancy category D; small amounts excreted into breast milk; compatible with breast feeding (oral absorption poor)

SIDE EFFECTS/ADVERSE REACTIONS

CNS: Confusion, depression, numbness, tremors, ***seizures,*** muscle twitching, ***neurotoxicity***

CV: Hypotension, myocarditis, palpitations

EENT: ***Ototoxicity (especially vestibular toxicity),*** deafness, visual disturbances

GI: Nausea, vomiting, anorexia

GU: ***Oliguria, hematuria, renal damage, azotemia, renal failure, nephrotoxicity***

HEME: ***Agranulocytosis, thrombocytopenia, leukopenia, eosinophilia***

SKIN: Rash, burning, urticaria, dermatitis, alopecia

▼ DRUG INTERACTIONS

Drugs

- *Amphotericin B, cephalosporins, cyclosporine, NSAIDs:* Increased nephrotoxicity
- *Ethacrynic acid, other aminoglycosides:* Increased ototoxicity
- *Extended spectrum penicillins:* Inactivation of aminoglycoside
- *Neuromuscular blocking agents:* Respiratory depression
- *Oral anticoagulants:* Enhanced hypoprothrombinemic response

SPECIAL CONSIDERATIONS

MONITORING PARAMETERS

- Serum drug levels; therapeutic peak levels 20-30 μg/ml, toxic peak levels (1 hr after IM administration) >50 μg/ml
- Keep patient well hydrated

succimer

(sux'sim-mer)

Chemet

Chemical Class: Analog of dimercaprol

Therapeutic Class: Heavy metal chelating agent

CLINICAL PHARMACOLOGY

Mechanism of Action: Forms water soluble chelates with heavy metals which are excreted renally

Pharmacokinetics

PO: Rapidly but incompletely absorbed; peak 1-2 hr; metabolized to mixed succimer-cysteine disulfides; $t_{1/2}$ 2 days; excreted in urine, mostly as metabolite, and feces

INDICATIONS AND USES: Treatment of lead poisoning in children with blood levels >45 μg/dL; not for prophylaxis; may be of benefit in mercury* and arsenic* poisoning

DOSAGE

Adult and Child

- PO 10 mg/kg/dose q8h for 5 days, then 10 mg/kg/dose q12h for 14 days; may repeat if indicated by blood lead level; allow 2 wk between courses

$ AVAILABLE FORMS/COST OF THERAPY

- Cap, Gel—Oral: 100 mg, 100's: **$318.00**

CONTRAINDICATIONS: Hypersensitivity

PRECAUTIONS: Reduced renal function, history of liver disease, children <1 yr age

PREGNANCY AND LACTATION: Pregnancy category C; excretion in breast milk unknown, discourage mothers from breast feeding during therapy

SIDE EFFECTS/ADVERSE REACTIONS

CNS: Drowsiness, dizziness, paresthesias, headache

GI: Nausea, vomiting, diarrhea, anorexia, metallic taste

GU: Voiding difficulty, proteinuria

SKIN: Rash, pruritis, mucocutaneous eruptions

RESP: Cough

MISC: Chills, fever, flu-like symptoms

▼ **DRUG INTERACTIONS**

Drugs

- *Other chelators (e.g., EDTA):* Co-administration not recommended

Labs

- *Increase:* LFT's, cholesterol
- *False positive:* Urinary ketones
- *False decrease:* Serum uric acid, CPK

SPECIAL CONSIDERATIONS

PATIENT/FAMILY EDUCATION

- In children unable to swallow capsule, separate capsule and sprinkle beads on food or on spoon followed by fruit drink

MONITORING PARAMETERS

- Serum transaminases at start of therapy then qwk during therapy
- After therapy monitor for rebound (because of redistribution of lead from bound stores to soft tissues, blood) qwk until stable

sucralfate

(soo-kral′ fate)

Carafate, Sulcrate ♣

Chemical Class: Aluminum salt of sulfated sucrose

Therapeutic Class: Antiulcer agent, gastric mucosa protectant

CLINICAL PHARMACOLOGY

Mechanism of Action: Forms a complex that adheres to ulcer site, protects against acid, pepsin, bile salts

Pharmacokinetics

PO: Minimally absorbed; duration up to 5 hr; excreted in feces (90%)

INDICATIONS AND USES: Duodenal ulcer, gastric ulcers,* reflux esophagitis,* NSAID-induced GI symptoms,* prevention of stress ulcers,* oral and esophageal radiation-induced ulcers (suspension)*

DOSAGE

Adult

- *Active ulcer:* PO 1 g qid 1 hr ac, hs for 4-8 wk
- *Maintenance:* PO 1 g bid

$ **AVAILABLE FORMS/COST OF THERAPY**

- Susp—Oral: 1 g/10 ml, 420 ml: **$29.02**
- Tab, Uncoated—Oral: 1 g, 100's: **$73.69-$84.00**

CONTRAINDICATIONS: Hypersensitivity

PRECAUTIONS: Renal failure, dialysis (small amounts aluminum absorbed with sucralfate)

PREGNANCY AND LACTATION: Pregnancy category B; little systemic absorption so minimal, if any, excretion into milk expected

SIDE EFFECTS/ADVERSE REACTIONS

CNS: Drowsiness, dizziness, headache, vertigo

EENT: ***Laryngospasm***
GI: Dry mouth, constipation, nausea, gastric pain, vomiting, diarrhea, indigestion
SKIN: Urticaria, rash, pruritus

▼ **DRUG INTERACTIONS**

Drugs

• *Quinolones:* Reduced antibiotic levels

---

sufentanil

(soo-fen′ ta-nil)
Sufenta

Chemical Class: Opiate, synthetic
Therapeutic Class: Narcotic analgesic, anesthetic
DEA Class: Schedule IV

CLINICAL PHARMACOLOGY

Mechanism of Action: Inhibits ascending pain pathways in CNS, increases pain threshold, alters pain perception

Pharmacokinetics

IV: Onset 1.3-3 min; $t_{1/2}$ 2½ hr; metabolized by liver, excreted in urine; crosses placenta

INDICATIONS AND USES: Primary anesthetic (doses ≥8 µg/kg), adjunct to general anesthetic (doses ≤8 µg/kg)

DOSAGE

Adult

• Use lean body weight in patients >20% above ideal body weight to calculate dose

• *Primary anesthetic:* IV 8-30 µg/kg given with 100% O_2, a muscle relaxant

• *Adjunct:* IV 2-8 µg/kg given with nitrous oxide/O_2

Children (<12 yr)

• *Induction anesthesia:* IV 10-25 µg/kg with 100% O_2

• *Maintenance of anesthesia:* IV Supplemental doses of 25-50 µg recommended, based on response

$ AVAILABLE FORMS/COST OF THERAPY

• Inj, Sol—IM;IV: 50 µg/ml, 1 ml: **$13.57**

CONTRAINDICATIONS: Hypersensitivity, acute asthma, upper airway obstruction

PRECAUTIONS: Substance abuse, increased intracranial pressure, MI (acute), cardiogenic shock, hypovolemia, COPD, cor pulmonale, hepatic disease, renal disease, child <18 yr

PREGNANCY AND LACTATION: Pregnancy category C; embryocidal effects in animal models; may enter breast milk

SIDE EFFECTS/ADVERSE REACTIONS

CNS: Drowsiness, dizziness, confusion, headache, sedation, euphoria
CV: Palpitations, bradycardia, ***cardiac arrest, hypotension***
EENT: Tinnitus, blurred vision, miosis, diplopia
GI: Nausea, vomiting, anorexia, constipation, cramps
GU: Increased urinary output, dysuria, urinary retention
MS: Intraoperative muscle movement
RESP: ***Respiratory depression***
SKIN: Rash, urticaria, bruising, flushing, diaphoresis, pruritus

▼ **DRUG INTERACTIONS**

Drugs

• *Nitrous oxide:* Cardiovascular depression with high dose sufentanil

Labs

• *Increase:* Amylase, lipase

sulfacetamide

(sul-fa-see'ta-mide)

AK-Sulf, Bleph-10, Cetamide, Isopto Cetamide, Ocusulf-10, Ophthacet, Sebizon, Sodium Sulamyd, Soss-10, Sulf-10, Sulf-15, Sulfair 15

Chemical Class: Sulfonamide
Therapeutic Class: Antibiotic

CLINICAL PHARMACOLOGY

Mechanism of Action: Inhibits bacterial synthesis of dihydrofolic acid by preventing the condensation of the pteridine with aminobenzoic acid through competitive inhibition of the enzyme dihydropteroate synthetase; bacteriostatic

Pharmacokinetics

OPHTH: Some systemic absorption, excreted mostly unchanged in urine, $t_{1/2}$ 7-13 hr

INDICATIONS AND USES: Conjunctivitis, corneal ulcer, superficial ocular infections, trachoma (adjunct to systemic sulfonamide therapy), seborrheic dermatitis, seborrhea sicca (dandruff), secondary bacterial infections of skin

DOSAGE

Adult and child >2 mo (>12 yr for TOP lotion)

• *Conjunctivitis/corneal ulcer:* OPHTH instill 1 gtt in lower conjunctival sac(s) q1-3h according to severity of infection; apply ¼″ ribbon of ointment to lower conjunctival sac(s) 1-4 times/d and hs

• *Trachoma:* OPHTH instill 2 gtt of 30% sol q2h (in conjunction with systemic sulfonamide therapy)

• *Seborrheic dermatitis/dandruff:* TOP apply lotion hs and allow to remain overnight; may use bid for severe cases with crusting, heavy scaling, and inflammation

$ AVAILABLE FORMS/COST OF THERAPY

• Oint—Ophth: 10%, 3.5 g: **$1.30-$14.86**

• Sol—Ophth: 10%, 5, 15 ml:**$4.17-$18.16;** 15%, 15 ml: **$1.63-$16.13;** 30%, 15 ml: **$5.06-$19.26**

• Lotion—Top: 10%, 85 g: **$18.25**

CONTRAINDICATIONS: Hypersensitivity to sulfonamides; infants <2 mo; epithelial herpes simplex keratitis, vaccinia, varicella, and many other viral diseases of the cornea and conjunctiva; mycobacterial infection or fungal diseases of the ocular structures

PRECAUTIONS: Severe dry eye, children

PREGNANCY AND LACTATION: Pregnancy category B (category D if used near term); compatible with breast feeding in healthy, full-term infants

SIDE EFFECTS/ADVERSE REACTIONS

CNS: Headache, fever

EENT: Blurred vision (especially with ointment), local irritation, itching, transient epithelial keratitis, reactive hyperemia, conjunctival edema, burning, transient stinging, browache

METAB: ***Bone marrow depression***

SKIN: ***Stevens-Johnson syndrome, exfoliative dermatitis, toxic epidermal necrolysis,*** photosensitivity, rash

▼ DRUG INTERACTIONS

Drugs

• *Silver preparations:* Incompatible with sulfacetamide

SPECIAL CONSIDERATIONS

PATIENT/FAMILY EDUCATION

• May cause sensitivity to bright light

• Do not touch tip of container to any surface

sulfadiazine

(sul-fa-dye'a-zeen)
Microsulfon
Chemical Class: Sulfonamide
Therapeutic Class: Antibiotic

CLINICAL PHARMACOLOGY

Mechanism of Action: Interferes with bacterial synthesis of folic acid (pteroylglutamic acid) from aminobenzoic acid through competitive inhibition of the enzyme dihydropteroate synthetase; bacteriostatic

Pharmacokinetics

PO: Peak 3-6 hr, 32%-56% bound to plasma proteins, metabolized by N-acetylation, excreted in urine as unchanged drug (43%-60%) and metabolites (15%-40%), $t_{1/2}$ 10 hr

INDICATIONS AND USES: Chancroid, trachoma, inclusion conjunctivitis, nocardiosis, UTIs (primarily pyelonephritis, pyelitis, and cystitis), toxoplasmosis (adjunctive therapy with pyrimethamine), malaria (adjunctive therapy for chloroquine-resistant strains of *Plasmodium falciparum*), meningococcal meningitis prophylaxis (when sulfonamide-sensitive group A strains prevail), meningococcal meningitis (when organism has been demonstrated susceptible), acute otitis media due to *Haemophilus influenzae* (when used concomitantly with penicillin or erythromycin), rheumatic fever prophylaxis (alternative to penicillin), *H. influenzae* meningitis (adjunctive therapy with parenteral streptomycin)

Antibacterial spectrum usually includes:

- Gram-positive organisms: Some strains of staphylococci, streptococci, *Bacillus anthracis, Clostridium tetani, C. perfringens,* many strains of *Nocardia asteroides* and *N. brasiliensis*
- Gram-negative organisms: *Enterobacter, Escherichia coli, Klebsiella, Proteus mirabilis, P. vulgaris, Salmonella, Shigella*
- Miscellaneous organisms: *Toxoplasma gondii, Plasmodium*

DOSAGE

Adult

- PO 2-4 g initially, followed by 2-4 g/d divided in 3-6 doses
- *Rheumatic fever prophylaxis:* PO 1 g qd (should not be used for treatment)
- *Nocardiosis:* PO 4-8 g/d in divided doses for minimum of 6 wk
- *Meningococcal meningitis prophylaxis:* PO 1 g bid for 2 days
- *Malaria:* PO 500 mg qid for 5 days in conjunction with quinine and pyrimethamine
- *Toxoplasmosis:* PO 2-8 g/d in divided doses in conjunction with pyrimethamine for 3-4 wk (up to 6 mo may be required in immunocompromised patients)

Child >2 mo

- PO 75 mg/kg initially followed by 150 mg/kg/d in 4-6 divided doses; do not exceed 6 g/d
- *Rheumatic fever prophylaxis:* PO (<30 kg) 500 mg qd
- *Meningococcal meningitis prophylaxis:* PO 1-12 yr 500 mg bid for 2 days; 2-12 mo 500 mg qd for 2 days
- *Malaria:* PO 25-50 mg/kg qid for 5 days; do not exceed 2 g/d
- *Toxoplasmosis:* PO 100-200 mg/kg/d in divided doses

$ AVAILABLE FORMS/COST OF THERAPY

- Tab, Uncoated—Oral: 500 mg, 100's: **$16.50-$50.25**

CONTRAINDICATIONS: Hypersensitivity to sulfonamides, infants <2 mo, porphyria

PRECAUTIONS: Group A β-hemolytic streptococcal infections (do not use for treatment), renal or hepatic function impairment, allergy or asthma, G-6-PD deficiency

PREGNANCY AND LACTATION: Pregnancy category B (category D if used near term); may cause jaundice, hemolytic anemia and kernicterus in newborns; excreted into breast milk in low concentrations, compatible with breast feeding in healthy, full-term infants

SIDE EFFECTS/ADVERSE REACTIONS

CNS: Headache, peripheral neuropathy, mental depression, ***seizures,*** ataxia, hallucinations, insomnia, drowsiness, transient lesions of posterior spinal column, transverse myelitis, apathy

CV: ***Allergic myocarditis***

EENT: Conjunctival and scleral injection, tinnitus, vertigo, hearing loss

GI: Nausea, vomiting, abdominal pains, diarrhea, anorexia, ***pancreatitis,*** stomatitis, ***hepatitis, hepatocellular necrosis, pseudomembranous colitis,*** glossitis

GU: ***Crystalluria, hematuria, proteinuria,*** elevated creatinine, ***nephrotic syndrome, toxic nephrosis with oliguria and anuria***

HEME: ***Agranulocytosis, aplastic anemia, thrombocytopenia, leukopenia, hemolytic anemia, methemoglobinemia, megaloblastic anemia,*** purpura

MS: Arthralgia

RESP: Transient pulmonary changes, pulmonary infiltrates

SKIN: Erythema multiforme, ***Stevens-Johnson syndrome, exfoliative dermatitis,*** photosensitivity

▼ **DRUG INTERACTIONS**

Drugs

• *Antidiabetics:* Enhanced hypoglycemic effects of oral antidiabetic agents

• *Cyclosporine:* Additive nephrotoxicity; reduced plasma concentrations of cyclosporine

• *PABA:* PABA may interfere with antibacterial activity of sulfonamides

Labs

• *False positive:* Urinary glucose tests (Benedict's method)

SPECIAL CONSIDERATIONS

PATIENT/FAMILY EDUCATION

• Avoid prolonged exposure to sunlight

• Notify physician of blood in urine, rash, ringing in ears, difficulty breathing, fever, sore throat, chills, blister on mucous membrane

• Ensure adequate fluid intake

• Administer with full glass of water

MONITORING PARAMETERS

• CBC, renal function tests, urinalysis

---

sulfamethizole

(sul-fa-meth'i-zole)

Thiosulfil Forte

Chemical Class: Sulfonamide

Therapeutic Class: Antibiotic

CLINICAL PHARMACOLOGY

Mechanism of Action: Interferes with bacterial synthesis of folic acid (pteroylglutamic acid) from aminobenzoic acid through competitive inhibition of the enzyme dihydropteroate synthetase; bacteriostatic

Pharmacokinetics

PO: Peak 2 hr, 90% bound to plasma proteins, metabolized by acetylation (2%-9%), excreted in urine (90%-95% unchanged)

INDICATIONS AND USES: UTIs caused by susceptible strains of the following organisms: *E. coli, Klebsiella, Enterobacter, Staphylococcus aureus, Proteus mirabilis,* and *P. vulgaris*

DOSAGE

Adult

• PO 0.5-1 g tid-qid

S

Child >2 mo

• PO 30-45 mg/kg/d divided qid

$ AVAILABLE FORMS/COST OF THERAPY

• Tab, Uncoated—Oral: 0.5 g, 100's: **$57.33**

CONTRAINDICATIONS: Hypersensitivity to sulfonamides, infants <2 mo, porphyria

PRECAUTIONS: Renal or hepatic function impairment, allergy or asthma, G-6-PD deficiency

PREGNANCY AND LACTATION: Pregnancy category B (category D if used near term); may cause jaundice, hemolytic anemia and kernicterus in newborns; excreted into breast milk in low concentrations, compatible with breast feeding in healthy, full-term infants

SIDE EFFECTS/ADVERSE REACTIONS

CNS: Headache, peripheral neuropathy, mental depression, ***seizures,*** ataxia, hallucinations, insomnia, drowsiness, transient lesions of posterior spinal column, transverse myelitis, apathy

CV: ***Allergic myocarditis***

EENT: Conjunctival and scleral injection, tinnitus, vertigo, hearing loss

GI: Nausea, vomiting, abdominal pains, diarrhea, anorexia, ***pancreatitis,*** stomatitis, ***hepatitis, hepatocellular necrosis, pseudomembranous colitis,*** glossitis

GU: ***Crystalluria, hematuria, proteinuria,*** elevated creatinine, ***nephrotic syndrome, toxic nephrosis with oliguria and anuria***

HEME: ***Agranulocytosis, aplastic anemia, thrombocytopenia, leukopenia, hemolytic anemia, methemoglobinemia, megaloblastic anemia,*** purpura

MS: Arthralgia

RESP: Transient pulmonary changes, pulmonary infiltrates

SKIN: Erythema multiforme, ***Stevens-Johnson syndrome, exfoliative dermatitis,*** photosensitivity

▼ DRUG INTERACTIONS

Drugs

• *Antidiabetics:* Enhanced hypoglycemic effects of oral antidiabetic agents

• *Cyclosporine:* Additive nephrotoxicity; reduced plasma concentrations of cyclosporine

• *PABA:* PABA may interfere with antibacterial activity of sulfonamides

Labs

• *False positive:* Urinary glucose tests (Benedict's method); urinary protein (sulfosalicylic acid test)

• *Interference:* Urobilistix test

SPECIAL CONSIDERATIONS

PATIENT/FAMILY EDUCATION

• Avoid prolonged exposure to sunlight

• Notify physician of blood in urine, rash, ringing in ears, difficulty breathing, fever, sore throat, chills, blister on mucous membrane

• Ensure adequate fluid intake

• Administer with full glass of water

---

sulfamethoxazole

(sul-fa-meth-ox'a-zole)

Gantanol, Urobak

Chemical Class: Sulfonamide

Therapeutic Class: Antibiotic

CLINICAL PHARMACOLOGY

Mechanism of Action: Inhibits bacterial synthesis of folic acid (pteroylglutamic acid) from aminobenzoic acid through competitive inhibition of the enzyme dihydropteroate synthetase; bacteriostatic

Pharmacokinetics

PO: Peak 3-4 hr, widely distributed into most body tissues, 50%-70% bound to plasma proteins, metabolized in liver by acetylation (inactive metabolite contributes to nephrotoxicity), excreted mainly in urine

(20% unchanged, 70% acetylated metabolite), $t_{1/2}$ 7-12 hr (prolonged in renal failure)

INDICATIONS AND USES: Chancroid, trachoma, inclusion conjunctivitis, nocardiosis, UTIs (primarily pyelonephritis, pyelitis, and cystitis), toxoplasmosis (adjunctive therapy with pyrimethamine), malaria (adjunctive therapy of chloroquine-resistant strains of *Plasmodium falciparum),* meningococcal meningitis prophylaxis (when sulfonamide-sensitive group A strains prevail), acute otitis media due to *Haemophilus influenzae* (when used concomitantly with penicillin or erythromycin)

Antibacterial spectrum usually includes:

• Gram-positive organisms: Some strains of staphylococci, streptococci, *Bacillus anthracis, Clostridium tetani, C. perfringens,* many strains of *Nocardia asteroides* and *N. brasiliensis*

• Gram-negative organisms: *Enterobacter, Escherichia coli, Klebsiella, Proteus mirabilis, P. vulgaris, Salmonella, Shigella*

• Miscellaneous organisms: *Toxoplasma gondii, Plasmodium*

DOSAGE

Adult

• PO, Mild to moderate infections, 2 g initially, then 1 g bid; severe infections, 2 g initially, then 1 g tid

Child >2 mo

• PO 50-60 mg/kg initially, then 25-30 mg/kg bid; do not exceed 75 mg/kg/d

$ AVAILABLE FORMS/COST OF THERAPY

• Tab, Uncoated—Oral: 500 mg, 100's: **$11.30-$50.81**

CONTRAINDICATIONS: Hypersensitivity to sulfonamides, infants < 2 mo, porphyria

PRECAUTIONS: Group A β-hemolytic streptococcal infections (do not use for treatment), renal or hepatic function impairment, allergy or asthma, G-6-PD deficiency

PREGNANCY AND LACTATION: Pregnancy category B (category D if used near term); may cause jaundice, hemolytic anemia and kernicterus in newborns; excreted into breast milk in low concentrations, compatible with breast feeding in healthy, full-term infants

SIDE EFFECTS/ADVERSE REACTIONS

CNS: Headache, peripheral neuropathy, mental depression, ***seizures,*** ataxia, hallucinations, insomnia, drowsiness, transient lesions of posterior spinal column, transverse myelitis, apathy

CV: ***Allergic myocarditis***

EENT: Conjunctival and scleral injection, tinnitus, vertigo, hearing loss

GI: Nausea, vomiting, abdominal pains, diarrhea, anorexia, ***pancreatitis,*** stomatitis, ***hepatitis, hepatocellular necrosis, pseudomembranous colitis,*** glossitis

GU: ***Crystalluria, hematuria, proteinuria,*** elevated creatinine, ***nephrotic syndrome, toxic nephrosis with oliguria and anuria***

HEME: ***Agranulocytosis, aplastic anemia, thrombocytopenia, leukopenia, hemolytic anemia, methemoglobinemia, megaloblastic anemia,*** purpura

MS: Arthralgia

RESP: Transient pulmonary changes, pulmonary infiltrates

SKIN: Erythema multiforme, ***Stevens-Johnson syndrome, exfoliative dermatitis,*** photosensitivity

▼ DRUG INTERACTIONS

Drugs

• *Antidiabetics:* Enhanced hypoglycemic effects of oral antidiabetic agents

• *Cyclosporine:* Additive nephro-

toxicity; reduced plasma concentrations of cyclosporine
• *PABA:* PABA may interfere with antibacterial activity of sulfonamides

Labs
• *False positive:* Urinary glucose tests (Benedict's method)

SPECIAL CONSIDERATIONS

PATIENT/FAMILY EDUCATION
• Avoid prolonged exposure to sunlight
• Notify physician of blood in urine, rash, ringing in ears, difficulty breathing, fever, sore throat, chills, blister on mucous membrane
• Ensure adequate fluid intake
• Administer with full glass of water

MONITORING PARAMETERS
• CBC, renal function tests, urinalysis

---

sulfanilamide

(sul-fa-nil'a-mide)
AVC, Avitrol
Chemical Class: Sulfonamide
Therapeutic Class: Vaginal antiinfective

CLINICAL PHARMACOLOGY
Mechanism of Action: Inhibits bacterial synthesis of folic acid (pteroylglutamic acid) from aminobenzoic acid through competitive inhibition of the enzyme dihydropteroate synthetase; bacteriostatic

INDICATIONS AND USES: *Candidia albicans* vulvovaginitis

DOSAGE

Adult
• VAG (supp) insert 1 suppository qd-bid, continue for 30 days; (cream) 1 applicatorful qd-bid, continued through 1 complete menstrual cycle

$ **AVAILABLE FORMS/COST OF THERAPY**
• Cre—Vag: 15%, 120 g: **$10.52-$28.92**
• Supp—Vag: 1.05 g, 16's: **$31.50**

CONTRAINDICATIONS: Hypersensitivity to sulfonamides, kidney disease, pregnancy at term

PRECAUTIONS: Children

PREGNANCY AND LACTATION: Pregnancy category B (category D if used near term); may cause jaundice, hemolytic anemia, and kernicterus in newborns; excreted into breast milk in low concentrations, compatible with breast feeding in healthy, full-term infants

SIDE EFFECTS/ADVERSE REACTIONS
GU: Local irritation
HEME: ***Agranulocytosis***
SKIN: ***Stevens-Johnson syndrome*** (rare)
MISC: Allergic reactions

SPECIAL CONSIDERATIONS

PATIENT/FAMILY EDUCATION
• Insert high into vagina
• Do not engage in vaginal intercourse during treatment
• Complete full course of therapy

---

sulfasalazine

(sul-fa-sal'a-zeen)
Azulfidine, Azulfidine EN-Tabs, Salazopyrin 🍁
Chemical Class: Sulfonamide; salicylate
Therapeutic Class: Antiinflammatory

CLINICAL PHARMACOLOGY
Mechanism of Action: Precise mechanism of action unknown, diazo bond cleaved *in vivo* by colonic flora to provide sulfapyridine and 5-aminosalicylic acid (mesalamine); therapeutic action may be result of antibacterial action of sulfapyridine or antiinflammatory action of 5-aminosalicylic acid on the colon

Pharmacokinetics

PO: Unchanged drug 10%-15% absorbed; sulfapyridine rapidly absorbed, only small portion of 5-aminosalicylic acid absorbed, peak 1.5-6 hr (EC 3-12 hr), sulfapyridine distributed to most body tissues, sulfapyridine metabolized via acetylation in liver, most of sulfasalazine excreted in urine (unchanged 15%, sulfapyridine and metabolites 60%, 5-aminosalicylic acid and metabolites 20%-33%), unabsorbed 5-aminosalicylic acid excreted in feces, $t_{1/2}$ 8.4-10.4 hr

INDICATIONS AND USES: Ulcerative colitis, acute Crohn's disease,* rheumatoid arthritis,* granulomatous colitis,* scleroderma,* collagenous colitis*

DOSAGE

Adult

- PO 1 g tid-qid; do not exceed 6 g/d; maintenance 2 g/d divided q6h

Child >2 yr

- PO 40-60 mg/kg/d in 3-6 divided doses; maintenance 30 mg/kg/d in 4 divided doses

$ AVAILABLE FORMS/COST OF THERAPY

- Tab, Uncoated—Oral: 500 mg, 100's: **$11.63-$20.50**
- Tab, Enteric Coated—Oral: 500 mg, 100's: **$24.56**

CONTRAINDICATIONS: Hypersensitivity to sulfonamides, infants <2 yr, porphyria, intestinal or urinary tract obstructions, hypersensitivity to salicylates

PRECAUTIONS: Renal or hepatic function impairment, allergy or asthma, G-6-PD deficiency, blood dyscrasias

PREGNANCY AND LACTATION: Pregnancy category B (category D if used near term); kernicterus and severe neonatal jaundice have not been reported following maternal use even when given up to time of delivery; may adversely affect spermatogenesis in male patients with inflammatory bowel disease; excreted into breast milk, should be given to nursing mothers with caution because significant adverse effects (bloody diarrhea) may occur in some nursing infants

SIDE EFFECTS/ADVERSE REACTIONS

CNS: Headache, fever, transverse myelitis, ***convulsions, meningitis,*** transient lesions of the posterior spinal column, cauda equina syndrome, ***Guillain-Barre syndrome,*** peripheral neuropathy, mental depression, vertigo, insomnia, ataxia, hallucinations, drowsiness

CV: Vasculitis, ***pericarditis with or without tamponade, allergic myocarditis***

EENT: Periorbital edema, hearing loss, conjunctival and scleral injection, tinnitus

GI: Anorexia, nausea, vomiting, gastric distress, ***hepatitis, hepatic necrosis, pancreatitis,*** bloody diarrhea, impaired folic acid absorption, stomatitis, diarrhea, abdominal pains, neutropenic enterocolitis

GU: Reversible oligospermia, ***toxic nephrosis with oliguria and anuria, nephritis, nephrotic syndrome, hematuria, crystalluria, proteinuria, hemolytic-uremic syndrome***

HEME: ***Heinz body anemia, hemolytic anemia, aplastic anemia, agranulocytosis, leukopenia, megaloblastic (macrocytic) anemia,*** purpura, ***thrombocytopenia, hypoprothrombinemia, methemoglobinemia, congenital neutropenia, myelodysplastic syndrome***

MS: ***Rhabdomyolysis,*** arthralgias

RESP: Pneumonitis with or without eosinophilia, fibrosing alveolitis, pleuritis, ***cyanosis***

SKIN: Skin rash, pruritus, urticaria, erythema multiforme, ***Stevens-***

S

Johnson syndrome, exfoliative dermatitis, epidermal necrolysis (Lyell's syndrome) with corneal damage, parapsoriasis varioliformis acuta (Mucha-Habermann syndrome), photosensitization, alopecia

MISC: ***Anaphylaxis,*** serum sickness syndrome, polyarteritis nodosa

▼ **DRUG INTERACTIONS**

Drugs

- *Antidiabetics:* Enhanced hypoglycemic effects of oral antidiabetic agents
- *Beta blockers:* Reduced serum beta-blocker concentrations, separate doses by 2-3 hr
- *Cyclosporine:* Additive nephrotoxicity; reduced plasma concentrations of cyclosporine
- *Digitalis glycosides:* Reduced serum digoxin concentrations

Labs

- *False positive:* Urinary glucose tests (Benedict's method)

SPECIAL CONSIDERATIONS

PATIENT/FAMILY EDUCATION

- Take each dose with a full glass of water to avoid crystalluria
- Avoid prolonged exposure to sunlight
- Notify physician if skin rash, sore throat, fever, mouth sores, unusual bruising, bleeding occur

MONITORING PARAMETERS

- CBC, renal function tests, urinalysis

sulfathiazole/ sulfacetamide/ sulfabenzamide (triple sulfa)

(sul-fa-thye'a-zole/sul-fa-see'ta-mide/sul-fa-ben'za-mide)

Dayto Sulf, Gyne-Sulf, Sultrin Triple Sulfa, Trysul, V.V.S

Chemical Class: Sulfonamide

Therapeutic Class: Vaginal anti-infective

CLINICAL PHARMACOLOGY

Mechanism of Action: Inhibits bacterial synthesis of folic acid (pteroylglutamic acid) from aminobenzoic acid through competitive inhibition of the enzyme dihydropteroate synthetase; bacteriostatic

INDICATIONS AND USES: *Gardnerella vaginalis* vaginitis

DOSAGE

Adult

- VAG (tabs) insert 1 tab QAM and QPM for 10 days, repeat prn; (cream) insert 1 applicatorful bid for 4-6 days; treatment can then be reduced 50%-25%, repeat prn

$ **AVAILABLE FORMS/COST OF THERAPY**

- Cre—Vag: 3.7% sulfabenzamide/ 2.86% sulfacetamide/3.42% sulfathiazole, 78 g: **$4.04-$28.68**
- Tab, Uncoated—Vag: 184 mg sulfabenzamide/143.75 mg sulfacetamide/172.5 mg sulfathiazole, 20's: **$31.20**

CONTRAINDICATIONS: Hypersensitivity to sulfonamides, kidney disease, pregnancy at term

PRECAUTIONS: Children

PREGNANCY AND LACTATION: Pregnancy category B (category D if used near term); may cause jaundice, hemolytic anemia, and kernicterus in newborns; excreted into breast milk in low concentrations, compatible with breast feeding in healthy, full-term infants

SIDE EFFECTS/ADVERSE REACTIONS

GU: Local irritation

HEME: ***Agranulocytosis***

SKIN: ***Stevens-Johnson syndrome*** (rare)

MISC: Allergic reactions

SPECIAL CONSIDERATIONS

PATIENT/FAMILY EDUCATION

- Insert high into vagina
- Do not engage in vaginal intercourse during treatment
- Complete full course of therapy

---

sulfinpyrazone

(sul-fin-pyr′a-zone)

Anturan, ✤ Anturane

Chemical Class: Pyrazolidine derivative

Therapeutic Class: Uricosuric

CLINICAL PHARMACOLOGY

Mechanism of Action: Inhibits tubular reabsorption of uric acid; also has antithrombotic and platelet inhibitory effects; lacks antiinflammatory and analgesic properties

Pharmacokinetics

PO: Well absorbed, 98%-99% bound to plasma proteins, 50% excreted in urine unchanged, $t_{1/2}$ 2.2-3 hr

INDICATIONS AND USES: Chronic and intermittent gouty arthritis, prevention of recurrent MI (further study indicated),* prevention of systemic embolism in rheumatic mitral stenosis*

DOSAGE

Adult

- PO 200-400 mg/d in 2 divided doses initially, increase to 400-800 mg/d in 2 divided doses; use lowest dose that will control blood uric acid level

$ **AVAILABLE FORMS/COST OF THERAPY**

- Cap, Gel—Oral: 200 mg, 100's: **$28.13-$54.80**
- Tab, Uncoated—Oral: 100 mg, 100's: **$13.49-$34.04**

CONTRAINDICATIONS: Active peptic ulcer, symptoms of GI inflammation or ulceration, hypersensitivity to phenylbutazone or other pyrazoles, blood dyscrasias

PRECAUTIONS: Renal function impairment, healed peptic ulcer, dehydration, acute gout attack

PREGNANCY AND LACTATION: Pregnancy category C

SIDE EFFECTS/ADVERSE REACTIONS

GI: Upper GI disturbances, aggravation or reactivation of peptic ulcer

HEME: ***Anemia, leukopenia, agranulocytosis, thrombocytopenia, aplastic anemia***

RESP: Bronchoconstriction (patients with aspirin-induced asthma)

SKIN: Rash

▼ **DRUG INTERACTIONS**

Drugs

- *Antidiabetics:* Increased hypoglycemic effects
- *Beta blockers:* Reduced hypotensive effects of beta-blockers
- *Oral anticoagulants+:* Marked increases in hypoprothrombinemic response to oral anticoagulants
- *Probenecid:* Increased serum sulfinpyrazone concentrations, clinical importance unknown
- *Salicylates:* Inhibited uricosuric effect of sulfinpyrazone

SPECIAL CONSIDERATIONS

PATIENT/FAMILY EDUCATION

- Take with food, milk, or antacids to decrease stomach upset
- Avoid aspirin and other salicylate-containing products
- Drink plenty of fluids

MONITORING PARAMETERS
- Serum uric acid concentrations, renal function, CBC

sulfisoxizole

(suf-fi-sox'a-zole)
Gantrisin, Novosoxazole ♣
Chemical Class: Sulfonamide
Therapeutic Class: Antibiotic

CLINICAL PHARMACOLOGY
Mechanism of Action: Inhibits bacterial synthesis of folic acid (pteroylglutamic acid) from aminobenzoic acid through competitive inhibition of the enzyme dihydropteroate synthetase; bacteriostatic
Pharmacokinetics
PO: Peak 1-4 hr, 85% bound to plasma proteins, parent drug and acetylated metabolites excreted in urine, $t_{1/2}$ 4.6-7.8 hr
INDICATIONS AND USES: Chancroid, trachoma, inclusion conjunctivitis, nocardiosis, UTIs (primarily pyelonephritis, pyelitis, and cystitis), toxoplasmosis (adjunctive therapy with pyrimethamine), malaria (adjunctive therapy of chloroquine-resistant strains of *Plasmodium falciparum),* meningococcal meningitis prophylaxis (when sulfonamide-sensitive group A strains prevail), meningococcal meningitis (when organism has been demonstrated susceptible), acute otitis media due to *Haemophilus influenzae* (when used concomitantly with penicillin or erythromycin), *H. influenzae* meningitis (adjunctive therapy with parenteral streptomycin), recurrent otitis media*
Antibacterial spectrum usually includes:
- Gram-positive organisms: some strains of staphylococci, streptococci, *Bacillus anthracis, Clostridium tetani, C. perfringens,* many strains of *Nocardia asteroides* and *N. brasiliensis*
- Gram-negative organisms: *Enterobacter, Escherichia coli, Klebsiella, Proteus mirabilis, P. vulgaris, Salmonella, Shigella*
- Miscellaneous organisms: *Toxoplasma gondii, Plasmodium*

DOSAGE
Adult
- PO 4-8 g/d in 4-6 divided doses

Child >2 mo
- PO 75 mg/kg initially, then 120-150 mg/kg/d in 4-6 divided doses; max 6 g/d

$ **AVAILABLE FORMS/COST OF THERAPY**
- Tab, Uncoated—Oral: 500 mg, 100's: **$9.99-$22.94**
- Susp—Oral: 500 mg/5ml, 120 ml: **$11.64**

CONTRAINDICATIONS: Hypersensitivity to sulfonamides, infants <2 mo, porphyria
PRECAUTIONS: Group A β-hemolytic streptococcal infections (do not use for treatment), renal or hepatic function impairment, allergy or asthma, G-6-PD deficiency
PREGNANCY AND LACTATION: Pregnancy category B (category D if used near term); may cause jaundice, hemolytic anemia, and kernicterus in newborns; excreted into breast milk in low concentrations, compatible with breast feeding in healthy, full-term infants
SIDE EFFECTS/ADVERSE REACTIONS
CNS: Headache, peripheral neuropathy, mental depression, ***seizures,*** ataxia, hallucinations, insomnia, drowsiness, transient lesions of posterior spinal column, transverse myelitis, apathy
CV: ***Allergic myocarditis***
EENT: Conjunctival and scleral infection, tinnitus, vertigo, hearing loss
GI: Nausea, vomiting, abdominal

pains, diarrhea, anorexia, ***pancreatitis,*** stomatitis, ***hepatitis, hepatocellular necrosis, pseudomembranous colitis,*** glossitis
GU: ***Crystalluria, hematuria, proteinuria,*** elevated creatinine, ***nephrotic syndrome, toxic nephrosis with oliguria and anuria***
HEME: ***Agranulocytosis, aplastic anemia, thrombocytopenia, leukopenia, hemolytic anemia, methemoglobinemia, megaloblastic anemia,*** purpura
MS: Arthralgia
RESP: Transient pulmonary changes, pulmonary infiltrates
SKIN: Erythema multiforme, ***Stevens-Johnson syndrome, exfoliative dermatitis,*** photosensitivity

▼ **DRUG INTERACTIONS**

Drugs

- *Antidiabetics:* Enhanced hypoglycemic effects of oral antidiabetic agents
- *Cyclosporine:* Additive nephrotoxicity; reduced plasma concentrations of cyclosporine
- *PABA:* PABA may interfere with antibacterial activity of sulfonamides

Labs

- *False positive:* Urinary glucose tests (Benedict's method); urinary protein (sulfosalicylic acid test)
- *Interference:* Urobilistix test

SPECIAL CONSIDERATIONS

PATIENT/FAMILY EDUCATION

- Avoid prolonged exposure to sunlight
- Notify physician of blood in urine, rash, ringing in ears, difficulty breathing, fever, sore throat, chills, blister on mucous membrane
- Ensure adequate fluid intake
- Administer with full glass of water

MONITORING PARAMETERS

- CBC, renal function tests, urinalysis

sulindac

(sul-in'dak)
Clinoril, Novosudac ♣
Chemical Class: Acetic acid derivative
Therapeutic Class: Nonsteroidal antiinflammatory drug (NSAID)

CLINICAL PHARMACOLOGY

Mechanism of Action: Sulfide metabolite inhibits cyclooxygenase activity and prostaglandin synthesis; other mechanisms such as inhibition of lipoxygenase, leukotriene synthesis, lysosomal enzyme release, neutrophil aggregation, and various cell-membrane functions may exist as well

Pharmacokinetics

PO: Onset of antirheumatic action within 7 days, peak 1-2 wk, peak serum levels 2-4 hr, sulindac is inactive until metabolized to active sulfide metabolite, excreted in urine primarily in biologically inactive forms (may possibly affect renal function to lesser extent than other NSAIDs), 25% excreted in feces, $t_{1/2}$ 7.8 hr (sulfide metabolite 16.4 hr)

INDICATIONS AND USES: Rheumatoid arthritis, osteoarthritis, ankylosing spondylitis, tendinitis, bursitis, acute painful shoulder, acute gout, juvenile rheumatoid arthritis,* sunburn*

DOSAGE

Adult

- PO 150-200 mg bid with food; max 400 mg/d

Child

- PO dose not established although 4 mg/kg/d divided bid have been used

$ **AVAILABLE FORMS/COST OF THERAPY**

- Tab, Uncoated—Oral: 150 mg,

100's: **$25.13-$97.35;** 200 mg, 100's: **$29.25-$119.64**

CONTRAINDICATIONS: Hypersensitivity to NSAIDs or aspirin

PRECAUTIONS: Bleeding tendencies, peptic ulcer, renal/hepatic function impairment, elderly, CHF, hypertension

PREGNANCY AND LACTATION: Pregnancy category B (category D if used in 3rd trimester); could cause constriction of the ductus arteriosus *in utero,* persistent pulmonary hypertension of the newborn or prolonged labor

SIDE EFFECTS/ADVERSE REACTIONS

CNS: Dizziness, headache, lightheadedness

CV: ***CHF,*** hypotension, hypertension, palpitation, dysrhythmias, tachycardia, edema, chest pain

EENT: Visual disturbances, photophobia, dry eyes, hearing disturbances, tinnitus

GI: Nausea, vomiting, diarrhea, constipation, abdominal cramps, *dyspepsia,* flatulence, ***gastric or duodenal ulcer with bleeding or perforation,*** occult blood in stool, ***hepatitis, pancreatitis***

HEME: ***Neutropenia, eosinophilia, leukopenia, pancytopenia, thrombocytopenia, agranulocytosis***

GU: ***Acute renal failure***

METAB: Hyperglycemia, hypoglycemia, hyperkalemia, hyponatremia

RESP: Dyspnea, bronchospasm, pulmonary infiltrates

SKIN: Rash, urticaria, photosensitivity

▼ **DRUG INTERACTIONS**

Drugs

• *Aminoglycosides:* Reduction of aminoglycoside clearance in premature infants

• *Furosemide:* Reduced diuretic and antihypertensive response to furosemide

• *Hydralazine:* Reduced antihypertensive response to hydralazine

• *Methotrexate:* Reduced renal clearance of methotrexate, increased toxicity

• *Oral anticoagulants:* Increased risk of bleeding due to adverse effects on GI mucosa and platelet function

• *Potassium sparing diuretics:* Acute renal failure

Labs

• *Increase:* Bleeding time

SPECIAL CONSIDERATIONS

PATIENT/FAMILY EDUCATION

• Avoid aspirin and alcoholic beverages

• Take with food, milk, or antacids to decrease GI upset

• Notify physician if edema, black stools, or persistent headache occurs

• Antirheumatic action may not be apparent for several weeks

MONITORING PARAMETERS

• CBC, BUN, serum creatinine, LFTs, occult blood loss

sumatriptan

(soo-ma-trip'tan)

Imitrex

Chemical Class: Serotonin agonist

Therapeutic Class: Anti-migraine

CLINICAL PHARMACOLOGY

Mechanism of Action: Selectively activates vascular 5-HT_1 receptors in cranial arteries causing vasoconstriction, an action correlating with the relief of migraine in humans

Pharmacokinetics

PO: Onset 1-1½ hr, peak 2-2½ hr

SC: Onset within 1 hr, peak 12 min Metabolized by microsomal monoamine oxidase (MAO), excreted in urine (60%) and feces (40%), $t_{1/2}$ 2½ hr

INDICATIONS AND USES: Acute migraine headache with or without aura, cluster headache*

DOSAGE

Adult

- SC 6 mg at first sign of headache or after completion of aura; may repeat if partial relief after 1 hr; max 12 mg/24 hr
- PO 25-100 mg at first sign of headache; may repeat q2h prn up to 300 mg/24 hr max; no evidence that doses larger than 25 mg provide substantially greater relief
- PO following SC single tablets (25-50 mg) may be repeated at 2 hr intervals up to 200 mg/24 hr max

$ AVAILABLE FORMS/COST OF THERAPY

- Inj, Sol—SC: 6 mg/0.5ml, 2's: **$70.22**
- Tab, Film Coated—Oral: 25 mg, 9's: **$96.60;** 50 mg, 9's: **$193.20**

CONTRAINDICATIONS: Hemiplegic or basilar migraine, IV inj (potential for coronary vasospasm), ischemic heart disease, Prinzmetal's angina, uncontrolled hypertension, hypersensitivity, within 24 hr of ergotamine-containing products

PRECAUTIONS: Atypical headache, renal or hepatic function impairment, elderly, children

PREGNANCY AND LACTATION: Pregnancy category C; excreted in breast milk in animals, no data in humans

SIDE EFFECTS/ADVERSE REACTIONS

CNS: Dizziness, drowsiness, headache, anxiety, fatigue

CV: Chest discomfort, ***dysrhythmia, coronary ischemia,*** hypertension, hypotension

EENT: Throat discomfort, vertigo, sinus discomfort, vision alterations

GI: Discomfort of mouth/tongue, reflux, diarrhea

MS: Weakness, neck pain/stiffness, myalgias, muscle cramps, jaw discomfort

SKIN: Inj site reaction, flushing, sweating

MISC: Atypical sensations, (tingling, warm/hot sensation, burning sensation, feeling of heaviness, pressure sensation, feeling of tightness, numbness, feeling strange, tight feeling in head, cold sensation)

▼ DRUG INTERACTIONS

Drugs

- *MAOIs:* Increased sumatriptan concentrations; clinical importance unestablished

SPECIAL CONSIDERATIONS

- First inj should be administered under medical supervision

PATIENT/FAMILY EDUCATION

- Use only to treat an actual migraine headache

suprofen

(soo-pro'fen)

Profenal

Chemical Class: Phenylalkanoic acid

Therapeutic Class: Ophthalmic nonsteroidal antiinflammatory drug (NSAID)

CLINICAL PHARMACOLOGY

Mechanism of Action: Inhibits miosis induced during ocular surgery by inhibiting the actions of prostaglandins which constrict the iris sphincter independently of cholinergic mechanisms

INDICATIONS AND USES: Inhibition of intraoperative miosis

DOSAGE

Adult

- OPHTH 2 gtt in conjunctival sac

3, 2, and 1 hr prior to surgery; may also instill 2 gtt q4h while awake the day preceding surgery

$ AVAILABLE FORMS/COST OF THERAPY

• Sol, Ophth—Top: 10 mg/ml, 2.5 ml: **$107.87**

CONTRAINDICATIONS: Epithelial herpes simplex keratitis, hypersensitivity

PRECAUTIONS: Known bleeding tendencies, concurrent use of anticoagulants, children

PREGNANCY AND LACTATION: Pregnancy category C

SIDE EFFECTS/ADVERSE REACTIONS

EENT: Transient burning and stinging, discomfort, itching, redness, iritis, pain, chemosis, photophobia, irritation, punctate epithelial staining

sutilains

(soo'ti-lains)

Travase

Chemical Class: Concentrate of proteolytic enzymes

Therapeutic Class: Topical debridement agent

CLINICAL PHARMACOLOGY

Mechanism of Action: Selectively digests necrotic soft tissues by proteolytic action; facilitates removal of necrotic tissues and purulent exudates that otherwise impair formation of granulation tissue and delay wound healing

Pharmacokinetics

TOP: Onset 60 min, peak effect 5-12 days with continuous use, duration 8-12 hr

INDICATIONS AND USES: Adjunct to established methods of wound care for biochemical debridement of second and third degree burns, decubitus ulcers, incisional, traumatic, and pyogenic wounds, ulcers secondary to peripheral vascular disease

DOSAGE

Adult and child

• TOP Thoroughly cleanse and irrigate wound then apply thin layer extending ¼"-½" beyond tissue being debrided; apply loose moist dressing; repeat tid-qid

$ AVAILABLE FORMS/COST OF THERAPY

• Oint—Top: 82,000 U/g, 14.2 g: **$43.69**

CONTRAINDICATIONS: Wounds communicating with major body cavities, wounds containing exposed major nerves or nervous tissue, fungating neoplastic ulcers, hypersensitivity

PRECAUTIONS: Application to >10%-15% of burned area at one time, children

PREGNANCY AND LACTATION: Pregnancy category B

SIDE EFFECTS/ADVERSE REACTIONS

SKIN: Mild transient pain, paresthesias, bleeding, transient dermatitis

SPECIAL CONSIDERATIONS

• A topical anti-infective should be used concurrently

PATIENT/FAMILY EDUCATION

• Discontinue use if bleeding or dermatitis occurs

• Avoid contact with eyes

tacrine

(tack'rin)

Cognex

Chemical Class: Cholinesterase inhibitor

Therapeutic Class: Dementia treatment

CLINICAL PHARMACOLOGY

Mechanism of Action: Centrally acting cholinesterase inhibitor; presumably elevates acetylcholine concentrations, a deficiency of acetylcholine may account for some clinical manifestations of mild to moderate dementia

Pharmacokinetics

PO: Rapidly absorbed, 55% bound to plasma proteins, metabolized by cytochrome P450 system in liver, elimination $t_{1/2}$ 2-4 hr

INDICATIONS AND USES: Treatment of mild to moderate dementia in Alzheimer's disease

DOSAGE

Adult

- PO 10 mg qid for 6 wk, then 20 mg qid for 6 wk, increase at 6-wk intervals if patient tolerating drug well, to dose of 120-160 mg/d in divided doses

$ AVAILABLE FORMS/COST OF THERAPY

- Cap, Gel—Oral: 10, 20, 30, 40 mg, 100's: **$119.69**

CONTRAINDICATIONS: Hypersensitivity to this drug or acridine derivatives, patients treated with this drug who developed jaundice (total bilirubin >3 mg/dl)

PRECAUTIONS: Sick sinus syndrome, history of ulcers, GI bleeding, hepatic disease, bladder obstruction, asthma

PREGNANCY AND LACTATION: Pregnancy category C; excretion into breast milk unknown

SIDE EFFECTS/ADVERSE REACTIONS

CNS: Dizziness, confusion, insomnia, tremor, ataxia, somnolence, anxiety, agitation, depression, hallucinations, hostility, abnormal thinking, chills, fever

CV: Hypotension, hypertension, bradycardia

GI: Nausea, vomiting, anorexia, transaminase elevation, dyspepsia, flatulence, *diarrhea,* ***hepatotoxicity***

GU: Frequency, UTI, incontinence

MS: Myalgia

SKIN: Rash, flushing

RESP: Rhinitis, URI, cough, pharyngitis, asthma

▼ DRUG INTERACTIONS

Drugs

- *Anticholinergics:* Inhibits anticholinergic effect, centrally acting anticholinergics may inhibit effect of tacrine
- *Beta blockers:* Additive bradycardia
- *Cholinergics:* Increased cholinergic effects
- *Cimetidine:* Increased tacrine levels
- *Levodopa:* Decreased levodopa effect
- *Neuromuscular blockers:* Prolonged effect of depolarizing neuromuscular blockers and antagonism of nondepolarizing agents
- *Quinolones:* Inhibition of tacrine metabolism
- *Smoking:* Markedly reduces tacrine levels

SPECIAL CONSIDERATIONS

- Transaminase elevation is the most common reason for withdrawal of drug (8%); monitor ALT q wk for first 18 weeks, then decrease to q 3 mo; when dose is increased monitor q wk for 6 weeks
- If elevations occur, modify dose as follows: ALT ≤3 times upper limit normal (ULN) continue current dose; ALT >3 to ≤5 times ULN reduce dose by 40 mg qd and resume dose titration when within normal limits; ALT >5 times ULN stop treatment; rechallenge may be tried if ALT is <10 times ULN
- Do not rechallenge if clinical jaundice develops

T

tamoxifen

(ta-mox'i-fen)

Nolvadex, Tamofen, ✤ Tamone ✤

Chemical Class: Nonsteroidal antiestrogen

Therapeutic Class: Antineoplastic

CLINICAL PHARMACOLOGY

Mechanism of Action: Competes with estrogen for receptor sites

Pharmacokinetics

PO: Extensively metabolized; peak 4-7 hr, $t_{1/2}$ 14 days (active metabolite), excreted primarily in feces

INDICATIONS AND USES: Adjuvant therapy of breast cancer of node-positive postmenopausal women; treatment of metastatic breast cancer in both women and men; most beneficial in estrogen receptor positive tumors; also used in mastalgia,* gynecomastia,* studies underway for use as prophylaxis in women at high risk for breast cancer*

DOSAGE

Adult

- PO 10-20 mg bid

$ AVAILABLE FORMS/COST OF THERAPY

- Tab, Uncoated—Oral: 10 mg, 60's: **$81.74-$86.14**

CONTRAINDICATIONS: Hypersensitivity

PRECAUTIONS: Leukopenia, thrombocytopenia, cataracts, liver disease, hypercalcemia, undiagnosed abnormal vaginal bleeding

PREGNANCY AND LACTATION: Pregnancy category D; excretion into breast milk unknown

SIDE EFFECTS/ADVERSE REACTIONS

CNS: Hot flashes, headache, lightheadedness, depression

CV: Chest pain

EENT: Ocular lesions, retinopathy, corneal opacity, blurred vision (high doses)

GI: Nausea, vomiting, altered taste, anorexia, abnormal liver function tests, ***hepatic necrosis***

GU: Vaginal bleeding, pruritus vulvae, irregular menses, ***endometrial cancer***

HEME: ***Thrombocytopenia, leukopenia, deep vein thrombosis***

METAB: Hypercalcemia

RESP: ***Pulmonary embolism***

SKIN: Rash, alopecia

▼ DRUG INTERACTIONS

Drugs

- Aminoglutethimide: Reduces tamoxifen concentrations

Labs

- *Increase:* Serum Ca, bilirubin, AST

teicoplanin

(tye-ko-pla'nin)

Targocid

Chemical Class: Glycopeptide structurally related to vancomycin

Therapeutic Class: Antibiotic

CLINICAL PHARMACOLOGY

Mechanism of Action: Interferes with cell wall synthesis by inhibiting peptidoglycan polymerization; bactericidal

Pharmacokinetics

PO: Minimally absorbed

IM: Peak 2-4 hr

Excreted unchanged in urine; terminal elimination $t_{1/2}$ 45-70 hr

INDICATIONS AND USES: Psuedomembranous colitis (PO), serious infections (skin and soft tissue, septicemia, bone and joint, endocarditis, respiratory tract, indwelling catheter-related infections, CAPD peritonitis) by gram positive bacteria including: *S. aureus,* and *S. epidermidis* (both methicillin-sensitive and -resistant strains), streptococci (viridans, groups B, D. F, G), *Enterococcus* (vancomycin sensitive strains), *Clostridium difficile, C. perfringens, Listeria monocytogenes, Corynebacterium jeikeium;* synergistic with aminoglycosides and imipenem, additive with rifampin

DOSAGE

• IM/IV Loading dose 6 mg/kg followed by 3 mg/kg/24 hr

• In renal insufficiency reduce dose or interval: for CrCl 40-60 ml/min halve dose or double interval; CrCl <40 ml/min, one third the dose or triple interval

• Dosage may need to be increased in children and in treatment of endocarditis

$ AVAILABLE FORMS/COST OF THERAPY

Due to be released early 1996 but release on hold as of 2/96

PRECAUTIONS: Renal insufficiency, hearing loss, liver disease, diabetes and immunocompromised patient (reduced efficacy)

SIDE EFFECTS/ADVERSE REACTIONS

CNS: Fatigue, headache

EENT: High frequency hearing loss (may be irreversible)

GI: Diarrhea, LFT elevation

GU: ***Nephrotoxicity***

HEME: Eosinophilia, ***reversible neutropenia,*** thrombocytosis

RESP: Bronchospasm

SKIN: Inj site pain, pruritis, urticaria, rash

MISC: ***Anaphylaxis***

▼ DRUG INTERACTIONS

Drugs

• *Aminoglycosides, imipenem:* Synergistic

• *Rifampin:* Additive

temazepam

(te-maz′e-pam)

Restoril

Chemical Class: Benzodiazepine

Therapeutic Class: Sedative-hypnotic

DEA Class: Schedule IV

CLINICAL PHARMACOLOGY

Mechanism of Action: Produces CNS depression at limbic, thalamic, hypothalamic levels of the CNS; may be mediated by neurotransmitter γ aminobutyric acid (GABA); results are sedation, hypnosis, skeletal muscle relaxation, anticonvulsant activity, anxiolytic action

Pharmacokinetics: Onset 30-45 min, peak 2-4 hr, duration 6-8 hr, $t_{1/2}$ 9.5-10.4 hr; metabolized by liver, excreted by kidneys, crosses placenta, excreted in breast milk

INDICATIONS AND USES: Insomnia

DOSAGE

Adult

• PO 15-30 mg hs

$ AVAILABLE FORMS/COST OF THERAPY

• Cap, Gel—Oral: 15 mg, 100's: **\$4.73-\$105.24;** 30 mg, 100's: **\$5.40-\$74.28**

CONTRAINDICATIONS: Hypersensitivity to benzodiazepines

PRECAUTIONS: Anemia, hepatic disease, renal disease, suicidal individuals, drug abuse, elderly, depression, psychosis, children <18 yr, acute narrow-angle glaucoma, seizure disorders, lung disease

PREGNANCY AND LACTATION: Pregnancy category X; may cause sedation and poor feeding in nursing infant

SIDE EFFECTS/ADVERSE REACTIONS

CNS: Lethargy, drowsiness, daytime sedation, dizziness, confusion, light-

T

headedness, headache, anxiety, irritability, rebound insomnia

CV: Chest pain, tachycardia, ***hypotension***

GI: Nausea, vomiting, diarrhea, heartburn, abdominal pain, constipation, anorexia

HEME: ***Leukopenia, granulocytopenia*** (rare)

RESP: ***Sleep apnea, respiratory depression***

▼ **DRUG INTERACTIONS**

Drugs

- *Cimetidine, disulfiram:* Increased benzodiazepine levels
- *Clozapine:* Possible increased risk of cardiorespiratory collapse
- *Ethanol:* Adverse psychomotor effects
- *Rifampin:* Reduced benzodiazepine levels

SPECIAL CONSIDERATIONS

PATIENT/FAMILY EDUCATION

- Withdrawal symptoms may occur if administered chronically and discontinued abruptly; symptoms include dysphoria, abdominal and muscle cramps, vomiting, sweating, tremor, and seizure
- May cause impairment the day following administration, exercise caution with hazardous tasks and driving

---

terazosin

(ter-a'zoe-sin)

Hytrin

Chemical Class: Quinazoline derivative, Alpha$_1$-adrenergic blocker

Therapeutic Class: Antihypertensive

CLINICAL PHARMACOLOGY

Mechanism of Action: Produces peripheral alpha$_1$-adrenergic blockade; reduces smooth muscle tone in prostate and bladder neck; reduces total peripheral resistance, lowering blood pressure

Pharmacokinetics

PO: Completely absorbed, peak 1 hr, $t_{1/2}$ 12 hr, excreted in urine (40%) and feces (60%), 70% as metabolites

INDICATIONS AND USES: Hypertension, benign prostatic hypertrophy (BPH)

DOSAGE

Adult

- *BPH:* PO 1 mg hs, increase to 2 mg, 5 mg, 10 mg/d (usual dose); not to exceed 20 mg/d; treatment at dose of 10 mg qd for 4-6 weeks necessary to determine response
- *Hypertension:* PO 1 mg hs; increase to desired response, usual dose 1-5 mg qd, max 20 mg/d; measure BP at end of dosing interval to determine if bid dose needed

$ AVAILABLE FORMS/COST OF THERAPY

- Cap, Gel—Oral: 1, 2, 5, 10 mg, 100's: **$126.99-$135.55**

CONTRAINDICATIONS: Hypersensitivity

PRECAUTIONS: Patients needing to perform hazardous tasks where syncope or dizziness could be dangerous

PREGNANCY AND LACTATION: Pregnancy category C; excretion into breast milk unknown

SIDE EFFECTS/ADVERSE REACTIONS

CNS: Dizziness, syncope (especially first days of therapy), *drowsiness,* depression, vertigo, weakness, fatigue, *headache,* paresthesia

CV: Palpitations, *postural hypotension,* hypotension, edema

EENT: Blurred vision, epistaxis, tinnitus, dry mouth, red sclera, *nasal congestion, sinusitis*

GI: Nausea

GU: Urinary frequency, incontinence, impotence

RESP: Dyspnea
MISC: Weight gain, ***anaphylaxis***

SPECIAL CONSIDERATIONS

• Marked lowering of BP with postural hypotension and syncope can occur ("first-dose" effect), especially during first week of therapy and after increases in dose; incidence of postural hypotension 4-5%
• Does not affect plasma PSA levels

PATIENT/FAMILY EDUCATION

• Always begin treatment at bedtime

terbinafine

(ter-been'a-feen)
Lamisil
Chemical Class: Synthetic allylamine derivative
Therapeutic Class: Topical antifungal

CLINICAL PHARMACOLOGY

Mechanism of Action: Inhibits fungal sterol biosynthesis, causing accumulation of squalene within the fungal cell and cell death
Pharmacokinetics: Small amounts absorbed systemically; metabolites excreted in urine

INDICATIONS AND USES: Tinea cruris, tinea corporis, tinea pedis, tinea versicolor;* active against *Epidermophyton floccosum, Trichophyton mentagrophytes, Trichophyton rubrum*

DOSAGE

Adult

• *Tinea pedis:* TOP apply bid for 1-4 weeks, until symptoms resolved
• *Tinea cruris/corporis:* TOP apply qd-bid for 1-4 weeks

$ AVAILABLE FORMS/COST OF THERAPY

• Cre—Top: 1%, 30 g: **$43.26**

CONTRAINDICATIONS: Hypersensitivity

PRECAUTIONS: Children <12 (safety and efficacy not established)

PREGNANCY AND LACTATION: Pregnancy category B; small amounts excreted into breast milk when administered orally; avoid application to the breast when breast feeding

SIDE EFFECTS/ADVERSE REACTIONS

SKIN: Irritation, burning, itching, dryness

terbutaline

(ter-byoo'te-leen)
Brethaire, Brethine, Bricanyl
Chemical Class: Selective $beta_2$-agonist
Therapeutic Class: Bronchodilator, tocolytic

CLINICAL PHARMACOLOGY

Mechanism of Action: Relaxes bronchial smooth muscle by direct action on $beta_2$-adrenergic receptors through accumulation of cAMP at beta-adrenergic receptor sites

Pharmacokinetics

PO: Onset ½ hr, peak 1-2 hr, duration 4-8 hr
SC: Onset 5-15 min, peak ½-1 hr, duration 1 ½-4 hr
INH: Onset 5-30 min, peak 1-2 hr, duration 3-6 hr
Excreted into breast milk.

INDICATIONS AND USES: Bronchospasm, premature labor*

DOSAGE

Adult

• *Bronchospasm:* INH 2 puffs separated by 1 minute, then q4-6h; PO 2.5-5 mg q8h to max 15 mg qd; SC 0.25 mg, may repeat once in 15-30 min
• *Premature labor:* SC 0.25 mg qh; IV INF 0.01 mg/min, increased by 0.005 mg q10min, not to exceed 0.025 mg/min; PO 5 mg q4h for 48 hr, then 5 mg q6h as maintenance for above doses

Child

• INH 1-2 puffs q 4-6h; PO 0.05 mg/kg/dose q8h, increased gradually to 0.15 mg/kg/dose to max daily dose 5 mg (<12 yr); SC 0.005-0.01 mg/kg/dose to max 0.4 mg/kg/dose q 15-20 min for 2 doses

$ **AVAILABLE FORMS/COST OF THERAPY**

• Inj, Sol—SC: 1 mg/ml, 1 ml: **$1.86-$2.62**

• Inh: 0.2 mg/spray, 7.5 ml:**$18.35-$20.75**

• Tab, Uncoated—Oral: 2.5 mg, 100's: **$25.39-$306.18;** 5 mg, 100's: **$36.56-$440.60**

CONTRAINDICATIONS: Hypersensitivity to sympathomimetics, narrow-angle glaucoma, tachydysrhythmias

PRECAUTIONS: Cardiac disorders, hyperthyroidism, diabetes mellitus, prostatic hypertrophy, lactation, elderly, hypertensive, glaucoma

PREGNANCY AND LACTATION: Pregnancy category B; compatible with breast feeding

SIDE EFFECTS/ADVERSE REACTIONS

CNS: Tremor, anxiety, insomnia, *headache, dizziness, shakiness, nervousness*

CV: Palpitations, tachycardia, hypertension, ***dysrhythmias, cardiac arrest, angina***

GI: Nausea, vomiting, elevated liver enzymes

terconazole

(ter-kon'a-zole)

Terazol 3, Terazol 7

Chemical Class: Triazole derivative

Therapeutic Class: Antifungal

CLINICAL PHARMACOLOGY

Mechanism of Action: Uncertain; may disrupt fungal cell membrane permeability

Pharmacokinetics Systemic absorption 5%-16%

INDICATIONS AND USES: Vulvovaginal candidiasis

DOSAGE

Adult

• VAG (Cream) 5 g (1 applicator) qhs for 3 (0.8%) or 7 (0.4%) days

• VAG (Supp) 1 qhs for 3 days

$ **AVAILABLE FORMS/COST OF THERAPY**

• Cre—Vag: 0.4%, 45 g: **$23.34;** 0.8%, 20 g: **$23.24**

• Supp—Vag: 80 mg, 3's: **$23.24**

CONTRAINDICATIONS: Hypersensitivity

PREGNANCY AND LACTATION: Pregnancy category C, systemic absorption occurs; excretion into breast milk unknown

SIDE EFFECTS/ADVERSE REACTIONS

CNS: Headache

GI: Abdominal pain

GU: Genital pain, vulvovaginal burning, itching, burning

SKIN: Photosensitivity reactions with repeated application under artificial UV light

terfenadine

(ter-fen'a-deen)

Seldane

Chemical Class: Butyrophenone derivative

Therapeutic Class: Antihistamine

CLINICAL PHARMACOLOGY

Mechanism of Action: Competes with histamine for H_1-receptor sites; prevents allergic responses mediated by histamine; no significant anticholinergic activity

Pharmacokinetics

PO: Onset of action 72 min, peak

effect 3-4 hr, duration of action >12 hr, $t_{1/2}$ 20.3 hr, 97% protein bound, eliminated in feces

INDICATIONS AND USES: Rhinitis, allergy symptoms

DOSAGE

Adult

- PO 60 mg bid

Child

- PO 30 mg bid (6-12 yr), 15 mg bid (3-6 yr)

$ **AVAILABLE FORMS/COST OF THERAPY**

- Tab, Plain Coated—Oral: 60 mg, 30's: **$36.78**

CONTRAINDICATIONS: Hypersensitivity, severe hepatic disease

PRECAUTIONS: Children <12 yr

PREGNANCY AND LACTATION: Pregnancy category C; excretion into breast milk unknown

SIDE EFFECTS/ADVERSE REACTIONS

CNS: Dizziness, poor coordination

CV: ***Life-threatening dysrhythmias*** (rare)

GI: Anorexia, increased liver function tests, dry mouth

GU: Urinary retention

RESP: Increased thick secretions

▼ **DRUG INTERACTIONS**

Drugs

- *Erythromycin+ clarithromycin, fluvoxamine, ketoconazole+, itraconazole, troleandomycin:* Increased terfenadine levels, prolonged QT interval, cardiac dysrythmias

Labs

- *False negative:* Skin allergy tests

testosterone

(tess-toss'ter-one)

Testoserone: Histerone-100, Tesamone, Testandro, Testosterone Aqueous

Testosterone cypionate: Dep-Andro 200, Depo-Testosterone, Depotest 200, Depotest 100, Duratest-200, Duratest-100

Testosterone enanthate: Andro L.A. 200, Andropository 200, Delatest, Delatestadiol, Delatestryl, Durathate-200

Testosterone propionate: Androlan, Testex

Methyltestosterone: Android, Oreton Methyl, Testred, Virilon

Transdermal System: Testoderm

Chemical Class: Testosterone and derivatives

Therapeutic Class: Androgenic anabolic steroid, antineoplastic

CLINICAL PHARMACOLOGY

Mechanism of Action: Increases weight by building body tissue, increases potassium, phosphorus, chloride, nitrogen levels, increases bone development

Pharmacokinetics: 98% protein bound, metabolized in liver, excreted in urine, breast milk; crosses placenta

Testosterone: IM $t_{1/2}$ 10-100 min TRANSDERM Peak 2-4 hr, returns to baseline 2 hr after removal

Testosterone cypionate: IM $t_{1/2}$ 8 days

Methyltestosterone: PO Peak concentration 1-2 hr; $t_{1/2}$ 2½-3½ hrs

INDICATIONS AND USES: Female breast cancer, eunuchoidism, male climacteric, oligospermia, impotence, osteoporosis, male hypogonadism, delayed male puberty

T

DOSAGE

Adult

• *Oligospermia:* IM 100-200 mg q4-6wk (cypionate or enanthate)

• *Breast cancer:* IM 50-100 mg 3 times/wk (propionate) or 200-400 mg q2-4wk (cypionate or enanthate); PO 50-200 mg qd, SUBLING 25-100 mg qd

• *Male climacteric/eunuchoidism/eunuchism/post pubertal cryptorchism:* IM 10-25 mg 2-4 times/wk (propionate), 50-400 mg q2-4 wk (cypionate or enanthate); PO 10-50 mg qd, SUBLING 5-25 mg qd, TRANSDERM place on scrotal skin, 6 mg/24 h

Child

• *Male hypogonadism:* Initiation of pubertal growth, IM 40-50 mg/m^2/dose (cypionate or enanthate) qmo until growth rate falls to prepubertal levels; terminal growth phase, IM 100 mg/m^2/dose (cypionate or enanthate) qmo until growth ceases, then twice/mo maintenance

• *Delayed puberty:* IM 40-50 mg/m^2/dose (cypionate or enanthate) qmo

$ AVAILABLE FORMS/COST OF THERAPY

Testosterone

• Film, Continuous Release—Percutaneous: 4 mg/24hr, 6 mg/24 hr, 30's: **$67.68**

• Inj, Susp—IM: 25 mg/ml, 10 ml: **$1.60-$4.90;** 50 mg/ml, 10 ml: **$2.40-$8.50;** 100 mg/ml, 10 ml: **$3.80-$18.38**

• Pellet—IV: 75 mg, 10's: **$150.00**

Testosterone cypionate

• Inj, Sol—IM: 100 mg/ml, 10 ml: **$6.65-$32.04;** 200 mg/ml, 10 ml: **$10.21-$57.48**

Testosterone enanthate

• Inj, Sol—IM: 100 mg/ml, 10 ml: **$10.90;** 200 mg/ml, 10 ml: **$10.31-$17.50**

Testosterone propionate

• Inj, Sol—IM: 25 mg/ml, 10 ml: **$1.60;** 50 mg/ml, 10 ml: **$2.40-$15.29;** 100 mg/ml, 10 ml: **$3.80-$17.40**

Methyltestosterone

• Tab, Uncoated—Oral: 10 mg, 100's: **$2.80-$130.06;** 25 mg, 100's: **$6.72-$325.13**

• Cap, Gel—Oral: 10 mg, 100's: **$43.20-$130.06**

• Tab, SL: 10 mg, 100's: **$5.00**

CONTRAINDICATIONS: Severe renal disease, severe cardiac disease, severe hepatic disease, hypersensitivity, genital bleeding (abnormal), male breast cancer, prostate cancer

PRECAUTIONS: Diabetes mellitus, CV disease, MI

PREGNANCY AND LACTATION: Pregnancy category X; excretion into breast milk unknown

SIDE EFFECTS/ADVERSE REACTIONS

CNS: Dizziness, headache, fatigue, tremors, paresthesias, flushing, sweating, anxiety, lability, insomnia, carpal tunnel syndrome, aggressive behavior, depression

CV: Increased B/P, edema, ***CHF***

EENT: Conjunctional edema, nasal congestion, deepening of voice

GI: Nausea, vomiting, constipation, weight gain, ***cholestatic jaundice, hepatocellular neoplasm***

GU: Amenorrhea, vaginitis, increased/decreased libido, decreased breast size, clitoral hypertrophy, testicular atrophy, priapism, gynecomastia

HEME: Polycythemia

METAB: Hyperglycemia, ***hypercalcemia*** (in breast cancer)

SKIN: Rash, acneiform lesions, oily hair and skin, flushing, sweating, acne vulgaris, alopecia, hirsutism

▼ DRUG INTERACTIONS

Drugs

• *Oral anticoagulants+:* Increased hypoprothrombinemic response

Labs

- *Increase:* Serum cholesterol, blood glucose, urine glucose
- *Decrease:* Serum Ca, serum K, T_4, T_3, thyroid ^{131}I uptake test, urine 17-OHCS, 17-KS, PBI

tetracaine

(tet'ra-cane)

Pontocaine; "Magic Numbing Solution" or TAC Solution (epinephrine 1:2,000, tetracaine 0.5%, cocaine 11.8%); LET Solution (lidocaine 4%, epeinephrine 0.1%, tetracaine 0.5%)

Chemical Class: PABA derivative ester

Therapeutic Class: Anesthetic

CLINICAL PHARMACOLOGY

Mechanism of Action: Decreases neuronal membrane permeability to sodium ions, blocking nerve impulses

Pharmacokinetics

INJ: Onset of action rapid, duration 2-3 hr

OPHTH: Onset of action 15 sec, duration 10-20 min

OPHTH, TOP: Onset of action 3-10 min, duration 30-60 min

TOP: Peak 3-8 min, duration 30-60 min

Hydrolyzed by plasma esterases, excreted by kidney

INDICATIONS AND USES: TOP: Pruritus, sunburn, toothache, sore throat, cold sores, oral pain, rectal pain and irritation, control of gagging; OPHTH: Cataract extraction, tonometry, gonioscopy, removal of foreign objects, corneal suture removal, glaucoma surgery; IV: Regional anesthesia; TOP TAC ("Magic Numbing Solution")/LET SOL: Topical anesthetic sol for repair of minor lacerations, especially in pediatric patients

DOSAGE

Adult and Child

- TOP Apply to affected area
- OPHTH Instill 1-2 gtt before procedure; TOP 0.5-1′ applied to lower conjunctival sac
- TOP TAC/LET Sol Apply 2-10 cc for 5-10 min (TAC) or 15 min (LET) with swab, cotton, gauze; tape or hold in place
- INJ 0.2%-0.3% sol for spinal anesthesia; for prolonged anesthesia (2-3 hr) 1% sol

$ **AVAILABLE FORMS/COST OF THERAPY**

- Inj, Sol—IV 1%, 2 ml: **$5.14;** 0.2%, 2 ml: **$5.01;** 0.3%, 2 ml: **$6.40**
- Sol—Ophth: 0.5%, 15 ml: **$2.31-$16.78**
- Sol—Top: 2%, 30 ml: **$22.04**
- Gel—Top: 2%, 60 g: **$7.10**

CONTRAINDICATIONS: Hypersensitivity to ester anesthetics, infants less than 1 yr, application to large areas, PABA allergies

PRECAUTIONS: Child <6 yr, sepsis, denuded skin

PREGNANCY AND LACTATION: Pregnancy category C; excretion into breast milk unknown

SIDE EFFECTS/ADVERSE REACTIONS

SKIN: Rash, irritation, sensitization burning, stinging, tenderness

▼ **DRUG INTERACTIONS**

Drugs

- *Sulfonamides:* Tetracaine metabolite inhibits sulfonamide action

T

tetracycline

(tet-ra-sye'kleen)

Systemic: Achromycin, Achromycin V, Cefracycline, ♣ Medicycline, ♣ Neo-Tetrine, ♣ Nor-Tet, Novotetra, ♣ Panmycin, Robitet, Sumycin 250, Sumycin 500, Sumycin Syrup, Teline, Teline 500, Tetracap, Tetracyn, Tetralan 250, Tetralan 500, Tetralan Syrup, Tetralean, ♣ Tetram

Ophthalmic: Achromycin Ophthalmic

Topical: Topicycline

Chemical Class: Tetracycline

Therapeutic Class: Broad-spectrum antibiotic

CLINICAL PHARMACOLOGY

Mechanism of Action: Inhibition of protein synthesis; bacteriostatic

Pharmacokinetics

PO: Peak 2-3 hr, duration 6 hr, t½ 6-10 hr; excreted in urine (60% unchanged), crosses placenta, excreted in breast milk, 20%-60% protein bound

INDICATIONS AND USES: Acne (systemic and topical); eye infection, ophthalmia neonatorum (ophthal); Infections caused by *Rickettsiae, Mycoplasma pneumoniae, Chlamydia trachomatis,* agents of psittacosis and ornithosis, agents of lymphogranuloma venereum and granuloma inguinale, the spirochetes *Borrelia recurrentis, Treponema pallidum* and *T. pertenue (yaws), Listeria monocytogenes, Bacillus anthracis, Haemophilus ducreyi, Yersinia pestis* and *Francisella tularensis, Bartonella bacilliformis,* Bacteroides sp, *Vibrio cholerae, Campylobacter fetus, Brucella* sp, *Neisseria gonorrhea;* adjunct to treatment of intestinal amebiasis; spectrum may include the following if susceptibility demonstrated: Gram-positive organisms, gram-negative organisms, some strains of *Streptococcus pyogenes, Str. faecalis,* Group A beta hemolytic-streptococci; *E. coli, Enterobacter aerogenes, Shigella, H. influenzae, Klebsiella* sp

DOSAGE

Adult

- PO 250-500 mg q6h; IM 250 mg/day or 150 mg q12h; IV 250-500 mg q8-12h
- *Gonorrhea:* PO 1.5 g, then 500 mg qid for a total of 9 g
- *Chlamydia:* PO 500 mg qid for 7 days
- *Syphilis:* PO 2-3 g in divided doses for 10-15 days; if syphilis duration >1 yr, must treat 30 days
- *Brucellosis:* PO 500 mg qid for 3 wk with 1 g streptomycin IM bid for 1 wk, and qd the second wk
- *Acne:* PO 250 mg qid; maintenance 125-500 mg qd; TOP Apply sol bid to affected area
- *Eye infection:* Instill sol or ointment bid-qid

Child (>8 yr)

- PO 25-50 mg/kg/d in divided doses q6h; IM 15-25 mg/kg/d in divided doses q8-12h; IV 10-20 mg/kg/d in divided doses q12h
- *Ophthalmia neonatorum* (neonate): TOP 1-2 gtt each eye post delivery

$ **AVAILABLE FORMS/COST OF THERAPY**

- Cap, Gel—Oral: 250 mg, 100's: **$3.30-$10.47;** 500 mg, 100's: **$4.88-$19.02**
- Tab, Coated—Oral: 250 mg, 100's: **$5.61;** 500 mg, 100's: **$10.91**
- Syr—Oral: 125 mg/5 ml, 480 ml: **$8.85-$10.85**
- Sol—Top: 2.2 mg/ml, 70 ml: **$49.55**
- Sol—Ophth: 1%, 4 ml: **$18.41**
- Oint—Ophth: 1%, 3 g: **$11.58**

• Inj, Dry-Sol—IM: 250 mg/vial: **$12.17;** 500 mg/vial: **$19.77**

CONTRAINDICATIONS: Hypersensitivity to tetracyclines, children <8 yr (systemic)

PRECAUTIONS: Renal disease, hepatic disease

PREGNANCY AND LACTATION: Pregnancy category D (systemic), category B (topical); systemic tetracycline excreted into breast milk in low concentrations; theoretically dental staining could occur but serum levels in infants undetectable and so considered compatible with breast feeding

SIDE EFFECTS/ADVERSE REACTIONS

CNS: Fever, headache ***(pseudotumor cerebri),*** paresthesia

CV: Pericarditis

EENT: Dysphagia, glossitis, decreased calcification of deciduous teeth, oral candidiasis, oral ulcers, esophagitis, poor corneal wound healing (ophth)

GI: Nausea, abdominal pain, *vomiting, diarrhea,* anorexia, enterocolitis, ***hepatotoxicity,*** flatulence, abdominal cramps, epigastric burning, stomatitis

GU: Increased BUN

HEME: ***Eosinophilia, neutropenia, thrombocytopenia, hemolytic anemia***

SKIN: Rash, urticaria, photosensitivity, increased pigmentation, ***exfoliative dermatitis,*** pruritus, ***angioedema,*** *stinging* (top)

▼ DRUG INTERACTIONS

Drugs

• *Antacids+, bismuth subsalicylate, food or products containing calcium+, magnesium+, zinc+, iron, sodium bicarbonate:* Reduced tetracycline concentrations

• *Oral contraceptives:* Possible decreased contraceptive effect

• *Methoxyflurane+:* Increased renal toxicity

• *Penicillin:* Impaired efficacy of penicillin

Labs

• *False negative:* Urine glucose with Clinistix or Tes-Tape

• *False increase:* Urinary catecholamines

SPECIAL CONSIDERATIONS

PATIENT/FAMILY EDUCATION

• Avoid milk products, antacids, or separate by 2 hr; take with a full glass of water

• Use in children ≤8 yr causes permanent discoloration of teeth, enamel hypoplasia, and retardation of skeletal development; risk greatest for children <4 yrs and receiving high doses

• Side effects noted for systemic administration not observed with topical formulations

tetrahydrozoline

(tet-ra-hi-droz′o-leen)

Ophthalmic: Collyrium Fresh Eye Drops, Eyesine, Murine Plus Eye Drops, Optigene 3 Eye Drops, Soo Drops, Visine Eye Drops

Nasal: Tyzine HCl, Tyzine Pediatric

Chemical Class: Direct sympathomimetic amine

Therapeutic Class: Ophthalmic and nasal vasoconstrictor

CLINICAL PHARMACOLOGY

Mechanism of Action: Produces vasoconstriction of eye and nasal arterioles

Pharmacokinetics

TOP: Duration 2-3 hr

INDICATIONS AND USES: Nasal sol: Decongestion of nasal and nasopharyngeal mucosa; Ophthal sol:

Ocular congestion, irritation, itching, redness

DOSAGE

Adult

- Nasal sol, instill 2-4 gtt/sprays 0.1% sol in each nostril q 4-8 h
- Ophthal sol, instill 1-2 gtt in affected eye up to qid

Child (2-6 yr)

- Nasal sol, instill 2-3 gtt 0.05% sol in each nostril q4-6h

$ AVAILABLE FORMS/COST OF THERAPY

- Aer, Spray—Nasal: 0.1%, 15 ml: **$9.01**
- Sol—Nasal: 0.05%, 15 ml: **$8.82;** 0.1%, 30 ml: **$11.04**
- Sol—Ophth: 0.05%, 30 ml: **$2.50**

CONTRAINDICATIONS: Hypersensitivity, narrow-angle glaucoma

PRECAUTIONS: Severe hypertension, diabetes, hyperthyroidism, elderly, severe arteriosclerosis, cardiac disease, infants, diabetes, asthma, CAD

PREGNANCY AND LACTATION: Pregnancy category C; excretion into breast milk unknown

SIDE EFFECTS/ADVERSE REACTIONS

CNS: Headache, dizziness, weakness

CV: Reflex bradycardia, hypertension, dysrhythmias, tachycardia, ***CV collapse,*** palpitation

EENT: Stinging, lacrimation, blurred vision, conjunctival allergy

▼ DRUG INTERACTIONS

Drugs

- *MAOI inhibitors:* Possible increased risk of hypertensive crisis

theophylline

(thee-off'i-lin)

Accurbron, Aerolate III, Aerolate Jr., Aerolate Slo-Phyllin, Aerolate Sr., Aquaphyllin, Asmalix, Bronkodyl, Constant-T, Elixomin, Elixophyllin, Elixophyllin SR, Lanophyllin, Quibron-T Dividose, Quibron-T/SR Dividose, Respid, Slo-Bid Gyrocaps, Slo-Phyllin Gyrocaps, Sustaire, Theolair-SR, Theo-24, Theobid Duracaps, Theobid Jr. Duracaps, Theochron, Theoclear-80, Theoclear L.A., Theo-Dur, Theo-Dur Sprinkle, Theolair, Theolair-SR, Theophylline Extended Release, Theophylline Oral, Theophylline S.R., Theo-Sav, Theospan-SR, Theostat 80, Theovent, Theox, T-Phyl, Uniphyl

Chemical Class: Methylxanthine

Therapeutic Class: Bronchodilator

CLINICAL PHARMACOLOGY

Mechanism of Action: Directly relaxes bronchial and pulmonary blood vessel smooth muscle, stimulates CNS, induces diuresis, increases gastric acid secretion, lowers lower esophageal sphincter pressure; is a central respiratory stimulant; exact mechanism unproven

Pharmacokinetics

PO: Well absorbed from GI tract, absorption altered by food; peak 2 hr; crosses placenta, excreted into breast milk; metabolized in liver, excreted (15% unchanged) in urine; $t_{1/2}$ 3-15 hr in non-smokers, 4-5 hr in smokers, 1-9 hr in children, 20-30 hr in premature neonates (who may accumulate the caffeine metabolite)

INDICATIONS AND USES: Bronchial asthma, reversible bronchospasm of chronic bronchitis and emphysema, apnea and bradycardia of prematurity*

DOSAGE

(Based on ideal body weight) When converting to sustained release products total daily dose remains the same.

Adult

• *Acute symptoms:* PO 5 mg/kg load; maintenance 3 mg/kg q8h (non-smokers), 3 mg/kg q6h (smokers), 2 mg/kg q8h (older patients), 1-2 mg/kg q12h (CHF)

• *Slow titration:* PO initial dose 16 mg/kg/24h or 400 mg/24 hr, whichever is less, doses divided q6-8h

• IV 5 mg/kg load over 20 min; maintenance 0.2 mg/kg/h (CHF, elderly), 0.43 mg/kg/h (non-smokers), 0.7 mg/kg/h (young adult smokers); measure serum level for patients currently receiving theophylline; approx 0.5 mg/kg theophylline increases serum level 1 μg/ml

Child

• 9-16 yr: PO 5 mg/kg load, maintenance 3 mg/kg q6h; IV 5 mg/kg load over 20 min, maintenance 0.7 mg/kg/h

• 1-9 yr: PO 5 mg/kg load, maintenance 4 mg/kg q6h; IV 5 mg/kg load over 20 min, maintenance 0.8 mg/kg/h

• Infants: PO $\{(0.2 \times \text{age in weeks}) + 5\} \times \text{kg} = 24$ hr dose in mg; divide into q8h dosing (6wk-6mo), q6h dosing (6-12 mo); IV 5 mg/kg load over 20 min, maintenance dose in mg/kg/h $\{(.0008 \times \text{age in weeks}) + 0.21\}$

• Premature infants: IV 1 mg/kg q 12h (≤24 days postnatal), 1.5 mg/kg q12h (>24 days postnatal)

• *PO dosage adjustment after serum theophylline measurement:*

• Serum level 5-10 μg/ml, increase dose by 25% at 3 day intervals;

• Serum level 10-20 μg/ml, maintain dosage if tolerated, recheck level q6-12mo;

• Serum level 20-25 μg/ml, decrease dose by 10%, recheck level in 3 days;

• Serum level 25-30 μg/ml, skip next dose, decrease dose by 25%, recheck level in 3 days;

• Serum level >30 μg/ml: skip next 2 doses, decrease dose by 50%, recheck level in 3 days

$ AVAILABLE FORMS/COST OF THERAPY

• Cap, Elastic—Oral: 100 mg, 100's **$19.61-$47.10;** 125 mg, 100's: **$22.87-$25.84;** 200 mg, 100's: **$29.23-$62.59;** 300 mg, 100's: **$34.82-$48.75;** 400 mg, 100's: **$55.19-$59.33**

• Cap, Gel, Sust Action—Oral: 50 mg, 100's: **$17.33-$20.91;** 60 mg, 100's: **$27.59;** 65 mg, 100's: **$17.00;** 75 mg, 100's: **$19.75-$22.20;** 100 mg, 100's, **$20.73-$25.83;** 125 mg, 100's: **$22.51-$58.91;** 130 mg, 100's: **$12.89-$18.25;** 200 mg, 100's: **$23.45-36.30;** 250 mg, 100's: **$45.07-$72.80;** 260 mg, 100's: **$20.00-$22.50;** 300 mg, 100's: **$42.17-$43.15**

• Tab, Coated, Sust Action—Oral: 100 mg, 100's: **$6.38-$27.45;** 200 mg, 100's: **$9.38-$20.78;** 250 mg, 100's: **$31.03-$33.78;** 300 mg, 100's: **$12.00-$40.50;** 400 mg, 100's: **$66.64-$87.00;** 450 mg, 100's: **$27.75-$53.77;** 500 mg, 100's: **$44.88-$95.00**

• Tab, Uncoated—Oral: 100 mg, 100's: **$19.56-$19.65;** 125 mg, 100's: **$33.06;** 250 mg, 100's: **$51.30;** 300 mg, 100's: **$36.07**

• Susp—Oral: 300 mg/15 ml, 240 ml: **$10.75**

• Elixir—Oral: 80 mg/15 ml, 120 ml: **$0.66-$1.45**

• Sol—Oral: 80 mg/15 ml, 480 ml: **$26.16**

• Syr—Oral: 80 mg/15 ml, 480 ml: **$12.30-$22.48**
• Inj, Sol—IV: 0.4 mg/ml, 1000 ml: **$15.92;** 0.8 mg/ml, 1000 ml: **$17.14;** 1.6 mg/ml, 500 ml: **$15.24;** 2 mg/ml, 100 ml: **$13.18;** 4 mg/ml, 100 ml: **$13.59**

CONTRAINDICATIONS: Hypersensitivity to xanthines, tachydysrhythmias, as sole treatment of status asthmaticus

PRECAUTIONS: Elderly, CHF, cor pulmonale, hepatic disease, active peptic ulcer disease, diabetes mellitus, hyperthyroidism, hypertension, active alcoholism, children, neonates

PREGNANCY AND LACTATION: Pregnancy category C; no reports of malformations; compatible with breast feeding with precaution that rapidly absorbed preparations may cause irritability in the infant

SIDE EFFECTS/ADVERSE REACTIONS

CNS: Anxiety, restlessness, insomnia, dizziness, ***seizure,*** headache, light-headedness, muscle twitching

CV: ***Palpitations, sinus tachycardia, hypotension, other dysrhythmias,*** fluid retention with tachycardia, pounding heartbeat

GI: Nausea, vomiting, anorexia, diarrhea, bitter taste, dyspepsia, GE reflux

RESP: Increased rate

SKIN: Flushing, urticaria

▼ DRUG INTERACTIONS

Drugs

• *Allopurinol, beta blockers, calcium channel blockers, cimetidine, ciprofloxacin, disulfiram, enoxacin, erythromycin, fluoxamine, interferon alpha, mexiletine, pefloxacin, pentoxifylline, propafenone, radioactive iodine, thiabendazole, ticlopidine, troleandomycin:* Increased theophylline levels
• *Barbiturates, carbamazapine, phenytoin, rifampin:* Reduced theophylline levels
• Lithium: Reduced lithium levels

SPECIAL CONSIDERATIONS

PATIENT/FAMILY EDUCATION

• Contents of beaded capsules may be sprinkled over food for children

MONITORING PARAMETERS

• Blood levels; therapeutic level is 10-20 µg/ml (6-14 µg/ml for apnea/bradycardia of prematurity); toxicity may occur with small increase above 20 µg/ml and occasionally at levels below this; obtain serum levels 1-2 hr after administration for immediate release products and 5-9 hr after the AM dose for sustained release formulations
• Signs of toxicity include nausea, vomiting, anxiety, insomnia, seizures, ventricular dysrythmias

---

thiabendazole

(thye-a-ben'da-zole)
Mintezol

Chemical Class: Benzimadazole derivative
Therapeutic Class: Anthelmintic

CLINICAL PHARMACOLOGY

Mechanism of Action: Precise mode of action unknown, but may inhibit the helminth-specific enzyme, fumarate reductase

Pharmacokinetics

PO: Peak 1-2 hr
Metabolized completely to 5-hydroxy form, excreted in urine as glucuronide or sulfate conjugates, most within 24 hr

INDICATIONS AND USES: Vermicidal and/or vermifugal against *Enterobius vermicularis* (pinworm), *Ascaria lumbricoides* (roundworm), *Strongyloides stercoralis* (threadworm), *Trichuris trichiura* (whipworm), trichinosis, *Ancylostoma duodenale* (hookworm), *Necator*

* = non-FDA-approved use + = major clinical significance

americanus, Ancylostoma braziliense (dog and cat hookworm)

DOSAGE

Adult and Child: PO 25 mg/kg in 2 doses qd × 2-5 days, not to exceed 3 g/d; strongyloidiasis 2 days; cutaneous larva migrans 2 consecutive days; visceral larva migrans 7 successive days; trichinosis, 2-4 successive days per response; roundworms, including ascariasis, uncinariasis, and trichuriasis 2 successive days

$ AVAILABLE FORMS/COST OF THERAPY

- Susp—Oral: 500 mg/5 ml, 120 ml: **$21.06**
- Tab, Chewable—Oral: 500 mg, 36's: **$36.25**

CONTRAINDICATIONS: Hypersensitivity

PRECAUTIONS: Severe malnutrition, hepatic disease, renal disease, anemia, severe dehydration, child <14 kg

PREGNANCY AND LACTATION: Pregnancy category C

SIDE EFFECTS/ADVERSE REACTIONS

CNS: Dizziness, headache, drowsiness, fever, flushing, ***convulsions,*** behavioral changes

CV: Hypotension, bradycardia

EENT: Tinnitus, blurred vision, xanthopsia

GI: Nausea, vomiting, anorexia, diarrhea, jaundice, liver damage, epigastric distress

GU: Hematuria, ***nephrotoxicity,*** enuresis, abnormal smell of urine

SKIN: Rash, pruritus, erythema, ***Stevens-Johnson syndrome***

MISC: ***Anaphylaxis***

▼ DRUG INTERACTIONS

Drugs

- *Theophylline:* May inhibit metabolism of xanthines, potentially elevating serum concentrations

Labs

- Increase: SGOT

SPECIAL CONSIDERATIONS

PATIENT/FAMILY EDUCATION

- Take after meals if possible; chew before swallowing
- Dietary restriction, complementary medications, and cleansing enemas are not needed
- Proper hygiene after BM, including handwashing technique; change bed linen
- Use caution, may alter mental alertness

---

thiamine

Betaxin, ✤ Betalin S, Biamine, Revitonus, Thiamilate

Chemical Class: Water soluble vitamin

Therapeutic Class: Vitamin B_1

CLINICAL PHARMACOLOGY

Mechanism of Action: Acts as coenzyme, as oxidation-reduction agent, or possibly as mitochondrial agent in pyruvate metabolism

Pharmacokinetics

PO/IM: Rapid and complete absorption, widely distributed (highest concentrations in liver, brain, kidney, and heart), rapidly metabolized, excess excreted in urine; body depletion of vitamin B_1 can occur after approx 3 wk of total absence of thiamine in the diet

INDICATIONS AND USES: Vitamin B_1 deficiency or polyneuritis, beriberi, pellagra, Wernicke-Korsakoff syndrome, metabolic disorders (maple syrup urine disease, subacute necrotizing encephalitis); parenteral thiamine is recommended in all patients presenting with coma or hypothermia of unknown etiology; essential component of total parenteral nutrition therapy

DOSAGE

Adult

- *Beriberi:* IM 10-500 mg tid × 2 wk, then 5-10 mg qd × 1 mo
- *Beriberi with cardiac failure:* IV 100-500 mg
- *Anemia/pellagra:* PO 100 mg qd
- *Wernicke's encephalopathy:* IV 500 mg or less, then 100 mg bid

Child

- *Beriberi:* IM 10-50 mg qd × 4-6 wk
- *Anemia/pellagra:* PO 10-50 mg qd in divided doses
- *Beriberi with cardiac failure:* IV 100-500 mg

$ AVAILABLE FORMS/COST OF THERAPY

- Inj, Sol—IM; IV: 100 mg/ml, 10 ml: **$0.88**
- Tab—Oral: 50 mg, 100's: **$2.17-$7.00;** 100 mg, 100's: **$1.65-$4.68;** 250 mg, 100's: **$3.90**

CONTRAINDICATIONS: Hypersensitivity

PREGNANCY AND LACTATION: Pregnancy category A; excreted into breast milk; American RDA for thiamine during lactation is 1.5-1.6 mg; supplement women with inadequate intake; compatible with breast feeding

SIDE EFFECTS/ADVERSE REACTIONS

CNS: Weakness, restlessness

CV: ***Collapse, pulmonary edema,*** hypotension

EENT: Tightness of throat

GI: Hemorrhage, *nausea, diarrhea*

SKIN: ***Angioneurotic edema,*** cyanosis, sweating, warmth, pruritus, urticaria, cyanosis

MISC: ***Anaphylaxis***

SPECIAL CONSIDERATIONS

- Worsening of Wernicke's encephalopathy following glucose administration, administer thiamine before or along with dextrose containing fluids
- Single vitamin B_1 deficiency is rare—suspect multiple vitamin deficiencies

thiethylperazine

(thye-eth-il-per′azeen)

Torecan, Norzine

Chemical Class: Phenothiazine, piperazine derivative

Therapeutic Class: Antiemetic

CLINICAL PHARMACOLOGY

Mechanism of Action: Acts centrally by blocking chemoreceptor trigger zone and vomiting center

Pharmacokinetics

PO: Onset 45-60 min; duration 4 hr

Metabolized by liver, excreted by kidneys, crosses placenta

INDICATIONS AND USES: Nausea, vomiting

DOSAGE

Adult

- PO/IM 10 mg qd-tid

$ AVAILABLE FORMS/COST OF THERAPY

- Inj, Sol—IV: 5 mg/ml, 2 ml × 20: **$105.63**
- Tab, Uncoated—Oral: 10 mg, 100's: **$54.30**

CONTRAINDICATIONS: Hypersensitivity to phenothiazines, coma, seizure, encephalopathy, bone marrow depression

PRECAUTIONS: Children <2 yr, elderly

PREGNANCY AND LACTATION: Pregnancy category C

SIDE EFFECTS/ADVERSE REACTIONS

CNS: Euphoria, depression, restlessness, tremor, EPS, ***convulsions,*** drowsiness

CV: ***Circulatory failure, tachycardia,*** postural hypotension, ECG changes

GI: Anorexia, dry mouth, diarrhea, constipation, weight loss, metallic taste, cramps
GU: Urinary retention, dark urine
RESP: ***Respiratory depression***

▼ **DRUG INTERACTIONS**

- *Anticholinergics, antiparkinson drugs, antidepressants:* Increased anticholinergic action
- *Barbiturates:* Induction, decreased effect of thiethylperazine
- *Beta blockers:* Augmented pharmacologic action of both drugs
- *Bromocriptine:* Neuroleptic drugs inhibit bromocriptine's ability to lower prolactin concentration
- *Epinephrine:* Reversed pressor response
- *Levodopa:* Inhibited antiparkinsonian effect
- *Lithium:* Lowered serum concentration of both drugs in combination
- *Narcotic analgesics:* Hypotension with meperidine, caution with other narcotic analgesics
- *Orphenadrine:* Lower thiethylperazine concentration and excessive anticholinergic effects

SPECIAL CONSIDERATIONS

- Effective antiemetic agent for the treatment of postoperative nausea and vomiting, nausea and vomiting secondary to mildly emetic chemotherapeutic agents, and vomiting secondary to radiation therapy and toxins
- No comparisons with prochlorperazine
- More extrapyramidal reactions than chlorpromazine, promazine (preferable in patients where the occurrence of a dystonic reaction would be hazardous i.e., head and neck surgery patients, patients with severe pulmonary disease, patients with a history of dyskinetic reactions)

PATIENT/FAMILY EDUCATION

- Avoid hazardous activities, activities requiring alertness

MONITORING PARAMETERS

- Respiratory status initially

thioridazine

(thye-or-rid'a-zeen)
Mellaril, Mellaril-S, Novoridazine ♣
Chemical Class: Phenothiazine, piperidine
Therapeutic Class: Antipsychotic/neuroleptic

CLINICAL PHARMACOLOGY

Mechanism of Action: Depresses cerebral cortex, hypothalamus, limbic system, blocks neurotransmission produced by dopamine at synapse; reduces excitement, hypermotility, abnormal initiative, affective tension, and agitation; exhibits strong alpha-adrenergic, anticholinergic blocking action; minimal antiemetic and minimal extrapyramidal stimulation, notably pseudoparkinsonism

Pharmacokinetics

PO: Onset erratic, peak 2-4 hr
Metabolized by liver, excreted in urine, crosses placenta, $t_{1/2}$ 26-36 hr

INDICATIONS AND USES: Psychotic disorders, schizophrenia, behavioral problems in children (combativeness, explosive hyperexcitable behavior), alcohol withdrawal as adjunct, short term treatment of anxiety, major depressive disorders, organic brain syndrome

DOSAGE

Adult

- *Psychosis:* PO 25-100 mg tid, max dose 800 mg/d; dose is gradually increased to desired response, then reduced to min maintenance
- *Depression/behavioral problems/ organic brain syndrome:* PO 25 mg

tid, range from 10 mg bid-qid to 50 mg tid-qid

Child 2-12 yr

• PO 0.5-3 mg/kg/d in divided doses

$ AVAILABLE FORMS/COST OF THERAPY

• Conc—Oral: 30 mg/ml, 120 ml: **$11.23-$30.78;** 100 mg/ml, 120 ml: **$36.89-$80.40**

• Tab, Coated—Oral: 10 mg, 100's: **$3.69-$30.60;** 15 mg, 100's: **$4.82-$33.60;** 25 mg, 100's: **$5.03-$40.08;** 50 mg, 100's: **$7.13-$48.66;** 100 mg, 100's: **$11.18-$59.22;** 150 mg, 100's: **$21.47-$75.18;** 200 mg, 100's: **$24.23-$85.68**

• Susp—Oral: 25 mg/ml, 480 ml: **$45.72;** 100 mg/ml, 480 ml: **$94.02**

CONTRAINDICATIONS: Hypersensitivity, blood dyscrasias, coma, severe CNS depression, child <2 yr, brain damage, bone marrow depression, Parkinson's disease, liver damage, severe hypertension/hypotension

PRECAUTIONS: Seizure disorders, hypertension, hepatic disease, cardiac disease

PREGNANCY AND LACTATION: Pregnancy category C

SIDE EFFECTS/ADVERSE REACTIONS

CNS: EPS (rare) including *pseudoparkinsonism, akathisia, dystonia, tardive dyskinesia;* ***seizures,*** *headache,* confusion

CV: Orthostatic hypotension, ***cardiac arrest,*** ECG changes, ***tachycardia***

EENT: Blurred vision, glaucoma, dry eyes, pigmentary retinopathy

GI: Dry mouth, nausea, vomiting, anorexia, constipation, diarrhea, jaundice, weight gain

GU: Urinary retention, urinary frequency, enuresis, impotence, amenorrhea, gynecomastia, galactorrhea

HEME: Anemia, ***leukopenia, leukocytosis, agranulocytosis***

RESP: ***Laryngospasm,*** dyspnea, ***respiratory depression***

SKIN: Rash, photosensitivity, dermatitis

▼ DRUG INTERACTIONS

Drugs

• *Anticholinergics, antiparkinson drugs, antidepressants:* Increased anticholinergic action

• *Barbiturates:* Induction, decreased effect of thioridazine

• *Beta blockers:* Augmented pharmacologic action of both drugs

• *Bromocriptine:* Neuroleptic drugs inhibit bromocriptine's ability to lower prolactin concentration; reverse not common

• *Epinephrine:* Reversed pressor response

• *Levodopa:* Inhibited antiparkinsonian effect

• *Lithium:* Lowered serum concentration of both drugs in combination

• *Narcotic analgesics:* Hypotension with meperidine, caution with other narcotic analgesics

• *Orphenadrine:* Lower thioridazine concentration and excessive anticholinergic effects

• *Phenylpropanolamine:* Patient on thioridazine died after single dose of phenylpropanolamine, causal relationship not established

Labs

• *Increase:* Liver function tests, cardiac enzymes, cholesterol, blood glucose, *prolactin,* bilirubin, cholinesterase

• *False positive:* Pregnancy tests, PKU

• *False negative:* Urinary steroids, pregnancy tests

SPECIAL CONSIDERATIONS

• Phenothiazine with weak potency, low incidence of EPS, but high incidence of sedation, anticholinergic effects, and cardiovascular effects

PATIENT/FAMILY EDUCATION

• Orthostatic hypotension

- Avoid abrupt withdrawal
- Use a sunscreen during sun exposure
- Caution with activities requiring complete mental alertness (e.g., driving), may cause sedation
- Full information on risks of tardive dyskinesia

thiothixene

(thye-oh-thix'een)

Navane

Chemical Class: Thioxanthene

Therapeutic Class: Antipsychotic/neuroleptic

CLINICAL PHARMACOLOGY

Mechanism of Action: Depresses cerebral cortex, hypothalamus, limbic system, which control activity, aggression; blocks neurotransmission produced by dopamine at synapse; exhibits α-adrenergic blocking properties, anticholinergic activity

Pharmacokinetics

PO: Onset slow, peak 2-8 hr, duration up to 12 hr

IM: Onset 15-30 min, peak 1-6 hr, duration up to 12 hr

Metabolized by liver, excreted in urine, crosses placenta, $t_{1/2}$ 34 hr

INDICATIONS AND USES: Psychotic disorders, schizophrenia, acute agitation

DOSAGE

Adult

- PO 2-5 mg bid-qid depending on severity of condition; dose gradually increased to 15-30 mg if needed
- IM 4 mg bid-qid; max dose 30 mg qd; administer PO dose as soon as possible

$ AVAILABLE FORMS/COST OF THERAPY

- Cap, Gel—Oral: 1 mg, 100's: **$9.75-$38.02;** 2 mg, 100's: **$12.75-$51.26;** 5 mg, 100's: **$18.23-$80.17;** 10 mg, 100's: **$26.93-$110.50;** 20 mg, 100's: **$5.07-$155.04**
- Conc—Oral: 5 mg/ml, 120 ml: **$25.13-$81.79**
- Inj, Sol—IM: 5 mg/ml, 10 mg × 10: **$35.35**

CONTRAINDICATIONS: Hypersensitivity (caution to phenothiazine hypersensitivity cross-over), blood dyscrasias, child <12 yr, bone marrow depression, blood dyscrasias, circulatory collapse, CNS depression, coma, alcoholism, CV disease, hepatic disease, Reye's syndrome, narrow-angle glaucoma

PRECAUTIONS: Lactation, seizure disorders, hypertension, hepatic disease, cardiovascular disease

PREGNANCY AND LACTATION: Pregnancy category C

SIDE EFFECTS/ADVERSE REACTIONS

CNS: EPS including *pseudoparkinsonism, akathisia, dystonia, tardive dyskinesia;* ***seizures;*** *headache*

CV: Orthostatic hypotension, hypertension, ***cardiac arrest,*** ECG changes, ***tachycardia***

EENT: Blurred vision, glaucoma

GI: Dry mouth, anorexia, constipation, diarrhea, jaundice, weight gain

GU: Urinary retention, urinary frequency, enuresis, impotence, amenorrhea, gynecomastia, galactorrhea

HEME: Anemia, ***leukopenia, leukocytosis, agranulocytosis***

RESP: ***Laryngospasm,*** dyspnea, ***respiratory depression***

SKIN: Rash, photosensitivity, dermatitis

MISC: Neuroleptic malignant syndrome

▼ DRUG INTERACTIONS

Drugs

- *Anticholinergics, antiparkinson drugs, antidepressants:* Increased anticholinergic action
- *Barbiturates:* Induction, decreased effect of thiothixene

T

• *Beta blockers:* Augmented pharmacologic action of both drugs
• *Bromocriptine:* Thiothixene inhibits bromocriptine's ability to lower prolactin concentration; reverse not common
• *Epinephrine:* Reversed pressor response
• *Levodopa:* Inhibited antiparkinsonian effect
• *Lithium:* Lowered serum concentration of both drugs in combination
• *Narcotic analgesics:* Hypotension with meperidine, caution with other narcotic analgesics
• *Orphenadrine:* Lower thiothixene concentration and excessive anticholinergic effects

Labs

• *Increase:* Liver function tests, cardiac enzymes, cholesterol, blood glucose, prolactin, bilirubin, cholinesterase
• *Decrease:* Uric acid

SPECIAL CONSIDERATIONS

• High-potency antipsychotic with a relatively high incidence of EPS, but a low incidence of sedation, anticholinergic effects, and cardiovascular effects

PATIENT/FAMILY EDUCATION

• Informed consent regarding risks of tardive dyskinesia; orthostatic hypotension

thyroid

(thye′roid)

Armour Thyroid, Cholaxin, ✱ S-P-T, Thyrar, Thyroid Strong

Chemical Class: Active thyroid hormone in natural state (porcine) and ratio (38 μg levothyroxine (T_4) and 9 μg liothyronine (T_3) per grain of thyroid)
Therapeutic Class: Thyroid hormone

CLINICAL PHARMACOLOGY

Mechanism of Action: Increases metabolic rate, increases cardiac output, O_2 consumption, body temperature, blood volume, growth, development at cellular level, metabolism of carbohydrates, lipids, and proteins; exerts profound influence on every organ system, especially CNS

Pharmacokinetics

PO: Peak 12-48 hr

Partially absorbed (48%-79%, T_3>T_4), 99% bound to plasma proteins, deiodinated in liver, kidney, enterohepatically circulated, neither T_3 or T_4 cross placenta; $t_{1/2}$ 6-7 days

INDICATIONS AND USES: Replacement or supplemental therapy (hypothyroidism, cretinism, myxedema); pituitary TSH suppressants in the treatment or prevention of various types of euthyroid goiters, including thyroid nodules, subacute or chronic lymphocytic thyroiditis (Hashimoto's), multinodal goiter and in the management of thyroid cancer; diagnostic agents in suppression tests to differentiate suspected mild hyperthyroidism or thyroid gland autonomy

DOSAGE

Adult

• *Hypothyroidism:* PO 65 mg qd, increased by 65 mg q30d until desired response; maintenance dose 65-120 mg qd
• *Myxedema:* After stabilization with IV levothyroxine or liothyronine and concurrent correction of electrolyte disturbances and administration of corticosteroids switch to PO thyroid; initial PO 15 mg qd, double dose q2wk, maintenance 65-120 mg/d
• *Thyroid cancer, thyroid suppression therapy:* TSH should be suppressed to low or undetectable lev-

els; therefore, larger doses of thyroid hormone than those used for replacement therapy are required.

- *Geriatric:* PO 7.5-15 mg qd, double dose q4-6wk until desired response/maintenance dose

Child

- *Cretinism/juvenile hypothyroidism:* [age, mg/d (mg/kg/d)]: 0-6 mo, 15-30 mg (4.8-6 mg); 6-12 mo, 30-45 mg (3.6-4.8 mg); 1-5 yr, 45-60 mg (3-3.6 mg); 6-12 yr, 60-90 mg (2.4-3 mg); >12 yr, >90 mg (1.2-1.8 mg)

$ AVAILABLE FORMS/COST OF THERAPY

- Tab, Uncoated—Oral: 15 mg, 100's: **$7.87;** 30 mg, 100's: **$4.50-$9.22;** 60 mg, 100's: **$5.89-$10.25;** 65 mg: **$4.80-$5.50;** 90 mg: **$16.19;** 130 mg: **$5.95;** 180 mg, 100's: **$7.95-$30.10;** 240 mg, 100's: **$45.10;** 300 mg, 100's: **$55.10**

CONTRAINDICATIONS: Adrenal insufficiency (uncorrected), thyrotoxicosis, hypersensitivity

PRECAUTIONS: Elderly, MI, angina pectoris, hypertension, ischemia, cardiac disease

PREGNANCY AND LACTATION: Pregnancy category A; excreted into breast milk in low concentrations (inadequate to protect a hypothyroid infant; too low to interfere with neonatal thyroid screening programs)

SIDE EFFECTS/ADVERSE REACTIONS

CNS: Insomnia, tremors, headache, thyroid storm

CV: Tachycardia, palpitations, angina, dysrhythmias, hypertension, ***cardiac arrest***

GI: Nausea, diarrhea, increased or decreased appetite, cramps

MS: Bone demineralization (osteoporosis)

MISC: Menstrual irregularities, weight loss, sweating, heat intolerance, fever

▼ DRUG INTERACTIONS

Drugs

- *Carbamazepine:* Increases elimination of thyroid hormones; may increase dosage requirements
- *Cholestyramine, colestipol:* Decreased absorption
- *Oral anticoagulants+:* Adjustments in anticoagulant dosage are likely if thyrometabolic status changes; thyroid hormones increase catabolism of vitamin K-dependent clotting factors
- *Phenytoin:* Phenytoin may increase thyroid replacement dosage requirements

Labs

- *Increase:* CPK, LDH, AST, PBI, blood glucose
- *Decrease:* TSH, ^{131}I uptake test, uric acid, triglycerides

SPECIAL CONSIDERATIONS

- Individualize dose by patient response and lab findings
- Although used traditionally, natural hormones less clinically desirable due to varying potencies, inconsistent clinical effects, and more adverse stimulatory effects; synthetic derivatives (i.e., levothyroxine) preferred

ticarcillin ticarcillin/clavulanic acid

(tye-kar-sill'in)

Ticaripen, 🍁 Ticar

Ticarcillin/clavulanic acid: Timentin

Chemical Class: Extended-spectrum penicillin; clavulanic acid is β-lactamase inhibitor

Therapeutic Class: Broad-spectrum, β-lactam antibiotic

CLINICAL PHARMACOLOGY

Mechanism of Action: Interferes with cell wall replication of susceptible organisms; bacteriocidal

Pharmacokinetics

IM: Peak ½-1 hr (63 μg/ml after 2 g IM), duration 4-6 hr

IV: Peak 30-45 min, (327 μg/ml after 5 g IV) duration 4 hr

$t_{1/2}$ 70 min; protein binding 45%, small amount metabolized in liver; excreted in urine (glomerular filtration and tubular secretion); addition of clavulanic acid doesn't affect pharmacokinetics of ticarcillin

INDICATIONS AND USES: Infections of the respiratory tract, soft tissue, urinary tract, and bacterial septicemia caused by susceptible organisms

Antibacterial spectrum usually includes:

- Gram-positive organisms: *Staphylococcus aureus, Streptococcus faecalis, Streptococcus pneumoniae*
- Gram-negative organisms: *Neisseria gonorrhoeae, Escherichia coli, Proteus mirabilis, Salmonella, Morganella morganii, Providencia rettgeri, Enterobacter, Pseudomonas aeruginosa, Serratia*
- Anaerobes: *Bacteroides* sp including *Bacteroides fragilis; Fusobacterium* sp; *Veillonella* sp; *Clostridium; Eubacterium* sp; *Peptococcus* sp; *Peptostreptococcus* sp

Ticarcillin/clavulanic acid: Addition of clavulanic acid expands spectrum to include bacteria caused by β-lactamase-producing strains of above organisms and also includes:

- Gram-positive organisms: *Staphylococcus epidermidis*
- Gram-negative organisms: *Klebsiella* sp, *Hemophilus influenzae, Citrobacter* sp, *Serratia marcescens*
- Anaerobes: *Bacteroides melaninogenicus*

DOSAGE

Adult

- IV/IM 12-24 g/d in divided doses q3-6h; infuse over ½-2 hr (usual dose 3 g q4h or 4 g q6h); dosage adjustments for decreased clearance: for CrCl (ml/min): >60, 3 g q4h; 30-60, 2 g q4h; 10-30, 2 g q8h; <10, 2 g q12h; <10 with hepatic dysfunction, 2 g q24h; peritoneal dialysis, 3 g q12h; hemodialysis, 2 g q12h supplemented with 3 g after each dialysis

Child

- IV/IM 50-300 mg/kg/d in divided doses q4-8h

Neonates

- IV INF 75-100 mg/kg/8-12 hr
- Ticarcillin/Clavulanic Acid: 3.1 g (contains 3 g ticarcillin, 100 mg clavulanic acid)

$ AVAILABLE FORMS/COST OF THERAPY

- Inj, Dry-Sol—IM;IV: 1 g/vial: **$0.34;** 3 g/vial: **$0.96;** 6 g/vial: **$1.75**

Ticarcillin/Clavulanic acid:

- Inj, Dry-Sol—IV: 0.1 g/3 g: **$1.37**

CONTRAINDICATIONS: Hypersensitivity to penicillins

PRECAUTIONS: Hypersensitivity to cephalosporins

PREGNANCY AND LACTATION: Pregnancy category B; excreted into breast milk in low concentrations; compatible with breast feeding. Note potential to modify bowel flora, cause allergic reactions, and interfere with culture results of fever workup

SIDE EFFECTS/ADVERSE REACTIONS

CNS: Lethargy, hallucinations, anxiety, depression, twitching, ***coma, convulsions***

GI: Nausea, vomiting, diarrhea, increased AST, ALT, abdominal pain, glossitis, colitis

GU: Oliguria, proteinuria, hematuria, *vaginitis, moniliasis,* ***glomerulonephritis, pseudomembranous colitis***

HEME: Anemia, increased bleeding time, ***bone marrow depression, granulocytopenia***

METAB: Hypokalemia

SKIN: Rash, pruritus, urticaria

MISC: Hypersensitivity, drug fever, local reactions (phlebitis)

▼ **DRUG INTERACTIONS**

Drugs

• *Aminoglycosides:* Inactivation of aminoglycosides in vitro and in vivo, reducing the aminoglycoside effect

• *Aspirin, probenecid:* Increased ticarcillin concentrations

Labs

• *False positive:* Urine glucose, urine protein

SPECIAL CONSIDERATIONS

• Synergistic with aminoglycosides; not stable in the presence of penicillinase

• Sodium content, 5.2 mEq/1 g ticarcillin

ticlopidine

(tye-klo'pa-deen)

Ticlid

Chemical Class: Thienpyridine

Therapeutic Class: Platelet aggregation inhibitor

CLINICAL PHARMACOLOGY

Mechanism of Action: Interferes with platelet membrane function by inhibiting ADP-induced platelet-fibrinogen binding and subsequent platelet-platelet interactions; time and dose-dependent inhibition of platelet aggregation and release of platelet granule constituents; prolongation of bleeding time; effects on platelet function irreversible for the life of the platelet

Pharmacokinetics

PO: Peak 2 hr

Rapidly absorbed (decreased 20% by meals), 98% bound to plasma proteins, extensively hepatically metabolized, excreted in urine, nonlinear pharmacokinetics (clearance decreases on repeated dosing), $t_{1/2}$ after a single 250 mg dose, 12.6 hr, with repeat dosing at 250 mg BID, $t_{1/2}$ rises to 4-5 days (steady state levels after approximately 14-21 days)

INDICATIONS AND USES: Reducing the risk of thrombotic stroke in aspirin intolerant or aspirin failures

DOSAGE

Adult

• PO 250 mg bid with food

$ **AVAILABLE FORMS/COST OF THERAPY**

• Tab, Uncoated—Oral: 250 mg, 30's: **$42.59**

CONTRAINDICATIONS: Hypersensitivity, active liver disease, current blood dyscrasia (neutropenia, thrombocytopenia), hemostatic disorder or active pathological bleeding (such as bleeding peptic ulcer or intracranial bleeding) patients with severe liver impairment

PRECAUTIONS: Past liver disease, renal disease, elderly, children, increased bleeding risk (trauma, surgery, or pathological conditions, dental procedures)

PREGNANCY AND LACTATION: Pregnancy category B

SIDE EFFECTS/ADVERSE REACTIONS

GI (40% have GI effects): Nausea, vomiting, diarrhea, GI discomfort, ***cholestatic jaundice, hepatitis,*** increased cholesterol, LDL, VLDL

HEME: ***Bleeding (epistaxis, hematuria, conjunctival hemorrhage, GI bleeding), agranulocytosis, neutropenia, thrombocytopenia***

T

SKIN: Rash, pruritus

▼ **DRUG INTERACTIONS**

Drugs

- *Theophylline:* Increased theophylline level via inhibition of metabolism, increased risk of toxicity

Labs

- Total cholesterol increases 8-10%
- *Increase:* LFTs

SPECIAL CONSIDERATIONS

- Due to the risk of life-threatening neutropenia or agranulocytosis and cost, ticlopidine should be reserved for patients intolerant to aspirin;

MONITORING PARAMETERS

- CBC qwk from 3 wk through 3 mo of therapy

---

timolol

(tim'oh-loll)

Blocadren (PO), Timoptic (Ophth)

Chemical Class: Nonselective, β-adrenergic blocker

Therapeutic Class: Antihypertensive, anti-glaucomatous agent

CLINICAL PHARMACOLOGY

Mechanism of Action: OPHTH reduces intraocular pressure via reduction in production of aqueous humor; PO non-selective adrenergic receptor blocking agent, no significant intrinsic sympathomimetic, direct myocardial depressant, or local anesthetic activity, decreases positive chronotropic, positive inotropic, bronchodilator, and vasodilator responses to β-adrenergic receptor agonists

Pharmacokinetics

OPHTH: Onset 15-30 min, peak 1-2 hr, duration 24 hr

PO: Peak 2 hr

Rapidly/completely absorbed, excreted 30%-45% unchanged; 60%-65% metabolized by liver; $t_{1/2}$, 4 hr

INDICATIONS AND USES: OPHTH: Ocular hypertension, chronic open-angle glaucoma, secondary glaucoma, aphakic glaucoma; PO: Hypertension, post-MI mortality reduction, migraine headache, sinus tachycardia,* persistent atrial extrasystoles,* tachydysrhythmias,* prophylaxis of angina pectoris*

DOSAGE

Adult

- OPHTH 1 gtt 0.25% sol in affected eye(s) bid, then 1 gtt for maintenance; may increase to 1 gtt 0.5% sol bid if needed
- *Hypertension:* PO 10 mg bid initially, usually maintenance 20-40 mg/d divided bid; not to exceed 60 mg/d
- *Post-MI prophylaxis:* PO 10 mg bid
- *Migraine:* 10 g bid, up to 30 mg qd divided bid

$ **AVAILABLE FORMS/COST OF THERAPY**

- Sol—Ophth: 0.25%, 5 ml: **$14.99;** 0.5%, 5 ml: **$17.73**
- Jel—Ophth: 0.25%, 5 ml: **$21.78;** 0.5%, 5 ml: **$25.86**
- Tab, Uncoated—Oral: 5 mg, 100's: **$16.50-$42.74;** 10 mg, 100's: **$22.50-$52.85;** 20 mg, 100's: **$53.33-$97.48**

CONTRAINDICATIONS: Hypersensitivity, asthma, 2nd or 3rd degree heart block, sinus bradycardia, right ventricular failure, congenital glaucoma (infants), COPD

PRECAUTIONS: Nonallergic bronchospasm, diabetes mellitus, pregnancy, children, myasthenia gravis

PREGNANCY AND LACTATION: Pregnancy category C; excreted into breast milk

SIDE EFFECTS/ADVERSE REACTIONS

CNS: Weakness, fatigue, depression, anxiety, headache, confusion, *in-*

somnia, dizziness, hallucinations
CV: Bradycardia, hypotension, dysrhythmias, syncope, heart block, ***CHF,*** edema claudication
EENT: Eye irritation, conjunctivitis, keratitis, *visual changes,* sore throat, *double vision,* dry burning eyes
GI: Nausea, anorexia, dyspepsia, ***ischemic colitis,*** diarrhea, abdominal pain, ***mesenteric arterial thrombosis***
GU: Impotence, frequency
HEME: ***Agranulocytosis, thrombocytopenia, purpura***
METAB: Hyperglycemia, hyperglycemia
MS: Joint pain
RESP: ***Bronchospasm,*** dyspnea, cough, rales
SKIN: Rash, urticaria, alopecia, pruritus, fever

▼ **DRUG INTERACTIONS**

Drugs

- *Amiodarone:* Combined therapy may lead to bradycardia, cardiac arrest, or ventricular dysrhythmia
- *Antidiabetics:* Beta-blockers increase blood glucose and impair peripheral circulation; altered response to hypoglycemia by prolonging the recovery of normoglycemia, causing hypertension, and blocking tachycardia
- *Barbiturates:* Reduced concentrations of timolol
- *Calcium channel blockers:* Additive hypotension (kinetic and dynamic)
- *Clonidine:* Hypertension occurring upon withdrawal of clonidine may be exacerbated by timolol
- *Disopyramide:* Additive negative inotropic cardiac effects
- *Epinephrine+:* Enhanced pressor response (hypertension and bradycardia)
- *Fluoxetine:* Increased beta blocking effects with potential for cardiac toxicity)
- *Isoproterenol:* Reduced isoproterenol efficacy in asthma
- *Local anesthetics:* Enhanced sympathomimetic side effects, especially if anesthetic combined with epinephrine; acute discontinuation of timolol before local anesthesia increases risk of anesthetic side effects
- *Methyldopa:* Potential for development of hypertension in the presence of increased catecholamines
- *Neuroleptics:* Increased plasma concentrations of each other, with potential for accentuated responses of both drugs
- *Nonsteroidal antiinflammatory drugs:* Reduced antihypertensive effects of timolol
- *Phenylephrine:* Potential for hypertensive episodes when administered together
- *Prazosin:* First dose response to prazosin may be enhanced by beta blockade
- *Rifampin:* Reduced timolol concentrations
- *Tacrine:* Additive bradycardia
- *Theophylline:* Antagonistic pharmacodynamic effects

Labs

- *Increase:* LFTs, RFTs, K, uric acid, LDL, TGs
- *Decrease:* Hct, Hgb, HDL

SPECIAL CONSIDERATIONS

- Currently available beta blockers appear to be equally effective; cardioselective or combined alpha- and beta-adrenergic blockade are less likely to cause undesirable effects and may be preferred

PATIENT/FAMILY EDUCATION

- Do not discontinue abruptly, taper over 2 wk; may cause precipitate angina

tioconazole

(tyeo-con'a-zole)
Vagistat-1
Chemical Class: Imidazole
Therapeutic Class: Antifungal

CLINICAL PHARMACOLOGY
Mechanism of Action: Alteration of the fungal cell membrane; fungicidal against *Candida*
Pharmacokinetics
PV: Negligible systemic absorption
INDICATIONS AND USES: Local treatment of vulvovaginal candidiasis
DOSAGE
Adult
• INSERT 1 applicatorful PV hs × 1
$ **AVAILABLE FORMS/COST OF THERAPY**
• Oint—Vag: 6.5%, 4.6 g single dose: **$24.19**
CONTRAINDICATIONS: Hypersensitivity
PRECAUTIONS: Discontinue if irritation or sensitization occurs; chronic or recurrent candidiasis may be a symptom of unrecognized diabetes or a compromised immune system
PREGNANCY AND LACTATION: Pregnancy category C
SIDE EFFECTS/ADVERSE REACTIONS
GU: Irritation, burning, itching, irritation, discharge, vulvar edema, vaginal pain, dysuria, nocturia, dryness of vaginal secretions, desquamation
▼ **DRUG INTERACTIONS**
Drugs
• *Cyclosporine:* Increased cyclosporine blood levels, resulting in increased toxicity via decreased metabolism or increased absorption of cyclosporine
SPECIAL CONSIDERATIONS
• Similar in efficacy to miconazole, econazole, and clotrimazole for the topical management of fungal skin infections; choice determined by cost and availability; additional efficacy vs. trichomoniasis with longer course of therapy

tiopronin

(tye-o-pro'nen)
Thiola
Chemical Class: Thiol compound
Therapeutic Class: Orphan drug: active reducing and complexing compound for the prevention of cysteine kidney stones

CLINICAL PHARMACOLOGY
Mechanism of Action: Undergoes thiol-disulfide exchange with cysteine to form a mixed, water-soluble disulfide of tiopronin-cysteine; the amount of sparingly soluble cysteine is reduced
Pharmacokinetics: 48% appears in urine in 4 hr; 78% by 72 hr; reduction of urinary cysteine of 250-500 mg on 1-2 g/d may be expected; rapid onset and offset of action
INDICATIONS AND USES: Prevention of kidney stone formation in patients with severe homozygous cystinuria with urinary cysteine greater than 500 mg/d, who are resistant to conservative treatment
DOSAGE
Adult
• PO 800-1000 mg/d, given in divided doses tid at least 1 hr before or 2 hr after meals
Child
• PO 15 mg/kg/d, given in divided doses tid at least 1 hr before or 2 hr after meals
$ **AVAILABLE FORMS/COST OF THERAPY**
• Tab, Uncoated—Oral: 100 mg, 100's: **$48.00**

CONTRAINDICATIONS: History of agranulocytosis, thrombocytopenia, aplastic anemia on this medication
PRECAUTIONS: Goodpasture's syndrome, children <9 yr
PREGNANCY AND LACTATION: Pregnancy category C
SIDE EFFECTS/ADVERSE REACTIONS
CNS: Drug fever
METAB: Vit B_6 deficiency
SKIN: Erythema, maculopapular rash, wrinkling skin, lupus like syndrome (fever, arthralgia, lymphadenopathy), pruritus
MISC: Blunting of taste

SPECIAL CONSIDERATIONS

• Equally effective to penicillamine

---

tobramycin

(toe-bra-mye'sin)
Nebcin
Tobrex, AKTob (OPHTH)
Chemical Class: Aminoglycoside
Therapeutic Class: Antibiotic

CLINICAL PHARMACOLOGY
Mechanism of Action: Interferes with protein synthesis in bacterial cell by binding to ribosomal subunit, causing inaccurate peptide sequence to form in protein chain; bactericidal
Pharmacokinetics
IM: Onset rapid, peak 30-90 min, peak urine concentration after 1 mg/kg IM dose, 75-100 µg/ml
IV: Onset immediate, peak 1 hr
$t_{1/2}$ 2-3 hr; not metabolized, excreted unchanged in urine (clearance proportional to creatinine), crosses placental barrier
INDICATIONS AND USES: Severe systemic infections of CNS, respiratory, GI, urinary tract, bone, skin, soft tissues caused by susceptible organisms
Antibacterial spectrum usually includes:
• Gram-positive aerobes: *S. aureus*
• Gram-negative aerobes: *Citrobacter* sp, *Enterobacter* sp, *Escherichia coli; Klebsiella* sp, *Morganella morganii, Pseudomonas aeruginosa, Proteus mirabilis, P. vulgaris, Providencia* sp, *Serratia* sp
• Low order of activity against most gram-positive organisms, including *Str. pyogenes, Str. pneumoniae,* and enterococci
• OPHTH: Ocular infections, bacterial blepharitis, blepharoconjunctivitis, bacterial conjunctivitis, dacrycystitis, bacterial keratitis
DOSAGE
Base dosage calculations on lean body weight
Adult
• IM/IV 3 mg/kg/d in divided doses q8h; may give up to 5 mg/kg/d in divided doses q6-8h
Child
• IM/IV 6-7.5 mg/kg/d in 3-4 equal divided doses
Neonates <1 wk
• IM up to 4 mg/kg/d in divided doses q12h; IV up to 4 mg/kg/d in divided doses q12h diluted in 50-100 mg NS or D_5W; give over 30-60 min
• OPHTH: Oint 1.25 cm to conjunctiva q8-12h; Sol: 1 drop q4h
$ AVAILABLE FORMS/COST OF THERAPY
• Inj, Dry-Sol—IV: 20 mg/vial: **$3.65-$4.50;** 60 mg/vial: **$6.92-$9.50;** 80 mg/vial: **$7.76**
• Sol—Ophth: 0.3%, 5 ml: **$9.90-$18.13**
• Oint—Ophth; Top: 0.3%, 3.5 g: **$18.12**
CONTRAINDICATIONS: Severe renal disease, hypersensitivity to any

T

aminoglycoside of sulfites (contains sodium bisulfite)

PRECAUTIONS: Neonates, mild renal disease, myasthenia gravis, hearing deficits, Parkinson's disease, extensive burns (altered pharmacokinetics)

PREGNANCY AND LACTATION: Pregnancy category D (OPHTH category B); excreted into breast milk; following 80 mg IM dose trace (0.52 μg/ml) over 8 hrs; given poor oral absorption, toxicity minimal; limited to modification of bowel flora and interference with interpretation of culture results if fever workup required

SIDE EFFECTS/ADVERSE REACTIONS

CNS: Confusion, depression, numbness, tremors, ***convulsions,*** muscle twitching, ***neurotoxicity,*** dizziness, vertigo

CV: Hypotension, hypertension, palpitation

EENT: ***Ototoxicity,*** deafness, visual disturbances, tinnitus; OPHTH, blurred vision, burning, stinging of eyes

GI: Nausea, vomiting, anorexia, increased ALT, AST, bilirubin, hepatomegaly, ***hepatic necrosis,*** splenomegaly

GU: ***Oliguria, hematuria, renal damage, azotemia, renal failure, nephrotoxicity***

HEME: ***Agranulocytosis, thrombocytopenia, leukopenia, eosinophilia,*** anemia

SKIN: Rash, burning, urticaria, dermatitis, alopecia

▼ DRUG INTERACTIONS

Drugs

- *Amphotericin B:* Additive nephrotoxicity
- *Cephalosporins:* Additive nephrotoxicity
- *Cyclosporine:* Additive nephrotoxicity
- *Ethacrynic acid+:* Additive ototoxicity
- *Extended spectrum penicillins:* Inactivate aminoglycosides in vitro and in vivo
- *Neuromuscular blocking agents+:* Potentiate respiratory depression
- *NSAIDs:* Reduced renal clearance of aminoglycosides in premature infants, resulting in increased serum concentrations
- *Oral anticoagulants:* Enhanced hypoprothrombinemic response to oral anticoagulants

SPECIAL CONSIDERATIONS

- Gentamicin is first-line aminoglycoside of choice; differences in toxicity between gentamicin and tobramycin not likely to be clinically important in most patients with normal renal function given short courses of treatment; consider tobramycin in patients who are more likely to develop toxicity (prolonged and/or recurrent aminoglycoside therapy, those with renal failure, and those infected with *Pseudomonas aeruginosa* because of increased antibacterial activity

MONITORING PARAMETERS

- Serum Ca, Mg, Na; peak (30 min following IV inf or 1 hr after IM inj) and trough (just prior to next dose); prolonged concentrations above 12 μg/ml or trough levels above 2 μg/ml may indicate tissue accumulation); such accumulation, advanced age, and cumulative dosage may contribute to ototoxicity and nephrotoxicity; perform serum level assays after 2 or 3 doses, so that the dosage can be adjusted if necessary, and at 3- to 4-day intervals during therapy; in the event of changing renal function, more frequent serum levels should be obtained and the dosage or dosage interval adjusted according to more detailed guidelines

tocainide

(toe-kay'nide)
Tonocard
Chemical Class: Lidocaine analog
Therapeutic Class: Antidysrhythmic (Class IB)

CLINICAL PHARMACOLOGY
Mechanism of Action: Decreases sodium and potassium, resulting in decreased excitability of myocardial cells
Pharmacokinetics
PO: Peak ½-2 hr
Oral bioavailability, 100%, $t_{1/2}$ 10-17 hr; metabolized by liver (negligible first pass metabolism), excreted in urine
INDICATIONS AND USES: Life threatening ventricular dysrhythmias (i.e., sustained ventricular tachycardia)
DOSAGE
Adult
• PO initial 400 mg q8h; usual maintenance dose 1200 and 1800 mg/d in a three dose daily divided regimen
$ AVAILABLE FORMS/COST OF THERAPY
• Tab, Plain Coated—Oral: 400 mg, 100's: **$80.42;**; 600 mg, 100's: **$102.50**
CONTRAINDICATIONS: Hypersensitivity to amides, severe heart block
PRECAUTIONS: Children, renal disease, liver disease, CHF, respiratory depression, myasthenia gravis, blood dyscrasias
PREGNANCY AND LACTATION: Pregnancy category C
SIDE EFFECTS/ADVERSE REACTIONS
CNS: Headache, dizziness, involuntary movement, confusion, psychosis, restlessness, irritability, paresthesias, tremors, ***seizures***
CV: Hypotension, bradycardia, angina, PVCs, ***heart block, cardiovascular collapse, arrest, CHF,*** chest pain, tachycardia, ***prodyshythmic effect***
EENT: Tinnitus, blurred vision, hearing loss
GI: Nausea, vomiting, anorexia, diarrhea, hepatitis
HEME: ***Blood dyscrasias: leukopenia, agranulocytosis, hypoplastic anemia, thrombocytopenia***
MS: Lupus-like illness, positive ANA
RESP: Dyspnea, ***respiratory depression, pulmonary fibrosis***
SKIN: Rash, urticaria, edema, swelling
▼ DRUG INTERACTIONS
Drugs
• *Propranolol, quinidine and all other antidysrhythmics:* Increased effects
Labs
• *Increase:* CPK
SPECIAL CONSIDERATIONS
• Oral lidocaine, antidysrhythmic drugs have not been shown to improve survival in patients with ventricular dysrhythmias; class I antidysrhythmic drugs (eg, tocainide) have increased the risk of death when used in patients with non-life-threatening dysrhythmias
MONITORING PARAMETERS
• Blood levels (therapeutic level 4-10 μg/ml)

T

tolazamide

(tole-az'a-mide)
Tolamide, Tolinase
Chemical Class: Sulfonylurea (1st generation)
Therapeutic Class: Antidiabetic

CLINICAL PHARMACOLOGY
Mechanism of Action: Causes

functioning β-cells in pancreas to release insulin; may improve binding to insulin receptors or increase the number of insulin receptors with prolonged administration; may also reduce basal hepatic glucose secretion; not effective without functioning β-cells

Pharmacokinetics

PO: Onset 4-6 hr, peak 4-8 hr, duration 12-24 hr

Completely absorbed by GI route, $t_{1/2}$ 7 hr; metabolized in liver, excreted in urine (active metabolites), highly protein bound

INDICATIONS AND USES: Type II (NIDDM) diabetes mellitus, adjunct to insulin in selected patients*

DOSAGE

Adult

• PO 100 mg/day for FBS <200 mg/dl or 250 mg/d for FBS >200 mg/dl; dose should be titrated to patient response, Divide doses >500 mg/d bid; max dose 1 g or less/d

$ AVAILABLE FORMS/COST OF THERAPY

• Tab, Uncoated—Oral: 100 mg, 100's: **$5.93-$28.12;** 250 mg, 100's: **$9.38-$59.37;** 500 mg, 100's: **$17.93-$113.92**

CONTRAINDICATIONS: Hypersensitivity to sulfonylureas, juvenile or brittle diabetes

PRECAUTIONS: Elderly, cardiac disease, thyroid disease, severe hypoglycemic reactions, renal disease, hepatic disease

PREGNANCY AND LACTATION: Pregnancy category C

SIDE EFFECTS/ADVERSE REACTIONS

CNS: Headache, weakness, fatigue, lethargy, dizziness, vertigo, tinnitus

GI: Nausea, vomiting, diarrhea, constipation, gas, ***hepatotoxicity, jaundice,*** heartburn

HEME: ***Leukopenia, thrombocytopenia, agranulocytosis, aplastic anemia, pancytopenia, hemolytic anemia***

METAB: ***Hypoglycemia***

SKIN: Rash, (rare) allergic reactions, pruritus, urticaria, eczema, photosensitivity, erythema

▼ DRUG INTERACTIONS

Drugs

• *Anabolic steroids:* Enhanced hypoglycemic effects

• *Beta blockers:* Alter response to hypoglycemia, increase blood glucose concentrations

• *Chloramphenicol:* Enhanced hypoglycemic effects

• *Clofibrate:* Enhanced hypoglycemic effects

• *Clonidine:* Diminished symptoms of hypoglycemia

• *Colestipol:* Sulfonylureas inhibit the response to colestipol

• *Corticosteroids:* Increase blood glucose in diabetics

• *Ethanol+:* Altered glycemic control, usually hypoglycemia; "Antabuse"-like reaction

• *Halofenate:* Increased serum concentrations of tolbutamide and other sulfonylureas

• *MAOIs: Hypoglycemia+:* Increased hypoglycemic action

• *Oral anticoagulants:* Dicoumarol, not warfarin, enhances hypoglycemic response

• *Oral contraceptives:* Impaired glucose tolerance

• *Rifampin:* Reduced serum levels, reduced hypoglycemic activity

• *Smoking:* Increased glucose concentrations

• *Sulfonamides:* Enhanced hypoglycemic effects

• *Thiazide diuretics:* Increased blood glucose and antidiabetic drug dosage requirements

SPECIAL CONSIDERATIONS

PATIENT/FAMILY EDUCATION

• Home blood glucose monitoring

• Symptoms of hypoglycemia, hyperglycemia

MONITORING PARAMETERS

• Blood glucose, glycated hemoglobin

tolazoline

(toe-laz'a-leen)

Priscoline

Chemical Class: Imidoline derivative

Therapeutic Class: Peripheral vasodilator

CLINICAL PHARMACOLOGY

Mechanism of Action: Peripheral vasodilation occurs by direct relaxation of vascular smooth muscle; also has weak α adrenergic blocking properties

Pharmacokinetics

IM/SC: Peak 30-60 min, duration 3-4 hr Excreted in urine, $t_{½}$ 3-10 hr

INDICATIONS AND USES: Persistent pulmonary hypertension of newborn; also hypoxic pulmonary hypertension, arterial trauma,* clonidine overdose,* cor pulmonale,* lumbar puncture headache,* peripheral vascular disease,* spasmodic torticollis*

DOSAGE

Newborn

• IV 1-2 mg/kg via scalp vein

• IV INF 1-2 mg/kg/hr

$ AVAILABLE FORMS/COST OF THERAPY

• Inj, Repository—IM; IV; SC: 25 mg/ml, 4 ml: **$47.87**

CONTRAINDICATIONS: Hypersensitivity, CVA, CAD

PRECAUTIONS: Active peptic ulcer, mitral stenosis

PREGNANCY AND LACTATION: Pregnancy category C

SIDE EFFECTS/ADVERSE REACTIONS

CV: Orthostatic hypotension, ***tachycardia,*** dysrhythmias, hypertension, ***cardiovascular collapse***

RESP: ***Pulmonary hemorrhage***

GU: Edema, oliguria, hematuria

GI: Nausea, vomiting, diarrhea, peptic ulcer, ***GI hemorrhage, hepatitis***

SKIN: Flushing, tingling, rash, chills, sweating, increased pilomotor activity

HEME: ***Thrombocytopenia, leukopenia***

▼ DRUG INTERACTIONS

Drugs

• *Epinephrine, norepinephrine, phenylephrine:* Decrease B/P, rebound hypertension

• *Ethanol, beta-blockers:* Increased effects

• *H_2-blockers: Decreased effects*

tolbutamide

(tole-byoo'ta-mide)

Mobenol, ♣ Novobutamide, ♣ Orinase, Tolbutone ♣

Chemical Class: Sulfonylurea (1st generation)

Therapeutic Class: Oral antidiabetic

CLINICAL PHARMACOLOGY

Mechanism of Action: Causes functioning β-cells in pancreas to release insulin; may improve binding to insulin receptors or increase the number of insulin receptors with prolonged administration; may also reduce basal hepatic secretion; not effective if patient lacks functioning β-cells

Pharmacokinetics

PO: Onset 30-60 min, peak 3-5 hr, duration 6-12 hr Completely absorbed by GI route; $t_{½}$ 4-5 hr; metabolized in liver; excreted in urine (active metabolites), 90% -95% plasma protein bound

INDICATIONS AND USES: PO,

Type II (NIDDM) diabetes mellitus; IV, diagnostic test (Fajan's test) for pancreatic islet cell adenoma

DOSAGE

Adult

- PO 1-2 g/d in divided doses, titrated to patient response
- Diagnostic test: 1 g at constant rate over 2-3 min

$ **AVAILABLE FORMS/COST OF THERAPY**

- Tab, Uncoated—Oral: 250 mg, 100's: **$12.00;** 500 mg, 100's: **$2.95-$27.20**
- Inj, Lyphl-Sol—IV: 1 g/vial, 20 ml: **$54.92**

CONTRAINDICATIONS: Hypersensitivity to sulfonylureas, juvenile or brittle diabetes

PRECAUTIONS: Elderly, cardiac disease, thyroid disease, severe hypoglycemic reactions, renal disease, hepatic disease

PREGNANCY AND LACTATION: Pregnancy category C; excreted into breast milk; M:P ratio 0.09-0.4; caution re: jaundice in neonate, otherwise compatible with breast feeding

SIDE EFFECTS/ADVERSE REACTIONS

CNS: Headache, weakness, paresthesia, tinnitus, dizziness, vertigo

GI: Nausea, fullness, heartburn, ***hepatotoxicity, cholestatic jaundice,*** taste alteration, diarrhea

HEME: ***Leukopenia, thrombocytopenia, agranulocytosis, aplastic anemia,*** increased AST, ALT, alk phosphatase

METAB: ***Hypoglycemia***

MS: Joint pains

SKIN: Rash, allergic reactions, pruritus, urticaria, eczema, photosensitivity, erythema

▼ **DRUG INTERACTIONS**

Drugs

- *Anabolic steroids:* Enhanced hypoglycemic effects
- *Beta blockers:* Alter response to hypoglycemia, increase blood glucose concentrations
- *Chloramphenicol:* Enhanced hypoglycemic effects
- *Clonidine:* Diminished symptoms of hypoglycemia
- *Colestipol:* Sulfonylureas inhibit the response to colestipol
- *Corticosteroids:* Increase blood glucose in diabetics
- *Ethanol+:* Altered glycemic control, usually hypoglycemia; "Antabuse"-like reaction
- *Halofenate:* Increased serum concentrations of tolbutamide and other sulfonylureas
- *MAOIs:* Hypoglycemia
- *NSAIDs +: Increased hypoglycemic action*
- *Oral anticoagulants:* Dicoumarol, not warfarin, enhances hypoglycemic response
- *Oral contraceptives:* Impaired glucose tolerance
- *Rifampin:* Reduced serum levels, reduced hypoglycemic activity
- *Smoking:* Increased glucose concentrations
- *Sulfonamides:* Enhanced hypoglycemic effects
- *Thiazide diuretics:* Increased blood glucose and antidiabetic drug dosage requirements

Labs

- *Decrease:* RAIU test
- *Interference:* Urinary albumin

SPECIAL CONSIDERATIONS

- Sulfonylurea derivatives interchangable; possible differences exist for tolbutamide (short duration of action, hepatic clearance), potential preferred choice in older patients with poor general physical status and renal impairment

PATIENT/FAMILY EDUCATION

- Hypoglycemia symptoms

MONITORING PARAMETERS

• Blood glucose, glycated hemoglobin

tolmetin

(tole'met-in)

Tolectin DS, Tolectin

Chemical Class: Pyrrole acetic acid derivative

Therapeutic Class: Nonsteroidal antiinflammatory

CLINICAL PHARMACOLOGY

Mechanism of Action: Inhibits prostaglandin synthesis by inhibiting cyclooxygenase, an enzyme needed for biosynthesis; analgesic, antiinflammatory, antipyretic

Pharmacokinetics

PO: Peak 2 hr $t_{1/2}$ 3-3 ½ hr; metabolized in liver, excreted in urine (metabolites), 99% protein binding

INDICATIONS AND USES: Mild to moderate pain, osteoarthritis, rheumatoid arthritis, ankylosing spondylitis juvenile rheumatoid arthritis*

DOSAGE

Adult

• PO 400 mg tid-qid, not to exceed 2 g/d

Child >2 yr

• PO 15-30 mg/kg/d in 3 or 4 divided doses

$ **AVAILABLE FORMS/COST OF THERAPY**

• Cap, Gel—Oral: 200 mg, 100's: **$46.09-$64.06;** 400 mg, 100's: **$32.63-$101.63;** 600 mg, 100's: **$85.92-$123.32**

CONTRAINDICATIONS: Hypersensitivity, asthma, severe renal disease, severe hepatic disease, ulcer disease

PRECAUTIONS: Children, bleeding disorders, GI disorders, cardiac disorders, hypersensitivity to other antiinflammatory agents, peptic ulcer disease

PREGNANCY AND LACTATION: Pregnancy category B; excreted into breast milk, M:P ratio 0.005-0.007, compatible with breast feeding

SIDE EFFECTS/ADVERSE REACTIONS

CNS: Dizziness, drowsiness, fatigue, tremors, confusion, insomnia, anxiety, depression

CV: Tachycardia, peripheral edema, palpitations, dysrhythmias, hypertension

EENT: Tinnitus, hearing loss, blurred vision

GI: Nausea, anorexia, vomiting, diarrhea, jaundice, ***cholestatic hepatitis,*** constipation, flatulence, cramps, dry mouth, peptic ulcer, ulceration, bleeding, perforation

GU: ***Nephrotoxicity: dysuria, hematuria, oliguria, azotemia, pseudoproteinuria***

HEME: ***Blood dyscrasias***

SKIN: Purpura, rash, pruritus, sweating

▼ **DRUG INTERACTIONS**

Drugs

• *Antidiabetics+:* Protein binding displacement potential, increased concentration of oral hypoglycemics

• *Aminoglycosides:* Reduced clearance of aminoglycosides with increased antibiotic concentrations

• *Angiotensin-converting inhibitors:* Inhibit the antihypertensive effects of ACE inhibitors

• *Beta blockers:* Reduced hypotensive effects of beta blockers

• *Binding resins:* Potential to delay absorption of NSAID

• *Cyclosporine:* Other NSAIDs increase cyclosporin concentrations

• *Furosemide:* Reduces the diuretic and hypotensive effects of furosemide

• *Hydralazine:* Reduced hypotensive effects of hydralazine

- *Lithium:* Increased lithium concentrations with most NSAIDs
- *Methotrexate:* Potentially increase methotrexate concentrations and toxicity
- *Potassium-sparing diuretics:* Potential for acute renal failure i.e., indomethacin and triamterene

Labs

- False positive: Occult fecal blood, proteinuria

SPECIAL CONSIDERATIONS

- May interact less with the oral anticoagulants than the other NSAIDs (along with ibuprofen and naproxen); has also been used for ankylosing spondylitis and juvenile rheumatoid arthritis

tolnaftate

(tole-naf'tate)

Absorbine Antifungal, Absorbine Jock Itch, Absorbine Jr. Antifungal, Aftate, Genaspor, NP-27, Quinsana Plus, Tinactin, Ting, Zeasorb-AF

Chemical Class: Carbamothioic acid

Therapeutic Class: Topical antifungal

CLINICAL PHARMACOLOGY

Mechanism of Action: Fungicidal

INDICATIONS AND USES: Topical fungal infections (tinea pedis, tinea manuum, tinea cruris, tinea corporis, tinea capitis, tinea versicolor) due to susceptible strains of the following dermatophytes: *Trichophyton rubrum, T. mentagrophytes, T. tonsurans, Microsporum canis, M. audouinii Epidermophyton floccosum, Pityrosporon orbiculare*

DOSAGE

Adult and child

- TOP apply to affected area bid for 2-6 wk

$ AVAILABLE FORMS/COST OF THERAPY

- Powder: 100 g: **$4.50**
- Cre—Top: 1%, 15 g: **$2.85-$5.11**
- Sol—Top: 10 ml: **$4.50**

CONTRAINDICATIONS: Hypersensitivity, nail infections

PREGNANCY AND LACTATION: Pregnancy category C

SIDE EFFECTS/ADVERSE REACTIONS

SKIN: Rash, urticaria, stinging

SPECIAL CONSIDERATIONS

- Nonprescription topical antifungal agent not effective in the treatment of deeper fungal infections of the skin nor is it reliable in the treatment of fungal infections involving the scalp or nail beds; *Candida* is resistant; useful for patients desiring self-medication of mild tinea infections; patients must be advised of limitations

torsemide

(tor'se-mide)

Demadex

Chemical Class: Pyridine-sulfonylurea class

Therapeutic Class: Loop diuretic

CLINICAL PHARMACOLOGY

Mechanism of Action: Inhibits the $Na^+/K^+/Cl^-$ carrier system in the thick ascending portion of the loop of Henle where it increases urinary excretion of Na, Cl, and water, but does not significantly alter glomerular filtration rate, renal plasma flow, or acid-base balance

Pharmacokinetics

IV: Onset 10 min, peak 1 hr

PO: Onset 1 hr, peak 1-2 hr

Bioavailability 80%, minimal first-pass metabolism, volume of distribution 12-15 L (doubled in CHF, renal failure), $t_{1/2}$ 3½ hrs, cleared via hepatic metabolism (80%) and renal excretion (20%)

INDICATIONS AND USES: Edema associated with CHF, hepatic cirrhosis and renal disease, hypertension

DOSAGE

Adult

• Note: Because of high bioavailability, IV and PO doses are interchangable

• *CHF, chronic renal failure:* 10-20 mg qd, titrate upward to response (usually doubling) to max 200 mg/d

• *Cirrhosis:* 5-10 mg qd (usually with aldosterone antagonist or potassium-sparing diuretic), titrate upward to response (usually by doubling) to max 40 mg/d

• *Hypertension:* 5-10 mg qd

$ AVAILABLE FORMS/COST OF THERAPY

• Inj, Sol—IV: 10 mg/ml, 2 ml: **$3.58**

• Tab, Uncoated—Oral: 5 mg, 100's: **$43.75;** 10 mg, 100's: **$48.75;** 20 mg, 100's: **$52.50;** 100 mg, 100's: **$216.25**

CONTRAINDICATIONS: Hypersensitivity, anuric patients

PRECAUTIONS: Dehydration, hepatic cirrhosis and ascites, impaired renal function, electrolyte imbalance

PREGNANCY AND LACTATION: Pregnancy category B

SIDE EFFECTS/ADVERSE REACTIONS

CNS: Headache, dizziness, asthenia, insomnia, nervousness

CV: ECG abnormality, sore throat, chest pain

GI: Diarrhea, constipation, dyspepsia, edema

METAB: Hypokalemia, hypocalcemia, hypomagnesemia, increases in BUN, creatinine, uric acid, glucose, total cholesterol,

MS: Arthralgia, myalgia

RESP: Rhinitis, cough

SKIN: Rash

▼ DRUG INTERACTIONS

Drugs

• *ACE inhibitors:* Initiation of ACE inhibitor in the presence of intensive diuretic therapy may result in precipitous fall in blood pressure; ACE inhibitors may induce renal insufficiency in the presence of diuretic-induced sodium depletion

• *Bile acid binding resins:* Reduced bioavailability and diuretic response of torsemide

• *Clofibrate:* Enhanced effects of both drugs especially in patients with hypoalbuminemia

• *Digitalis glycosides:* Diuretic-induced hypokalemia may increase risk of digitalis toxicity

• *NSAIDs:* Reduced diuretic and antihypertensive efficacy of torsemide

• *Phenytoin:* Reduced diuretic response to torsemide

SPECIAL CONSIDERATIONS

• Offers potential advantages over other loop diuretics, including a longer duration of action and less adverse electrolyte/metabolic effects; available data not extensive or convincing enough at present to recommend replacement of standard loop diuretic (furosemide); considered alternative in refractory patients

tramadol

(traah'ma-doll)

Ultram

Chemical Class: trans-2-(dimethylamino methyl)-1-(m-methoxyphenyl)-cyclohexanol hydrochloride

Therapeutic Class: Centrally acting synthetic opioid-type analgesic

CLINICAL PHARMACOLOGY

Mechanism of Action: Complementary binding to μ-opiate receptors and inhibition of reuptake of norepinephrine and serotonin

Pharmacokinetics

PO: Onset 1 hr, peak 2-3 hr; rapid/complete absorption, $t_{1/2}$ 6-7 hr, volume of distribution 2.6-2.9 L/kg, 20% protein binding, extensively metabolized, mostly inactive metabolites, 60% excreted in urine

INDICATIONS AND USES: Moderate to moderately severe pain management

DOSAGE

Adult

- 50-100 mg q4-6h, not to exceed 400 mg/day; not necessary to reduce dose for elderly (<300 mg/d suggested); renal impairment, CrCl <30 ml/min, extend dosing interval q12h; hepatic impairment (cirrhosis) 50 mg q12h

$ AVAILABLE FORMS/COST OF THERAPY

- Tab, Uncoated—Oral: 50 mg, 100's: **$60.00**

CONTRAINDICATIONS: Hypersensitivity, acute intoxication with alcohol, hypnotics, centrally acting analgesics, opioids or psychotropic drugs

PRECAUTIONS: Respiratory depression, increased intracranial pressure or head trauma, acute abdominal conditions, opioid dependence, drug abuse and dependence, seizure disorder

PREGNANCY AND LACTATION: Pregnancy category C; minimal lactation data available; after 100 mg single IV dose, 100 μg (0.1% of maternal dose) and metabolites were excreted into breast milk

SIDE EFFECTS/ADVERSE REACTIONS

CNS: Dizziness, vertigo, headache, somnolence, CNS stimulation, asthenia, anxiety, confusion, coordination disturbance, euphoria, nervousness, sleep disorder

CV: Vasodilation,

EENT: Visual disturbance

GI: Nausea, constipation, vomiting, dyspepsia, dry mouth, diarrhea, abdominal pain, anorexia, flatulence

GU: Urinary retention/frequency, menopausal symptoms

SKIN: Pruritus, rash

▼ DRUG INTERACTIONS

Drugs

- *Carbamazepine:* Increased tramadol metabolism, may require significantly increased tramadol dosing for equianalgesic effects
- *MAOI:* Potential exaggerated norepinephrine and serotonin effects, as tramadol inhibits reuptake

Labs

- *Increase:* Creatinine, LFTs
- *Decrease:* Hemoglobin

SPECIAL CONSIDERATIONS

- Expensive, non-narcotic, "narcotic"/tricyclic antidepressant combination analgesic; potential use in chronic pain; demonstrated efficacy in a variety of pain syndromes*; minimal cardiovascular and respiratory side effects and low potential for abuse and psychological/physical dependence, based on limited and non-comparative data
- Does not completely bind to opioid receptors, caution in addicted patients

tranylcypromine

(tran-ill-sip'roe-meen)

Parnate

Chemical Class: Non hydrazine

Therapeutic Class: MAOI antidepressant

CLINICAL PHARMACOLOGY

Mechanism of Action: Increases concentrations of endogenous epinephrine, norepinephrine, serotonin, dopamine in storage sites in CNS by inhibition of MAO

Pharmacokinetics

PO: Onset 10 days

Well absorbed, metabolized by liver, excreted by kidneys (within 24 hr), MAO activity is recovered in 3-5 days (possibly up to 10 days) after withdrawal

INDICATIONS AND USES: Atypical exogenous depression, bulimia,* panic disorder with agoraphobia*

DOSAGE

Adult

- PO 10 mg bid; may increase to 30 mg/d after 2 wk; max 60 mg/d

$ AVAILABLE FORMS/COST OF THERAPY

- Tab, Plain Coated—Oral: 10 mg, 100's: **$45.80**

CONTRAINDICATIONS: Hypersensitivity, elderly, hypertension, CHF, severe hepatic disease, pheochromocytoma, severe renal disease, severe cardiac disease

PRECAUTIONS: Suicidal patients, convulsive disorders, severe depression, schizophrenia, hyperactivity, diabetes mellitus

PREGNANCY AND LACTATION: Pregnancy Category C

SIDE EFFECTS/ADVERSE REACTIONS

CNS: Dizziness, drowsiness, confusion, headache, anxiety, tremors, stimulation, weakness, hyperreflexia, mania, insomnia, fatigue, weight gain

CV: Orthostatic hypotension, hypertension, dysrhythmias, hypertensive crisis

EENT: Blurred vision

GI: Constipation, dry mouth, nausea, vomiting, *anorexia,* diarrhea, weight gain

GU: Change in libido, frequency

HEME: Anemia

METAB: ***SIADH-like syndrome***

SKIN: Rash, flushing, increased perspiration

▼ DRUG INTERACTIONS

Drugs

- *Amphetamines+:* Severe hypertensive reactions
- *Antidiabetics:* Prolonged hypoglycemia
- *Barbiturates:* Prolonged effect of barbiturates
- *Ephedrine+:* Severe hypertension
- *Ethanol:* With tyramine, hypertensive response
- *Fluoxetine+:* Severe or fatal reactions, serotonin related
- *Levodopa:* Hypertensive response; carbidopa minimizes the reaction
- *Lithium:* Hyperpyrexia with phenelzine
- *Meperidine+:* Serotonin accumulation—agitation, blood pressure elevations, hyperpyrexia, convulsions
- *Metaraminol+:* Hypertensive response
- *Phenylephrine+:* Hypertensive reactions
- *Phenylpropanolamine+:* Hypertensive reactions
- *Pseudoephedrine+:* Hypertensive reactions
- *Sertraline+:* Severe or fatal reactions, serotonin related
- *Sumatriptan:* Increased sumatriptan concentrations, possible toxicity

Labs

- Decrease: Glucose (stimulation of insulin, lower blood glucose levels), urine vanillylmandelic acid

SPECIAL CONSIDERATIONS

- Irreversible nonselective MAOI effective for typical and atypical depression; equal efficacy to other MAOIs with quicker onset of action, and an amphetamine-like activity with a higher potential for

T

abuse; no anticholinergic or cardiac effects

PATIENT/FAMILY EDUCATION

• Therapeutic effects may take 1-4 wk

• Avoid alcohol ingestion, CNS depressants, OTC medications (cold, weight loss, hay fever, cough syrup)

• Prodromal signs of hypertensive crisis are increased headache, palpitations; discontinue drug immediately

• Do not discontinue medication quickly after long-term use

• Avoid high-tyramine foods (aged cheese, sour cream, beer, wine, pickled products, liver, raisins, bananas, figs, avocados, meat tenderizers, chocolate, yogurt)

---

trazodone

(tray'zoe-done)

Desyrel

Chemical Class: Triazolopyridine

Therapeutic Class: Antidepressant

CLINICAL PHARMACOLOGY

Mechanism of Action: Mechanism not fully understood; selectively inhibits serotonin uptake by brain synaptosomes and potentiates behavioral changes induced by serotonin precursor, 5-hydroxytryptophan; cardiac conduction effects qualitatively dissimilar and quantitatively less pronounced than those seen with tricyclic antidepressants

Pharmacokinetics

PO: Peak plasma levels 1-2 hr, onset of therapeutic effect 2-4 wk, 85%-95% bound to plasma proteins, extensively metabolized in liver (active metabolite m-chlorophenylpiperazine), excreted mainly in urine with some fecal elimination, $t_{1/2}$ 4-7½ hr

INDICATIONS AND USES: Depression, aggressive behavior,* panic disorder,* agoraphobia with panic attacks,* insomnia*

DOSAGE

Adult

• PO 150 mg/d divided tid initially, increase by 50 mg/d q3-4d; adjust dose to lowest effective level; max 400 mg/d (outpatients), 600 mg/d (inpatients)

Child 6-18 yr

• PO 1.5-2 mg/kg/d in divided doses initially, increase gradually q3-4d as needed; max 6 mg/kg/d divided tid

$ **AVAILABLE FORMS/COST OF THERAPY**

• Tab, Plain Coated—Oral: 50, 100, 150, 300 mg, 100's: **$7.73-$349.66**

CONTRAINDICATIONS: Hypersensitivity

PRECAUTIONS: Preexisting cardiac disease, initial recovery phase of MI, children <18 yr, suicidal ideation, electroconvulsive therapy

PREGNANCY AND LACTATION: Pregnancy category C; excreted into human breast milk, effects on nursing infant unknown, but of possible concern

SIDE EFFECTS/ADVERSE REACTIONS

CNS: Anger, hostility, nightmares/vivid dreams, confusion, disorientation, decreased concentration, *dizzines,* lightheadedness, *drowsiness,* excitement, fatigue, headache, insomnia, impaired memory, nervousness, incoordination, paresthesia, tremors, hallucinations, psychosis, hypomania, mania, impaired speech, akathisia, numbness, delusions, agitation, weakness, ***seizures,*** EPS, ***tardive dyskinesia,*** stupor

CV: Edema, hypertension, hypotension, syncope, tachycardia, palpitations, chest pain, ***MI,*** ventricular ectopic activity, vasodilation, conduc-

tion block, orthostatic hypotension, bradycardia, ***cardiac arrest,*** atrial fibrillation, ***dysrhythmias***
EENT: Vertigo, tinnitus, blurred vision, red eyes, nasal/sinus congestion, diplopia
GI: Abdominal/gastric disorder, bad taste in mouth, *dry mouth,* nausea, vomiting, *diarrhea,* constipation, flatulence, hypersalivation, inappropriate ADH syndrome, liver enzyme alterations, intrahepatic cholestasis, hyperbilirubinemia, jaundice
GU: Hematuria, delayed urine flow, increased urinary frequency, urinary incontinence/retention
METAB: Decreased/increased libido, impotence, ***priapism,*** retrograde ejaculation, early menses, missed periods, breast enlargement and engorgement, lactation
MS: Aches and pains, muscle twitches, ataxia
RESP: Shortness of breath, apnea
SKIN: Rash, pruritis, urticaria, sweating, clamminess, alopecia
MISC: Decreased appetite, weight gain or loss, malaise

▼ **DRUG INTERACTIONS**

Drugs

- *Anticholinergics:* Excessive anticholinergic effects
- *Ethanol:* Additive impairment of motor skills; abstinent alcoholics may eliminate cyclic antidepressants more rapidly than non-alcoholic
- *Fluoxetine:* Increased plasma trazodone concentrations

Labs

- *Increase:* Serum bilirubin, blood glucose, alk phosphatase
- *False increase:* Urinary catecholamines
- *Decrease:* VMA, 5-HIAA

SPECIAL CONSIDERATIONS

PATIENT/FAMILY EDUCATION

- Take with food; use caution driving or performing other tasks requiring alertness
- Male patients with prolonged, inappropriate, and painful erections should immediately discontinue drug and consult prescriber

---

tretinoin

(tret'i-noyn)
Retin-A, Stievaa ♣
Chemical Class: Vitamin A derivative
Therapeutic Class: Acne product

CLINICAL PHARMACOLOGY

Mechanism of Action: Exact mode of action unknown; decreases cohesiveness of follicular epithelial cells with decreased microcomedone formation; stimulates mitotic activity and increases turnover of follicular epithelial cells causing extrusion of comedones

INDICATIONS AND USES: Topical treatment of acne vulgaris, lamellar ichthyosis,* mollusca contagiosa,* verrucae plantaris,* verrucae planae juveniles,* ichthyosis vulgaris,* bullous congenital icthyosiform and pityriasis rubra pilaris,* improvement of photoaged skin (especially wrinkling and liver spots)*

DOSAGE

Adult and child >12 yr

- TOP apply qd before retiring; begin therapy with 0.025% cream or 0.1% gel and increase concentration as tolerated; if stinging or irritation develops, decrease frequency of application

$ AVAILABLE FORMS/COST OF THERAPY

- Cre—Top: 0.025%, 20, 45 g: **$26.10-$49.44;** 0.05%, 20, 45 g: **$27.06-$50.82;** 0.10%, 20, 45 g: **$31.56-$59.28;** 0.010%, 15, 45 g:

$21.00-$49.74; 0.025%, 15, 45 g: **$21.24-%50.16**

• Liq—Top: 0.05%, 28 ml: **$41.58**

CONTRAINDICATIONS: Hypersensitivity

PRECAUTIONS: Eczematous skin, sunburned skin (do not use until skin is fully recovered)

PREGNANCY AND LACTATION: Pregnancy category B; teratogenic risk when used topically is thought to be close to zero; minimal absorption occuring after topical application probably precludes detection of clinically significant amounts in breast milk

SIDE EFFECTS/ADVERSE REACTIONS

SKIN: Irritation, excessive dryness, erythema, edema, blistering, crusting, temporary hyperpigmentation or hypopigmentation, photosensitivity, *initial acne flare up*

▼ **DRUG INTERACTIONS**

Drugs

• *Sulfur, resorcinol, benzoyl peroxide, salicylic acid:* Concomitant topical acne products may cause significant skin irritation

SPECIAL CONSIDERATIONS

PATIENT/FAMILY EDUCATION

• Keep away from eyes, mouth, angles of nose, and mucous membranes

• Avoid excessive exposure to ultraviolet light

• Acne may worsen transiently

• Normal use of cosmetics is permissible

triamcinolone

(trye-am-sin'oh-lone)

Oral: Aristocort, Atolone, Kenacort

Injectable: Amcort, Aristocort, Aristocort Forte, Aristospan, Ariculose L.A., Cenocort Forte, Tac, Kenalog, Cenocort A, Kenaject, Traiam-A, Tri-Kort, Triam Forte, Triamolone, Trilog, Trilone, Tristoject

Inhalation: Azmacort

Nasal: Nasacort

Topical: Aristocort, Aristocort A, Delta-Tritex, Flutex, Kenalog, Kenalog-H, Kenalog in Orabase, Kenonel, Oradent Dental, Triacet, Triderm

Chemical Class: Synthetic fluorinated adrenal corticosteroid; medium-high potency (topical)

Therapeutic Class: Antiinflammatory agent; inhaled corticosteroid; topical corticosteroid; systemic corticosteroid

CLINICAL PHARMACOLOGY

Mechanism of Action: Decreases inflammation by suppression of migration of polymorphonuclear leukocytes and reversal of increased capillary permeability; suppresses immune system by reducing activity and volume of lymphatic system

Pharmacokinetics

TOP: Absorbed through the skin (increased by inflammation and occlusive dressings)

IM: Peak within 8-10 hr

Metabolized in liver, excreted in urine and bile, biologic $t_{1/2}$ 18-36 hr

INDICATIONS AND USES: (Systemic) Antiinflammatory or immunosuppressant agent in the treatment of a variety of diseases including those of hematologic, allergic, inflammatory, neoplastic, and autoimmune origin: (topical) psoriasis, eczema, contact dermatitis, pruritis; (nasal) seasonal or perennial rhinitis, nasal polyps,* (inhalation) control of bronchial asthma, related corticosteroid-responsive bronchospastic states

DOSAGE

Adult

- PO 4-60 mg/d
- IM (diacetate) 40 mg per wk; (acetonide) 2.5-60 mg/d
- Intra-articular/intrasynovial/intralesional/sublesional (acetonide) 2.5-5 mg (small joints), 5-15 mg (large joints), 1 mg/inj site using only 3 mg/ml or 10 mg/ml strength (intradermal); (diacetate) 5-40 mg, do not use more than 12.5 mg/inj site, usual dose is 25 mg/lesion (intralesional or sublesional); (hexacetonide) 2-20 mg (intra-articular); 10-20 mg (large joints); 2-6 mg (small joints); up to 0.5 mg/in^2 of affected area (intralesional or sublesional)
- TOP apply to affected area bid-tid
- INH 2 inhalations tid-qid up to 16 inh/d
- NASAL 2 sprays in each nostril qb-bid

Child

- IM (acetonide or hexacetonide) 0.03-0.2 mg/kg at 1-7 day intervals
- INH 1-2 inhalation tid-qid up to 12 inh/d
- Intraarticular/intrasynovial/intralesional/sublesional 2.5-15 mg, repeated prn
- TOP apply bid-tid

$ **AVAILABLE FORMS/COST OF THERAPY**

- Tab, Uncoated—Oral: 1 mg, 50's: **$17.23;** 2 mg, 100's: **$72.52;** 4 mg, 100's: **$6.75-$131.23;** 8 mg, 50's: **$96.49-$107.57**
- Cre (acetonide)—Top: 0.025%, 15, 30, 60, 80, 454 g: **$1.04-34.05;** 0.1%, 15, 30, 60, 80, 240, **$0.90-$68.88;** 0.5%, 15, 20, 30, 240, 454 g: **$2.80-$88.98**
- Inj, Susp (acetonide)—Intraarticular; IM: 40 mg/ml, 1 ml: **$4.46;** 40 mg/ml, 5 ml: **$4.92-$31.65**
- Inj, Susp (diacetate)—Intraarticular; IM: 40 mg/ml, 5 ml: **$11.50**
- Inj, Sol (acetonide)—IV: 40 mg/ml, 5 ml: **$6.50-$19.20**
- Inj, Sol (diacetate)—IV: 25 mg/ml, 5 ml **$20.30**
- Inj, Sol (hexacetonide)—IV: 5 mg/ml, 5 ml: **$11.94;** 20 mg/ml, 5 ml: **$18.40**
- Inj, Susp (acetonide)—Intraarticular; Intrasynovial; ID: 10 mg/ml, 5 ml: **$6.95**
- Inj, Susp (acetonide)—ID: 3 mg/ml, 5 ml: **$8.95**
- Inj, Sol (diacetate)—IM; IV; SC: 40 mg/ml, 5 ml: **$3.70-$26.10**
- Lotion (acetonide)—Top: 0.025%, 60 ml: **$6.67-$30.75;** 0.1%, 60 ml: **$6.90-$34.52**
- Oint (acetonide)—Top: 0.025%, 15, 80, 454 g: **$1.04-$34.05;** 0.05%, 454 g: **$24.45;** 0.1%, 15, 30, 60, 80, 240, 454 g: **$1.13-$34.05;** 0.5%, 15, 20, 240 g: **$3.09-$209.56**
- Paste (acetonide)—Dental: 0.1%, 5 g: **$4.38-$12.33**
- Aer (acetonide)—Inh: 100 μg, 100 spr's: **$43.36**
- Aer (acetonide)—Nasal: 55 μg, 10 g: **$39.18**
- Aer, spray (acetonide)—Top: 3.3 mg/50 g, 63 g: **$24.27**
- Syr (diacetate)—Oral: 2 mg/5 ml, 120 ml: **$20.21;** 4 mg/5 ml, 120 ml: **$33.25**

CONTRAINDICATIONS: Systemic fungal infections, hypersensitivity, idiopathic thrombocytopenic purpura (IM); bacterial infection of nose (nasal); status asthmaticus (inhalation)

PRECAUTIONS: Psychosis, acute glomerulonephritis, amebiasis, ce-

T

rebral malaria, child <2 yr, elderly, AIDS, tuberculosis, diabetes mellitus, glaucoma, osteoporosis, ulcerative colitis, CHF, myasthenia gravis, renal disease, esophagitis, peptic ulcer, ocular herpes simplex, live virus vaccines, hypertension; quiescent tuberculosis infections of the respiratory tract (inhalation); nasal septal ulcers, recurrent epistaxis, nasal surgery or trauma (nasal); viral infections, bacterial infections, children, use on face, groin, or axilla (topical)

PREGNANCY AND LACTATION: Pregnancy category C; may appear in breast milk and could suppress growth, interfere with endogenous corticosteroid production, or cause unwanted effects in the nursing infant

SIDE EFFECTS/ADVERSE REACTIONS

CNS: Depression, vertigo, ***convulsions,*** headache, *mood changes*

CV: Hypertension, ***thromboembolism,*** tachycardia, CHF

EENT: Increased intraocular pressure, blurred vision, cataract; hoarseness, *Canadida* infection of oral cavity, *sore throat,* hoarseness/dysphonia (inhalation); nasal irritation and stinging, dryness, rebound congestion, epistaxis, sneezing (nasal)

GI: Diarrhea, nausea, abdominal distension, ***GI hemorrhage,*** increased appetite, ***pancreatitis***

METAB: Cushingoid state, growth suppression in children, HPA suppression, decreased glucose tolerance

MS: Fractures, osteoporosis, aseptic necrosis of femoral and humeral heads, weakness, muscle mass loss

SKIN: Acne, poor wound healing, ecchymosis, bruising, petechiae, striae, thin fragile skin, suppression of skin test reactions; burning, dryness, itching, irritation, acne, folliculitis, hypertrichosis, perioral dermatitis, hypopigmentation, atrophy, miliaria, allergic contact dermatitis, secondary infection (topical)

MISC: Systemic absorption of topical corticosteroids has produced reversible HPA axis suppression (more likely with occlusive dressings, prolonged administration, application to large surface areas, liver failure and in children)

▼ DRUG INTERACTIONS

Drugs

- *Aminoglutethamide:* Enhanced elimination of triamcinolone; marked reduction in corticosteroid response
- *Antidiabetics:* Increased blood glucose in patients with diabetes
- *Barbiturates, carbamazepine:* Reduced serum concentrations of corticosteroids
- *Cholestyramine:* Possible reduced absorption of corticosteroids
- *Estrogens:* Enhanced effects of corticosteroids
- *Isoniazid:* Reduced plasma concentrations of isoniazid
- *Phenytoin:* Reduced therapeutic effect of corticosteroids
- *Rifampin:* Reduced therapeutic effect of corticosteroids
- *Salicylates:* Enhanced elimination of salicylates; subtherapeutic salicylate concentrations possible

Labs

- *Increase:* Cholesterol, blood glucose, urine glucose
- *Decrease:* Calcium, potassium, T_4, T_3, thyroid ^{131}I uptake test
- *False Negative:* Skin allergy tests

SPECIAL CONSIDERATIONS

PATIENT/FAMILY EDUCATION

- May cause GI upset, take with meals or snacks
- Take single daily doses in AM
- Notify physician if unusual weight gain, swelling of lower extremities, muscle weakness, black tarry stools,

vomiting of blood, puffing of the face, menstrual irregularities, prolonged sore throat, fever, cold, or infection occurs
• Signs of adrenal insufficiency include fatigue, anorexia, nausea, vomiting, diarrhea, weight loss, weakness, dizziness, and low blood sugar, notify physician if these signs and symptoms appear following dose reduction or withdrawal of therapy
• Avoid abrupt withdrawal of therapy following high dose or long-term therapy
• To be used on a regular basis, not for acute symptoms (nasal and inhalation)
• Use bronchodilators before oral inhaler (for patients using both)
• Nasal sol may cause drying and irritation of nasal mucosa
• Clear nasal passages prior to use of nasal sol

MONITORING PARAMETERS
• Potassium and blood sugar during long-term therapy
• Edema, blood pressure, cardiac symptoms, mental status, weight
• Observe growth and development of infants and children on prolonged therapy

triamterene
(trye-am′ter-een)
Dyrenium
Chemical Class: Pteridine derivative
Therapeutic Class: Potassium-sparing diuretic

CLINICAL PHARMACOLOGY
Mechanism of Action: Inhibits reabsorption of sodium ions in exchange for potassium and hydrogen ions at the distal tubule; degree of natriuresis and diuresis produced by inhibition of the exchange mechanism is limited
Pharmacokinetics
PO: Onset 2-4 hr, peak 3 hr, duration 7-9 hr, primarily metabolized to sulfate conjugate of hydroxytriamterene (active), 21% excreted in urine unchanged, $t_{1/2}$ 1½-2 hr

INDICATIONS AND USES: Edema associated with CHF, cirrhosis of the liver, and the nephrotic syndrome; steroid-induced edema, idiopathic edema, and edema due to secondary hyperaldosteronism; may be used alone or with other diuretics either for its added diuretic effect or its potassium-conserving potential

DOSAGE
Adult
• PO 100 mg bid pc; do not exceed 300 mg/d; when combined with other diuretics or antihypertensives, decrease total daily dosage initially and adjust to patient's needs
Child
• PO 2-4 mg/kg/d in 1-2 divided doses; max 6 mg/kg/d or 300 mg/d

$ AVAILABLE FORMS/COST OF THERAPY
• Cap, Gel—Oral: 50 mg, 100's: **$34.15;** 100 mg, 100's: **$42.90**

CONTRAINDICATIONS: Anuria, severe or progressive kidney disease or dysfunction (with possible exception of nephrosis), severe hepatic disease, hypersensitivity, preexisting elevated serum potassium, patients receiving spironolactone or amiloride

PRECAUTIONS: Diabetes, renal function impairment, hepatic function impairment, children, electrolyte imbalance, renal stones, predisposition to gouty arthritis

PREGNANCY AND LACTATION: Pregnancy category D (category B according to manufacturer); many investigators consider diuretics contraindicated in pregnancy, except for

T

patients with heart disease; may decrease placental perfusion; excreted in cow's milk, no human data

SIDE EFFECTS/ADVERSE REACTIONS

CNS: Dizziness, headache

GI: Diarrhea, nausea, vomiting, jaundice, liver enzyme abnormalities, dry mouth

GU: Elevated BUN and creatinine, has been found in renal stones, ***interstitial nephritis***

HEME: ***Thrombocytopenia, megaloblastic anemia***

METAB: Electrolyte imbalance, ***hyperkalemia,*** hypokalemia

SKIN: Photosensitivity, rash

MISC: Fatigue, weakness, ***anaphylaxis***

▼ **DRUG INTERACTIONS**

Drugs

- *ACE inhibitors:* Hyperkalemia in predisposed patients
- *NSAIDs:* Acute renal failure with indomethacin and possibly other NSAIDs
- *Potassium+:* Hyperkalemia in predisposed patients

Labs

- *Interference:* Serum quinidine levels

SPECIAL CONSIDERATIONS

PATIENT/FAMILY EDUCATION

- Take with meals
- Avoid prolonged exposure to sunlight
- Take single daily doses in AM

MONITORING PARAMETERS

- ECG if hyperkalemia suspected
- Serum potassium, BUN, serum creatinine
- Liver function tests

---

triazolam

(trye-ay′zoe-lam)

Halcion

Chemical Class: Benzodiazepine

Therapeutic Class: Sedative/hypnotic

DEA Class: Schedule IV

CLINICAL PHARMACOLOGY

Mechanism of Action: Facilitates the inhibitory effect of α-aminobutyric acid (GABA) on neuronal excitability by increasing membrane permeability to chloride ions

Pharmacokinetics

PO: Onset 15-30 min, peak 42 min, duration 6-7 hr, 89% bound to plasma proteins, extensively metabolized in liver, excreted in urine as unchanged drug and metabolites, $t_{1/2}$ 1.7-5 hr

INDICATIONS AND USES: Short-term treatment of insomnia (generally 7-10 days); use for more than 2-3 weeks requires complete reevaluation of the patient

DOSAGE

Adult

- PO 0.125-0.5 mg hs

Elderly or debilitated patients

- PO 0.125-0.25 mg hs; initiate with 0.125 mg until individual response is determined

$ **AVAILABLE FORMS/COST OF THERAPY**

- Tab, Plain Coated—Oral: 0.125 mg, 100's: **$56.37-$67.83**; 0.25 mg, 100's: **$61.65-$74.15**

CONTRAINDICATIONS: Hypersensitivity to benzodiazepines, narrow angle glaucoma, psychosis, children <18 yr

PRECAUTIONS: Elderly, debilitated, hepatic disease, renal disease, history of drug abuse, abrupt withdrawal, respiratory depression, prolonged use

PREGNANCY AND LACTATION: Pregnancy category X (according to manufacturer); no congenital anomalies have been attributed to use during human pregnancies, other benzodiazepines have been suspected of producing fetal malformations after 1st trimester exposure

SIDE EFFECTS/ADVERSE REACTIONS

CNS: Somnolence, asthenia, hypokinesia, hangover, abnormal thinking, anxiety, agitation, anterograde amnesia, early morning insomnia, apathy, emotional lability, hostility, ***seizure,*** sleep disorder, stupor, ataxia, decreased libido, decreased reflexes, neuritis

CV: ***Dysrhythmia,*** syncope

EENT: Ear pain, eye irritation/pain/swelling, photophobia, pharyngitis, rhinitis, sinusitis, epistaxis

GI: Dyspepsia, decreased/increased appetite, flatulence, gastritis, enterocolitis, melena, mouth ulceration, abdominal pain, increased AST

GU: Frequent urination, menstrual cramps, urinary hesitancy/urgency, vaginal discharge/itching, hematuria, nocturia, oliguria, penile discharge, urinary incontinence

HEME: ***Agranulocytosis***

MS: Lower extremity pain, back pain

RESP: Cold symptoms, asthma, cough, dyspnea, hyperventilation

SKIN: Urticaria, acne, dry skin, photosensitivity

▼ DRUG INTERACTIONS

Drugs

- *Cimetidine, erythromycin, ketoconazole, oral contraceptives, troleandomycin:* Increased plasma triazolam concentrations
- *Clozapine:* Cardiorespiratory collapse
- *Ethanol:* Enhanced adverse psychomotor effects of benzodiazepines

Labs

- *Increase:* AST/ALT, serum bilirubin
- *False increase:* 17-OHCS
- *Decrease:* RAIU

SPECIAL CONSIDERATIONS

Prescriptions should be written for short-term use (7-10 days); drug should not be prescribed in quantities exceeding a 1-mo supply

PATIENT/FAMILY EDUCATION

- Avoid alcohol and other CNS depressants
- Do not discontinue abruptly after prolonged therapy
- May cause drowsiness or dizziness, use caution while driving or performing other tasks requiring alertness
- May be habit forming

tridihexethyl chloride

(trye-dye-hex′eth-ill)

Pathilon

Chemical Class: Quaternary ammonium compound

Therapeutic Class: Gastrointestinal antimuscarinic/antispasmodic

CLINICAL PHARMACOLOGY

Mechanism of Action: Inhibits GI motility and diminishes gastric acid secretion

Pharmacokinetics

PO: Onset within 1 hr, peak effect 2 hr, duration 4-8 hr

INDICATIONS AND USES: Adjunctive therapy in peptic ulcer treatment; functional GI disorders (diarrhea, pylorospasm, hypermotility, neurogenic colon);* irritable bowel syndrome (spastic colon, mucous colitis);* acute enterocolitis,* ulcerative colitis,* diverticulitis,* mild dysenteries,* pancreatitis,* splenic flexure syndrome*

T

DOSAGE

Adult

- PO 25-50 mg tid-qid, ac and hs; hs dose 50 mg

$ AVAILABLE FORMS/COST OF THERAPY

- Tab, Coated—Oral: 25 mg, 100's: **$66.32**

CONTRAINDICATIONS: Hypersensitivity to anticholinergic drugs, narrow-angle glaucoma, obstructive uropathy, obstructive disease of the GI tract, paralytic ileus, intestinal atony, unstable cardiovascular status in acute hemorrhage, severe ulcerative colitis, toxic megacolon complicating ulcerative colitis, myasthenia gravis

PRECAUTIONS: Hyperthyroidism, CAD, dysrhythmias, CHF, ulcerative colitis, hypertension, hiatal hernia, hepatic disease, renal disease, urinary retention, prostatic hypertrophy, elderly, children, glaucoma

PREGNANCY AND LACTATION: Pregnancy category C; excretion into breast milk unknown, although would be expected to be minimal due to quaternary structure

SIDE EFFECTS/ADVERSE REACTIONS

CNS: Confusion, stimulation (especially in elderly), headache, insomnia, dizziness, drowsiness, anxiety, weakness, hallucination

CV: Palpitations, tachycardia

EENT: Blurred vision, photophobia, mydriasis, cycloplegia, increased ocular tension

GI: Dry mouth, constipation, ***paralytic ileus,*** heartburn, nausea, vomiting, dysphagia, absence of taste

GU: Hesitancy, retention, impotence

SKIN: Urticaria, rash, pruritus, anhidrosis, fever, allergic reactions

SPECIAL CONSIDERATIONS

PATIENT/FAMILY EDUCATION

- Usually taken 30-60 min before a meal
- May cause drowsiness, dizziness, or blurred vision; use caution while driving or performing other tasks requiring alertness
- Notify physician if eye pain occurs

---

trientine

(trye-en'teen)

Spyrine

Chemical Class: Thiol compound

Therapeutic Class: Chelating agent

CLINICAL PHARMACOLOGY

Mechanism of Action: Chelating agent that binds copper and facilitates its excretion from the body (cupriuresis)

INDICATIONS AND USES: Treatment of Wilson's disease in patients intolerant of penicillamine

DOSAGE

Adult

- PO 750-1250 mg/d divided bid-qid; may increase to max of 2 g/d

Child ≤12 yr

- PO 500-750 mg/d divided bid-qid; may increase to max of 1.5 g/d

$ AVAILABLE FORMS/COST OF THERAPY

- Cap, Gel—Oral: 250 mg, 100's: **$90.16**

CONTRAINDICATIONS: Hypersensitivity, cystinuria, rheumatoid arthritis, biliary cirrhosis

PRECAUTIONS: Iron deficiency anemia, children

PREGNANCY AND LACTATION: Pregnancy category C

SIDE EFFECTS/ADVERSE REACTIONS

GI: Heartburn, epigastric pain

HEME: Iron deficiency anemia

MS: Muscle pain, cramps
SKIN: Tenderness, thickening and fissuring of skin
MISC: Systemic lupus erytematosus, malaise

SPECIAL CONSIDERATIONS

PATIENT/FAMILY EDUCATION

- Take on empty stomach

MONITORING PARAMETERS

- Free serum copper (adequately treated patients will have <10 μg/dl), increase daily dose only when clinical response is not adequate or concentration of free serum copper is persistently above 20 μg/dl (determine optimal long-term maintenance dosage at 6-12 month intervals)
- 24 hr urinary copper analysis at 6-12 mo intervals (adequately treated patients will have 0.5-1 mg copper/24 hr collection of urine)

---

trifluoperazine

(trye-floo-oh-per′a-zeen)
Novoflurazine, ♣ Solazine, ♣ Stelazine
Chemical Class: Piperazine phenothiazine derivative
Therapeutic Class: Antipsychotic/neuroleptic

CLINICAL PHARMACOLOGY

Mechanism of Action: Blocks postsynaptic dopamine receptors in the basal ganglia, hypothalamus, limbic system, brain stem, and medulla; appears to act at both D_1 and D_2 receptors; also exerts α-adrenergic blocking effects; weak anticholinergic and sedative effects, strong extrapyramidal effects, strong antiemetic activity

Pharmacokinetics

PO: Peak 1½-4½ hr, duration ≥12 hr, ≥90% bound to plasma proteins, extensive liver metabolism, excreted in urine and bile, $t_{1/2}$ >24 hr with chronic use (7-18 hr after single dose)

INDICATIONS AND USES: Psychotic disorders, short-term treatment of nonpsychotic anxiety (not drug of choice in most patients)

DOSAGE

Adult

- *Psychotic disorders:* PO 2-5 mg bid; most patients show optimum response with 15-20 mg/d, some may require ≥40 mg/d; IM (for prompt control of symptoms) 1-2 mg q4-6h prn; doses >6 mg/24 hr are rarely necessary
- *Nonpsychotic anxiety:* PO 1-2 mg bid; do not administer >6 mg/day or for >12 wk

Child

- PO 1 mg qd-bid initially; usually not necessary to exceed 15 mg/d: IM 1 mg qd-bid (little experience in children)

$ AVAILABLE FORMS/COST OF THERAPY

- Conc—Oral: 10 mg/ml, 60 ml: **$56.74-$108.00**
- Tab, Plain Coated—Oral: 1 mg, 100's: **$7.98-$60.95;** 2 mg, 100's: **$9.25-$89.90;** 5 mg, 100's: **$10.60-$113.15;** 10 mg, 100's: **$13.55-$170.55**
- Inj, Sol—IM: 2 mg/ml, 10 ml: **$49.55**

CONTRAINDICATIONS: Hypersensitivity to phenothiazines, severe toxic CNS depression, coma, subcortical brain damage, bone marrow depression

PRECAUTIONS: Elderly, children <12 yr, prolonged use, severe cardiovascular disorders, epilepsy, hepatic or renal disease, glaucoma, prostatic hypertrophy, severe asthma, emphysema, hypocalcemia (increased susceptibility to dystonic reactions)

PREGNANCY AND LACTATION: Pregnancy category C; has been

T

used as an antiemetic during normal labor without producing any observable effect on newborn, bulk of evidence indicates safety for mother and fetus

SIDE EFFECTS/ADVERSE REACTIONS

CNS: *EPS (pseudoparkinsonism, akathisia, dystonia,* ***tardive dyskinesia****), drowsiness, headache,* ***seizures, neuroleptic malignant syndrome,*** confusion, insomnia, restlessness, anxiety, euphoria, agitation, depression, lethargy, vertigo, exacerbation of psychotic symptoms including hallucinations, catatonic-like behavioral states, heat or cold intolerance

CV: Tachycardia, hypotension, hypertension, ECG changes

EENT: Blurred vision, glaucoma, dry eyes, cataracts, retinopathy, pigmentation of retina or cornea

GI: Anorexia, constipation, diarrhea, hypersalivation, dyspepsia, *nausea,* vomiting, *dry mouth*

GU: Urinary retention, priapism

HEME: Transient leukopenia, leukocytosis, minimal decreases in red blood cell counts, anemia, ***agranulocytosis, aplastic anemia, hemolytic anemia***

METAB: Lactation, breast engorgement, mastalgia, menstrual irregularities, gynecomastia, impotence, increased libido, hyperglycemia, hypoglycemia, hyponatremia

RESP: ***Laryngospasm, bronchospasm,*** increased depth of respiration

SKIN: Maculopapular and acneiform skin reactions, photosensitivity, loss of hair, diaphoresis

▼ **DRUG INTERACTIONS**

Drugs

• *Anticholinergics:* Inhibited therapeutic response to antipsychotic; enhanced anticholinergic side effects
• *Antidepressants:* Increased serum concentrations of some cyclic antidepressants
• *Barbiturates:* Reduced effect of antipsychotic
• *Beta blockers:* Enhanced effects of both drugs
• *Bromocriptine, lithium:* Reduced effects of both drugs
• *Epinephrine:* Reversed pressor response to epinephrine
• *Guanethidine+:* Inhibited antihypertensive response to guanethidine
• *Levodopa:* Inhibited effect of levodopa on Parkinson's disease
• *Narcotic analgesics:* Excessive CNS depression, hypotension, respiratory depression
• *Orphenadrine:* Reduced serum neuroleptic concentrations, excessive anticholinergic effects

Labs

• *Increase:* Liver function tests, cardiac enzymes, cholesterol, blood glucose, prolactin, bilirubin, PBI, cholinesterase, ^{131}I
• *False positive:* Pregnancy tests, PKU
• *False negative:* Urinary steroids, 17-OHCS

SPECIAL CONSIDERATIONS

PATIENT/FAMILY EDUCATION

• Dilute concentrate in 60 ml of diluent just prior to administration (suggested diluents: tomato or fruit juice, milk, simple syrup, orange syrup, carbonated beverages, coffee, tea, or water)
• Contact prescriber if sore throat, or other signs of infection
• Arise slowly from reclining position
• Do not discontinue abruptly
• Use a sunscreen during sun exposure to prevent burns, take special precautions to stay cool in hot weather
• May cause drowsiness

MONITORING PARAMETERS

- Observe closely for signs of tardive dyskinesia
- Periodic CBC with platelets during prolonged therapy

triflupromazine

(trye-floo-proe'ma-zeen)

Vesprin

Chemical Class: Aliphatic phenothiazine derivative

Therapeutic Class: Antispychotic/neuroleptic; antiemetic

CLINICAL PHARMACOLOGY

Mechanism of Action: Blocks postsynaptic dopamine receptors in the basal ganglia, hypothalamus, limbic system, brain stem and medulla; appears to act at both D_1 and D_2 receptors; strong anticholinergic effects, moderate to strong extrapyramidal and sedative effects, strong antiemetic activity

Pharmacokinetics

IM: Onset 15-30 min, peak 1 hr, duration 4-6 hr, metabolized by liver, excreted in urine and feces

INDICATIONS AND USES: Psychotic disorders, control of severe nausea and vomiting

DOSAGE

Adult

- *Psychotic disorders:* IM 60 mg, up to max of 150 mg/d
- *Nausea and vomiting:* IV 1 mg up to a max total 3 mg/d; IM 5-15 mg as a single dose, may repeat q4h up to max of 60 mg/d

Elderly or debilitated patients

- *Nausea and vomiting:* IM 2.5 mg up to a max of 15 mg/d

Child >2 yr

- IM 0.2-0.25 mg/kg, up to max total dose of 10 mg/d

$ AVAILABLE FORMS/COST OF THERAPY

- Inj, Sol—IM; IV: 10 mg/ml, 10 ml: **$47.53;** 20 mg/ml, 1 ml: **$13.00**

CONTRAINDICATIONS: Hypersensitivity to phenothiazines, severe toxic CNS depression, coma, subcortical brain damage, bone marrow depression, narrow-angle glaucoma

PRECAUTIONS: Elderly, prolonged use, severe cardiovascular disorders, epilepsy, hepatic or renal disease, glaucoma, prostatic hypertrophy, severe asthma, emphysema, hypocalcemia (increased susceptibility to dystonic reactions)

PREGNANCY AND LACTATION: Pregnancy category C; bulk of evidence indicates phenothiazines are safe for mother and fetus

SIDE EFFECTS/ADVERSE REACTIONS

CNS: EPS (pseudoparkinsonism, akathisia, dystonia, ***tardive dyskinesia),*** *drowsiness, headache,* ***seizures, neuroleptic malignant syndrome,*** confusion, insomnia, restlessness, anxiety, euphoria, agitation, depression, lethargy, vertigo, exacerbation of psychotic symptoms including hallucinations, catatonic-like behavioral states, heat or cold intolerance

CV: Tachycardia, hypotension, hypertension, ECG changes

EENT: Blurred vision, glaucoma, dry eyes, cataracts, retinopathy, pigmentation of retina or cornea

GI: Anorexia, constipation, diarrhea, hypersalivation, dyspepsia, *nausea,* vomiting, *dry mouth*

GU: Urinary retention, priapism

HEME: Transient leukopenia, leukocytosis, minimal decreases in red blood cell counts, anemia, ***agranulocytosis, aplastic anemia, hemolytic anemia***

METAB: Lactation, breast engorgement, mastalgia, menstrual irregularities, gynecomastia, impotence,

T

increased libido, hyperglycemia, hypoglycemia, hyponatremia

RESP: ***Laryngospasm, bronchospasm,*** increased depth of respiration

SKIN: Maculopapular and acneiform skin reactions, photosensitivity, loss of hair, diaphoresis

▼ **DRUG INTERACTIONS**

Drugs

• *Anticholinergics:* Inhibited therapeutic response to antipsychotic; enhanced anticholinergic side effects

• *Antidepressants:* Increased serum concentrations of some cyclic antidepressants

• *Barbiturates:* Reduced effect of antipsychotic

• *Beta blockers:* Enhanced effects of both drugs

• *Bromocriptine, lithium:* Reduced effects of both drugs

• *Epinephrine:* Reversed pressor response to epinephrine

• *Guanethidine+:* Inhibited antihypertensive response to guanethidine

• *Levodopa:* Inhibited effect of levodopa on Parkinson's disease

• *Narcotic analgesics:* Excessive CNS depression, hypotension, respiratory depression

• *Orphenadrine:* Reduced serum neuroleptic concentrations, excessive anticholinergic effects

Labs

• *Increase:* Liver function tests, cardiac enzymes, cholesterol, blood glucose, prolactin, bilirubin, PBI, cholinesterase, ^{131}I

• *False positive:* Pregnancy tests, PKU

• *False negative:* Urinary steroids, 17-OHCS

SPECIAL CONSIDERATIONS

PATIENT/FAMILY EDUCATION

• Arise slowly from reclining position

• Do not discontinue abruptly

• Use a sunscreen during sun exposure to prevent burns, take special precautions to stay cool in hot weather

• May cause drowsiness

MONITORING PARAMETERS

• Observe closely for signs of tardive dyskinesia

• Periodic CBC with platelets during prolonged therapy

trifluridine

(trye-flure'i-deen)

Viroptic

Chemical Class: Fluorinated pyrimidine nucleoside

Therapeutic Class: Ophthalmic antiviral

CLINICAL PHARMACOLOGY

Mechanism of Action: Interferes with DNA synthesis in cultured mammalian cells; antiviral mechanism of action not completely known

Pharmacokinetics: Penetrates the intact cornea, systemic absorption following therapeutic dosing appears to be negligible

INDICATIONS AND USES: Primary keratoconjunctivitis and recurrent epithelial keratitis due to herpes simplex virus types 1 and 2; epithelial keratitis unresponsive to topical idoxuridine, or intolerance to idoxuridine; epithelial keratitis resistant to topical vidarabine

DOSAGE

Adult

• Instill 1 gtt onto cornea of affected eye(s) q2h while awake until ulcer has completely reepithelialized; max 9 gtt/d; after reepithelialization, 1 gtt q4h while awake for an additional 7 days; minimum 5 gtt/d; do not exceed 21 days due to potential for ocular toxicity

AVAILABLE FORMS/COST OF THERAPY

• Sol—Ophth: 10 mg/ml, 7.5 ml: **$48.29**

CONTRAINDICATIONS: Hypersensitivity

PRECAUTIONS: Prolonged use (>21 days); not effective for bacterial, fungal, or chlamydial infections of the cornea or trophic lesions

PREGNANCY AND LACTATION: Pregnancy category C

SIDE EFFECTS/ADVERSE REACTIONS

EENT: Burning, stinging, palpebral edema, superficial punctate keratopathy, epithelial keratopathy, hypersensitivity reaction, stromal edema, irritation, keratitis sicca, hyperemia, increased intraocular pressure

SPECIAL CONSIDERATIONS

PATIENT/FAMILY EDUCATION

• Notify prescriber if no improvement after 7 days

trihexyphenidyl

(trye-hex-ee-fen'i-dill)

Aparkane,♣ Aphen, Artane, Novohexidyl,♣ Trihexy

Chemical Class: Synthetic tertiary amine

Therapeutic Class: Anticholinergic; antiparkinson agent

CLINICAL PHARMACOLOGY

Mechanism of Action: Blocks striatal cholinergic receptors which helps balance cholinergic and dopaminergic activity

Pharmacokinetics

PO: Onset within 1 hr, peak effects last 2-3 hr, duration 6-12 hr, excreted in urine

INDICATIONS AND USES: Adjunctive treatment of all forms of Parkinson's syndrome; extrapyramidal effects (except tardive dyskinesia) and acute dystonic reactions due to neuroleptic drugs

DOSAGE

Adult

• *Parkinsonism:* PO 1-2 mg on first day, increase by 2 mg q3-5d to 6-10 mg/d divided tid-qid; postencephalitic patients may require 12-15 mg/d; when used with levodopa 3-6 mg/d in divided doses is usually adequate

• *Drug-induced extrapyramidal disorders:* PO 1 mg initially, progressively increase subsequent doses if reaction not controlled in a few hr; maintenance 5-15 mg/d in divided doses

AVAILABLE FORMS/COST OF THERAPY

• Elixir—Oral: 2 mg/5 ml, 480 ml: **$19.20-$32.94**

• Tab, Uncoated—Oral: 2 mg, 100's: **$12.36-$20.33;** 5 mg, 100's: **$20.25-$40.78**

CONTRAINDICATIONS: Hypersensitivity, narrow-angle glaucoma, myasthenia gravis, GI/GU obstruction, peptic ulcer, megacolon, prostatic hypertrophy

PRECAUTIONS: Elderly, tachycardia, liver or kidney disease, drug abuse history, dysrhythmias, hypotension, hypertension, psychosis, children, tardive dyskinesia

PREGNANCY AND LACTATION: Pregnancy category C

SIDE EFFECTS/ADVERSE REACTIONS

CNS: Confusion, anxiety, restlessness, irritability, delusions, hallucinations, headache, sedation, depression, incoherence, dizziness, memory loss

CV: Palpitations, tachycardia, hypotension, mild bradycardia, postural hypotension, flushing

EENT: Blurred vision, photophobia, dilated pupils, difficulty swallowing, dry eyes, mydriasis, increased

T

intraocular tension, angle-closure glaucoma
GI: Dry mouth, constipation, nausea, vomiting, abdominal distress, ***paralytic ileus,*** epigastric distress
GU: Hesitancy, retention, dysuria, erectile dysfunction
MS: Muscular weakness, cramping
SKIN: Rash, urticaria, other dermatoses
MISC: Decreased sweating, ***hyperthermia, heat stroke,*** numbness of fingers

▼ **DRUG INTERACTIONS**

Drugs

- *Amantadine:* Anticholinergic drugs may potentiate the side effects of amantadine
- *Cyclic antidepressants:* Excessive anticholinergic effects
- *Neuroleptics:* Inhibition of therapeutic response to neuroleptics; excessive anticholinergic effects

SPECIAL CONSIDERATIONS

PATIENT/FAMILY EDUCATION

- Do not discontinue abruptly
- Avoid driving or other hazardous activities, drowsiness may occur
- Use caution in hot weather, drug may increase susceptibility to heat stroke

---

trimeprazine

(trye-mep'ra-zeen)
Panectyl, ♣ Temaril
Chemical Class: Phenothiazine derivative
Therapeutic Class: Antihistamine

CLINICAL PHARMACOLOGY

Mechanism of Action: Blocks the effects of histamine by competing with histamine for H_1-receptor sites of effector cells; prevents but does not reverse responses mediated by histamine alone

INDICATIONS AND USES: Symptomatic treatment of various allergic conditions, pruritus associated with urticaria

DOSAGE

Adult

- PO 2.5 mg qid; PO SR 5 mg q12h

Child

- PO (6 mo-3 yr) 1.25 mg hs or tid prn; (>3 yr) 2.5 mg hs or tid prn; PO SR (>6 yr) 5 mg qd

$ **AVAILABLE FORMS/COST OF THERAPY**

- Syr—Oral: 2.5 mg/5 ml, 120 ml: **$20.40**
- Cap, Gel, Sust Action—Oral: 5 mg, 100's: **$105.13**
- Tab, Coated—Oral: 2.5 mg, 100's: **$65.43**

CONTRAINDICATIONS: Hypersensitivity to phenothiazines, narrow-angle glaucoma, comatose patients, jaundice, bone marrow depression, acutely ill or dehydrated children (increased susceptibility to dystonias)

PRECAUTIONS: Acute asthma, bladder neck obstruction, prostatic hypertrophy, predisposition to urinary retention, cardiovascular disease, glaucoma, hepatic function impairment, hypertension, history of peptic ulcer, seizure disorder, intestinal obstruction

PREGNANCY AND LACTATION: Pregnancy category C; excreted into breast milk at levels too low to produce effects in infant

SIDE EFFECTS/ADVERSE REACTIONS

CNS: Dizziness, drowsiness, poor coordination, fatigue, anxiety, euphoria, confusion, paresthesia, neuritis
CV: Hypotension, palpitations, tachycardia
EENT: Blurred vision, dilated pupils, tinnitus, nasal stuffiness, dry nose
GI: Constipation, dry mouth, nausea, vomiting, anorexia, diarrhea

GU: Urinary retention, dysuria
HEME: ***Thrombocytopenia, agranulocytosis, hemolytic anemia***
RESP: Increased thick secretions, wheezing, chest tightness
SKIN: Photosensitivity, rash, urticaria

▼ DRUG INTERACTIONS

Drugs

• *CNS depressants:* Additive sedative action

Labs

• *False positive:* Immunologic urinary pregnancy tests
• *Interference:* Blood grouping in the ABO system, flare response in intradermal allergen tests

SPECIAL CONSIDERATIONS

PATIENT/FAMILY EDUCATION

• Avoid prolonged exposure to sunlight
• May cause drowsiness, use caution driving or performing other tasks requiring alertness
• Avoid alcohol

---

trimethadione

(trye-meth-a-dye'one)
Tridione
Chemical Class: Oxazolidinedione derivative
Therapeutic Class: Anticonvulsant

CLINICAL PHARMACOLOGY

Mechanism of Action: Decreases seizures in cortex, basal ganglia; decreases synaptic stimulation to low-frequency impulses

Pharmacokinetics

PO: Peak 30-120 min, demethylated in liver to active metabolite (dimethadione), excreted by kidneys, $t_{1/2}$ 16-24 hr (dimethadione 6-13 days)

INDICATIONS AND USES: Refractory absence (petit mal) seizures

DOSAGE

Adult

• PO 300-600 mg tid-qid; give 900 mg/d initially, increase by 300 mg at weekly intervals until therapeutic results are seen or toxicity appears

Child

• PO 300-900 mg/d divided tid-qid

$ AVAILABLE FORMS/COST OF THERAPY

• Cap, Gel—Oral: 300 mg, 100's: **$42.69**
• Tab, Chewable—Oral: 150 mg, 100's: **$37.66**

CONTRAINDICATIONS: Hypersensitivity to oxazolidinediones

PRECAUTIONS: Hepatic disease, renal disease, abrupt discontinuation, diseases of retina or optic nerve, intermittant porphyria, myasthenia gravis

PREGNANCY AND LACTATION: Pregnancy category D; has demonstrated both clinical and experimental fetal risk greater than other anticonvulsants, avoid use in pregnancy if possible

SIDE EFFECTS/ADVERSE REACTIONS

CNS: Drowsiness, dizziness, fatigue, paresthesia, irritability, headache, insomnia
CV: Hypertension, hypotension
EENT: Photophobia, diplopia, epistaxis, retinal hemorrhage
GI: Abdominal pain, *nausea, vomiting,* bleeding gums, abnormal liver function tests
GU: Vaginal bleeding, albuminuria, nephrosis
HEME: ***Thrombocytopenia, agranulocytosis, leukopenia, neutropenia, hemolytic anemia, eosinophilia, aplastic anemia,*** increased prothrombin time
SKIN: ***Exfoliative dermatitis,*** rash, alopecia, petechiae, erythema

MISC: Lupus erythematosus

SPECIAL CONSIDERATIONS

PATIENT/FAMILY EDUCATION

- Take with food if GI upset occurs
- Avoid prolonged exposure to sunlight
- Use caution driving or performing other tasks requiring alertness

MONITORING PARAMETERS

- CBC at baseline and qmo thereafter; satisfactory control usually occurs when serum dimethadione levels are ≥700 μg/ml

---

trimethobenzamide

(trye-meth-oh-ben′za-mide)
Arrestin, T-Gen, Tebamide, Ticon, Tigan, Trimazide

Chemical Class: Substituted ethanolamine derivative
Therapeutic Class: Antiemetic

CLINICAL PHARMACOLOGY

Mechanism of Action: Exact mechanism unknown; appears to directly affect the medullary chemoreceptor trigger zone (CTZ) by inhibiting stimuli at the CTZ

Pharmacokinetics

PO: Onset 10-40 min, duration 3-4 hr

IM: Onset 15-35 min, duration 2-3 hr

Exact metabolic fate unclear, 30%-50% excreted unchanged in urine

INDICATIONS AND USES: Control of nausea and vomiting (less effective than phenothiazines)

DOSAGE

Adult

- PO 250 mg tid-qid; PR/IM 200 mg tid-qid

Child

- PO (13.6-45 kg) 100-200 mg tid-qid; PR (<13.6 kg) 100 mg tid-qid; (13.6-45 kg) 100-200 mg tid-qid

$ AVAILABLE FORMS/COST OF THERAPY

- Inj, Sol—IM: 100 mg/ml, 20 ml: **$8.68-$22.05**
- Cap, Gel—Oral: 100 mg, 100's: **$39.15;** 250 mg, 100's: **$34.55-$47.20**
- Supp—Rect: 100 mg, 10's: **$3.70-$15.05;** 200 mg, 10's: **$4.08-$17.85**

CONTRAINDICATIONS: Hypersensitivity to trimethobenzamide, benzocaine, or similar anesthetics; parenteral use in children; suppositories in premature infants or neonates

PRECAUTIONS: Acute febrile illness, encephalitis, Reye's syndrome, gastroenteritis, dehydration, electrolyte imbalance

PREGNANCY AND LACTATION: Pregnancy category C; has been used to treat nausea and vomiting during pregnancy

SIDE EFFECTS/ADVERSE REACTIONS

CNS: Parkinson-like symptoms, ***coma, seizures,*** depression, disorientation, dizziness, *drowsiness,* headache, dystonic reactions

CV: Hypotenstion (IM)

EENT: Blurred vision

GI: Diarrhea, ***jaundice***

HEME: ***Blood dyscrasias***

MS: Muscle cramps

SKIN: Allergic-type skin reactions, burning and stinging at inj site (IM)

MISC: Hypersensitivity

---

trimethoprim

(trye-meth′oh-prim)
Proloprim, Trimpex

Chemical Class: Synthetic folate-antagonist
Therapeutic Class: Antibiotic

CLINICAL PHARMACOLOGY

Mechanism of Action: Selectively interferes with bacterial biosynthesis of nucleic acids and proteins by blocking production of tetrahydrofolic acid from dihydrofolic acid via binding to and reversibly inhibiting the required enzyme, dihydrofolate reductase; binding much stronger for bacterial enzyme than for corresponding mammalian enzyme

Pharmacokinetics

PO: Peak 1-4 hr, widely distributed into body tissues and fluids, 42%-46% bound to plasma proteins, metabolized in liver to oxide and hydroxylated metabolites, excreted in urine (80% unchanged), $t_{1/2}$ 8-11 hr (prolonged in renal failure)

INDICATIONS AND USES: Acute uncomplicated UTI, prophylaxis of chronic and recurrent UTI,* *Pneumocystis carinii* pneumonia (in conjunction with dapsone or sulfamethoxazole),* travelers' diarrhea*

Antibacterial spectrum usually includes:

- Gram-positive organisms: *Streptococcus pneumoniae,* group A β-hemolytic streptococci, coagulase-negative staphylococci
- Gram-negative organisms: *Acinetobacter, Citrobacter, Enterobacter, Escherichia coli, Klebsiella pneumoniae, Proteus mirabilis, Salmonella, Shigella, Haemophilus influenzae*

DOSAGE

Adult

- PO 100 mg q12h or 200 mg q24h, each for 10 days
- Dosing in renal failure (CrCl 15-30 ml/min): PO 50 mg q12h

$ **AVAILABLE FORMS/COST OF THERAPY**

- Tab, Uncoated—Oral: 100 mg, 100's: **$17.03-$75.23;** 200 mg, 100's: **$27.75-$150.47**

CONTRAINDICATIONS: Hypersensitivity, megaloblastic anemia due to folate deficiency, infants <2 mo, serum creatinine <15 ml/min

PRECAUTIONS: Renal or hepatic impairment, children <12 yr, folate deficiency (folates may be administered concurrently without interfering with antibacterial action)

PREGNANCY AND LACTATION: Pregnancy category C; because trimethoprim is a folate antagonist, caution should be used during the 1st trimester; excreted into breast milk in low concentrations, compatible with breast feeding

SIDE EFFECTS/ADVERSE REACTIONS

CNS: Fever

GI: Epigastric distress, *nausea, vomiting,* glossitis, elevation of serum transaminases and bilirubin

GU: Increased BUN and serum creatinine

HEME: ***Thrombocytopenia, leukopenia, neutropenia, megaloblastic anemia, methemoglobinemia***

SKIN: Rash, pruritus, ***exfoliative dermatitis***

▼ **DRUG INTERACTIONS**

Drugs

- *Dapsone:* Increased serum concentrations of both drugs
- *Procainamide:* Increased serum concentrations of procainamide and N-acetylprocainamide

SPECIAL CONSIDERATIONS

PATIENT/FAMILY EDUCATION

- Complete full course of therapy

trimipramine

(trye-mip'ra-meen)

Surmontil

Chemical Class: Tertiary amine

Therapeutic Class: Antidepressant (tricyclic)

CLINICAL PHARMACOLOGY

Mechanism of Action: Inhibits the reuptake of norepinephrine and serotonin at the presynaptic neuron prolonging neuronal activity; inhibition of histamine and acetylcholine activity; mild peripheral vasodilator effects and possible "quinidine-like" actions

Pharmacokinetics

PO: Peak within 6 hr, 95% bound to plasma proteins, metabolized in liver to desmethlytrimipramine, excreted in urine, $t_{1/2}$ 20-26 hr

INDICATIONS AND USES: Relief of symptoms of depression, peptic ulcer disease,* chronic urticaria and angioedema,* nocturnal pruritus in atopic eczema*

DOSAGE

Adult

• PO 75-100 mg/d in divided doses initially, increase to 150-200 mg/d; max 300 mg/d

Adolescent and Elderly

• PO 50 mg/d initially, increase to 100 mg/d

$ AVAILABLE FORMS/COST OF THERAPY

• Cap, Gel—Oral: 25 mg, 100's: **$62.99;** 50 mg, 100's: **$103.09;** 100 mg, 100's: **$149.86**

CONTRAINDICATIONS: Hypersensitivity to tricyclic antidepressants, acute recovery phase of MI, concurrent use of MAOIs

PRECAUTIONS: Suicidal patients, convulsive disorders, prostatic hypertrophy, psychiatric disease, severe depression, increased intraocular pressure, narrow-angle glaucoma, urinary retention, cardiac disease, hepatic disease/renal disease, hyperthyroidism, electroshock therapy, elective surgery, elderly, abrupt discontinuation

PREGNANCY AND LACTATION: Pregnancy category C; excreted into breast milk, effect on nursing infant unknown but may be of concern

SIDE EFFECTS/ADVERSE REACTIONS

CNS: Dizziness, drowsiness, confusion (especially in elderly), headache, anxiety, nervousness, panic, tremors, stimulation, weakness, fatigue, insomnia, nightmares, EPS (elderly), increased psychiatric symptoms, memory impairment,

CV: Orthostatic hypotension, ***ECG changes,*** tachycardia, ***dysrhythmias,*** hypertension, palpitations, syncope

EENT: Blurred vision, tinnitus, mydriasis, ophthalmoplegia, nasal congestion

GI: Constipation, dry mouth, nausea, vomiting, ***paralytic ileus,*** increased appetite, cramps, epigastric distress, jaundice, ***hepatitis,*** stomatitis, diarrhea

GU: Urinary retention

HEME: ***Agranulocytosis, thrombocytopenia, eosinophilia, leukopenia***

SKIN: Rash, urticaria, sweating, pruritus, photosensitivity

▼ DRUG INTERACTIONS

Drugs

• *Amphetamines:* Theoretical increase in effect of amphetamines, clinical evidence lacking

• *Anticholinergics:* Excessive anticholinergic effects

• *Barbiturates, carbamazepine:* Reduced serum concentrations of cyclic antidepressants

• *Bethanidine:* Reduced antihypertensive effect of bethanidine

• *Clonidine:* Reduced antihypertensive response to clonidine; enhanced hypertensive response with abrupt clonidine withdrawal

• *Debrisoquin:* Inhibited antihypertensive response of debrisoquin

• *Epinephrine+:* Markedly enhanced pressor response to IV epinephrine

• *Ethanol:* Additive impairment of motor skills; abstinent alcoholics may eliminate cyclic antidepressants more rapidly than nonalcoholics

• *Fluoxetine:* Marked increases in

cyclic antidepressant plasma concentrations
- *Guanethidine:* Inhibited antihypertensive response to guanethidine
- *MAOIs:* Excessive sympathetic response, mania or hyperpyrexia possible
- *Moclobemide+:* Potential association with fatal or non-fatal serotonin syndrome
- *Neuroleptics:* Increased therapeutic and toxic effects of both drugs
- *Norepinephrine+:* Markedly enhanced pressor response to norepinephrine
- *Phenylephrine:* Enhanced pressor response to IV phenylephrine
- *Phenytoin:* Altered seizure control; decreased cyclic antidepressant serum concentrations
- *Propoxyphene:* Enhanced effect of cyclic antidepressants
- *Quinidine:* Increased cyclic antidepressant serum concentrations

Labs
- *Increase:* Serum bilirubin, blood glucose, alk phosphatase
- *Decrease:* VMA, 5-HIAA
- *False increase:* Urinary catecholamines

SPECIAL CONSIDERATIONS

PATIENT/FAMILY EDUCATION
- Therapeutic effects may take 2-3 wk
- Use caution in driving or other activities requiring alertness
- Avoid rising quickly from sitting to standing, especially elderly
- Avoid alcohol ingestion, other CNS depressants
- Do not discontinue abruptly after long-term use

MONITORING PARAMETERS
- CBC
- Weight
- ECG
- Mental status: mood, sensorium, affect, suicidal tendencies

trioxsalen

(trye-ox'a-len)
Trisoralen
Chemical Class: Psoralen derivative
Therapeutic Class: Pigmenting agent

CLINICAL PHARMACOLOGY

Mechanism of Action: Exact mechanism unknown; may involve increased tyrosinase activity in melanin-producing cells, as well as inhibition of DNA synthesis, cell division, and epidermal turnover; successful pigmentation requires the presence of functioning melanocytes

Pharmacokinetics

PO: Onset 1-2 hr, maximal effects 2-4 hr, duration 7-8 hr, 80% appears in urine within 8 hr as hydroxylated or glucuronide derivatives

INDICATIONS AND USES: Repigmentation in the treatment of vitiligo, in conjunction with UVA—treatment known as PUVA (psoralen plus ultraviolet light A); increasing tolerance to sunlight and enhancing pigmentation (in conjunction with controlled exposure to UVA light or sunlight)

DOSAGE

Adult and Child >12 yr
- *Idiopathic vitiligo:* PO 5-10 mg qd 2-4 hr before measured periods of sunlight or UVA exposure; if necessary may increase in 10 mg increments to max of 80 mg/day; successful treatment usually requires 6-9 mo
- *Other uses:* PO 10 mg qd 2 hr before measured periods of sunlight or UVA exposure; do not exceed 14 days of therapy or 140 mg total dose

T

AVAILABLE FORMS/COST OF THERAPY

• Tab, Uncoated—Oral: 5 mg, 100's: **$200.13**

CONTRAINDICATIONS: Hypersensitivity to psoralens, diseases associated with photosensitivity, melanoma, invasive squamous cell carcinoma, aphakia (oral)

PRECAUTIONS: Cardiac disease, hepatic disease, children <12 yr, contains tartrazine (FD&C #5), photosensitizing agents

PREGNANCY AND LACTATION: Pregnancy category C

SIDE EFFECTS/ADVERSE REACTIONS

CNS: Nervousness, insomnia, psychological depression, dizziness, headache, malaise

CV: Edema, hypotension

EENT: Cataract formation

GI: Nausea

MS: Leg cramps

SKIN: ***Severe burns,*** basal cell epitheliomas, hypopigmentation, vesiculation and bullae formation, nonspecific rash, herpes simplex, urticaria, folliculitis, cutaneous tenderness, extension of psoriasis, *pruritus, erythema*

▼ **DRUG INTERACTIONS**

Drugs

• *Anthralin, coal tar, griseofulvin, phenothiazines, nalidixic acid, halogenated salicylanilides, sulfonamides, tetracyclines, thiazides:* Increased photosensitivity

SPECIAL CONSIDERATIONS

PATIENT/FAMILY EDUCATION

• Do not sunbathe during 24 hr prior to ingestion and UVA exposure

• Wear UVA-absorbing sunglasses for 24 hr following treatment to prevent cataract

• Avoid sun exposure for at least 8 hr after ingestion

• Take with food or milk

• Avoid furocoumarin-containing foods (e.g., limes, figs, parsley, parsnips, mustard, carrots, celery)

• Repigmentation may require 6-9 mo

---

tripelennamine

(tri-pel-enn'a-meen)

PBZ, PBZ-SR, Pelamine

Chemical Class: Ethylenediamine derivative

Therapeutic Class: Antihistamine

CLINICAL PHARMACOLOGY

Mechanism of Action: Competes with histamine for H_1-receptor sites on effector cells in the GI tract, blood vessels, and respiratory tract; antagonizes most of pharmacological effects of histamine; also has anticholinergic, antipruritic, and sedative effects

Pharmacokinetics

PO: Onset within 30 min, duration 4-6 hr (SR 8 hr), metabolized in liver, excreted in urine

INDICATIONS AND USES: Perennial and seasonal allergic rhinitis and other allergic symptoms including urticaria

DOSAGE

Adult

• PO 25-50 mg q4-6h, max 600 mg/d; PO SR 100 mg bid; may also be given q8h in difficult cases

Child

• PO 5 mg/kg/d or 150 mg/m^2/d in 4-6 divided doses; max 300 mg/d

AVAILABLE FORMS/COST OF THERAPY

• Tab, Uncoated—Oral: 25 mg, 100's: **$14.28;** 50 mg, 100's: **$6.23-$21.67**

• Tab, Coated, Sust Action—Oral: 100 mg, 100's: **$35.69**

CONTRAINDICATIONS: Hypersensitivity, narrow-angle glaucoma, bladder neck obstruction

PRECAUTIONS: Liver disease, elderly, increased intraocular pressure, hyperthyroidism, cardiovascular disease, hypertension, urinary retention, renal disease, stenosed peptic ulcers

PREGNANCY AND LACTATION: Pregnancy category B; manufacturer considers the drug contraindicated in nursing mothers, possibly due to increased sensitivity of newborn or premature infants to antihistamines

SIDE EFFECTS/ADVERSE REACTIONS

CNS: Dizziness, drowsiness, poor coordination, fatigue, anxiety, euphoria, confusion, paresthesia, neuritis

CV: Hypotension, palpitations, tachycardia

EENT: Blurred vision, dilated pupils, tinnitus, nasal stuffiness, dry nose, throat

GI: Dry mouth, nausea, vomiting, anorexia, *constipation,* diarrhea

GU: Retention, dysuria, frequency, impotence

HEME: ***Thrombocytopenia, agranulocytosis, hemolytic anemia***

RESP: Increased thick secretions, wheezing, chest tightness

SKIN: Photosensitivity

▼ DRUG INTERACTIONS

Labs

• *False negative:* Skin allergy tests

SPECIAL CONSIDERATIONS

PATIENT/FAMILY EDUCATION

• Avoid driving or other hazardous activities if drowsiness occurs

triprolidine

(trye-proe'li-deen)

Actidil, Myidil

Chemical Class: Alkylamine derivative

Therapeutic Class: Antihistamine

CLINICAL PHARMACOLOGY

Mechanism of Action: Competes with histamine for H_1-receptor sites on effector cells in the GI tract, blood vessels, and respiratory tract; antagonizes most pharmacological effects of histamine; also has anticholinergic, antipruritic, and sedative effects

Pharmacokinetics

PO: Onset 20-60 min, duration 8-12 hr, metabolized in liver, excreted in urine

INDICATIONS AND USES: Perennial and seasonal allergic rhinitis and other allergic symptoms including urticaria

DOSAGE

Adult

• PO 2.5 mg q4-6h

Child 6-12 yr

• PO 1.25 mg q4-6h

$ AVAILABLE FORMS/COST OF THERAPY

• Syr—Oral: 1.25 mg/5 ml, 480 ml: **$4.80**

• Tab, Uncoated—Oral: 2.5 mg, 100's: **$2.63**

CONTRAINDICATIONS: Hypersensitivity, narrow-angle glaucoma, bladder neck obstruction

PRECAUTIONS: Liver disease, elderly, increased intraocular pressure, hyperthyroidism, cardiovascular disease, hypertension, urinary retention, newborn or premature infants, renal disease, GI outlet obstruction

T

PREGNANCY AND LACTATION: Pregnancy category C; manufacturer claims that no reports of teratogenicity have been received in over 20 years of marketing; excreted into breast milk, compatible with breast feeding

SIDE EFFECTS/ADVERSE REACTIONS

CNS: Dizziness, drowsiness, poor coordination, fatigue, anxiety, euphoria, confusion, paresthesia, neuritis

CV: Hypotension, palpitations, tachycardia

EENT: Blurred vision, dilated pupils, tinnitus, nasal stuffiness, dry nose, throat

GI: Dry mouth, nausea, vomiting, anorexia, *constipation,* diarrhea

GU: Retention, dysuria, frequency, impotence

HEME: ***Thrombocytopenia, agranulocytosis, hemolytic anemia***

RESP: Increased thick secretions, wheezing, chest tightness

SKIN: Photosensitivity

▼ DRUG INTERACTIONS

Drugs

• *Barbiturates:* Excessive CNS depression

Labs

• *False negative:* Skin allergy tests

SPECIAL CONSIDERATIONS

PATIENT/FAMILY EDUCATION

• Avoid driving or other hazardous activities if drowsiness occurs

tromethamine

(troe-meth'a-meen)

Tham

Chemical Class: Organic amine buffer

Therapeutic Class: Alkalinizer

CLINICAL PHARMACOLOGY

Mechanism of Action: Acts as a proton acceptor preventing or correcting acidosis by actively binding hydrogen ions (H^+); binds cations of fixed or metabolic acids, and hydrogen ions of carbonic acid, thus increasing bicarbonate anion (HCO_3^-); also acts as an osmotic diuretic, increasing urine flow, urinary pH, and excretion of fixed acids, carbon dioxide, and electrolytes

Pharmacokinetics

IV: Rapidly eliminated by kidney (75% or more appears in the urine after 8 hr), urinary excretion continues over a period of 3 days

INDICATIONS AND USES: Metabolic acidosis associated with cardiac bypass surgery and cardiac arrest; correction of acidity of acid citrate dextrose (ACD) blood in cardiac bypass surgery

DOSAGE

Dosage may be estimated from the buffer base deficit of extracellular fluid (mEq/L) using the following formula as a general guide: ml of 0.3 M tromethamine solution = body weight (kg) × base deficit (mEq/L) × 1.1

Adult

• *Acidosis during cardiac bypass surgery:* IV INF total single dose of 500 ml (150 mEq or 10 g) is adequate for most adults; larger single doses (up to 1000 ml) may be required in severe cases; do not exceed individual doses of 500 mg/kg over a period of not less than 1 hr

• *Acidity of ACD priming blood:* Use from 0.5-2.5 g (15-77 ml) added to each 500 ml of ACD blood; 62 ml added to 500 ml of ACD blood is usually adequate

• *Acidosis associated with cardiac arrest:* IV 3.6-10.8 g (111-333 ml) into large peripheral vein; if chest is open, inject 2-6 g (62-185 ml) directly into ventricular cavity

AVAILABLE FORMS/COST OF THERAPY

- Inj, Sol—IV: 36 mg/ml (0.3 M), 500 ml: **$140.41**

CONTRAINDICATIONS: Anuria, uremia

PRECAUTIONS: Respiratory depression, perivascular infiltration, neonates, renal function impairment, children

PREGNANCY AND LACTATION: Pregnancy category C

SIDE EFFECTS/ADVERSE REACTIONS

GI: ***Hemorrhagic hepatic necrosis***
METAB: Transient depression of blood glucose, hypovolemia
RESP: ***Respiratory depression***
SKIN: Local reactions (febrile response, infection, venous thrombosis or phlebitis)

SPECIAL CONSIDERATIONS

- Avoid overdosage and alkalosis

MONITORING PARAMETERS

- Pretreatment and subsequent blood gas values
- Urinary output
- ECG
- Serum potassium, glucose, and electrolytes before, during, and after administration
- Experience limited to short-term use; administer for >1 day in life-threatening situation

---

tropicamide

(troe-pik'a-mide)

Mydriacyl Ophthalmic, Tropicacyl, Opticyl

Chemical Class: Amide-type derivative of tropic acid
Therapeutic Class: Mydriatic; cytoplegic

CLINICAL PHARMACOLOGY

Mechanism of Action: Blocks responses of the sphincter muscle of the iris and the accommodative muscle of the ciliary body to stimulation by acetylcholine, dilation of the pupil (mydriasis) and paralysis of accommodation (cytoplegia) result

Pharmacokinetics: Peak mydriasis 20-40 min, recovery 0.25 days; peak cycloplegia 20-35 min, recovery <0.25 days

INDICATIONS AND USES: Mydriasis and cycloplegia for diagnostic purposes

DOSAGE

Adult and Child

- *Refraction:* Instill 1-2 gtt of 1% sol into eye(s); repeat in 5 min; an additional gtt may be instilled after 20-30 min to prolong effect if needed
- *Examination of fundus:* Instill 1-2 gtt of 0.5% sol 15-20 min prior to examination

AVAILABLE FORMS/COST OF THERAPY

- Sol—Ophth: 0.5%, 15 ml: **$5.04-$27.28;** 1%, 15 ml: **$6.30-$32.06**

CONTRAINDICATIONS: Hypersensitivity to belladonna alkaloids, adhesions between the iris and the lens, primary glaucoma, narrow anterior chamber angle

PRECAUTIONS: Elderly, small children, and infants

PREGNANCY AND LACTATION: Pregnancy category C

SIDE EFFECTS/ADVERSE REACTIONS

CNS: Confusion, somnolence, headache, visual hallucinations, fever
CV: Tachycardia, vasodilation
EENT: Blurred vision, photophobia, increased intraocular pressure, irritation, edema
GI: Dry mouth, abdominal distension in infants, decreased GI motility
GU: Urinary retention
SKIN: Rash, dry skin

SPECIAL CONSIDERATIONS

- Individuals with heavily pig-

T

mented irides may require larger doses

PATIENT/FAMILY EDUCATION

- Do not drive or engage in any hazardous activities while pupils are dilated
- May cause sensitivity to light, protect eyes from bright light
- To minimize systemic effects, compress the lacrimal sac for several min following instillation

undecylenic acid

(un-de-sye-len'ik)

Caldesene, Cruex, Decylenes, Desenex, Desenex Maximum Strength, Fungoid Topical Solution, Protectol

Chemical Class: Hendecenoic acid

Therapeutic Class: Antifungal

CLINICAL PHARMACOLOGY

Mechanism of Action: Interferes with fungal cell membrane permeability, fungistatic

Pharmacokinetics: Improvement may be seen within 1 wk

INDICATIONS AND USES: Tinea cruris, tinea pedis, tinea corporis, diaper rash; newer topical antifungal agents more effective

DOSAGE

Adult and Child

- TOP apply to affected areas bid for 2-4 wk

$ AVAILABLE FORMS/COST OF THERAPY

- Aer—Top: 1.5 oz: **$5.11**
- Cre—Top: 0.5 oz: **$4.55**
- Liq—Top: 10%, 100 ml: **$7.20**
- Oint—Top: 30 g: **$1.80-$4.55**
- Powder—Top: 1.5 oz: **$3.74**
- Soap—Top: 3.25 oz: **$2.36**
- Spray—Top: 3 oz: **$4.31**

CONTRAINDICATIONS: Hypersensitivity

PRECAUTIONS: Impaired circulation; diabetes mellitus; broken, pustular skin; puncture wounds, children <2 yr

PREGNANCY AND LACTATION: Problems not documented in breast feeding

SIDE EFFECTS/ADVERSE REACTIONS

SKIN: Skin irritation

urea

(yoor-ee'a)

Parenteral: Ureaphil

Topical: Aquacare, Carmol, Carmol 10, Gordon's Urea 40%, Gormel Creme, Lanaphilic, Nutraplus, Ureacin-10, Ureacin-20, Ureacin-40, Ultra Mide 25

Chemical Class: Carbonic acid diamide salt

Therapeutic Class: Diuretic, osmotic agent, antiglaucoma agent

CLINICAL PHARMACOLOGY

Mechanism of Action: Elevates plasma osmolality, increasing flow of water into tissues, including the brain and the eye

Pharmacokinetics

IV: Onset of action 10 min, peak effect 1-2 hr, duration of action 3-10 hr (diuresis and decreased CSF pressure), 5-6 hr (reduced intraocular pressure); excreted in urine, crosses placenta, excreted in breast milk

INDICATIONS AND USES: Parenteral: cerebral edema, glaucoma; has been used for induction of abortion by intra-amniotic injection; Topical: Emollient, hydration and removal of hyperkeratotic skin

DOSAGE

Adult and Child >2 yr

- IV 0.5-1.5 g/kg as 30% sol in 5% or 10% dextrose over ½-2 hr at rate not exceeding 4 ml/min, max 2 g/kg/d

• TOP apply bid-qid

Child <2 yrs

• IV 0.1-1.5 g/kg as sol as described and administered for adults

$ AVAILABLE FORMS/COST OF THERAPY

• Inj, Dry-Sol—IV: 40 g: **$70.25**

• Lot—Top: 10%, 240 ml: **$5.00-$6.54;** 25%, 8 oz: **$8.89**

• Cre—Top: 20%, 2.5 oz: **$4.75;** 10%, 3.0 oz: **$6.12**

CONTRAINDICATIONS: Severe renal disease, active intracranial bleeding (except during craniotomy), severe dehydration, liver failure

PRECAUTIONS: Hepatic disease, renal disease, electrolyte imbalances, cardiac disease, CHF, hypovolemia

PREGNANCY AND LACTATION: Pregnancy category C; no data on breastfeeding available

SIDE EFFECTS/ADVERSE REACTIONS

Systemic use:

CNS: Dizziness, headache, disorientation, fever, syncope, *headache*

CV: Postural hypotension, tachycardia

GI: Nausea, vomiting

HEME: ***Hemolysis, intraocular bleeding***

METAB: Hypokalemia, hyponatremia, dehydration

SKIN: Venous thrombosis, phlebitis, extravasation

SPECIAL CONSIDERATIONS

• To prepare 135 ml of a 30% sol, mix 40 g urea with 105 ml diluent

• Do not infuse into lower extremity veins

• Monitor for extravasation, tissue necrosis may occur

urokinase

(yoor-oh-kine'ase)

Abbokinase, Abbokinase Open-Cath (not for systemic administration)

Chemical Class: Enzyme produced by the kidney

Therapeutic Class: Thrombolytic agent

CLINICAL PHARMACOLOGY

Mechanism of Action: Promotes thrombolysis by directly converting plasminogen to plasmin

Pharmacokinetics: Onset of fibrinolysis is rapid; $t_{1/2}$ 10-20 min, duration ≥ 4 hr; cleared by liver, small amount excreted in urine and bile, unknown if crosses placenta or if excreted in breast milk

INDICATIONS AND USES: Venous thrombosis, pulmonary embolism, arterial thrombosis, arterial embolism, arteriovenous cannula occlusion, lysis of coronary artery thrombi after MI, thrombotic stroke*

DOSAGE

Adult/Child

• *Pulmonary embolism/arterial or venous thrombosis:* IV 4400 IU/kg over 10 min followed by 4400 IU/kg/hr for 12 hr; after thrombin time has decreased to less than twice normal control value (approx 3-4 hr) begin heparin (no loading dose)

• *Venous catheter occlusion:* INSTILL into catheter a volume of urokinase (5000 IU/ml) equal to the internal volume of catheter over 1-2 min; aspirate from catheter 1-4 hr later, flush catheter with saline, may repeat with 10,000 U/ml sol if not cleared

• *Coronary artery thrombosis (adult):* IC (following IV heparin bolus) 6000 IU/min for up to 2 hr (average dose 500,000 IU); repeat

U

angiography q15min until artery maximally opened; continuing heparin therapy recommended

$ AVAILABLE FORMS/COST OF THERAPY

• Inj, Lyphl-Sol—IV: 5000 U/ml, 1 ml: **$49.04** (not for systemic administration); 9000 U/vial: **$85.52** (not for systemic administration); 250,000 U/vial: **$397.73**

CONTRAINDICATIONS: (Systemic therapy only, no contraindications for catheter use.) Hypersensitivity, active bleeding, intraspinal surgery, CNS neoplasms, ulcerative colitis/enteritis, coagulation defects, rheumatic valvular disease, cerebral embolism/thrombosis/hemorrhage within 2 mo; intraarterial diagnostic procedure, surgery, or trauma within 10 days; severe hypertension

PRECAUTIONS: Moderate hypertension, recent lumbar puncture, patients receiving IM medications, renal disease, hepatic disease, childbirth within 10 days, diabetic retinopathy, age >75 yr

PREGNANCY AND LACTATION: Pregnancy category B; no data available on breast feeding

SIDE EFFECTS/ADVERSE REACTIONS

CV: Transient hypertension or hypotension, tachycardia, ***MI***

GI: Nausea, vomiting

HEME: ***Internal bleeding (GI, GU, vaginal, IM, retroperitoneal or intracranial sites),*** surface bleeding

METAB: Acidosis

RESP: Dyspnea, hypoxemia, ***bronchospasm***

SKIN: Rash

MISC: Chills, fever

▼ DRUG INTERACTIONS

Drugs

• *Anticoagulants and antiplatelet agents:* Bleeding complications

SPECIAL CONSIDERATIONS

MONITORING PARAMETERS

• Prior to therapy check coagulation tests such as PT, APTT, TT, fibrinogen, and FDP, Hct, platelet count, bleeding time (some sources recommend not administering urokinase if >15 min)

• Proceed with therapy before results known in therapy for acute coronary artery occlusion

• During therapy continue to monitor coagulation tests and/or tests of fibrinolytic activity; results do not reliably predict efficacy or risk of bleeding

• Treat bleeding with cryoprecipitate or fresh frozen plasma

ursodiol

(your-soo'dee-ol)

Actigall

Chemical Class: Ursodeoxycholic acid

Therapeutic Class: Gallstone dissolution agent

CLINICAL PHARMACOLOGY

Mechanism of Action: Decreases cholesterol content of bile and bile stones by reducing hepatic cholesterol secretion and reabsorption of cholesterol by the intestine

Pharmacokinetics: 90% absorption from small bowel, first pass hepatic clearance, conjugates secreted into bile, peak concentration 1-3 hr, $t_{1/2}$ 100 hr

INDICATIONS AND USES: Dissolution of radiolucent, noncalcified gallbladder stones (<20 mm in diameter) in which surgery is not indicated, chronic cholestatic liver disease*

DOSAGE

Adult

• PO 8-10 mg/kg/d in 2-3 divided doses using gallbladder ultrasound

* = non-FDA-approved use + = major clinical significance

q6mo; determine if stones have dissolved; if so, continue therapy, repeat ultrasound within 1-3 mo; maintenance therapy 250 mg qhs for 6-12 mo, use beyond 24 mo not established

Child

• *Cholestatic liver disease:* 10-18 mg/kg/d

$ AVAILABLE FORMS/COST OF THERAPY

• Cap, Gel—Oral: 300 mg, 100's: **$207.57**

CONTRAINDICATIONS: Calcified cholesterol stones, radiopaque stones, stones >20 mm in diameter, bile pigment stones, patients with compelling reasons for cholecystectomy (cholangitis, biliary obstruction), hypersensitivity

PRECAUTIONS: Children, chronic liver disease, non-visualizing gall bladder

PREGNANCY AND LACTATION: Pregnancy category B; excretion into breast milk unknown

SIDE EFFECTS/ADVERSE REACTIONS

CNS: Headache, anxiety, depression, insomnia, fatigue

EENT: Rhinitis, metallic taste

GI: Diarrhea, nausea, vomiting, abdominal pain, constipation, stomatitis, flatulence, dyspepsia, biliary pain

MS: Arthralgia, myalgia, back pain

RESP: Cough

SKIN: Pruritus, rash, urticaria, dry skin, sweating, alopecia

▼ DRUG INTERACTIONS

Drugs

• *Aluminum containing antacids, cholestyramine, colestipol, clofibrate, estrogens, neomycin, progestins:* Decreased effectiveness of ursodiol

SPECIAL CONSIDERATIONS

• Complete dissolution may not occur; likelihood of success is low if partial stone dissolution not seen by 12 mo

• Stones recur within 5 yr in 50% of patients

PATIENT/FAMILY EDUCATION

• Administer with food to facilitate dissolution in the intestine

---

valacyclovir

(val-a-sye'kloe-ver)

Valtrex

Chemical Class: Derivative of acylovir

Therapeutic Class: Antiviral

CLINICAL PHARMACOLOGY

Mechanism of Action: Converted to acyclovir triphosphate *in vitro;* stops viral replication by interfering with viral DNA synthesis

Pharmacokinetics

PO: Rapidly absorbed from GI tract and converted to acylovir by first-pass intestinal or hepatic metabolism; plasma protein binding 14%-18%; excreted in urine (89%) and feces; $t_{1/2}$ of acyclovir 2.5-3.3 hr (14 hr in end stage renal disease)

INDICATIONS AND USES: Herpes zoster in immunocompetent adults

DOSAGE

• PO 1 g tid for 7 days within 72 hr of onset of rash; for CrCl 30-49 ml/min give 1 g q12h, CrCl 10-29 ml/min 1 g q24h, CrCl < 10 ml/min 500 mg q24h

$ AVAILABLE FORMS/COST OF THERAPY

• Cap—Oral: 500 mg, 100's: **$178.21**

CONTRAINDICATIONS: Hypersensitivity to valacylovir or acyclovir, immunocompromised patients

PRECAUTIONS: Renal insufficiency, hepatic insufficiency, elderly, children

PREGNANCY AND LACTATION: Pregnancy category B; acyclovir excreted into breast milk, safety not established

SIDE EFFECTS/ADVERSE REACTIONS

CNS: Headache, dizziness

GI: Nausea, vomiting, diarrhea, constipation, abdominal pain, anorexia

GU: ***Renal dysfunction, hemolytic uremic syndrome***

HEME: ***Thrombotic thrombocytopenic purpura***

▼ **DRUG INTERACTIONS**

Drugs

• *Cimetidine, probenecid:* Reduced rate but not extent of conversion of valacyclovir to acyclovir

---

valproate/divalproex

(val-proe'ate)

Valproic acid: Depakene

Divalproex: Depakote, Depakote Sprinkle, Epival ♣

Chemical Class: Carboxylic acid derivative

Therapeutic Class: Anticonvulsant

CLINICAL PHARMACOLOGY

Mechanism of Action: Increases levels of γ-aminobutyric acid (GABA, inhibitory neurotransmitter) in brain; divalproex dissociates to the valproate ion in the GI tract

Pharmacokinetics

PO: Onset 15-30 min, peak 1-5 hr (slower absorption with sprinkles and food), $t_{1/2}$ 6-16hr; (shorter with younger age and serum levels lower in polytherapy; 40-60 hr in newborns)

REC: Onset slow, duration 4-6 hr, $t_{1/2}$ 6-16 hr

Metabolized by liver, excreted by kidneys and in feces, crosses placenta, excreted into breast milk

INDICATIONS AND USES: Simple, complex (petit mal) absence, mixed, tonic-clonic (grand mal) seizures, mania in bipolar disorders in adults (divalproex sodium)*

DOSAGE

Adult

• PO for monotherapy 5-15 mg/kg/d divided in 1-3 doses, may increase by 5-10 mg/kg/d qwk; for polytherapy initial dose 10-30 mg/kg/d; If dose exceeds 250 mg qd divide into 2 or more doses; max 60 mg/kg/d

Child

• PO same as adult; children receiving polytherapy may require doses up to 100 mg/kg/d in 3-4 divided doses

• REC dilute syr 1:1 with water; give loading dose 17-20 mg/kg once as retention enema; maintenance 10-15 mg/kg/dose q8h

$ **AVAILABLE FORMS/COST OF THERAPY**

Valproic acid:

• Cap, Elastic—Oral: 250 mg, 100's: **$15.75-$116.34**

• Syr—Oral: 250 mg/5 ml, 480 ml: **$37.27-$118.90**

Divalproex sodium:

• Cap, Enteric Coated (Sprinkle)—Oral: 125 mg, 100's: **$31.11-$32.89**

• Tab, Enteric Coated—Oral: 125 mg, 100's: **$30.95-$32.73;** 250 mg, 100's: **$60.76-$62.55;** 500 mg, 100's: **$112.08-$113.86**

CONTRAINDICATIONS: Hypersensitivity, hepatic disease

PRECAUTIONS: Renal disease, Addison's disease, blood dyscrasias; children < 2 yr, patients with organic brain disease and patients on multiple anticonvulsants (polytherapy) at increased risk of hepatotoxicity

PREGNANCY AND LACTATION: Pregnancy category D, teratogenic; increased risk of neural tube defects (1%-2% when used between day

17-30 after fertilization); compatible with breast feeding

SIDE EFFECTS/ADVERSE REACTIONS

CNS: Sedation, drowsiness, dizziness, headache, incoordination, paresthesia, depression, hallucinations, behavioral changes, tremors, aggression, weakness, ataxia, nystagmus, diplopia, ***encephalopathy, coma***

GI: Nausea, vomiting, constipation, diarrhea, heartburn, anorexia, cramps, ***hepatic failure, pancreatitis,*** stomatitis

GU: Enuresis, irregular menses, amenorrhea, breast enlargement, galactorrhea

HEME: ***Thrombocytopenia, leukopenia,*** lymphocytosis, ***hypofibrinogenemia,*** anemia

METAB: Abnormal thyroid function tests, SIADH, hyponatremia, hyperammonemia, hyperglycemia, carnitine deficiency

SKIN: Rash, alopecia, pruritis, ***erythema multiforme, Stevens-Johnson syndrome***

▼ DRUG INTERACTIONS

Drugs

• *Carbamazepine, phenytoin:* Increase, decrease, or no effect on carbamazepine levels

• *Phenobarbital, primidone:* Increased phenobarbital levels

• *Salicylates:* Increased valproate levels

• *Zidovudine* Increased zidovudine levels

Labs

• *False positive:* Urinary ketones

SPECIAL CONSIDERATIONS

PATIENT/FAMILY EDUCATION

• Administer with food to decrease GI side effects

• Do not administer with carbonated beverages or milk

• May mix sprinkle capsules with soft foods but do not chew sprinkle beads

MONITORING PARAMETERS

• Therapeutic levels (draw just before next dose) 50-100 μg/ml; toxic levels >100-150 μg/ml

• Perform LFTs, coagulation studies, and platelet count prior to therapy and monitor during therapy, especially first 6 mo

• Minor elevations in SGOT, SGPT are frequent and dose related

vancomycin

(van-koe-mye'sin)

Lyphocin, Vancocin, Vancoled

Chemical Class: Tricyclic glycopeptide

Therapeutic Class: Antibacterial

CLINICAL PHARMACOLOGY

Mechanism of Action: Inhibits bacterial cell wall synthesis, cell membrane permeability, and RNA synthesis; bactericidal against Gram-positive organisms, bacteriostatic against enterococci

Pharmacokinetics

PO: Absorption poor

IV: 15mg/kg dose over 60 min yields mean plasma concentration of 63, 23, and 8 μg/ml immediately, 2 hr, and 8 hr after inf; penetrates inflamed meninges, and into inflamed pleural, pericardial, ascitic, and synovial fluids, urine, peritoneal dialysis fluid, atrial appendage tissue, and bile; 55% protein bound; $t_{1/2}$ 4-8 hr; excreted in urine (active form) linearly associated with creatinine clearance; therapeutic serum concentrations, peak 25-40 μg/ml; trough <5-10 μg/ml

INDICATIONS AND USES: Serious or severe Gram-positive infections not treatable with other antimicrobials, including penicillins and cephalosporins caused by susceptible organisms

Antibacterial spectrum usually includes:

- Severe staphylococcal infections (including methicillin-resistant staphylococci) including endocarditis, bone infections, lower respiratory tract infections, septicemia, and skin and skin structure infections
- Endocarditis; staphylococcal—vancomycin alone; streptococcal (S. viridans, *S. bovis*)—vancomycin alone or in combination with an aminoglycoside; enterococcal endocarditis requires combination vancomycin and aminoglycoside; diphtheroid—with rifampin, an aminoglycoside, or both; prophylactic
- Penicillin-allergic patient with valvular heart disease undergoing dental procedures or surgical procedures of the upper respiratory tract; pseudomembranous colitis (*Clostridium difficile,* oral dosing ONLY)

DOSAGE (Note: administer IV doses over 60 min; prevents "red-neck syndrome")

Adult

- *Serious staphylococcal infections:* IV 500 mg q6h or 1 g q12h
- *Pseudomembranous/staphylococcal enterocolitis:* PO 500 mg -2 g/d in 3-4 divided doses for 7-10 days
- *Endocarditis prophylaxis:* IV 1 g over 1 hr, 1 hr before dental procedure; repeat in 8 hrs; add aminoglycoside for GI and GU procedures
- *Dosage adjustment for renal impairment:* After initial loading dose of 750 mg -1 g, CrCl 50-80 ml/min 1 g q1-3d; CrCl 10-50 ml/min 1 g q3-7d; CrC1 <10 1 g q7-14d, guided by serum vancomycin concentrations.

Child

- *Serious staphylococcal infections:* IV 40 mg/kg/d divided q6h

Neonates

- IV 15 mg/kg initially followed by 10 mg/kg q8-12h
- *Pseudomembranous/staphylococcal enterocolitis:* PO 40 mg/kg/d divided q6h, not to exceed 2 g/d
- *Endocarditis prophylaxis:* 20 mg/kg over 1 hr, 1 hr before dental procedure; repeat in 8 hr; add aminoglycoside for GI and GU procedures

$ AVAILABLE FORMS/COST OF THERAPY

- Inj, Conc-Sol—IV: 500 mg/vial: **$8.56-$11.32;** 1 g/vial: **$11.51-$22.62**
- Cap, Gel—Oral: 125 mg, 20's: **$94.50;** 250 mg, 20's: **$189.01**

CONTRAINDICATIONS: Hypersensitivity, decreased hearing

PRECAUTIONS: Renal disease, elderly, neonates

PREGNANCY AND LACTATION: Pregnancy category C (oral), B (IV); excreted into breast milk, milk level 4 hr after steady state dose, 12.7 μg/ml (similar to mother's trough level), poorly absorbed orally, systemic absorption not expected, problems limited to modification of bowel flora, allergic sensitization, and interference with interpretation of culture results during fever workup

SIDE EFFECTS/ADVERSE REACTIONS

CV: ***Cardiac arrest, vascular collapse***

EENT: ***Ototoxicity, permanent deafness,*** tinnitus

HEME: ***Leukopenia, eosinophilia, neutropenia***

GI: ***Nausea***

GU: ***Nephrotoxicity, increased BUN, creatinine, albumin, fatal uremia***

RESP: Wheezing, dyspnea

SKIN: Chills, fever, rash, thrombophlebitis at inj site, urticaria, pruritus, necrosis with extravasation (Red man's syndrome or "red-neck syndrome")

MISC: ***Anaphylaxis***

▼ **DRUG INTERACTIONS**

Drugs

• *Aminoglycosides, cephalosporins, colistin, polymyxin, bacitracin, cisplatin, amphotericin B:* Ototoxicity or nephrotoxicity

Labs

• Increase: Red blood cell aggregation (produce false-positive direct antiglobulin tests)

SPECIAL CONSIDERATIONS

MONITORING PARAMETERS

• Audiograms, RFTs, serum concentrations

• Should not be routinely included in empirical antibiotic regimens for febrile neutropenic patients because of resistance; reserve for patients with a high clinical index of suspicion or in centers with a high incidence of methicillin-resistant *S. aureus,* clostridial infections, or enterococcus

vasopressin

(vay-soe-press'in)

Pitressin Synthetic

Chemical Class: Lysine vasopressin

Therapeutic Class: Pituitary hormone

CLINICAL PHARMACOLOGY

Mechanism of Action: Vasopressor and antidiuretic hormone (ADH) activity

Pharmacokinetics

IM/SQ: Antidiuretic activity duration 2-8 hr

Metabolized or destroyed in liver, kidneys, excreted in urine, $t_{1/2}$ 15 min

INDICATIONS AND USES: Diabetes insipidus (non nephrogenic/non psychogenic), abdominal distension postoperatively, bleeding esophageal varices*

DOSAGE

Adult

• *Diabetes insipidus:* IM/SC 5-10 U bid-qid as needed; IM/SC 2.5-5 units q2-3d (Pitressin Tannate) for chronic therapy

• *Abdominal distension:* IM 5 U, then q3-4h, increasing to 10 U if needed (aqueous)

• *Esophageal varices:* IV or selective intra-arterial: 0.2 U/min initially, increased to 0.4 U/min if bleeding continues (max 0.9 U/min)

Child

• *Diabetes insipidus:* IM/SC 2.5-10 U bid-qid as needed; IM/SC 1.25-2.5 U q2-3d (Pitressin Tannate) for chronic therapy

$ **AVAILABLE FORMS/COST OF THERAPY**

• Inj, Sol—IM; SC: 20 U/ml, 1 ml: **$3.22**

CONTRAINDICATIONS: Hypersensitivity, chronic nephritis

PRECAUTIONS: Vascular disease (especially CAD), epilepsy, migraine, asthma, CHF

PREGNANCY AND LACTATION: Pregnancy category B; breast feeding reported without complications

SIDE EFFECTS/ADVERSE REACTIONS

CNS: Drowsiness, headache, lethargy, flushing, tremor, vertigo

CV: Increased B/P, ***cardiac arrest,*** circumoral pallor, ***dysrhythmias,*** decreased cardiac output, ***angina, MI,*** peripheral vasoconstriction, gangrene

GI: Nausea, vomiting, heartburn, cramps, flatus

GU: Vulval pain, uterine cramping

RESP: Bronchial constriction

SKIN: Vasoconstriction/necrosis with extravasation, sweating, urticaria

MISC: Water intoxication (drowsiness, listlessness, headaches, coma, convulsions), ***anaphylaxis,*** urticaria, bronchial constriction

▼ **DRUG INTERACTIONS**

Drugs

• *Carbamazepine:* Potentiates ADH, may potentiate the effects of vasopressin

• *Chlorpropamide:* Potentiates ADH, may potentiate the effects of vasopressin

Labs

• Increase: Cortisol, serum

SPECIAL CONSIDERATIONS

• Routine use has diminished because of the availability of other, longer-acting agent

PATIENT/FAMILY EDUCATION

• Common adverse effects (skin blanching, abdominal cramps, and nausea may be reduced by taking 1-2 glasses of water with the dose of vasopressin; self limited in minutes

MONITORING PARAMETERS

• ECG, fluid and electrolyte status

venlafaxine

(ven-la-fax'een)

Effexor

Chemical Class: Substituted cyclohexanol

Therapeutic Class: Antidepressant

CLINICAL PHARMACOLOGY

Mechanism of Action: Potentiation of neurotransmitter activity in the CNS by strong inhibition of neuronal serotonin and norepinephrine reuptake and weak inhibition of dopamine reuptake

Pharmacokinetics

PO: Peak level 1-2 hr, steady-state level of drug and active metabolites achieved in 3 days; absorption 92% (no change with food); protein binding 27%; metabolized by cytochrome P450 system in liver; unchanged drug and metabolites excreted in urine, elimination $t_{1/2}$ 3-7 hr for drug, 9-13 hr for active metabolites; clearance of drug and active metabolites reduced by 50% in cirrhotics, reduced by 25% if CrCl 10-70 ml/min, and reduced by 60% in dialysis patients

INDICATIONS AND USES: Depression, obsessive-compulsive disorder*

DOSAGE

Adult

• PO starting dose 75 mg qd, given bid or tid; increase daily dose by 75 mg up to 225 mg qd, given bid or tid (375 mg qd for severe depression) at intervals of no less than 4 days

• Reduce total daily dose 25% in patients with mild to moderate renal impairment, by 50% in patients with severe renal impairment; dialysis patients should receive dose after dialysis; reduce total daily dose by 50% in patients with moderate hepatic impairment

• When discontinuing drug, taper over 2 wk

$ **AVAILABLE FORMS/COST OF THERAPY**

• Tab, Uncoated—Oral: 25 mg, 100's: **$88.88;** 37.5 mg, 100's: **$91.54;** 50 mg, 100's: **$94.28;** 75 mg, 100's: **$99.94;** 100 mg, 100's: **$105.94**

CONTRAINDICATIONS: Concurrent use of MAOIs (at least 14 days should elapse between discontinuation of an MAOI and initiation of venlafaxine; at least 7 days should be allowed after stopping venlafaxine before starting an MAOI), age <18 yrs

PRECAUTIONS: Hypertension, anxiety, seizures, aggravation of bipolar disorder (0.5%)

PREGNANCY AND LACTATION: Pregnancy category C; excretion into breast milk unknown

SIDE EFFECTS/ADVERSE REACTIONS

CNS: Anxiety, dizziness, insomnia, nervousness, ***seizures (0.3%),*** somnolence, tremor

CV: Hypertension (dose dependent; frequency 3%-13%), *vasodilation*

EENT: Blurred vision, dry mouth, dysgeusia, mydriasis, tinnitus

GI: Anorexia, dyspepsia, *nausea,* vomiting

GU: Abnormal ejaculation/orgasm, impotence, urinary retention

RESP: Yawning

SKIN: Sweating

MISC: Asthenia

▼ **DRUG INTERACTIONS**

Drugs

- *Cimetidine:* Reduces venlafaxine clearance

Labs

- *Increase:* Cholesterol (mean 3 mg/dl)

SPECIAL CONSIDERATIONS

- Do not stop medication abruptly

---

verapamil

(ver-ap'a-mill)

Calan, Calan SR, Isoptin, Isoptin SR, Verelan

Chemical Class: Phenylalkylamine

Therapeutic Class: Calcium channel blocker

CLINICAL PHARMACOLOGY

Mechanism of Action: Inhibits calcium ion influx across cell membrane during cardiac depolarization; produces relaxation of coronary vascular smooth muscle; dilates coronary arteries; decreases SA/AV node conduction; dilates peripheral arteries

Pharmacokinetics

IV: Onset 3 min, peak 3-5 min, duration 10-20 min

PO: Onset variable (30 min from non-sustained release preparations, peak 1-2.2 hr, duration 17-24 hr 90% absorption, extensive first-pass metabolism, bioavailability 20%-35%; 83%-90% protein bound, metabolized by liver (norverapamil 20% activity of verapamil), excreted in urine (96% as metabolites), $t_{1/2}$ (biphasic) 4 min, 3-7 hr (terminal)

INDICATIONS AND USES: Chronic stable angina pectoris, vasospastic angina, unstable angina, dysrhythmias, hypertension, migraine headaches,* cardiomyopathy*

DOSAGE

Adult

- *Angina:* PO initial, 80-120 mg tid, titrate to 480 mg weekly based on response
- *Dysrhythmias (atrial fibrillation/digitalized):* PO 240-320 mg/d in tid or qid dosage
- *Dysrhythmias (SVT):* IV BOL initial 5-10 mg over 2 min; repeat dose 10 mg, 30 min after 1st if ineffective
- *Hypertension:* PO initial 80 mg tid or 240 mg SR; daily doses 320-480 mg/d

Child 0-1 yr

- *Dysrhythmias (SVT):* IV BOL 0.1-0.2 mg/kg over >2 min with ECG monitoring, repeat if necessary in 30 min

Child 1-15 yr

- IV BOL 0.1-0.3 mg/kg over >2 min, repeat in 30 min, not to exceed 10 mg in a single dose

$ **AVAILABLE FORMS/COST OF THERAPY**

- Inj, Sol—IV: 2.5 mg/ml, 2 ml: **$2.35-$12.99**
- Tab, Coated, Sust Action—Oral:

V

180 mg, 100's: **$97.28-$112.86;** 240 mg, 100's: **$96.45-$129.12**

- Tab, Plain Coated—Oral: 40 mg, 100's: **$4.15-$33.17;** 80 mg, 100's: **$5.63-$44.23;** 120 mg, 100's: **$8.25-$59.80**

CONTRAINDICATIONS: Sick sinus syndrome, 2nd or 3rd degree heart block, hypotension less than 90 mm Hg systolic, cardiogenic shock, severe CHF, hypersensitivity

PRECAUTIONS: CHF, hypotension, hepatic injury, children, renal disease, concomitant IV beta blocker therapy, cirrhosis, Duchenne's muscular dystrophy

PREGNANCY AND LACTATION: Pregnancy category C; excreted in breast milk, (Case report) approx. 25% of maternal serum, serum level in infant 2.1 μg/ml, but undetectable at 38 hr; compatible with breast feeding

SIDE EFFECTS/ADVERSE REACTIONS

CNS: Dizziness, lightheadedness, headache, asthenia

CV: Edema, ***CHF,*** bradycardia, hypotension, palpitations, AV block

GI: Nausea, *constipation*

GU: Nocturia, polyuria

SKIN: Rash

▼ DRUG INTERACTIONS

Drugs

- *Barbiturates:* Reduced plasma concentrations of verapamil
- *Benzodiazepines:* Marked increase in midazolam concentrations, increased sedation likely to result
- *Beta blockers:* Beta blocker serum concentrations increased, bradycardia or hypotension possible
- *Carbamazepine:* Increased carbamazepine toxicity when verapamil added to chronic anticonvulsant regimens, reduced metabolism
- *Cimetidine:* Increased verapamil concentrations and effect by cimetidine
- *Digitalis glycosides:* Increased digoxin concentrations by approximately 70%
- *Neuromuscular blocking agents:* Prolonged neuromuscular blockade
- *Quinidine:* Quinidine toxicity via inhibition of metabolism
- *Rifampin:* Induced metabolism, reduced verapamil concentrations
- *Theophylline:* Verapamil inhibits metabolism, increases theophylline levels

Labs

- Increased: Liver function tests
- *Interference:* Pituitary LH and FSH (inhibition of release normally stimulated by gonadotropin releasing hormone)

SPECIAL CONSIDERATIONS

- Appropriate calcium channel blocker choice in the treatment of atrial fibrillation, atrial flutter, paroxysmal supraventricular tachycardia, and hypertension; diltiazem has relatively lower incidence of adverse effects
- Nifedipine preferred over verapamil and diltiazem in patients with sinus bradycardia, conduction disturbances, and left ventricular dysfunction and for combination with a beta-blocker

---

vidarabine

(vye-dare'a-been)

Vira-A

Therapeutic Class: Antibacterial, antiviral

Chemical Class: Purine nucleoside

CLINICAL PHARMACOLOGY

Mechanism of Action: Inhibits bacterial/viral replication by preventing DNA synthesis, as does active metabolite

Pharmacokinetics

OPHTH: Minimal systemic absorption

INDICATIONS AND USES: Ocular infections caused by susceptible organisms; antiviral spectrum usually includes Herpes simplex virus 1 and 2, varicella zoster, and vaccinia viruses; except for rhabdovirus and oncornavirus, minimal activity against other RNA or DNA viruses; Indications: acute keratoconjunctivitis and recurrent epithelial keratitis, superficial keratitis

DOSAGE

Adult and Child

- OPHTH: 0.5″ to lower lid 5 times daily (q3h); after re-epithelialization, treat for 7 more days at bid

$ AVAILABLE FORMS/COST OF THERAPY

- Oint—Ophth: 3%, 3.5g: **$19.78**

CONTRAINDICATIONS: Hypersensitivity

PREGNANCY AND LACTATION: Pregnancy category C

SIDE EFFECTS/ADVERSE REACTIONS

EENT: Burning, stinging, photophobia, pain, temporary visual haze, edema

SPECIAL CONSIDERATIONS

- Trifluridine is more effective; vidarabine is not the drug of choice in any viral infections; however, it may be a useful alternative in patients who cannot tolerate or have failed other antiviral therapy

vitamin A

Aquasol A, Del-Vi-A, Vitamin A

Chemical Class: Retinol

Therapeutic Class: Vitamin, fat soluble

CLINICAL PHARMACOLOGY

Mechanism of Action: Involved in bone and tooth development, visual dark adaptation, skin disease, mucosa tissue repair, assists in production of adrenal steroids, cholesterol, RNA

Pharmacokinetics

PO/IM: Stored in liver, kidneys, fat; transported in plasma as retinol, bound to retinol-binding protein, excreted (metabolites) in bile bound to glucuronide and small amount in urine; normal serum vitamin A level is 80-200 IU/ml

INDICATIONS AND USES: Vitamin A deficiency

DOSAGE

Adult and Child > 8 yr

- PO 100,000-500,000 IU qd × 3d, then 50,000 qd × 2 wk; dose based on severity of deficiency; maintenance 10,000-20,000 IU for 2 mo

Child 1-8 yr

- IM 5,000-15,000 IU qd × 10 days; then maintenance as follows:

Child 4-8 yr

- IM 15,000 IU qd × 2mo

Child < 4 yr

- IM 10,000 IU qd × 2 mo

Infants < 1 yr

- IM 5,000-15,000 IU × 10 days

$ AVAILABLE FORMS/COST OF THERAPY

- Cap, Elastic—Oral: 25,000 U, 100's: **$2.25-$41.61;** 50,000 U, 100's: **$2.50-$72.36**
- Inj, Sol—IM: 50,000 U/ml, 2 ml: **$19.73**

CONTRAINDICATIONS: Hypersensitivity to Vit A, malabsorption syndrome (PO)

PRECAUTIONS: Impaired renal function

PREGNANCY AND LACTATION: Pregnancy category A; safety of exceeding 5000/6000 IU PO/IV (RDA) not established; naturally present in breast milk, deficiency rare, RDA during lactation is 6000 IU; danger of higher doses unknown

SIDE EFFECTS/ADVERSE REACTIONS

CNS: Headache, increased intracranial pressure, intracranial hypertension, lethargy, malaise

EENT: Gingivitis, papilledema, exophthalmos, inflammation of tongue and lips

GI: Nausea, vomiting, anorexia, abdominal pain, ***jaundice***

METAB: Hypomenorrhea, hypercalcemia

MS: Arthralgia, retarded growth, hard areas on bone

SKIN: Drying of skin, pruritus, increased pigmentation, night sweats, alopecia

▼ **DRUG INTERACTIONS**

Drugs

- *Mineral oil, cholestyramine, colestipol:* Decreased absorption of Vit A
- *Corticosteroids, oral contraceptives:* Increased levels of Vit A

Labs

- *False increase:* Bilirubin, serum cholesterol

SPECIAL CONSIDERATIONS

PATIENT/FAMILY EDUCATION

- Administer with food for better PO absorption
- Foods high in vitamin A: yellow and dark green vegetables, yellow/orange fruits, A-fortified foods, liver, egg yolks
- Vit A deficiency: decreased growth, night blindness, dry, brittle nails, hair loss, urinary stones, increased infection, hyperkeratosis of skin, drying of cornea
- Single Vit A deficiency is rare

vitamin D (cholecalciferol, vitamin D_3; ergocalciferol, vitamin D_2)

(cole'ee-cal-sif'er-ol; er'go-cal-sif'erol)

Calciferol, Deltalin, Drisdol, Hytakerol, Radiostol, ✤ Radiostol Forte ✤

Chemical Class: Fat soluble vitamin

Therapeutic Class: Vitamin D

CLINICAL PHARMACOLOGY

Mechanism of Action: Participates in regulation of calcium, phosphate, bone development, parathyroid activity, neuromuscular functioning; synthesis in two steps: hydroxylation in the liver (to 25-hydroxy vitamin D) and in the kidneys (to 1,25-dihydroxy vitamin D); parathyroid hormone is responsible for regulation of metabolism in the kidneys

Pharmacokinetics

PO/INJ: Lag of 10 to 24 hr between the administration of vitamin D and the initiation of its action in the body due to the necessity of synthesis of these active metabolites; max hypercalcemic effects at 4 weeks; duration 2 mo; readily absorbed from small intestine (bile is essential for adequate absorption); $t_{1/2}$ 7-12 hr; stored in liver; excreted in bile (metabolites) and urine

INDICATIONS AND USES: Dietary supplement, Vit D deficiency, refractory rickets, renal osteodystrophy, hypoparathyroidism, hypophosphatemia, hypocalcemic tetany

DOSAGE (Note: The range between therapeutic and toxic doses is narrow. Calcium intake should be adequate. Cholecalciferol 1 mg provides 40,000 U Vit D activity; ergocalciferol 1.25 mg provides 50,000 IU of Vit D activity)

Adult

- *Vit D deficiency:* PO/IM 12,000 IU qd, then increased to 500,000 IU/day
- *Vit D-resistant rickets:* 12,000 to 500,000 USP units daily
- *Hypoparathyroidism:* 50,000 to 200,000 USP units daily concomitantly with calcium lactate 4 g, administered 6 times/day

Child

- *Vit D deficiency:* PO/IM 1500/5000 IU qd × 2-4 wk, may repeat after 2 wk or 600,000 IU as single dose
- *Hypoparathyroidism:* PO/IM 200,000 IU qd given with 4 g Ca tab

$ AVAILABLE FORMS/COST OF THERAPY

- Cap, Elastic—Oral: 50,000 U D_2, 50's: **$1.23-$45.74**
- Liq—Oral: 8000 U/ml D_2, 60 ml: **$61.88**
- Tab—Oral: 400 IU D_3, 250's: **$8.50**
- Inj—IM: 500,000 IU/ml, 1 ml amp: **$14.62**

CONTRAINDICATIONS: Hypersensitivity, hypercalcemia, renal dysfunction, hyperphosphatemia, abnormal sensitivity to the toxic effects of Vit D and hypervitaminosis D

PRECAUTIONS: Cardiovascular disease, renal calculi

PREGNANCY AND LACTATION: Pregnancy Category A (400 USP U/d); Category C (pharmacologic doses), associated with supravalvular aortic stenosis, elfin facies, and mental retardation; caution should be exercised when ergocalciferol is administered to nursing women; Vit D and metabolites appear in breast milk and have caused infant hypercalcemia

SIDE EFFECTS/ADVERSE REACTIONS

CNS: Fatigue, weakness, drowsiness, ***convulsions,*** headache, psychosis

CV: Hypertension, dysrhythmias

GI: Nausea, vomiting, anorexia, cramps, diarrhea, constipation, metallic taste, dry mouth

GU: Polyuria, nocturia, ***hematuria, albuminuria, renal failure,*** decreased libido

MS: Decreased bone growth, early joint pain, early muscle pain

SKIN: Pruritus, photophobia

▼ DRUG INTERACTIONS

Drugs

- *Cholestyramine, colestipol, mineral oil:* Decreased Vit D absorption
- *Thiazide diuretics:* Hypercalcemia

SPECIAL CONSIDERATIONS

MONITORING PARAMETERS

- Serum calcium and phosphorus levels (Vit D levels also helpful, although less frequently)
- Height and weight in children

---

vitamin E

Amino-Opti-E, Aquasol E, Daltose, ♣ E-Complex-600, E-Ferol, E-Vitamin Succinate, E-200 I.U. Softgels, Gordo-Vite E, Tocopherol, Vita-Plus E Softgells, Vitec

Chemical Class: Fat soluble vitamin

Therapeutic Class: Vitamin E

CLINICAL PHARMACOLOGY

Mechanism of Action: Involved in digestion and metabolism of polyunsaturated fats, decreases platelet aggregation, decreases blood clot formation, promotes normal growth and development of muscle tissue, prostaglandin synthesis

Pharmacokinetics
PO: Metabolized in liver, excreted in bile
INDICATIONS AND USES: Vit E deficiency, impaired fat absorption,* hemolytic anemia in premature neonates,* prevention of retrolental fibroplasia,* sickle cell anemia,* supplement in malabsorption syndrome*
DOSAGE
Adult
• PO/IM 60-75 IU qd, not to exceed 300 IU/d
Child
• PO/IM 1 mg/0.6 g of dietary fat
$ AVAILABLE FORMS/COST OF THERAPY
• Cap, Gel—Oral: 100 IU, 100's: **$1.75-$4.00;** 200 IU, 100's: **$2.20-$3.78;** 400 IU, 100's: **$2.90-$5.58;** 600 IU, 100's: **$8.98-$15.00;** 1000 IU, 100's: **$12.98**
• Sol, Drops—Oral: 50 IU/ml, 12 ml: **$10.06**
PREGNANCY AND LACTATION: Pregnancy category A (C if used above RDA doses), RDA in pregnancy is 15 IU; excreted into breast milk, 5 times richer in vitamin E than cow's milk, American RDA of vitamin E during lactation is 16 IU
SIDE EFFECTS/ADVERSE REACTIONS
METAB: Altered metabolism of hormones, thyroid, pituitary, adrenal, altered immunity
MS: Weakness
CNS: Headache, fatigue
GI: Nausea, cramps, diarrhea
GU: Gonadal dysfunction
CV: Increased risk thrombophlebitis
EENT: Blurred vision
SKIN: Sterile abscess, contact dermatitis
▼ DRUG INTERACTIONS
Drugs
• *Oral anticoagulants:* Increased action
• *Cholestyramine, colestipol, mineral oil, sucralfate:* Decreased absorption
Labs
• *Increase:* CPK (serum and urine) suggest muscle damage by vitamin E
SPECIAL CONSIDERATIONS
• RDA adult male 15 IU, adult female 12 IU

warfarin
(war'far-in)
Carfin, Coumadin, Panwarfin, Sofarin, Warfilone Sodium, ♣ Warnerin ♣
Chemical Class: Coumarin derivative
Therapeutic Class: Anticoagulant

CLINICAL PHARMACOLOGY
Mechanism of Action: Inhibits synthesis of vitamin K dependent coagulation factors causing sequential depression of Factors VII, IX, X, and II activity in a dose-dependent manner; has no direct effect on established thrombus; prevents further extension of formed clot and prevents secondary thromboembolic complications
Pharmacokinetics
PO: Rapidly and completely absorbed, peak activity 1½-3 days, duration 2-5 days, 97%-99% bound to plasma proteins, metabolized by hepatic microsomal enzymes, excreted in urine and feces (inactive metabolites), $t_{1/2}$ 1-2½ days
INDICATIONS AND USES: Prophylaxis and treatment of venous thrombosis, pulmonary embolism, atrial fibrillation with embolism, thromboembolic complications associated with cardiac valve replacement and systemic embolism after MI; recur-

rent transient ischemic attack,* hypercoagulable states*

DOSAGE

Adult

- PO initiate with 5-10 mg qd for 2-4 days; adjust dosage according to INR determinations; usual maintenance dose 2-10 mg qd, based on INR determinations

Child

- PO 0.1 mg/kg/d with a range of 0.05-0.34 mg/kg/d; adjust dosage according to INR determinations; consistent anticoagulation may be difficult to maintain in children <5 yr

$ AVAILABLE FORMS/COSTS OF THERAPY

- Tab, Uncoated—Oral: 1 mg, 100's: **$52.32;** 2 mg, 100's: **$14.84-$54.60;** 2.5 mg, 100's: **$17.61-$56.28;** 4 mg, 100's: **$56.70;** 5 mg, 100's: **$30.90-$57.12;** 7.5 mg, 100's: **$86.22;** 10 mg, 100's: **$88.80**

CONTRAINDICATIONS: Active bleeding, hemorrhagic blood dyscrasias; hemorrhagic tendencies (e.g., hemophilia, polycythemia vera, purpura, leukemia); history of bleeding diathesis; recent cerebral hemorrhage; active ulceration of the GI tract; ulcerative colitis; open traumatic or surgical wounds; recent or contemplated brain, eye, spinal cord surgery or prostatectomy; regional or lumbar block anesthesia; continuous tube drainage of the small intestine; severe renal or hepatic disease; subacute bacterial endocarditis; pericarditis; polyarthritis; diverticulitis; visceral carcinoma; severe or malignant hypertension; eclampsia or preeclampsia; threatened abortion; emaciation; malnutrition; vitamin C or K deficiencies; pregnancy; breastfeeding; history of warfarin-induced necrosis

PRECAUTIONS: Trauma, infection, renal insufficiency, hypertension, vasculitis, indwelling catheters, severe diabetes, active tuberculosis, postpartum, protein C deficiency, hepatic insufficiency, elderly, children, hyperthyroidism, hypothyroidism, CHF

PREGNANCY AND LACTATION: Pregnancy category X; use in 1st trimester carries significant risk to the fetus; exposure in the 6th-9th wk of gestation may produce a pattern of defects termed the fetal warfarin syndrome with an incidence up to 25% in some series; compatible with breast feeding for normal, full-term, infants

SIDE EFFECTS/ADVERSE REACTIONS

GI: ***Hepatotoxicity, cholestatic jaundice,*** nausea, vomiting, anorexia, sore mouth, mouth ulcers, ***paralytic ileus***

GU: ***Renal tubular necrosis,*** albuminuria, anuria, red-orange urine

HEME: ***Hemorrhage, leukopenia,*** anemia

SKIN: Dermatitis, urticaria, alopecia, ***necrosis or gangrene of skin and other tissues, exfoliative dermatitis***

MISC: ***Systemic cholesterol microembolization ("purple toes" syndrome)***

▼ DRUG INTERACTIONS

Drugs

- *Allopurinol, azapropazone, binding resins, cimetidine, ciprofloxacin, clofibrate+, co-trimoxazole+, danazol+, dextrothyroxine+, disulfiram+, erythromycin, fluconazole, glucagon, itraconazole, ketoconazole, metronidazole+, miconazole, naladixic acid, norfloxacin, propafenone, sulfamethizole, sulfinpyrazone+, testosterone+, triclofos, vitamin E:* Enhanced hypoprothrombinemic response to warfarin
- *Aminoglutethimide, barbiturates+, carbamazepine, glutethimide+, gris-*

W

eofulvin, rifampin+: Reduced hypoprothrombinemic response to warfarin
• *Antidiabetics:* Potential enhanced hypoprothrombinemic response to warfarin with some sulfonylureas
• *Cephalosporins:* Enhanced hypoprothrombinemic response to warfarin with moxalactam, cefoperazone, cefamandole, cefotetan, and cefmetazole
• *Chloral hydrate:* Transient increase of hypoprothrombinemic response to warfarin
• *Ethanol:* Enhanced hypoprothrombinemic response to warfarin with acute ethanol intoxication
• *Heparin:* Prolonged activated partial thromboplastin time in patients receiving heparin; prolonged prothrombin times in patients receiving warfarin
• *NSAIDs:* Increased risk of bleeding in anticoagulated patients
• *Phenytoin:* Transient increase in hypoprothrombinemic response to warfarin with initiation of phenytoin therapy, followed within 1-2 wk by inhibition of hypoprothrombinemic response to warfarin
• *Salicylates+:* Increased risk of bleeding in anticoagulated patients; enhanced hypoprothrombinemic response to warfarin with large salicylate doses

Labs

• *Interference:* May cause orange-red discoloration of urine which may interfere with some lab tests

SPECIAL CONSIDERATIONS

PATIENT/FAMILY EDUCATION

• Strict adherence to prescribed dosage schedule is necessary
• Avoid alcohol, salicylates, and drastic changes in dietary habits
• May cause orange-red discoloration of urine
• Notify physician of unusual bleeding or bruising, red or dark brown urine, red or tar black stools
• Do not change from one brand to another without consulting physician

MONITORING PARAMETERS

• INR q4-6 wk once stabilized, more frequently if INR out of range
• Hct, urinalysis, stool guaiac, sign and symptoms of bleeding

xylometazoline

(zye-loe-met-az'oh-leen)
Otrivin

Chemical Class: Imidazoline derivative
Therapeutic Class: Nasal decongestant

CLINICAL PHARMACOLOGY

Mechanism of Action: Vasoconstriction through a local adrenergic mechanism on dilated nasal mucosal blood vessels

Pharmacokinetics

Onset 5-10 min, duration 5-6 hr, occasionally enough drug is absorbed to produce systemic effects

INDICATIONS AND USES: Relief of nasal congestion associated with acute or chronic rhinitis, common cold, sinusitis, and hay fever or other allergies

DOSAGE

Adult

• Instill 2-3 gtt or sprays of 0.1% sol into each nostril q8-10h; do not exceed 3 administrations in 24 hr; should not be used for longer than 3-5 days

Child 2-12 yr

• Instill 2-3 gtt or sprays of 0.05% sol into each nostril q8-10h; do not exceed 3 administrations in 24 hr; should not be used for longer than 3-5 days

* = non-FDA-approved use + = major clinical significance

AVAILABLE FORMS/COST OF THERAPY

• Sol, Drops—Nasal: 0.05%, 25 ml: **$5.38;** 0.1%, 25 ml: **$6.24**

• Sol, Spray—Nasal: 0.1%, 20 ml: **$2.50-$4.88**

CONTRAINDICATIONS: Hypersensitivity, angle-closure glaucoma

PRECAUTIONS: Children <2 yr, hyperthyroidism, heart disease, hypertension, diabetes mellitus

PREGNANCY AND LACTATION: Pregnancy category C

SIDE EFFECTS/ADVERSE REACTIONS

CNS: Headache, nervousness, dizziness, weakness

CV: Hypertension, cardiac irregularities

EENT: Transient burning, stinging, dryness, ulceration of nasal mucosa, sneezing, anosmia; rebound congestion/hyperemia

GI: Nausea

SKIN: Sweating

SPECIAL CONSIDERATIONS

PATIENT/FAMILY EDUCATION

• May produce increased nasal congestion if overused

• Do not use longer than 3-5 days unless under the direction of a physician

yohimbine

(yoe-him'been)

Aphrodyne, Dayto Himbin, Yocon, Yohimex

Chemical Class: Indolalkylamine alkaloid

Therapeutic Class: Agent for impotence

CLINICAL PHARMACOLOGY

Mechanism of Action: Blocks presynaptic α_2-adrenergic receptors; increases parasympathetic (cholinergic) and decreases sympathetic (adrenergic) activity in peripheral autonomic nervous system; may theoretically increase penile inflow, decrease penile blood outflow or both; exerts no significant influence on cardiac stimulation; effect on blood pressure, if any, would be to lower it (some reports indicate an increase in blood pressure)

Pharmacokinetics

No data available

INDICATIONS AND USES: Impotence of vascular or diabetic origins (data are sparse),* sexual dysfunction caused by selective serotonin reuptake inhibitors,* orthostatic hypotension (much more research needed)*

DOSAGE

Adult

• *Impotence:* PO 5.4 mg tid

• *Orthostatic hypotension:* PO 12.5 mg/d in divided doses

AVAILABLE FORMS/COST OF THERAPY

• Tab, Uncoated—Oral: 5.4 mg, 100's: **$10.25-$37.32**

CONTRAINDICATIONS: Hypersensitivity, renal disease, children

PRECAUTIONS: History of gastric or duodenal ulcer; generally not for use in females

PREGNANCY AND LACTATION: Do not use during pregnancy

SIDE EFFECTS/ADVERSE REACTIONS

CNS: Central excitation, increased motor activity, nervousness, irritability, tremor, dizziness, headache

CV: Increased or decreased blood pressure, increased heart rate

GI: Nausea, vomiting

GU: Anti-diuresis

SKIN: Sweating, skin flushing

zalcitabine (ddC)

(zal-site'a-been)
Hivid

Chemical Class: Synthetic pyrimidine nucleoside analog
Therapeutic Class: Antiviral

CLINICAL PHARMACOLOGY

Mechanism of Action: Converted to active metabolite, dideoxycytidine 5'-triphosphate (ddCTP), by cellular enzymes; ddCTP serves as an alternative substrate to deoxycytidine triphosphate (dCTP) for HIV-reverse transcriptase and inhibits the *in vitro* replication of HIV-1 by inhibition of viral DNA synthesis; incorporation into growing DNA chain leads to premature chain termination; ddCTP serves as a competitive inhibitor of the natural substrate, dCTP, for the active site of DNA polymerase further inhibiting viral as well as cellular DNA synthesis

Pharmacokinetics

PO: Absolute bioavailability 80% (reduced by food), <4% bound to plasma proteins, phosphorylated intracellularly to ddCTP, excreted in urine, $t_{1/2}$ 1-3 hr

INDICATIONS AND USES: Combination therapy with zidovudine in advanced HIV infection (CD4 cell count ≤300/mm^3 with significant clinical or immunologic deterioration)

DOSAGE

Adult >30 kg

• PO 0.75 mg with 200 mg zidovudine q8h; interrupt therapy with zalcitabine if signs and symptoms of peripheral neuropathy appear, reinstitute at 0.375 mg q8h if all findings related to peripheral neuropathy improve to mild symptoms

• Renal function impairment: PO (CrCl 10-40 ml/min) 0.75 mg q12h; (CrCl <10 ml/min) 0.75 mg q24h

$ **AVAILABLE FORMS/COST OF THERAPY**

• Tab, Uncoated—Oral: 0.375 mg, 100's: **$183.42;** 0.750 mg, 100's: **$229.92**

CONTRAINDICATIONS: Hypersensitivity

PRECAUTIONS: Low CD4 cell counts (<50/mm^3), existing peripheral neuropathy, history of pancreatitis, ethanol abuse, cardiomyopathy, congestive heart failure, renal or hepatic function impairment, children <13 yr

PREGNANCY AND LACTATION: Pregnancy category C

SIDE EFFECTS/ADVERSE REACTIONS

CNS: Headache, dizziness, *peripheral neuropathy,* fever

EENT: Pharyngitis

GI: Oral ulcers, nausea, dysphagia, anorexia, abdominal pain, vomiting, constipation, diarrhea, ***pancreatitis, exacerbation of hepatic dysfunction,*** dry mouth, esophageal ulcers, dyspepsia, glossitis

MS: Myalgia, arthralgia

SKIN: Rash, pruritus, night sweats

MISC: Fatigue, weight decrease

▼ **DRUG INTERACTIONS**

Drugs

• *Chloramphenicol, cisplatin, dapsone, disulfiram, ethionamide, glutethimide, gold, hydralazine, iodoquinol, isoniazid, metronidazole, nitrofurantoin, phenytoin, ribavirin, vincristine:* Increased risk of peripheral neuropathy

• *Pentamidine:* Increased risk for pancreatitis

• *Food:* Decreased zalcitabine concentrations

SPECIAL CONSIDERATIONS

PATIENT/FAMILY EDUCATION

- Report early symptoms of peripheral neuropathy or pancreatitis

MONITORING PARAMETERS

- Periodic CBC, serum chemistry tests
- Serum amylase and triglyceride concentrations in patients with history of elevated amylase, pancreatitis, ethanol abuse, or receiving parenteral nutrition
- Signs and symptoms of peripheral neuropathy (numbness, tingling, hypesthesias, burning or shooting pains of the lower or upper extremities, loss of vibratory sense or ankle reflex
- Liver function tests

zidovudine

(zyde-o'vue-deen)

Retrovir

Chemical Class: Thymidine analog

Therapeutic Class: Antiviral

CLINICAL PHARMACOLOGY

Mechanism of Action: Converted by cellular thymidine kinase to zidovudine monophosphate which is further converted to diphosphate by cellular thymidylate kinase and to triphosphate derivative by other cellular enzymes; triphosphate interferes with the HIV viral RNA dependent DNA polymerase (reverse transcriptase) inhibiting viral replication

Pharmacokinetics

PO: Peak 30-90 min, 25%-38% bound to plasma proteins, metabolized in liver to inactive metabolites, 63%-95% excreted in urine as metabolites and unchanged drug, terminal $t_{1/2}$ 60 min

INDICATIONS AND USES: Initial treatment of HIV-infected adults with CD4 cell counts ≤500 cells/mm^3; HIV-infected children >3 mo who have HIV-related symptoms or who are asymptomatic with abnormal laboratory values indicating significant HIV-related immunosuppression; prevention of maternal-fetal HIV transmission; combination with zalcitabine for treatment of selected patients with advanced HIV disease (CD4 cell count ≤300 cells/mm^3)

DOSAGE

Adult

- *Asymptomatic HIV infection:* PO 100 mg q4h while awake (500 mg/day); IV 1 mg/kg/dose infused over 1 hr q4h while awake (5 mg/kg/d)
- *Symptomatic HIV infection:* PO 100 mg q4h (600 mg/d); IV 1-2 mg/kg/dose infused over 1 hr q4h
- *Maternal-fetal HIV transmission:* Maternal dose (>14 weeks of pregnancy) PO 100 mg 5 times/day until start of labor; during labor and delivery, IV zidovudine should be administered at 2 mg/kg (total body weight) over 1 hr followed by continuous IV inf of 1 mg/kg/hr (total body weight) until clamping of the umbilical cord; infant dose PO 2 mg/kg q6h starting within 12 hr after birth and continuing through 6 wk of age; IV 1.5 mg/kg, infused over 30 min, q6h
- *Combination therapy with zalcitabine:* PO 200 mg with zalcitabine 0.75 mg q8h

Child 3 mo-12 yr

- PO 90-180 mg/m^2/dose q6h; max 200 mg q6h; IV INF 0.5-1.8 mg/kg/hr; IV 100 mg/m^2/dose q6h

$ **AVAILABLE FORMS/COST OF THERAPY**

- Cap, Gel—Oral: 100 mg, 100's: **$154.80**
- Inj, Conc, W/Buf—IV: 10 mg/ml, 20 ml: **$16.74**

• Syr—Oral: 50 mg/5 ml, 240 ml: **$37.15**

CONTRAINDICATIONS: Hypersensitivity

PRECAUTIONS: Bone marrow compromise (granulocyte count <1000 cells/mm^3 or Hgb <9.5 g/dl); hepatomegaly, hepatitis, or other known risk factor for liver disease; severely impaired renal or hepatic function; children

PREGNANCY AND LACTATION: Pregnancy category C; indicated for pregnant women >14 wk gestation for prevention of maternal-fetus HIV transmission

SIDE EFFECTS/ADVERSE REACTIONS

CNS: Fever, headache, dizziness, *insomnia,* paresthesia, somnolence, chills, tremor, twitching, anxiety, confusion, depression, emotional lability, loss of mental acuity

EENT: Vertigo, hearing loss, photophobia

GI: Nausea, vomiting, diarrhea, anorexia, cramps, *dyspepsia,* constipation, dysphagia, flatulence, rectal bleeding, mouth ulcer, taste change, ***cholestatic hepatitis***

GU: Dysuria, polyuria, urinary frequency or hesitancy

HEME: ***Granulocytopenia, anemia, thrombocytopenia, leukopenia***

MS: Myalgia, arthralgia, muscle spasm

RESP: Dyspnea

SKIN: Diaphoresis, rash, acne, pruritus, urticaria, pigmentation of nails (blue)

MISC: Malaise

▼ **DRUG INTERACTIONS**

Drugs

• *Food:* Taking zidovudine with meals lowers plasma concentrations

• *Ganciclovir+:* Increased hematologic toxicity

• *Interferon, probenecid, valproic acid:* Increased plasma concentrations of zidovudine

• *Rifampin:* Reduced plasma concentrations of zidovudine

SPECIAL CONSIDERATIONS

PATIENT/FAMILY EDUCATION

• Close monitoring of blood counts is extremely important; does not reduce risk of transmitting HIV to others through sexual contact or blood contamination

MONITORING PARAMETERS

• CBC with differential and platelets q2wk

---

zinc sulfate

Eye-Sed Ophthalmic, Orazinc, Scrip Zinc, Verazinc, Zinca-Pak, Zincate, Zinc 15, Zinc-220

Chemical Class: Zinc product
Therapeutic Class: Ophthalmic astringent; trace element

CLINICAL PHARMACOLOGY

Mechanism of Action: Vasoconstriction occurs by action on conjunctiva; needed for adequate healing, bone and joint development

Pharmacokinetics

PO: Poorly absorbed, excreted mainly through the intestine

INDICATIONS AND USES: Dietary supplement, treatment or prevention of zinc deficiency; temporary relief of minor eye irritation (ophthalmic)

DOSAGE

Adult

• PO 110-220 mg (15-50 mg zinc) qd; RDA 66 mg (15 mg zinc) qd; IV 2.5-4 mg/d in metabolically stable adults (add 2 mg/d for acute catabolic states)

• *Minor eye irritation:* Instill 1 gtt bid-tid

Child
• PO 0.3 mg/kg/d
• *Minor eye irritation:* Instill 1 gtt bid-tid

$ AVAILABLE FORMS/COST OF THERAPY
• Sol—Ophth: 0.25%, 15 ml: **$2.72**
• Tab—Oral: 66 mg (15 mg zinc), 100's: **$1.45;** 110 mg (25 mg zinc), 100's: **$3.89;** 200 mg (45 mg zinc), 1000's: **$10.73**
• Cap, Gel—Oral: 220 mg, 100's: **$7.70-$13.31**
• Inj, Sol—IV: 1 mg/ml, 10 ml: **$44.38;** 5 mg/ml, 5 ml: **$61.25**

CONTRAINDICATIONS: Hypersensitivity

PRECAUTIONS: Narrow-angle gaucoma (ophthalmic), excessive doses

PREGNANCY AND LACTATION: Pregnancy category A (in doses not exceeding RDA)

SIDE EFFECTS/ADVERSE REACTIONS
EENT: Eye irritation, burning (ophthalmic)
GI: Nausea, vomiting

▼ DRUG INTERACTIONS
Drugs
• *Ciprofloxacin:* Reduced serum ciprofloxacin concentrations, clinical significance appears to be minimal
• *Food:* Bran products may decrease zinc absorption
• *Tetracycline:* Reduced serum tetracycline concentrations

SPECIAL CONSIDERATIONS

PATIENT/FAMILY EDUCATION
• Take with food if GI upset occurs

zolpidem

(zole-pi'dem)
Ambien
Chemical Class: Imidazopyridine derivative
Therapeutic Class: Sedative/hypnotic
DEA Class: Schedule IV

CLINICAL PHARMACOLOGY
Mechanism of Action: Subunit modulation of the GABA receptor chloride channel macromolecular complex is hypothesized to be responsible for pharmacologic effects; selective binding to the omega$_1$ receptor may explain the preservation of deep sleep (stages 3 and 4) in human studies
Pharmacokinetics
PO: Peak 1.6 hr, 92.5% bound to plasma proteins, converted to inactive metabolites, eliminated primarily by renal excretion, $t_{1/2}$ 2½ hr

INDICATIONS AND USES: Short-term treatment of insomnia

DOSAGE
Adult
• PO 5-10 mg immediately hs; do not exceed 10 mg/d

$ AVAILABLE FORMS/COST OF THERAPY
• Tab, Uncoated—Oral: 5 mg, 100's: **$124.50;** 10 mg, 100's: **$153.14**

CONTRAINDICATIONS: Hypersensitivity

PRECAUTIONS: Psychiatric disorders, elderly and/or debilitated patients, depression, abrupt discontinuation, concomitant systemic illness, compromised respiratory function, hepatic impairment, history of drug abuse, children <18 yr

PREGNANCY AND LACTATION: Pregnancy category B; excreted into breast milk in small amounts

SIDE EFFECTS/ADVERSE REACTIONS

CNS: Daytime drowsiness, dizziness, amnesia, headache, lethargy, confusion, lightheadedness, anxiety, irritability, poor coordination
CV: Chest pain, palpitation
GI: Diarrhea, nausea, vomiting, heartburn, abdominal pain, constipation
HEME: ***Leukopenia, granulocytopenia (rare)***

SPECIAL CONSIDERATIONS

PATIENT/FAMILY EDUCATION

- Take immediately prior to retiring
- Avoid alcohol
- Use caution driving or performing other tasks requiring alertness

Appendix A

Comparative Tables

The following comparative drug tables were developed by practicing physicians to assist providers in choosing medications of a given therapeutic class. These tables allow clinicians to compare drugs on the basis of important pharmacologic or clinical characteristics. Whenever possible, the information is based on definitive drug data and should help the reader obtain maximal therapeutic effect with minimal adverse effects. When applicable, accepted practice guidelines have been incorporated into the tables.

Acid Secretion Inhibitors

Drug Name	Trade Name	Usual Adult Starting Oral Dose	Nonprescription Strength	Cost	Drug Interactions	Dose Adjustment in Renal Dysfunction
H2 Blockers						
Cimetidine	Tagamet	300 mg qid or 800 mg hs	100 mg	$1.50 (300 mg)	Benzodiazepines, beta adrenergic blockers, itraconazole, ketoconazole, lidocaine, meperidine, nifedipine, phenytoin, procainamide, quinidine, tacrine, tricyclic antidepressants, warfarin	Yes (CrCl <30 ml/min)
Famotidine	Pepcid	20 mg bid or 40 mg hs	10 mg	$1.54 (20 mg)	Itraconazole, ketoconazole, nifedipine, quinolone antibiotics	Yes (CrCl <50 ml/min)
Nizatidine	Axid	150 mg bid or 300 mg hs	NA	$1.54 (150 mg)	Itraconazole, ketocoazole, nifedipine, quinolone antibiotics	Yes (CrCl <50 ml/min)
Ranitidine	Zantac	150 mg bid or 300 mg hs	75 mg	$1.59 (150 mg)	Itraconazole, ketoconazole, nifedipine, quinolone antibiotics	Yes (CrCl <50 ml/min)
Proton Pump Inhibitors						
Lansoprazole	Prevacid	15-30 mg qd	NA	$3.25 (15 mg)	Theophylline, iron, ketoconazole, amoxicillin, digoxin	No
Omeprazole	Prilosec	20 mg qd	NA	$3.60 (20 mg)	Diazepam, warfarin, phenytoin, iron, ketoconazole, amoxicillin, digoxin	No

Nonnarcotic Analgesics

Drug Name	Trade Name	Usual Adult Dose (mg)	Maximum Adult Daily Dose (mg)	Oral Dose Forms (mg)	Nonprescription Strength (mg)	Chemical Class	Comment
Acetaminophen	Tylenol	325-650 q4-6h	4000	80, 160, 325, 500, 650	All forms	Aminophenol	Hepatotoxicity if overdosed and in persons with cirrhosis
Salicylates							
Acetylsalicylic acid	Aspirin	325-975 q4h	6000	81, 165, 325, 500, 650, 975	All forms	Salicylate	Antagonizes effect of probenecid; increases effect of sulfonylureas; reduces renal clearance of methotrexate
Choline magnesium trisalicylate	Trilisate	500-1000 q12h	3000	500, 750, 1000	NA	Salicylate	Antagonizes effect of probenecid; increases effect of sulfonylureas; reduces renal clearance of methotrexate
Salsalate	Disalcid	500-1000 q8h 750-1500 q12h	3000	500, 750, 1000	NA	Salicylate	Antagonizes effect of probenecid; increases effect of sulfonylureas; reduces renal clearance of methotrexate
Short-acting NSAIDs							
Diclofenac	Cataflam	50 tid	200	25, 50	NA	Acetic acid	Formulation is immediate release
Diclofenac	Voltaren	25-75 bid-tid	200	25, 50, 75	NA	Acetic acid	Formulation is delayed release
Fenoprofen	Nalfon	300-600 q6h	3200	200, 300, 600	NA	Propionic acid	Highly protein bound (to albumin)
Ibuprofen	Motrin, Rufen	400-600 q6h	3200	200, 300, 400, 600, 800	200	Propionic acid	Also approved for primary dysmenorrhea
Indomethacin	Indocin, Indocin SR	25-50 q8h or 75 q12h (sustained release)	200	25, 50, 75 (sustained release)	NA	Acetic acid	Available in suppository, suspension, and sustained-release forms

Continued.

Nonnarcotic Analgesics—cont'd

Drug Name	Trade Name	Usual Adult Dose (mg)	Maximum Adult Daily Dose (mg)	Oral Dose Forms (mg)	Nonprescription Strength (mg)	Chemical Class	Comment
Ketoprofen	Orudis	50-75 q6-8h	300	12.5, 25, 50, 75, 200 (sustained release)	12.5	Propionic acid	High rate of dyspepsia (11%), available in sustained-release form
Ketorolac	Toradol	10 q4-6h	40	10	NA	Acetic acid	100% bioavailable; indicated only as continuation of parenteral ketorolac, short term
Meclofenamate	Meclomen	50-100 q6h	400	50, 100	NA	Anthranilic acid	High rate of diarrhea (10%-33%)
Mefenamic acid	Ponstel	500, then 250 q6h	1000	250	NA	Anthranilic acid	Also approved for primary dysmenorrhea
Tolmetin	Tolectin	400 q6-8h	2000	200, 400, 600	NA	Acetic acid	High rate of nausea (11%)
Intermediate-acting NSAIDs							
Diflunisal	Dolobid	500 q12h	1500	250, 500	NA	Salicylate derivative	Not metabolized to salicylate; increases acetaminophen level by 50% when coadministered
Etodolac	Lodine	200-400 bid-qid	1200	200, 300	NA	Acetic acid	Antacids reduce peak concentration by 20%
Flurbiprofen	Ansaid	50-100 bid-tid	300	50, 100	NA	Propionic acid	May cause CNS stimulation
Naproxen	Naprosyn	250-500 q8-12h	1250	220, 250, 375, 500		Propionic acid	Approved for acute gout; may increase effect of protein-bound drugs such as phenytoin, sulfonylureas, and warfarin

Nonnarcotic Analgesics

Drug Name	Trade Name	Usual Adult Dose (mg)	Maximum Adult Daily Dose (mg)	Oral Dose Forms (mg)	Nonprescription Strength (mg)	Chemical Class	Comment
Naproxen	Anaprox	275-550 q8-12h	1375	275, 550	220	Propionic acid	Approved for acute gout; may increase effect of protein-bound drugs such as phenytoin, sulfonylureas, and warfarin
Sulindac	Clinoril	150-200 q12h	400	150, 200	NA	Acetic acid	Approved for acute gout
Long-acting NSAIDs							
Nabumetone	Relafen	500-750 bid; 1000-1500 qd	1500	500, 750	NA	Nonacidic	High rate of diarrhea (14%)
Piroxicam	Feldene	10-20 qd	20	10, 20	NA	Oxicam	High rate of dyspepsia (20%); may increase effect of protein-bound drugs such as phenytoin, sulfonylureas, and warfarin
Oxaprozin	Daypro	1200 qd	1800	600		Proprionic acid	
Parenteral NSAID							
Ketorolac	Toradol	30 or 60 initially, then 15-30 q6h (all IM)	150 1st day, then 120 qd	15, 30, 60	NA	Acetic acid	Total duration of treatment should not exceed 5 days; 30 mg equal to 6-12 mg morphine sulfate but 10 times as expensive

Narcotic and Narcotic-like Analgesics

Drug Name	Trade Name	Usual Adult Dose (mg) and Routes	Parenteral Dose (mg) Equal to 10 mg Morphine Sulfate IM	Oral Dose (mg) Equal to Listed Parenteral Dose	Comment
Narcotic-like agents					
Buprenorphine	Buprenex	0.3 q6h IM	0.3	NA	Mixed agonist-antagonist; schedule V controlled substance
Butorphanol	Stadol	1-4 q3-4h IM, Nasal	2-3	NA	Mixed agonist-antagonist; not a controlled substance
Nalbuphine	Nubain	10 q6h IM, IV, or SC	10	NA	Mixed agonist-antagonist; not a controlled substance
Tramadol	Ultram	50-100 q4-6h PO	NA	NA	100 mg equinalagesic to 60 mg codeine; use not associated with dependence but long term data limited
Narcotics					
Fentanyl	Sublimaze, Duragesic (transdermal)	0.05-0.1 q1-2h IM or IV; 25-100 µg/h transdermal (base dose on total morphine dose); 0.2-0.4 as lozenge	0.125	NA	Primary use is IV or epidural for perioperative or patient-controlled analgesia; transdermal form available but costly
Oxymorphone	Numorphan	1-1.5 q4-6h IM; 5 q4-6h PR	1	NA	Major use is perioperative
Hydromorphone	Dilaudid	2 q4-6h PO; 1-2 q4-6h IM; 3 q6-8h PR	1.5	7.5	High abuse potential
Levorphanol	Levo-Dromoran	2 q6-8h PO	NA	4	Long acting
Methadone	Dolophine	5-10 q4-6h PO	NA	20	Different $t_{1/2}$ for analgesia and prevention of opiate withdrawal

Continued.

Narcotic and Narcotic-like Analgesics—cont'd

Drug Name	Trade Name	Usual Adult Dose (mg) and Routes	Parenteral Dose (mg) Equal to 10 mg Morphine Sulfate IM	Oral Dose (mg) Equal to Listed Parenteral Dose	Comment
Morphine sulfate	Roxanol	5-20 q4h IM; 5-20 q6h PR; 10 q4h SL; 10-30 mg q4h PO	10	60 (single dose)	Oral bioavailability poor; sublingual form useful for breakthrough pain
Morphine, sustained release	MS Contin	15-60 q6-12h PO	NA	30 (repeated doses)	Not appropriate for prn use
Oxycodone	Percocet, Percodan, Tylox	5-10 q4-6h PO	NA	25	Often combined with aspirin (Percodan) or acetaminophen (Percocet, Tylox)
Hydrocodone	Vicodin	5-10 q4-6h PO	NA	30	Only available combined with acetamino-phen or aspirin
Pentazocine	Talwin	30-60 q3-4h IM; 50-100 q4h PO	45	135	Mixed agonist-antagonist
Meperidine	Demerol	50-125 q3-4h IM; 50-100 q4h PO	75	250	May be used IV; metabolite normeperidine may accumulate with prolonged use causing excitation or seizures
Codeine	Codeine	15-60 q4h PO	130	200	Schedule II unless combined with acetamin-ophen or aspirin; used as cough suppressant
Propoxyphene	Darvon	32-100 q4h PO	180	360	Less abuse potential than codeine at usual doses

Cephalosporin Antibiotics

Drug Name (Generation in Parentheses)	Trade Name	Usual Adult Dose (g)	Adjust Dose for Renal Insufficiency	Comment
Oral				
Cefadroxil (1)	Duricef	0.5-1.0 q12-24h	Y	
Cephalexin (1)	Keflex	0.25-0.5 q6h	Y	Cheapest in its therapeutic class
Cephradine (1)	Velosef	0.5 q6h	Y	
Cefaclor (2)	Ceclor	0.25-0.5 q8h	N	
Cefpodoxime (2)	Vantin	0.1-0.4 q12h	Y	
Cefprozil (2)	Cefzil	0.25-0.5 q12h	Y	
Cefuroxime axetil (2)	Ceftin	0.25-0.5 q12h	Y	
Cefixime (3)	Suprax	0.4 q24h	Y	Single dose therapy for gonococcal genital and pharyngeal infections
Parenteral (IV/IM)				
Cefazolin (1)	Ancef, Kefzol	1-2 q6-8h	Y	
Cephalothin (1)	Keflin	1-2 q4-6h	Y	
Cephapirin (1)	Cefadyl	1 q4-6h	Y	
Cefamandole (2)	Mandol	0.5-1.0 q4-8h	Y	
Cefmetazole (2)	Zefazone	2 q6-12h	Y	
Cefonicid (2)	Monocid	1-2 q24h	Y	May be useful in outpatient therapy of endocarditis

Continued.

Cephalosporin Antibiotics—cont'd

Drug Name (Generation in Parentheses)	Trade Name	Usual Adult Dose (g)	Adjust Dose for Renal Insufficiency	Comment
Ceforanide (2)	Precef	0.5-1.0 q12h	Y	
Cefotetan (2)	Cefotan	1-2 q12h	Y	Covers GI anaerobes
Cefoxitin (2)	Mefoxin	1-2 q4-6h	Y	Covers GI anaerobes
Cefuroxime (2)	Zinacef	0.75-1.5 q8h	Y	Crosses blood-brain barrier
Cefoperazone (3)	Cefobid	1-2 q8-12h	N	
Cefotaxime (3)	Claforan	1-2 q4-6h	Y	Crosses blood-brain barrier
Ceftazidine (3)	Fortaz	1-2 q6-8h	Y	
Ceftizoxime (3)	Cefizox	1-2 q6-8h	Y	Crosses blood-brain barrier
Ceftriaxone (3)	Rocephin	1-2 q12-24h	N	May be useful in outpatient therapy of endocarditis; single-dose (250 mg IM) therapy for gonococcal genital and pharyngeal infections; crosses blood-brain barrier

Macrolide Antibiotics

Drug Name	Trade Name	Usual Adult Dose (mg)	Comment
Azithromycin	Zithromax	500, followed by 250 q24h	Single dose therapy for chlamydial urethritis or cervicitis (1000 mg); antibacterial spectrum includes *Hemophilus influenzae*
Clarithromycin	Biaxin	250-500 q12h	Antibacterial spectrum includes *Mycobacterium avium-intracellulare, Helicobacter pylori*, and *H. influenzae*
Dirithromycin	Dynabac	500 q24h	Antibacterial spectrum includes *H. influenzae*
Erythromycin	Erythromycin	250-500 q6-12h	Available as combination product with sulfisoxazole (extends spectrum to include *H. influenzae*)

Penicillin Antibiotics

Drug Name	Trade Name	Usual Adult Dose (g)	Comment
ORAL			
Penicillin V	Penicillin VK	0.25-0.5 q6h	
Broad Spectrum Penicillins			
Amoxicillin	Amoxicillin	0.25-0.5 q8h	
Amoxicillin-Clavulanate	Augmentin	One tablet (0.25 or 0.5 amoxicillin/0.125 clavulanate) q8h	Spectrum extended to include beta-lactamase producers such as *Hemophilus influenza, Moraxella catarrhalis, Staphylococcus aureus* (except MRSA), and *Escherichia coli*
Ampicillin	Ampicillin	0.5-1.0 q6h	Gives higher and more sustained serum levels of ampicillin
Bacampicillin	Spectrobid	0.4-0.8 q12h	
Penicillinase Resistant Penicillins			
Cloxacillin	Tegopen	0.25-0.5 q6h	Oral penicillin of choice for *S. aureus* (except MRSA)
Dicloxacillin	Dycill	0.25-0.5 q6h	Oral penicillin of choice for *S. aureus* (except MRSA)
PARENTERAL (IV)			
Penicillin G	Penicillin	1-3 million U q4-6h	Procaine and benzathine forms available for IM use
Broad Spectrum Penicillins			
Ampicillin	Ampicillin	1-2 q4-6h	
Ampicillin-Sulbactam	Unasyn	1-2/0.5-1.0 q6h	Spectrum extended to include beta-lactamase producers such as *H. influenza, M. catarrhalis, S. aureus* (except MRSA), and *E. coli*
Carbenicillin	Geopen	4-5 q4-6h	
Ticarcillin	Ticar	2-3 q4-6h	

Continued.

Penicillin Antibiotics—cont'd

Drug Name	Trade Name	Usual Adult Dose (g)	Comment
Ticarcillin-Clavulanic Acid	Timentin	3.1 (3.0 ticarcillin, 0.1 clavulanate potassium) q4-6h	Spectrum extended to include beta-lactamase producers such as *S. aureus* (except MRSA), *E. coli, Klebsiella* sp, and *Bacteroides fragilis*
Azlocillin	Azlin	2-3 q4-6h	Spectrum includes enterococci, *Klebsiella, Enterobacter,* and *Serratia* sp
Mezlocillin	Mezlin	2-4 q4-8h	Spectrum includes enterococci, *Klebsiella, Enterobacter,* and *Serratia* sp
Piperacillin	Pipracil	3-4 q4-6h	Spectrum includes enterococci, *Klebsiella, Enterobacter, Acinetobacter,* and *Serratia* sp
Piperacillin-Tazobactam	Zosyn	3.375 (3.0 piperacillin, 0.375 tazobactam) q4-6h	Spectrum includes enterococci, *Klebsiella, Enterobacter, Acinetobacter,* and *Serratia* sp; extended to include beta-lactamase producers such as *S. aureus* (except MRSA) and *B. fragilis*
Penicillinase Resistant Penicillins			
Methicillin	Methicillin	1-2 q4-6h	Parenteral penicillin of choice for *S. aureus* (except MRSA)
Nafcillin	Nafcillin	0.5-2.0 q4-6h	Parenteral penicillin of choice for *S. aureus* (except MRSA)
Oxacillin	Oxacillin	0.5-2.0 q4-6h	Parenteral penicillin of choice for *S. aureus* (except MRSA)

Note: MRSA = Methicillin resistant *S. aureus.*

Quinolone Antibiotics

Drug Name	Trade Name	Usual Adult Dose (mg)	Cost (10 Days of Oral Therapy)	Comment
Cinoxacin	Cinobac	PO: 250 q6h or 500 q12h	$38	Approved only to treat UTIs; *Enterococcus, Staphylococcus,* and *Pseudomonas* sp are resistant
Ciprofloxacin	Cipro	PO: 250-750 q12h IV: 200-400 q12h	$63	Available for ophthalmic use; useful in oral therapy of osteomyelitis; approved for *Campylobacter, Salmonella,* and *Shigella* infections; antibacterial spectrum includes *Mycobacterium avium-intracellulare*
Enoxacin	Penetrex	PO: 400 q12h	$57	Approved only to treat UTIs
Lomefloxacin	Maxaquin	PO: 400 q24h	$61	Not effective for *Pseudomonas aeruginosa* infections outside of the urinary tract
Norfloxacin	Noroxin	PO: 400 q12h	$52	Available for ophthalmic use; approved only to treat UTIs and conjunctivitis
Ofloxacin	Floxin	PO: 200-400 q12h IV: 200-400 q12h	$76	Available for ophthalmic use

Sulfonamide Antibiotics

Drug Name	Trade Name	Usual Adult Dose	Comment
SYSTEMIC			
Sulfamethoxazole	Gantanol	PO: 500-1000 mg q12h	Primary use is for UTIs
Sulfamethoxazole-trimethoprim	Septra, Septra DS, Bactrim, Bactrim DS, Co-trimoxazole	PO: 800 mg/160 mg q12h IV: 10-20 mg/kg/d based on trimethoprim component divided into q6-12h schedule	First line therapy for *Pneumocystis carinii* pneumonia
Sulfadiazine	Sulfadiazine	PO: 500-1000 mg q6h	Used with pyrimethamine to treat toxoplasmosis
Sulfisoxazole	Gantrisin	PO: 500-1000 mg q6h	Available in combination with erythromycin ethylsuccinate for oral use
TOPICAL			
Silver sulfadiazine	Silvadene	TOP: 1% cream to affected area qd-bid (desired thickness 1-2 mm)	Primary use is for 2nd and 3rd degree burns
Sodium sulfacetamide	Sodium Sulamyd	OPHTH: 10% sol in affected eye q2-4h; 10% oint; 0.5 inch into lower conjunctival sac QID	Primary indication is bacterial conjunctivitis

Systemic Antifungal Antibiotics

Drug Name	Trade Name	Usual Adult Dose	Common Indications	Comment
Amphotericin B	Fungizone	IV: 0.4-0.6 mg/kg/d for 8-10 wk	Histoplasmosis, blastomycosis, candidiasis, cryptococcosis, coccidioidomycosis, aspergillosis, mucormycosis	Used topically in bladder; causes multiple electrolyte abnormalities (hypokalemia, renal tubular acidosis, hypomagnesemia, azotemia); give 1 mg test dose prior to giving full dose
Fluconazole	Diflucan	PO or IV: 100-400 qd	Blastomycosis, histoplasmosis, candidiasis, coccidioidomycosis	Increases serum rifabutin levels and toxicity; increases effect of cyclosporine, terfenadine, astemizole, warfarin, sulfonylureas, and others; single dose treatment for vaginal infection (po)
Flucytosine	Ancobon	PO: 12.5-37.5 mg/kg q6h	Cryptococcosis, candidiasis, chromoblastomycosis	Usually used in combination with amphotericin B (allows lower dose); converted to 5-fluorouracil in fungal cell
Griseofulvin	Fulvicin, Gris-PEG	PO: 500 mg qd-bid (microcrystalline) PO: 330 mg qd-bid (ultra microcrystalline)	Dermatophytes	Hepatic mixed function oxidase inducer; absorption enhanced when taken with fatty foods
Itraconazole	Sporanox	PO: 100-200 mg qd-bid	Onychomycosis, blastomycosis, histoplasmosis, candidiasis, coccidioidomycosis, sporotrichosis, cryptococcosis, aspergillosis	Hepatic mixed function oxidase inhibitor (cytochrome P450 3A—affects cyclosporine, terfenadine, astemizole, warfarin, sulfonylureas, and others)
Ketoconazole	Nizoral	PO: 200-400 mg qd-bid	Blastomycosis, histoplasmosis, candidiasis, coccidioidomycosis, dermatophytes	Hepatic mixed function oxidase inhibitor (cytochrome P450 3A—affects cyclosporine, terfenadine, astemizole, warfarin, sulfonylureas, and others); requires acid pH for absorption; reduces testosterone synthesis; available in topical form
Miconazole	Monistat	IV: 200-1200 mg q8h	Coccidioidomycosis, candidiasis, cryptococcosis	Increases warfarin and sulfonylurea effect; used topically for cutaneous and vaginal infections

Selective Serotonin Reuptake Inhibitor (SSRI) Antidepressants

Drug Name	Brand Name	Usual Adult Dose (mg/d)	Drug and Active Metabolite ($t_{1/2}$ (hr)	Serotonin Reuptake Inhibition	Anticholinergic Effect	Drowsiness	Degree of Cytochrome P450 System Inhibition	Comment
Fluoxetine	Prozac	20-40 (starting dose 10 in elderly)	24-72 (acute); 96-144 (chronic); (norfluoxetine: 96-384)	3+	0	0	2-3+	Up to 60 mg/d for obsessive-compulsive disorder
Fluvoxamine	Luvox	50-300	15-26 (no active metabolite)	3+	0	1+	2+	Only indicated for obsessive-compulsive disorder
Paroxetine	Paxil	20-50 (starting dose 10 in elderly)	21 (no active metabolite)	4+	1+	1+	2+	May cause weight gain
Sertraline	Zoloft	50-200 (starting dose 12.5-25 in elderly)	26 (desmethylsertraline: 62-104)	4+	0	0	1+	Metabolite weakly active

Tricyclic and Tetracyclic Antidepressants

Drug Name	Brand Name	Usual Adult Dose (mg) for Acute Therapy (Maintenance Dose is ½-⅔ of this; lower doses recommended for elderly persons)	Relative Sedation	Relative Anticholinergic Effect	Relative Delay of Cardiac Conduction	Relative Postural Hypotension	Comment
TRICYCLIC							
Amitriptyline	Elavil	75-300	3+	2+	3+	3+	Used for chronic pain
Clomipramine	Anafranil	25-250	2+	2+	2+	2+	Primary use is for obsessive-compulsive disorder; may lower seizure threshold; may increase plasma concentration of protein bound drugs (e.g., digoxin, warfarin)
Desipramine	Norpramin	75-300	1+	1+	3+	1+	Used for chronic pain; metabolite of imipramine
Doxepin	Sinequan	75-300	3+	3+	1+	3+	Potent antihistamine
Imipramine	Tofranil	50-300	2+	2+	3+	2+	Used for chronic pain, panic disorder, and headache
Nortriptyline	Pamelor	50-150	1+	1+	2+	2+	Used for chronic pain, panic disorder, and headache; metabolite of amitriptyline
Protriptyline	Vivactil	15-60	0+	2+	2+	1+	
Trimipramine	Surmontil	50-300	2+	2+	3+	2+	

Continued.

Tricyclic and Tetracyclic Antidepressants—cont'd

Drug Name	Brand Name	Usual Adult Dose (mg) for Acute Therapy (Maintenance Dose is $\frac{1}{2}$-$\frac{2}{3}$ of this; lower doses recommended for elderly persons)	Relative Sedation	Relative Anticholinergic Effect	Relative Delay of Cardiac Conduction	Relative Postural Hypotension	Comment
TETRACYCLIC							
Amoxapine	Asendin	200-600	2+	1+	1+	1+	Metabolite has neuroleptic side effect
Maprotiline	Ludiomil	75-300	2+	1+	1+	1+	May lower seizure threshold
HETEROCYCLIC							
Nefazodone	Serzone	200-600	2+	1+	0+	1+	Divided doses on bid schedule; do not administer with terfenadine or astemizole; may increase plasma concentration of protein bound drugs (e.g., digoxin, warfarin)
Trazodone	Desyrel	150-600	3+	1+	0+	2+	Risk of priapism in males and similar phenomenon in females; may increase plasma concentration of protein bound drugs (e.g., digoxin, warfarin); should be given as divided doses

Miscellaneous Antidepressants, Including Foods That Interact With MAOIs

Drug Name	Brand Name	Usual Adult Dose (mg/d)	Anticholinergic Effect	Drowsiness	Orthostatic Hypotension	Cardiac Dysrhythmias	Comment
Bupropion	Wellbutrin	300-450	0	0	0	1+	Single dose should not exceed 150 mg; inhibits dopamine reuptake; given bid or tid
Venlafaxine	Effexor	75-375	1+	1+	0	1+	Inhibits serotonin and norepinephrine reuptake; given bid or tid
Monoamine oxidase inhibitors (MAOIs)							Avoid foods rich in amines (see below) and selected medications while taking MAOI and for 14 days after last dose
Isocarboxazid	Marplan	10-30	2+	2+	3+	1+	May be given as single daily dose
Phenelzine	Nardil	15-90	2+	2+	3+	1+	Given in divided doses
Tranylcypromine	Parnate	30-60	2+	1+	3+	1+	Given in divided doses

Avoid the following foods if taking MAOIs (contain tyramine and other amines, often as a result of aging or fermenting): broad beans; red wines; yeast extracts; beer with yeast; chicken or beef liver; caviar, anchovies, and pickled herring; fermented sausages (bologna, pepperoni, salami, and summer sausage); and aged cheeses (Boursault, Brie, Camembert, cheddar, Emmenthaler, Gruyere, mozzarella, parmesan, romano, Roquefort, and Stilton).

Insulins

Drug Name	Time to Onset of Effect (hr) for SC	Time to Peak Effect (hr) for SC	Duration of Effect (hr) for SC	Routes of Administration
Regular insulin (SC)	½-1	3-8	6-12	SC
Regular insulin (IV)	⅙-½	¼-½	½-1	IV, IM
NPH Insulin	2-4	4-12	24	SC
Lente Insulin	1-3	5-14	24	SC
Protamine Zinc Insulin (PZI)	4-8	14-24	36	SC
Ultralente Insulin	4-8	10-30	36	SC
50/50 Insulin	½-1	4-8	24	SC
70/30 Insulin	½-1	4-8	24	SC

Notes:
1. Most insulin types are available as beef, pork, or human types. Onset of action is faster and duration is shorter with human insulin preparations.
2. Insulin is available in U-100 (100 units per ml) and U-500 (500 units per ml) forms. Duration of action of U-500 forms is longer than U-100 forms.

Appendix B

Bibliography

Physicians GenRx, St. Louis, 1996, Mosby–Year Book.

Briggs GG, Freeman RK, Yaffe SJ: *Drugs in pregnancy and lactation,* ed 4, Baltimore, 1994, Williams and Wilkins.

Shepard TH: *Catalog of teratogenic agents,* ed 7, Baltimore, 1992, Johns Hopkins University Press.

Hansten PD, Horn JR: *Drug interactions and updates quarterly,* Vancouver, Wash, 1996, Applied Therapeutics.

Drug facts and comparisons, St. Louis, 1996, Facts and Comparisons.

McEvoy GK, American Hospital Formulary Service: *Drug Information,* Bethesda, Md, 1995, American Society of Hospital Pharmacists.

Taketomo CK, Hodding JH, Kraus DM: *Pediatric dosage handbook,* ed 3, Hudson, Ohio, 1996, Lexicomp.

Doherty MC: *Drug topics red book 1995,* Montvale, NJ, 1995, Medical Economics Data Production.

United States Pharmacopeial Convention: USP dispensing information, Vol I, *Drug information for the health care professional,* ed 16, Easton, Penn, 1996, Mack Publishing.

Index

A

Abbokinase, 849-850
A/B Otic, 55-56
Absorbine, 820
acarbose, 1
Accupril, 727-728
Accurbron, 798-800
Accutane, 443-444
acebutolol, 2-3
Acephen, 3-4
Aceta, 3-4
acetaminophen, 3-4
Acetazolam, 5-6
acetazolamide, 5-6
acetic acid, 6-7
acetohexamide, 7-8
acetohydroxamic acid, 8-9
Acetosol, 6-7
acetylcholine, 9
acetylcysteine, 9-10
Aches-N-Pain, 419-420
Achromycin, 796-797
Acidulated Phosphate Fluoride, 759-761
Aci-Jel, 6-7
Acloderm, 13-14
Aclosone, 13-14
Aclovate, 13-14
Acne-10, 83-84
Acnigel, 83-84
Acrocillin, 643-645
ACT, 759-761
ACTH, 213-214
Acthar, 213-214
Acticort 100, 409-411
Actidil, 845-846
Actidose-Aqua, 158-159
Actigall, 850-851
Actilyse, 18-19
Actimmune, 430-431
Activase, 18-19
activated charcoal/charcoal, 158-159
Acular, 452-453
Acutrim, 668-669
acyclovir, 10-11
Adalat, 594-595
Adapin, 292-294
Adenocard, 11-12
adenosine, 11-12
Adipex-P, 663-664
Adipost, 657
Adphen, 657
Adrenalin Chloride, 311-313
Adsorbocarpine, 673-674
Adsorbonac Ophthalmic Solution, 757-758
Advil, 419-420
AeroBid, 354-355
Aerolate, 798-800
Aeroseb-Dex, 244-246
Aeroseb-HC, 409-411
Aerosporin, 682-683
Afrin, 628-629
Afrin Children's Nose Drops, 628-629
Afrin Saline Mist, 757-758
Aftate, 820
A-Hydrocort, 409-411
Airbron, 9-10
Akaprine, 673-674
AK-Chlor, 161-163
AK-Con, 583
Ak-Dex Ophthalmic, 244-246
Ak-Dilate, 667-668
AK-Fluor, 357-358
AK-Homatropine, 403-404
Akineton, 94-95
AK-Mycin, 318-320
AK-NaCl, 757-758
Ak-Nefrin, 667-668
Akne-Mycin, 318-320
AK-Pentolate, 221
AK-Pred, 693-695
AK-Sulf, 773

Entries can be identified as follows: generic name, Trade Name.

AK-Taine, 710-711
AKTob, 813-814
Ak-Tracin, 75-76
Ak-Zol, 5-6
Ala-Cort, 409-411
Ala-Scalp, 409-411
Albalon, 583
albuterol, 12-13
Alcaine, 710-711
alclometasone, 13-14
Alconefrin, 667-668
Aldactone, 765-766
Aldomet, 536-538
Aleve, 584-585
Alfenta, 14-15
alfentanil, 14-15
Alferon N, 429
Algesic, 110
Alka-Mints, 116-119
Aller-Chlor, 171-172
Allerdryl, 280-281
Allerest Eye Drops, 583
Allerest 12 Hour Nasal, 628-629
Allergen, 55-56
Allergia-C, 280-281
allopurinol, 15-16
Alphaderm, 409-411
Alphamul, 132
alphaRedisol, 414-415
Alphatrex, 89-91
alprazolam, 16-17
alprostadil, 17-18
Altace, 733-734
Altaflor, 759-761
alteplase, 18-19
AlternaGEL, 20-22
Alu-Cap, 20-22
Alugel, 20-22
aluminum acetate, 19-20
aluminum chloride hexahydrate, 20
aluminum hydroxide, 20-22
aluminum salts, 20-22
Alupent, 514-515
Alurate, 57-58
Alu-Tab, 20-22
Alzapam, 477-478
amantadine, 22-23
Amaphen, 110
ambenonium, 23-24
Ambien, 869-870
amcinonide, 24-25
Amcort, 826-829
Amen, 495-496
Americaine, 82
Americet, 110
A-methaPred, 541-542
Amicar, 27-28
Amicill, 48-49
Amigesic, 744-745
amikacin, 25-26
Amikin, 25-26
amiloride, 26-27
aminocaproic acid, 27-28
aminoglutethimide, 28-29
Amino-Opti-E, 861-862
aminophylline (theophylline ethylenediamine), 29-32
aminosalicylate, 32
amiodarone, 33-34
Amitone, 116-119
amitriptyline, 34-36
amlodipine, 36-37
ammonium chloride, 37-38
amobarbital, 38-40
Amodopa, 536-538
Amonidrin, 391-392
amoxapine, 40-42
amoxicillin, 42-43
amoxicillin/clavulanate, 43-45
Amoxil, 42-43
amphetamine, 45-46
Amphojel, 20-22
amphotericin B, 46-48
ampicillin, 48-49
amrinone, 49-50
amyl nitrite, 50-51
Amytal Sodium, 38-40
Anacaine, 82
Anacin-3, 3-4
Anadrol-50, 629-630
Anafranil, 197-199
Anapolon 50, 629-630
Anaprox, 584-585
Anaspaz, 419
Ancasal, 59-61
Ancef, 136-137
Ancobon, 352-353
Ancotil, 352-353
Android, 543-544, 793-795
Andro LA 200, 793-795

Entries can be identified as follows: generic name, Trade Name.

Androlan, 793-795
Androlone-D 200, 581-583
Andropository 200, 793-795
Anergan, 707-708
Anestacon, 466-467
Anexsia, 407-408
Anhydron, 225-226
anisindione, 51-52
anisolyated plasminogen activator complex (APSAC), 53-54
anistreplase, 53-54
Anolor 300, 110
Anoquan, 110
Anorex, 657
Ansaid, 365-366
Antabuse, 285-286
Anthra-Derm, 54-55
anthralin, 54-55
Antilirium, 671-672
Antiminth, 719-720
antipyrine and benzocaine, 55-56
Antispas, 260
Anti-tuss, 391-392
Antivert, 492-493
Antrizine, 492-493
Anturan, 781-782
Anturane, 781-782
Anucort-HC, 409-411
Anxanil, 418-419
Apacet, 3-4
Aparkane, 837-838
Aphen, 837-838
Aphrodyne, 865-866
Apoallopurinol, 15-16
Apo-alpraz, 16-17
Apo-Atenol, 62-64
Apo-Bisacodyl, 95-96
Apo-C, 58-59
Apo-Carbamazepine, 122-124
Apo-Diazepam, 250-252
APO-Diltiaz, 275-276
Apo-Doxy, 294-296
Apo-Meprobamate, 509-510
Apo-Methyldopa, 536-538
Apo-metoprolol, 549-551
Apo-Metronidazole, 551-553
Apo-Oxazepam, 623-624
Apo-Pen-VK, 643-645
Apo-Perphenazine, 653-655
Apo-sulfatrim, 207-208
Apresoline, 405-406
aprobarbital, 57-58
APSAC (anisolyated plasminogen activator complex), 53-54
Aquacare, 848-849
Aquachloral Supprettes, 160-161
AquaMEPHYTON, 672-673
Aquaphyllin, 798-800
Aquasol A, 859-860
Aquasol E, 861-862
Aquatensen, 534-536
Aquest, 328-329
Aralen, 166-167
Aramine, 515-516
Aredia, 634
Argesic-SA, 744-745
Ariculose LA, 826-829
Aristocort, 826-829
Aristospan, 826-829
Arm-a-char, 158-159
Arm-a-Med, 435-436
Arm-a-Med Metaproterenol Sulfate, 514-515
Armour Thyroid, 806-807
Arrestin, 840
Artane, 837-838
Artha-G, 744-745
Arthritis Pain Formula, 3-4
Arthropan, 181-182
Articulose, 693-695
A.S.A., 59-61
Asacol, 510-511
ascorbic acid (vitamin C), 58-59
Ascorbicap, 58-59
Asendin, 40-42
Asmalix, 798-800
Aspergum, 59-61
aspirin, 59-61
Aspirin Free Pain Relief, 3-4
astemizole, 61-62
AsthmaHaler Mist, 311-313
AsthmaNefrin, 311-313
Astromorph PF, 567-569
Atarax, 418-419
Atasol, 3-4
atenolol, 62-64
Ativan, 477-478
Atolone, 826-829
atovaquone, 64-65
Atozine, 418-419

Entries can be identified as follows: generic name, Trade Name.

Atromid-S, 195-196
Atropair, 65-67
Atropen, 65-67
atropine, 65-67
Atropisol, 65-67
Atrovent, 433
A/T/S, 318-320
Audifluor, 759-761
Augmentin, 43-45
Auralgan, 55-56
auranofin, 67
Aureomycin, 177
Aurodex, 55-56
Auro Ear Drops, 124
Aurolate, 68-69
aurothioglucose/gold sodium thiomalate, 68-69
Auroto, 55-56
AVC, 778
Aventyl, 606-608
Avitrol, 778
Avlosulfan, 232
Axid, 601-602
Aygestin, 603-604
Ayr, 757-758
Azactam, 73-74
azatadine, 69-70
azathioprine, 70
azithromycin, 71
Azlin, 72-73
azlocillin, 72-73
Azmacort, 826-829
Azo-Standard, 656
aztreonam, 73-74
Azulfidine, 778-780

B

B-A-C, 110
bacampicillin, 74-75
Bacarate, 657
Baci-Rx, 75-76
bacitracin, 75-76
baclofen, 76-77
Bacticin, 75-76
Bactine Hydrocortisone, 409-411
Bactrim, 207-208
Bactroban, 569
Bactrocill, 618-520
Baldex, 244-246
BAL in Oil, 278
Bancap HC, 407-408
Banesin, 3-4
Banflex, 618
Banlin, 709-710
Banophen, 280-281
Banthine, 521-522
Barbased, 108-109
Barbita, 659-661
Baridium, 656
Basalijel, 20-22
Basaljel, 20-22
Bayer, 59-61
Bayer Children's Aspirin, 59-61
beclomethasone, 77-78
Beclovent, 77-78
Beconase, 77-78
Bedoz, 218-219
Beef NPH Iletin II, 426-427
Beef Regular Iletin II, 426-427
Beesix, 723-724
Beldin, 280-281
Belix, 280-281
belladonna alkaloids, 78-79
belladonna and opium, 79-80
Bellafoline, 78-79
Bena-D-10, 280-281
Benadryl, 280-281
Benahist, 280-281
Ben-Aqua, 83-84
Benasept, 81-82
Ben-A-Vance, 280-281
benazepril, 80-81
Bendramine, 280-281
Benemid, 698-699
Benoject, 280-281
Benoquin, 566
Ben-Rex, 280-281
Bensylate, 85-86
Bentyl, 260
Bentylol, 260
Benuryl, 698-699
Benylin DM, 249-250
Benza, 81-82
Benzac, 83-84
Benzagel, 83-84
benzalkonium chloride, 81-82
Benzashave, 83-84
benzathine penicillin, 643-645
benzocaine, 82
benzocaine and antipyrine, 55-56

Entries can be identified as follows: generic name, Trade Name.

benzonatate, 83
Benzotic, 55-56
benzoyl peroxide, 83-84
benzquinamide, 84-85
benztropine, 85-86
benzylpenicilloylpolylysine, 86-87
bepridil, 87-88
beractant, 88-89
Beta-2, 435-436
Betalin S, 801-802
Betaloc, 549-551
betamethasone, 89-91
Betapen-VK, 643-645
Betaseron, 429-430
Betaspace, 763-764
Betatrex, 89-91
Beta-Val, 89-91
Betaxin, 801-802
betaxolol, 91-93
bethanechol, 93-94
Bethaprim, 207-208
Betoptic, 91-93
Biamine, 801-802
Biaxin, 187-188
Bicillin, 643-645
Bicitra, 758-759
Biltricide, 691
Biocal, 116-119
Biocef, 153-155
Biomox, 42-43
Bio-Statin, 608-609
Bio-Tab, 294-296
biperiden, 94-95
Bisac-Evac, 95-96
bisacodyl, 95-96
Bisacodyl Uniserts, 95-96
Bisco-Lax, 95-96
bismuth subsalicylate, 96-97
bisoprolol, 97-98
bitolterol, 98-99
Black Draught, 751-752
Bleph-10, 773
Blocadren, 810-811
Bluboro Powder, 19-20
Bonamine, 492-493
Bonine, 492-493
Bontril PDM, 657
Boropak Powder, 19-20
B & O Suppositories, 79-80
Breathe Free, 757-758
Breonesin, 391-392
B_{12} Resin, 218-219
Brethaire, 791-792
Brethine, 791-792
Bretylate, 99-100
bretylium, 99-100
Bretylol, 99-100
Brevibloc, 321-322
Brevicon, 615-617
Brevoxyl, 83-84
Bricanyl, 791-792
British Anti-Lewisite, 278
Bromfed DM, 249-250
bromocriptine, 100-101
Bromphen, 101-102
brompheniramine, 101-102
Bronitin Mist, 311-313
Bronkaid Mist, 311-313
Bronkephrine, 338
Bronkodyl, 798-800
Bronkometer, 435-436
Bronkosol, 435-436
Bucladin-S Softabs, 102-103
buclizine, 102-103
bumetanide, 103-104
Bumex, 103-104
bupivacaine, 104-105
Buprenex, 105-106
buprenorphine, 105-106
bupropion, 106-107
Burcillin-G, 643-645
Burow's Solution, 19-20
BuSpar, 107-108
buspirone, 107-108
butabarbital, 108-109
Butace, 110
Butalan, 108-109
butalbital/acetaminophen/caffeine, 110
butalbital/aspirin/caffeine, 110
Butalbital Compound, 110
Butal Compound, 110
Butalgen, 110
Butatran, 108-109
Butazolidin, 665
Buticaps, 108-109
Butisol Sodium, 108-109
butoconazole, 111
butorphanol, 111-112

Entries can be identified as follows: generic name, Trade Name.

Byclomine, 260
Bydramine, 280-281

C

Caffedrine, 112-113
caffeine, 112-113
Calan, 857-858
Cal Carb-HD, 116-119
Calcibind, 153
Calci-Chew, 116-119
Calciday, 116-119
calcifediol, 113-114
Calciferol, 313-314, 860-861
Calcijex, 115-116
Calcimar, 114-115
Calci-Mix, 116-119
calcitonin, 114-115
calcitriol (1,25-dihydroxychole-calciferol), 115-116
calcium acetate, 116-119
calcium carbonate, 116-119
calcium chloride, 116-119
calcium citrate, 116-119
Calcium Disodium Versenate, 300-301
calcium glubionate, 116-119
calcium gluconate, 116-119
calcium salts, 116-119
Caldecort Anti-Itch, 409-411
Calderol, 113-114
Caldesene, 848
Cal-Guard, 116-119
Calm-X, 277-278
Cal Plus, 116-119
Cal-Plus, 116-119
Caltrate, 116-119
Campain, 3-4
Canesten, 203-204
Cantil, 502-503
Capastat, 119-120
Capitrol, 170
Capoten, 120-121
capreomycin, 119-120
captopril, 120-121
Carafate, 771-772
carbachol, 122
carbamazepine, 122-124
carbamide peroxide, 124
carbenicillin, 125-126
carbidopa-levodopa, 126-127
carbinoxamine/pseudoephedrine, 127-128
Carbocaine, 508-509
Carbolith, 472-473
carboprost, 128-129
Cardene, 591-592
Cardilate, 317
Cardioquin, 730-732
Cardizem, 275-276
Cardura, 292
Carfin, 862-864
carisoprodol, 129
Carmol, 848-849
carteolol, 130-131
Carter's Little Pills, 95-96
Cartrol, 130-131
Cascara, 131-132
cascara sagrada, 131-132
castor oil, 132
Cataflam, 255-256
Catapres, 200-202
C-Crystals, 58-59
Cebid Timecelles, 58-59
Ceclor, 132-133
Cecon, 58-59
cefaclor, 132-133
cefadroxil, 133-134
Cefadyl, 156-157
cefamandole, 134-136
Cefanex, 153-155
cefazolin sodium, 136-137
cefixime, 137-138
Cefizox, 149-150
cefmetazole, 138-139
Cefobid, 140-141
cefonicid, 139-140
cefoperazone, 140-141
ceforanide, 141-142
Cefotan, 143-144
cefotaxime, 142-143
cefotetan, 143-144
cefoxitin sodium, 144-145
cefpodoxime, 145-147
cefprozil, 147
Cefracycline, 796-797
ceftazidime, 148
Ceftin, 151-153
ceftizoxime, 149-150
ceftriaxone, 150-151
cefuroxime, 151-153

Entries can be identified as follows: generic name, Trade Name.

Cefzil, 147
Celestone, 89-91
CellCept, 570-571
cellulose sodium phosphate (CSP), 153
Celontin, 533-534
Celstone Soluspan, 89-91
Cel-U-Jec, 89-91
Cenafed, 718-719
Cena-K, 684-686
Cenocort, 826-829
Cenolate, 58-59
Centrax, 690-691
cephalexin, 153-155
cephalothin, 155-156
cephapirin, 156-157
cephradine, 157-158
Cephulac, 455-456
Ceporex, 153-155
Ceptaz, 148
Cerespan, 635-636
C.E.S., 327-328
Cetacort, 409-411
Cetamide, 773
Cetane, 58-59
Cetazol, 5-6
Cevalin, 58-59
Cevi-Bid, 58-59
Ce-Vi-Sol, 58-59
Charcoaide, 158-159
charcoal/activated charcoal, 158-159
CharcoCaps, 158-159
Charcodote, 158-159
Chealamide, 301-302
Checkmate, 759-761
Chemet, 770-771
Chenix, 159-160
chenodiol, 159-160
Chibroxin Ophthalmic, 604-605
Children's Advil, 419-420
Children's Feverall, 3-4
Children's Hold, 249-250
Chlo-Amine, 171-172
Chlor-100, 171-172
chloral hydrate, 160-161
chloramphenicol, 161-163
Chlorate, 171-172
chlordiazepoxide, 163-164
chlorhexidine, 164-165
chlormezanone, 165
Chloromycetin Kapseals, 161-163
Chloromycetin Ophthalmic, 161-163
Chloromycetin Otic, 161-163
Chloromycetin Palmitate, 161-163
Chloromycetin Sodium Succinate, 161-163
Chloromycetin (topical), 161-163
Chloronase, 174-175
chloroprocaine, 165-166
Chloroptic, 161-163
chloroquine, 166-167
chlorothiazide, 167-169
chlorotrianisene, 169-170
chloroxine, 170
Chlorphed-LA, 628-629
chlorphenesin, 170-171
chlorpheniramine, 171-172
Chlor-Pro, 171-172
Chlorpromanyl, 172-174
chlorpromazine, 172-174
chlorpropamide, 174-175
chlorprothixene, 175-177
Chlorspan-12, 171-172
Chlortab-4, 171-172
Chlortab-B, 171-172
chlortetracycline, 177
chlorthalidone, 177-178
Chlor-Trimeton, 171-172
chlorzoxazone, 178-179
Cholac, 455-456
Cholaxin, 806-807
cholecalciferol, 860-861
Choledyl, 625-626
cholestyramine, 179-180
choline magnesium trisalicylate, 180-181
choline salicylate, 181-182
Cholybar, 179-180
Chooz, 116-119
Chronulac, 455-456
Cibacalcin, 114-115
Cibalith-S, 472-473
ciclopirox, 182-183
cimetidine, 183-184
Cinobac, 185
cinoxacin, 185
Cipro, 185-187
ciprofloxacin, 185-187
cisapride, 187
Citracal, 116-119

Entries can be identified as follows: generic name, Trade Name.

Citra pH, 758-759
Citratred Caffeine, 112-113
citric acid and sodium citrate, 758-759
Citrolith, 758-759
Citroma, 483-484
Citro-Nesia, 483-484
Citrucel, 536
Claforan, 142-143
Claripen, 195-196
Claripex, 195-196
clarithromycin, 187-188
Claritin, 476-477
clavulanate/amoxicillin, 43-45
clavulanic acid/ticarcillin, 807-809
Clavulin, 43-45
Clear Eyes, 583
Clearplex, 83-84
clemastine, 189
Cleocin, 190-192
clidinium, 189-190
Climestrone, 324-325
Clinda-Derm, 190-192
clindamycin, 190-192
Clinoril, 783-784
clioquinol (iodochlorhydroxyquin), 192
Clistin, 127-128
clobetasol, 192-193
clocortolone, 193-194
Cloderm, 193-194
clofazimine, 194-195
clofibrate, 195-196
Clomid, 196-197
clomiphene, 196-197
clomipramine, 197-199
clonazepam, 199-200
clonidine, 200-202
Clopra, 546-547
clorazepate, 202-203
clotrimazole, 203-204
cloxacillin, 204-205
Cloxapen, 204-205
clozapine, 205-207
Clozaril, 205-207
Cobex, 218-219
codeine, 209-210
Codimal-A, 101-102
Codroxomin, 414-415
Cogentin, 85-86
Co-Gesic, 407-408
Cognex, 786-787
Colace, 287-288
colchicine, 210-211
Colestid, 211
colestipol, 211
colfosceril, 212
colistin, 212-213
Collyrium Fresh Eye Drops, 797-798
Colonaid, 282
Colsalide Improved, 210-211
Coly-Mycin S Oral, 212-213
Coly-Mycin S Otic, 212-213
Combantrin, 719-720
Comfort Eye Drops, 583
Comoxol, 207-208
Compazine, 702-704
Compound W, 742-743
Condylox, 681
Congestion Relief, 718-719
Conjugated Estrogens, 327-328
Constant-T, 798-800
Constilac, 455-456
Constulose, 455-456
Control, 668-669
Cophene-B, 101-102
Cordarone, 33-34
Cordran, 363-364
Corgard, 572-574
Corophyllin, 29-32
Correctol Extra Gentle, 287-288
Cortaid, 409-411
Cort-Dome, 409-411
Cortef, 409-411
Cortef Feminine Itch, 409-411
Cortenema, 409-411
Corticotropin, 213-214
corticotropin (ACTH), 213-214
Cortifoam, 409-411
cortisone, 214-215
Cortizone, 409-411
Cortone, 214-215
Cortril, 409-411
Cortrosyn, 216
cosyntropin, 216
Cotazym, 635
Cotrim, 207-208
co-trimoxazole (sulfamethoxazole and trimethoprim), 207-208

Entries can be identified as follows: generic name, Trade Name.

Coumadin, 862-864
Cozaar, 478
Creon, 635
Crolom, 216-217
cromolyn, 216-217
crotamiton, 217-218
Cruex, 848
Crystamine, 218-219
Crystapen, 643-645
Crysti-12, 218-219
Crysticillin A.S., 643-645
Crystodigin, 268-269
C-Solve 2, 318-320
CSP (cellulose sodium phosphate), 153
Cuprimine, 642-643
Curretab, 495-496
Cyanabin, 218-219
cyanide antidote, 218
cyanocobalamin (vitamin B_{12}), 218-219
Cyanoject, 218-219
Cyclan, 219-220
cyclandelate, 219-220
cyclobenzaprine, 220-221
Cyclocort, 24-25
Cyclogyl, 221
cyclopentolate, 221
cyclophosphamide, 222-223
cycloserine, 223-224
Cyclospasmol, 219-220
cyclosporine, 224-225
cyclothiazide, 225-226
Cycrin, 495-496
Cylert, 640
Cyomin, 218-219
cyproheptadine, 226-227
Cystospaz, 419
Cytadren, 28-29
cytarabine, 227-228
Cytomel, 469-470
Cytosar, 227-228
Cytotec, 562
Cytovene, 376-377
Cytoxan, 222-223

D

Dalalone, 244-246
Dalcaine, 466-467
Dalgan, 250
Dalmane, 364-365
Daltose, 861-862
D-Amp, 48-49
danazol, 228-230
Danocrine, 228-230
Dantrium, 230-231
dantrolene, 230-231
Dapa, 3-4
Dapex 37.5, 663-664
dapiprazole, 231-232
dapsone, 232
Daranide, 254-255
Daraprim, 724-726
Darvon, 711-712
Datril, 3-4
Daypro, 622-623
Dayto Himbin, 865-866
Dayto Sulf, 780-781
Dazamide, 5-6
DC Softgels, 287-288
DDAVP, 239-240
ddC (zalcitabine), 866-867
ddI, 261-262
Debrox, 124
Decaderm, 244-246
Decadron, 244-246
Decadron Phosphate, 244-246
Decadron Phosphate Ophthalmic, 244-246
Decadron Phosphate Turbinaire, 244-246
Deca-Durabolin, 581-583
Decaject, 244-246
Decaspray, 244-246
Declomycin, 236-237
Decofed Syrup, 718-719
Decon Otic Ear Drops, 55-56
Decylenes, 848
DeFed-60, 718-719
deferoxamine, 233-234
Degest 2, 583
Dehist, 101-102
Delacort, 409-411
Deladiol-40, 325-326
Delatest, 793-795
Delatestadiol, 793-795
Delatestryl, 793-795
Delcort, 409-411
Delsym, 249-250
Delta-Cortef, 693-695

Entries can be identified as follows: generic name, Trade Name.

Deltalin, 313-314, 860-861
Deltapen, 643-645
Deltasone, 695-696
Delta-Tritex, 826-829
Del-Vi-A, 859-860
Demadex, 820-821
demecarium bromide, 234-235
demeclocycline, 236-237
Demerol, 503-504
Demser, 553-554
Demulen, 615-617
Deoestrogen, 325-326
Depakene, 852-853
Depakote, 852-853
Dep-Andro 200, 793-795
Depen, 642-643
depGynogen, 325-326
depMedalone, 541-542
Depo-Estradiol, 325-326
Depogen, 325-326
Depoject, 541-542
Depo-Medrol, 541-542
Deponit, 598-600
Depopred, 541-542
Depo-Predate, 541-542
Depo-Provera, 495-496
Depotest, 793-795
Depo-Testosterone, 793-795
Dermacort, 409-411
Derma-Smoothe/FS, 355-356
Dermicort, 409-411
Dermolate Anti-Itch, 409-411
Dermtex HC, 409-411
DES, 264-265
Desenex, 848
Desferal, 233-234
desipramine, 237-239
desmopressin, 239-240
Desogen, 615-617
desonide, 241
DesOwen, 241
desoximetasone, 242
Desoxyn, 520-521
desoxyribonuclease, 242-243
Desquam, 83-84
Desyrel, 824-825
Detue, 373-374
Dexacen, 244-246
Dex-A-Diet, 668-669
dexamethasone, 244-246
Dexasone, 244-246
Dexatrim, 668-669
Dexchlor, 246-247
dexchlorpheniramine, 246-247
Dex-Cpm, 246-247
Dexedrine, 248-249
Dexitac, 112-113
Dexone, 244-246
Dexotic, 244-246
dexrazoxane, 247-248
dextroamphetamine, 248-249
dextromethorphan, 249-250
Dextrostat, 248-249
Dey-Lute Metaproterenol Sulfate, 514-515
Dey-Pak Sodium Chloride 3% and 10%, 757-758
dezocine, 250
D.H.E. 45, 272-273
DHPG (ganciclovir), 376-377
DHT, 273-274
DiaBeta, 383-384
Diabinese, 174-175
Diachlor, 167-169
Dialose, 287-288
Dialume, 20-22
Diamine T.D., 101-102
Diamox, 5-6
Diapid, 481
Diaqua, 406-407
Di-Atro, 282
diazepam, 250-252
diazoxide, 252-253
Dibenil, 280-281
Dibent, 260
Dibenzyline, 661-662
dibucaine, 253
Dicarbosil, 116-119
dichlorphenamide, 254-255
diclofenac, 255-256
diclonine, 256
dicloxacillin, 257
dicumarol, 258-259
dicyclomine, 260
didanosine, 261-262
Dideoxyinosine, 261-262
Didronel, 339-340
dienestrol, 262-263
Diet-Aid-Efed II Yellow, 668-669
diethylpropion, 263-264

Entries can be identified as follows: generic name, Trade Name.

diethylstilbestrol, 264-265
difenoxin, 265
diflorasone, 266
Diflucan, 351-352
diflunisal, 266-268
Digibind, 271-272
digitoxin, 268-269
digoxin, 269-271
digoxin immune FAB, 271-272
dihydroergotamine, 272-273
dihydrotachysterol, 273-274
dihydroxyaluminum sodium carbonate, 274-275
1,25-dihydroxycholecalciferol, 115-116
Dilacor XR, 275-276
Dilantin, 669-670
Dilatair, 667-668
Dilatrate-SR, 441-442
Dilaudid, 413-414
Dilocaine, 466-467
Dilor, 298
diltiazem, 275-276
Dimelor, 7-8
dimenhydrinate, 277-278
dimercaprol, 278
Dimetabs, 277-278
Dimetane, 101-102
Dimetane DX, 249-250
Dimotal, 282
Dinate, 277-278
dinoprostone, 278-279
Diocto, 287-288
Diodoquin, 432
Dioeze, 287-288
Dioval, 325-326
Dipentum, 612
Diphen, 280-281
Di-Phen, 669-670
Diphenacen-50, 280-281
Diphenatol, 282
Diphenhist, 280-281
diphenhydramine, 280-281
diphenidol, 281
diphenoxylate, 282
Diphenoxylate W/Atropine, 282
Diphenylan, 669-670
dipivefrin, 282-283
Diprosone, 89-91
dipyridamole, 283-284
dirithromycin, 284
Disalcid, 744-745
Disodium EDTA, 301-302
Disonate, 287-288
disopyramide, 284-285
Disotate, 301-302
Di-Spaz, 260
Dispos-a-Med Isoproterenol, 439-440
Distamine, 642-643
disulfiram, 285-286
Ditropan, 626-627
Diucardin, 411-412
Diulo, 547-549
Diuril, 167-169
divalproex, 852-853
divalproex/valproate, 852-853
Dixarit, 200-202
Dizmiss, 492-493
Doan's pills, 484-486
dobutamine, 286-287
Dobutrex, 286-287
docusate, 287-288
DOK, 287-288
Dolacet, 407-408
Dolene, 711-712
Dolenex, 3-4
Dolmar, 110
Dolobid, 266-268
Dolophine, 518-519
Domeboro, 19-20
Dommanate, 277-278
Dopamet, 536-538
dopamine, 288-289
Dopar, 461-462
Dopastat, 288-289
Dopram, 290-292
Doral, 726-727
Dorcol Children's Decongestant, 718-719
Dorcol Children's Fever and Pain Reliever, 3-4
Doriden, 382-383
Doriglute, 382-383
Dorimide, 382-383
dornase alfa, 289-290
Doryx, 294-296
dorzolamide, 290
DOS Softgel, 287-288
doxapram, 290-292

Entries can be identified as follows: generic name, Trade Name.

doxazosin, 292
doxepin, 292-294
Doxinate, 287-288
Doxy, 294-296
Doxychel Hyclate, 294-296
Doxycin, 294-296
doxycycline, 294-296
Dramamine, 277-278
Dramanate, 277-278
Dramocen, 277-278
Dramoject, 277-278
Dr. Caldwell's Senna Laxative, 751-752
Drisdol, 313-314, 860-861
Dristan Long Lasting, 628-629
Dristan Saline, 757-758
Drithocreme, 54-55
Dritho-Scalp, 54-55
dronabinol, 296-297
droperidol, 297-298
Dr. Scholl's Wart Remover, 742-743
Drysol, 20
D-S-S, 287-288
Dulcolax, 95-96
Dull-C, 58-59
DuoCet, 407-408
DuoFilm, 742-743
DuoPlant, 742-743
Duo-Trach Kit, 466-467
Duotrate, 645-646
Duphalac, 455-456
Durabolin, 581-583
Duracillin A.S., 643-645
Duradyne DHC, 407-408
Dura-Estrin, 325-326
Duragen, 325-326
Duragesic, 346-347
Duralith, 472-473
Duralone, 541-542
Duralutin, 417-418
Duramist Plus, 628-629
Duramorph, 567-569
Duranest, 338-339
Duratest, 793-795
Durathate-200, 793-795
Duration, 628-629, 667-668
Durel, 418-419
Duricef, 133-134
Duvoid, 93-94
DV, 262-263
Dycill, 257
Dyclone, 256
Dyflex, 298
Dylline, 298
Dymelor, 7-8
Dymenate, 277-278
Dynabac, 284
Dynacin, 559-561
DynaCirc, 445-446
Dynapen, 257
dyphylline, 298
Dyrenium, 829-830
Dyrexan-OD, 657
Dytuss, 280-281

E

Easprin, 59-61
E-Base, 318-320
echothiophate iodide, 298-299
EC-Naprosyn, 584-585
E-Complex-600, 861-862
econazole, 299-300
Econopred, 693-695
Ecotrin, 59-61
E-Cypionate, 325-326
Edecrin, 330-331
Edecrin Sodium, 330-331
edetate calcium disodium, 300-301
edetate disodium, 301-302
edrophonium, 302-303
E.E.S., 318-320
E-Ferol, 861-862
Effer-K, 684-686
Effer-Syllium, 719
Effexor, 856-857
Efidac 24, 718-719
eflornithine, 303-304
8-Hour Bayer Timed Release, 59-61
E-200 I.U. Softgels, 861-862
Elase, 242-243
Elavil, 34-36
Eldepryl, 749-750
Eldopaque, 414
Eldoquin, 414
Elimite, 652-653
Elixomin, 798-800
Elixophyllin, 798-800
Elocon, 565-566
Emete-Con, 84-85
emetine, 304-305

Entries can be identified as follows: generic name, Trade Name.

Emex, 546-547
Eminase, 53-54
Empirin, 59-61
Emulsoil, 132
E-Mycin, 318-320
enalapril/enalaprilat, 305-306
encainide, 307-308
En-DeKay, 759-761
Endep, 34-36
Endolor, 110
Endrate, 301-302
Enduron, 534-536
Ener-B, 218-219
Enkaid, 307-308
Enlon, 302-303
Enovil, 34-36
enoxacin, 308-309
enoxaparin, 309-310
Enulose, 455-456
E-Pam, 250-252
ephedrine, 310-311
Epifrin, 311-313
epinephrine, 311-313
Epi-Pen, 311-313
EpiPen Jr., 311-313
Epitol, 122-124
Epival, 852-853
Epogen, 320-321
Epsom Salts, 483-484
Equanil, 509-510
Equi-Cet, 110
Equilet, 116-119
Eramycin, 318-320
Ergamisol, 460-461
ergocalciferol, 313-314, 860-861
ergoloid, 314-315
ergonovine, 315-316
Ergostat, 316-317
ergotamine, 316-317
Ergotrate Maleate, 315-316
Eridium, 656
Eryc, 318-320
Erycette, 318-320
Eryderm, 318-320
Erygel, 318-320
Erymax, 318-320
Eryped, 318-320
Ery-Tab, 318-320
erythrityl tetranitrate, 317
erythromycin, 318-320
erythropoietin, 320-321
Eserine Salicylate, 671-672
Eserine Sulfate Ointment, 671-672
Esgic, 110
Esidrix, 406-407
Eskalith, 472-473
esmolol, 321-322
E-Solve 2, 318-320
Esoterica, 414
estazolam, 323-324
esterified estrogens, 324-325
Estinyl, 333-335
Estrace, 325-326
Estra-D, 325-326
Estraderm, 325-326
estradiol, 325-326
Estradiol LA, 325-326
Estra-L, 325-326
Estratab, 324-325
Estraval, 325-326
Estro-Cyp, 325-326
Estrofem, 325-326
estrogens, conjugated, 327-328
Estroject-LA, 325-326
estrone, 328-329
Estrone-5, 328-329
Estrone Aqueous, 328-329
Estronol, 328-329
Estronol-LA, 325-326
estropipate, 329-330
Estrovis, 728-729
ethacrynic acid, 330-331
ethambutol, 331-332
Ethamolin, 332
ethanolamine oleate, 332
ethchlorvynol, 333
ethinyl estradiol, 333-335
ethionamide, 335
Ethmozine, 566-567
ethosuximide, 335-336
ethotoin, 336-338
ethylnorepinephrine, 338
Etibi, 331-332
etidocaine, 338-339
etidronate, 339-340
etodolac, 340-341
etretinate, 341-342
ETS-2%, 318-320
Eulexin, 367
Eurax, 217-218

Entries can be identified as follows: generic name, Trade Name.

Evac-Q-Mag, 483-484
E-Vista, 418-419
E-Vitamin Succinate, 861-862
Excedrin IS, 419-420
Exosurf Neonatal, 212
Exsel, 750-751
Extra Strength Gas-X, 754
Eye-Sed Ophthalmic, 868-869
Eyesine, 797-798
Ezol, 110

F

Factrel (HCl), 387-388
famotidine, 342-343
Farbital, 110
Fastin, 663-664
Feldene, 679-680
felodipine, 343-344
Femazole, 551-553
Fembutal, 110
FemCare, 203-204
Femcet, 110
Feminone, 333-335
Femiron, 347-348
Femogen Forte, 328-329
Femstat, 111
Fenesin, 391-392
fenfluramine, 344-345
fenoprofen, 345-346
fentanyl, 346-347
Fentanyl Oralet, 346-347
Feosol, 347-348
Feostat, 347-348
Feratab, 347-348
Fergon, 347-348
Fer-In-Sol, 347-348
Fer-Iron, 347-348
Fero-Gradumet, 347-348
Ferospace, 347-348
Ferralet, 347-348
Ferralyn, 347-348
Ferra-TD, 347-348
Ferrets, 347-348
ferrous salts, 347-348
Fiberall, 719
finasteride, 348-349
Fiorex, 110
Fiorgen, 110
Fioricet, 110
Fiorinal, 110
Fiormor, 110
Fisostin, 671-672
Flagyl, 551-553
Flarex, 358-359
Flavorcee, 58-59
flavoxate, 349
flecainide, 349-350
Fleet Babylax, 385-386
Fleet Bisacodyl Laxit, 95-96
Fleet Castor Oil, 132
Fleet Relief, 688-689
Fletcher's Castoria, 751-752
Flexeril, 220-221
Flexoject, 618
Flexon, 618
Florical, 116-119
Florinef Acetate, 353
Florone, 266
Floropryl, 436-437
Floxin, 610-612
fluconazole, 351-352
flucytosine, 352-353
fludrocortisone, 353
Fluidil, 225-226
Flumadine, 741
flumazenil, 353-354
flunisolide, 354-355
fluocinolone, 355-356
fluocinonide, 356-357
Fluoen, 759-761
Fluonex, 356-357
Fluonid, 355-356
Fluorabon, 759-761
Fluor-A-Day, 759-761
fluorescein, 357-358
Fluorescite, 357-358
Fluorets, 357-358
Fluorigard, 759-761
Fluorineed, 759-761
Fluorinse, 759-761
Fluor-I-Strip, 357-358
Fluoritab, 759-761
Fluorodex, 759-761
fluorometholone, 358-359
Fluor-Op, 358-359
Fluotic, 759-761
fluoxetine, 359-360
fluoxymesterone, 360-361
fluphenazine, 361-363
Flura, 759-761

Entries can be identified as follows: generic name, Trade Name.

flurandrenolide, 363-364
flurazepam, 364-365
flurbiprofen, 365-366
Flurosyn, 355-356
flutamide, 367
Flutex, 826-829
fluvoxamine, 367-368
FML, 358-359
Folex PFS, 527-529
folic acid, 368-369
Folvite, 368-369
Formulex, 260
Fortabs, 110
Fortaz, 148
foscarnet, 369-370
Foscavir, 369-370
fosinopril, 370-372
Fostex, 742-743
4-Way Long Lasting Nasal, 628-629
Freezone, 742-743
Froben, 365-366
FS Shampoo, 355-356
Ful-Glo, 357-358
Fulvicin, 390-391
Fumasorb, 347-348
Fumerin, 347-348
Funduscein, 357-358
Fungizone IV, 46-48
Fungizone (topical), 46-48
Fungoid Topical Solution, 848
Furacin, 598
Furadantin, 596-598
furazolidone, 372
Furocot, 373-374
furosemide, 373-374
Furoxone, 372
Fynex, 280-281

G

G-1, 110
gabapentin, 374-375
gallium nitrate, 375-376
gamma benzene hexachloride, 468-469
ganciclovir (DHPG), 376-377
Ganite, 375-376
Gantanol, 776-778
Gantrisin, 782-783
Garamycin, 378-380
Garamycin Ophthalmic, 378-380
Gastrocrom, 216-217
Gastrosed, 419
Gas-X, 754
gBh, 468-469
Gee-Gee, 391-392
Gel II, 759-761
Gelcalc, 116-119
Gel-Kam, 759-761
Gel-Tin, 759-761
gemfibrozil, 377-378
Genabid, 635-636
Genahist, 280-281
Genapap, 3-4
Genaphed, 718-719
Genasal, 628-629
Genaspor, 820
Genatuss, 391-392
Genebs, 3-4
gen K, 684-686
Genoptic Gentacidin, 378-380
Gen-optic Ophthalmic, 378-380
Genora, 615-617
Genpril, 419-420
Genprin, 59-61
Gentak, 378-380
Gent-AK, 378-380
gentamicin, 378-380
Gentlax, 751-752
Gen-Xene, 202-203
Geocillin, 125-126
Geone, 110
Geopen, 125-126
Geridium, 656
Gerimal, 314-315
Germicin, 81-82
Gesterol 50, 705-707
Gesterol L.A. 250, 417-418
GG-Cen, 391-392
Glaucon, 311-313
glipizide, 380-381
glucagon, 381-382
Glucophage, 516-517
Glucotrol, 380-381
glutethimide, 382-383
Glyate, 391-392
glyburide, 383-384
glycerin, 385-386
Glycerin USP, 385-386
Glycerol, 385-386
glycopyrrolate, 386-387

Entries can be identified as follows: generic name, Trade Name.

Glycotuss, 391-392
Glynase Prestab, 383-384
Glytuss, 391-392
G-Myticin, 378-380
gold sodium thiomalate/
aurothioglucose, 68-69
gonadorelin, 387-388
Gordofilm, 742-743
Gordon's Urea 40%, 848-849
Gordo-Vite E, 861-862
Gormel Creme, 848-849
goserelin, 388-389
granisetron, 389-390
Gravol, 277-278
Grifulvin V, 390-391
Grisactin, 390-391
griseofulvin, 390-391
Gris-PEG, 390-391
guaifenesin, 391-392
guanabenz, 392-393
guanadrel, 393-394
guanethidine, 394-395
guanfacine, 395-396
Guiatuss, 391-392
G-Well, 468-469
Gyne-Lotrimin, 203-204
Gynergen, 316-317
Gyne-Sulf, 780-781
Gynogen LA, 325-326

H

Habitrol, 593-594
halazepam, 396-397
halcinonide, 397-398
Halcion, 830-831
Haldol, 399-401
Haldol Decanoate, 399-401
Halenol, 3-4
halobetasol, 398-399
Halofed, 718-719
Halog, 397-398
haloperidol, 399-401
haloprogin, 401
Halotestin, 360-361
Halotex, 401
Halotussin, 391-392
Haltran, 419-420
1% HC, 409-411
Head and Shoulders Intensive
Treatment, 750-751
Hemocyte, 347-348
Hemorrhoidal HC, 409-411
heparin, 401-403
Herplex, 420-421
Hexa-Betalin, 723-724
Hexadrol Phosphate, 244-246
HiCor 1.0, 409-411
Hi-Cor 2.5, 409-411
Hip-Rex, 523-524
Hiprex, 523-524
Hismanal, 61-62
Histaject, 101-102
Histerone-100, 793-795
Hivid, 866-867
HMS Liquifilm, 496-497
Hold DM, 249-250
Homatrine, 403-404
homatropine hydrobromide, 403-404
Honvol, 264-265
Hormogen Depot, 325-326
Humatin, 638-639
Humatrope, 762
Humegon, 501-502
Humibid, 391-392
HuMist, 757-758
Humorsol, 234-235
Humulin, 426-427
hyaluronidase, 404
Hybolin Decanoate, 581-583
Hybolin Improved, 581-583
Hycort, 409-411
Hydeltrasol, 693-695
Hydeltra-T.B.A., 693-695
Hydergine, 314-315
Hydextran, 433-434
hydralazine, 405-406
Hydramine, 280-281
Hydrate, 277-278
Hydril, 280-281
Hydrobexan, 414-415
Hydrocet, 407-408
Hydro-Chlor, 406-407
hydrochlorothiazide, 406-407
Hydrocil, 719
Hydro-Cobex, 414-415
hydrocodone, 407-408
hydrocortisone, 409-411
Hydrocortone, 409-411
Hydrocortone Acetate, 409-411
Hydrocortone Phosphate, 409-411

Entries can be identified as follows: generic name, Trade Name.

Hydro-Crysti-12, 414-415
HydroDiuril, 406-407
hydroflumethiazide, 411-412
Hydromal, 406-407
hydromorphone, 413-414
hydroquinone, 414
Hydro-T, 406-407
HydroTex, 409-411
Hydroxacen, 418-419
hydroxocobalamin (vitamin B_{12}), 414-415
hydroxychloroquine, 415-417
hydroxyprogesterone, 417-418
hydroxyzine, 418-419
Hydroxyzine HCl, 418-419
Hydroxyzine Pamoate, 418-419
Hy-Gestrone, 417-418
Hygroton, 177-178
Hylidone, 177-178
Hylorel, 393-394
Hylutin, 417-418
hyoscyamine, 419
Hyperstat, 252-253
Hy-Phen, 407-408
Hyprogest 250, 417-418
Hyrexin, 280-281
Hysterone, 360-361
Hytakerol, 273-274, 860-861
Hytone, 409-411
Hytrin, 790-791
Hytuss, 391-392
Hyzine-50, 418-419

I

Ibuprin, 419-420
ibuprofen, 419-420
Ibuprohm, 419-420
IBU-Tab, 419-420
Ide-Cet, 110
Idenal, 110
idoxuridine, 420-421
I-Homatrine, 403-404
Iletin NPH, 426-427
Iletin II U-500, 426-427
Ilosone, 318-320
Ilotycin, 318-320
Ilozyme, 635
Imdur, 441-442
I-methasone, 244-246
Imferon, 433-434
imipenem, 421-422
imipramine, 422-423
Imitrex, 784-785
Imodium, 475
Impril, 422-423
Imuran, 70
Inapsine, 297-298
indapamide, 423-424
Inderal, 712-714
Indocin, 424-425
indomethacin, 424-425
Inflamase, 693-695
Infumorph, 567-569
INH, 77-78
Inocor, 49-50
Insulatard NPH, 426-427
insulin, 426-427
Intal, 216-217
interferon alfa-2a/2b, 427-429
interferon alfa-n 3, 429
interferon beta, 429-430
interferon gamma, 430-431
Intron-a (interferon alfa-2b), 427-429
Intropin, 288-289
Inversine, 491-492
iodinated glycerol, 431
iodochlorhydroxyquin, 192
iodoquinol, 432
Ionamin, 663-664
Iophen, 431
Iosat, 686-687
ipecac, 432-433
I-Phrine, 667-668
ipratroplum, 433
Ircon, 347-348
iron dextran, 433-434
Ismelin, 394-395
ISMO, 441-442
Ismotic, 440-441
Iso-Bid, 441-442
Isobutal, 110
Isocaine HCl, 508-509
isocarboxazid, 434-435
Isocet, 110
Isocom, 437
isoetharine, 435-436
isoflurophate, 436-437
Isolin, 110
Isoltyl, 110

Entries can be identified as follows: generic name, Trade Name.

isometheptene, 437
isoniazid, 437-439
Isopap, 110, 437
isophane suspension (NPH) insulin, 426-427
isoproterenol, 439-440
Isoptin, 857-858
Isopto Atropine, 65-67
Isopto Carbachol, 122
Isopto Carpine, 673-674
Isopto Cetamide, 773
Isopto Eserine Solution, 671-672
Isopto Frin, 667-668
Isopto Homatropine, 403-404
Isopto Hyoscine, 746-747
Isordil, 441-442
isosorbide, 440-441
isosorbide dinitrate/mononitrate, 441-442
Isotrate Timecelles, 441-442
isotretinoin, 443-444
isoxuprine, 444-445
isradipine, 445-446
Isuprel, 439-440
Itch-X, 688-689
itraconazole, 446-447
I-Tropine, 65-67

J
Janimine, 422-423
Jenamicin, 378-380
Jenest-28, 615-617

K
K+10, 684-686
Kabikinase, 768-769
Kainair, 710-711
Kalcinate, 116-119
kanamycin, 447-448
Kantrex, 447-448
Kaochlor, 684-686
Kaodene, 448-449
kaolin-pectin, 448-449
Kaon, 684-686
Kaopectate, 448-449
Kapectolin, 448-449
Karidium, 759-761
Karigel, 759-761
Kasof, 287-288
Kato, 684-686
Kay Ciel, 684-686
Kayexalate, 761
Kaylizer, 684-686
K+ Care, 684-686
K-Dur, 684-686
Keflex, 153-155
Keflin, 155-156
Keftab, 153-155
Kefurox, 151-153
Kefzol, 136-137
Kemadrin, 704-705
Kenacort, 826-829
Kenaject, 826-829
Kenalog, 826-829
Kenonel, 826-829
Keralyt, 742-743
Kerlone, 91-93
Kestrone-5, 328-329
ketoconazole, 449-451
ketoprofen, 451-452
ketorolac, 452-453
Key-Pred, 693-695
K-Feron, 433-434
K-G Elixir, 684-686
Kidkare Decongestant Drops, 718-719
K-Lease, 684-686
Klonopin, 199-200
K-lor, 684-686
Klor-Con, 684-686
Klorvess, 684-686
Klotrix, 684-686
K-Lyte, 684-686
K-Lyte/Cl, 684-686
K-Norm, 684-686
Kolyum, 684-686
Konakion, 672-673
Kondon's Nasal, 310-311
Konsyl, 719
K-P, 448-449
K-Pek, 448-449
K-tab, 684-686
Ku-Zyme HP, 635
Kwell, 468-469
Kwellada, 468-469
Kytril, 389-390

L
LA-12, 414-415
labetalol, 453-455

Entries can be identified as follows: generic name, Trade Name.

Lacticare-HC, 409-411
lactulose, 455-456
LAE 20, 325-326
Lamictal, 456-457
Lamisil, 791
lamotrigine, 456-457
Lamprene, 194-195
Lanaphilic, 848-849
Laniazid, 437-439
Laniroif, 110
Lanophyllin, 798-800
Lanorinal, 110
Lanoxicaps, 269-271
Lanoxin, 269-271
lansoprazole, 457
Lariam, 498-499
Larodopa, 461-462
Lasan, 54-55
Lasix, 373-374
L-Caine, 466-467
Ledercillin-VK, 643-645
Lentard Monotard, 426-427
Lente Ile I, 426-427
Lente Iletin II, 426-427
Lente Insulin, 426-427
Lente Purified Pork Insulin, 426-427
LET Solution, 795
leucovorin, 458-459
leuprolide, 459-460
levamisole, 460-461
Levate, 34-36
Levatol, 641-642
Levlen, 615-617
levodopa, 461-462
Levo-Dromoran, 463-464
levonorgestrel, 462-463
Levophed, 602-603
Levoprome, 529-530
Levora, 615-617
levorphanol, 463-464
Levo-T, 464-466
Levothroid, 464-466
levothyroxine, 464-466
Levoxine, 464-466
Levsin, 419
Levsinex Timecaps, 419
Libritabs, 163-164
Librium, 163-164
Lidemol, 356-357
Lidex, 356-357
Lidocaine HCl, 466-467
lidocaine (local, topical), 466-467
lidocaine (systemic), 467-468
Lidoject, 466-467
Lidopen Auto-Injector, 467-468
lindane (gamma benzene hexachloride), 468-469
Lioresal, 76-77
liothyronine (T3), 469-470
Liquaemin, 401-403
Liqu-Char, 158-159
Liquid Pred, 695-696
Liqui-Flur, 759-761
Liquiprin, 3-4
lisinopril, 470-472
Listermint with Fluoride, 759-761
Lithane, 472-473
lithium, 472-473
Lithobid, 472-473
Lithonate, 472-473
Lithostat, 8-9
Lithotabs, 472-473
Locoid, 409-411
Lodine, 340-341
Loestrin Fe, 615-617
Lofene, 282
Logen, 282
Lomanate, 282
lomefloxacin, 473-474
Lomocot, 282
Lomodix, 282
Lomotil, 282
Lomoxate, 282
Loniten, 561-562
Lonox, 282
Lo/ovral, 615-617
loperamide, 475
Lopid, 377-378
Lopresor, 549-551
Lopressor, 549-551
Loprox, 182-183
Lopurin, 15-16
Lorabid, 475-476
loracarbef, 475-476
loratadine, 476-477
Loraz, 477-478
lorazepam, 477-478
Lorazepam Intensol, 477-478
Lorcet, 407-408

Entries can be identified as follows: generic name, Trade Name.

Lorelco, 699-700
Lo-Rex, 282
Lortab, 407-408
losartan, 478
Lotabs, 282
Lotensin, 80-81
Lotrimin, 203-204
Lo-Trol, 282
lovastatin, 479
Lovenox, 309-310
Low-Quel, 282
Lowsium, 482
Loxapax, 480-481
loxapine, 480-481
Loxapine Succinate, 480-481
Loxitane IM, 480-481
Loxitane/Loxitane-C, 480-481
Lozide, 423-424
Lozol, 423-424
Loz-Tabs, 759-761
Ludiomil, 488-489
Lufyllin, 298
Lugol's Solution, 686-687
Lumicaine, 20
Luminal, 659-661
Lupron, 459-460
Luramide, 373-374
Luride, 759-761
Lutrepulse, 387-388
Luvox, 367-368
Lyphocin, 853-855
lypressin, 481

M

Macrobid, 596-598
Macrodantin, 596-598
mafenide, 481-482
magaldrate, 482
Magan, 484-486
Magic Numbing Solution (TAC Solution), 795
magnesium, 483-484
magnesium citrate, 483-484
magnesium gluconate, 483-484
magnesium hydroxide, 483-484
magnesium oxide, 483-484
magnesium salicylate, 484-486
magnesium sulfate, 483-484
Magnesium Sulfate Injection, 483-484
Magonate, 483-484
Mag-Ox 400, 483-484
malathion, 486
Mallamint, 116-119
Malotuss, 391-392
Mandameth, 523-524
Mandelamine, 523-524
Mandol, 134-136
mannitol, 487-488
Maolate, 170-171
Maox, 483-484
maprotiline, 488-489
Marbaxin, 526-527
Marcaine, 104-105
Marflex, 618
Margesic, 110
Marinol, 296-297
Marmine, 277-278
Marnal, 110
Marplan, 434-435
Maxair, 678
Maxaquin, 473-474
Maxeran, 546-547
Maxidex, 244-246
Maxiflor, 266
Maximum Bayer, 59-61
Maximum Strength Wart Remover, 742-743
Maxivate, 89-91
Maxolon, 546-547
Mazanor, 489-490
Mazepine, 122-124
mazindol, 489-490
Mebaral, 506-508
mebendazole, 490-491
mecamylamine, 491-492
Meclan, 493
meclizine, 492-493
meclocycline, 493
meclofenamate, 493-494
Meclomen, 493-494
Meda Tab, 3-4
Medicycline, 796-797
Medigesic, 110
Medihaler-Epi, 311-313
Medihaler Ergotamine, 316-317
Medihaler-Iso, 439-440
Medilium, 163-164
Mediplast, 742-743
Medipren, 419-420

Meditran, 509-510
Medralone, 541-542
Medrol, 541-542
medroxyprogesterone, 495-496
medrysone, 496-497
mefenamic acid, 497-498
mefloquine, 498-499
Mefoxin, 144-145
Megace, 499-500
Megacillin, 643-645
megestrol, 499-500
Melanex, 414
Melfiat, 657
Mellaril, 803-805
menadiol, 500-501
Menadol, 419-420
Menest, 324-325
Meni-D, 492-493
menotropins, 501-502
mepenzolate, 502-503
meperidine, 503-504
mephentermine, 504-505
mephenytoin, 505-506
mephobarbital, 506-508
Mephyton, 672-673
mepivacaine, 508-509
meprobamate, 509-510
Mepron, 64-65
Meprospan, 509-510
Meravil, 34-36
mesalamine, 510-511
Mesantoin, 505-506
mesna, 511-512
Mesnex, 511-512
mesoridazine, 512-514
Mestinon, 721-722
Metamucil, 719
Metaprel, 514-515
metaproterenol, 514-515
metaraminol, 515-516
metaxalone, 516
metformin, 516-517
methacholine, 517-518
methadone, 518-519
Methadose, 518-519
methamphetamine, 520-521
methantheline, 521-522
methazolamide, 522-523
methenamine, 523-524
Methergine, 539
methicillin, 524-525
methimazole, 525-526
methocarbamol, 526-527
methotrexate, 527-529
Methotrexate LPF, 527-529
methotrimeprazine, 529-530
methoxamine, 530-531
methoxsalen, 531-532
methscopolamine, 532-533
methsuximide, 533-534
methylcelluose, 536
methylclothiazide, 534-536
methyldopa, 536-538
methylene blue, 538-539
methylergonovine, 539
Methylone, 541-542
methylphenidate, 539-540
methylprednisolone, 541-542
methyltestosterone, 543-544, 793-795
methysergide, 544-545
Meticorten, 695-696
metipranolol, 545-546
Metizol, 551-553
metoclopramide, 546-547
metolazone, 547-549
metoprolol, 549-551
Metra, 657
Metric 21, 551-553
Metro IV, 551-553
metronidazole, 551-553
Metryl, 551-553
metyrosine, 553-554
Mevacor, 479
Meval, 250-252
mexiletine, 554-555
Mexitil, 554-555
Mezlin, 555-556
mezlocillin, 555-556
Miacalcin, 114-115
Micatin, 556-557
miconazole, 556-557
Micro-K, 684-686
Micronase, 383-384
microNefrin, 311-313
Micronor, 603-604
Microsulfon, 774-775
Midamor, 26-27
midazolam, 558
Midchlor, 437

Entries can be identified as follows: generic name, Trade Name.

Midol-200, 419-420
Midrin, 437
Migratine, 437
Milk of Magnesia, 483-484
Milontin Kapseals, 662-663
Milophene, 196-197
milrinone, 559
Miltown, 509-510
Minims-Atropine, 65-67
Minipress, 692
Minitran, 598-600
Minocin, 559-561
minocycline, 559-561
Minodyl, 561-562
Minotal, 110
minoxidil, 561-562
Mintezol, 800-801
Minute-Gel, 759-761
Miocarpine, 673-674
Miochol, 9
Miostat, 122
Miradon, 51-52
misoprostol, 562
Mithracin, 680-681
mithramycin, 680-681
Mitran, 163-164
Mixtard 70/30, 426-427
Moban, 564-565
Mobenol, 817-819
Mobidin, 484-486
Modane Bulk, 719
Modane Soft, 287-288
Modicon, 615-617
Modified Burow's Solution, 19-20
Modified Shohl's solution, 758-759
moexipril, 562-563
molindone, 564-565
Mol-Iron, 347-348
mometasone, 565-566
Monistat, 556-557
Monitan, 2-3
monobenzone, 566
Monocid, 139-140
Monodox, 294-296
Mono-Gesic, 744-745
Monoket, 441-442
Monopril, 370-372
8-Mop, 531-532
moricizine, 566-567
morphine, 567-569
Mosco, 742-743
Motofen, 265
Motrin, 419-420
MS Contin, 567-569
MSIR, 567-569
Mucomyst, 9-10
Mucosil, 9-10
mupirocin, 569
Murine Ear Drops, 124
Murine Plus Eye Drops, 797-798
muromonab-CD3, 569-570
Muro-128 Ophthalmic, 757-758
Muroptic-S, 757-758
Myambutol, 331-332
Myapap, 3-4
Mycelex, 203-204
Mycifradin, 578-588
Myciguent, 578-588
Mycobutin, 738-739
mycophenolate, 570-571
Mycostatin, 608-609
Mydfrin, 667-668
Mydriacyl Ophthalmic, 847-848
Mygracet, 110
Myidil, 845-846
Mykrox, 547-549
Mylaramine, 246-247
Mylicon, 754
Myolin, 618
Myotonachol, 93-94
Myotrol, 618
Mytelase, 23-24
Mytussin, 391-392
MZM, 522-523

N

nabumetone, 571-572
nadolol, 572-574
Nadostine, 608-609
nafarelin, 574-575
Nafazair, 583
Nafcil, 575-576
nafcillin sodium, 575-576
Nafrinse, 759-761
naftifine, 576-577
Naftin, 576-577
nalbuphine, 577-578
Naldecon DX, 249-250
Naldecon Senior EX, 391-392
Nalfon, 345-346

Entries can be identified as follows: generic name, Trade Name.

nalidixic acid, 578
Nallpen, 575-576
nalmefene, 578-579
naloxone, 579-580
naltrexone, 580-581
Nandrobolic, 581-583
nandrolone, 581-583
naphazoline, 583
Naphcon, 583
Naprosyn, 584-585
naproxen, 584-585
Narcan, 579-580
Nardil, 658-659
Nasacort, 826-829
Nasahist-B, 101-102
NaSal, 757-758
NASAL, 77-78
Nasalcrom, 216-217
Nasalide, 354-355
Nasal Relief, 628-629
Natacyn, 585-586
natamycin, 585-586
Navane, 805-806
ND Stat, 101-102
Nebcin, 813-814
NebuPent, 647-648
nedocromil, 586
N.E.E. 1/35, 615-617
nefazodone, 586-587
NegGram, 578
Nelova, 615-617
Nembutal, 649-651
Neo-Calgucon, 116-119
Neo-calme, 250-252
Neocyten, 618
Neo-Durabolic, 581-583
Neo-Estrone, 324-325
Neo-Fradin, 578-588
Neoloid, 132
Neo-Metric, 551-553
neomycin, 578-588
Neopap, 3-4
Neoquess, 260, 419
Neoral, 224-225
Neosar, 222-223
Neo-Synephrine 12 Hour, 628-629
Neo-Synephrine (nasal), 667-668
Neo-Synephrine (ophthalmic), 667-668
Neo-Synephrine (systemic), 665-666
Neo-Tabs, 578-588
Neo-Tetrine, 796-797
Neothylline, 298
Nephro-Calci, 116-119
Nephro-Fer, 347-348
Nephron Inhalant, 311-313
Neptazane, 522-523
Nervocaine, 466-467
Nesacaine, 165-166
Nestrex, 723-724
netilmicin, 589-590
Netromycin, 589-590
Neuramate, 509-510
Neurontin, 374-375
Neutracare, 759-761
Nia-Bid, 590-591
Niac, 590-591
Niacels, 590-591
niacin (vitamin B_3; nicotinic acid), 590-591
Niacor, 590-591
nicardipine, 591-592
N'ice Vitamin C Drops, 58-59
Nico-400, 590-591
Nicobid, 590-591
Nicoderm, 593-594
Nicolar, 590-591
Nicorette, 593-594
nicotine, 593-594
Nicotinex, 590-591
nicotinic acid, 590-591
Nicotrol, 593-594
Nico-Vert, 277-278
nifedipine, 594-595
Niloric, 314-315
Nilstat, 608-609
nimodipine, 596
Nimotop, 596
Nipride, 600-601
Nisaval, 724
Nitro-Bid, 598-600
Nitrocine Timecaps, 598-600
Nitrodisc, 598-600
Nitro-Dur, 598-600
nitrofurantoin, 596-598
nitrofurazone, 598
Nitrogard, 598-600
nitroglycerin, 598-600
Nitroglyn, 598-600
Nitrol, 598-600

Nitrolingual, 598-600
Nitrong, 598-600
Nitropress, 600-601
nitroprusside, 600-601
Nitrostat, 598-600
Nix, 652-653
nizatidine, 601-602
Nizoral, 449-451
Nobesine, 263-264
Noctec, 160-161
No-Doz, 112-113
Nolvadex, 788
Noradryl, 280-281
Norafed, 280-281
Norcet 5 mg, 407-408
Nordette, 615-617
Nordryl, 280-281
norepinephrine, 602-603
Norethin, 615-617
norethindrone, 603-604
Norflex, 618
norfloxacin, 604-605
norgestrel, 605-606
Norinyl, 615-617
Norlutate, 603-604
Norlutin, 603-604
Nor-Mil, 282
Normodyne, 453-455
Noroxin, 604-605
Norpace, 284-285
Norplant System, 462-463
Norpramin, 237-239
Nor-Q.D., 603-604
Nor-Tet, 796-797
nortriptyline, 606-608
Norvasc, 36-37
Norwich Extra-Strength, 59-61
Norzine, 802-803
Nostril, 667-668
Nostrilla, 628-629
Novapurol, 15-16
Nova-Rectal, 649-651
Novo-alprazol, 16-17
Novobutamide, 817-819
Novocaine, 701-702
Novocarbamaz, 122-124
Novochlorhydrate, 160-161
Novochloroquine, 166-167
Novocimetine, 183-184
Novoclopate, 202-203
Novocloxin, 204-205
Novodipam, 250-252
Novoflurazine, 833-835
Novofolacid, 368-369
Novofuran, 596-598
Novohexidyl, 837-838
Novolexin, 153-155
Novolin, 426-427
Novolorazem, 477-478
Novomedopa, 536-538
Novomepro, 509-510
Novometoprol, 549-551
Novonidazole, 551-553
Novopen G, 643-645
Novopramine, 422-423
Novopropamide, 174-175
Novop VK, 643-645
Novoreserpine, 736
Novoridazine, 803-805
Novorythro, 318-320
Novosalmol, 12-13
Novosemide, 373-374
Novosoxazole, 782-783
Novospiroton, 765-766
Novosudac, 783-784
Novotetra, 796-797
Novothalidone, 177-178
Novotriphyl, 625-626
Novotriptyn, 34-36
Novoxapam, 623-624
Nozinan, 529-530
NP-27, 820
NPH Iletin, 426-427
NPH Insulin, 426-427
NPH Purified Pork, 426-427
NTZ, 628-629
Nu-alpraz, 16-17
Nu-Amp, 48-49
Nubain, 577-578
Nu-Cephalex, 153-155
Nuclox, 204-205
Numorphan, 630-631
Nupercainal, 253
Nuprin, 419-420
Nutracort, 409-411
Nutraplus, 848-849
Nutropin, 762
Nydrazid, 437-439
nystatin, 608-609

Entries can be identified as follows: generic name, Trade Name.

Nystat-Rx, 608-609
Nystex, 608-609

O

Obalan, 657
Obe-Nix, 663-664
Obephen, 663-664
Obermine, 663-664
Obestin-30, 663-664
Obeval, 657
Occlusal-HP, 742-743
Ocean, 757-758
Octamide PFS, 546-547
Octocaine HCl, 466-467
octreotide, 609-610
Ocu-Caine, 710-711
Ocu-Carpine, 673-674
Ocu-Clear, 628-629
Ocufen, 365-366
Ocuflox, 610-612
Ocugestrin, 667-668
Ocu-Phrin Sterile Eye Drops/ Ophthalmic Solution, 667-668
Ocupress, 130-131
Ocusert Pilo, 673-674
Ocusulf-10, 773
Ocu-Tracin, 75-76
Ocu-Tropine, 65-67
Off-Ezy Wart Remover, 742-743
O-Flex, 618
ofloxacin, 610-612
olsalazine, 612
omeprazole, 612-613
Omnipen, 48-49
OMS Concentrate, 567-569
ondansetron, 613-614
Ophthacet, 773
Ophthaine, 710-711
Ophthalgan Ophthalmic, 385-386
Ophthetic, 710-711
Ophthifluor, 357-358
opium, 614-615
opium and belladonna, 79-80
Opium Tincture Deodorized, 614-615
Opticrom, 216-217
Opticyl, 847-848
Optigene 3 Eye Drops, 797-798
Optimine, 69-70
Optipranolol, 545-546
Oracit, 758-759
Oradent Dental, 826-829
oral contraceptives, 615-617
Oraminic II, 101-102
Oramorph SR, 567-569
Orap, 674
Oraphen-PD, 3-4
Orasone, 695-696
Orazinc, 868-869
Oretic, 406-407
Oreton, 543-544
Oreton Methyl, 793-795
Organidin, 431
Orinase, 817-819
Ormazine, 172-174
Ornidyl, 303-304
orphenadrine, 618
Orphenate, 618
Ortho-Cept, 615-617
Orthoclone OKT3, 569-570
Ortho-Cyclen, 615-617
Ortho Dienestrol, 262-263
Ortho-Novum, 615-617
Ortho Tri-Cyclen, 615-617
OR-Tyl, 260
Orudis, 451-452
Oruvail, 451-452
Os-Cal, 116-119
Osmitrol, 487-488
Osmoglyn, 385-386
Otocain, 82
Otrivin, 864-865
Ovcon, 615-617
Ovide, 486
Ovol, 754
Ovral, 615-617
Ovrette, 605-606
oxacillin, 618-520
oxamniquine, 620
Oxandrin, 621-622
oxandrolone, 621-622
oxaprozin, 622-623
oxazepam, 623-624
oxiconazole, 624-625
Oxistat, 624-625
Ox-Pam, 623-624
Oxsoralen, 531-532
oxtriphylline, 625-626
oxybutynin, 626-627
oxycodone, 627-628

Entries can be identified as follows: generic name, Trade Name.

Oxydess II, 248-249
oxymetazoline, 628-629
oxymetholone, 629-630
oxymorphone, 630-631
oxytetracycline, 631-633
oxytocin, 633-634
Oysco, 116-119
Oyst-Cal, 116-119
Oystercal, 116-119
Oyster Shell Calcium, 116-119

P

Pacaps, 110
Palaron, 29-32
Pamelor, 606-608
pamidronate, 634
Pamine, 532-533
Pamprin-IB, 419-420
Panadol, 3-4
Panasol-S, 695-696
Pancrease, 635
pancrelipase, 635
Panectyl, 838-839
Panex, 3-4
Panmycin, 796-797
Pan-Oxyl, 83-84
Panscol, 742-743
Pantopon, 614-615
Panwarfin, 862-864
papaverine, 635-636
Paraflex, 178-179
Parafon Forte DSC, 178-179
Paral, 636-637
paraldehyde, 636-637
Parapectolin, 448-449
Paregique, 637-638
paregoric, 637-638
Par Glycerol, 431
Parlodel, 100-101
Parnate, 822-824
paromomycin, 638-639
paroxetine, 639-640
Pathilon, 831-832
Pathocil, 257
Pavabid, 635-636
Pavarine Spancaps, 635-636
Pavased, 635-636
Pavatine, 635-636
Pavatym, 635-636
Paverolan Lanacaps, 635-636
Pavusule, 635-636
Paxil, 639-640
Paxipam, 396-397
PBZ, 844-845
PCE Dispertab, 318-320
Pedia Care Allergy Formula, 171-172
PediaCare Infant's Decongestant Pseudo, 718-719
Pediadent, 759-761
Pediaflor, 759-761
PediaPatch, 742-743
Pediapred, 693-695
PediaProfen, 419-420
Pedi-Boro Soak Paks, 19-20
Peganone, 336-338
Pelamine, 844-845
pemoline, 640
Penapar-VK, 643-645
penbutolol, 641-642
Pendramine, 642-643
Penecort, 409-411
Penetrex, 308-309
Penglobe, 74-75
penicillamine, 642-643
penicillin, 643-645
penicillin G potassium, 643-645
penicillin G procaine, 643-645
penicillin G sodium, 643-645
penicillin V potassium, 643-645
Pentacarinat, 647-648
Pentacef, 148
pentaerythritol tetranitrate, 645-646
Pentam 300, 647-648
pentamidine, 647-648
Pentasa, 510-511
Pentazine, 707-708
pentazocine, 648-649
Pentids, 643-645
pentobarbital, 649-651
Pentogen, 649-651
pentoxifylline, 651-652
Pentylan, 645-646
Pen-Vee K, 643-645
Pepcid, 342-343
Pepto-Bismol, 96-97
Peptol, 183-184
Perdiem, 719
pergolide, 652
Pergonal, 501-502

Entries can be identified as follows: generic name, Trade Name.

Periactin, 226-227
Peridex, 164-165
Periogard, 164-165
Peritrate, 645-646
Permapen, 643-645
Permax, 652
permethrin, 652-653
Permitil, 361-363
Pernavite, 218-219
Peroxin, 83-84
perphenazine, 653-655
Persa-Gel, 83-84
Persantine, 283-284
Pertofrane, 237-239
Pertussin, 249-250
P.E.T.N., 645-646
Pfeiffer's Allergy, 171-172
Pfizerpen, 643-645
Pfizerpien, 643-645
Pharm-A-Dry, 280-281
Pharmaflur, 759-761
Pharmagesic, 110
Phazyme, 754
phenacemide, 655-656
Phenameth, 707-708
Phenaphen, 3-4
Phenazine, 653-655, 707-708
Phenazo, 656
Phenazodine, 656
phenazopyridine, 656
phendimetrazine, 657
phenelzine, 658-659
Phenergan, 707-708
Phenetron, 171-172
phenobarbital, 659-661
Phenoject-50, 707-708
phenoxybenzamine, 661-662
Phenpropionate, 581-583
phensuximide, 662-663
phentermine, 663-664
phentolamine, 664-665
Phentride, 663-664
Phentrol, 663-664
Phenurone, 655-656
phenylbutazone, 665
Phenyldrine, 668-669
phenylephrine (systemic), 665-666
phenylephrine (topical), 667-668
phenylpropanolamine, 668-669
phenytoin, 669-670
Phenytoin Oral Suspension, 669-670
Phenzine, 657
Phos-Ex, 116-119
Phos-Flur, 759-761
PhosLo, 116-119
Phospholine Iodide, 298-299
Phyllocontin, 29-32
physostigmine, 671-672
phytonadione (vitamin K_1), 672-673
Pilagan, 673-674
Pilocar, 673-674
pilocarpine, 673-674
Pilocarpine HCl, 673-674
Pilopine HS, 673-674
Piloptic, 673-674
Pilostat, 673-674
Pima, 686-687
pimozide, 674
pindolol, 675-676
Pink Bismuth, 96-97
Pin-Rid, 719-720
Pin-X, 719-720
piperacillin, 676-677
piperacillin/tazobactam, 676-677
piperazine, 677-678
Pipracil, 676-677
pirbuterol, 678
piroxicam, 679-680
Pitocin, 633-634
Pitressin Synthetic, 855-856
Placidyl, 333
Plaquenil, 415-417
Plegine, 657
Plendil, 343-344
plicamycin (mithramycin), 680-681
PMS Carbamazepine, 122-124
PMS-Metronidazole, 551-553
Podoben, 681-682
Podocon, 681-682
Pododerm, 681-682
Podofilm, 681-682
podofilox, 681
podophyllum, 681-682
Point-Two, 759-761
Poladex, 246-247
Polaramine, 246-247
Polargen, 246-247
Polocaine, 508-509
Polycillin, 48-49
Polycitra, 758-759

Entries can be identified as follows: generic name, Trade Name.

Polymox, 42-43
polymyxin B, 682-683
Poly-Rx, 682-683
polythiazide, 683-684
Pondimin, 344-345
Ponstel, 497-498
Pontocaine, 795
Porcelana, 414
Pork NPH Iletin II, 426-427
Pork Regular Iletin II, 426-427
Posture, 116-119
Potasalan, 684-686
potassium chloride, 684-686
potassium citrate and sodium citrate, 758-759
potassium gluconate, 684-686
potassium iodide, 686-687
potassium salts, 684-686
pralidoxime, 687-688
PrameGel, 688-689
pramoxine, 688-689
Pravachol, 689
pravastatin, 689
Prax, 688-689
prazepam, 690-691
praziquantel, 691
prazosin, 692
Precef, 141-142
Precose, 1
Predaject, 693-695
Predalone, 693-695
Predcor, 693-695
Pred Forte, 693-695
Predicort, 693-695
Pred Mild, 693-695
Prednicen-M, 695-696
prednisolone, 693-695
Prednisol TBA, 693-695
prednisone, 695-696
Prednisone Intensol Concentrate, 695-696
Prefrin Liquifilm, 667-668
Prelone, 693-695
Prelu-2, 657
Premarin, 327-328
Premphase, 327-328
Prempro, 327-328
Pre-Pen, 86-87
Prepidil Gel, 278-279
Pretz, 757-758
Pretz-D, 310-311
Prevacid, 457
Prevident, 759-761
Prilosec, 612-613
Primacor, 559
primaquine, 697-698
Primaquine phosphate, 697-698
Primatene Mist, 311-313
Primaxin, 421-422
Prinivil, 470-472
Priscoline, 817
Privine, 583
Pro 50, 707-708
Probalan, 698-699
Pro-Banthine, 709-710
probenecid, 698-699
probucol, 699-700
procainamide, 700-701
procaine, 701-702
Pro-Cal-Sof, 287-288
Procan SR, 700-701
Procardia, 594-595
prochlorperazine, 702-704
Procrit, 320-321
ProctoFoam, 688-689
Procyclid, 704-705
procyclidine, 704-705
Procytox, 222-223
Pro-Depo, 417-418
Prodrox 250, 417-418
Profenal, 785-786
Progestaject, 705-707
Progestasert, 705-707
progesterone, 705-707
Proglycem, 252-253
Prolamine, 668-669
Prolixin, 361-363
Prolixin Decanoate, 361-363
Prolixin Enanthate, 361-363
Proloprim, 840-841
Prometh-50, 707-708
promethazine, 707-708
Promine, 700-701
Pronestyl, 700-701
propafenone, 708-709
Propagest, 668-669
propantheline, 709-710
proparacaine, 710-711
Propine, 282-283
propoxyphene, 711-712

Entries can be identified as follows: generic name, Trade Name.

propranolol, 712-714
Propulsid, 187
propylthiouracil (PTU), 714-715
Propyl-Thyracil, 714-715
Prorex, 707-708
Proscar, 348-349
Pro-Sof, 287-288
ProSom, 323-324
Prostaphlin, 618-520
ProStep, 593-594
Prostin E_2, 278-279
Prostin/15 M, 128-129
Prostin VR, 17-18
protamine, 715-716
Protamine Zinc Insulin Suspension (PZI), 426-427
Protectol, 848
Prothiazine, 707-708
Protilase, 635
Protopam Chloride, 687-688
Protophylline, 298
Protostat, 551-553
protriptyline, 716-718
Protropin, 762
Proventil, 12-13
Provera, 495-496
Provocholine, 517-518
Prozac, 359-360
pseudoephedrine, 718-719
pseudoephedrine/carbinoxamine, 127-128
PseudoGest, 718-719
Psorcon, 266
Psorion, 89-91
P&S Shampoo, 742-743
psyllium, 719
PTU, 714-715
Pulmozyme, 289-290
Purimol, 15-16
PVFK, 643-645
Pyopen, 125-126
pyrantel, 719-720
pyrazinamide, 720-721
Pyridiate, 656
Pyridium, 656
pyridostigmine, 721-722
pyridoxine (vitamin B_6), 723-724
pyrilamine, 724
pyrimethamine, 724-726
PZI, 426-427

Q

Q-Pam, 250-252
Quarzan, 189-190
quazepam, 726-727
Questran, 179-180
Quibron-T, 798-800
Quick Pep, 112-113
Quiess, 418-419
Quinaglute Dura-Tabs, 730-732
Quinalan, 730-732
quinapril, 727-728
quinestrol, 728-729
Quinidex Extentabs, 730-732
quinidine, 730-732
quinine, 732-733
Quinora, 730-732
Quinsana Plus, 820

R

Racepinephrine, 311-313
Radiostol, 860-861
ramipril, 733-734
ranitidine, 734-735
Rapifen, 14-15
Reclomide, 546-547
Redisol, 218-219
Redoxon, 58-59
Reese's Pinworm, 719-720
Regibon, 263-264
Regitine, 664-665
Reglan, 546-547
Regonol, 721-722
Regular Purified Pork, 426-427
Regulex SS, 287-288
Reguloid, 719
Regutol, 287-288
Rela, 129
Relafen, 571-572
Relief Eye Drops for Red Eyes, 667-668
Remular-S, 178-179
Renese, 683-684
Repan, 110
Rep-Pred, 541-542
Resectial, 487-488
reserpine, 736
Respid, 798-800
Resposans-10, 163-164
Restoril, 789-790
Retin-A, 825-826

Retrovir, 867-868
Reversol, 302-303
Revex, 578-579
Rev-Eyes, 231-232
ReVia, 580-581
Revimine, 288-289
Revitonus, 801-802
R-Gen, 431
Rheumatrex Dose Pack, 527-529
Rhinall-10, 667-668
Rhindecon, 668-669
Rhythmin, 700-701
ribavirin, 737-738
riboflavin (vitamin B_2), 738
Ridaura, 67
rifabutin, 738-739
Rifadin, 739-740
rifampin, 739-740
Rimactane, 739-740
rimantadine, 741
Rinlaxer, 170-171
Riopan, 482
Risperdal, 741-742
risperidone, 741
Ritalin, 539-540
Rival, 250-252
RMS, 567-569
Robaxin, 526-527
Robicillin-V, 643-645
Robigesic, 3-4
Robimycin Robitabs, 318-320
Robinul, 386-387
Robitet, 796-797
Robitussin, 391-392
Robitussin Cough Calmers, 249-250
Robitussin Pediatric, 249-250
Robomol, 526-527
Rocaltrol, 115-116
Rocephin, 150-151
Rodex TD, 723-724
Rofact, 739-740
Roferon-a (interferon alfa-2a), 427-429
Rogaine, 561-562
Rogesic, 110
Rogitine, 664-665
Rolaids, 116-119, 274-275
Rolavil, 34-36
Romazicon, 353-354
Romotil, 282
Rounax, 3-4
Rowasa, 510-511
Roxanol, 567-569
Roxicodone, 627-628
Rubesol-1000, 218-219
Rubion, 218-219
Rubramin PC, 218-219
Rufen, 419-420
Rum-K, 684-686
Ru-Vert-M, 492-493
Rx Otic Drops, 55-56
Rythmol, 708-709

S

S-2, 311-313
St. Joseph Aspirin-Free for Children, 3-4
St. Joseph Children's, 59-61
St. Joseph Cough Suppressant, 249-250
St. Joseph Measured Dose, 667-668
Sal-Acid, 742-743
Salactic Film, 742-743
Salagen, 673-674
Salazopyrin, 778-780
Salbutamol, 12-13
Saleto, 419-420
Salflex, 744-745
salicylic acid, 742-743
SalineX, 757-758
salmeterol, 743-744
Sal-Plant, 742-743
salsalate, 744-745
Salsitab, 744-745
Sal-Tropine, 65-67
Saluron, 411-412
Sandimmune, 224-225
Sandostatin, 609-610
Sani-Supp, 385-386
Sanorex, 489-490
Sansert, 544-545
Sarisol, 108-109
Satric, 551-553
Scabene, 468-469
scopolamine, 746-747
Scot-Tussin Expectorant, 391-392
Scrip Zinc, 868-869
SeaMist, 757-758
Sebizon, 773
secobarbital, 747-749

Secogen, 747-749
Seconal, 747-749
Secretin-Ferring, 747-749
Sectral, 2-3
Seffin, 155-156
Seldane, 792-793
selegiline, 749-750
selenium sulfide, 750-751
Selestoject, 89-91
Selsun, 750-751
Selsun Blue, 750-751
Semilente Iletin I, 426-427
Semilente Insulin, 426-427
Senexon, 751-752
senna, 751-752
Senna-Gen, 751-752
Senokot, 751-752
Senolax, 751-752
Sensorcaine, 104-105
Septra, 207-208
Seral, 747-749
Serax, 623-624
Serentil, 512-514
Serevent, 743-744
Seromycin, 223-224
Serophene, 196-197
sertraline, 752
Serutan, 719
Serzone, 586-587
Seudotabs, 718-719
Shodryl, 280-281
Shohl's Solution, Modified, 758-759
Siblin, 719
Silvadene, 753-754
silver nitrate, 752-753
silver sulfadiazine, 753-754
simethicone, 754
Simron, 347-348
simvastatin, 754-755
Sinemet, 126-127
Sinequan, 292-294
Sinex, 667-668
Sinex Long-Acting, 628-629
Sinumist-SR, 391-392
Skelaxin, 516
Slo-Bid Gyrocaps, 798-800
Slo-Niacin, 590-591
Slow-Fe, 347-348
Slow-K, 684-686
Slyn-LL, 657
Snaplets-FR granules, 3-4
sodium bicarbonate, 755-757
sodium chloride, 757-758
sodium citrate and citric acid, 758-759
sodium citrate and potassium citrate, 758-759
sodium fluoride, 759-761
Sodium P.A.S., 32
sodium polystyrene sulfonate, 761
Sodium Sulfamyd, 773
Sofarin, 862-864
Solaquin, 414
Solazine, 833-835
Solfoton, 659-661
Solganal/Myochrysine, 68-69
Solium, 163-164
Solu-Cortef, 409-411
Solu-Flur, 759-761
Solu-Medrol, 541-542
Solurex, 244-246
Soma, 129
somatrem, 762
somatropin, 762
Somnol, 364-365
Soo Drops, 797-798
Soprodol, 129
sorbitol, 762-763
Sorbitrate, 441-442
Soss-10, 773
sotalol, 763-764
Spancap #1, 248-249
Span-FF, 347-348
Spasmoject, 260
Spectazole, 299-300
spectinomycin, 764-765
Spectro-Atropine, 65-67
Spectro-Bacitracin, 75-76
Spectrobid, 74-75
spironolactone, 765-766
Sporanox, 446-447
SPS Suspension, 761
S-P-T, 806-807
Spyrine, 832-833
SSD, 753-754
SSKI, 686-687
Stadol, 111-112
stanozolol, 766-767
Staphcillin, 524-525
Staticin, 318-320

Entries can be identified as follows: generic name, Trade Name.

Statobex, 657
stavudine, 767-768
Stay Trim Diet Gum, 668-669
S-T Cort, 409-411
Stelazine, 833-835
Stemetil, 702-704
Sterapred, 695-696
Stievaa, 825-826
Stilboestrol, 264-265
Stilphostrol, 264-265
Stimute, 239-240
Stoxil, 420-421
Streptase, 768-769
streptokinase, 768-769
streptomycin, 769-770
Strong Iodine Solution (Lugol's Solution), 686-687
Sublimaze, 346-347
Sub-Quin, 700-701
succimer, 770-771
sucralfate, 771-772
Sucrets Cough Control, 249-250
Sudafed, 718-719
Sufenta, 772
sufentanil, 772
Sulcrate, 771-772
Sulf, 773
sulfacetamide, 773
sulfadiazine, 774-775
Sulfair 15, 773
Sulfalax Calcium, 287-288
sulfamethizole, 775-776
Sulfamethoprim, 207-208
sulfamethoxazole, 776-778
sulfamethoxazole and trimethoprim, 207-208
Sulfamylon, 481-482
sulfanilamide, 778
sulfasalazine, 778-780
sulfathiazole/sulfacetamide/sulfabenzamide (triple sulfa), 780-781
Sulfatrim, 207-208
sulfinpyrazone, 781-782
sulfisoxizole, 782-783
Sulftrin Triple Sulfa, 780-781
sulindac, 783-784
sumatriptan, 784-785
Sumycin, 796-797
Supasa, 59-61
Superchar, 158-159
Supeudol, 627-628
Suppress, 249-250
Suprax, 137-138
suprofen, 785-786
Surfak, 287-288
Surmontil, 841-843
Survanta, 88-89
Sus-Phrine, 311-313
Sustaire, 798-800
sutilains, 786
Syllact, 719
Symadine, 22-23
Symmetrel, 22-23
Synacort, 409-411
Synalar, 355-356
Synarel, 574-575
Synemol, 355-356
Synkavite, 500-501
Synkayvite, 500-501, 672-673
Synthroid, 464-466
Synthrox, 464-466
Syntocinon, 633-634
Syoxin, 83-84
Sytobex, 218-219

T

T3, 469-470
Tac, 826-829
TAC Solution, 795
TACE, 169-170
Tacet, 110
tacrine, 786-787
Tagamet, 183-184
Talwin, 648-649
Tambocor, 349-350
Tamofen, 788
Tamone, 788
tamoxifen, 788
Tapazole, 525-526
Tarabine PFS, 227-228
Taractan, 175-177
Targocid, 788-789
Tavist, 189
Tazicef, 148
Tazidime, 148
tazobactam/piperacillin, 676-677
T-Diet, 663-664
Tebamide, 840
Tebrazid, 720-721

Entries can be identified as follows: generic name, Trade Name.

Teejel, 181-182
Tega-Cort, 409-411
Tega Dryl, 280-281
Tegison, 341-342
Tegopen, 204-205
Tegretol, 122-124
teicoplanin, 788-789
Telachlor, 171-172
Teladar, 89-91
Teldrin, 171-172
Teline, 796-797
Temaril, 838-839
temazepam, 789-790
Temovate, 192-193
Tempra, 3-4
Tencet, 110
Tenex, 395-396
Ten-K, 684-686
Tenormin, 62-64
Tensilon, 302-303
Tenuate, 263-264
Tepanil, 263-264
Terazol, 792
terazosin, 790-791
terbinafine, 791
Terbutaline, 791-792
terconazole, 792
terfenadine, 792-793
Terramycin, 631-633
Tesamone, 793-795
Tessalon Perles, 83
Testandro, 793-795
Testex, 793-795
Testoderm, 793-795
testosterone, 793-795
Testosterone Aqueous, 793-795
testosterone cypionate, 793-795
testosterone enanthate, 793-795
testosterone propionate, 793-795
Testred, 543-544, 793-795
tetracaine, 795
Tetracap, 796-797
tetracycline, 796-797
Tetracyn, 796-797
tetrahydrozoline, 797-798
Tetralan, 796-797
Tetralean, 796-797
Tetram, 796-797
Texacort, 409-411
T-Gen, 840
Thalitone, 177-178
Tham, 846-847
Theelin Aqueous, 328-329
Theo-24, 798-800
Theobid, 798-800
Theochron, 798-800
Theoclear, 798-800
Theo-Dur, 798-800
Theolair, 798-800
theophylline, 798-800
theophylline ethylenediamine, 29-32
Theo-Sav, 798-800
Theospan-SR, 798-800
Theostat 80, 798-800
Theovent, 798-800
Theox, 798-800
TheraFlu, 249-250
Thera-Flur, 759-761
Theramycin Z, 318-320
Therapy Bayer, 59-61
Theroxide, 83-84
thiabendazole, 800-801
Thiamilate, 801-802
thiamine, 801-802
thiethylperazine, 802-803
Thiola, 812-813
thioridazine, 803-805
Thiosulfil Forte, 775-776
thiothixene, 805-806
Thiuretic, 406-407
Thorazine, 172-174
Thyrar, 806-807
Thyro-Block, 686-687
thyroid, 806-807
Thyroid Strong, 806-807
Ticar, 807-809
ticarcillin, 807-809
ticarcillin/clavulanic acid, 807-809
Ticaripen, 807-809
Ticlid, 809-810
ticlopidine, 809-810
Ticon, 840
Tigan, 840
Tilade, 586
Timentin, 807-809
timolol, 810-811
Timoptic, 810-811
Tinactin, 820
Ting, 820
tioconazole, 812

tiopronin, 812-813
Tirend, 112-113
Titralac, 116-119
tobramycin, 813-814
Tobrex, 813-814
tocainide, 815
Tocopherol, 861-862
Tofranil, 422-423
Tolamide, 815-817
tolazamide, 815-817
tolazoline, 817
tolbutamide, 817-819
Tolbutone, 817-819
Tolectin, 819-820
Tolinase, 815-817
tolmetin, 819-820
tolnaftate, 820
Tonocard, 815
Topicort, 242
Topicycline, 796-797
Toprol XL, 549-551
Toradol, 452-453
Torecan, 802-803
Tornalate, 98-99
torsemide, 820-821
Totacillin, 48-49
TPA, 18-19
T-Phyl, 798-800
tramadol, 821-822
Trancopal, 165
Trandate, 453-455
Transderm-Nitro, 598-600
Transderm-Scop, 746-747
Trans-Plantar, 742-743
Trans-Ver-Sal, 742-743
Tranxene, 202-203
tranylcypromine sulfate, 822-824
Travase, 786
trazodone, 824-825
Trecator-SC, 335
Trendar, 419-420
Trental, 651-652
tretinoin, 825-826
Triacet, 826-829
Triad, 110
Triadapin, 292-294
Triam-A, 826-829
triamcinolone, 826-829
Triam Forte, 826-829
Triaminic DM, 249-250
Triamolone, 826-829
triamterene, 829-830
triazolam, 830-831
Tri-B3, 590-591
tricalcium phosphate, 116-119
Triderm, 826-829
Tridesilon, 241
tridihexethyl chloride, 831-832
Tridil, 598-600
Tridione, 839-840
trientine, 832-833
trifluoperazine, 833-835
triflupromazine, 835-836
trifluridine, 836-837
Trihexy, 837-838
trihexyphenidyl, 837-838
Tri-K, 684-686
Tri-Kort, 826-829
Trilafon, 653-655
Tri-Levlen, 615-617
Trilisate, 180-181
Trilog, 826-829
Trilone, 826-829
Trimazide, 840
Trimcaps, 657
trimeprazine, 838-839
trimethadione, 839-840
trimethobenzamide, 840
trimethoprim, 840-841
trimethoprim and sulfamethoxazole, 207-208
trimipramine, 841-843
Trimox, 42-43
Trimpex, 840-841
Trimstat, 657
Trimtabs, 657
Tri-Norinyl, 615-617
Triostat, 469-470
trioxsalen, 843-844
tripelennamine, 844-845
Triphasic, 615-617
Triphasil, 615-617
triprolidine, 845-846
triple sulfa, 780-781
Triptil, 716-718
Triptone Caplets, 277-278
Trisoralen, 843-844
Tristoject, 826-829
Trobicin, 764-765
Trochal, 249-250

tromethamine, 846-847
Tronolane, 688-689
Tronothane, 688-689
Tropicacyl, 847-848
tropicamide, 847-848
Truphylline, 29-32
Trusopt, 290
Truxadryl, 280-281
Trysul, 780-781
T-Stat, 318-320
Tums, 116-119
Tusstat, 280-281
12 Hour Nasal, 628-629
12 Hour Sinarest, 628-629
Twice-A-Day, 628-629
Twin-K, 684-686
Two-Dyne, 110
Tylenol, 3-4
Tyzine, 797-798

U

Uad Dryl, 280-281
U-Cort, 409-411
Ultracef, 133-134
Ultralente, 426-427
Ultralente Iletin I, 426-427
Ultralente Insulin, 426-427
Ultram, 821-822
Ultra Mide 25, 848-849
Ultrase MT, 635
Ultravate, 398-399
undecylenic acid, 848
Unicaine, 701-702
Uni-Lom, 282
Unipen, 575-576
Uniphyl, 798-800
Uni Sed, 718-719
Unitrol, 668-669
Uni-Tussin, 391-392
Univasc, 562-563
urea, 848-849
Ureacin, 848-849
Ureaphil, 848-849
Urecholine, 93-94
Urex, 523-524
Urispas, 349
Uri-Tet, 631-633
Uritol, 373-374
Urobak, 776-778
Urodine, 656
Urogesic, 656
urokinase, 849-850
Urolene Blue, 538-539
Uro-Mag, 483-484
Uroplus, 207-208
ursodiol, 850-851
Uticillin-VK, 643-645
Uticort, 89-91

V

Vagistat-1, 812
valacyclovir, 851-852
Valadol, 3-4
Valergen, 325-326
Valison, 89-91
Valium, 250-252
valproate/divalproex, 852-853
valproic acid, 852-853
Valrelease, 250-252
Valtrex, 851-852
Vamate, 418-419
Vancenase, 77-78
Vanceril, 77-78
Vancocin, 853-855
Vancoled, 853-855
vancomycin, 853-855
Vansil, 620
Vantin, 145-147
Vaponefrin, 311-313
Vascor, 87-88
VasoClear, 583
Vasocon Regular, 583
Vasodilan, 444-445
vasopressin, 855-856
Vasotec, 305-306
Vasoxyl, 530-531
V-Cillin K, 643-645
Veetids, 643-645
Velosef, 157-158
Velosulin, 426-427
Veltane, 101-102
venlafaxine, 856-857
Ventolin, 12-13
verapamil, 857-858
Verazinc, 868-869
Verelan, 857-858
Vermizine, 677-678
Vermox, 490-491
Versed, 558
Vertab, 277-278

Entries can be identified as follows: generic name, Trade Name.

Vesprin, 835-836
V-Gan, 707-708
Vi-Atro, 282
Vibramycin, 294-296
Vibra-Tabs, 294-296
Vibutal, 110
Vicks Formula 44, 249-250
Vicks Vatronol, 310-311
Vicodin, 407-408
vidarabine, 858-859
Videx, 261-262
Vigopen, 575-576
Vimicon, 226-227
Vinafluor, 759-761
Vioform, 192
Viokase, 635
Vira-A, 858-859
Virazole, 737-738
Virilon, 543-544, 793-795
Viroptic, 836-837
Viserol, 260
Visine Eye Drops, 797-798
Visine LR, 628-629
Visken, 675-676
Vistacon, 418-419
Vistaject, 418-419
Vistaquel 50, 418-419
Vistaril, 418-419
Vistazine 50, 418-419
Vita-C, 58-59
vitamin A, 859-860
vitamin B_2, 738
vitamin B_3, 590-591
vitamin B_6, 723-724
vitamin B_{12}, 218-219, 414-415
vitamin C, 58-59
vitamin D, 860-861
vitamin D_2, 860-861
vitamin D_3, 860-861
vitamin E, 861-862
vitamin K_1, 672-673
Vita-Plus E Softgells, 861-862
Vitec, 861-862
Vivactil, 716-718
Vivarin, 112-113
Vivol, 250-252
V-Lax, 719
Volmax, 12-13
Voltaren, 255-256
Vontrol, 281
VoSol, 6-7
Votaren SR, 255-256
Voxsuprine, 444-445
V.V.S., 780-781

W

warfarin, 862-864
Warfilone Sodium, 862-864
Warnerin, 862-864
Wart-Off, 742-743
Wart Remover, 742-743
Wehdryl, 280-281
Wehless, 657
Weightrol, 657
Wellbutrin, 106-107
Wellcovorin, 458-459
Westcort, 409-411
Winstrol, 766-767
Wyamine, 504-505
Wyamycin S, 318-320
Wycillin, 643-645
Wydase, 404
Wymox, 42-43
Wytensin, 392-393

X

Xanax, 16-17
Xerac Ac, 20
Xylocaine for Cardiac Arrhythmias (systemic), 467-468
Xylocaine HCl (local), 466-467
Xylocaine (topical), 466-467
xylometazoline, 864-865

Y

Yocon, 865-866
Yodoxin, 432
yohimbine, 865-866
Yohimex, 865-866

Z

zalcitabine (ddC), 866-867
Zantac, 734-735
Zapex, 623-624
Zarontin, 335-336
Zaroxolyn, 547-549
Zeasorb-AF, 820
Zebeta, 97-98
Zefazone, 138-139

Entries can be identified as follows: generic name, Trade Name.

Zephiran, 81-82
Zerit (d4T), 767-768
Zeroxin, 83-84
Zestril, 470-472
zidovudine, 867-868
Zinacef, 151-153
Zinc, 868-869
Zinca-Pak, 868-869
Zincate, 868-869
zinc sulfate, 868-869
zinc suspension insulin, 426-427
Zinecard, 247-248
Zithromax, 71
Zocor, 754-755
Zofran, 613-614
Zoladex, 388-389
Zolicef, 136-137
Zoloft, 752
zolpidem, 869-870
Zonalon, 292-294
ZORprin, 59-61
Zosyn, 676-677
Zovirax, 10-11
Zydone, 407-408
Zyloprim, 15-16
Zymafluor, 759-761
Zymase, 635

Conversion Information

WEIGHTS AND MEASURES

PREFIXES FOR FRACTIONS

deci = 10^{-1}
centi = 10^{-2}
milli = 10^{-3}
micro = 10^{-6}
nano = 10^{-9}
pico = 10^{-12}

TEMPERATURE MEASURES

°C = 5/9 × (°F −32)
°F = 9/5 × (°C +32)

PERCENTAGE EQUIVALENTS

0.1% solution contains: 1 mg per ml
1% solution contains: 10 mg per ml
10% solution contains: 100 mg per ml

MILLIEQUIVALENT CONVERSIONS

1 mEq Na = 23 mg Na = 58.5 mg NaCl
1 g Na = 2.54 g NaCl = 43 mEq Na
1 g NaCl = 0.39 g Na = 17 mEq Na

1 mEq K = 39 mg K = 74.5 mg KCl
1 g K = 1.91 g KCl = 26 mEq K
1 g KCl = 0.52 g K = 13 mEq K

1 mEq Ca = 20 mg Ca
1 g Ca = 50 mEq Ca

1 mEq Mg = 0.12 g $MgSO_4 \cdot 7H_2O$
1 g Mg = 10.2 g $MgSO_4 \cdot 7H_2O$ = 82 mEq Mg

10 mmol P_i = 0.31 g P_i = 0.95 g PO_4
1 g P_i = 3.06 g PO_4 = 32 mmol P_i